WHAT'S A SERVING SIZE?

FRUITS

1 serving of fruit looks like:

1 medium peach

or

1 mango

1 medium apple **or** 1 cup chopped apples **or**

1 8-inch banana

compa
with

1 cup (8 fl. oz) 100% fruit juice

VEGETABLES

1 serving of vegetables looks like:

2 cups lettuce **or**

1 cup cooked broccoli **or**

7 baby carrots | 1 large bell pepper

DAIRY

1 serving of dairy looks like:

8 oz yogurt

1 cup (8 fl. oz) milk

compa
with

How Much Do I E...

When you're creating a healthful diet for yourself, doing a diet assessment project, it's important to keep in mind not only the types of foods you eat, but also how much. However, it can be difficult to know what a particular number of cups, ounces, or ounce-equivalents looks like. Here is a visual tip sheet that will help you translate the food on your plate into common serving sizes. Tear it out and bring it with you to the dining hall, the café, or the kitchen table.

A "Hand-y" Way to Estimate Serving Size

The following photos show how to judge serving sizes with something you always have with you—your hand.

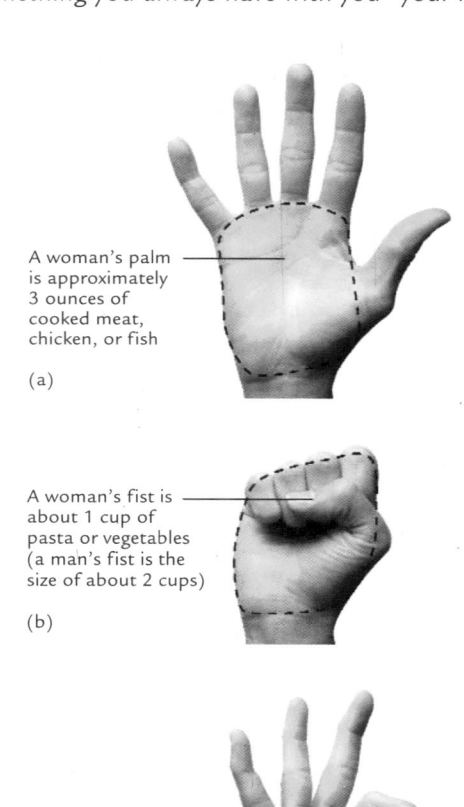

A woman's palm is approximately 3 ounces of cooked meat, chicken, or fish

(a)

A woman's fist is about 1 cup of pasta or vegetables (a man's fist is the size of about 2 cups)

(b)

About 1 tbsp. of vegetable oil

(c)

GRAINS

1 serving of grains looks like:

	or		or		=	
1/2 cup rice		1/2 cup pasta		1/2 cup oatmeal		1/2 baseball

| 1 slice bread | 1 cup cereal | 1 piece cornbread | one 6-inch tortilla | one 3-inch (mini) bagel |

MEAT & BEANS

1 serving of meat or beans looks like:

	or		or		or		=	
3 oz chicken		5 oz steak		4 oz pork		6 oz tofu		mouse

		=	
	3 oz fish		checkbook

	or		=	
1/2 cup garbanzo beans		1/2 cup pinto beans		light bulb

	or		or		=	
1 oz peanuts		1 oz almonds		2 T. peanut butter		ping pong ball

FATS

1 serving of fats looks like:

				or		=	
1 t. butter	1 oz potato chips	1 T. salad dressing	2 T. cream cheese		2 T. olive oil		ping pong ball

ALCOHOL

One "drink" of alcohol is defined as the amount of a beverage that provides 1/2 fl. oz of alcohol, which normally equals 1-1/2 oz of distilled spirits, 5 oz of wine, or 12 oz of beer or wine cooler.

TOLERABLE UPPER INTAKE LEVELS (UL[a])

Vitamins

Life-Stage Group	Vitamin A (µg/d)[b]	Vitamin C (mg/d)	Vitamin D (µg/d)	Vitamin E (mg/d)[c,d]	Niacin (mg/d)[d]	Vitamin B6 (mg/d)	Folate (µg/d)[d]	Choline (g/d)
Infants								
0–6 mo	600	ND[e]	25	ND	ND	ND	ND	ND
7–12 mo	600	ND	25	ND	ND	ND	ND	ND
Children								
1–3 y	600	400	50	200	10	30	300	1.0
4–8 y	900	650	50	300	15	40	400	1.0
Males, Females								
9–13 y	1,700	1,200	50	600	20	60	600	2.0
14–18 y	2,800	1,800	50	800	30	80	800	3.0
19–70 y	3,000	2,000	50	1,000	35	100	1,000	3.5
>70 y	3,000	2,000	50	1,000	35	100	1,000	3.5
Pregnancy								
≤18 y	2,800	1,800	50	800	30	80	800	3.0
19–50 y	3,000	2,000	50	1,000	35	100	1,000	3.5
Lactation								
≤18 y	2,800	1,800	50	800	30	80	800	3.0
19–50 y	3,000	2,000	50	1,000	35	100	1,000	3.5

Elements

Life-Stage Group	Boron (mg/d)	Calcium (g/d)	Copper (µg/d)	Fluoride (mg/d)	Iodine (µg/d)	Iron (mg/d)	Magnesium (mg/d)[f]	Manganese (mg/d)	Molybdenum (µg/d)	Nickel (mg/d)	Phosphorus (g/d)	Selenium (µg/d)	Vanadium (mg/d)[g]	Zinc (mg/d)	Sodium (g/d)	Chloride (g/d)
Infants																
0–6 mo	ND	ND	ND	0.7	ND	40	ND	ND	ND	ND	ND	45	ND	4	ND	ND
7–12 mo	ND	ND	ND	0.9	ND	40	ND	ND	ND	ND	ND	60	ND	5	ND	ND
Children																
1–3 y	3	2.5	1,000	1.3	200	40	65	2	300	0.2	3	90	ND	7	1.5	2.3
4–8 y	6	2.5	3,000	2.2	300	40	110	3	600	0.3	3	150	ND	12	1.9	2.9
Males, Females																
9–13 y	11	2.5	5,000	10	600	40	350	6	1,100	0.6	4	280	ND	23	2.2	3.4
14–18 y	17	2.5	8,000	10	900	45	350	9	1,700	1.0	4	400	ND	34	2.3	3.6
19–70 y	20	2.5	10,000	10	1,100	45	350	11	2,000	1.0	4	400	1.8	40	2.3	3.6
>70 y	20	2.5	10,000	10	1,100	45	350	11	2,000	1.0	3	400	1.8	40	2.3	3.6
Pregnancy																
≤18 y	17	2.5	8,000	10	900	45	350	9	1,700	1.0	3.5	400	ND	34	2.3	3.6
19–50 y	20	2.5	10,000	10	1,100	45	350	11	2,000	1.0	3.5	400	ND	40	2.3	3.6
Lactation																
≤18 y	17	2.5	8,000	10	900	45	350	9	1,700	1.0	4	400	ND	34	2.3	3.6
19–50 y	20	2.5	10,000	10	1,100	45	350	11	2,000	1.0	4	400	ND	40	2.3	3.6

Sources: Adapted from the Dietary Reference Intakes series, National Academies Press. Copyright 1997, 1998, 2000, 2001, by the National Academy of Sciences. These reports may be accessed via www.nap.edu. Courtesy of the National Academies Press, Washington, D.C.

[a] UL = The maximum level of daily nutrient intake that is likely to pose no risk of adverse effects. Unless otherwise specified, the UL represents total intake from food, water, and supplements. Due to lack of suitable data, ULs could not be established for vitamin K, thiamin, riboflavin, vitamin B12, pantothenic acid, biotin, or carotenoids. In the absence of ULs, extra caution may be warranted in consuming levels above recommended intakes.

[b] As preformed vitamin A only.

[c] As α-tocopherol; applies to any form of supplemental α-tocopherol.

[d] The ULs for vitamin E, niacin, and folate apply to synthetic forms obtained from supplements, fortified foods, or a combination of the two.

[e] ND = Not determinable due to lack of data of adverse effects in this age group and concern with regard to lack of ability to handle excess amounts. Source of intake should be from food only to prevent high levels of intake.

[f] The ULs for magnesium represent intake from a pharmacological agent only and do not include intake from food and water.

[g] Although vanadium in food has not been shown to cause adverse effects in humans, there is no justification for adding vanadium to food, and vanadium supplements should be used with caution. The UL is based on adverse effects in laboratory animals, and this data could be used to set a UL for adults but not children and adolescents.

NUTRITION, HEALTH & WELLNESS: AN APPLIED APPROACH

SECOND EDITION

Compiled by

Abour H. Cherif, Dianne M. Jedlicka, Betsy A. Hornick, Sujata Verma, Robert D. Aron, and Bashar W. Hanna

Excerpts taken from:

Nutrition: An Applied Approach, Second Edition
by Janice Thompson and Melinda Manore

Total Fitness and Wellness, Media Update, Fifth Edition
by Scott K. Powers, Stephen L. Dodd, Erica M. Jackson

Decisions for Healthy Living
by B.E. Pruitt and Jane J. Stein

Nutrition and Diet Therapy for Nurses
by Sheila Buckley Tucker and Vera Dauffenbach

Access to Health, Green Edition
by Rebecca J. Donatelle

Nutrition: Core Concepts for Good Health & You
by Joan Salge Blake

Learning Solutions

New York   Boston   San Francisco
London   Toronto   Sydney   Tokyo   Singapore   Madrid
Mexico City   Munich   Paris   Cape Town   Hong Kong   Montreal

Nutrition, Health, and Wellness: An Applied Approach
Second Edition
Published in 2010

Cover Art: Untitled Symphony—Rosemary Broton Broyle

Taken from:

Nutrition: An Applied Approach, Second Edition
by Janice Thompson and Melinda Manore
Copyright © 2009 by Pearson Education, Inc.
Published by Benjamin Cummings
San Francisco, California 94111

Total Fitness and Wellness, Media Update, Fifth Edition
by Scott K. Powers, Stephen L. Dodd, Erica M. Jackson
Copyright © 2011, 2009, 2006 by Pearson Education, Inc.
Published by Benjamin Cummings

Decisions for Healthy Living
by B.E. Pruitt and Jane J. Stein
Copyright © 2004 by Pearson Education, Inc.
Published by Benjamin Cummings

Nutrition and Diet Therapy for Nurses
by Sheila Buckley Tucker and Vera Dauffenbach
Copyright © 2011 by Pearson Education, Inc.
Published by Prentice Hall
Upper Saddle River, New Jersey 07458

Access to Health, Green Edition
by Rebecca J. Donatelle
Copyright © 2011 by Pearson Education, Inc.
Published by Benjamin Cummings

Nutrition: Core Concepts for Good Health & You
by Joan Salge Blake
Copyright © 2011 by Pearson Education, Inc.
Published by Benjamin Cummings

Pearson Learning Solutions, 501 Boylston Street, Suite 900, Boston, MA 02116
A Pearson Education Company
www.pearsoned.com

Printed in the United States of America

2 3 4 5 6 7 8 9 10 V011 15 14 13 12

000200010270614446

SB/LP

ISBN 10: 0-558-86595-X
ISBN 13: 978-0-558-86595-5

Dedicated to Faculty who teach Nutrition, Health, and Wellness throughout the world for giving unstintingly of their time, effort, and commitment to help and support students.

Physical health
includes nutrition
and physical activity

Occupational health
meaningful work
or vocation

Social health
includes family,
community, and
social environment

Spiritual health
spiritual values
and beliefs

Emotional health
includes positive
feelings about
oneself and life

Many factors contribute to an individual's wellness. Primary among these are a nutritious diet and regular physical activity.

FIRST EDITION PREFACE

Welcome to *Nutrition, Health, and Wellness: An Applied Approach*

Nutrition, health, and wellness receives a lot of press. Pick up a magazine and you'll read the latest debate over high-protein/low-carbohydrate diets. Turn on the TV and you'll hear a Hollywood star describe how she lost 50 pounds without exercising. Scan the newspaper and you'll discover the politics surrounding the creation of the new food guide pyramid. How can you evaluate these sources of nutrition information and find out whether the advice they provide is reliable? How do you navigate through the endless recommendations and come up with a way of living that's right for you—one that supports your physical activity, allows you to maintain a healthful weight, and helps you to avoid chronic disease?

Nutrition, Health, and Wellness: An Applied Approach is an exciting book that is scientific in its approach. In addition to being a great nutrition text, it also includes outstanding elements of wellness, health and physical fitness. Wellness and physical fitness are as important for a healthy body as the foods that go into the body, and we have tried to integrate these concepts and their explanations with the traditional nutrition coverage and to do so in a manner that is easy to read, comprehend, and apply.

Today's nursing and college level nutrition courses must include wellness, health, and physical fitness in order to prepare students for both their professions and their lives. However, while traditional nutrition books may mention wellness and physical fitness, their coverage is typically light. For example, mental health is often a brief topic, if covered at all. In *Nutrition, Health, and Wellness,* we have included several chapters that address the growing concern for mental health in our modern, technologically advanced society. We have also addressed the issues associated with drug and substance abuse by including chapters on this important topic. Finally, traditional Nutrition books may mention fitness plans and activities, but *Nutrition, Health, and Wellness* includes two chapters devoted to caloric input, types of activities and anatomical and physiological changes during exercise.

Nutrition, Health, and Wellnes, imparts knowledge, understanding and the ability to communicate information regarding the effects of food, vitamins, clean water, exercise, mood or happiness, crowding, and disease. While this is positive at both the personal and professional levels, we hope that students will also take the time to extend the knowledge and applications covered in the text to a broader theatre—the impact of the global economy, food abundance, food scarcity, and food distribution on nutrition, health, and wellness. Our planet can produce an abundance of foods. However, the objectives of good nutrition, health, and wellness remain at risk in the face of two major problems: (1) food distribution; and (2) education about food choices. Achieving appropriate distribution requires complex logistical and political solutions, but even in their absence, the many peoples and nations of the world can benefit from a better understanding of nutrition, wellness, health, and physical fitness.

We live in an age of technology, computers, new scientific advancements, and other technological tools. In addition to delivering a sound, scientifically based course, the Editors believe that it is important to educate this generation in a manner they find both comfortable and easy to understand. The text has many accompanying study aids that are in tune with the current technologies. In particular, we would like to call your attention to **MyNutritionLab.** This online standard course management system is loaded with teaching and learning resources that make giving assignments and tracking student progress easy. **MyNutritionLab,** powered by CourseCompass, features a wealth of pre-loaded content for instructors, including PowerPoint slides, Test Bank questions, Instructor's Manual material, and more. Features for students include interactive label activities, animations, and drag-and-drop activities. Research Navigator, which provides three databases of credible and reliable source materials, is also included. This learning management system, in conjunction with the *Nutrition, Health, and Wellness* text, bridges the gaps found in introductory and intermediate college level texts and programs and offers college students, including undergraduate nursing students, a sound, scientifi-cally oriented course focusing on Nutrition, Health, and Wellness.

Abour H. Cherif, Ph.D.
Dianne M. Jedlicka, Ph.D.
Sujata Verma, Ph.D.
Robert D. Aron, Ph.D.
Bashar Hanna, Ph.D.

SECOND EDITION PREFACE

The first edition of *Nutrition, Health, and Wellness: An Applied Approach* was a remarkable success, and the courses that used it prospered as well. For example, DeVry University's SCI-228 Nutrition, Health, and Wellness, which was designed to fulfill the school's science requirement, grew substantially, and then grew again when students from Chamberlain College of Nursing began to take the course as part of their program of study. Many factors contributed to create this success, including content, design, and supportive print and web-base materials for both instructors and students. However, most important of all, was the manner in which the editors of the text were able to assemble and integrate the three main topics of the text—nutrition, health, and wellness—in a creative, effective, and inviting way. Building on this success, we are very excited to intro-duce the second edition of *Nutrition, Health, and Wellness: An Applied Approach,* including additional resources, updated information, revised chapters, inte-grated labs (wet and web-based), and a revised custom edition of *MyNutritionLab* (MNL), which includes materials from *MyHealthLab* and *MyFitnessLab*.

The custom version of *MyNutritionLab*, powered by CourseCompass, features everything needed to teach introductory nutrition, health and wellness in one convenient place, including PowerPoine slides, Test Bank questions, Instructor's Manual materials, and more. Features for students include:

- Updated and highly sophisticated web-based animations and activities;
- ABC News videos;
- Tutorials, exercises, and practice exams;
- Interactive drag-and-drop activities;

- Nutrition Debate activities that can be emailed to professors;
- Case studies; and
- Answers to the Nutri-Cases, Find the Quack, and end-of-chapter Review Questions. Research Navigator, which provides three databases of creditable and reliable source materials, is included.

The new second edition of the text includes the following changes:

1. Updated information and data;
2. Updated case studies and review questions;
3. The deletion of several chapters;
4. The addition of new chapters; and
5. The addition of student labs, which are included at the back of the text.

In addition to the text and *MyNutritionLab*, the following items are available:

Cases on the Web: Nutrition

Additional real case scenarios, intended for student use, are available electronically on the web;

EvaluEat Dietary Analysis Software

EvaluEat diet analysis software is accurate, use friendly, and comprehensive and contains a food database of 6,200 foods. Students can use the software to create a variety of reports, calculate how many calories they're consuming versus how many they're expending in exercise, and determine whether they're meeting the DRIs for various vitamins and minerals.

Live Right! Beating Stress in College and Beyond

Live Right! gives students useful tips for coping with stressful life challenges both during college and for the rest of their lives. Topics include sleep, managing finances, time management, coping with academic pressure, and relationships.

Eat Right! Healthy Eating in College and Beyond

Eat Right!, a handy, full-color 80-page booklet, provides students with practical guidelines, tips, shopper's guides and recipes that turn healthy eating principles into blueprints for action. Topics include healthy eating in the cafeteria, dorm room, and fast-food restaurants; planning meals on a budget; weight management; vegetarian alternatives; and the effects of alcohol on health.

In response to faculty and student suggestions, we have deleted the chapters on "The Health Effect of Smoking and Drinking", and "Understanding The Dangers of Drug Use". In addition, we have replaced several chapters as follows:

1. "The Biomechanics of Physical Exercise" with "Personal Fitness";
2. "Managing Stress", with "Stress management";
3. "Understanding the Dangers of Drug Use" with "Total Fitness Addiction and Substance Abuse"; and
4. "Nutrient Values of Foods" with "Complementary and Alternative Medicine".

Finally, based on faculty and student recommendations, we have made two other additions:

1. We have added a Diet Therapy Module. The Diet Therapy Module consists of *Nursing and Nutrition Care*, *Diet Therapy in Disease Management*, and Case Studies. In each of the end-of-chapter case studies (2–3 per chapter), students will complete a nutrition assessment, diagnosis, recommended intervention, and a plan for monitoring/evaluation; and

2. We have added laboratories and a suggested list of chapters where they can be best be used and have placed those laboratories at the end of the text in a ready-to-use format. We purposely provided a variety of laboratory alternatives under most categories to offer faculty and instructors the flexibility and freedom to select the labs that they prefer. In addition, it's important to note that we have included these laboratories with the textbook because we want to emphasize for both students and faculty that this is a lab course and to make the labs available so that they can easily be used.

As always, we are so thankful to all the faculty, instructors, and students at both DeVry University System and Chamberlain College of Nursing who have provided us with priceless feedback, suggestions and recommendations since the publication of the first edition of *Nutrition, Health, and Wellness: An Applied Approach* was published. In particular, we would like to thank Associate Professor Carole L. Keeth, Ph.D., RN, of the Addison, Illinois campus of Chamberlain College of Nursing for her time, effort, and detailed review of Chapter 23, *Nursing and Nutrition Care,* and Chapter 24, *Diet Therapy in Disease Management.* Her suggestions have made those chapters better. We hope that this 2nd edition will enjoy the same success as the first edition.

Abour Cherif, Ph.D.
National Associate Dean
Math and Science Curriculum
DeVry University
Downers Grove, Illinois, USA
August 2010

FIRST EDITION ACKNOWLEDGMENTS

It is eye opening to author a textbook and to realize that the work of so many people contributes to the final product. There are numerous people to thank and we'd like to begin by extending our gratitude to our contributors, Cindy Beck of Evergreen State College, Kendra Golden of Whitman College, and Patricia Ketcham of Oregon State University. Cindy, Kendra, and Patricia wrote Chapters, and their efforts are greatly appreciated. In addition we offer our sincere thanks to Judy Sheeshka, of the University of Guelph, who created the Canadian Recommendations and Guidelines appendix for this book, and Patricia Brown, of Cuesta College, for her consultation on the Nutrient Values of Common Foods table that also appears as an appendix.

Our goal of meeting instructor and student needs could not have been realized without the team of educators and editorial staff who worked on the substantial supplements package for *Nutrition*. Dr. Kim Aaronson of Truman College wrote the inventive and useful Student Study Guide; Ruth Reilly and Jesse Morell, both of the University of New Hampshire, created a comprehensive Test Bank; and Linda Flemming of Middlesex Community College, authored the wonderful Instructor's Manual; all of which were managed by editor Ziki Dekel. Ryan Shaw, Assistant Editor, and Dr. Amy Marion of New Mexico State University worked on the Instructor's Resource CD-ROM and PowerPoint lecture slides. Alex Levering, Media Producer, headed up the coordination and development of the companion website to the text, working with content contributors Marie Dunford; Judy Kaufman of Monroe Community College; Colleen Kvaska of Mt. San Antonio College; Kristy Long; Wendy Cunningham of California State University of Sacramento; Andria Pescatello of University of California, Irvine; Priya Venkatesan of Pasadena City College; Sandra Weatherilt of Mt. San Antonio College; and Jennifer Weddig of Metropolitan State College of Denver.

SECOND EDITION ACKNOWLEDGMENTS

It is eye-opening to author a textbook and to realize that the work of so many people contributes to the final product. There are numerous people to thank, and we'd like to begin by extending our gratitude to our contributors. John Fishback of Ozarks Technical and Community College revised Chapters 1 and 7, and Tara Barber of East Carolina University revised Chapter 8. Linda Vaughan, of Arizona State University, revised our life cycle chapters and wrote the new *In Depth* features on alcohol and on vitamins and minerals. Annie Wetter of University of Wisconsin–Stevens Point wrote the new *In Depth* on phytochemicals and functional foods. Thanks also goes to previous contributors Cindy Beck of Evergreen State College and Kendra Golden of Whitman College, who wrote the original versions of Chapters 14 and 15, respectively; their efforts are greatly appreciated. In addition, we offer our sincere thanks to Patricia Brown, of Cuesta College, for her consultation on the Nutrient Values of Common Foods table that also appears as an appendix.

We would like to thank the fabulous staff at Benjamin Cummings for their incredible support and dedication to this book. Our past and current Acquisitions Editors, Deirdre Espinoza and Sandra Lindelof, respectively, have provided unwavering support and guidance throughout the entire process of writing and publishing this book. We could never have written this text without the exceptional editing skills of Laura Bonazzoli, our Developmental Editor. In addition to providing content guidance, she wrote the chapter-opening stories, the Find the Quack features, and the Nutri-Cases. Laura's energy, enthusiasm, and creativity significantly enhanced the quality of this textbook. We are also deeply indebted to Art Development Editor Laura Southworth. She developed a spectacular art program and guided two non-artists through the arduous process of creating informative and attractive textbook illustrations. Our Project Editor, Marie Beaugureau, kept us on course, kept us sane with her sense of humor and excellent organizational skills, and made revising this book a pleasure instead of a chore. Jacob Evans, Editorial Assistant, provided us with editorial and administrative support that we would have been lost without.

Multiple talented players helped build this book in the production and design processes as well. Beth Masse, Production Supervisor, and Brandi Nelson, Eric Arima, and the whole group at Elm Street Publishing Services kept manuscripts moving through the entire process, and they never lost track of the minute details. Donna Kalal, Art and Photo Coordinator, supervised the art and photo programs. Yvo Riezebos created a beautiful text design. Jeanne Calabrese designed the stunning cover. Kristin Piljay performed research for hundreds and hundreds of photos.

We can't go without thanking the marketing and sales teams, especially Neena Bali, Marketing Manager, who coordinated nutrition forums and extensive market research to ensure that we directed our writing efforts to meet the needs of students and instructors, and who has been working incredibly hard to get this book out to those who will benefit most from it.

Our goal of meeting instructor and student needs could not have been realized without the team of educators and editorial staff who worked on the substantial supplements package for *Nutrition: An Applied Approach.* Dr. Kim Aaronson of Truman College wrote the inventive and useful Student Study Guide; Ruth Reilly and Jesse Morell, both of University of New Hampshire, created a comprehensive Test Bank; and Linda Fleming, of Middlesex Community College, authored the wonderful Instructor's Manual; all of whom were managed by editor Jennifer Cassidento. Alex Streczyn, Assistant Editor, coordinated the creation of the Instructor's Media Manager, including the PowerPoint lecture slides created by Dr. James Bailey of University of Tennessee, Knoxville and the clicker questions and quiz show questions, written by Franca Alphin of Duke University. Jacob Evans, Editorial Assistant, headed up the coordination and development of the companion website to the text, working with content contributors Marie Dunford, Elizabeth Quintana of West Virginia University, and Carol Friesen of Ball State University.

We would also like to thank the many colleagues, friends, and family members who helped us along the way. Janice would like to thank her colleagues at both the University of New Mexico Office of Native American Diabetes Programs and the University of Bristol. Their unflagging support and interest helped her to maintain her energy and enthusiasm while editing this book. She would also like to thank her family and friends, who have been so incredibly supportive throughout her career. They are always there to offer a sympathetic ear and endless encouragement.

Melinda would specifically like to thank her husband, Steve Carroll, for the patience and understanding he has shown through this process—once again. He has learned that there is always another chapter due! Melinda would also like to thank her family, friends, graduate students, and professional colleagues for their support and listening ear throughout this whole process. They all helped make life a little easier during this incredibly busy time. Finally, she would like to thank Janice, a great friend and colleague, who makes working on the book fun and rewarding.

REVIEWERS

Jan Adair
Minnesota State University

Helen Alexanderson-Lee
California State University, Long Beach

Robert Alman II
Indiana University of Pennsylvania

Janet Anderson
Utah State University

Barbara Anton
Minnesota State University

Laura Avila
Glendale Community College

James Bailey
University of Tennessee, Knoxville

Bobby Baldridge
Asbury College

Jeremy Barnes
Southeast Missouri State University

Robert B. Beavers
Benedict College

Beverly Benes
University of Nebraska, Lincoln

Ethan Bergman
Central Washington University

Nancy Berkoff
Los Angeles Trade Technical College

Jaqueline Berning
University of Colorado, Colorado Springs

Carlton Bessinger
Winthrop University

Jill Black
Cleveland State University

Gregory Blake Biren
Rowan University

M. Ann Bock
New Mexico State University

Roger Bounds
Sam Houston State University

Nancy Bradley
Central Florida Community College, Ocala

Ellen Brennan
San Antonio College

K. Shane Broughton
University of Wyoming

Liz Brown
Rose State College

Ardith Brunt
North Dakota State University

Laura J. Burger
Grossmont College

Joanne Burke
Boston College

John Capeheart
University of Houston, Downtown

Denise Cazes
University of Houston, Clearlake

Dorothy Chen-Maynard
California State University, San Bernardino

Kim Clark
California State University San Bernadino

Debbie Cohen
Southeast Missouri State University

Priscilla Connors
University of North Texas

Margaret Craig-Schmidt
Auburn University

Wendy Cunningham
California State University, Sacramento

Diane Dembicki
Dutchess County Community College

Richard Dowdy
University of Missouri, Columbia

Jean Dunlap
Rose State College

Mandi Dupain
Millersville University

Craig Elder
Southeast Missouri State University

Richard Mark Ellington
University of North Carolina-Wilmington

Virginia Englert
Colorado State University

Bruce Evans
Huntington College

Farahnaz
Veterinary College, London

Sally Feltner
Western Carolina University

Rosemary Ferguson
University of North Carolina-Wilmington

Gary Fosmire
Pennsylvania State University

Bernard Frye
University of Texas, Arlington

Peggy Gorbach
Evergreen Valley College

Cynthia Gossage
Prince George's Community College

Sandra Gross
Westchester University

Nancy Harris
East Carolina University

William Helferich
University of Illinois, Urbana-Champaign

Loretta R. Herrin
Benedict College

Beckee Hobson
College of the Sequoias

Carolyn Holcroft
Foothill College

J. David Holland
Springfield College, Illinois

Claire Hollenbeck
San Jose State University

Gwendolyn Holmes
Norfolk State University

Peter Horvath
State University of New York, Buffalo

Cara Hoyt
California State University, Hayward

Holli Hudson
Berea College

Jasminka Ilich
University of Connecticut

Loeen Irons
Baylor University

Rao Ivaturi
Indiana State University

Thunder Jalili
University of Utah

Catherine Jen
Wayne State University

Jay Kandiah
Ball State University

Judy Kaufman
Monroe Community College

Margaret Kessel
Ohio State University

Karl Kleinkopf
College of Idaho

Robert Kostelnik
Indiana University of Pennsylvania

Laura Kruskall
University of Nevada, Las Vegas

Melody Kyzer
University of North Carolina, Wilmington

Larry Lanciotti
Morton College

Deirdre Larkin
California State University, Northridge

Rebecca, Leas
Clarion University

Ellen Lee
California State University-Fullerton

Barbara Lohse
Kansas State University

Greg Lonning
Luther College

Linda Ludovico
Tyler Junior College

Bonnie Luft
Baylor University

Bernadene Magnuson
University of Maryland, College Park

Teresa Marcus
Chattanooga State Technical Community College

Rose Martin
Pennsylvania State University

Karen Mason
Western Kentucky University

Marlene McCall
Community College of Allegheny County

Jaqueline McClelland
North Carolina State University

Shelley McGuire
Washington State University

Glen McNeil
Fort Hays State University

Renee Melton
State University of New York, Buffalo

Sharon Michael
Tacoma Community College

Danyte Mockus
San Diego State University

Helene Monthley
Pennsylvania State University

Gina Marie Morris
Frank Phillips College

Donna Mueller
Drexel University

Mary Murimi
Louisiana Tech University

Michelle Neyman
California State University, Chico

Valorie Nybo
Western Carolina University

Irene O'Boyle
Central Michigan University

Anne O'Donnell
Santa Rosa Junior College

Millie Owens
College of the Sequoias

Miguel Perez
California State University Fresno

Erwina Peterson
Yakima Valley Community College

Roseanne Poole
Tallahassee Community College

Pat Rada-Sidinger
Colorado Mountain College

Ann Raithel
Deaconess College of Nursing

Linda Rankin
Idaho State University

Ruth Reed
Juniata College

Amy Reeder
University of Utah

Larry Reichard
Maple Woods Community College

Ruth Reilly
University of New Hampshire

Raylene Reimer
University of Calgary

Tonia Reinhard
Wayne State College

Bob Reynolds
University of Illinois, Chicago

Nuha Rice
University of Phoenix

Jennifer Ricketts
University of Arizona

José E. Rivera
Indiana University of Pennsylvania

Leah Robinson
Bucks County Community College

Judith Rodriguez
University of North Florida

George Rosales
Ventura College

Julie Sammarco Henderson
University of Utah

Lisa Sasson
New York University

Susan Saylor
University of Alabama

Monique Schaefer
El Camino College

Donal Scheidel
University of South Dakota

Connie Vinton Schoepske
Iowa Central Community College

Jiri Seltzer
Valdosta State University

Terry Shaw
Austin Community College

Tina Shepard
Arizona State University East

Sarah Short
Syracuse University

Kathryn Silliman
California State University, Chico

Clifford Singh
California State University, San Bernardino

Neeta Singh
University of the Incarnate Word

Elizabeth Skendzic
University of Wisconsin, Parkside

Carole Sloan
Henry Ford Community College

Mollie Smith
California State University, Fresno

Anastasia Snelling
American University

Diana Marie Spillman
Miami University

Stasinos Stavrianeas
Williamette University

Jiri Stelzer
Valdosta State University

Tammy Stephenson
University of Kentucky

Lianne Summerfield
Marymount University

Steven Swoap
Williams College

Robin Sytsma
Solano Community College

Elsie Takeguchi
Sacramento City College

Norman Temple
Athabasca University

Ann Thompson
South Plains College

Linda Vaughn
Arizona State University

Priya Venkatesan
Pasadena City College

Robert Walker
John Brown University

Daryle Wane
Pasco-Hernando Community College

Beverly Webber
University of Utah

Jennifer Weddig
Metropolitan State College of Denver

Sally Weerts
University of North Florida

Stacie Wing
University of Utah

Cynthia Wright
Southern Utah University

Gloria Young
Virginia State University

Maureen Zimmerman
Mesa Community College

Donna Zoss
Purdue University

Nutrition Forum and Focus Group Participants

Amy Allen-Chabot
Anne Arundel Community College

Janet Anderson
Utah State University

James Bailey
University of Tennessee, Knoxville

Beverly Benes
University of Nebraska, Lincoln

Patricia Brown
Cuesta College

Alison Campbell
Brigham Young University

Paula Cochrane
TVI Community College

Priscilla Connors
University of North Texas

Robert Cullen
Illinois State University

Earlene Davis
Bakersfield College

Linda Davis
Virginia Polytechnic Institute and State University

Gail Frank
California State University, Long Beach

Bernard Frye
University of Texas, Arlington

Art Gilbert
University of California, Santa Barbara

Cynthia Gossage
Prince Georges Community College

Lisa Gurule
TVI Community College

Beckee Hobson
College of the Sequoias

Clarie Hollenbeck
San Jose State University

Thunder Jalili
University of Utah

Mary Kelso
Antelope Valley College

Laura Kruskall
University of Nevada, Las Vegas

Renee Melton
SUNY Buffalo

Debra Pearce
Northern Kentucky University

Ruth Reilly
University of New Hampshire

Nidia Romer
Miami Dade College

Margaret Craig Schmidt
Auburn University

Roseann Schnoll
Brooklyn College

Sarah Short
Syracuse University

Priya Venkatesan
Pasadena City College

Jennifer Weddig
Metropolitan College of Denver

Sally Weerts
University of North Florida

Jurist Willis-Morris
Miami Dade College

Cynthia Wright
Southern Utah University

Research Consultants

The authors wish to thank the following individuals who provided research materials for their consultation. Their contributions helped ensure the exceptional currency and accuracy of the textbook.

Janet Anderson
Utah State University

Beverly Benes
University of Nebraska, Lincoln

Ethan Bergman
Central Washington University

Priscilla Connors
University of North Texas

Stacy Gehrig
Illinois Central College

Silvia Giraudo
University of Georgia

David Holben
Ohio University

Clarie Hollenbeck
San Jose State University

Peter Horvath
SUNY Buffalo

Thunder Jalili
University of Utah

Laura Kruskall
University of Nevada, Las Vegas

Janet Sundberg
Southern Illinois University

Class Testers

Kim Aaronson
Truman College

Kwaku Addo
University of Kentucky

Amy Allen-Chabot
Anne Arundel Community College

Julianne Arient
Triton College

Jennifer Asher
Southeast Missouri State University

Garry Auld
Colorado State University

James Bailey
University of Tennessee, Knoxville

Susan Balinsky
College of Charleston

Sharon Barron
Brevard Community College

Cynthia Beck
Evergreen State College

Nancy Berkoff
LA Trade Technical College

Jean Boone
Palm Beach Community College

Ardith Brunt
North Dakota State University

Alison Campbell
Brigham Young University

Nancy Canolty
University of Georgia

Catherine Christie
University of North Florida

Elizabeth Chu
San Diego Mesa College

Debbie Cohen
Southeast Missouri State University

Fabio Comona
San Diego State University

Rhena Cooper
North Idaho College

Wendy Cunningham
California State University, Sacramento

Noemi Custodia-Lora
Northern Essex Community College

Earlene Davis
Bakersfield College

Cindy Dostal
Hawkeye Community College

Sally Feltner
Western Carolina University

Brian Findley
Palm Beach Community College

Anthony Giusti
American River College

Cynthia Gonzalez
Santa Monica College

Peggy Gorbach
Evergreen Valley College

Meledath Govindan
Fitchburg State College

Carolyn Holcroft
Foothill College

Julie Hood
Central Oregon Community College

Debra Hook
California State University, San Bernardino

Brian Hug
Olivet College

Linda Ibarra–Gonzalez
Palo Alto College

Thunder Jalili
University of Utah

James Kahora
Middlesex Community College

Judy Kaufman
Monroe Community College

Susan Kazen
Palo Alto College

Mary Kelso
Antelope Valley College

Linda Kollett
Massasoit Community College

Dorothy Koteski
Community College of Philadelphia

Laura Kruskall
University of Nevada, Las Vegas

Alison Leahy
Shoreline Community College

Jeannie Luther
Albuquerque Technical Vocational Institute

Susan Meyers
Miami Dade College

Lauren Morgan
Gloucester County College

Gina Marie Morris
Frank Phillips College

Rose Ann Neff
Lock Haven University of Pennsylvania

Terry O'Toole
Lynchburg College

Anna Page
Johnson County Community College

Stephanie Perry
University of North Florida

Roseann Poole
Tallahassee Community College

Ralph Price
University of Arizona

Peggy Ramsey
University of California, Irvine

Linda Rankin
Idaho State University

Ruth Reilly
University of New Hampshire

Carol Reynolds
Fullerton College

Tom Richard
Keene State College

Christian Roberts
University of California, Los Angeles

Leah Robinson
Bucks County Community College

Nidia Romer
Miami Dade College

Donal Scheidel
University of South Dakota

Connie Schneider
California State University, Fresno

Roseanne Schnoll
Brooklyn College

A.I. Clifford Singh
California State University, San Bernardino

Neeta Singh
University of the Incarnate Word

Lorraine Siniscaro
Herkimer County Community College

Eleanor Skelley
Palo Alto College

Mollie Smith
California State University, Fresno

Debra St. George
Massasoit Community College

Ann Thompson
South Plains College

Joan Thompson
Weber State University

Alan Titchenal
University of Hawaii, Manoa

Simin Vaghefi
University of North Florida

Linda Vaughan
Arizona State University

Marva Volk
Tulsa Community College

Sandra Weatherilt
Mt. San Antonio College

Jennifer Weddig
Metropolitan College of Denver

Sally Weerts
University of North Florida

Kathy White
St. Philips College

Jurist Willis-Morris
Miami Dade College

Jean York
Mt. San Antonio College

Wendy Zins
Anoka Ramsey Community College

Franca Alphin
Duke University School of Medicine

James Bailey
University of Tennessee, Knoxville

Virginia A. Bennett
Central Washington University

Joye M. Bond
Minnesota State University, Mankato

Patricia B. Brevard
James Madison University

John Capeheart
University of Houston, Downtown

Paula K. Cochrane
Albuquerque TVI Community College

John Fishback
Ozarks Technical and Community College

Carol Friesen
Ball State University

Nancy Harris
East Carolina University

James Hollis
Purdue University

Ann Hunter
Wichita State University

Teresa Johnson
Troy State University

Danita Kelley
Western Kentucky University

Kris Levy
Columbus State Community College

Susan L. Meacham
University of Nevada, Las Vegas

Anne F. Miller
De Anza College

Candi Possinger
SUNY Buffalo

Bassam M. Salameh
California State University, Bakersfield

Vicki Schwartz
Drexel University

Janet Tou
West Virginia University

Priya Venkatesan
Pasadena City College

John P. Warber
Morehead State University

Jennifer Weddig
Metropolitan College of Denver

Christopher Wendtland
Monroe Community College

BRIEF CONTENTS

CONTENTS

CHAPTER 15 Disordered Eating   580

CHAPTER 20 Nutrition Through the Life Cycle: Childhood to Late Adulthood 738

Chapters 1–11, 13, 15, 18–20, 23, 24, Appendices, Glossary, and Answers taken from: *Nutrition: An Applied Approach,* Second Edition, by Janice Thompson and Melinda Manore; Chapters 12, 22 taken from: *Access to Health,* Green Edition, by Rebecca J. Donatelle; Chapters 16, 21 taken from: *Decisions for Healthy Living,* by B.E. Pruitt and Jane J. Stein; and Chapters 14, 17, and Lab Assignments taken from *Total Fitness Update,* Media Update, Fifth Edition, by Scott K. Powers, Stephen L. Dodd, Erica M. Jackson.

LABORATORY ASSIGNMENTS CHART

Laboratory Name	Laboratory Usage: Recommended Chapter(s)
Lifestyle Assessment Inventory	1
Assessing Nutritional Habits	1
Analyzing Your Diet	1 or 2
Setting Goals for a Healthy Diet	1, 2, or 3
Planning a New Diet	1, 2, or 3
What Triggers Your Eating	3
Estimating Daily Caloric Expenditure and the Caloric Deficit Required to Lose 1 Pound of Fat per Week	4
Finding Your Cholesterol Plan	4
Assessing Body Image	5
Weight-Loss Goals and Progress Report	5 and 6 and 11
Wellness Profile	7, 8, 9, 10, or 13
Determining Ideal Body Weight Using Percent Body Fat and the Body Mass Index	11
Warming Up	12
Which Physical Activities Work Best for You?	11, 12, or 13
Using a Pedometer to Count Your Steps	11, 12, or 13
Measuring Cardiorespiratory Fitness: The 1.5-Mile Run Test	11, 12, or 13
Measuring Cardiorespiratory Fitness: The 1-Mile Walk Test	11, 12, or 13
Measuring Cardiorespiratory Fitness: Submaximal Cycle Test	11, 12, or 13
Measuring Cardiorespiratory Fitness: Step Test	11, 12, or 13
Determining Target Heart Rate	11, 12, or 13
Developing Your Personal Exercise Prescription	11, 12, or 13
Determining Rate of Perceived Exertion	11, 12, or 13
Evaluating Fitness Products	13
Managing Time and Establishing Priorities	14
Assessing Your Personality Behavior Pattern	14

NUTRITION, HEALTH, AND WELLNESS: AN APPLIED APPROACH

CHAPTER 1

CHAPTER OBJECTIVES

After reading this chapter you will be able to:

1. Define the term *nutrition*, p. 4.

2. Discuss why nutrition is important to health, pp. 4–7.

3. Identify the six classes of nutrients essential for health, pp. 8–9.

4. Compare and contrast the three energy nutrients, pp. 8–12.

5. Explain how vitamins and minerals differ from each other, pp. 12–13.

6. Identify the Dietary Reference Intakes for nutrients, pp. 14–17.

7. Describe the four steps of the scientific method, p. 19.

8. List at least four sources of reliable and accurate nutrition information, pp. 24–27.

TEST YOURSELF TRUE OR FALSE?

1. Calories are a measure of the amount of fat in foods. **T or F**

2. Proteins are not a primary source of energy for our bodies. **T or F**

3. All vitamins must be consumed daily to support good health. **T or F**

4. The Recommended Dietary Allowance is the maximum amount of nutrients that people should consume to support normal body functions. **T or F**

5. Federal agencies in the United States are typically poor sources of reliable nutrition information. **T or F**

Test Yourself answers can be found after the Chapter Summary.

The Role of Nutrition in Our Health

miguel hadn't expected that college life would make him feel so tired. After classes, he just wanted to go back to his dorm and sleep. Plus, he had been having difficulty concentrating and was worried that his first-semester grades would be far below those he'd achieved in high school. Scott, his roommate, had little sympathy. "It's all that junk food you eat!" he insisted. "Let's go down to the organic market for some real food." Miguel dragged himself to the market with Scott but rested at the juice counter while his roommate went shopping. A middle-aged woman wearing a white lab coat approached him and introduced herself as the market's staff nutritionist. "You're looking a little pale," she said. "Anything wrong?" Miguel explained that he had been feeling tired lately. "I don't doubt it," the woman answered. "I can see from your skin tone that you're anemic. You need to start taking an iron supplement." She took a bottle of pills from a shelf and handed it to him. "This one is the easiest for you to absorb, and it's on special this week. Take it twice a day, and you should start feeling better in a day or two." Miguel purchased the supplement and began taking it that night with the meal his roommate prepared. He took it twice the next day as well, just as the nutritionist had recommended, but didn't feel any better. After 2 more days, he visited the university health clinic, where a nurse drew some blood for testing. When the results of the blood tests came in, the physician told him that his thyroid gland wasn't making enough of the hormone that he needed to keep his body functioning properly. She prescribed a medication and congratulated Miguel for catching the problem early. "If you had waited," she said, "it would only have gotten worse, and you could have become seriously ill." Miguel asked if he should continue taking his iron supplements. The physician looked puzzled. "Where did you get the idea that you needed iron supplements?"

Like Miguel, you've probably been offered nutrition-related advice from well-meaning friends and self-professed "experts." Perhaps you found the advice helpful, or maybe, as in Miguel's case, it turned out to be all wrong. Where can you go for reliable advice about nutrition? What exactly *is* nutrition anyway, and why does what we eat have such an influence on our health? In this chapter, we'll begin to answer these questions, and you'll gain a deeper understanding as you work through the rest of this book. Our goal is that, by the time you finish this course, you'll be the expert on your own nutritional needs!

What Is Nutrition?

If you think that the word *nutrition* means pretty much the same thing as *food,* you're right—partially. But the word has a broader meaning that will gradually become clear as you make your way in this course. Specifically, **nutrition** is the science that studies food and how food nourishes our bodies and influences our health. It encompasses how we consume, digest, metabolize, and store nutrients and how these nutrients affect our bodies. Nutrition also involves studying the factors that influence our eating patterns, making recommendations about the amount we should eat of each type of food, attempting to maintain food safety, and addressing issues related to the global food supply. You can think of nutrition, then, as the discipline that encompasses everything about food.

Nutrition is a relatively new scientific discipline. Although food has played a defining role in the lives of humans since the evolution of our species, the importance of nutrition to our health has only been formally recognized and studied over the past 100 years or so. Early research in nutrition focused on making the link between nutrient deficiencies and illness. For instance, the cause of scurvy, which is a vitamin C deficiency, was discovered in the mid-1700s. At that time, however, vitamin C had not been identified—what was known was that some ingredient found in citrus fruits could prevent scurvy. Another example of early discoveries in nutrition is presented in the accompanying Highlight box on early nutrition research into a disease called pellagra. As is the case with scurvy and vitamin C, this early research was able to pinpoint a deficiency disease and foods that could prevent it; it would only be later in the 20th century that the exact nutrient responsible for the deficiency symptoms would be discovered. Thus, unlike sciences such as physics and mathematics, the majority of discoveries in the field of nutrition are relatively recent, and we still have much to learn.

Why Is Nutrition Important?

Think about it: if you eat three meals a day, then by this time next year, you'll have had more than a thousand chances to influence your body's makeup! As you'll learn in this text, you are what you eat: the substances you take into your body are broken down and reassembled into your brain cells, bones, muscles—all of your tissues and organs. The foods you eat also provide your body with the energy it needs to function properly. In addition, we know that proper nutrition can help us improve our health, prevent certain diseases, achieve and maintain a desirable weight, and maintain our energy and vitality. More surprisingly, in the Nutrition Debate at the end of this chapter you'll find out that food can influence not only your own health but also the health of any children you might have. Let's take a closer look at how nutrition supports health and wellness.

Nutrition Is One of Several Factors Contributing to Wellness

Wellness can be defined in many ways. Traditionally considered simply the absence of disease, wellness has been redefined as we have learned more about our bodies and what it means to live a healthful lifestyle. Wellness is now considered to be a multidimensional process, one that includes physical, emotional, social, occupational,

Nutrition is the science that studies all aspects of food.

nutrition The science that studies food and how food nourishes our bodies and influences our health.

wellness A multidimensional, lifelong process that includes physical, emotional, and spiritual health.

HIGHLIGHT

Early Nutrition Research: Solving the Mystery of Pellagra

In the first few years of the 20th century, Dr. Joseph Goldberger successfully controlled outbreaks of several fatal infectious diseases, from yellow fever in Louisiana to typhus in Mexico. So it wasn't surprising that, in 1914, the Surgeon General of the United States chose him to tackle another disease thought to be infectious that was raging throughout the South. Called pellagra, the disease was characterized by

Pellagra is often characterized by a scaly skin rash.

a skin rash, diarrhea, and mental impairment. At the time, it afflicted more than 50,000 people each year, and in about 10% of cases, it resulted in death.

Goldberger began studying the disease by carefully observing its occurrence in groups of people. He asked, if it is infectious, then why would it occur in prison inmates, yet leave their guards unaffected? Why, in fact, did it overwhelmingly affect impoverished Southerners, while leaving their affluent (and well-fed) neighbors healthy? Could a dietary deficiency cause pellagra? Before he could confirm his hunch, he first had to prove that pellagra was not spread by germs. To do so, he and his colleagues deliberately injected or ingested patients' scabs or bodily fluids. When he and his team remained healthy, he conducted a series of experiments in which he fed his patients different nutrient-rich foods. Finally he found an inexpensive and widely available substance—brewer's yeast—that cured the disease. Shortly after Goldberger's death in 1937, scientists identified the precise nutrient that was deficient in the diet of pellagra patients: niacin, one of the B vitamins, which is plentiful in brewer's yeast.

Source: Based on Markel, H. 2003. The New Yorker who changed the diet of the South. *New York Times,* August 12, section D5.

and spiritual health **(FIGURE 1.1)**. Wellness is not an endpoint in our lives, but is an active process we work on every day.

In this book, we focus on two critical aspects of physical health: nutrition and physical activity. The two are so closely related that you can think of them as two sides of the same coin: our overall state of nutrition is influenced by how much energy we expend doing daily activities, and our level of physical activity has a major impact on how we use the nutrients in our food. We can perform more strenuous activities for longer periods of time when we eat a nutritious diet, whereas an inadequate or excessive food intake can make us lethargic. A poor diet, inadequate or excessive physical activity, or a combination of these also can lead to serious health problems. Finally, several studies have suggested that healthful nutrition and regular physical activity can increase feelings of well-being and reduce feelings of anxiety and depression. In other words, wholesome food and physical activity just plain feel good!

A Healthful Diet Can Prevent Some Diseases and Reduce Your Risk for Others

Early work in the area of nutrition focused on nutrient deficiencies and how we can prevent them. As you read in the Highlight box on pellagra, nutrient deficiencies can cause serious, even life-threatening

Occupational health meaningful work or vocation

Physical health includes nutrition and physical activity

Social health includes family, community, and social environment

Spiritual health spiritual values and beliefs

Emotional health includes positive feelings about oneself and life

FIGURE 1.1 Many factors contribute to an individual's wellness. Primary among these are a nutritious diet and regular physical activity.

TABLE 1.1 Ten Leading Causes of Death in the United States for People of All Ages

Rank	Cause of Death	Number of Deaths
1	Heart disease	696,947
2	Cancer	557,271
3	Stroke	162,672
4	Chronic lower respiratory disease	124,816
5	Accidents (unintentional injuries)	106,742
6	Diabetes	73,249
7	Influenza/pneumonia	65,681
8	Alzheimer's disease	58,866
9	Nephritis, nephrotic syndrome, and nephrosis	40,974
10	Septicemia	33,865

Source: National Center for Health Statistics. 2004. Fast Stats A to Z. Deaths—Leading Causes. www.cdc.gov/nchs/fastats/lcod.htm.

diseases; scurvy, goiter, and rickets are other examples discussed in this book. The discoveries of the causes of such diseases have helped nutrition experts develop guidelines for healthful diets that can prevent them. An ample food supply and fortifying foods with nutrients have ensured that the majority of nutrient deficiency diseases are no longer of concern in developed countries. However, these diseases are still major problems in many developing nations.

In addition to preventing nutrient deficiency diseases, a healthful diet can reduce your risk for *chronic* diseases, that is, diseases that come on slowly and persist for years (if not for life), often despite treatment. Nutrition is strongly associated with four chronic diseases that are among the top ten causes of death in the United States (Table 1.1): heart disease, cancer, cerebrovascular disease (which causes strokes), and type 2 diabetes. Obesity, which increases our risk for all of these diseases, is significantly affected by nutrition and activity: consuming too much food and exercising too little are factors in obesity. In the United States and many developed nations, the prevalence of obesity (FIGURE 1.2) and these four chronic diseases has dramatically increased over the past 16 years. Throughout this text, we will discuss in more detail how nutrition and physical activity affect the development of obesity and other chronic diseases.

In short, nutrition appears to play a role in a variety of diseases. Its role can vary from mild influence, to a strong association, to directly causing a disease (FIGURE 1.3). The strength of the association between nutrition and various diseases will continue to be modified as nutrition research continues.

> RECAP: *Nutrition is the science that studies food and how food affects our body and our health. Nutrition is an important component of wellness and is strongly associated with physical activity. One goal of a healthful diet is to prevent nutrient deficiency diseases such as scurvy and pellagra; a second goal is to lower the risk for chronic diseases such as type 2 diabetes and heart disease.*

What Are Nutrients?

A glass of milk or a spoonful of peanut butter may seem to be all one substance, but in reality most foods are made up of many different chemicals. Some of these chemicals are not useful to the body, whereas others are critical to human growth and function. These latter chemicals are referred to as **nutrients.** The six groups of nutrients found in the foods we eat are (FIGURE 1.4):

- carbohydrates
- fats and oils (two types of lipids)
- proteins
- vitamins
- minerals
- water

As you may know, the term *organic* is commonly used to describe foods that are grown without the use of non-natural fertilizers or chemicals. But when scientists describe individual nutrients as **organic,** they mean that these nutrients contain an element called carbon that is an essential component of all living organisms. Carbohydrates, lipids, proteins, and vitamins are organic because they contain carbon.

nutrients Chemicals found in foods that are critical to human growth and function.

organic A substance or nutrient that contains the element carbon.

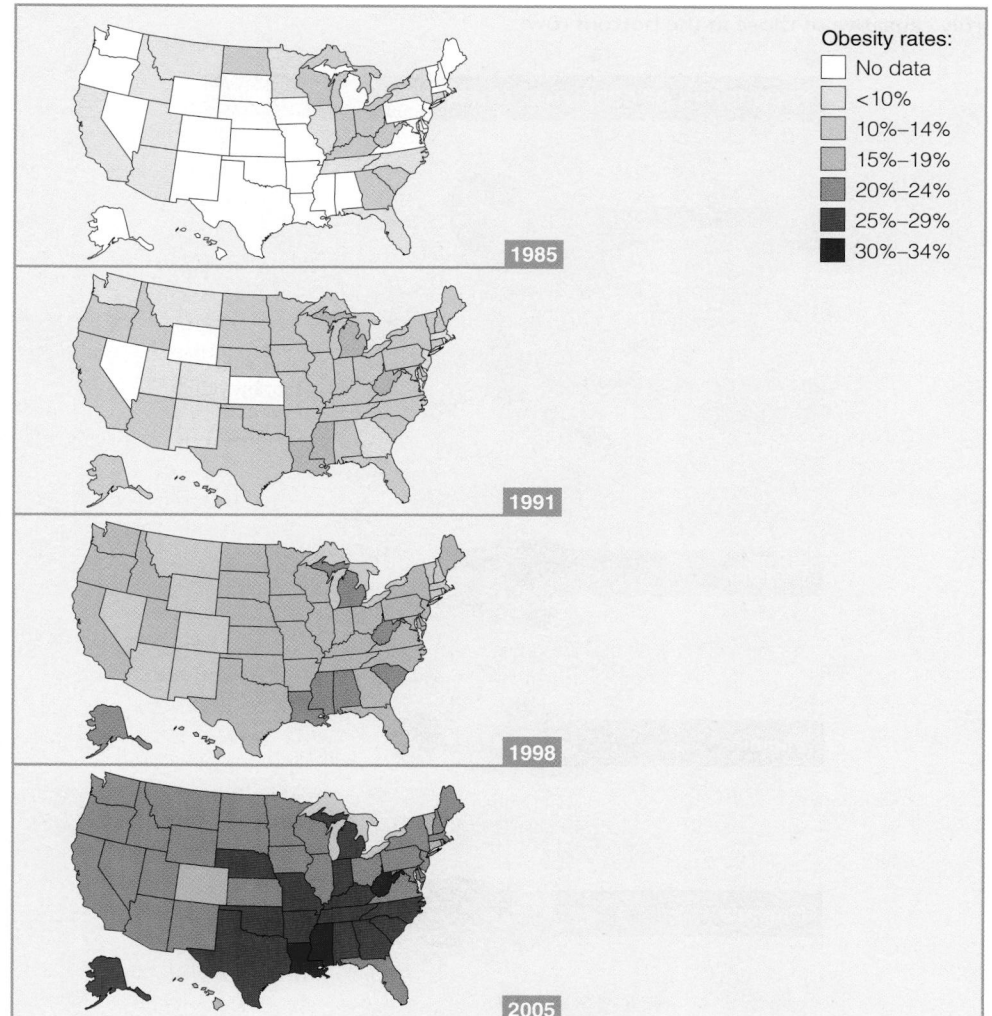

FIGURE 1.2   These diagrams illustrate the increase in obesity rates across the United States from 1985 to 2005 as documented in the Behavioral Risk Factor Surveillance Survey. Obesity is defined as a body mass index greater than or equal to 30, or approximately 30 pounds overweight for a 5'4" woman. (Data from Mokdad, A. H., et al. 1999. *JAMA* 282:16; Mokdad, A. H., et al. 2001. *JAMA* 286:10. Graphics from Centers for Disease Control and Prevention, U.S. Obesity Trends 1985 to 2005.)

Diseases in which nutrition plays some role	Osteoporosis Osteoarthritis Some forms of cancer
Diseases with a strong nutritional component	Type 2 diabetes Heart disease High blood pressure Obesity
Diseases caused by nutritional deficiencies or toxicities	Pellagra Scurvy Iron-deficiency anemia Other vitamin and mineral deficiencies Nutrient toxicities

FIGURE 1.3   The relationship between nutrition and human disease. Notice that, whereas nutritional factors are only marginally implicated in the diseases of the top row, they are strongly linked to the development of the diseases in the middle row, and truly causative of those in the bottom row.

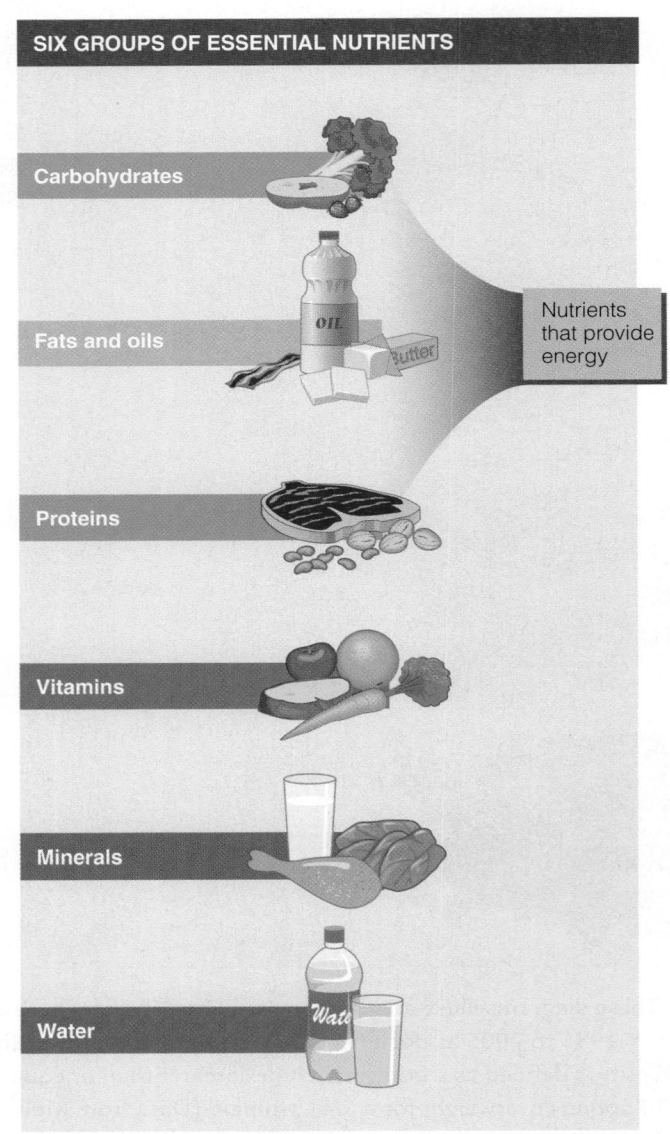

FIGURE 1.4   The six groups of essential nutrients found in the foods we consume.

HIGHLIGHT

What Is a Kilocalorie?

Have you ever wondered what the difference is between the terms *energy, kilocalories,* and *calories*? Should these terms be used interchangeably, and what do they really mean? The brief review provided in this highlight should broaden your understanding. First, some precise definitions:

- *Energy* is defined as the capacity to do work. We derive energy from the energy-containing nutrients in the foods we eat, namely, carbohydrates, fats, and proteins.
- A *kilocalorie* (kcal) is the amount of heat required to raise the temperature of 1 kilogram (about 2.2 pounds) of water by 1 degree Celsius. It is a unit of measurement we use to quantify the amount of energy in food that can be supplied to the body. For instance, we can say

that the energy found in 1 gram of carbohydrate is equal to 4 kcal.
- A *calorie* (cal) is also a unit of measurement: technically, 1 kilocalorie is equal to 1,000 calories. *Kilo-* is a prefix used in the metric system to indicate 1,000 (think of *kilometer* or *kilobytes*). However, for the sake of simplicity, nutrition labels use the term *calories* to indicate kilocalories. Thus, if the wrapper on an ice cream bar states that it contains 150 calories, it actually contains 150 kilocalories.

In this textbook, we use the term *energy* when referring to the general concept of energy intake or energy expenditure. We use the term *kilocalories* (or *kcal*) when discussing units of energy. We use the term *calories* only when reviewing information about food labels.

Minerals and water are **inorganic** because they do not contain carbon. Organic and inorganic nutrients are equally important for sustaining life but differ in their structures, functions, and basic chemistry.

Carbohydrates, Fats, and Proteins Are Nutrients That Provide Energy

Carbohydrates, fats, and proteins are the only nutrients that provide energy. By this we mean that our bodies break down these nutrients and reassemble into a fuel that supports physical activity and basic functioning. Although taking a multivitamin and a glass of water might be beneficial in other ways, it will not provide you with the energy you need to do your 20 minutes on the stair-climber! The energy nutrients are also referred to as **macronutrients.** *Macro* means "large," and our bodies need relatively large amounts of these nutrients to support normal function and health.

Alcohol is a chemical commonly consumed in beverage form and may also be added to some foods as a flavoring or preservative—but it is not considered a nutrient. This is because it does not support the regulation of body functions or the building or repairing of tissues. In fact, alcohol is considered to be both a drug and a toxin.

We express energy in units of *kilocalories* (kcal). Refer to the Highlight box What Is a Kilocalorie? for an explanation of energy and kilocalories. Both carbohydrates and proteins provide 4 kcal per gram, alcohol provides 7 kcal per gram, and fats provide 9 kcal per gram. Thus, for every gram of fat we consume, we obtain more than twice the energy as compared to a gram of carbohydrate or protein. Refer to the You Do the Math box on page 10 to learn how to calculate the energy contribution of carbohydrates, fats, and proteins in a given food.

Carbohydrates Are a Primary Fuel Source

Carbohydrates are the primary source of fuel for our bodies, particularly for our brain and during physical exercise (FIGURE 1.5). A close look at the word "carbohydrate" reveals the chemical structure of this nutrient. *Carbo-* refers to carbon, and *-hydrate* refers to water. You may remember that water is made up of hydrogen and oxygen. Thus, carbohydrates are composed of chains of carbon, hydrogen, and oxygen.

Carbohydrates are the primary source of fuel for our bodies, particularly for our brain.

inorganic A substance or nutrient that does not contain carbon.

macronutrients Nutrients that our bodies need in relatively large amounts to support normal function and health. Carbohydrates, fats, and proteins are macronutrients.

carbohydrates The primary fuel source for our bodies, particularly for our brain and for physical exercise.

YOU DO THE MATH

Calculating the Energy Contribution of Carbohydrates, Fats, and Proteins

The energy in food is used for everything from maintaining normal body functions—such as breathing, digesting food, and repairing damaged tissues and organs—to enabling you to perform physical activity and even to read this text. So how much energy is produced from the foods you eat?

Carbohydrates are the main energy source for your body and should make up the largest percentage of your nutrient intake, about 45–65%; they provide 4 kcal of energy per gram of carbohydrate consumed. Proteins also provide 4 kcal of energy per gram, but they should be limited to no more than 10–35% of your daily energy intake. Fats provide the most energy, 9 kcal per gram. Fats should make up approximately 20–35% of your total energy intake per day. In order to figure out whether you're taking in the appropriate percentages of carbohydrates, fats, and proteins, you will need to use a little math.

1. Let's say you have completed a personal diet analysis, and you consume 2,500 kcal per day. From your diet analysis you also find that you consume 300 g of carbohydrates, 90 g of fat, and 123 g of protein.
2. To calculate your percentage of total energy that comes from carbohydrate, you must do two things:
   a. Take your total grams of carbohydrate and multiply by the energy value for carbohydrate to give you how many kcal of carbohydrate you have consumed.

   300 g of carbohydrate × 4 kcal/g
   = 1,200 kcal of carbohydrate

   b. Take the kcal of carbohydrate you have consumed, divide this number by the total number of kcal you consumed, and multiply by 100. This will give you the percentage of the total energy you consume that comes from carbohydrate.

   (1,200 kcal/2,500 kcal) × 100 = 48% of total energy comes from carbohydrate

3. To calculate your percentage of total energy that comes from fat, you follow the same steps but incorporate the energy value for fat:
   a. Take your total grams of fat and multiply by the energy value for fat to find the kcal of fat consumed.

   90 g of fat × 9 kcal/g = 810 kcal of fat

   b. Take the kcal of fat you have consumed, divide this number by the total number of kcal you consumed, and multiply by 100 to get the percentage of total energy you consume that comes from fat.

   (810 kcal/2,500 kcal) × 100 = 32.4% of total energy comes from fat

Now try these steps to calculate the percentage of the total energy you consume that comes from protein.

Also, have you ever heard that alcohol provides "empty calories"? Alcohol contributes 7 kcal per gram. You can calculate the percentage of kcal from alcohol in your daily diet, but remember that it is not considered an energy nutrient.

These calculations will be very useful throughout this course as you learn more about how to design a healthful diet and how to read labels to assist you in meeting your nutritional goals. Later in this book, in Chapter 11, you will learn how to estimate your unique energy needs and determine the ideal amount of energy you need from carbohydrates, fats, and proteins.

FIGURE 1.5 Carbohydrates are a primary source of energy for our bodies and are found in a wide variety of foods.

Carbohydrates

- Primary source of energy for body
- Composed of carbon, hydrogen, and oxygen

Carbohydrates encompass a wide variety of foods; rice, wheat, and other grains as well as vegetables are carbohydrates, and fruits contain natural sugars that are carbohydrates. Carbohydrates are also found in legumes (including lentils, dry beans, and peas), milk and other dairy products, seeds, and nuts. Carbohydrates and their role in health are the subject of Chapter 4.

Fats Provide Energy and Other Essential Nutrients

Fats are another important source of energy for our bodies (FIGURE 1.6). They are a type of *lipids*, a diverse group of organic substances that are insoluble in water. Like carbohydrates, fats are composed of carbon, hydrogen, and oxygen; however, they contain proportionally much less oxygen and water than carbohydrates do. This quality allows them to pack together tightly, which explains why they yield more energy per gram than either carbohydrates or proteins.

Fats are an important energy source for our bodies at rest and during low-intensity exercise. Our bodies are capable of storing large amounts of fat as adipose tissue. These fat stores can then be broken down for energy during periods when we are not eating; for example, while we are asleep. Foods that contain fats are also important in providing fat-soluble vitamins and essential fatty acids.

Dietary fats come in a variety of forms. Solid fats include such things as butter, lard, and margarine. Liquid fats, referred to as *oils*, include vegetable oils such as canola and olive oils. Cholesterol is a form of lipid that our bodies can make independently, and it can also be consumed in the diet. Chapter 5 provides a thorough discussion of lipids.

Proteins Support Tissue Growth, Repair, and Maintenance

Proteins also contain carbon, hydrogen, and oxygen, but they are different from carbohydrates and fats in that they contain the element *nitrogen* (FIGURE 1.7). Within proteins, these four elements assemble into small building blocks known as amino acids. We break down dietary proteins into amino acids and reassemble them to build our own body proteins—for instance, the proteins in our muscles and blood.

Although proteins can provide energy, they are not a primary source of energy for our bodies. Instead, the main role of proteins is in building new cells and tissues,

fats An important energy source for our bodies at rest and during low-intensity exercise.

proteins The only macronutrient that contains nitrogen; the basic building blocks of proteins are amino acids.

FIGURE 1.6 Fats are an important energy source during rest and low-intensity exercise. Foods containing fat also provide other important nutrients.

Fats and oils
- Important source of energy at rest and during low-intensity exercise
- Composed of carbon, hydrogen, and oxygen
- Foods containing fats also provide fat-soluble vitamins and essential fatty acids

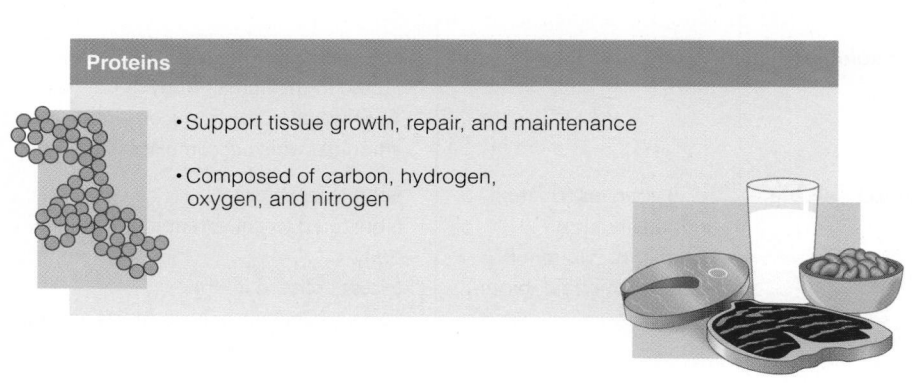

Proteins
- Support tissue growth, repair, and maintenance
- Composed of carbon, hydrogen, oxygen, and nitrogen

FIGURE 1.7 Proteins contain nitrogen in addition to carbon, hydrogen, and oxygen. Proteins support the growth, repair, and maintenance of body tissues.

Fat-soluble vitamins are found in a variety of fat-containing foods, including dairy products.

vitamins Organic compounds that assist us in regulating our bodies' processes.

metabolism The process by which large molecules such as carbohydrates, fats, and proteins are broken down via chemical reactions into smaller molecules that can be used as fuel, stored, or assembled into new compounds the body needs.

micronutrients Nutrients needed in relatively small amounts to support normal health and body functions. Vitamins and minerals are micronutrients.

fat-soluble vitamins Vitamins that are not soluble in water, but are soluble in fat. These include vitamins A, D, E, and K.

water-soluble vitamins Vitamins that are soluble in water. These include vitamin C and the B vitamins.

minerals Inorganic substances that are not broken down during digestion and absorption and are not destroyed by heat or light. Minerals assist in the regulation of many body processes and are classified as major minerals or trace minerals.

both for growth and for repair. Proteins are also important in regulating the breakdown of foods and our fluid balance.

Proteins are found in many foods. Meats and dairy products are our primary sources, but we also obtain small amounts of protein from vegetables and whole grains. Seeds, nuts, and legumes are good sources of protein. Proteins are reviewed in detail in Chapter 6.

> RECAP: *The six essential nutrient groups found in foods are carbohydrates, fats, proteins, vitamins, minerals, and water. Carbohydrates, fats, and proteins are referred to as the energy nutrients, as they provide our bodies with the energy necessary to thrive. Carbohydrates are the primary energy source for our bodies; fats provide fat-soluble vitamins and essential fatty acids and act as energy storage molecules; and proteins support tissue growth, repair, and maintenance.*

Vitamins Assist in the Regulation of Biological Processes

Vitamins are organic compounds that help regulate our bodies' functions. Contrary to popular belief, vitamins do not contain energy (or kilocalories); however, they are essential to energy **metabolism,** the process by which the macronutrients are broken down into smaller molecules that our body can absorb and use. As you'll learn in Chapter 10, vitamins assist with releasing and using the energy found in all three macronutrients: carbohydrates, fats, and proteins. They are also critical in building and maintaining healthy bone, muscle, and blood, supporting our immune system so we can fight infection and disease, and ensuring healthy vision. Because we need relatively small amounts of these nutrients to support normal health and body functions, the vitamins (in addition to minerals) are referred to as **micronutrients.**

Vitamins are classified as two types: **fat soluble** and **water soluble** (Table 1.2). This classification is based upon their solubility in water, which affects how vitamins are absorbed, transported, and stored in our bodies. As our bodies cannot synthesize most vitamins, we must consume them in our diets. Both types of vitamins are essential for our health and are found in a variety of foods. Learn more about vitamins in the *In Depth* look on pages 252–263. Chapters 7 through 10 discuss individual vitamins in detail.

Minerals Assist in the Regulation of Many Body Functions

Minerals are inorganic substances, meaning that they do not contain carbon. Some important dietary minerals include sodium, potassium, calcium, magnesium, and iron. Minerals are different from the macronutrients and vitamins in that they are

TABLE 1.2 Overview of Vitamins

Type	Names	Distinguishing Features
Fat soluble	A, D, E, and K	Soluble in fat Stored in the human body Toxicity can occur from consuming excess amounts, which accumulate in the body
Water soluble	C, B vitamins (thiamin, riboflavin, niacin, vitamin B_6, vitamin B_{12}, pantothenic acid, biotin, and folate)	Soluble in water Not stored to any extent in the human body Excess excreted in urine Toxicity generally only occurs as a result of vitamin supplementation

TABLE 1.3 Overview of Minerals

Type	Names	Distinguishing Features
Major minerals	Calcium, phosphorus, sodium, potassium, chloride, magnesium, sulfur	Needed in amounts greater than 100 mg/day in our diets Amount present in the human body is greater than 5 g (or 5,000 mg)
Trace minerals	Iron, zinc, copper, manganese, fluoride, chromium, molybdenum, selenium, iodine	Needed in amounts less than 100 mg/day in our diets Amount present in the human body is less than 5 g (or 5,000 mg)

not broken down during digestion or when our bodies use them to promote normal function; they are also not destroyed by heat or light. Thus, all minerals maintain their structure no matter what environment they are in. This means that the calcium in our bones is the same as the calcium in the milk we drink, and the sodium in our cells is the same as the sodium in our table salt.

Minerals have many important functions in our bodies. They assist in fluid regulation and energy production, are essential to the health of our bones and blood, and help rid our body of harmful by-products of metabolism.

Minerals are classified according to the amounts we need in our diet and according to how much of the mineral is found in our bodies. The two categories of minerals in our diets and bodies are the **major minerals** and the **trace minerals** (Table 1.3). Learn more about minerals in the *In Depth* look on pages 252–263. Chapters 7 through 10 discuss individual minerals in detail.

Water Supports All Body Functions

Water is an inorganic nutrient that is vital for our survival. We consume water in its pure form; in juices, soups, and other liquids; and in solid foods such as fruits and vegetables. Adequate water intake ensures the proper balance of fluid both inside and outside of our cells, and also assists in the regulation of nerve impulses, muscle contractions, nutrient transport, and excretion of waste products. Because of the key role that water plays in our health, Chapter 7 focuses on water and its function in our bodies.

Peanuts are a good source of magnesium and phosphorus, which play important roles in the formation and maintenance of our skeleton.

> RECAP: *Vitamins are organic compounds that assist in breaking down the macronutrients for energy, and in maintaining the health of body tissues, the immune system, and vision. Minerals are inorganic elements that maintain their structure throughout the processes of digestion, absorption, and metabolism. They play critical roles in virtually all aspects of human health and function. Water is critical for our survival and is important for regulating nervous impulses, muscle contractions, nutrient transport, and excretion of waste products.*

How Can I Figure Out My Nutrient Needs?

Now that you know what the six classes of nutrients are, you are probably wondering how much of each you need each day. But before you can learn more about specific nutrients and how to plan your own healthful diet, you need to become familiar with current dietary standards and how these standards shape nutrition recommendations.

Use the Dietary Reference Intakes to Check Your Nutrient Intake

In the past, the dietary standards in the United States were referred to as the *Recommended Dietary Allowances (RDAs)*, and the standards in Canada were termed the *Recommended Nutrient Intakes (RNIs)*. These standards define recommended

major minerals Minerals we need to consume in amounts of at least 100 mg per day and of which the total amount in our bodies is at least 5 g.

trace minerals Minerals we need to consume in amounts less than 100 mg per day and of which the total amount in our bodies is less than 5 g.

intake values for various nutrients and can be used to plan diets for both individuals and groups. They were developed from the perspective of preventing nutrient deficiency diseases; however, in developed countries like the United States and Canada, these diseases are now extremely rare. Thus, much of our current work in nutrition is focused on the associations between nutrition and wellness. We want to learn more about the role of nutrition in reducing our risk for chronic diseases and to design diets that promote optimal health. In response to these changes in focus, a new set of reference values was developed to replace and expand upon the RDAs and RNIs. These new reference values in both the United States and Canada are termed the **Dietary Reference Intakes (DRIs)** (FIGURE 1.8).

The DRIs are dietary standards for healthy people only; they do not apply to people with diseases or those who are suffering from nutrient deficiencies. Like the RDAs and RNIs, they identify the amount of a nutrient needed to prevent deficiency diseases in healthy individuals, but they also consider how much of this nutrient may reduce the risk for chronic diseases in healthy people. The DRIs also establish an upper level of safety for nutrients.

The DRIs for most nutrients consist of four values:

- Estimated Average Requirement (EAR)
- Recommended Dietary Allowance (RDA)
- Adequate Intake (AI)
- Tolerable Upper Intake Level (UL)

For total energy and the macronutrients, different standards are used. These include the Estimated Energy Requirement (EER) and the Acceptable Macronutrient Distribution Ranges (AMDRs). Let's now define each of these DRI values.

The Estimated Average Requirement Guides the Recommended Dietary Allowance

Dietary Reference Intakes (DRIs)
A set of nutritional reference values for the United States and Canada that applies to healthy people.

Estimated Average Requirement (EAR) The average daily nutrient intake level estimated to meet the requirement of half of the healthy individuals in a particular life stage or gender group.

The **Estimated Average Requirement (EAR)** represents the average daily nutrient intake level estimated to meet the requirement of half of the healthy individuals in a particular life stage or gender group.[1] FIGURE 1.9 provides a graph representing this value. As an example, the EAR for phosphorus for women between the ages of 19 and 30 years represents the average daily intake of phosphorus that meets the requirement of half of the women in this age group. The EAR is used by scientists to define the Recommended Dietary Allowance (RDA) for a given nutrient. Obviously, if the EAR meets the needs of only half the people in a group, then the recommended intake will be higher.

FIGURE 1.8 The Dietary Reference Intakes (DRIs) for all nutrients. Note that the Estimated Energy Requirement (EER) only applies to energy, and the Acceptable Macronutrient Distribution Range (AMDR) only applies to the macronutrients and alcohol.

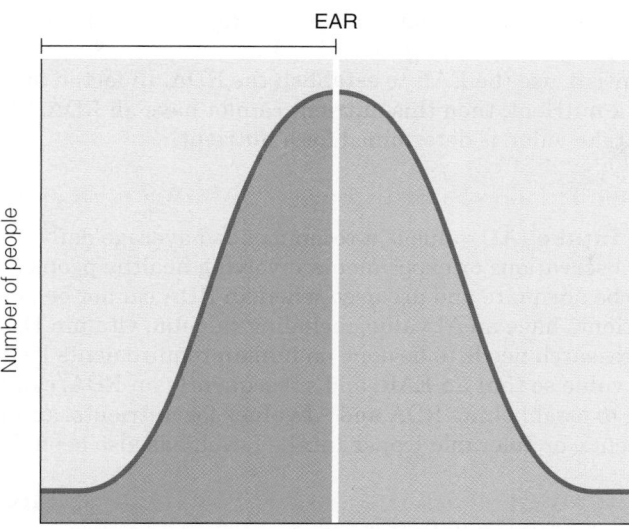

FIGURE 1.9 The Estimated Average Requirement (EAR) represents the average daily nutrient intake level that meets the requirements of half of the healthy individuals in a given group.

The Recommended Dietary Allowance Meets the Needs of Nearly All Healthy People

As previously stated, the term **Recommended Dietary Allowance (RDA)** used to refer to all nutrient recommendations in the United States. Now, the RDA is only one of many reference standards within the larger umbrella of the DRIs. The RDA represents the average daily nutrient intake level that meets the requirements of 97–98% of healthy individuals in a particular life stage and gender group (FIGURE 1.10).[1] For example, the RDA for phosphorus is 700 mg per day for women between the ages of

Recommended Dietary Allowance (RDA) The average daily nutrient intake level that meets the nutrient requirements of 97–98% of healthy individuals in a particular life stage and gender group.

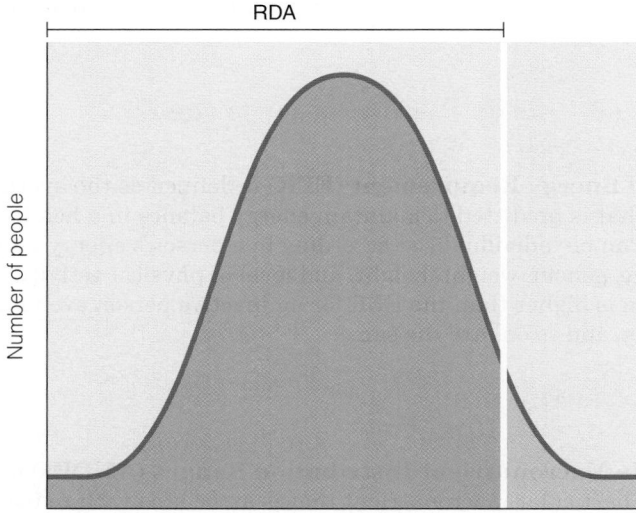

FIGURE 1.10 The Recommended Dietary Allowance (RDA) represents the average daily nutrient intake level that meets the requirements of almost all (97–98%) healthy individuals in a given life stage or gender group.

Knowing your daily Estimated Energy Requirement (EER) is a helpful way to maintain a healthy body weight. Your EER is defined by your age, gender, weight, height, and physical activity level.

19 and 30 years. This amount of phosphorus will meet the nutrient requirements of almost all women in this age category.

Again, scientists use the EAR to establish the RDA. In fact, if an EAR cannot be determined for a nutrient, then this nutrient cannot have an RDA. When this occurs, an Adequate Intake value is determined for a nutrient.

The Adequate Intake Is Based on Estimates of Nutrient Intakes

The **Adequate Intake (AI)** value is a recommended average daily nutrient intake level based on observations or experiments involving healthy people. These estimates are assumed to be adequate and are used when an RDA cannot be determined.[1] Numerous nutrients have an AI value, including calcium, vitamin D, vitamin K, and fluoride. More research needs to be done on human requirements for the nutrients assigned an AI value so that an EAR, and subsequently an RDA, can be established.

In addition to establishing RDA and AI values for nutrients, an upper level of safety for nutrients, or Tolerable Upper Intake Level, has also been defined.

The Tolerable Upper Intake Level Is the Highest Level That Poses No Health Risk

The **Tolerable Upper Intake Level (UL)** is the highest average daily nutrient intake level likely to pose no risk of adverse health effects to almost all individuals in a particular life stage and gender group.[1] This does not mean that we should consume this intake level or that we will receive more benefits from a nutrient by meeting it. Rather, as our intake of a nutrient increases in amounts above the UL, the potential for toxic effects and health problems increases. The UL value is a helpful guide to assist you in determining the highest average intake level that is deemed safe for a given nutrient.

> RECAP: *The Dietary Reference Intakes (DRIs) are dietary standards for nutrients established for healthy people in a particular life stage or gender group. The Estimated Average Requirement (EAR) represents the nutrient intake level that meets the requirement of half of the healthy individuals in a group. The Recommended Dietary Allowance (RDA) represents the nutrient intake level that meets the requirements of 97–98% of healthy individuals in a group. The Adequate Intake (AI) is a recommended nutrient intake level used when there is not enough information to set an RDA. The Tolerable Upper Intake Level (UL) is the highest daily nutrient intake level that likely poses no risk of adverse health effects.*

Adequate Intake (AI) A recommended average daily nutrient intake level based on observed or experimentally determined estimates of nutrient intake by a group of healthy people.

Tolerable Upper Intake Level (UL) The highest average daily nutrient intake level likely to pose no risk of adverse health effects to almost all individuals in a particular life stage and gender group.

Estimated Energy Requirement (EER) The average dietary energy intake that is predicted to maintain energy balance in a healthy adult.

Acceptable Macronutrient Distribution Range (AMDR) A range of intakes for a particular energy source that is associated with reduced risk of chronic disease while providing adequate intakes of essential nutrients.

The Estimated Energy Requirement Is the Intake Predicted to Maintain a Healthy Weight

The **Estimated Energy Requirement (EER)** is defined as the average dietary energy intake that is predicted to maintain energy balance in a healthy adult. This dietary intake can be individualized according to a person's energy intake, energy expenditure, age, gender, weight, height, and level of physical activity.[2] The EER for an active person is higher than the EER for an inactive person even if all other factors (age, gender, and so on) are the same.

The Acceptable Macronutrient Distribution Ranges Are Associated with Reduced Risk for Chronic Diseases

The **Acceptable Macronutrient Distribution Ranges (AMDRs)** define a range of intakes for a particular macronutrient that is associated with reduced risk of chronic disease but also provides adequate levels of essential nutrients.[2] The AMDR is expressed as a percentage of total energy or as a percentage of total kilocalories. The AMDR also has a lower and upper boundary; if we consume nutrients above or below this range, there is a potential for increasing our risk for chronic diseases and for increasing our risk of consuming inadequate levels of nutrients essential for health. The AMDRs for carbohydrate, fat, and protein are listed in Table 1.4.

TABLE 1.4   Acceptable Macronutrient Distribution Ranges (AMDRs) for Healthful Diets

Nutrient	AMDR*
Carbohydrate	45–65%
Fat	20–35%
Protein	10–35%

*AMDR values are expressed as percent of total energy or as percent of total calories.
Source: Institute of Medicine, Food and Nutrition Board. 2005. *Dietary Reference Intakes for Energy, Carbohydrates, Fiber, Fat, Fatty Acids, Cholesterol, Protein, and Amino Acids (Macronutrients)*. Washington, DC: National Academies Press. Reprinted by permission.

Calculating Your Unique Nutrient Needs

The primary goal of dietary planning is to develop a diet or eating plan that is nutritionally adequate, meaning that the chances of consuming too little or too much of any nutrient are very low. By eating foods that give you nutrient intakes that meet the DRI values, you help your body to maintain a healthful weight, support your daily physical activity, prevent nutrient deficiencies and toxicities, and reduce your risk for chronic disease.

The DRI values are listed in a table on the inside cover of this book; they are also reviewed with each nutrient as it is introduced throughout this text. Find your life stage group and gender in the left-hand column, then simply look across to see each nutrient's value for you. Using the DRI values in conjunction with diet-planning tools such as MyPyramid or the Dietary Guidelines for Americans will ensure a healthful and adequate diet. Chapter 2 provides details on how you can use these tools to develop a healthful diet.

RECAP: *The Estimated Energy Requirement (EER) is the average daily energy intake that is predicted to maintain energy balance in a healthy adult. The EER is defined by a person's age, gender, weight, height, and physical activity level. The Acceptable Macronutrient Distribution Ranges (AMDRs) define ranges of intakes for a particular macronutrient that are associated with reduced risk of chronic disease but also provide adequate levels of essential nutrients. The DRI values can be used to plan diets that are nutritionally adequate and healthful.*

Research Study Results: Who Can We Believe?

"Eat more carbohydrates! Fats cause obesity!"
"Eat more protein and fat! Carbohydrates cause obesity!"

Do you ever feel overwhelmed by the abundant and often conflicting advice in media reports related to nutrition? If so, you are not alone. In addition to the "high-carb, low-carb" controversy, we've been told that calcium supplements are essential to prevent bone loss and that calcium supplements have no effect on bone loss; that high fluid intake prevents constipation and that high fluid intake has no effect on constipation. For years, we were told that coffee and tea could be bad for our health; now, it appears that both may actually contain nutrients that are beneficial! How can you navigate this sea of changing information? What constitutes valid, reliable evidence, and how can you determine whether or not research findings apply to you?

To become a more educated consumer and informed critic of nutrition reports in the media, you need to understand the research process and how the results of different types of studies should be interpreted. Let's now learn more about research.

Research Involves Applying the Scientific Method

When confronted with a claim about any aspect of our world, from "The Earth is flat" to "Carbohydrates cause obesity," scientists, including nutritionists, must first consider whether or not the claim can be tested. In other words, can evidence be presented to substantiate the claim, and if so, what data would qualify as evidence? Scientists worldwide use a standardized method of looking at evidence called the *scientific method*. This method ensures that certain standards and processes are used in evaluating claims. The scientific method usually includes the following steps, which are described in more detail below and summarized in FIGURE 1.11:

- The researcher makes an *observation* and description of a phenomenon.
- The researcher proposes a *hypothesis* or educated guess to explain why the phenomenon occurs.
- The researcher develops an *experimental design* that will test the hypothesis.
- The researcher *collects and analyzes data* that will either support or reject the hypothesis.
- If the data are rejected, then an *alternative hypothesis* is proposed and tested.
- If the data support the original hypothesis, then a *conclusion* is drawn.

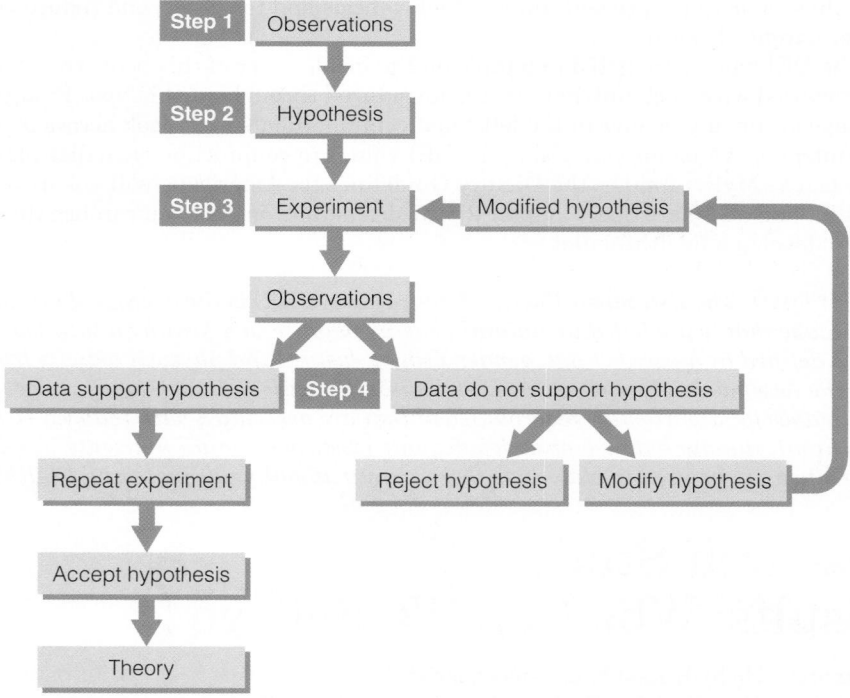

FIGURE 1.11   The scientific method, which forms the framework for scientific research. Step 1: Observations are made regarding some phenomenon, which lead the researcher to ask a question. Step 2: A hypothesis is generated to explain the observations. Step 3: An experiment is conducted to test the hypothesis. Observations are made during the experiment, and data are generated and documented. Step 4: The data may either support or refute the hypothesis. If the data support the hypothesis, more experiments are conducted to test and confirm support for the hypothesis. A hypothesis that is supported after repeated testing may be called a theory. If the data do not support the hypothesis, the hypothesis is either rejected or modified and then retested.

- The experiment must be *repeatable*, so other researchers can obtain similar results.

- Finally, a *theory* is proposed offering a conclusion drawn from repeated experiments that have supported the hypothesis time and time again.

Observation of a Phenomenon Initiates the Research Process

The first step in the scientific method is the observation and description of a phenomenon. As an example, let's say you are working in a healthcare office that caters to mostly elderly clients. You have observed that many of the elderly have high blood pressure, but there are some who have normal blood pressure. After talking with a large number of elderly clients, you notice a pattern developing in that the clients who report being more physically active are also those having lower blood pressure readings. This observation leads you to question the relationship that might exist between physical activity and blood pressure. Your next step is to develop a *hypothesis,* or possible explanation for your observation.

A Hypothesis Is a Possible Explanation for an Observation

A **hypothesis** is also referred to as a research question. In this example, your hypothesis would be, "If elderly people exercise regularly, then their blood pressure will decrease." Your hypothesis must be written in a way so that it can be evaluated as either true or false. To evaluate a hypothesis you must collect data and use a reliable method of analyzing that data. When determining whether a hypothesis is correct or not, three criteria must be met: the hypothesis is testable, unbiased, and repeatable. Determining whether a hypothesis is valid requires a well-thought-out experimental design.

An Experiment Is Designed to Test the Hypothesis

An *experiment* is a scientific study that is conducted to test a hypothesis. A well-designed experiment should include several key elements:

- The *sample size* or the number of people being studied should be adequate to ensure that the results obtained are not due to chance alone. For example, would you be more likely to believe a study that tested five people or five hundred?

- Having a *control group* is essential for comparing treated and untreated individuals. A control group is a group of people who are as much like the treated group as possible except with respect to the variable being tested, for instance, elderly people who do not exercise. Using a control group helps a researcher to judge whether a particular treatment has worked or not. One way scientists compare data between the experimental and control groups is by plotting variables on a graph. The *independent variable* is controlled or manipulated by the experimenter, for example, 45 minutes of aerobic exercise a day. The *dependent variable* is not manipulated, but simply observed or measured by the experimenter. In the case of your study, this would be the participants' blood pressure readings. The independent variable is plotted on the horizontal axis (or x-axis) and the dependent variable on the vertical axis (or y-axis).

- A good experimental design also attempts to control for other variables that may coincidentally influence the results. For example, what if someone in your study was on a diet, smoked, or took blood pressure–lowering medication? Since any of these factors could affect the results, researchers try to design experiments that have as many *constants* as possible. In doing so, they increase the chance that their results will be valid. To use an old saying, you can think of validity as "Comparing apples to apples."

Data Is Collected and Analyzed to Determine Whether It Supports or Rejects the Hypothesis

As part of the design of the experiment, the researcher must determine what kind of data is to be collected and how it will be collected. For example, in your study the data being collected are the blood pressures of various elderly individuals. These values

hypothesis An educated guess as to why a phenomenon occurs.

could be collected by a person or a machine. An automatic blood pressure gauge would provide the most reliable and consistent data as opposed to blood pressure measurements taken by an individual or several individuals. Consider that the data you're collecting is evidence that will be closely scrutinized by other scientists.

Once the data or evidence has been collected, it must be interpreted or analyzed. Often, the data will begin to make sense only after it has been organized and put into different forms such as tables or graphs that reveal patterns that at first were not obvious.

Most scientific results must have a quantitative aspect to them; in other words, the results have to be measurements that can be compared. In the case of your study you can compare blood pressure readings from both your study participants and the control group to see whether there is a significant difference between the two groups. Results must show a certain *confidence level* or *statistical significance*. Most scientists insist on a significance level of 95%, which means that the result obtained has a 95% chance of being true. So if you found that the blood pressure numbers in your experimental group and your control group were significantly different at the 95% level you could be fairly certain that exercising regularly can lower blood pressure.

Most Hypotheses Need to Be Refined

Remember that a hypothesis is basically a guess as to what causes a particular phenomenon. Rarely do scientists get it right the first time. The original hypothesis is often refined after the initial results are obtained, usually because the answer to the question is not clear and leads to more questions. When this happens an alternative hypothesis is proposed, a new experiment is designed, and the new hypothesis is tested. It is important to emphasize that one research study does not prove or disprove a hypothesis. Ideally, multiple experiments are conducted over many years to thoroughly examine a hypothesis. Science exists to allow us to continue to challenge existing hypotheses and expand what we currently know.

An Experiment Must Be Repeatable

As we just said, one research study does not prove or disprove a hypothesis. Unfortunately, media reports on the findings of a research study that has just been published rarely include a thorough review of the other studies conducted on that topic. Thus, one article in a newspaper or magazine should never be taken as absolute fact on any topic. Repeatability is a cornerstone of scientific investigation. Scientists and skeptics alike must be able to replicate an experiment and arrive at similar conclusions or the hypothesis becomes invalid.

The experimental design plays a key role in repeatability. Other investigators must follow the design of the experiment as closely as possible, using sample sizes and subjects as well as equipment and control measures similar to those used by the initial investigators. Have you ever wondered why the measurements used in scientific textbooks are always in the metric system? The answer is repeatability. Scientists use the metric system because it is a universal system. It is this element of the scientific method—repeatability—that allows scientists to form theories.

A Theory May Be Developed Following Extensive Research

If the results of multiple experiments consistently support a hypothesis, then it is possible to develop a **theory.** A theory represents a hypothesis or group of related hypotheses that has been confirmed through repeated scientific experiments. Theories are strongly accepted principles, but they can be challenged and changed as a result of applying the scientific method. Remember that, centuries ago, it was theorized that the Earth was flat. People were so convinced of this that they refused to sail beyond known boundaries because they believed they would fall off the edge of the Earth. Only after multiple explorers challenged this theory was it discovered that the Earth is round. We continue to apply the scientific method today to test hypotheses and challenge theories.

theory A conclusion drawn from repeated experiments.

RECAP: *The steps in the scientific method are 1) observing a phenomenon, 2) creating a hypothesis, 3) designing and conducting an experiment, and 4) collecting and analyzing data that support or refute the hypothesis. If the data are rejected, then an alternative hypothesis is proposed and tested. If the data support the original hypothesis, then a conclusion is drawn. A hypothesis that is supported after repeated experiments may be called a theory.*

Various Types of Research Studies Tell Us Different Stories

You have just learned how the scientific method is applied to test a hypothesis. Establishing nutrition guidelines and understanding the role of nutrition in health involve constant experimentation. Depending on how the research study is designed, we can gather information that tells us different stories. Let's now learn more about the different types of research conducted and what they tell us.

Epidemiological Studies Inform Us of Existing Relationships

Epidemiological studies are also referred to as observational studies. These types of studies involve assessing nutritional habits, disease trends, or other health phenomena of large populations and determining the factors that may influence these phenomena. However, these studies can indicate only relationships between factors, not specifically a cause-and-effect relationship. For example, let's say that an epidemiological study finds that the blood pressure values of physically active elderly people are lower than those of inactive elderly people. These results do not indicate that regular physical activity reduces blood pressure or that inactivity causes high blood pressure. All these results can tell us is that there is a relationship between higher physical activity and lower blood pressure in elderly people.

Model Systems

Humans are not very good experimental models because it is difficult to control for all of the variables that affect their lives. Humans also have long life spans, so it would take a long time to determine the effects of certain nutritional studies. For this reason laboratory studies generally involve experiments with animals. In many cases, animal studies provide preliminary information that can assist us in designing and implementing human studies. Animal studies also are used to conduct research that cannot be done with humans. For instance, it is possible to study nutritional deficiencies in animals by causing a deficiency and studying its adverse health effects over the life span of the animal; this type of experiment is not acceptable to do in humans.

Animals with relatively short reproduction times can be studied when researchers need to look at the effects of specific drugs or treatments over many generations. Such animals can also be bred so they display specific traits such as certain diseases or metabolic conditions. One drawback to animal studies is that the results may not apply directly to humans. Another drawback is the ethical implications of studies involving animals, especially when the research reduces the animals' quality of life.

Human Studies

The two primary types of studies conducted with humans include case control studies and clinical trials. *Case control studies* are epidemiological studies done on a smaller scale. Case control studies involve comparing a group of individuals with a particular condition (for instance, elderly with high blood pressure) to a similar group without this condition (for instance, elderly with low blood pressure). This comparison allows the researcher to identify factors other than the defined condition that differ between the two groups. By identifying these factors, researchers can gain a better understanding of things that may cause and help prevent disease. In the case of your experiment, you may find that elderly with low blood pressure not only are more physically active, but also eat more fruits and vegetables and less sodium.

Epidemiological studies indicate relationships between factors, such as between exercise and blood pressure in older adults, but cannot prove cause and effect.

These findings would indicate that other factors in addition to physical activity may play a role in affecting the blood pressure levels of elderly people.

Clinical trials are tightly controlled experiments in which an intervention is given to determine its effect on a certain disease or health condition. Interventions may include medications, nutritional supplements, controlled diets, or exercise programs. Clinical trials include the experimental group, who are given the intervention, and the control group, who are not given the intervention. The responses of the intervention group are compared to those of the control group. In the case of your experiment, you could assign one group of elderly people with high blood pressure to an exercise program and assign a second group of elderly people with high blood pressure to a program in which no exercise is done. After the intervention phase was completed, you could compare the blood pressure of the elderly people who exercised to that of those who did not. If the blood pressure of the intervention group decreased and the blood pressure of the control group did not, and if the amount of the decrease was statistically significant, then you could propose that the exercise program caused a decrease in blood pressure.

There are other important things to consider when conducting a quality clinical trial. Ideally, it is best to randomly assign research participants to intervention and control groups. Randomizing participants is like flipping a coin or drawing names from a hat; doing this reduces prejudice or bias to the assignment of each group. If possible, it is also important to "blind" both researchers and participants to the treatment being given. A *double-blind experiment* is one in which neither researchers nor participants know which group is really getting the treatment. Blinding helps prevent the researcher from seeing only the results he or she wants to see.

In testing the effectiveness of a medication or nutritional supplement, the blinding process can be assisted by the use of a placebo. A *placebo* is an imitation treatment that has no scientifically recognized therapeutic value, for instance, a sugar pill that looks, feels, smells, and tastes identical to the medication being tested. In this case, neither the researcher giving the medication nor the study participant receiving it knows whether the pill being administered is the medication being tested or a placebo.

Another important variable that cannot be overlooked in clinical trials is the effect of participation in the study on the participant's state of mind. This is known as the *psychosomatic effect* or *placebo effect*. Sometimes, just knowing they're in a study will cause participants to experience physiological changes that they may interpret as therapeutic. For example, since the elderly people in your study know they are part of a study concerning high blood pressure, they may subconsciously be more relaxed and content because they feel validated and important. They may therefore show a decrease in blood pressure.

Use Your Knowledge of Research to Help You Evaluate Media Reports

How can all of this research information assist you in becoming a better consumer and critic of media reports? By having a better understanding of the research process and types of research conducted, you are more capable of discerning the truth or fallacy within media reports. Keep the following points in mind when examining any media report:

- Who is reporting the information? Is it an article in a newspaper, in a magazine, or on the Internet? If the report is made by a person or group who may financially benefit from you buying their products, you should be skeptical of the reported results. Also, many people who write for popular magazines and newspapers are not trained in science and are capable of misinterpreting research results.

- Who conducted the research, and who paid for it? Was the study funded by a company that stands to profit from certain results? Are the researchers receiving goods, personal travel funds, speaking fees, or other perks from the research sponsor, or do they have investments in companies or products related to their study? If the answer to these questions is yes, there exists a conflict of interest between the researchers and the funding agency. If a conflict of interest does exist, it may seriously compromise the researchers' ability to conduct unbiased research and report the results in an accurate and responsible manner.

- Is the report based on reputable research studies? Did the research follow the scientific method, and were the results reported in a reputable scientific journal? Ideally, the journal is peer-reviewed; that is, the articles are critiqued by other specialists working in the same scientific field. A reputable report should include the reference, or source of the information, and should identify researchers by name. This allows the reader to investigate the original study and determine its merit. Reputable journals include the *American Journal of Clinical Nutrition, Journal of Nutrition, Journal of the American Dietetic Association,* the *New England Journal of Medicine,* and the *Journal of the American Medical Association* (*JAMA*).

To become a more educated consumer and informed critic of nutrition reports in the media, you need to understand the research process and how study results should be interpreted.

- Is the report based on testimonials about personal experiences? Are sweeping conclusions made from only one study? Be aware of personal testimonials, as they are fraught with bias. In addition, one study cannot answer all of our questions or prove any hypothesis, and the findings from individual studies should be placed in their proper perspective.

- Are the claims in the report too good to be true? Are claims made about curing disease or treating a multitude of conditions? If something sounds too good to be true, it probably is. Claims about curing diseases or treating many conditions with one product should be a signal to question the validity of the report.

Throughout this text we provide you with information to assist you in becoming a more educated consumer regarding nutrition. You will learn about labeling guidelines, the proper use of supplements, and whether various nutrition topics are myths or facts. We'll also test your knowledge at the end of every chapter with a feature called *Find the Quack*. As you may know, *quackery* is the misrepresentation of a product, program, or service for financial gain. For example, a high-priced supplement may be marketed as uniquely therapeutic when in fact it is only as effective as much less expensive remedies commonly available. Many manufacturers of such products describe them as "patented," but this means only that the product has been registered with the United States Patent Office, for a fee. It provides no guarantee of the product's effectiveness or its safety. After considering the information presented in each *Find the Quack* feature, you'll have a chance to decide for yourself: Is this a legitimate product or service, or is it quackery? Armed with the information in this book, plus plenty of opportunities to test your knowledge, you will become more confident when trying to evaluate nutrition claims.

RECAP: *Epidemiological studies involve large populations, model studies involve animals, and human studies include case control studies and clinical trials. Each type of study can be used to gather a different kind of data. When evaluating media reports, consider who is reporting the information, who conducted and paid for the research, whether or not the research was published in a reputable journal, and whether it involves testimonials or makes claims that sound too good to be true. Quackery is the misrepresentation of a product, program, or service for financial gain.*

Nutrition Advice: Who Can You Trust?

After reading this chapter, you can see that one of the major nutritional concerns in the United States is our high risk for certain chronic diseases. One result of this concern has been the publication of an almost overwhelming quantity of nutritional information on television shows, Web sites, newspapers, magazines, newsletters, journals, and many other forums. In addition to this information overload, we continually discover that the nutritional messages from these supposedly "expert" sources are confusing, dissimilar, or even contradictory. On certain issues, even nutrition scientists and physicians cannot seem to agree! If you are wondering how to determine whether or not an "expert" is trustworthy, the following discussion should help.

Trustworthy Experts Are Educated and Credentialed

The number of health professionals and organizations who provide reliable nutrition information is considerable, so it's not possible to identify them all in this chapter. The following is a list of a few of the most important groups that provide reputable nutrition information:

- Registered dietitian (or RD): A registered dietitian is an individual who possesses at least a baccalaureate (bachelor's) degree and has completed a defined content of course work and experience in nutrition and dietetics. This individual has also successfully completed the Registration Exam for Dietitians. For a list of individuals who are registered dietitians in your community, you can look in the yellow pages of your phone book or contact the American Dietetic Association at **www.eatright.org**.

- Licensed nutritionist: A licensed nutritionist is an individual who is educated, is trained, and holds a professional license in nutrition. This individual may also be a registered dietitian, but a person can be a licensed nutritionist independent of being an RD. Each state in the United States has its own laws regulating dietitians or nutritionists. These laws specify which types of licensure or registration a nutrition professional must obtain in order to provide nutrition services or advice to individuals. Individuals who practice nutrition and dietetics without the required license or registration can be prosecuted for breaking the law.

- Nutritionist: This term generally has no definition or laws regulating it. It may refer to anyone who thinks he or she is knowledgeable about nutrition. To make sure the person is a legitimate nutrition professional, ask whether they are registered with the American Dietetic Association (ADA). The ADA will certify only those individuals who have at least a bachelor's degree with training in the field of nutrition.

- Professional with an advanced degree (a master's degree [MA or MS] or doctoral degree [Ph.D.]) in nutrition): Many individuals, including many registered dietitians, hold an advanced degree in nutrition. Some teach at community colleges and universities, and others work in fitness and healthcare settings. Professionals with advanced degrees who are not licensed nutritionists or registered dietitians are not certified to provide clinical dietary counseling or treatment for individuals with diseases or illnesses; however, they are still very knowledgeable about nutrition and health.

- Medical doctor: A medical doctor, also called a physician or MD, is educated, trained, and licensed to practice medicine in the United States. This individual typically has limited experience and training in the area of nutrition. However, if you become ill, the medical doctor is usually one of the first health professionals to see for an accurate medical diagnosis. If you require a dietary plan to treat an illness or disease, most medical doctors will refer you to an RD or licensed nutritionist to assist you in meeting your dietary needs.

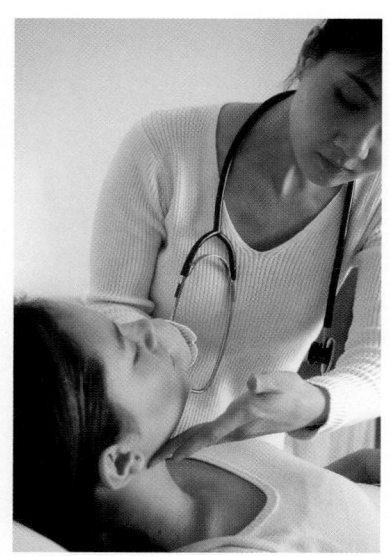

Your medical doctor may have limited experience and training in the area of nutrition but can refer you to a registered dietitian (RD) or licensed nutritionist to assist you in meeting your dietary needs.

Remember that, as an educated consumer, it is important to seek out individuals who can provide you with reliable nutrition information. Even highly educated and credentialed people have limits on their knowledge and can make mistakes. Seeking a second opinion about nutrition information that affects your health is strongly advised.

Government Sources of Information Are Usually Trustworthy

Many government health agencies have come together in the last 20 years to address the growing problem of nutrition-related disease in the United States. These organizations are funded with taxpayer dollars, and many of these agencies provide financial support for research in the areas of nutrition and health. Thus, these agencies have the resources to organize and disseminate the most recent and reliable information related to nutrition and other areas of health and wellness. A few of the most recognized and respected of these government agencies are discussed here.

The Centers for Disease Control and Prevention Protects the Health and Safety of Americans

The **Centers for Disease Control and Prevention (CDC)** is considered to be the leading federal agency in the United States that protects human health and safety. Located in Atlanta, Georgia, the CDC works in the areas of health promotion, disease prevention and control, and environmental health. The CDC's mission is to promote health and quality of life by preventing and controlling disease, injury, and disability. Among its many activities, the CDC supports two large national surveys that provide us with important nutrition and health information. These surveys are discussed below. To learn more about the CDC, go to **www.cdc.gov**.

The National Health and Nutrition Examination Survey. The **National Health and Nutrition Examination Survey (NHANES)** is a survey conducted by the National Center for Health Statistics and the CDC that tracks the nutrient consumption of Americans. Nutrition and other health information is gathered during an interview conducted in a person's household and during an examination in a mobile unit. The nutritional data is gathered using a tool called the **24-hour recall** interview, which is a data collection tool that assesses everything a person has consumed over the past 24 hours. The database for the NHANES survey is extremely large, and an abundance of research papers have been generated from it. To learn more about the NHANES and other national health surveys, go to the Web site for the National Center for Health Statistics at **www.cdc.gov/nchs/express.htm**.

The Behavioral Risk Factor Surveillance System. The **Behavioral Risk Factor Surveillance System (BRFSS)** was established by the CDC. The world's largest telephone survey, it tracks lifestyle behaviors that increase our risk for chronic disease. The BRFSS includes questions related to injuries, infectious diseases, and chronic diseases. This survey places a particularly strong focus on the health behaviors that increase our risk for the nation's leading killers: heart disease, stroke, cancer, and diabetes. These health behaviors include:[3]

- Lack of adequate physical activity
- Consuming a diet that is low in fiber and high in fat
- Using tobacco and alcohol
- Not getting medical care that is known to save lives; includes regular Pap smears, mammograms, flu shots, and screening for cancer of the colon and rectum

These behaviors have garnered significant interest because it is estimated that four out of ten deaths (or 40%) in the United States can be attributed to smoking, alcohol misuse, lack of physical activity, and eating an unhealthful diet.[3]

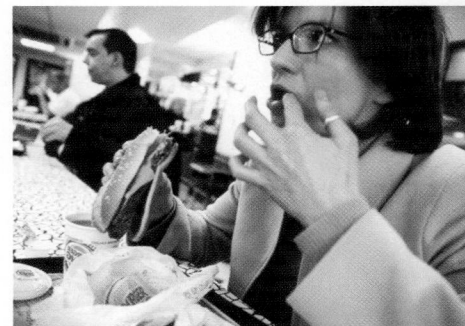

Lifestyle behaviors, such as eating an unhealthful diet, can increase your risk for chronic disease.

Centers for Disease Control and Prevention (CDC) The leading federal agency in the United States that protects the health and safety of people. Its mission is to promote health and quality of life by preventing and controlling disease, injury, and disability.

National Health and Nutrition Examination Survey (NHANES) A survey conducted by the National Center for Health Statistics and the CDC; this survey tracks the nutrient and food consumption of Americans.

24-hour recall A data collection tool that assesses everything a person has consumed over the past 24 hours.

Behavioral Risk Factor Surveillance System (BRFSS) The world's largest telephone survey that tracks lifestyle behaviors that increase our risks for chronic diseases.

The National Institutes of Health Is the Leading Medical Research Agency in the World

The **National Institutes of Health (NIH)** is the world's leading medical research center, and it is the focal point for medical research in the United States. The NIH is one of the agencies of the Public Health Services, which is part of the U.S. Department of Health and Human Services. The mission of the NIH is to uncover new knowledge that leads to better health for everyone. This mission is accomplished by support of medical research throughout the world and by fostering communication of medical information. The NIH has many institutes and centers that focus on a broad array of nutrition-related health issues. Some of these institutes include:

- National Cancer Institute (NCI)
- National Eye Institute (NEI)
- National Heart, Lung, and Blood Institute (NHLBI)
- National Institute of Diabetes and Digestive and Kidney Diseases (NIDDK)
- National Center for Complementary and Alternative Medicine (NCCAM)

NIH headquarters are located in Bethesda, Maryland. To find out more about the NIH, go to **www.nih.gov**.

Professional Organizations Provide Reliable Nutrition Information

There are a number of professional organizations whose members are qualified nutrition professionals, scientists, and educators. These organizations publish cutting-edge nutrition research studies and educational information in journals that are accessible in most university and medical libraries. Some of these organizations include:

- The American Dietetic Association (ADA): This is the largest organization of food and nutrition professionals in the United States. The mission of this organization is to promote nutrition, health, and well-being. The ADA publishes a professional journal called the *Journal of the American Dietetic Association*; information about ADA can be found at **www.eatright.org**.
- The American Society for Nutrition (ASN): The ASN is a research society whose goal is to improve the quality of life through the science of nutrition. The ASN publishes a professional journal called the *American Journal of Clinical Nutrition*; information about the ASN can be found at **www.nutrition.org**.
- The Society for Nutrition Education (SNE): The SNE is dedicated to promoting healthy, sustainable food choices in communities through nutrition research and education. The primary goals of SNE are to educate individuals, communities, and professionals about nutrition education and to influence policy makers about nutrition, food, and health. The professional journal of SNE is the *Journal of Nutrition Education and Behavior*. Information about SNE can be found at **www.sne.org**.
- The American College of Sports Medicine (ACSM): The ACSM is the leading sports medicine and exercise science organization in the world. Many members are nutrition professionals who combine their nutrition and exercise expertise to promote health and athletic performance. *Medicine and Science in Sports and Exercise* is the professional journal of the ACSM. You can learn more about the ACSM at **www.acsm.org**.

RECAP: *The Centers for Disease Control and Prevention is the leading federal agency in the United States that protects the health and safety of people. The CDC supports two large national surveys that provide important nutrition and health information: the National Health and Nutrition Examination Survey (NHANES) and the Behavioral Risk Factor Surveillance System (BRFSS). The National Institutes of Health is the leading medical research agency in the world. The American Dietetic Association, the American Society for Clinical Nutrition, the Society for Nutrition Education, and the American College of Sports Medicine are examples of professional organizations that provide reliable nutrition information.*

National Institutes of Health (NIH) The world's leading medical research center and the focal point for medical research in the United States.

NUTRI-CASE YOU PLAY THE EXPERT!

A multitude of features throughout this book challenge you to think about how the various recommendations of the so-called "experts" apply to you. In contrast, our Nutri-Case feature gives you the chance to play the expert by offering nutritional advice to five individuals who are seeking advice from a variety of sources—some reliable and others questionable. As you do this, keep in mind that these case scenarios are offered to assist you in gaining a more complete understanding of the nutrition information presented. In the real world, only properly trained and licensed health professionals are qualified to offer nutritional advice. The people presented in these scenarios represent a wide range of personal backgrounds and nutritional challenges. You will learn more about each of these people in subsequent chapters, and they briefly introduce themselves here.

" I'm Hannah and I'm 12 years old and I go to Valley Middle School. I get really good grades, especially in science. It's my favorite class. Last week, our science teacher taught us about what we're supposed to eat, and then the school nurse weighed us. She said I weigh more than a kid my age should, and I need to play outside more and eat less. I told my mom about it, but she said that's just the way I'm built and we don't have lots of money to eat fancy stuff anyway. I wish I knew what to do, because I feel kind of bad when we go swimming at the YMCA and I see kids staring at me. I always wonder if they're thinking how fat I am.

" I'm Judy, Hannah's mother, and I'm a nurse's aide at Valley Hospital. Back when Hannah was a baby, I dreamed of going to college so I could be a registered nurse. But then my ex and I split up, and Hannah and me, we've been in survival mode ever since. I'm proud to be raising my daughter without any hand-outs, and I do good work, but the pay never goes far enough and it's exhausting. I guess that's partly because I'm out of shape, and my blood sugar's high, too. Most nights, I'm so tired at the end of my shift that I just pick up some fast food for supper. I know I should be feeding Hannah home-cooked meals, but like I said, I'm in survival mode.

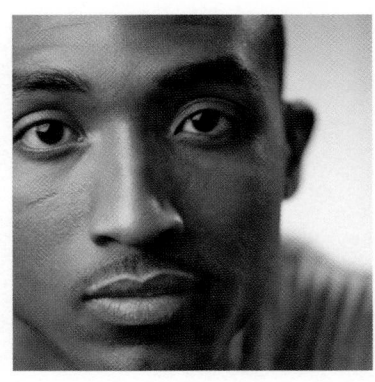

" Hi, I'm Theo. Let's see, I'm 21, and my parents moved to the Midwest from Nigeria 11 years ago. The first time I ever played basketball, in junior high, I was hooked. I won lots of awards in high school and then got a full scholarship to the state university, where I'm a sophomore studying political science. I decided to take a nutrition course because, in my freshman year, I had a hard time making it through the playing season, plus keeping up with my classes and homework. I want to have more energy and keep my weight up, so I thought a nutrition class might help me find out if I'm eating right. I really want to figure out this food thing before basketball season starts again.

"I'm Liz, I'm 20, and I'm a dance major at the School for Performing Arts. Last year, two other dancers from my class and I won a state championship and got to dance in the New Year's Eve celebration at the Governor's mansion. This spring, I'm going to audition for the City Ballet, so I have to be in top condition. I wish I had time to take a nutrition course, but I'm too busy with dance classes and rehearsals and teaching a class for kids. But it's okay, because I get lots of tips from other dancers and from the Internet. Like last week, I found a Web site especially for dancers that explained how to get rid of bloating before an audition. I'm going to try it for my audition with the City Ballet!

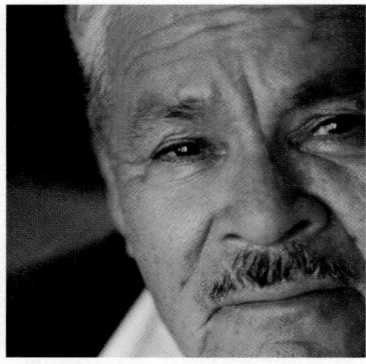

"Hello. My name is Gustavo. Almost 60 years ago, when I was 13, I came to the U.S. from Mexico with my father and mother and three sisters to pick crops in California, and now I manage a vineyard. They ask me when I'm going to retire, but I can still work as hard as a man half my age. Health problems? None. Well, my doctor tells me my blood pressure is high, but that's normal for my age! I guess what keeps me going is thinking about how my father died 6 months after he retired, of colon cancer, and he never knew he had it until it was too late. Anyway, I watch the nightly news and read the papers, so I keep up on what's good for me, eating less fat and salt and all that. I'm doing fine.

Throughout this text you will interact with these five characters as they are dealing with nutrition-related challenges in their lives. As you do, you might find that they remind you of people you know, and you may also discover you have something in common with one or more of them. Think about how much you differ from each one in regard to your age, developmental stage, family and personal history, food issues, physical activity level, and nutrition and health goals. Our hope is that these characters and their challenges will assist you in applying the nutrition knowledge you acquire in this course not only to their situation, but also to your own life.

CHAPTER SUMMARY

- Nutrition is the scientific study of food and how food nourishes the body and influences health.

- Nutrition is an important component of wellness. A healthful diet plays a critical role in eliminating nutritional deficiency disease and can help reduce our risks for various chronic diseases.

- Nutrients are chemicals found in food that are critical to human growth and function.

- The six essential nutrients found in the foods we eat are carbohydrates, fats, proteins, vitamins, minerals, and water.

- The nutrients that provide energy for our bodies are the macronutrients: carbohydrates, fats, and proteins.

- Carbohydrates are composed of carbon, hydrogen, and oxygen. They are the primary energy source for our bodies, particularly our brains.

- Fats store large quantities of energy and provide us with fat-soluble vitamins and essential fatty acids.

- Proteins can provide energy if needed, but they are not a primary fuel source. Proteins support tissue growth, repair, and maintenance.

- Vitamins are organic substances found in minute amounts in foods. They assist with the regulation of body processes.

- Minerals are inorganic substances found in foods and are critical to human health and function. Unlike the macronutrients and vitamins, minerals are not changed by digestion or other metabolic processes.

- Water is critical to support numerous body functions, including fluid balance, conduction of nervous impulses, and muscle contraction.

- The Dietary Reference Intakes (DRIs) are reference standards for nutrient intakes for healthy people in the United States and Canada.

- The DRIs include the Estimated Average Requirement, the Recommended Dietary Allowance, the Adequate Intake, the Tolerable Upper Intake Level, the Estimated Energy Requirement, and the Acceptable Macronutrient Distribution Ranges.

- The steps in the scientific method are 1) observing a phenomenon, 2) creating a hypothesis, 3) designing and conducting an experiment, and 4) collecting and analyzing data that support or refute the hypothesis. If the data are rejected, then an alternative hypothesis is proposed and tested. If the data support the original hypothesis, then a conclusion is drawn.

- A scientific theory represents a conclusion drawn from repeated experimentation.

- Different types of studies, from epidemiological studies involving large populations, to studies involving smaller groups of animals or humans, can be used to gather different types of data.

- Quackery is the misrepresentation of a product, program, or service for financial gain.

- Potentially good sources of reliable nutrition information include individuals who are registered dietitians, who are licensed nutritionists, or who hold an advanced degree in nutrition.

- The Centers for Disease Control and Prevention (CDC) is the leading federal agency that protects human health and safety.

- The National Health and Nutrition Examination Survey (NHANES) is a survey conducted by the CDC and the National Center for Health Statistics that tracks the nutritional status of people in the United States.

- The Behavioral Risk Factor Surveillance System (BRFSS) was established by the CDC and is the world's largest telephone survey; the BRFSS tracks the health behaviors and risks of Americans.

- The National Institutes of Health (NIH) is the leading medical research agency in the world. The mission of NIH is to uncover new knowledge that leads to better health for everyone.

TEST YOURSELF ANSWERS

1. **False.** Calories are a measure of the energy in foods. More precisely, a kilocalorie is the amount of heat required to raise the temperature of 1 kilogram of water by 1 degree Celsius.

2. **True.** Carbohydrates and fats are the primary energy sources for our bodies.

3. **False.** Most water-soluble vitamins need to be consumed daily. However, we can consume foods that contain fat-soluble vitamins less frequently because our bodies can store these vitamins.

4. **False.** The Recommended Dietary Allowance is the average daily nutrient intake level that meets the nutrient requirements of 97–98% of healthy individuals in a particular life stage and gender group.

5. **False.** Other good sources are professional organizations in the field of nutrition research and education and individuals who are licensed or registered as nutrition professionals.

REVIEW QUESTIONS

1. Vitamins A and C, thiamin, calcium, and magnesium are considered
   a. water-soluble vitamins.
   b. fat-soluble vitamins.
   c. energy nutrients.
   d. micronutrients.

2. The world's leading medical research center is the
   a. Centers for Disease Control.
   b. National Institutes of Health.
   c. American Medical Association.
   d. National Health and Nutrition Examination Survey.

3. Ten grams of fat
   a. contain 40 kcal of energy.
   b. constitute the Dietary Reference Intake for an average adult male.
   c. contain 90 kcal of energy.
   d. constitute the Tolerable Upper Intake Level for an average adult male.

FIND THE QUACK

Since she was a little girl, LaVeeta has imagined her wedding day with the same essential detail: walking down the aisle in her mother's wedding dress. Now her wedding is just 6 months away, and to fit into that dress, she'll need to lose a whole dress size. It's not surprising, then, that when she sees a weight-loss booth at a bridal show, LaVeeta stops in. A slender young woman introduces herself as Amy, and listens closely as LaVeeta explains why she simply must lose 30 pounds in the next 6 months. Amy smiles reassuringly: "You've come to the right place! Your goal of losing 30 pounds in 6 months is closer than you ever imagined with Mini Mix, my patented minimizer-formula weight-loss powder. Mixed with 8 ounces of skim milk, it's a complete low-calorie breakfast, and it curbs your appetite for the rest of the day! It's full of vitamins and minerals, so you won't need to worry when you just don't feel like eating anything else all day—Mini Mix meets your nutritional needs for up to 24 hours!"

LaVeeta notices the price on the stack of cans of the powder: $49 for a can that says it's "a 30-day supply." She quickly calculates: $300 seems like a lot of money for 6 months' worth of powdered vitamins. How can she tell whether or not the product is legit? While she is trying to decide, another customer approaches the booth, and Amy begins to chat with her. LaVeeta uses the opportunity to look around the booth. She notices on the wall a framed certificate. Beneath Amy's name is the title Certified Nutrition Consultant, and beneath that is the name of a professional-sounding association of "Nutrition Consultants." LaVeeta then picks up a can of Mini Mix. On the label, she reads the following:

- Consumed as recommended with 8 ounces of skim milk, Mini Mix provides 100% of the recommended intake of 1 day's micronutrient needs for just 150 calories.

- One scoop of Mini Mix powder also contains a precise blend of natural appetite suppressants from around the world, including willow bark from Germany and guarana from Brazil. Mini Mix also contains all-natural vanilla or chocolate flavoring.

- Drinking one Mini Mix shake per day will curb your appetite for the rest of the day. Because you won't feel hungry, you won't be tempted to overeat. You'll lose weight quickly, and keep it off for life!

1. The certificate on the wall of the Mini Mix booth states that Amy is a Certified Nutrition Consultant. Does this mean that Amy has graduated from an educational institution with a degree in nutrition? If not, what does it mean?

2. The Mini Mix label says that the product "provides 100% of the recommended intake of 1 day's micronutrient needs for just 150 calories." Amy claims that, "It's full of vitamins and minerals, so you won't need to worry when you just don't feel like eating anything else all day—Mini Mix meets your nutritional needs for up to 24 hours!" Are these claims essentially identical? Could they be true? Why or why not?

3. Mini Mix contains "willow bark from Germany and guarana from Brazil." Look up these plants on a reputable online encyclopedia such as Britannica. What substances do they contain?

4. Mini Mix costs $49 for a 30-day supply. Should LaVeeta purchase a can? Why or why not?

Answers can be found at www.aw-bc.com/thompson.

4. Which of the following statements about hypotheses is true?

   a. Hypotheses can be proven by clinical trials.

   b. "Many inactive people have high blood pressure" is an example of a hypothesis.

   c. If the results of multiple experiments consistently support a hypothesis, it is confirmed as fact.

   d. "A high-protein diet increases the risk for porous bones" is an example of a hypothesis.

5. Which of the following foods contains all six nutrient groups?

   a. strawberry ice cream

   b. an egg-salad sandwich

   c. creamy tomato soup

   d. all of the above

6. True or false? Fat-soluble vitamins provide energy.

7. True or false? The Recommended Dietary Allowance represents the average daily intake level that meets the requirements of almost all healthy individuals in a given life stage or gender group.

8. True or false? Nutrition significantly affects a person's risk for heart disease.

9. True or false? Nutrition-related reports in the *American Journal of Clinical Nutrition* are usually trustworthy.

10. True or false? Carbohydrates, fats, and proteins all contain carbon, hydrogen, and oxygen.

11. Explain the difference between a hypothesis and a theory.

12. Compare the Estimated Average Requirement to the Recommended Dietary Allowance.

13. Your uncle has learned that you are taking a nutrition course and says, "How can I find reliable nutrition information?" How would you answer?

14. Your mother, who is a self-described "chocolate addict," phones you. She has read in the newspaper a summary of a research study suggesting that the consumption of a moderate amount of bittersweet chocolate reduces the risk of heart disease in older women. You ask her who funded the research. She says she doesn't know and asks you why it would matter. Explain why such information is important.

15. Intrigued by the idea of a research study on chocolate, you obtain a copy of the full report. In it, you learn that:
    • twelve women participated in the study;
    • the women's ages ranged from 65 to 78;
    • the women had all been diagnosed with high blood pressure;
    • they all described themselves as sedentary; and
    • six of the twelve smoked at least half a pack of cigarettes a day, but the others did not smoke.

Your mother is 51 years old, walks daily, and takes a weekly swim class. Her blood pressure is on the upper end of the normal range. She does not smoke. Identify at least three aspects of the study that would cause you to doubt its relevance to your mother.

WEB LINKS

www.eatright.org
American Dietetic Association (ADA)

Obtain a list of registered dietitians in your community from the largest organization of food and nutrition professionals in the United States.

www.cdc.gov
Centers for Disease Control and Prevention (CDC)

Visit this site for additional information about the leading federal agency in the United States that protects the health and safety of people.

www.cdc.gov/nchs/express.htm
National Center for Health Statistics

Go to this site to learn more about the National Health and Nutrition Examination Survey (also referred to as NHANES) and other national health surveys.

www.nih.gov
National Institutes of Health (NIH)

Find out more about the National Institutes of Health, an agency under the U.S. Department of Health and Human Services.

www.nutrition.org
The American Society for Nutrition (ASN)

Learn more about the American Society for Nutrition and its goal to improve the quality of life through the science of nutrition.

www.sne.org
Society for Nutrition Education (SNE)

Go to this site for further information about the Society for Nutritional Education and its goals to educate individuals, communities, and professionals about nutrition education and influence policy makers about nutrition, food, and health.

www.acsm.org
American College of Sports Medicine (ACSM)

Obtain information about the leading sports medicine and exercise science organization in the world.

REFERENCES

1. Institute of Medicine, Food and Nutrition Board. 2003. *Dietary Reference Intakes: Applications in Dietary Planning.* Washington, DC: National Academies Press.

2. Institute of Medicine, Food and Nutrition Board. 2002. *Dietary Reference Intakes for Energy, Carbohydrates, Fiber, Fat, Protein and Amino Acids (Macronutrients).* Washington, DC: National Academies Press.

3. U.S. Department of Health and Human Services. Centers for Disease Control and Prevention. 2007. CDC at a Glance. Health Risks in America: Behavioral Risk Factor Surveillance System 2007. www.cdc.gov/nccdphp/publications/aag/brfss.htm. (Accessed May 2007.)

4. Watters, E. 2006. DNA is not destiny. *Discover* 27(11):32–75.

5. The NCMHD Center of Excellence for Nutritional Genomics. Retrieved April 2007, from http://nutrigenomics.ucdavis.edu.

6. Johnson, N., and J. Kaput. 2003. Nutrigenomics: an emerging scientific discipline. *Food Technology* 57(4):60–67.

7. Grierson, B. 2003. What your genes want you to eat. *New York Times*, May 4.

8. Underwood, A., and J. Adler. 2005. Diet and genes. *Newsweek*, January 17, p. 40.

9. Wallace, K. 2007. Diet, exercise may lower colon cancer risk [television broadcast]. CBS News, March 15.

10. Kaput, J., and R. Rodriguez. 2004. Nutritional genomics: the next frontier in the postgenomic era. *Physiological Genomics* 16:166–177.

NUTRITION DEBATE

Nutrigenomics: Personalized Nutrition or Pie in the Sky?

agouti mice are specifically bred for scientific studies. These mice are normally yellow in color, obese, and prone to cancer and diabetes, and they typically have a short life span. When agouti mice breed, these traits are passed on to their offspring. Look at the picture of the agouti mice on this page; do you see a difference? The mouse on the right is obviously brown and of normal weight, but what you can't see is that it did not inherit its parents' susceptibility to disease and therefore will live a longer, healthier life. What caused this dramatic difference between parent and offspring? The answer is diet![4]

With only a change in diet, inbred agouti mice (left) gave birth to young mice (right) that differed not only in appearance but also in their susceptibility to disease.

In 2000, researchers at Duke University found that when they changed the mother's diet just before conception, they could "turn off" the agouti gene, and any offspring born to that mother would appear normal.[4] As you might know, a *gene* is a segment of DNA, a molecule in the nucleus of cells. DNA is responsible for inheritance, or the passing on of traits from parents to offspring. The diet researchers fed the mother was high in methyl donors, chemical compounds that attached to the agouti gene and turned it off.[4] These studies were some of the first to directly link a dietary intervention to a genetic modification, and led to the emerging science of *nutrigenomics* (or *nutritional genomics*).

What Is Nutrigenomics?

Nutrigenomics is a scientific discipline studying the interactions between genes, the environment, and nutrition.[5,6] For decades, the conventional wisdom has been that the genes a person is born with determine that person's fate. But the theory behind nutrigenomics is that our genes might not matter as much as what we eat or expose our body to.

Scientists have known for some time that diet and environmental factors can contribute to disease, but what has not been understood before is *how* these factors contribute to disease, namely, by altering how our genes are expressed. Nutrigenomics proposes that foods and environmental factors can act like a switch in body cells, turning on some genes while turning off others. When a gene is activated, it will instruct the cell to create a protein that will show up as a physical characteristic or functional ability, such as a pigment that makes the agouti's fur yellow or a protein that facilitates the storage of fat. When a gene is switched off, the cell will not create that protein, and the organism's form or function will differ. Factors thought most likely to affect gene activation include smoking, drug and alcohol use, exposure to carcinogens, radiation, stress, physical activity level,

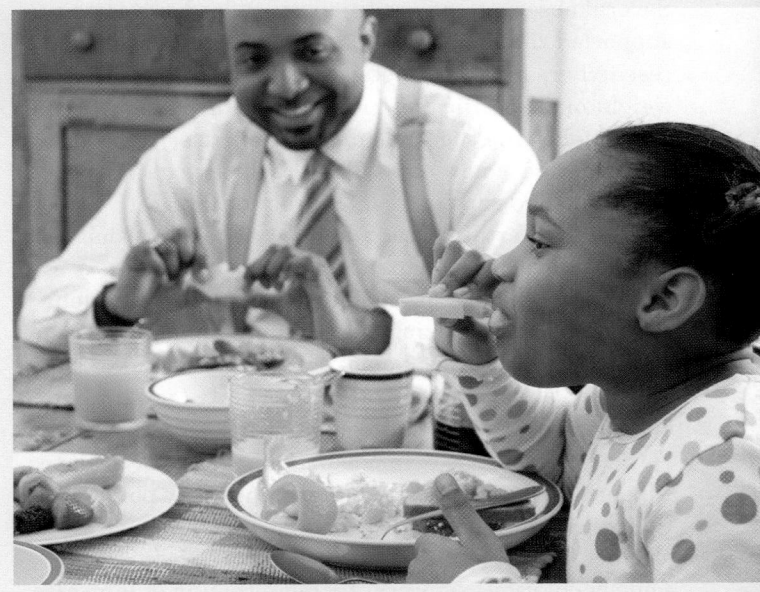

Nutrigenomics suggests that food and environmental factors can either activate or turn off the genes a person inherits from his or her parents.

33

One example of a research area in nutrigenomics is the study of whether leafy green vegetables can interact with a gene that suppresses cancerous tumors.

socioeconomic status, and particularly nutrition, since our genes are continually exposed to the components of our diet.[5,6]

In addition, nutrigenomics scientists are discovering that what we expose our genes to—food, smoke, etc.—can affect gene expression not only in the exposed organism, but also in his or her offspring.[4] In the Duke University study, switching off the agouti gene caused beneficial changes. But sometimes flipping the switch can be harmful, as when paternal exposure to radiation causes changes in sperm cells that increase the likelihood of birth defects in the offspring.

In short, nutrigenomics proposes that foods and environmental factors can influence not only our own genes, but also the genes of our children. It's an intriguing theory—but is there any real evidence to support it?

Evidence for Nutrigenomics

Several observations over many decades have certainly supported the theory. For example, nutrition researchers have long noted that some people will lose weight on a specific diet and exercise program, whereas others following the same diet and exercise program will experience no weight loss or will even gain weight.[6,7] The varying results are now thought to depend to a certain extent on how the foods in that diet affect the study participants' genes.

Another example is smoking. Researchers have long understood that smoking is harmful to human health, but they now recognize that smokers with a particular genotype have a much higher rate of mortality (death) than smokers with a different genotype.[8]

Scientists also look to population studies for evidence supporting nutrigenomics. For example, they point out that when different ethnic groups are exposed to a western diet, the percentage of type 2 diabetes increases in some populations significantly more than in others. Also, the health disparities that exist between people in developed versus those in developing countries are known to

be due in large part to their different access to appropriate nutrition.[5]

Evidence of nutrigenomics influencing future generations includes the breakthrough study of agouti mice, as well as recent historical data that suggest a link between the availability of food and diabetes. Researchers have found that when one generation experiences a food surplus during critical periods of reproductive development, their offspring are more likely to develop diabetes.[4]

Promises of Nutrigenomics

Currently, researchers involved in nutrigenomics are making predictions not unlike that of the famous inventor Thomas Edison: "The doctor of the future will give no medicine but will interest his patients in the care of the human frame, in diet and in the cause and prevention of disease."

One promise of nutrigenomics is that it can assist people in optimizing their health by reducing their risk of developing diet-related diseases and possibly even by treating existing conditions through diet alone.[6] For example, some research studies how leafy green vegetables may turn on an important gene that suppresses cancerous tumors.[9]

Another promise of nutrigenomics is personalized nutrition. Today, dietary advice is based primarily on observations of large populations. Typically, these epidemiological studies do not consider genetic and cultural variations within the group.[5,6] But advice that is generally appropriate for a population might not be appropriate for every individual within that population. The field of nutrigenomics would eliminate this concern because each individual would have a personalized diet. In the future world of nutrigenomics, you could provide a tissue sample to a healthcare provider who would send it to a lab for genetic analysis. Then, the healthcare provider could tailor a diet to your specific genetic makeup. This "personalized diet" would identify both foods to eat and foods to avoid, thus turning on beneficial genes and turning off genes that may be detrimental.

Another promise of nutrigenomics is increased understanding of the role of physical activity in human health. Recent research shows that exercise can influence genes involved in certain diseases such as colon cancer. Dr. Anne McTiernan of the Fred Hutchinson Cancer Research Center in Seattle has found that exercise can reduce the risk of colon cancer by 50%. McTiernan has observed that study participants who exercise at least 4 hours a week turned abnormal-looking cells that had the potential to develop into polyps and even colon cancer into normal functioning cells.[9] Thus, nutrigenomics is finding that the conventional advice to "eat a balanced diet and exercise" holds true for the majority of people.

A final promise of nutrigenomics is reduction in the global problem of health disparities. Information gained from comparing nutrient/gene interactions as well as environmental factors in different populations may help scientists address the problem of global malnutrition and disease in both developed and developing countries.[5]

Challenges of Nutrigenomics

One obstacle in making nutrigenomic therapies a reality is determining what foods or supplements turn on or off specific genes in specific individuals. Genetic pathways are extremely complicated, and turning on a gene may have a beneficial effect on one body function but a harmful effect on another. To complicate the matter further, other factors such as age, gender, and lifestyle also affect how different foods interact with these different genetic pathways. In addition, dietary intervention to prevent or treat chronic diseases would be challenging because multiple genes may be involved, and environmental, emotional, and even social factors may also play a role.[10] The number of variables that have to be considered in order to develop a "personalized diet" is staggering.

Even by themselves, food interactions are extremely complicated because when one eats a meal, hundreds of nutrient compounds are consumed at one time. Think about all the ingredients found in just one food item, such as pancakes. Each one of these ingredients may affect gene expression directly or indirectly and may interact with a large number of genes in an uncontrollable and uncountable number of ways.[10] Scientists have determined that there are at least 150 different genes that are linked to type 2 diabetes and 300 or more that have been linked to obesity. Which of the ingredients consumed affect what gene and how? It will be years before researchers are capable of mapping out these complex interactions.[8]

Considering these challenges, regulation of the nutrigenomics industry is a growing concern. Safety will become a major issue as applications of nutrigenomics become a public reality. How this emerging industry is regulated will play an important role in how we protect ourselves from fraudulent or even dangerous dietary advice.[6]

A major challenge facing the field of nutrigenomics may already have been surmounted: Who should be able to gain access to an individual's DNA profile? On April 25, 2007, the U.S. House of Representatives passed a bill that would ban employers and insurance companies from discriminating against people based on their genetic makeup. Under this bill, genetic profiles could not be used by insurance companies to deny insurance coverage or raise premiums, nor could employers terminate individuals from their jobs for having a genetic mutation.

When Will Nutrigenomics Become Reality?

Delivering on the promises of nutrigenomics will require a multidisciplinary approach involving researchers in genetics, nutrition, chemistry, molecular biology, physiology, pathology, sociology, ethics, and many more fields. The number and complexity of nutritional, environmental, and genetic interactions these scientists will have to contend with are so staggering that decades may pass before nutrigenomics is a viable industry.

Consumers will probably first encounter nutrigenomics in diagnostic testing. In this process, a blood or tissue sample of DNA will be genetically analyzed to determine how food and food supplements interact with that individual's genes and how a change in diet might affect those interactions. Genetic counseling will be required to help consumers understand the meaning and recommendations suggested by their genetic profile.[6]

Second, consumers will probably begin to see more specialized foods promoted for specific conditions. For example, consumers currently have an array of foods they can choose from if they want to lower their cholesterol or enhance their bone health. More such foods will likely be developed, and food packages of the future might even be coded for certain genetic profiles.

We may be decades away from a "personalized diet," but one thing is clear right now: nutrigenomics is showing us the importance of nutrition and environmental factors in preserving our health. Nutrigenomics is sure to change not only the way we look at food but also the field of nutrition itself.

CHAPTER 2

CHAPTER OBJECTIVES

After reading this chapter, you will be able to:

1. Identify the characteristics of a healthful diet, pp. 38–40.

2. Name five components that must be included on food labels and use the Nutrition Facts Panel to determine the nutritional adequacy of a given food, pp. 40–43.

3. Describe the Dietary Guidelines for Americans and discuss how these Guidelines can be used to design a healthful diet, pp. 48–51.

4. Identify the food groups, number of servings, and serving sizes included in MyPyramid, pp. 52–55.

5. Explain how MyPyramid can be used to design a healthful diet, pp. 60–62.

6. Discuss the characteristics of the DASH diet plan, pp. 67–69.

7. Describe the components of the Exchange System, pp. 69–71.

8. List at least four ways to practice moderation and apply healthful dietary guidelines when eating out, pp. 72–73.

TEST YOURSELF TRUE OR FALSE?

1. A healthful diet should always include vitamin supplements. T or F

2. The Dietary Guidelines for Americans recommend that all Americans should consume alcohol sensibly. T or F

3. MyPyramid is limited in scope and cannot be used by most Americans to design a healthful diet. T or F

4. The DASH diet plan encourages us to eat 5 servings of fruits and 5 servings of vegetables each day. T or F

5. It is impossible to eat a healthful diet when eating out. T or F

Test Yourself answers can be found after the Chapter Summary.

Designing a Healthful Diet

Shivani and her parents moved to the United States from India when Shivani was 6 years old. Although delicate in comparison to her American peers, Shivani was healthy and energetic, excelling in school and riding her new bike in her suburban neighborhood. By the time Shivani entered high school, her weight had caught up to her American classmates. Now a college freshman, she has joined the more than 16% of U.S. teens who are overweight.[1,2] Shivani explains, "In India, the diet is mostly rice, lentils, and vegetables. Many people are vegetarians, and many others eat meat only once or twice a week, and very small portions. Desserts are only for special occasions. When we moved to America, I wanted to eat like all the other kids: hamburgers, French fries, sodas, and sweets. I gained a lot of weight on that diet, and now my doctor says my cholesterol, my blood pressure, and my blood sugar levels are all too high. I wish I could start eating like my relatives back in India again, but they don't serve rice and lentils at the dorm cafeteria."

What influence does diet have on health? What exactly qualifies as a "poor diet," and what makes a diet healthful? Is it more important to watch how much we eat, or what kinds of foods we choose? Is low-carb better, or low-fat? What do the national dietary guidelines advise, and do they apply to "real people" like you?

A healthful diet can help prevent disease.

Many factors contribute to uncertainty about the influence of nutrition on human health. First, nutrition is a relatively young science. In contrast to physics, chemistry, and astronomy, which have been studied for thousands of years, the science of nutrition emerged around 1900, with discovery of the first vitamin in 1897. The initial Recommended Dietary Allowance (RDA) values for the United States were published in 1941. Because nutritional research is in its infancy, new findings on the effects of foods and nutrients are discovered almost daily. These new findings contribute to regular changes in how we define a healthful diet.

Second, as stated in Chapter 1, the popular media typically report the results of only selected studies, usually the most recent. This practice does not give a complete picture of all the research conducted in any given area. Indeed, the results of a single study are often misleading.

Third, there is no one right way to eat that is healthful and acceptable for everyone. We are individuals with unique needs, food preferences, and cultural influences. For example, a person with diabetes may benefit from eating lower amounts of added sugars and higher amounts of protein than a person without diabetes. People following certain religious practices may limit or avoid foods like specific meats and dairy products. Thus, there are literally millions of different ways to design a healthful diet to fit individual needs.

Given all this potential confusion, it's a good thing there are nutritional tools to guide us in designing a healthful diet. In this chapter, we introduce these tools, including the Dietary Guidelines for Americans, the USDA Food Guide, and others. Before we explore the question of how to design a healthful diet, however, we should first make sure we understand what a healthful diet *is*.

What Is a Healthful Diet?

A **healthful diet** provides the proper combination of energy and nutrients. It has four characteristics: it is adequate, moderate, balanced, and varied. No matter if you are young or old, overweight or underweight, healthy or coping with illness, if you keep in mind these characteristics of a healthful diet, you will be able to consciously select foods that provide you with the optimal combination of nutrients and energy each day.

A Healthful Diet Is Adequate

An **adequate diet** provides enough of the energy, nutrients, and fiber to maintain a person's health. A diet may be inadequate in only one area. For example, many people in the United States eat plenty of breads, meats, fruits, and dairy products, but do not eat enough vegetables. Thus, their intake of many of the important nutrients found in vegetables, such as fiber, beta-carotene, and potassium, is likely to be inadequate. However, their intake of protein, fat, carbohydrate, and calcium may be adequate. In fact, many people who eat too few vegetables are overweight or obese, which means that they are eating a diet that exceeds their energy needs but may not be adequate in the nutrients found predominantly in vegetables.

On the other hand, a generalized state of undernutrition can occur if an individual's diet contains an inadequate level of several nutrients for a long period of time. This situation occurs when a person severely limits his or her intake of all foods to avoid gaining weight. For example, many teenage girls and college-aged women follow a very restrictive eating pattern to maintain a thin figure. These individuals may skip multiple meals each day, avoid foods that contain any fat, and limit their meals to only a few foods such as a bagel, a banana, a diet soda, or a small green salad. This type of restrictive eating pattern practiced over a prolonged period can cause low energy levels, loss of bone and hair, impaired memory and cognitive function, and menstrual dysfunction in women.

A diet that is adequate for one person may not be adequate for another. For example, a small woman who is lightly active may require approximately 1,700 to 2,000 kcal of energy each day to support her body's functions. In contrast, a highly active male athlete may require more than 4,000 kcal of energy each day to support his body's demands. These two individuals differ greatly in their activity level and in

healthful diet A diet that provides the proper combination of energy and nutrients and is adequate, moderate, balanced, and varied.

adequate diet A diet that provides enough of the energy, nutrients, and fiber to maintain a person's health.

A diet that is adequate for one person may not be adequate for another. A woman who is lightly active may require fewer kilocalories of energy per day than a highly active male.

their quantity of body fat and muscle mass, which means they require very different levels of fat, carbohydrate, protein, and other nutrients to support their daily needs.

A Healthful Diet Is Moderate

Moderation is the key to a healthful diet. **Moderation** refers to eating the right amounts of foods to maintain a healthy weight and to optimize the body's metabolic processes. If a person eats too much or too little of certain foods, healthful goals cannot be reached. For example, some people drink a lot of sugared soft drinks, as they enjoy the sweet taste and the energetic feeling produced by the caffeine in these drinks. It is not uncommon for people to drink at least 60 fl. oz (or three 20-oz bottles) of soft drinks on some days. Drinking this amount would contribute an extra 765 kcal of energy to a person's diet. In order to maintain weight, a person would need to compensate for the extra energy either by greatly increasing his or her physical activity or by reducing the amount of food consumed. This could lead to a person cutting healthful food choices from his or her diet. By reducing soft drink consumption, or switching to diet soft drinks or water, people can consume more healthful foods and maintain a healthy body weight.

A Healthful Diet Is Balanced

A **balanced diet** is one that contains the combinations of foods that provide the proper balance of nutrients. As you will learn in this course, our bodies need many types of foods in varying amounts to maintain health. For example, fruits and vegetables are excellent sources of fiber, vitamin C, beta-carotene, potassium, and magnesium. In contrast, meats are not good sources of these nutrients. However, meats are excellent sources of protein, iron, zinc, and copper. By eating the proper balance of all healthful foods, including fruits, vegetables, and meats (or meat substitutes), we can be confident that we are consuming the proper balance of the nutrients we need to maintain health.

A Healthful Diet Is Varied

Variety refers to eating a lot of different foods each day. Most U.S. supermarkets offer literally thousands of healthful foods we can choose from. Trying new foods on a regular basis can assist us in eating a more varied diet. Do not be afraid to eat a new

moderation Eating the right amounts of foods to maintain a healthy weight and to optimize our bodies' metabolic processes.

balanced diet A diet that contains the combinations of foods that provide the proper proportions of nutrients.

variety Eating a lot of different foods each day.

green vegetable each week. Or try putting spinach on your turkey sandwich in place of iceberg lettuce. By selecting a variety of foods, we optimize our chances of consuming the multitude of nutrients our bodies need. As an added benefit, eating a varied diet prevents boredom and helps us avoid getting into a "food rut." Later in this chapter, we provide suggestions for eating a varied diet.

> RECAP: *A healthful diet is adequate, moderate, balanced, and varied. It provides adequate nutrients and energy, and it includes sweets, fats, and salty foods in moderate amounts only. It includes an appropriate balance of foods and a wide variety of foods.*

What Tools Can Help Me Design a Healthful Diet?

Many people feel it is impossible to eat a healthful diet. They may mistakenly believe that the foods they would need to eat are too expensive or not available to them, or they may feel too busy to do the necessary planning, shopping, and cooking. Some people rely on dietary supplements to get enough nutrients instead of focusing on eating a variety of foods. But is it really that difficult to eat a healthful diet?

Although designing and maintaining a healthful diet is not as simple as eating whatever you want, most of us can do it with a little practice and a little help. Let's look now at some tools for designing a healthful diet.

Food Labels

An essential first step in designing and following a healthful diet is to learn how to read food labels. It may surprise you to discover that prior to 1973, there were no federal regulations for including nutrition information on food labels. In that year, the U.S. Food and Drug Administration (FDA) established an initial set of labeling regulations; however, they were not as specific as they are today and were not required for many foods. Throughout the 1970s and 1980s, consumer interest in food quality substantially grew, and many watchdog groups were formed to protect consumers from unclear labeling and false claims made by some manufacturers.

Public interest and concern about how food affects our health became so strong that in 1990, the U.S. Congress passed the Nutrition Labeling and Education Act. This act specifies which foods require a food label, provides detailed descriptions of the information that must be included on the food label, and describes the companies and food products that are exempt from publishing complete nutrition information on food labels. For example, detailed food labels are not required for meat or poultry, as these products are regulated by the U.S. Department of Agriculture, not the FDA. In addition, foods such as coffee and most spices are not required to follow the FDA labeling guidelines, as they contain insignificant amounts of all nutrients that must be listed in nutrition labeling.

Five Components Must Be Included on Food Labels

Five primary components of information must be included on food labels (FIGURE 2.1):

1. *A statement of identity:* The common name of the product or an appropriate identification of the food product must be prominently displayed on the label. This information tells us very clearly what the product is.

2. *The net contents of the package:* The quantity of the food product in the entire package must be accurately described. Information may be listed as weight (e.g., grams), volume (e.g., fluid ounces), or numerical count (e.g., 4 each).

3. *Ingredient list:* The ingredients must be listed by their common name, in descending order by weight. This means that the first product listed in the ingredient list is the predominant ingredient in that food. This information can be

FIGURE 2.1 The five primary components that are required for food labels. (© ConAgra Brands, Inc.)

very useful in many situations, such as when you are looking for foods that are lower in fat or sugar, or when you are attempting to identify foods that contain whole-grain flour instead of processed wheat flour. The ingredient list must also clearly state the presence of any of eight common food allergens, including peanuts, tree nuts, milk, wheat, eggs, soy, fish, and shellfish.

4. *The name and address of the food manufacturer, packer, or distributor:* This information can be used if you want to find out more detailed information about a food product and to contact the company if there is something wrong with the product or you suspect that the food product caused an illness.

5. *Nutrition information:* The Nutrition Facts Panel contains the nutrition information required by the FDA. This panel is the primary tool to assist you in choosing more healthful foods. An explanation of the components of the Nutrition Facts Panel follows.

How to Read and Use the Nutrition Facts Panel on Foods

FIGURE 2.2 shows an example of a **Nutrition Facts Panel,** which contains a variety of information that is useful when designing a healthful diet. You can use this information to learn more about an individual food or to compare one food to another. Let's start at the top of the panel and work our way down to better understand how to use this information.

1. *Serving size and servings per container:* Describes the serving size in a common household measure (e.g., cup), a metric measure (e.g., grams), and how many servings are contained in the package. The FDA has defined serving sizes based on the amounts people typically eat for each food. However, keep in mind that the serving size listed on the package may not be the same as the amount *you* eat. You must factor in how much of the food you eat when determining the amount of nutrients that this food contributes to your actual diet.

The serving size on a nutrition label may not be the same as the amount you eat.

Nutrition Facts Panel The label on a food package that contains the nutrition information required by the FDA.

FIGURE 2.2 The Nutrition Facts Panel contains a variety of information to help you select more healthful food choices.

2. *Calories and calories from fat per serving:* Describes the total number of calories and the total amount of calories that come from fat per one serving of that food. By looking at this section of the label, you can determine whether this food is relatively high in fat. For example, one serving of the food on this label (as prepared) contains 320 total calories, with 90 of those calories coming from fat. This means that this food contains 28% of its total calories as fat (90 fat calories ÷ 320 total calories), making it relatively low in fat.

3. *List of nutrients:* Describes various nutrients that are found in this food. Those nutrients listed toward the top, including total fat, saturated fat, *trans* fat, cholesterol, and sodium, are generally nutrients that we strive to limit in a healthful diet. Some of the nutrients listed toward the bottom are those we try to consume more of, including fiber, vitamins A and C, calcium, and iron.

4. ***Percent Daily Values (%DV):*** Tells you how much a serving of food contributes to your overall intake of nutrients listed on the label. For example, 10 grams of fat constitutes 15% of an individual's total daily recommended fat intake. Because we are all individuals with unique nutritional needs, it is impractical to

percent Daily Values (%DV) Information on a Nutrition Facts Panel that identifies how much a serving of food contributes to your overall intake of nutrients listed on the label; based on an energy intake of 2,000 calories per day.

include nutrition information that applies to each person consuming a food. That would require thousands of labels! Thus, when defining the %DV, the FDA based their calculations on a 2,000 calorie diet. Even if you do not consume 2,000 calories each day, you can still use the %DV to figure out whether a food is high or low in a given nutrient. For example, foods that contain less than 5% DV of a nutrient are considered low in that nutrient, while foods that contain more than 20% DV are considered high in that nutrient. If you are trying to consume more calcium in your diet, select foods that contain more than 20% DV for calcium. In contrast, if you are trying to consume lower fat foods, select foods that contain less than 5% or 10% fat. By comparing the %DV between foods for any nutrient, you can quickly decide which food is higher or lower in that nutrient without having to know anything about how many calories you need.

5. *Footnote* (or lower part of panel): Includes a footnote that must be present on all food labels. This footnote tells you that the %DV are based on a 2,000 calorie diet and that your needs may be higher or lower based on your caloric needs. The remainder of the footnote includes a table with values that illustrate the differences in recommendations between a 2,000 calorie and 2,500 calorie diet; for instance, someone eating 2,000 calories should strive to eat less than 65 grams of fat per day, whereas a person eating 2,500 calories should eat less than 80 grams of fat per day. The table may not be present if the food label is too small. The footnote and the table, when present, are always the same because the information refers to general dietary advice for all Americans rather than to a specific food.

By comparing labels from various foods, you can start designing a more healthful diet today. Try looking at the two labels in FIGURE 2.3 to decide which food is a more nutritious choice. First, you must decide which nutrients are more important for you. Let's assume you are trying to eat foods with more fiber and potassium. The food label on the left shows that cereal 1 contains 2 g of dietary fiber and 60 mg of potassium per serving. The food label on the right shows that cereal 2 contains 5 g of dietary fiber and 85 mg of potassium per serving if served with skim milk. For these two nutrients, cereal 2 on the right would be a more nutritious choice.

Food Labels Can Contain a Variety of Nutrient Claims

Although not required, food labels may also contain various claims related to nutrients and health. You have likely seen additional claims such as "This food is part of a heart healthy diet," or "This food is low in sodium." These claims may influence consumers to buy these foods even when they are not sure what the claims mean.

Food companies are allowed to make certain approved nutrient claims on food labels. Table 2.1 on page 45 includes the approved, regulated terms and their definitions. The Daily Values on the food labels serve as a basis for these claims. For instance, if the label states that a food is "low in sodium," this indicates that the particular food contains 140 mg or less of sodium per serving. It is prohibited for any company to list a nutrient or health claim on a label that is not approved by the FDA.

Companies are also allowed to make certain claims related to health and disease on food labels. The health claims that the FDA allows at the present time are listed in Table 2.2 on page 46. To help consumers gain a better understanding of nutritional information related to health, the FDA has developed a Health Claims Report Card (FIGURE 2.4 on page 46) that grades the level of confidence in a health claim based on current scientific evidence. For example, if current scientific evidence is not convincing, a particular health claim may have to include a disclaimer so that consumers are not misled. Complete the Nutrition Label Activity on page 47 to determine the strengths of certain health claims made on foods commonly consumed.

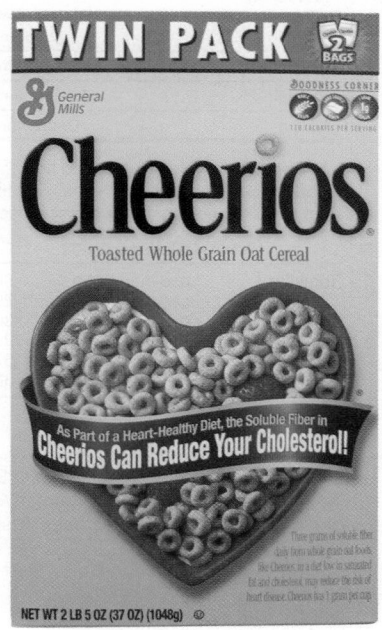

This Cheerios label is an example of an approved health claim.

Nutrition Facts

Serving Size 3/4 cup (27g)
Servings Per Container 13

Amount Per Serving

| | | With 1/2 Cup Vitamin A & D | |
	Cereal alone	Fortified Skim Milk	
Calories	90	130
Calories from Fat	10	10

	% Daily Value	
Total Fat 1g*	2%	2%
Saturated Fat 0g	0%	0%
Polyunsaturated Fat 0.5g		
Monounsaturated Fat 0.5g		
Trans Fat 0g		
Cholesterol 0mg	0%	0%
Sodium 190mg	8%	11%
Potassium 85mg	2%	8%
Total Carbohydrate 23g	8%	10%
Dietary Fiber 5g	20%	20%
Sugars 5g		
Protein 2g		
Vitamin A	0%	4%
Vitamin C	10%	15%
Calcium	0%	15%
Iron	2%	2%
Vitamin E	2%	2%

85mg Potassium
8% Daily Value
(with milk)

5g Dietary Fiber
20% Daily Value

* Amount in Cereal. One half cup skim milk con-tributes an additional 40 calories, 65mg Sodium, 190mg Potassium, 6g Total Carbohydrate (6g sugars), and 4g Protein.

* Percent Daily Values are based on a 2000 calorie diet. Your daily values may be higher or lower depending on your calorie needs:

		Calories	2,000	2,500
Total Fat	Less than		65g	80g
Sat. Fat	Less than		20g	25g
Cholesterol	Less than		300mg	300mg
Sodium	Less than		2,400mg	2,400mg
Total Carbohydrate			300g	375g
Dietary fiber			25g	30g

Calories per gram:
Fat 9 • Carbohydrate 4 • Protein 4

INGREDIENTS: Yellow Corn Flour, Corn Bran Flour, Unsulphured Molasses, Oat Flour, Expeller Pressed High Oleic Oil (Canola and/or Sunflower), Salt, Baking Soda, Natural Vitamin E, Vitamin C.

Nutrition Facts

Serving Size 1 cup (25g)
Servings Per Container 8.5

Amount Per Serving

Calories 70

Calories from Fat 5

	% Daily Value
Total Fat 0.5g	1%
Saturated Fat 0g	0%
Trans Fat 0g	
Cholesterol 0mg	0%
Sodium 0mg	0%
Potassium 60mg	2%
Total Carbohydrate 13g	4%
Dietary Fiber 2g	8%
Sugars 0g	
Protein 3g	

Vitamin A 0%	•	Vitamin C 0%
Calcium 0%	•	Iron 4%
Thiamin 2%	•	Riboflavin 2%
Niacin 4%	•	Phosphorus 6%

60mg Potassium
2% Daily Value

2g Dietary Fiber
8% Daily Value

* Percent Daily Values are based on a 2,000 calorie diet. Your daily values may be higher or lower depending on your calorie needs.

		Calories	2,000	2,500
Total Fat	Less than		65g	80g
Sat. Fat	Less than		20g	25g
Cholesterol	Less than		300mg	300mg
Sodium	Less than		2,400mg	2,400mg
Total Carbohydrate			300g	375g
Dietary fiber			25g	30g

Calories per gram:
Fat 9 • Carbohydrate 4 • Protein 4

INGREDIENTS: Whole Oats, Long Grain Brown Rice, Whole Rye, Whole Hard Winter Wheat, Whole Triticale, Whole Buckwheat, Whole Barley, Sesame Seeds.

(a)

(b)

FIGURE 2.3 Labels from two breakfast cereals. Note that there is less fiber and potassium in (**a**) cereal 1 than in (**b**) cereal 2.

TABLE 2.1 United States Food and Drug Administration (FDA)–Approved Nutrient-Related Terms and Definitions

Nutrient	Claim	Meaning
Energy	Calorie free	Less than 5 kcal per serving
	Low calorie	40 kcal or less per serving
	Reduced calorie	At least 25% fewer kcal than reference (or regular) food
Fat and Cholesterol	Fat free	Less than 0.5 g of fat per serving
	Low fat	3 g or less fat per serving
	Reduced fat	At least 25% less fat per serving than reference food
	Saturated fat free	Less than 0.5 g of saturated fat **AND** less than 0.5 g of *trans* fat per serving
	Low saturated fat	1 g or less saturated fat and less than 0.5 g *trans* fat per serving **AND** 15% or less of total kcal from saturated fat
	Reduced saturated fat	At least 25% less saturated fat **AND** reduced by more than 1 g saturated fat per serving as compared to reference food
	Cholesterol free	Less than 2 mg of cholesterol per serving **AND** 2 g or less saturated fat and *trans* fat combined per serving
	Low cholesterol	20 mg or less cholesterol **AND** 2 g or less saturated fat per serving
	Reduced cholesterol	At least 25% less cholesterol than reference food **AND** 2 g or less saturated fat per serving
Fiber and Sugar	High fiber	5 g or more fiber per serving*
	Good source of fiber	2.5 g to 4.9 g fiber per serving
	More or added fiber	At least 2.5 g more fiber per serving than reference food
	Sugar free	Less than 0.5 g sugars per serving
	Low sugar	Not defined; no basis for recommended intake
	Reduced/less sugar	At least 25% less sugars per serving than reference food
	No added sugars or without added sugars	No sugar or sugar-containing ingredient added during processing
Sodium	Sodium free	Less than 5 mg sodium per serving
	Very low sodium	35 mg or less sodium per serving
	Low sodium	140 mg or less sodium per serving
	Reduced sodium	At least 25% less sodium per serving than reference food
Relative Claims	Free, without, no, zero	No or a trivial amount of given nutrient
	Light (or lite)	This term can have three different meanings: 1) a serving provides ⅓ fewer kcal than or half the fat of the reference food; 2) a serving of a low-fat, low-calorie food provides half the sodium normally present; or 3) lighter in color and texture, with the label making this clear (for example, light molasses)
	Reduced, less, fewer	Contains at least 25% less of a nutrient or kcal than reference food
	More, added, extra, or plus	At least 10% of the Daily Value of nutrient as compared to reference food (may occur naturally or be added). May only be used for vitamins, minerals, protein, dietary fiber, and potassium
	Good source of, contains, or provides	10% to 19% of Daily Value per serving (may not be used for carbohydrate)
	High in, rich in, or excellent source of	20% or more of Daily Value per serving for protein, vitamins, minerals, dietary fiber, or potassium (may not be used for carbohydrate)

Source: U.S. Food and Drug Administration. Center for Food Safety and Applied Nutrition. 2004. A Food Labeling Guide. Appendix A and Appendix B. www.cfsan.fda.gov/~dms/flg-6a.html and www.cfsan.fda.gov/~dms/flg-6b.html.
*High fiber claims must also meet the definition of low fat; if not, then the level of total fat must appear next to the high fiber claim.

TABLE 2.2 U.S. Food and Drug Administration–Approved Health Claims on Labels

Disease/Health Concern	Nutrient	Example of Approved Claim Statement
Osteoporosis	Calcium	Regular exercise and a healthy diet with enough calcium help teens and young adult white and Asian women maintain good bone health and may reduce their high risk of osteoporosis later in life.
Coronary heart disease	Saturated fat and cholesterol Fruits, vegetables, and grain products that contain fiber, particularly soluble fiber Soluble fiber from whole oats, psyllium seed husk, and beta glucan soluble fiber from oat bran, rolled oats (or oatmeal), and whole oat flour Soy protein Plant sterol/stanol esters Whole-grain foods	Diets low in saturated fat and cholesterol and rich in fruits, vegetables, and grain products that contain some types of dietary fiber, particularly soluble fiber, may reduce the risk of heart disease, a disease associated with many factors.
Cancer	Dietary fat Fiber-containing grain products, fruits, and vegetables Fruits and vegetables Whole-grain foods	Low-fat diets rich in fiber-containing grain products, fruits, and vegetables may reduce the risk of sometypes of cancer, a disease associated with many factors.
Hypertension and stroke	Sodium Potassium	Diets containing foods that are a good source of potassium and that are low in sodium may reduce the risk of high blood pressure and stroke.*
Neural tube defects	Folate	Healthful diets with adequate folate may reduce a woman's risk of having a child with a brain or spinal cord defect.
Dental caries	Sugar alcohols	Frequent between-meal consumption of foods high in sugars and starches promotes tooth decay. The sugar alcohols in [name of food] do not promote tooth decay.

Source: U.S. Food and Drug Administration. Center for Food Safety and Applied Nutrition. 2005. A Food Labeling Guide. Appendix C. www.cfsan.fda.gov/~dms/flg-6c.html.
*Required wording for this claim. Wordings for other claims are recommended model statements but not required verbatim.

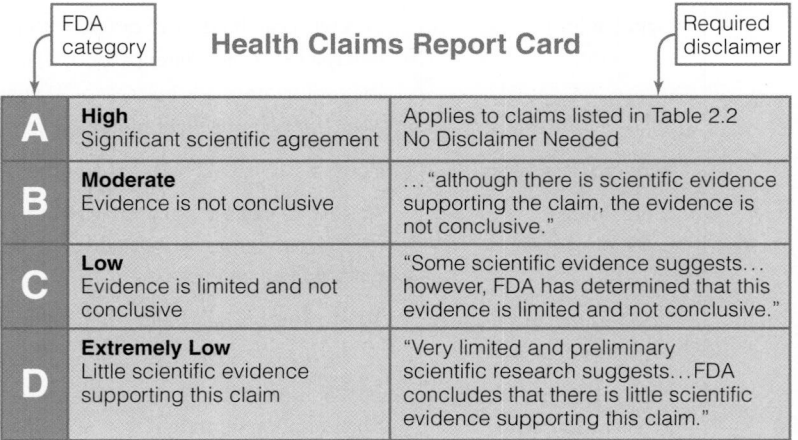

FIGURE 2.4 The U.S. Food and Drug Administration's Health Claims Report Card.

How Do Health Claims on Food Labels Measure Up?

The U.S. Food and Drug Administration has published a Health Claims Report Card to assist consumers in deciphering health claims on food labels (Figure 2.4). It is important to note that the claims made that are based on high scientific agreement do not require a label disclaimer. The claims reported in Table 2.2 are those that are based on high scientific agreement. Included below is a food label listing health claims. Look at this label: based on the Health Claims Report Card criteria listed in Figure 2.4, what level of confidence do scientists currently have about these health claims? Taking this level of confidence into consideration, would you recommend this product to relatives or friends if they were concerned with heart disease? Why or why not?

PATENTED BLEND TO HELP IMPROVE CHOLESTEROL*
U.S. Patents 5,578,334; 5,843,497 & 6,630,192   SEE NUTRITION INFORMATION FOR FAT AND SAT FAT CONTENT

HEART HEALTH NEWS SEE INSIDE PANEL

- 50% Less Fat & Calories than butter or margarine
- Vitamins A, B6, B12 & E Added
- No Hydrogenation
- Precisely Balanced Fats
- No Palm Kernel Oil
- Gluten & Gelatin Free
- Contains a _Full_ 16 oz.

NON-HYDROGENATED
SMART BALANCE *light*
Real Butter Taste!
BEST TASTE 2007 CHEFSBEST

BUTTERY SPREAD
37% VEGETABLE OIL

Lactose Free
No Trans Fatty Acids
Naturally!
Ⓤ PARVE

16 OZ. (1LB.) 454g

Smart Balance® Light Spread Offers:

Right Balance of Fats: Same precise balance as in regular Smart Balance.

No Trans Fatty Acids: Trans fats occur in foods containing partially hydrogenated oil.

No Hydrogenated Oil in this spread.

50% Less Fat & Calories than butter and regular margarine.

220mg Omega-3 per serving.

Lactose Free. Contains no dairy ingredients.

No Gelatin, Starch or Gums.

Nutrition Facts
Serving Size 1 Tbsp (14g)
Servings Per Container 32
Calories 45
Calories from Fat 45

*Percent Daily Values (DV) are based on a 2,000 calorie diet.

Amount/Serving	%DV*	Amount/Serving	% DV*
Total Fat 5g	8%	**Cholesterol** 0mg	0%
Sat Fat 1.5g	8%	**Sodium** 85mg	4%
Trans Fat 0g		**Total Carb.** 0g	0%
Poly Fat 1.5g		**Protein** 0g	
Mono Fat 2g			

Vitamin A 10% (15% as beta carotene)
Vitamin B6 35% • Vitamin B12 20% • Vitamin E 10%
Not a significant source of dietary fiber, sugars, Vitamin C, Calcium, and Iron.

Ingredients: water, Natural Oil Blend (palm fruit, soybean, canola and olive oils), contains less than 2% of salt, vegetable monoglycerides and sorbitan ester of fatty acids (emulsifiers), soybean lecithin, potassium sorbate, lactic acid (to protect freshness), natural and artificial flavor, calcium disodium EDTA, Vitamin E (dl-tocopherol acetate), Vitamin A palmitate, Vitamin B6, Vitamin B12 and beta-carotene color.

BUY BEFORE
FEB0908L11 06:37

*Natural oil blend helps enhance ratio of HDL "good" to LDL "bad" cholesterol.

The right balance of fats may improve the important cholesterol ratio when at least two-thirds of fat intake comes from this product or our Food Plan. Total fat intake should be limited to 30% of calories (65g/day), saturated fat to 10% (20g/day), dietary cholesterol to under 300mg per day and trans fatty acids reduced by avoiding foods with partially hydrogenated oils. Regular exercise is essential. Help balance your fat intake with the Smart Balance Food Plan. It's available free by mail or online at www.smartbalance.com.

0 33776 01150 5

Owned & Dist. by: HEART BEAT FOODS
DIV. GFA BRANDS INC., P.O. BOX 397
CRESSKILL, NJ 07626-0397
Visit our website at: www.smartbalance.com

• No Hydrogenated Oil • No Trans Fatty Acids • No Lactose

Keep Refrigerated - DO NOT FREEZE!
This spread has a very low fat content, freezing may cause grainy texture and/or separation (physical separation of oil and water is not harmful in any way). Store in Refrigerator up to 1 year.

Contents: A Full 16 oz.
Compared to other major brands which only contain 15 oz.

NUTRI-CASE GUSTAVO

"Until last night, I hadn't stepped inside of a grocery store for 10 years, maybe more. But then my wife fell and broke her hip and had to go to the hospital. On my way home from visiting her, I remembered that we didn't have much food in the house, so I thought I'd do a little shopping. Was I ever in for a shock. I don't know how my wife does it, choosing between all the different brands, reading those long labels. She never went to school past sixth grade, and she doesn't speak English very well either! I bought a frozen chicken pie for my dinner, but it didn't taste right. So I got the package out of the trash and read all the labels, and that's when I realized there wasn't any chicken in it at all! It was made out of tofu! This afternoon, my daughter is picking me up, and we're going to do our grocery shopping together!"

Given what you've learned about FDA food labels, what parts of a food package would you advise Gustavo to be sure to read before he makes a choice? What other advice might you give him to make his grocery shopping easier? Imagine that, like Gustavo's wife, you have only limited skills in mathematics and reading. In that case, what other strategies might you use when shopping for nutritious foods?

> RECAP: *Reading food labels is a necessary skill when planning a healthful diet. Food labels must list the identity of the food, the net contents of the package, the contact information for the food manufacturer or distributor, the ingredients in the food, and a Nutrition Facts Panel. The Nutrition Facts Panel provides specific information about calories, macronutrients, and select vitamins and minerals. Food labels may also contain claims related to nutrients and health.*

Dietary Guidelines for Americans

The **Dietary Guidelines for Americans** are a set of principles developed by the U.S. Department of Agriculture and the U.S. Department of Health and Human Services to assist Americans in designing a healthful diet and lifestyle.[3] They are updated every 5 years. The current Guidelines, which were published in 2005, can be viewed at **www.health.gov/dietaryguidelines**. These Guidelines identify both food choices and physical activity habits that can help reduce our risk for chronic diseases.

The United States is not the only country to develop dietary guidelines. Other countries, including Canada and the United Kingdom, also publish nutrition recommendations. Following is a brief description of each of the chapters and key recommendations of the Dietary Guidelines for Americans. Refer to Table 2.3 for specific examples of how you might alter your current diet and physical activity habits to meet some of these guidelines.

Adequate Nutrients Within Energy Needs

It is important to consume adequate nutrients to promote health while staying within your energy needs. Key recommendations include consuming a variety of nutrient-dense foods and beverages within and among the basic food groups while choosing foods that are limited in saturated and *trans* fats, cholesterol, added sugars, salt, and alcohol. You can meet your recommended intakes within energy needs by adopting a balanced eating pattern, such as the USDA Food Guide (MyPyramid) or the DASH eating plan, which are both discussed later in this chapter.

Dietary Guidelines for Americans
A set of principles developed by the U.S. Department of Agriculture and the U.S. Department of Health and Human Services to assist Americans in designing a healthful diet and lifestyle. These Guidelines are updated every 5 years.

TABLE 2.3 Ways to Incorporate the Dietary Guidelines for Americans into Your Daily Life

If You Normally Do This:	Try Doing This Instead:
Watch television when you get home at night	Do 30 minutes of stretching or lifting of hand weights in front of the television
Drive to the store down the block	Walk to and from the store
Go out to lunch with friends	Take a 15 or 30 minute walk with your friends at lunchtime 3 days each week
Eat white bread with your sandwich	Eat whole-wheat bread or some other bread made from whole grains
Eat white rice or fried rice with your meal	Eat brown rice or even try wild rice
Choose cookies or a candy bar for a snack	Choose a fresh nectarine, peach, apple, orange, or banana for a snack
Order French fries with your hamburger	Order a green salad with low-fat salad dressing on the side instead of French fries
Spread butter or margarine on your white toast each morning	Spread fresh fruit compote on whole-grain toast
Order a bacon double cheeseburger at your favorite restaurant	Order a turkey burger or grilled chicken sandwich without the cheese and bacon, and add lettuce and tomato
Drink nondiet soft drinks to quench your thirst	Drink water with a slice of lemon, diet soft drinks, or iced tea
Eat regular potato chips and pickles with your favorite sandwich	Eat carrot slices and crowns of fresh broccoli and cauliflower dipped in low-fat ranch dressing

Weight Management

Being overweight or obese increases our risk for many chronic diseases, including heart disease, type 2 diabetes, stroke, and some forms of cancer. Key recommendations include maintaining body weight in a healthful range by balancing energy from foods and beverages with energy expended. To prevent gradual weight gain over time, you should make small decreases in the amount of energy you consume and increase your physical activity.

Physical Activity

Key recommendations include engaging in regular physical activity and reducing sedentary activities to promote health, psychological well-being, and a healthy body weight. You are also encouraged to achieve physical fitness by including cardiovascular conditioning, stretching exercises for flexibility, and resistance exercises or calisthenics for muscle strength and endurance. By accumulating at least 30 minutes of moderate physical activity on most, preferably all, days of the week, you can reduce your risk for chronic diseases. Moderate physical activity includes walking, riding a bike, mowing the lawn with a push mower, or performing heavy yard work or housework. Other activities that are beneficial include those that build strength, such as lifting weights, groceries, or other objects, carrying your golf clubs while you walk around the course, and participating in yoga or other flexibility activities. The 30-minute guideline is a minimum; if you are already doing more activity than this, then continue on your healthy path. For most people, greater health benefits can be obtained by engaging in physical activity that is of more vigorous intensity or

Being physically active for at least 30 minutes each day can reduce your risk for chronic diseases.

longer duration. If you are currently inactive, 30 minutes is a realistic and healthful goal. Being physically active 60 to 90 minutes per day on most days of the week is recommended to prevent weight gain and to promote weight loss in those who are overweight.

Food Groups to Encourage

Eating a variety of fruits and vegetables is important to ensure that we consume the various nutrients we need to enhance health. A few of the nutrients provided by fruits and vegetables include vitamin A, beta-carotene, vitamin C, folate, and potassium. Key recommendations include consuming a sufficient amount of fruits and vegetables each day while staying within energy needs. In addition, we should choose a variety of fruits and vegetables, selecting from all five vegetable subgroups: dark-green, orange, legumes, starchy vegetables, and other vegetables. The Guidelines also encourage us to eat 3 or more oz of whole-grain foods each day and to consume 3 cups per day of low-fat or fat-free milk or equivalent milk products.

Fats

Fat is an important part of a healthful diet, as it provides energy and important nutrients such as essential fatty acids and fat-soluble vitamins. However, eating a diet high in total fat can lead to overweight and obesity. Eating foods high in saturated and *trans* fats causes an increase in our blood cholesterol levels, and high blood cholesterol levels increase our risk for heart disease. Thus, it is important to minimize your intake of saturated and *trans* fat. Key recommendations include consuming less than 10% of your total energy intake as saturated fatty acids and less than 300 mg/day of cholesterol. *Trans* fat intake should be as low as possible. Total fat intake should be 20% to 35% of total energy intake, with most fats coming from fish, nuts, and vegetable oils. The Guidelines also encourage us to select low-fat or fat-free meat and milk products.

Carbohydrates

Carbohydrates are an important source of energy and essential nutrients. Key recommendations include choosing fiber-rich fruits, vegetables, and whole grains often and choosing and preparing foods and beverages with little added sugars. It is important to moderate our intake of foods high in sugar and starch, as these foods promote tooth decay. To reduce the risk of dental caries (or cavities), the Guidelines recommend that we practice good oral hygiene and consume foods and beverages that contain sugar and starch less frequently.

Sodium and Potassium

Salt contains the mineral sodium, and eating a lot of sodium is linked to high blood pressure in some people. Potassium is linked with healthy blood pressure levels. Eating high amounts of sodium also can cause us to lose calcium from our bones, which could increase our risk for bone loss and bone fractures. Much of the salt we consume in our diets comes from processed and prepared foods. Key recommendations include consuming less than 2,300 mg (approximately 1 tsp. of salt) of sodium per day, choosing and preparing foods with little salt, and consuming potassium-rich foods such as fruits and vegetables. Ways to decrease our salt intake include eating fresh, plain frozen, or canned vegetables without salt added, limiting our intake of processed meats such as cured ham, sausage, bacon, and most canned meats, and looking for foods with labels that say "low-sodium." In addition, adding little or no salt to foods at home and limiting our intake of salty condiments such as ketchup, mustard, pickles, soy sauce, and olives can help reduce our sodium intake.

Alcoholic Beverages

Alcoholic beverages provide us with energy, but they do not contain any nutrients. Drinking alcoholic beverages in excess can lead to many health and social problems. Key recommendations for those who choose to drink include drinking sensibly and in moderation. Moderation is defined as no more than one drink per day for women and

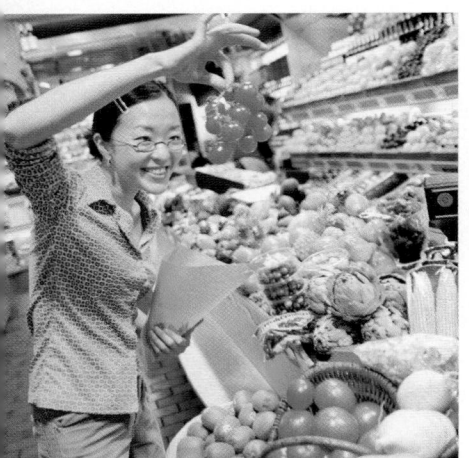

When grocery shopping, try to select a variety of fruits and vegetables.

Eating a diet rich in whole-grain foods and fiber-rich fruits and vegetables can enhance your overall health.

no more than two drinks per day for men. Those who should not drink any alcohol include those who cannot restrict their intake, women of childbearing age who may become pregnant, pregnant and lactating women, children and adolescents, individuals taking medications that can interact with alcohol, people with certain medical conditions, and people who are engaging in activities that require attention, skill, or coordination. To learn more about whether or not alcohol can be part of a healthful diet, refer to the *In Depth* look on alcohol on pages 160–169.

Food Safety

A healthful diet is one that is safe from foodborne illnesses like those caused by bacteria, viruses, and other toxins. Food safety is discussed in more detail in Chapter 18. Important tips to remember include storing and cooking foods at the proper temperatures, avoiding unpasteurized juices and milk products and raw or undercooked meats and shellfish, and washing your hands and cooking surfaces before cooking and after handling raw meats, shellfish, and eggs.

> RECAP: *The Dietary Guidelines for Americans emphasize healthful food choices and physical activity behaviors. The Guidelines include achieving a healthy weight, being physically active each day, using the USDA Food Guide or the DASH diet plan to select foods, eating whole-grain foods, fruits, and vegetables daily, keeping foods safe to eat, eating foods low in saturated and trans fat and cholesterol and moderate in total fat, moderating sugar intake, eating less salt, eating more potassium-rich foods, and drinking alcohol in moderation, if at all.*

MyPyramid: The Food Guide Pyramid

The U.S. Department of Agriculture (USDA) Food Guide Pyramid is another tool that can guide you in designing a healthful diet. It was created to provide a conceptual framework for the types and amounts of foods that make up a healthful diet. An evolving document, it will continue to change as we learn more about the roles of specific nutrients and foods in promoting health and preventing disease.

In 2005, a revised pyramid-based food guidance system was introduced by the USDA, called **MyPyramid** (FIGURE 2.5). This system is based on both the 2005 Dietary Guidelines for Americans and the Dietary Reference Intakes from the National Academy of Sciences. MyPyramid is an interactive, personalized guide that people can access on the Internet to assess their current diet and physical activity levels and to make changes in their food intake and physical activity patterns.

Components of MyPyramid

The graphic represents six components: activity, moderation, personalization, proportionality, variety, and gradual improvement.

The activity component of MyPyramid is represented by the steps and the person climbing them. This is a reminder for people to be physically active every day.

The moderation component of MyPyramid is represented by the narrowing of each food group from the bottom to the top of the pyramid. The wider base of each food group represents foods in that group of which a person should eat more, as they contain important nutrients and little or no solid fats or added sugars. The narrower area at the top of each food group stands for foods in that group of which a person should eat less, as they contain more solid fats and added sugars.

Personalization is represented by the person on the steps of MyPyramid, the slogan (MyPyramid.gov, "Steps to a Healthier You"), and the Web site. When you log onto **www.MyPyramid.gov**, you are prompted to enter your gender, age, and daily activity level. MyPyramid then assigns you a recommended kcal intake level, such as 1,800 kcal for a sedentary female adult, and shows you how much of each type of food you should eat each day to stay within that level. Since there are twelve different recommended kcal intake levels, ranging from 1,000 kcal/day to 3,200 kcal/day, twelve possible pyramids can be generated. This personalization helps you design a diet that meets your unique needs.

MyPyramid A revised pyramid-based food guidance system developed by the USDA and based on the 2005 Dietary Guidelines for Americans and the Dietary Reference Intakes from the National Academy of Sciences.

MyPyramid
STEPS TO A HEALTHIER YOU
MyPyramid.gov

GRAINS	VEGETABLES	FRUITS	MILK	MEAT & BEANS
Make half your grains whole	**Vary your veggies**	**Focus on fruits**	**Get your calcium-rich foods**	**Go lean with protein**
Eat at least 3 oz. of whole-grain cereals, breads, crackers, rice, or pasta every day 1 oz. is about 1 slice of bread, about 1 cup of breakfast cereal, or ¹/2 cup of cooked rice, cereal, or pasta	Eat more dark-green veggies like broccoli, spinach, and other dark leafy greens Eat more orange vegetables like carrots and sweet-potatoes Eat more dry beans and peas like pinto beans, kidney beans, and lentils	Eat a variety of fruit Choose fresh, frozen, canned, or dried fruit Go easy on fruit juices	Go low-fat or fat-free when you choose milk, yogurt, and other milk products If you don't or can't consume milk, choose lactose-free products or other calcium sources such as fortified foods and beverages	Choose low-fat or lean meats and poultry Bake it, broil it, or grill it Vary your protein routine—choose more fish, beans, peas, nuts, and seeds

For a 2,000-calorie diet, you need the amounts below from each food group. To find the amounts that are right for you, go to MyPyramid.gov.

Eat 6 oz. every day	Eat 2¹/2 cups every day	Eat 2 cups every day	Get 3 cups every day; for kids aged 2 to 8, it's 2	Eat 5¹/2 oz. every day

Find your balance between food and physical activity
- Be sure to stay within your daily calorie needs.
- Be physically active for at least 30 minutes most days of the week.
- About 60 minutes a day of physical activity may be needed to prevent weight gain.
- For sustaining weight loss, at least 60 to 90 minutes a day of physical activity may be required.
- Children and teenagers should be physically active for 60 minutes every day, or most days.

Know the limits on fats, sugars, and salt (sodium)
- Make most of your fat sources from fish, nuts, and vegetable oils.
- Limit solid fats like butter, margarine, shortening, and lard, as well as foods that contain these.
- Check the Nutrition Facts label to keep saturated fats, *trans* fats, and sodium low.
- Choose food and beverages low in added sugars. Added sugars contribute calories with few, if any, nutrients.

MyPyramid.gov
STEPS TO A HEALTHIER YOU

U.S. Department of Agriculture
Center for Nutrition Policy and Promotion
April 2005
CNPP-15

USDA

USDA is an equal opportunity provider and employer.

FIGURE 2.5 The USDA MyPyramid. This pyramid is an interactive food guidance system based on the 2005 Dietary Guide-lines for Americans and the Dietary Reference Intakes from the National Academy of Sciences. MyPyramid is a personalized guide that people can use to assess their current diet and physical activity levels and to make changes in their food intake and physical activity patterns. There are six components of this symbol, including activity, moderation, personalization, proportion-ality, variety, and gradual improvement. To learn more about this pyramid, go to www.MyPyramid.gov.

Proportionality is illustrated through the use of differing widths of the food group bands, or sections. The widths indicate how much food a person should consume from each group, in proportion to the other groups. To get an indication of the amount you should consume, you must log onto **www.MyPyramid.gov**.

The variety component of MyPyramid is represented by six longitudinally oriented, color-coded bands, or sections that represent five categories of foods and an oils category that should be eaten each day. The five food categories are grains, vegetables, fruits, milk, and meat and beans.

Gradual improvement is encouraged by the slogan "Steps to a Healthier You." This slogan suggests that people can benefit from taking small steps each day to improve their diet and lifestyle.

The overall framework of the MyPyramid food guidance system is designed to result in the following changes: 1) increase the intake of vitamins, minerals, dietary fiber, and other essential nutrients; 2) lower the intake of saturated fats, *trans* fats, and cholesterol and increase the intake of fruits, vegetables, and whole grains; and 3) balance energy intake with energy expenditure to prevent weight gain and/or to promote a healthy weight.

Food Groups in MyPyramid

Again, the food groups in MyPyramid are grains, vegetables, fruits, milk, and meat and beans, and there is an additional category for oils.

The grains section of MyPyramid emphasizes "making half your grains whole," meaning you should make sure at least half of the grains you eat each day come from whole-grain sources. People are advised to eat at least 3 oz of whole-grain bread, cereal, crackers, rice, or pasta each day. The foods in this group are clustered together because they provide fiber-rich carbohydrates and are good sources of the nutrients riboflavin, thiamin, niacin, iron, folate, zinc, protein, and magnesium.

The vegetables section of MyPyramid emphasizes "vary your veggies," meaning you should eat a variety of vegetables each day. Included in this message are recommendations to eat more dark-green and orange vegetables and more dry beans and peas.

The fruits section of MyPyramid emphasizes "focus on fruits," encouraging people to eat a variety of fruits (including fresh, frozen, canned, or dried) and to go easy on fruit juices. Although fruits and vegetables are good sources of many of the same nutrients, including carbohydrate, fiber, vitamins A and C, folate, potassium, and magnesium, the groups are separated in the pyramid because they do not contain all of the same nutrients. Thus, eating a variety of *both* fruits and vegetables is important in ensuring our consumption of many vital nutrients. Fruits and vegetables also contain differing amounts and types of naturally occurring *phytochemicals*, plant chemicals that enhance our health. An *In Depth* look at phytochemicals is provided on pages 350–359.

The oils section of MyPyramid is identified by the narrow yellow band. This section emphasizes "know your fats," encouraging people to select healthier forms of fat. These include fat from fish, nuts, and vegetable oils. The message also stresses limiting solid fats such as butter, stick margarine, shortening, lard, and visible fat on meat.

The milk section, which includes milk, yogurt, and cheese, emphasizes "get your calcium-rich foods." Low-fat or fat-free dairy products are suggested, and those who cannot consume dairy are encouraged to choose lower lactose and lactose-free dairy products or other calcium sources such as calcium-fortified juices and soy beverages. These foods are good sources of calcium, phosphorus, riboflavin, protein, and vitamin B_{12}; many of these foods are also fortified with vitamins D and A.

The meat and beans section, which includes meat, poultry, fish, dry beans, eggs, and nuts, emphasizes "go lean on protein." Low-fat or lean meats and poultry are encouraged, as is using cooking methods such as baking, broiling, or grilling. People are also encouraged to vary their meat choices to include more fish, beans, nuts, and seeds. This group is composed of foods that are good sources of protein, phosphorus, vitamin B_6, vitamin B_{12}, zinc, magnesium, iron, niacin, riboflavin, and thiamin. Notice that legumes, which include dried beans, peas, and lentils, are included both in the meat and beans section and in the vegetables section. This is because legumes are good sources of fiber and many of the vitamins found in vegetables, as well as of protein and some of the minerals found in meat and poultry.

Some of your daily fruit servings can come from canned fruits.

Discretionary Calories in MyPyramid

One new concept introduced in MyPyramid is that of **discretionary calories.** Discretionary calories represent the extra amount of energy you can consume after you have met all of your essential needs by consuming the recommended amounts and types of foods. The number of discretionary calories recommended depends on your age, gender, and physical activity level. For people who do not want to gain weight, it is typically small, between about 100 and 300 kcal/day.

Foods that some people may choose to use up their discretionary calories include butter, margarine, lard, salad dressings, oils, mayonnaise, sour cream, cream, and gravy. High-sugar foods such as candies, desserts, gelatin, soft drinks, and fruit drinks may also be consumed, and alcoholic beverages are also included in your discretionary calorie allowance. You can also use your discretionary calories to eat more healthful foods.

Number and Size of Servings in MyPyramid

As noted earlier, MyPyramid also helps you decide *how much* of each food you should eat. When you enter your gender, age, and activity level on the homepage, MyPyramid generates a table showing you the number of servings you should eat from each food group for your recommended kcal level. FIGURE 2.6 shows the recommendations for four different energy intake levels. As you can see in this table, people who expend more energy need to eat more foods from each food group.

A term used in this table that may be new to you is **ounce-equivalent** (or *oz-equivalent*). It identifies a serving size that is 1 oz, or equivalent to an ounce, for the grains and meats and beans group. For example, ½ cup of cooked brown rice is 1 oz-equivalent.

What is considered a serving size for the foods listed in MyPyramid? FIGURE 2.7 shows examples of the number of cups or oz-equivalents recommended for a 2,000 kcal food intake pattern and the amounts that are equal to 1 cup or 1 oz-equivalent for foods in each group. An oz-equivalent serving from the grains group is defined as one slice of bread, 1 cup of ready-to-eat cereal, or ½ cup of cooked rice, pasta, or cooked cereal. One cup of vegetables is equal to 2 cups of raw leafy vegetables such as spinach or equal to 1 cup of chopped raw or cooked vegetables such as broccoli. An oz-equivalent serving of meat is actually 1 oz; thus, 3 oz of meat is equal to 3 oz-equivalents. It may be helpful to learn that 3 oz of meat is approximately the size of a deck of cards. One egg, 1 tbsp. peanut butter, and ¼ cup cooked dry beans are also considered 1 oz-equivalents from the meat and beans group. Although it may

discretionary calories A term used in the MyPyramid food guidance system that represents the extra amount of energy you can consume after you have met all of your essential needs by consuming the most nutrient-dense foods that are low-fat or fat-free and that have no added sugars.

ounce-equivalent (or oz-equivalent) A term used to define a serving size that is 1 oz, or equivalent to 1 oz, for the grains group and the meats and beans group of MyPyramid.

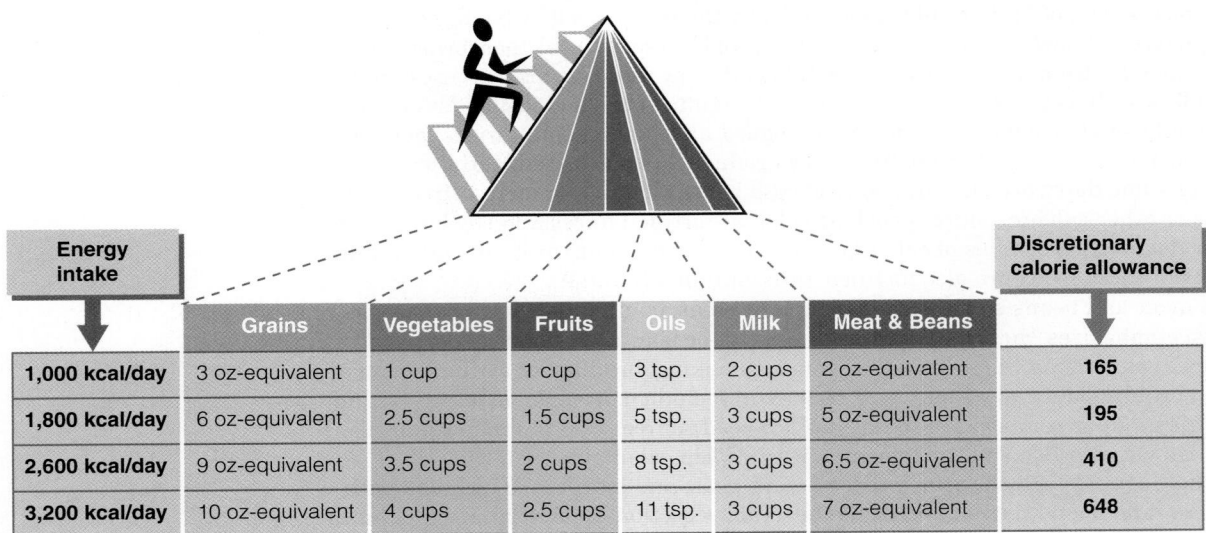

Energy intake	Grains	Vegetables	Fruits	Oils	Milk	Meat & Beans	Discretionary calorie allowance
1,000 kcal/day	3 oz-equivalent	1 cup	1 cup	3 tsp.	2 cups	2 oz-equivalent	165
1,800 kcal/day	6 oz-equivalent	2.5 cups	1.5 cups	5 tsp.	3 cups	5 oz-equivalent	195
2,600 kcal/day	9 oz-equivalent	3.5 cups	2 cups	8 tsp.	3 cups	6.5 oz-equivalent	410
3,200 kcal/day	10 oz-equivalent	4 cups	2.5 cups	11 tsp.	3 cups	7 oz-equivalent	648

FIGURE 2.6 Sample diets from MyPyramid at four different energy intakes.

Food group	Number of cups or oz-equivalents for a 2,000-kcal food intake pattern	Examples of amounts equal to 1 cup or 1 oz-equivalent			
Milk group	3 cups	1 cup (8 fl. oz) milk	1 cup (8 fl. oz) yogurt	1.5 oz hard cheese	1 cup of ice cream
Meat and beans group	5.5 oz-equivalents	1 oz pork loin chop	1 oz chicken breast without skin	1/4 cup pinto beans	1/2 oz almonds
Vegetables group	2.5 cups	1 cup (8 fl. oz) tomato juice	2 cups raw spinach	1 cup cooked broccoli	1 cup mashed potatoes
Fruits group	2 cups	1 cup (8 fl. oz) orange juice	1 cup strawberries	1 cup of pears	1/2 pink grapefruit
Grains group	6 oz-equivalents	1 (1 oz) slice of whole-wheat bread	1/2 cup (1 oz) cooked brown rice	1/2 regular hamburger bun	2 pancakes (4" diameter)

FIGURE 2.7 Examples of serving sizes for foods in each food group of MyPyramid for a 2,000 kcal food intake pattern. Here are some examples of household items that can help you to estimate serving sizes: 1.5 oz of hard cheese is equal to 4 stacked dice, 3 oz of meat is equal in size to a deck of cards, and half of a regular hamburger bun is the size of a yo-yo.

seem unnatural and inconvenient to measure our food servings, understanding the size of a serving is crucial to planning a nutritious diet.

It is important to understand that the serving sizes defined in MyPyramid are not standardized and may not correspond to serving sizes identified on food labels. For instance, the serving size for crackers in MyPyramid is 3 to 4 small crackers, whereas a serving size for crackers on a food label can range from 5 to 18 crackers, depending on the size and weight of the cracker. When comparing serving sizes from MyPyramid with serving sizes on packaged foods you eat, remember to check the Nutrition Fact Panels. Try the Nutrition Label Activity to determine whether the serving sizes listed on assorted food labels match the serving sizes that you normally consume.

NUTRITION LABEL ACTIVITY

How Realistic Are the Serving Sizes Listed on Food Labels?

Many people read food labels to determine the energy (that is, caloric) value of foods, but it is less common to pay close attention to the actual serving size that corresponds to the listed caloric value. To test how closely your "naturally selected" serving size meets the actual serving size of certain foods, try these label activities:

- Choose a breakfast cereal that you commonly eat. Pour the amount of cereal that you would normally eat into a bowl. Before adding milk to your cereal, use a measuring cup to measure the amount of cereal you poured. Now read the label of the cereal to determine the serving size (for example, ½ cup or 1 cup) and the caloric value listed on the label. How do your "naturally selected" serving size and the label-defined serving size compare?

- At your local grocery store, locate various boxes of snack crackers. Look at the number of crackers and total calories per serving listed on the labels of crackers such as regular Triscuits, reduced-fat Triscuits, Vegetable Thins, and Ritz crackers. How do the number of crackers and total calories per serving differ for the serving size listed on each box? How do the serving sizes listed in the Nutrition Facts Panel compare to how many crackers you would usually eat? These activities are just two examples of ways to understand how nutrition labels can assist the consumer with making balanced and healthful food choices. As many people do not know what constitutes a serving size, they are inclined to consume too much of some foods (such as snack foods and meat) and too little of other foods (such as fruits and vegetables).

For items consumed individually, such as muffins, frozen burgers, bottled juices, and so on, the serving sizes in MyPyramid are typically much smaller than the items we buy. In addition, serving sizes in restaurants, cafes, and movie theatres have grown substantially over the past 30 years.[4] This "super-sizing" phenomenon, now seen even at home, indicates a major shift in accessibility to foods and in accepted eating behaviors, and emphasizes the importance of becoming educated about portion size control.

In addition to being a potentially important contributor to the rise in obesity rates around the world, this increase in serving size leads to confusion among consumers. This confusion is illustrated by the results of a study conducted by Young and Nestle in which introductory nutrition students were asked to bring to class one sample of a "medium" bagel, baked potato, muffin, apple, or cookie.[5] The weights of these foods were measured, and most of the foods the students brought to class well exceeded the USDA's definition of a serving size. Young and Nestle report that the discrepancy in portion size of many common foods sold outside of the home in comparison to USDA standards is quite staggering—chocolate chip cookies are seven times larger than USDA standards, while steaks are more than twice as large, and a serving of cooked pasta in a restaurant is almost five times larger.[6] Thus, when using diet-planning tools like food labels and MyPyramid, it is essential to learn the definition of serving size for the tool you are using, and *then* measure your food intake to determine whether you are meeting the guidelines. Refer to the You Do the Math activity to estimate how much physical activity you would need to do in order to expend the excess energy you consume because of increasing food portion sizes.

> RECAP: *The USDA MyPyramid food guidance system can be used to plan a personalized, healthful, balanced diet that includes a variety of foods. The serving sizes of foods as defined in MyPyramid typically are smaller than the amounts we normally eat or are served, so it is important to learn the definitions of serving sizes when using MyPyramid to design a healthful diet.*

YOU DO THE MATH %

How Much Exercise Is Needed to Combat Increasing Food Portion Sizes?

Although the causes of obesity are complex and multifactorial, it is speculated that one reason obesity rates are rising around the world is a combination of increased energy intake due to expanding food portion sizes and a reduction in overall daily physical activity. This activity should help you to better understand how portion sizes have increased over the past 20 years and how much physical activity you would need to do to expend the excess energy resulting from these larger portion sizes.

The photos in Figure 2.8 give examples of foods whose portion sizes have increased substantially. A bagel 20 years ago had a diameter of approximately 3 inches and contained 140 kcal. A bagel in today's society is about 6 inches in diameter and contains 350 kcal. Similarly, a cup of coffee 20 years ago was 8 fl. oz and was typically served with a small amount of whole milk and sugar. It contained about 45 kcal. A standard coffee mocha commonly consumed today is 16 fl. oz and contains 350 kcal; this excess energy comes from the addition of sugar, milk, and flavored syrup.

On her morning break at work, Judy routinely consumes a bagel and a coffee drink like the ones described here. Judy has type 2 diabetes, and her doctor has advised her to lose weight. How much physical activity would Judy need to do to "burn" this excess energy? Let's do some simple math to answer this question.

1. Calculate the excess energy Judy consumes from both of these foods:
   a. Bagel: 350 kcal in larger bagel – 140 kcal in smaller bagel = 110 kcal extra
   b. Coffee: 350 kcal in large coffee mocha – 45 kcal in small regular coffee = 305 kcal extra

   Total excess energy for these two larger portions = 415 kcal

2. Judy has started walking each day in an effort to lose weight. Judy currently weighs 200 lb. Based on her relatively low fitness level, Judy walks at a slow pace (approximately 2 miles per hour); it is estimated that walking at this pace expends 1.2 kcal per pound of body weight per hour. How long does Judy need to walk each day to expend 415 kcal?

   a. First, calculate how much energy Judy expends if she walks for a full hour by multiplying her body weight by the energy cost of walking per hour = 1.2 kcal/lb body weight × 200 lb = 240 kcal

   b. Next, you need to calculate how much energy she expends each minute she walks by dividing the energy cost of walking per hour by 60 minutes = 240 kcal/hour ÷ 60 minutes/hour = 4 kcal/minute

   c. To determine how many minutes she would need to walk to expend 415 kcal, divide the total amount of energy she needs to expend by the energy cost of walking per minute = 415 kcal ÷ 4 kcal/minute = 103.75 minutes

   Thus, Judy would need to walk for approximately 104 minutes, or about 1 hour and 45 minutes, to expend the excess energy she consumes by eating the larger bagel and coffee. If she wanted to burn off all of the energy in her morning snack, she would have to walk even longer! Now use your own weight in these calculations to determine how much walking you would have to do if you consumed these same foods.

   For more information about large portion sizes and physical activities one needs to do to avoid weight gain, take the National Heart, Lung, and Blood Institute's Portion Distortion Quiz at **http://hp2010.nhlbihin.net/portion/index.htm**.

Variations of the Food Guide Pyramid

Because MyPyramid has just been released to the general public, there are not yet variations developed for diverse populations. However, you can easily select foods that may meet your specific ethnic, religious, or other lifestyle preferences and still follow the MyPyramid system. Using adaptations of the previous version of the USDA Food Guide Pyramid can provide guidance in meeting your dietary needs. For instance, Houtkooper modified the previous Food Guide Pyramid for athletes by including fluids as a new food category at the base of the pyramid, emphasizing the importance of daily fluid replacement for active people. There are also pyramids for children and for older adults.[7–9]

FIGURE 2.8 Examples of increases in food portion sizes over the past 20 years. **(a)** A bagel has increased in diameter from 3 inches to 6 inches; **(b)** a cup of coffee has increased from 8 fl. oz to 16 fl. oz, and now commonly contains calorie-dense flavored syrup as well as steamed whole milk.

20 years ago   **Today**

3-inch diameter, 140 calories   6-inch diameter, 350 calories

(a) Bagel

8 fluid ounces, 45 calories   16 fluid ounces, 350 calories

(b) Coffee

There are also many ethnic and cultural variations of the Food Guide Pyramid. As you know, the population of the United States is culturally and ethnically diverse, and this diversity influences our food choices. Foods that we may typically consider a part of an Asian, Latin American, or Mediterranean diet can also fit into a healthful diet. Variations of the previous USDA Food Guide Pyramid that have been introduced include the Vegetarian Diet Pyramid, the African American Diet Pyramid, the Latin American Diet Pyramid, and the Asian Diet Pyramid (FIGURE 2.9). There are also variations for Singapore, Malaysia, and Native American.[10] These variations illustrate that anyone can design a healthful diet to accommodate their individual food preferences.

Of these variations, the Mediterranean diet has enjoyed considerable popularity. Does it deserve its reputation as a healthful diet? Check out the Highlight box on page 61 to learn more about the Mediterranean diet.

Using MyPyramid to Design a Healthful Diet

At the beginning of this chapter, we identified four key characteristics of a healthful diet: adequacy, moderation, balance, and variety. Let's look at how we can use the principles in MyPyramid to design a diet with all four characteristics.

Eat an Adequate Diet. As we said earlier, an adequate diet provides enough of the energy, nutrients, and fiber to maintain a person's health. For example, MyPyramid suggests that adults eat 2 to 3 cups of milk or yogurt each day. That's because these foods are excellent sources of calcium, as well as several other nutrients. If you avoid dairy products, you will need to replace milk or yogurt with other foods that provide calcium, such as calcium-fortified orange juice and soy milk, turnip greens, broccoli, kale, black-eyed peas, or sardines. If you don't, your diet will be deficient in calcium, which puts you at risk for excessive bone loss and its related health consequences (see Chapter 9).

Eating an adequate diet also means practicing optimal energy control. Failing to eat enough energy deprives your body of adequate nutrients. Eating too much energy will eventually result in weight gain. Eating the number of calories and servings recommended in MyPyramid will help you maintain the proper balance of energy in your diet.

Eat in Moderation.   MyPyramid helps you eat moderately by recommending certain numbers of servings for you to consume each day. Eating too much of certain foods, such as those high in fat and added sugar, leads to weight gain and could prevent you from consuming adequate vitamins, minerals, and fiber. Practicing moderation allows you to eat more nutritious foods without overeating.

Eat a Balanced Diet.   MyPyramid can help you plan a diet that provides the proper balance of nutrients by eating the appropriate number of servings from each food group. If you are looking for foods high in protein, excellent sources are meat, poultry, fish, dry beans, eggs, nuts, milk, yogurt, and cheese. In general, meat, fish, and poultry are also high in iron and zinc, but dairy foods are low in these minerals. So if you use milk, yogurt, and cheese as your primary protein sources, you could develop a deficiency of zinc and iron over time. As you can see, designing a healthful diet is a balancing act: each of the food groups in MyPyramid is critical to a balanced diet, so no group should be completely substituted for another.

In addition to dairy products, kale is an excellent source of calcium.

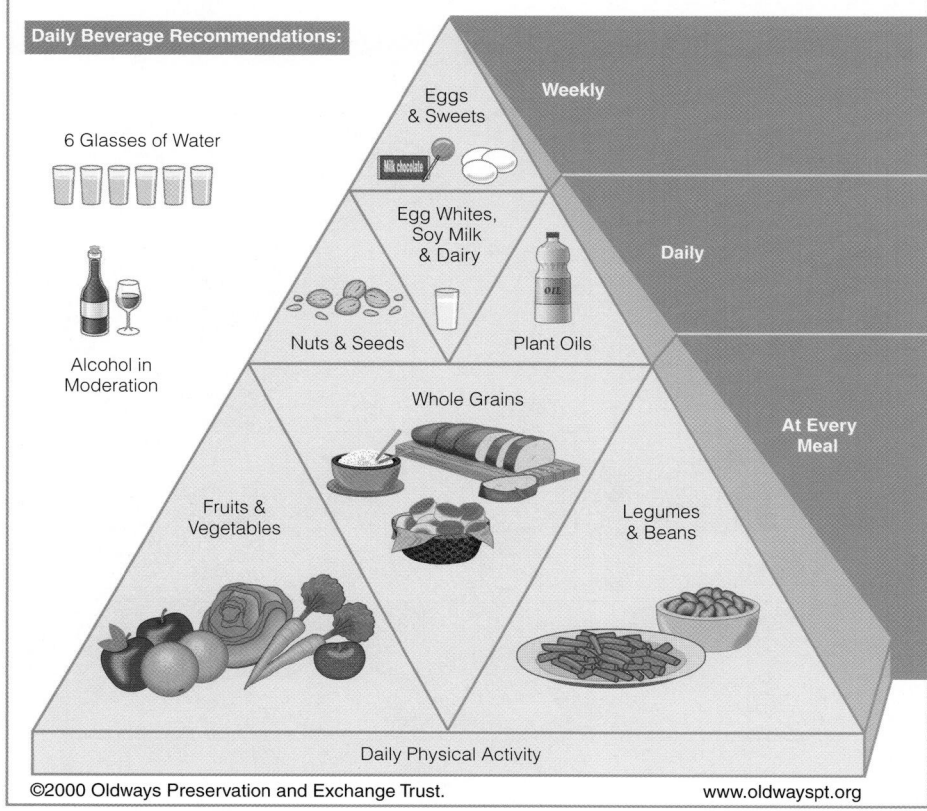

(a) Vegetarian diet pyramid

Daily Beverage Recommendations:

6 Glasses of Water

Alcohol in Moderation

Eggs & Sweets — Weekly

Egg Whites, Soy Milk & Dairy — Daily

Nuts & Seeds

Plant Oils

Whole Grains

Fruits & Vegetables

Legumes & Beans

At Every Meal

Daily Physical Activity

©2000 Oldways Preservation and Exchange Trust.   www.oldwayspt.org

FIGURE 2.9   Ethnic and cultural variations of an earlier version of the USDA Food Guide Pyramid. **(a)** The Vegetarian Diet Pyramid. **(b)** The Latin American Diet Pyramid. **(c)** The Asian Diet Pyramid. (© 2000 Oldways Preservation and Exchange Trust. The Food Issues Think Tank. Healthy Eating Pyramids & Other Tools. www.oldwayspt.org.)

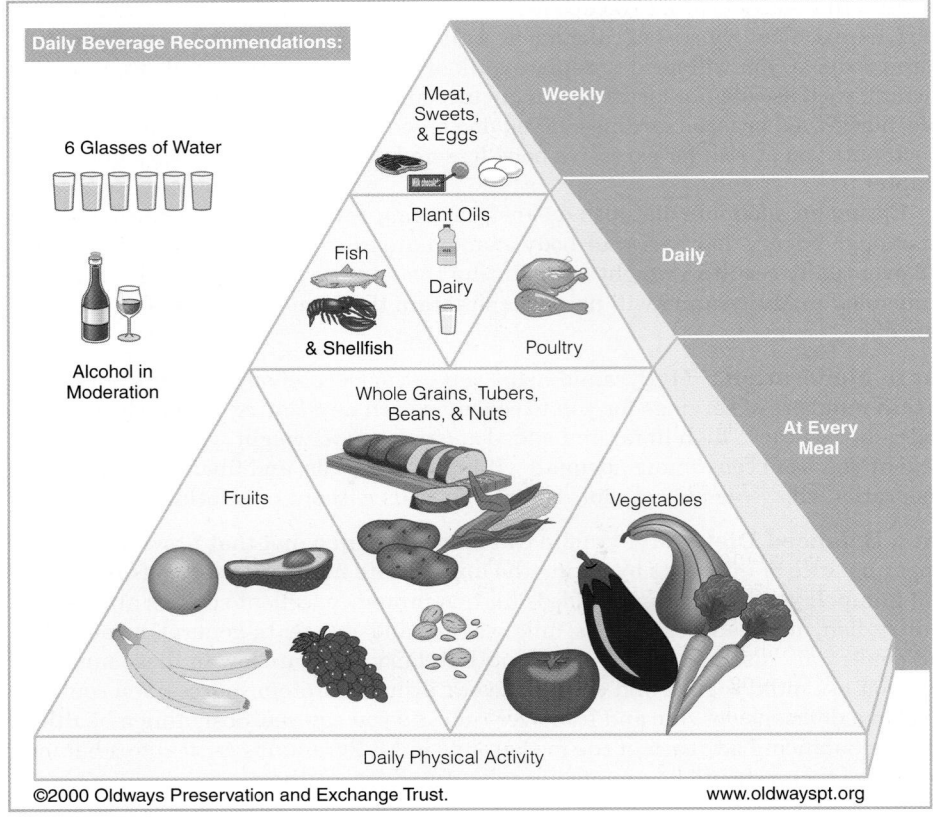

(b) Latin American diet pyramid

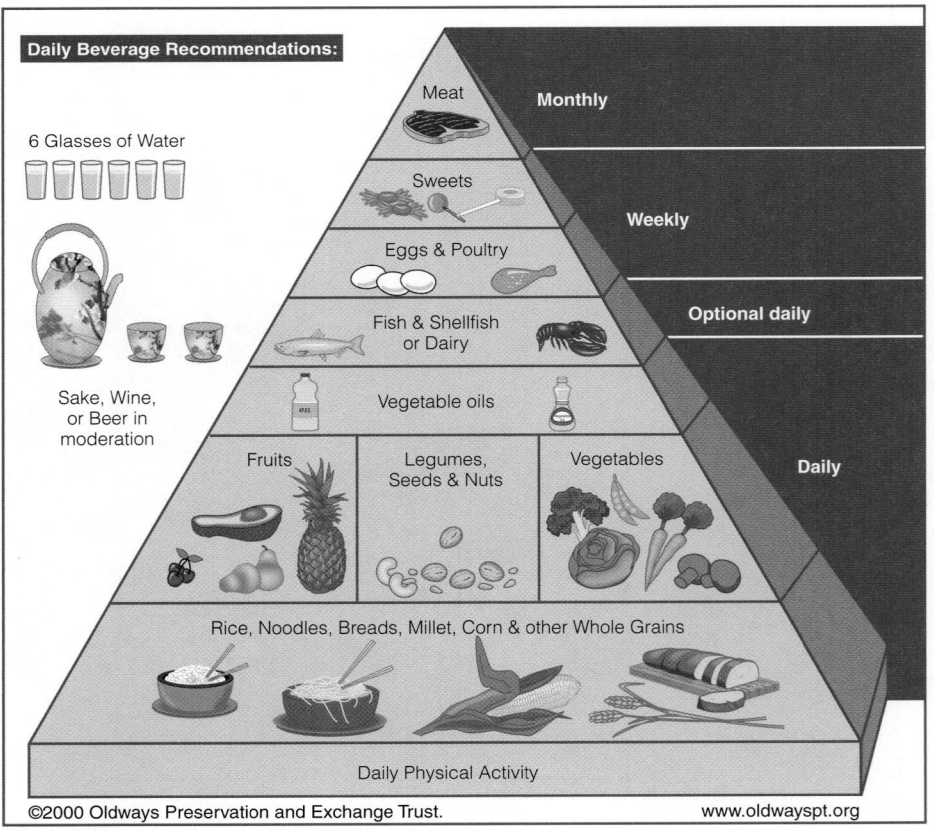

(c) Asian diet pyramid

HIGHLIGHT

The Mediterranean Diet and Pyramid

A Mediterranean-style diet has received significant attention in recent years, as the rates of cardiovascular disease in many Mediterranean countries are substantially lower than rates in the United States. There is actually not a single Mediterranean diet, as this region of the world includes Portugal, Spain, Italy, France, Greece, Turkey, and Israel. Each of these countries has different dietary patterns; however, there are similarities that have led nutrition researchers to speculate that this type of diet is more healthful than the typical U.S. diet:

- Meat is eaten monthly, and eggs, poultry, fish, and sweets are eaten weekly, making the diet low in saturated fats and refined sugars.

- The predominant fat used for cooking and flavor is olive oil, making the diet high in monounsaturated fats.

- Foods eaten daily include grains such as bread, pasta, couscous, and bulgur; fruits; beans and other legumes; nuts; vegetables; and cheese and yogurt. These choices make this diet high in fiber and rich in vitamins and minerals.

As you can see in Figure 2.10, the base of the Mediterranean Pyramid is similar to that of the previous U.S. Food Guide Pyramid, as it includes breads, cereals, and other grains. Another similarity is the daily intake of fruits and vegetables. The two pyramids differ in several important aspects. The Mediterranean Pyramid includes beans, other legumes, and nuts daily; fish, poultry, and eggs are eaten weekly (not daily); and red meat is eaten only about once each month. The Mediterranean Pyramid highlights cheese and yogurt as the primary dairy sources and recommends daily consumption of olive oil. Two unique features of the Mediterranean diet are the inclusion of wine and daily physical activity.

Interestingly, the Mediterranean diet is not lower in fat; in fact, about 40% of the total energy in this diet is derived from fat, which is much higher than the dietary fat recommendations made in the United States. This fact has led some nutritionists to criticize the Mediterranean diet. Supporters point out that the majority of fats in the Mediterranean diet are more healthful than the animal fats found in

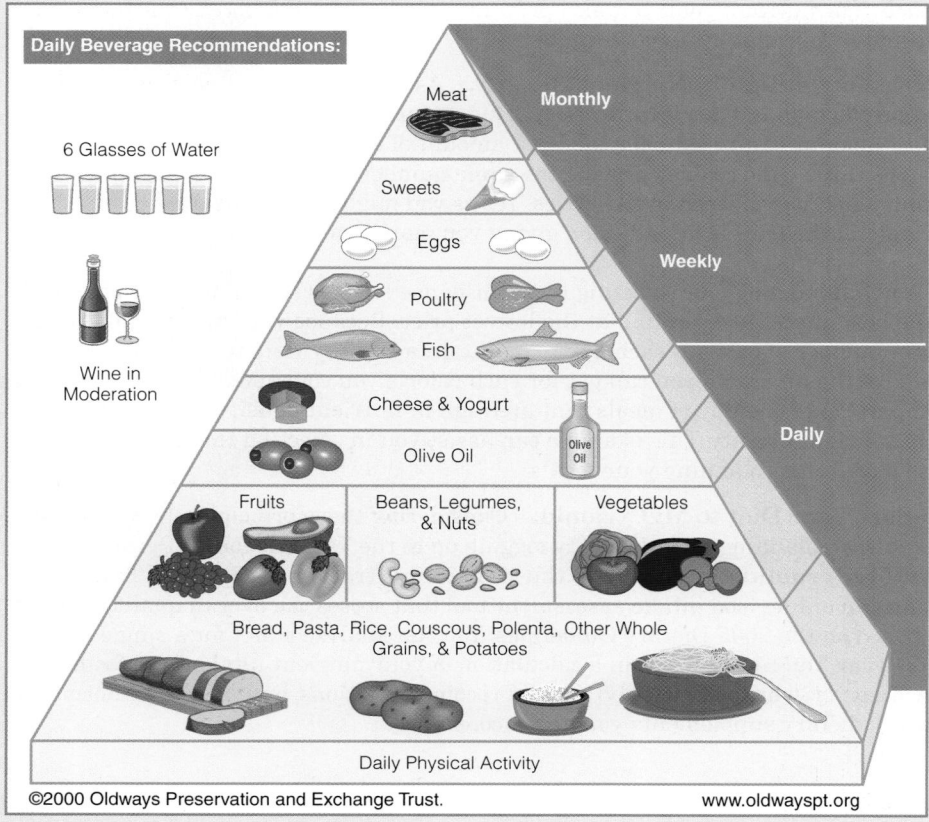

FIGURE 2.10 The Mediterranean Diet Pyramid. (© 2000 Oldways Preservation and Exchange Trust. The Food Issues Think Tank. Healthy Eating Pyramids & Other Tools. www.oldwayspt.org.)

(Continued)

The Mediterranean Diet and Pyramid—*Continued*

the U.S. diet, which makes the Mediterranean diet more protective against cardiovascular disease. The potential benefits of the Mediterranean diet in reducing our cholesterol levels and reducing our risk for heart disease are discussed in Chapter 5.

Can following a Mediterranean-style diet really improve your health? In June 1995, an entire supplement issue of the *American Journal of Clinical Nutrition* reviewed the most recent findings on the Mediterranean diet. Renaud et al.[11] studied the effects of a Mediterranean diet on individuals living in Crete who were recovering from a heart attack. These researchers found that those who ate a Mediterranean diet had a much lower risk of recurrent heart attack and prema-

ture death than individuals who followed the heart-healthy diet prescribed by their doctors. Tavani and La Vecchia reported that people from Italy who ate more fruits and vegetables as a part of a Mediterranean diet had significantly lower risks of some types of cancers, particularly cancers of the mouth, esophagus, stomach, lung, and intestines.[12] A more recent study found that people who consumed a Mediterranean diet were significantly less likely to be obese than people who did not.[13] These studies indicate that eating a Mediterranean-style diet that includes more fruits and vegetables, less meat, and few high-fat dairy products can reduce the risks for obesity, heart disease, and some cancers.

Seafood, meat, poultry, dry beans, eggs, and nuts are examples of foods that are high in protein.

nutrient density The relative amount of nutrients per amount of energy (or number of calories).

Eat a Variety of Foods. MyPyramid encourages you to eat a variety of foods. One way to see if you are varying your foods is to look at the colors on your plate. A healthful range of foods generally is represented by many colors, including green, red, deep yellow or orange, brown, and white. Eating a rainbow of foods not only helps you to reach your nutrient goals but also prevents you from feeling bored or deprived, as you could if your diet were more limited.

Choose Foods High in Nutrient Density. As a general guideline, you should choose foods high in **nutrient density.** This means eating foods that give you the highest amount of nutrients for the least amount of energy (or calories). As an example, three Oreo cookies provide the same number of calories as a medium banana and ½ cup of fresh blackberries. Yet as you might guess, the density of nutrients in the fruit is far superior, giving you more true nourishment per kcal (FIGURE 2.11).

A helpful analogy for selecting nutrient-dense foods is shopping: most of us look for the best quality we can find at the lowest price. Because you can only "afford" a certain number of calories each day to maintain a healthy weight, it makes sense to maximize the nutrients you can get for each calorie you consume. FIGURE 2.12 provides a comparison of one day of meals that are high in nutrient density to meals that are low in nutrient density. This example can assist you in selecting the most nutrient-dense foods when planning your meals.

Compare Your Diet to MyPyramid. Considering these principles, how can you proceed with planning your diet? Try logging on to the Web site for MyPyramid (**www.MyPyramid.gov**) and go to the MyPyramid Tracker. MyPyramid Tracker contains an online food intake assessment tool that scores the overall quality of your diet based on the 2005 Dietary Guidelines. You can analyze a diet for a single day or up to 1 year. You can also obtain a calculation of your nutrient intake from foods, a comparison of your diet with MyPyramid recommendations, and nutrient information from any dietary supplements you might consume.

(a)   (b)

FIGURE 2.11   Examples of foods that are low or high in nutrient density. **(a)** Three chocolate sandwich cookies. **(b)** The combination of one medium banana and ½ cup fresh blackberries. Each bowl of food provides approximately 140 kcal. The cookies provide 51.5 kcal from fat (5.72 g), 1 g of fiber, and very few vitamins and minerals. The fruit combination provides almost 7 g of fiber, 6.66 kcal from fat (0.74 g), and a significant amount of other nutrients such as potassium (539 mg), vitamin A (12 RAE), and vitamin C (25.4 mg). For our limited daily energy budget, the fruit is more nutrient dense and a more healthful choice. (Calculated using USDA National Nutrient Database for Standard Reference, Release 19, 2006, Nutrient Data Laboratory Home Page, http://www.ars.usda.gov/ba/bhnrc/ndl.)

NUTRI-CASE JUDY

" After she was diagnosed with type 2 diabetes, Judy used the MyPyramid Web site to analyze one day of her diet. Figure 2.13 shows the results of this analysis. As you can see, Judy's diet as compared to the 2005 Dietary Guidelines was too high in total fat, saturated fat, and sodium. Her intake did not match the recommended MyPyramid because she ate too few foods from the fruits, vegetables, meat and beans, and milk groups. What specific foods could Judy eat to improve the quality of her diet?

Limitations of MyPyramid

Although MyPyramid is a very useful tool that you can use when designing a healthful diet, it does have its limitations. These limitations are discussed in more detail in the Nutrition Debate at the end of this chapter. Briefly, as discussed in the previous section, the serving sizes as defined in MyPyramid are relatively small and do not always coincide with the standard amounts of food we buy, prepare, and serve. Some nutrition professionals believe these serving sizes are unrealistic, and it has been suggested that the serving sizes should be redefined to more closely match the amount of food people typically eat.

Another drawback of MyPyramid is that low-fat and low-calorie food choices are not clearly defined in each food category. For instance, 1 oz-equivalent servings of meat, poultry, fish, dry beans, eggs, and nuts are suggested in MyPyramid, but these

Meals with Foods High in Nutrient Density		Meals with Foods Low in Nutrient Density	

Breakfast
1 cup cooked oatmeal with
  1/2 cup skim milk
1 slice whole-wheat toast with
  1 tsp. butter
6 fl. oz grapefruit juice
			Breakfast
			1 cup puffed rice cereal with
			  1/2 cup whole milk
			1 slice white toast with
			  1 tsp. butter
			6 fl. oz grape drink

Snack 1 peeled orange 1 cup nonfat yogurt			**Snack** 1 12-oz can orange soft drink 1.5 oz cheddar cheese

Lunch
Turkey sandwich
  3 oz turkey breast
  2 slices whole-grain bread
  2 tsp. Dijon mustard
  3 slices fresh tomato
  2 leaves red leaf lettuce
1 cup baby carrots with
  broccoli crowns
20 fl. oz (2.5 cups) water
			Lunch
			Hamburger
			  3 oz regular ground beef
			  1 white hamburger bun
			  2 tsp. Dijon mustard
			  1 tbsp. tomato ketchup
			  2 leaves iceberg lettuce
			1 snack-sized bag potato chips
			20 fl. oz cola soft drink

Snack 1/2 whole-wheat bagel 1 tbsp. peanut butter 1 medium apple			**Snack** 3 chocolate sandwich cookies 1 12-oz can diet soft drink 10 Gummi Bears candy

Dinner
Spinach salad
  1 cup fresh spinach leaves
  1/4 cup diced tomatoes
  1/4 cup diced green pepper
  1/2 cup kidney beans
  1 tbsp. fat-free Italian
  salad dressing
3 oz broiled chicken breast
1/2 cup cooked brown rice
1/2 cup steamed broccoli
8 fl. oz (1 cup) skim milk
			Dinner
			Green salad
			  1 cup iceberg lettuce
			  1/4 cup diced tomatoes
			  1tsp. green onions
			  1/4 cup bacon bits
			  1 tbsp. regular Ranch
			  salad dressing
			3 oz beef round steak,
			  breaded and fried
			1/2 cup cooked white rice
			1/2 cup sweet corn
			8 fl. oz (1 cup) iced tea

FIGURE 2.12 A comparison of one day's meals that contain foods high in nutrient density to meals that contain foods low in nutrient density.

Here is the food displayed for Judy on 11/28/2006

Select your serving sizes and specify how many servings you consumed for each. When you are done, click on **Save & Analyze** to save your food entry information and to analyze your food intake. If you want to make more than one day's food entry, click on **Return to Login** to save a day's food entry information and make another day's food entry. For a record of today's food entry, click **Print Food Record** prior to saving food entry. To return to initial values, click **Reset Values**. To add or remove food items, click on **Enter Foods**.

Foods Consumed	Select Serving Size	Number of Servings (Enter a number (e.g. 1.5))
BAGEL, W/ RAISINS	1 large (3-1/2" to 3-3/4" dia) ▼	2
CREAM CHEESE	1 tablespoon ▼	2
WATER	1 fl oz ▼	16
APPLE (APPLES), FRESH	1 medium (2-3/4 dia) (approx 3 per lb) ▼	1
HAM, FRESH, LEAN ONLY	1 thin slice (approx 4-1/2 x 2-1/2 x 1/8) ▼	6
BREAD, MARBLE RYE & PUMPERNICKEL	1 regular slice ▼	2
MUSTARD	1 teaspoon ▼	2
MAYONNAISE, REGULAR	1 tablespoon ▼	1
RED LEAF LETTUCE	1 small leaf ▼	2
POTATO CHIPS, BAKED	10 chips ▼	3
LETTUCE SALAD, W/ CHEESE, TOMATO/CARROTS, NO DRESSING	1 cup ▼	2
SALAD DRESSING, LOW CALORIE	1 tablespoon ▼	2
HERSHEY BAR	1 Big Block bar (2.2 oz) ▼	1
COFFEE, MADE FROM GROUND, REGULAR, FLAVORED	1 fl oz ▼	20
CHEDDAR OR COLBY, LOWFAT CHEESE	1 slice (1 oz) ▼	1

| Save & Analyze | Enter Foods | Return to Login | Reset Values |

Print Food Record

(a) Judy's diet for one day

FIGURE 2.13 Analysis of 1 day of Judy's diet using MyPyramid Tracker. **(a)** This is a list of all the foods Judy ate and recorded for 1 day.

foods differ significantly in their fat content and in the type of fat they contain. Fish is well recognized for being low in fat and containing a healthier type of fat than that found in red meats. However, these two types of meat are treated equally in MyPyramid. Thus, the revised dietary guidelines and MyPyramid may not have gone far enough in encouraging people to consume more healthful foods.

In response to these limitations and others, researchers at the Harvard School of Public Health developed a Healthy Eating Pyramid (FIGURE 2.14). Following the

The 2005 Dietary Guidelines (DG) Recommendations
for Judy on 2/14/2007

Click directly on the 😊 😐 ☹️ emoticon (face) for more detailed dietary information.

Dietary Guidelines Recommendations	Emoticon	Number of cup/oz. Equ. Eaten	Number of cup/oz. Equ. Recommended
Grain	😊	7.5 oz equivalent	6 oz equivalent
Vegetable	😐	2 cup equivalent	2.5 cup equivalent
Fruit	☹️	0.1 cup equivalent	1.5 cup equivalent
Milk	☹️	1.2 cup equivalent	3 cup equivalent
Meat and Beans	😐	4.5 oz equivalent	5 oz equivalent

Dietary Guidelines Recommendations	Emoticon	Amount Eaten	Recommendation or Goal
Total Fat	☹️	41.1% of total calories	20% to 35%
Saturated Fat	☹️	14.4% of total calories	less than 10%
Cholesterol	😊	202 mg	less than 300 mg
Sodium	😐	2770 mg	less than 2300 mg
Oils	*	*	*
Discretionary calories (solid fats, added sugars, and alcohol)	*	*	*

* Calculations for oils and discretionary calories from foods are under revision.

More information about the Dietary Guidelines for Americans 2005
(To view this document you need Adobe Acrobat Reader)

(b) Judy's Tracker results

Comparison of Your Intake with
MyPyramid Recommendations for Judy

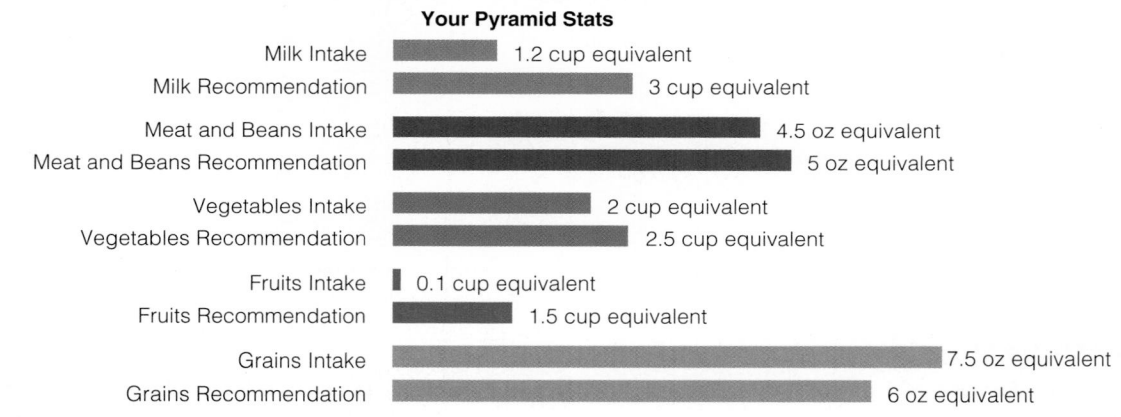

Your Pyramid Stats

- Milk Intake — 1.2 cup equivalent
- Milk Recommendation — 3 cup equivalent
- Meat and Beans Intake — 4.5 oz equivalent
- Meat and Beans Recommendation — 5 oz equivalent
- Vegetables Intake — 2 cup equivalent
- Vegetables Recommendation — 2.5 cup equivalent
- Fruits Intake — 0.1 cup equivalent
- Fruits Recommendation — 1.5 cup equivalent
- Grains Intake — 7.5 oz equivalent
- Grains Recommendation — 6 oz equivalent

Pyramid Categories	Percent Recommendation
Milk	40%
Meat and Beans	90%
Vegetables	80%
Fruits	7%
Grains	125%

Back   Nutrient Intakes   HEI Score   Calculate History

(c) Judy's comparison of nutrient intake to MyPyramid recommendations

FIGURE 2.13 *Continued.* **(b)** When Judy entered her diet into MyPyramid Tracker, her diet for this day was too low in fruit, grains, milk, and meat and beans and was too high in total and saturated fat. **(c)** As you can see, Judy's personal pyramid stats do not match the recommended MyPyramid guidelines as she ate too few foods from the fruits, grains, milk, and meat and beans groups. (*Source:* USDA, Center for Nutrition Policy and Promotion, www.MyPyramidtracker.gov.)

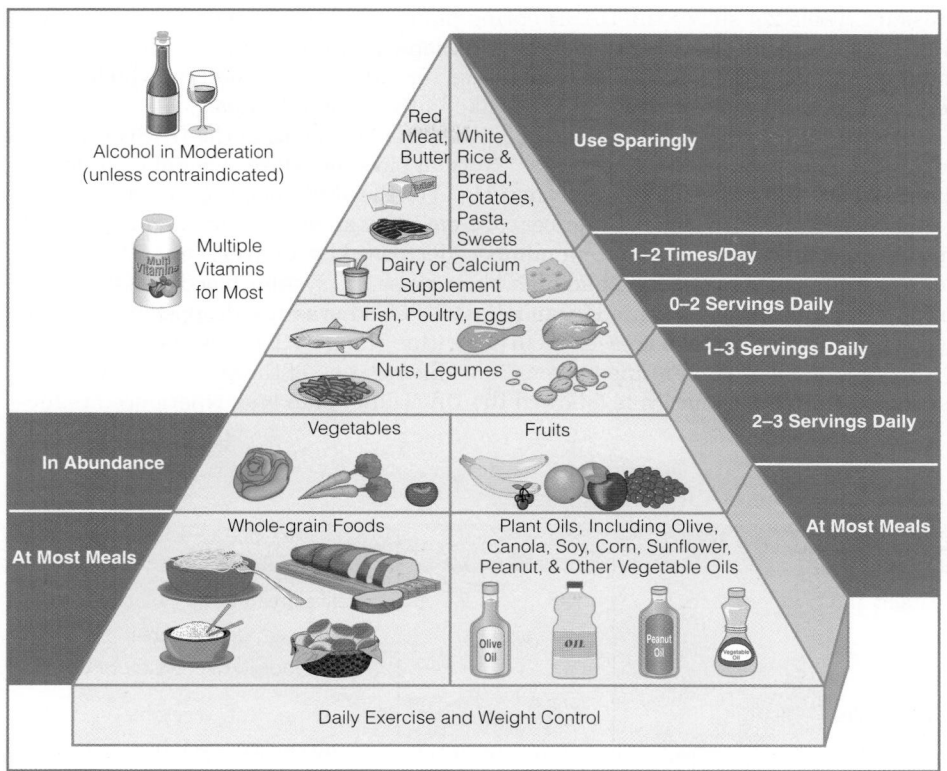

FIGURE 2.14 The Healthy Eating Pyramid. This pyramid was developed as a more healthful alternative to the previous USDA Food Guide Pyramid. (Reprinted with the permission of Simon & Schuster Adult Publishing Group from *Eat, Drink, and Be Healthy: The Harvard Medical School Guide to Healthy Eating* by Walter C. Willett, M.D. © 2001 by President and Fellows of Harvard College.)

design of the previous Food Guide Pyramid, the Healthy Eating Pyramid highlights healthful food choices and emphasizes daily exercise and weight control.

> RECAP: *There are many ethnic and cultural variations of the USDA Food Guide Pyramid. The flexibility inherent in both MyPyramid and the previous USDA Food Guide Pyramid allows anyone the ability to design a diet that meets the goals of adequacy, moderation, balance, variety, and nutrient density. Some of the limitations of MyPyramid include relatively small serving sizes and the failure to distinguish between higher fat and lower fat food choices within certain food groups.*

Eating Plans

As you already have learned, there is no single diet that is right for all individuals. By using MyPyramid, each of us can design a healthful diet that fits our personal preferences and lifestyle. That said, there are a few eating plans that can improve health for many people. The DASH diet and the exchange system are two such eating plans, and we review them here. Try one on for a while, and see if the design works for you!

The DASH Diet Plan

The **DASH diet** resulted from a large research study funded by the National Institutes of Health (NIH). DASH stands for "Dietary Approaches to Stop Hypertension"; thus, this study was designed to assess the effects of the DASH diet on high blood

DASH diet The diet developed in response to research into hypertension funded by the National Institutes of Health (NIH); stands for "Dietary Approaches to Stop Hypertension."

The DASH diet was created to reduce blood pressure.

pressure. Table 2.4 shows the DASH eating plan for a 2,000 kcal diet. This plan is similar to the goals of MyPyramid in that it is low in fat and high in fiber. The sodium content of the DASH diet is about 3 g (or 3,000 mg) of sodium, which is slightly less than the average sodium intake in the United States.

The results of this study convincingly illustrated that eating the DASH diet has a very positive impact on blood pressure.[14] Normal blood pressure is equal to, or lower than, 120/80 millimeters of mercury (mm Hg). For the study participants overall, systolic blood pressure (the top number) decreased by an average of 5.5 mm Hg, and diastolic blood pressure (the bottom number) decreased by an average of 3.0 mm Hg. For the study participants who had high blood pressure, systolic blood pressure dropped an average of 11.4 mm Hg, and diastolic blood pressure dropped by an average of 5.5 mm Hg. These decreases occurred within the first 2 weeks of eating the DASH diet and were maintained throughout the duration of the study. Researchers estimated that if all Americans followed the DASH diet plan and experienced reduc-

TABLE 2.4   The DASH Eating Plan

Food Group	Daily Servings	Serving Size
Grains and grain products	7–8	1 slice bread 1 cup ready-to-eat cereal* ½ cup cooked rice, pasta, or cereal
Vegetables	4–5	1 cup raw leafy vegetables ½ cup cooked vegetable 6 fl. oz vegetable juice
Fruits	4–5	1 medium fruit ¼ cup dried fruit ½ cup fresh, frozen, or canned fruit 6 fl. oz fruit juice
Low-fat or fat-free dairy foods	2–3	8 fl. oz milk 1 cup yogurt 1½ oz cheese
Lean meats, poultry, and fish	2 or less	3 oz cooked lean meats, skinless poultry, or fish
Nuts, seeds, and dry beans	4–5 per week	⅓ cup or 1½ oz nuts 1 tbsp. or ½ oz seeds ½ cup cooked dry beans
Fats and oils †	2–3	1 tsp. soft margarine 1 tbsp. low-fat mayonnaise 2 tbsp. light salad dressing 1 tsp. vegetable oil
Sweets	5 per week	1 tbsp. sugar 1 tbsp. jelly or jam ½ oz jelly beans 8 fl. oz lemonade

Note: The plan is based on 2,000 kcal/day. The number of servings in a food group may differ from the number listed, depending on your own energy needs.
*Serving sizes vary between ½ and 1¼ cups. Check the product's nutrition label.
† Fat content changes serving counts for fats and oils: For example, 1 tbsp. of regular salad dressing equals 1 serving; 1 tbsp. of a low-fat dressing equals ½ serving; 1 tablespoon of a fat-free dressing equals 0 servings.
Source: National Institutes of Health. Healthier Eating with DASH. www.nhlbi.nih.gov/health/public/heart/hbp/dash/new_dash.pdf.

tions in blood pressure similar to this study, then heart disease would be reduced by 15% and the number of strokes would be 27% lower.

Further study of the DASH diet has found that blood pressure decreases even more if sodium intake is reduced below 3,000 mg per day. A second study was conducted in which participants ate a DASH diet that provided either 3,300 mg (average U.S. intake), 2,400 mg (upper recommended intake), or 1,500 mg of sodium each day.[15] After 1 month on this diet, all people eating the DASH diet saw a significant decrease in their blood pressure; however, those who ate the lowest sodium version of the DASH diet experienced the largest decrease. These results indicate that eating a diet low in sodium and high in fruits and vegetables reduces blood pressure and decreases your risk for heart disease and stroke.

The Exchange System

The **Exchange System** is another tool that can be used to plan a healthful diet. The American Dietetic Association and the American Diabetes Association originally designed the Exchange System for people with diabetes. It has also been used successfully in weight-loss programs. Exchanges, or portions, are organized according to the amount of carbohydrate, protein, fat, and calories in each food. There are six food groups, or exchange lists, and these lists contain foods that are similar in calories, carbohydrate, fat, and protein content (Table 2.5). The six exchange lists are starch/bread, meat and meat substitutes, vegetables, fruits, milk, and fat. In addition to these lists, there are also other categories (not shown in Table 2.5) that can assist you in meal planning, including free foods (any food or drink with less than 20 calories per serving), combination foods (foods such as soups, casseroles, and pizza), and special-occasion foods (desserts such as cakes, cookies, and ice cream).

To use the Exchange System effectively, you must learn the portion sizes for each of the exchange lists. In addition, you must learn which foods fit into each exchange list. For instance, starchy vegetables such as corn, potatoes, peas, beans, and lentils are placed into the starch/bread exchange list, not the vegetable exchange list. The meat and meat substitute group classifies meat in three subcategories: lean, medium-fat, and high-fat meats. Whereas 1 oz of lean meat such as turkey breast without skin is 1 exchange of lean meat, a high-fat meat choice such as 1 Ball Park frank is 1 high-fat meat exchange and 1 fat exchange.

There are many advantages of using the Exchange System to plan a healthful diet. Because a portion of any food on a given exchange list has the same number of calories and macronutrients, you can easily exchange foods within each list to design a varied diet plan. In addition, the portion sizes defined in the Exchange System and the distinction between meats with different fat contents help you to better control energy and fat intakes. Once you have learned how to use the Exchange System, you can effectively design a healthful diet based on your energy needs. Refer to FIGURE 2.15 for an example of how a 2,600 calorie meal plan might look using the Exchange System.

Other Diet Plans

The DASH diet and the Exchange System are two programs that are linked to research studies showing healthful benefits, and both are endorsed by federal agencies. There are many other diet plans available to consumers, and many of these may or may not have been researched to determine their health benefits. Some of these plans, such as Weight Watchers, the Zone Diet, and the Ornish Program, have been marketed specifically for weight loss; many weight-loss plans can be adapted to achieve healthy weight maintenance. It is inappropriate to endorse one specific diet plan for all people, as our nutritional needs and preferences are diverse and cannot be met by a single plan. Each person must make his or her own decisions about healthful diet choices based on personal preferences, ethnic considerations, activity level, cost, and convenience.

When designing a healthful diet for yourself, you need to look closely at any diet plan to determine whether it meets the healthful guidelines reviewed in this book. You can use the Dietary Guidelines for Americans as a standard for comparison, and you can also check to see whether or not the diet emphasizes the principles of adequacy, moderation, balance, variety, and nutrient density. For a more detailed review of various diet plans and fad diets, see Chapter 11.

Exchange System A diet planning tool developed by the American Dietetic Association and the American Diabetes Association in which exchanges, or portions, are organized according to the amount of carbohydrate, protein, fat, and calories in each food.

TABLE 2.5 Exchange Groups and Their Energy and Macronutrient Content

Exchange List	Calories	Carbohydrate (g)	Fat (g)	Protein (g)	Serving Sizes
Starch/ Bread	80	15	Trace (0.5 to 1)	3	1 oz bread ¾ cup dry, unsweetened cereal ½ cup cooked cereal 4–5 snack crackers ½ cup pasta or starchy vegetable ⅓ cup rice, grains, stuffings 1 cup soup ⅓ cup cooked beans, peas, lentils 3 cups popcorn without added fat
Meat and Meat Substitutes					
Lean Meat	55	0	3	7	1 oz fish, poultry, lean beef (round sirloin, flank steak), processed hams, veal, cottage cheese, low-fat cheeses, lean luncheon meats
Medium-Fat Meat	75	0	5	7	1 oz of most beef and pork cuts, poultry with skin, skim-milk cheeses, 1 egg
High-Fat Meat	100	0	8	7	1 oz fried meats, poultry, or fish; 1 oz prime cuts of beef, corned beef, spareribs, regular cheeses, regular luncheon meats, sausages, hot dogs, and peanut butter
Vegetables	25	5	0	2	½ cup cooked vegetables ½ cup vegetable juice 1 cup raw vegetables
Fruits	60	15	0	0	1 small to medium fresh fruit ½ cup canned fruit ¼ cup dried fruit ⅓–½ cup fruit juice
Milk					
Nonfat and Very-Low-Fat Milk	90	12	0–3	8	1 cup skim, ½%, or 1% milk 1 cup nonfat or low-fat buttermilk ¾ cup (6 oz) plain nonfat yogurt 1 cup (8 oz) nonfat or low-fat artificially sweetened fruit flavored yogurt
Low-Fat Milk	120	12	5	8	1 cup 2% milk ¾ cup plain low-fat yogurt
Whole Milk	150	12	8	8	1 cup whole milk ½ cup evaporated whole milk
Fat	45	0	5	0	1 tsp. margarine or butter 1 tbsp. reduced-calorie margarine 1 tsp. mayonnaise or oil 1 tbsp. regular salad dressing 2 tbsp. low-calorie salad dressing 2 tbsp. sour cream

Meal	Starch/Bread	Lean Meat	Vegetable	Fruit	Nonfat Milk	Fat
Breakfast	2 slices whole-wheat toast 1/2 cup cooked oatmeal			1 cup orange juice	1 cup skim milk	2 tsp. margarine (spread on toast)
Snack	3 cups popcorn with no added fat 5 whole-wheat crackers			1 small banana		4 tsp. peanut butter (spread on crackers)
Lunch	2 slices rye bread 1/3 cup baked beans	3 oz lean sliced turkey ham	1 cup baby carrots 1 cup raw cauliflower 1/2 cup V8 juice	1 medium apple	1 cup nonfat strawberry yogurt sweetened with aspartame	2 tsp. mayonnaise (spread on rye bread) 1 tbsp. ranch dressing (for dipping vegetables)
Snack	16 animal crackers			1 small nectarine		
Dinner	1 large baked potato	4 oz broiled skinless chicken breast	2 cups butter lettuce with 1/4 cup each green onion, sweet red pepper, fresh tomatoes, and carrots		1 cup skim milk	2 tsp. butter (for potato) 2 tbsp. reduced fat Italian salad dressing (for salad)
Total Exchanges/day	13	7	6	5	3	10

FIGURE 2.15 Example of a 1-day meal plan for a 2,600-kcal diet using the Exchange System.

RECAP: *The DASH diet and the Exchange System are two examples of healthful food plans. The DASH diet includes 8 to 10 servings of fruits and vegetables and no more than 3,000 mg of sodium each day. It has been shown to significantly decrease blood pressure. The Exchange System was originally designed for people with diabetes. Exchanges, or portions, are organized according to the amount of carbohydrate, protein, fat, and calories in each food. One advantage of the Exchange System is that lean, medium-fat, and high-fat foods in the meat and dairy groups are clearly defined, which assists in controlling fat and energy intake.*

Can Eating Out Be Part of a Healthful Diet?

How many times each week do you eat out? A report from the Pew Research Center states that about one-third of Americans eat out once per week, while another one-third eat out two or more times per week.[16] Almost half (47%) of men and 35% of women surveyed report eating a meal at a fast-food restaurant at least once per week. Restaurant sales for 2003 exceeded $426 billion. Over the past 20 years, there has been phenomenal growth in the restaurant industry, particularly in the fast-food market. During this same time period, rates of obesity have increased by more than 60%, and now an estimated 66% of U.S. adults are either overweight or obese.[1]

The Hidden Costs of Eating Out

Table 2.6 shows an example of foods served at McDonald's and Burger King restaurants. As you can see, a regular McDonald's hamburger has only 270 kcal, whereas the Big Xtra with Cheese has 810 kcal. A meal of the Quarter Pounder with Cheese, large French fries, and a large Coke provides 1,340 kcal. This meal has almost enough energy to support an entire day's needs for a small, lightly active woman! Similar meals at Burger King and other fast-food chains are also very high in calories, not to mention total fat and sodium.

Fast-food restaurants are not alone in serving large portions. Most sit-down restaurants also serve large meals that may include bread with butter, a salad with dressing, sides of vegetables and potatoes, and free refills of sugar-filled drinks. Combined with a high-fat appetizer like potato skins, fried onions, fried mozzarella sticks, or buffalo wings, it is easy to eat more than 2,000 kcal at one meal!

Does this mean that eating out cannot be a part of a healthful diet? Not necessarily. By becoming an educated consumer and making wise meal choices while dining out, you can enjoy both a healthful diet and the social benefits of eating out.

The Healthful Way to Eat Out

Most restaurants, even fast-food restaurants, offer lower fat menu items that you can choose. For instance, eating a regular McDonald's hamburger, a small order of

Foods served at fast-food chains are often high in calories, total fat, and sodium. McDonald's popular sausage, egg, and cheese McGriddles breakfast sandwiches, for example, contain 550 kcal, 33 g of fat, and 1,290 mg of sodium.

TABLE 2.6 Nutritional Value of Selected Fast Foods

Menu Item	kcal	Fat (g)	Fat (% kcal)	Sodium (mg)
McDonald's				
Hamburger	270	9	29.6	600
Cheeseburger	320	13	37.5	830
Quarter Pounder	430	21	44.2	840
Quarter Pounder with cheese	530	30	50.9	1,310
Big Mac	570	32	49.1	1,100
Big Xtra	710	46	59.2	1,400
Big Xtra with cheese	810	55	60.5	1,870
French fries, small	210	10	42.8	135
French fries, medium	450	22	44.4	290
French fries, large	540	26	42.6	350
Burger King				
Hamburger	320	15	43.8	520
Cheeseburger	360	19	47.2	760
Whopper	660	40	54.5	900
Whopper with cheese	760	48	56.6	1,380
Double Whopper	920	59	57.6	980
Bacon Cheeseburger	400	22	50.0	940
Bacon Double Cheeseburger	620	38	54.8	1,230
French fries, small	250	13	48.0	550
French fries, medium	400	21	47.5	820
French fries, King Size	590	30	45.8	1,180

French fries, and a diet beverage or water provides 480 kcal and 19 g of fat (or 35% of kcal from fat). To provide some vegetables for the day, you could add a side salad with low-fat or nonfat salad dressing. Other fast-food restaurants also offer smaller portions, sandwiches made with whole-grain bread, grilled chicken or other lean meats, and side salads. Many sit-down restaurants offer "lite" menu items such as grilled chicken and a variety of vegetables, which are usually a much better choice than eating from the regular menu.

Here are some other suggestions on how to eat out in moderation. Practice some of these suggestions every time you eat out:

- Avoid coffee drinks made with syrups, as well as those made with cream, whipping cream, or whole milk; select reduced-fat or skim milk in your favorite coffee drink.

- Avoid eating appetizers that are breaded, fried, or filled with cheese or meat; you may want to skip the appetizer completely. Alternatively, you may want to order a healthful appetizer as an entrée instead of a larger meal.

- Share an entrée with a friend! Many restaurants serve entrées large enough for two people.

- Order broth-based soups instead of cream-based soups.

- Order any meat dish grilled or broiled, and avoid fried or breaded meat dishes.

- If you order a meat dish, select lean cuts of meat, such as chicken or turkey breast, extra-lean ground beef, pork loin chop, or filet mignon.

- Order a meatless dish filled with vegetables and whole grains. Avoid dishes with cream sauces and a lot of cheese.

- Order a salad with low-fat or nonfat dressing served on the side. Many restaurants smother their salads in dressing, and you will eat less by controlling how much you put on the salad.

- Order steamed vegetables on the side instead of potatoes or rice. If you order potatoes, make sure you get a baked potato (with very little butter or sour cream on the side).

- Order beverages with few or no calories, such as water, tea, or diet drinks.

- Eat no more than half of what you are served, and take the rest home for another meal.

- Skip dessert or share one dessert with a lot of friends! Another healthful alternative is to order fresh fruit for dessert.

Table 2.7 lists examples of low-fat foods you can choose when you eat out.[17] Although provided as examples for people with diabetes, they are useful for anyone

Eating out can be a part of a healthful diet, if you are careful to choose wisely.

When ordering your favorite coffee drink, avoid those made with flavored syrups, cream, or whipping cream and request reduced-fat or skim milk instead.

TABLE 2.7 Low-Fat Food Choices Available in Restaurants

Appetizers	Salads	Breads	Entrée	Fats	Desserts
Minestrone soup	Tossed with mixed greens, lettuce, tomato, cucumber	Whole-grain rolls	Baked halibut with thyme and fresh-squeezed lemon	Diet margarine	Fresh fruit
Chicken soup with vegetables		Corn tortillas		Low-fat/low-calorie salad dressing	Fruit sorbet
Raw celery and carrots with low-fat or nonfat ranch dressing	Spinach salad with crab meat, raw vegetables, and nonfat salad dressing	Whole-wheat or pumpernickel bread	Grilled skinless chicken breast with tomato salsa	Low-fat sour cream or yogurt	Fat-free or low-fat yogurt

Adapted from: American Diabetes Association. 2007. Your Guide to Eating Out. www.diabetes.org/nutrition-and-recipes/nutrition/eatingoutguide.jsp. Printed with permission.

who is interested in making more healthful food choices while eating out. By choosing healthful foods and appropriate portion sizes, you can eat out regularly and still maintain a healthful body weight.

[RECAP: *Healthful ways to eat out include choosing menu items that are smaller in size, ordering meats that are grilled or broiled, avoiding fried foods, choosing items with steamed vegetables, avoiding energy-rich appetizers and desserts, and eating less than half of the food you are served.*

CHAPTER SUMMARY

- A healthful diet provides adequate energy, nutrients, and fiber to maintain health.

- A healthful diet is moderate in the amounts of foods eaten. Foods that contain a lot of fat and sugar should be eaten only in moderation to maintain a healthy weight.

- A healthful diet contains the proper balance of food groups and nutrients to maintain health.

- A healthful diet provides a variety of foods every day.

- The FDA regulates the content of food labels; food labels must contain a statement of identity, the net contents of the package, the contact information of the food manufacturer or distributor, an ingredient list, and nutrition information.

- The Nutrition Facts Panel on a food label contains important nutrition information about serving size, servings per package, total calories and calories of fat per serving, a list of various macronutrients, vitamins, and minerals, and the % Daily Values for the nutrients listed on the panel.

- The Dietary Guidelines for Americans are general directives about healthful eating and physical activity. They include aiming for a healthy weight, being physically active each day, using MyPyramid or the DASH diet plan to select foods, eating whole-grain foods, fruits, and vegetables each day, keeping food safe to eat, choosing foods lower in saturated fat, *trans* fat, and cholesterol and moderate in total fat, moderating your intake of sugar, eating less salt, eating more potassium-rich foods, and drinking alcoholic beverages in moderation, if at all.

- MyPyramid is an interactive Web-based tool developed by the USDA that can be used to design a healthful diet. The groups in the pyramid include grains, fruits, vegetables, oils, milk, and meat and beans.

- Specific serving sizes are defined for foods in each group of MyPyramid. There is no standard definition for a serving size, and the serving sizes defined in the pyramid are generally smaller than those listed on food labels and than the servings generally sold to consumers.

- There are many ethnic and cultural variations of the previous USDA Food Guide Pyramid, including the Vegetarian, Mediterranean, African American, Latin American, and Asian Diet Pyramids.

- MyPyramid can be used to design a diet that meets the healthful goals of adequacy, moderation, balance, variety, and nutrient density.

- The limitations of MyPyramid include relatively small serving sizes that can be confusing to consumers, failure to clearly distinguish between high-fat and low-fat food choices within the food groups, and challenges to meeting all nutrient needs even if the recommended number of servings from each food group are consumed.

- The DASH diet (Dietary Approaches to Stop Hypertension) is high in fiber and low in fat and includes 8 to 10 servings of fruits and vegetables each day.

- Eating the DASH diet can significantly decrease blood pressure, with particular benefit to people with high blood pressure.

- The exchange system is another tool you can use to design a healthful diet. The American Diabetes Association and the American Dietetic Association originally designed this system as a plan for individuals with diabetes.

- The Exchange System includes the use of exchanges, or portions, that are organized based on amounts of carbohydrate, protein, fat, and calories.

- The six food groups, or exchange lists, are starch/bread, meat and meat substitutes, vegetables, fruits, milk, and fat.

- Two advantages of using the Exchange System are the ease of exchanging foods with each list, which allows for a great deal of variety, and the clear definition of portion sizes and lean, medium-fat, and high-fat food choices, which helps control energy and fat intake.

- Eating out is challenging because of the high fat content and large serving sizes of many fast-food and sit-down restaurant menu items.

- Behaviors that can improve the quality of your diet when eating out include choosing lower fat meats that are grilled or broiled, eating vegetables and salads as side or main dishes, asking for low-fat salad dressing on the side, skipping high-fat desserts and appetizers, and drinking low- or noncaloric beverages.

TEST YOURSELF ANSWERS

1. **False.** A healthful diet can be achieved by food alone; particular attention must be paid to adequacy, variety, moderation, and balance. However, some individuals may need to take vitamin supplements under certain circumstances.

2. **False.** The Dietary Guidelines for Americans recommend that people who choose to drink should do so sensibly and in moderation. Moderation is defined as no more than one drink per day for women and no more than two drinks per day for men.

3. **False.** Although MyPyramid does have its limitations, it can be used by most Americans to design a healthful diet. This tool is flexible and allows for modifications as needed; there are also many ethnic variations available.

4. **True.** The DASH diet plan recommends that people eat 4 to 5 fruits and 4 to 5 vegetables each day, for a total of 8 to 10 fruits and vegetables each day.

5. **False.** Eating out poses many challenges to healthful eating, but it is possible to eat a healthful diet when dining out. Ordering and/or consuming smaller portion sizes, selecting foods that are lower in fat and added sugars, and selecting eating establishments that serve more healthful foods can assist you in eating healthfully while dining out.

REVIEW QUESTIONS

1. The Nutrition Facts Panel identifies which of the following?
   a. All of the nutrients and calories in the package of food.
   b. The Recommended Dietary Allowance for each nutrient found in the package of food.
   c. A footnote identifying the Tolerable Upper Intake Level for each nutrient found in the package of food.
   d. The % Daily Values of select nutrients in a serving of the packaged food.

2. An adequate diet
   a. provides enough energy to meet minimum daily requirements.
   b. provides enough of the energy, nutrients, and fiber to maintain a person's health.
   c. provides a sufficient variety of nutrients to maintain a healthy weight.
   d. contains combinations of foods that provide healthful proportions of nutrients.

3. MyPyramid recommends eating
   a. at least half your grains as whole grains each day.
   b. 6 to 11 servings of milk, cheese, and yogurt each day.
   c. 200 kcal to 500 kcal of discretionary calories each day.
   d. 2 to 3 servings of fruit juice each day.

4. The Dietary Guidelines for Americans recommend which of the following?
   a. Choosing and preparing foods without salt.
   b. Consuming two alcoholic beverages per day.
   c. Being physically active each day.
   d. Following the Mediterranean diet.

5. What does it mean to choose foods for their nutrient density?
   a. Dense foods such as peanut butter or chicken are more nutritious choices than transparent foods such as mineral water or gelatin.
   b. Foods with a lot of nutrients per calorie such as fish are more nutritious choices than foods with fewer nutrients per calorie such as candy.
   c. Calorie-dense foods such as cheesecake should be avoided.
   d. Fat makes foods dense, and thus foods high in fat should be avoided.

6. True or false? The USDA has written a standardized definition for a serving size for most foods.

7. True or false? A drawback of MyPyramid is that low-fat and low-calorie food choices are not clearly defined in each food category.

8. True or false? The six exchange lists are grains, meat and meat substitutes, fruits and vegetables, dairy products, sweets, and fats.

9. True or false? The Healthy Eating Pyramid suggests that pasta be eaten sparingly.

10. True or false? The DASH diet plan was instituted by the American Diabetes Association.

11. Defend the statement that no single diet can be appropriate for every human being.

12. Explain why MyPyramid identifies a range in the number of suggested daily servings of each food group

instead of telling us exactly how many servings of each food to eat each day.

13. Compare and contrast MyPyramid and the DASH eating plan.

14. Identify at least six differences between MyPyramid and the Healthy Eating Pyramid.

15. Log onto **www.MyPyramid.gov** and find out how many kcal/day you should consume. Now look at Table

2.6. If you were to eat a Burger King Whopper, a small bag of French fries, and a 16-oz soda containing 190 kcal, what percentage of your daily kcal intake would this meal provide? Which of the MyPyramid food groups are entirely missing from this meal? Now look at the Healthy Eating Pyramid (Figure 2.15). Within what part of this pyramid does the entire meal belong?

FIND THE QUACK

Jimena is a 19-year-old sophomore in a small liberal arts college. Everyone in Jimena's family is either overweight or obese, but now that she is away from home and living at an out-of-state school, Jimena has become determined to break out of her "family pattern" and lose weight. In a fashion magazine, she reads about a grapefruit diet called the Mayo Clinic Diet. Jimena figures that any diet with a medical clinic behind it must be reputable, so she decides to try it. The diet requires that Jimena eat two eggs and two slices of bacon every morning with an 8-oz glass of grapefruit juice or half a grapefruit; eat a salad, red meat or poultry, and another serving of grapefruit at lunch; and eat a salad, red meat or poultry, and another serving of grapefruit at dinner. No snacks between meals are allowed. The diet is to be followed for 8 weeks: 12 days on the diet followed by 2 days off, then resumption of the diet again.

The magazine article claims:

• The consumption of grapefruit or grapefruit juice is absolutely essential because the grapefruit "is a catalyst that starts the fat-burning process."

• The consumption of the bacon and eggs at breakfast and salad at lunch and dinner is also absolutely essential because these foods combine to promote fat burning.

• Anyone following the diet will lose 52 lb in 8 weeks. No weight loss will occur during the first 4 days, but

the average weight loss for the remainder of the 8-week period will be 1 lb a day.

• The diet is safe and healthful if followed as described for 8 weeks.

1. Although you have not yet studied digestion and absorption of food, do you believe the article's claim that there is something unique about grapefruit that catalyzes (initiates and speeds up) fat burning? Why or why not?

2. If loss of 1 lb of body weight requires the body to expend 3,500 kcal more than it takes in, do you think it is possible for anyone trying the grapefruit diet to lose 52 lb in 56 days, without any prescribed physical activity, and consuming daily: two eggs, two strips of bacon, three servings of grapefruit, two salads, and two servings of meat or poultry? Why or why not?

3. What two food groups are entirely missing from this diet? Do you think this might be problematic for some dieters? Why or why not?

4. Do you believe that this grapefruit diet, which the article refers to as the Mayo Clinic Diet, is truly endorsed by the Mayo Clinic, the medical institution based in Rochester, Minnesota and known internationally for its quality healthcare? Go online and, using your favorite search engine, type in the search terms "grapefruit diet" and "Mayo Clinic." What do you discover?

Answers can be found at www.aw-bc.com/thompson.

WEB LINKS

www.fda.gov
U.S. Food and Drug Administration (FDA)

Learn more about the government agency that regulates our food and first established regulations for nutrition information on food labels.

www.health.gov/dietaryguidelines
Dietary Guidelines for Americans

Use these guidelines to make changes in your food choices and physical activity habits to help reduce your risk for chronic disease.

www.MyPyramid.gov
USDA MyPyramid Steps to a Healthier You

Use the MyPyramid Tracker on this Web site to assess the overall quality of your diet based on the USDA MyPyramid.

www.hc-sc.gc.ca
Health Canada

Learn more about Canadian's Food Guide to Healthy Eating and other Canadian health policies.

www.oldwayspt.org
Oldways Preservation and Exchange Trust

Find different variations of ethnic and cultural food pyramids.

www.5aday.gov
National Cancer Institute's 5-a-Day for Better Health Program

Learn more about the 5-a-Day Program, a major public health initiative for nutrition and cancer prevention.

www.nih.gov
The National Institutes of Health (NIH, part of the U.S. Department of Health and Human Services)

Search this site to learn more about the DASH (Dietary Approaches to Stop Hypertension) diet.

http://hin.nhlbi.nih.gov/portion
The National Institutes of Health (NIH) Portion Distortion Quiz

Take this short quiz to see if you know how today's food portions compare to those of 20 years ago.

www.diabetes.org/home.jsp
The American Diabetes Association

Find out more about the nutritional needs of people living with diabetes as well as meal planning exchange lists.

www.eatright.org
The American Dietetic Association

Visit the food and nutrition information section of this Web site for additional resources to help you achieve a healthy lifestyle.

www.hsph.harvard.edu
The Harvard School of Public Health

Search this site to learn more about the Healthy Eating Pyramid, an alternative to the USDA Food Guide Pyramid.

REFERENCES

1. Centers for Disease Control and Prevention. 2006. Prevalence of overweight and obesity among adults: United States, 2003–2004. http://www.cdc.gov/nchs/products/pubs/pubd/hestats/overweight/overwght_adult_03.htm.
2. Centers for Disease Control and Prevention. 2006. Prevalence of overweight among children and adolescents: United States, 2003–2004. http://www.cdc.gov/nchs/products/pubs/pubd/hestats/overweight/overwght_child_03.htm.
3. U.S. Department of Health and Human Services (USDHHS) and U.S. Department of Agriculture (USDA). 2005. Dietary Guidelines for Americans, 2005, 6th edn. Washington, DC: U.S. Government Printing Office. www.healthierus.gov/dietaryguidelines. (Accessed March 2007.)
4. Nielsen, S. J., and B. M. Popkin. 2003. Patterns and trends in food portion sizes, 1977–1998. *JAMA* 289(4):450–453.
5. Young, L. R., and M. Nestle. 1998. Variation in perceptions of a "medium" food portion: implications for dietary guidance. *J. Am. Diet. Assoc.* 98:458–459.
6. Young, L. R., and M. Nestle. 2002. The contribution of expanding portion sizes to the US obesity epidemic. *Am. J. Pub. Health* 92(2):246–249.
7. Houtkooper, L. 1994. *Winning Sports Nutrition Training Manual.* Tucson, AZ: University of Arizona Cooperative Extension.
8. U.S. Department of Agriculture (USDA). 2006. MyPyramid for Kids. http://mypyramid.gov/kids/index.html. (Accessed March 2007.)
9. Tufts University. 2002. Tufts Food Guide Pyramid for Older Adults. http://nutrition.tufts.edu/pdf/pyramid.pdf. (Accessed March 2007.)
10. Food and Nutrition Information Center. 2006. Dietary Guidance. Ethnic/Cultural Food Pyramid. http://fnic.nal.usda.gov/nal_display/index.php?info_center=4&tax_level=3&tax_subject=256&topic_id=1348&level3_id=5732. (Accessed March 2007.)
11. Renaud, S., M. de Lorgeril, J. Delaye, J. Guidollet, F. Jacquard, N. Mamelle, J.-L. Martin, I. Monjaud, P. Salen, and P. Toubol. 1995. Cretan Mediterranean diet for prevention of coronary heart disease. *Am. J. Clin. Nutr.* 61(suppl.):1360S–1367S.
12. Tavani, A., and C. La Vecchia. 1995. Fruit and vegetable consumption and cancer risk in a Mediterranean population. *Am. J. Clin. Nutr.* 61(suppl.):1374S–1377S.
13. Panagiotakos, D. B., C. Chrysohoou, C. Pitsavos, and C. Stefanadis. 2006. Association between the prevalence of obesity and adherence to the Mediterranean diet: the ATTICA study. *Nutrition* 22(5):449–456.
14. Appel, L. J., T. J. Moore, E. Obarzanek, W. M. Vollmer, L. P. Svetkey, F. M. Sacks, G. A. Bray, T. M. Vogt, J. A. Cutler, M. M. Windhauser, P.-H. Lin, and N. Karanja. 1997. A clinical trial of the effects of dietary patterns on blood pressure. *N. Engl. J. Med.* 336:1117–1124.
15. Sacks, F. M., L. P. Svetkey, W. M. Vollmer, L. J. Appel, G. A. Bray, D. Harsha, E. Obarzanek, P. R. Conlin, E. R. Miller III, D. G. Simons-Morton, N. Karanja, and P.-H. Lin. 2001. Effects on blood pressure of reduced dietary sodium and the Dietary Approaches to Stop Hypertension (DASH) diet. *N. Engl. J. Med.* 344:3–10.
16. Taylor, P., C. Funk, and P. Craighill. 2006. Eating More; Enjoying Less. Pew Research Center. A Social Trends Report. http://pewresearch.org/assets/social/pdf/Eating.pdf. (Accessed March 2007.)
17. American Diabetes Association. 2006. Your Guide to Eating Out. www.diabetes.org/nutrition-and-recipes/nutrition/eatingoutguide.jsp. (Accessed March 2007.)
18. McCullough, M. L., D. Feskanich, M. J. Stampfer, E. L. Giovannucci, E. B. Rimm, F. B. Hu, D. Spiegelman, D. J. Hunter, G. A. Colditz, and W. C. Willett. 2002. Diet quality and major chronic disease risk in men and women: moving toward improved dietary guidance. *Am. J. Clin. Nutr.* 76(6):1261–1271.

NUTRITION DEBATE

Will Revising the USDA Food Guide Pyramid Help Us Find the Perfect Diet?

as you learned in this chapter, the previous USDA Food Guide Pyramid (FGP) was revised in 2005. MyPyramid was developed to address many of the limitations of the previous FGP. For instance, one major criticism was that the FGP was overly simple and did not help consumers make appropriate choices within each food group. MyPyramid has addressed this concern by instructing consumers to choose foods that are lower in fat and added sugar and higher in fiber, and by providing many specific examples of healthful foods in each food group. Another criticism was that the USDA Food Guide Pyramid did not mention the need for regular physical activity. On the left side, MyPyramid includes a graphic of a person climbing stairs to emphasize the importance of daily physical activity.

Despite these improvements upon the FGP, MyPyramid's reception has been lukewarm. Indeed, many of the same criticisms once leveled at the FGP persist, as does a fundamental doubt that such a tool can really help Americans design and maintain a healthful diet. Let's explore some of the specific concerns nutrition and public health experts have raised since the release of MyPyramid.

One major criticism is that the serving sizes suggested in MyPyramid are unrealistic or do not coincide with typical serving sizes of foods listed on food labels. For instance, one serving of a muffin as defined in MyPyramid is 1 oz-equivalent, but most muffins available to consumers range from 2 oz to 8 oz! The way that foods are packaged is also confusing to consumers. Unless people read food labels carefully, it is easy to consume an entire package of a food that contains multiple servings and assume that the entire package is equal to one serving. For example, it is common to find soft drinks sold in 20 fl. oz bottles. Although the serving size listed on the label is

Although the serving size of a muffin in MyPyramid is 1 oz-equivalent, many muffins sold today range in size from 2 oz to 8 oz.

8 fl. oz, and total servings per bottle is listed as 2.5, most people just drink the entire bottle in one sitting and assume they had one soft drink.

A second criticism of MyPyramid is that it has not gone far enough to encourage people to consume more healthful foods. For instance, low-fat and low-calorie food choices are not clearly defined in each food category. The 1 oz-equivalent servings of meat, poultry, fish, dry beans, eggs, and nuts suggested in MyPyramid are not differentiated by their fat content or by the type of fat they contain. Fish is low in fat and contains a more healthful type of fat than that found in red meats. In addition, although nuts are relatively high in fat, the type of fat in nuts is more healthful than that found in meats. MyPyramid fails to point out these differences, treating all foods in the meat, poultry, fish, dry beans, eggs, and nuts group as equivalent choices. In addition, MyPyramid recommends that at least half the grains eaten each day should be from whole-grain sources, allowing for eating half of your grain sources from refined foods. In reality, it is more healthful to eat virtually all your grains from whole-grain foods.

A third criticism is that a person must have access to the Internet and the ability to maneuver through Web-based programming in order to effectively use MyPyramid. Although it may be hard for many people to imagine, there are still a considerable number of Americans who do not have access to the Internet, and many of those who do are not comfortable using interactive programming. MyPyramid is quite limited in its usefulness as a stand-alone graphic. Without the capacity to access and manipulate the interactive components on the Internet at www.MyPyramid.gov, individuals cannot personalize MyPyramid.

A fourth criticism is that MyPyramid does not graphically illustrate the principles it claims to represent. For example, by simply looking at the MyPyramid graphic, a consumer cannot know that the varying widths of bands represent how much of that food group to consume. In addition, varying the widths of each band from wider at the bottom to narrower at the top of MyPyramid is not a clear way to illustrate that we should eat more of certain foods and less of others in each of the food categories. Also, it is questionable whether consumers will notice the yellow band and link it with the oil drop below the graphic in the text. A number of nutrition experts feel

Problems with accessing or navigating the Internet can prevent people from using MyPyramid.

that the MyPyramid graphic on its own is not particularly useful, as it is difficult to understand how to use MyPyramid unless the graphic is linked with the text and supplemented with information provided on the Web site.

Because of these limitations and criticisms, there is considerable doubt among many nutrition experts that MyPyramid can halt the current obesity epidemic or significantly contribute to improving the health of Americans. Although MyPyramid is grounded in science, new research emphasizes the importance of eating specific nutrients and whole foods that promote health and prevent disease—concepts that MyPyramid does not adequately address. The Healthy Eating Pyramid (on page 67) has been identified as one example of a better tool for designing a healthful diet. In fact, a recent study shows that people eating a diet based on the Healthy Eating Pyramid reduced their risk for heart disease two times more than people eating a diet based on the previous FGP.[18] Because of the recent release of MyPyramid, no studies are yet available comparing the effectiveness of the Healthy Eating Pyramid to MyPyramid in reducing chronic disease risk.

As you can imagine, a great deal of time, effort, and money was invested in the new message, content, and design of MyPyramid. In making this investment, nutrition experts at the USDA intended that MyPyramid would help reduce the alarmingly high obesity rates in the United States. The primary assumption made by these experts was that people would actually use MyPyramid to design their diets. In fact, however, the extent to which people use MyPyramid in their daily lives is debatable.

Think about it; prior to taking this class, did you use the previous FGP or the new MyPyramid to help you design a healthful diet? It may be that you had not even seen these pyramids, or if you did, you had no idea how to use them. This is the case for many Americans. Our work with community members throughout the United States has shown us that some people have no idea what MyPyramid or the USDA Food Guide Pyramid are, and many of those who have seen these tools do not know how to use them. Others who have tried to use them find them confusing because of the limitations just discussed. In addition, the pyramid shape does not make sense to many consumers, and changing the orientation of the food groups from horizontal to vertical does not appear to have made things any clearer. Many people find these pyramids too vague: they need specific menus and recipes to follow and prefer to buy diet books that provide this information. Still others do not use the pyramids because they view them as another confusing mandate from experts who are out of touch with how "real" people eat and live their lives.

What do you think? Do you feel that the revised MyPyramid has adequately addressed the flaws of the previous USDA Food Guide Pyramid? Do you think that MyPyramid will help people to lose weight and assist us in the battle against obesity? It is obvious that we need to address the obesity epidemic effectively. In doing so, one of the major challenges we face is to design nutrition recommendations and tools that millions of Americans can, and will, use. Until easier-to-use and more accessible guidelines are available and their impact on the rates of obesity and chronic disease is assessed, this debate will continue.

Will MyPyramid help you select the most healthful option when you eat?

CHAPTER 3

CHAPTER OBJECTIVES

After reading this chapter you will be able to:

1. Distinguish between appetite and hunger, describing the mechanisms that stimulate each, pp. 82–85.

2. Describe what is meant by the saying "We are what we eat," pp. 87–90.

3. Identify two functions of the plasma membrane, p. 88.

4. Draw a picture of the gastrointestinal tract, labeling all major and accessory organs, p. 91.

5. Describe the contribution of each organ of the gastrointestinal system to the digestion, absorption, and elimination of food, pp. 91–100.

6. Identify the source and function of the key enzymes involved in digesting foods, pp. 94–96.

7. Discuss the causes, symptoms, and treatments of gastroesophageal reflux disease, ulcers, food allergies, celiac disease, diarrhea, constipation, and irritable bowel syndrome, pp. 102–110.

8. List several signs and symptoms of dehydration resulting from diarrhea, p. 108.

TEST YOURSELF TRUE OR FALSE?

1. Sometimes you may have an appetite even though you are not hungry. T or F

2. The entire process of digestion and absorption of one meal takes about 24 hours. T or F

3. Some types of bacteria actually help keep our digestive system healthy. T or F

4. Most ulcers result from a type of infection. T or F

5. Irritable bowel syndrome is a rare disease that mostly affects older people. T or F

Test Yourself answers can be found after the Chapter Summary.

The Human Body: Are We Really What We Eat?

two months ago, Andrea's lifelong dream of becoming a lawyer came one step closer to reality: she moved out of her parents' home in the Midwest to attend law school in Boston. Unfortunately, the adjustment to a new city, new friends, and her intensive coursework was more stressful than she'd imagined, and Andrea has been experiencing insomnia and exhaustion. What's more, her always "sensitive stomach" has been getting worse: after almost every meal, she gets cramps so bad she can't stand up, and twice she has missed classes because of sudden attacks of pain and diarrhea. She suspects that the problem is related to stress, and wonders if she is going to experience it throughout her life. She is even thinking of dropping out of school if that would make her feel well again.

Almost everyone experiences brief episodes of abdominal pain, diarrhea, or other symptoms from time to time. Such episodes are usually caused by food poisoning or an infection like influenza. But do you know anyone who experiences these symptoms periodically for days, weeks, or even years? If so, has it made you wonder why? What are the steps in normal digestion and absorption of food, and at what points can the process break down?

We begin this chapter with a look at some of the factors that make us feel as if we want to eat. We then discuss the physiologic processes by which the body digests and absorbs food and eliminates waste products. Finally, we look at some disorders that affect these processes.

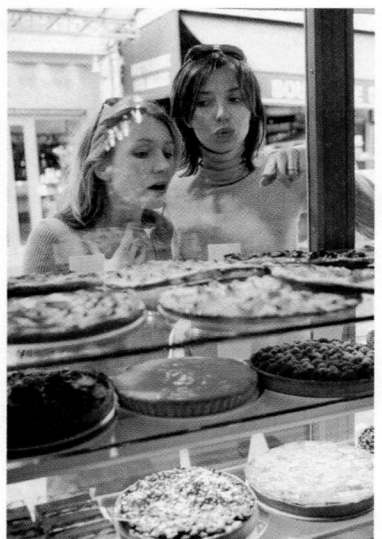

Food stimulates our senses.

Why Do We Want to Eat What We Want to Eat?

You've just finished eating at your favorite Thai restaurant. As you walk back to the block where you parked your car, you pass a bakery window displaying several cakes and pies, each of which looks more enticing than the last, and through the door wafts a complex aroma of coffee, cinnamon, and chocolate. You stop. You know you're not hungry . . . but you go inside and buy a slice of chocolate torte and an espresso anyway. Later that night, when the caffeine from the chocolate and espresso keeps you awake, you wonder why you succumbed.

Two mechanisms prompt us to seek food: **Hunger** is a physiologic drive for food that occurs when the body senses that we need to eat. The drive is *nonspecific*; when you're hungry, a variety of different foods could satisfy you. If you've recently finished a nourishing meal, then hunger probably won't compel you toward a slice of chocolate torte. Instead, the culprit is likely to be **appetite,** a psychological desire to consume *specific* foods. It is aroused when environmental cues—such as the sight of chocolate cake or the smell of coffee—stimulate our senses, prompting pleasant emotions and often memories.

People commonly experience appetite in the absence of hunger. That's why you can crave cake and coffee even after eating a full meal. On the other hand, it is possible to have a physiologic need for food yet have no appetite. This state, called **anorexia,** can accompany a variety of illnesses from infectious diseases to mood disorders. It can also occur as a side effect of certain medications, such as the chemotherapy used in treating cancer patients. Although in the following sections we describe hunger and appetite as separate entities, ideally the two states coexist: we seek specific, appealing foods to satisfy a physiologic need for nutrients.

hunger A physiologic sensation that prompts us to eat.

appetite A psychological desire to consume specific foods.

anorexia An absence of the appetite.

hypothalamus A region of forebrain above the pituitary gland where visceral sensations such as hunger and thirst are regulated.

The Hypothalamus Prompts Hunger in Response to Various Signals

Because hunger is a physiologic stimulus that drives us to find food and eat, it is often felt as a negative or unpleasant sensation. The primary organ producing that sensation is the brain. That's right—it's not our stomachs, but our brains that tell us when we're hungry. The region of brain tissue that is responsible for prompting us to seek food is called the **hypothalamus** (FIGURE 3.1). It's located above the pituitary gland in the forebrain, a region that regulates many types of involuntary activity. The hypothalamus triggers feelings of hunger or satiation (fullness) by integrating signals from nerve cells and chemicals throughout our bodies. Even the amount and type of food we eat influence the hypothalamus to cause us to feel hungry or full. Let's now review these three types of signals generated from nerve cells, hormones, and the food we eat.

The Role of Nerve Cells

One important signal comes from special cells lining the stomach and small intestine that detect changes in pressure according to whether the organ is empty or distended with food. The cells relay these data to the hypothalamus. For instance, if you have not eaten for many hours and your stomach and small intestine do not contain food, these data are sent to the hypothalamus, which in turn prompts you to experience the sensation of hunger.

The Role of Hormones

Hormones are chemical messengers that are secreted into the bloodstream by one of the many *glands* of the body. Their presence in the blood helps regulate one or more body functions. Insulin and glucagon are two hormones produced in the pancreas. They are

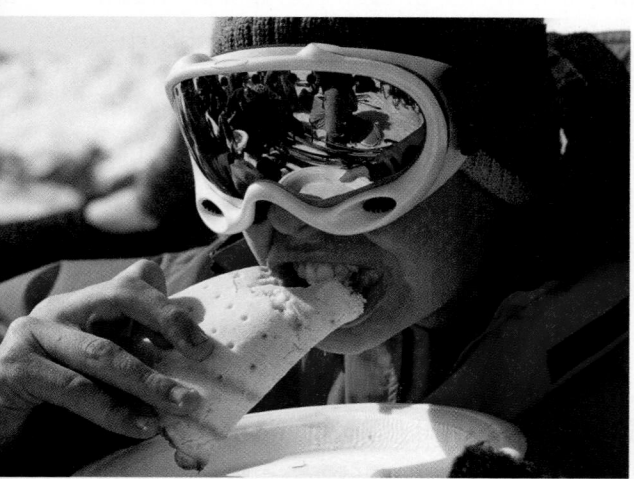

Hunger is a physiologic stimulus that prompts us to find food and eat.

FIGURE 3.1   The hypothalamus triggers hunger by integrating signals from nerve cells throughout the body as well as from messages carried by hormones.

responsible for maintaining blood glucose levels. Glucose is our bodies' most readily available fuel supply. It's not surprising, then, that its level in our blood is an important signal affecting hunger. When we have not eaten for a while, our blood glucose levels fall, prompting a change in the level of insulin and glucagon. This chemical message is relayed to the hypothalamus, which then prompts us to eat in order to supply our bodies with more glucose.

Some people get irritable or feel a little faint when their blood glucose drops to a certain point. At any given moment, the level of glucose in our blood reflects when we last ate, how much we ate, how active we are, and our individual rates of metabolism.

After we eat, the hypothalamus picks up the sensation of a distended stomach, other signals from the gut, and a rise in blood glucose levels. When it integrates these signals, you have the experience of feeling full, or *satiated*. However, as we have noted, even though our brain sends us clear signals about hunger, most of us become adept at ignoring them . . . and eat when we are not truly hungry.

In addition to insulin and glucagon, a variety of other hormones and hormone-like substances signal the hypothalamus to cause us to feel hungry or satiated. Examples of hormones and hormone-like substances that stimulate food intake include neuropeptide Y and galanin, while those that create feelings of satiety include leptin, cholecystokinin, and serotonin.[1] More details about the various hormones involved in digestion are provided later in this chapter. For more information about the role of hormones in weight management, see Chapter 11.

The Role of Amount and Type of Food

Foods containing protein have the highest satiety value.[1] This means that a ham and egg breakfast will cause us to feel satiated for a longer period of time than will pancakes with maple syrup, even if both meals have exactly the same number of calories. High-fat diets have a higher satiety value than high-carbohydrate diets.

Another factor affecting hunger is how bulky the meal is—that is, how much fiber and water is within the food. Bulky meals tend to stretch the stomach and small intestine, which sends signals back to the hypothalamus telling us that we are full, so we stop eating. Beverages tend to be less satisfying than semisolid foods, and semisolid foods have a lower satiety value than solid foods. For example, if you were to eat a bunch of grapes, you would feel a greater sense of fullness than if you drank a glass of grape juice.

hormone Chemical messenger that is secreted into the bloodstream by one of the many glands of the body and acts as a regulator of physiologic processes at a site remote from the gland that secreted it.

> RECAP: *In contrast to appetite, hunger is a physiologic sensation triggered by the hypothalamus in response to cues about stomach and intestinal distention and the levels of certain hormones and hormone-like substances. High-protein foods make us feel satiated for longer periods of time, and bulky meals fill us up quickly, causing the distention that signals us to stop eating.*

Environmental Cues Trigger Appetite

Whereas hunger is prompted by internal signals, appetite is triggered by aspects of our environment. The most significant factors influencing our appetite are sensory data, social and cultural cues, and learning (FIGURE 3.2).

The Role of Sensory Data

Foods stimulate our five senses. Foods that are artfully prepared, arranged, or ornamented, with several different shapes and colors, appeal to our sense of sight. Food producers know this and spend millions of dollars annually in the United States to promote and package their products in an appealing way.

The aromas of foods like freshly brewed coffee and baked goods can also be powerful stimulants. Interestingly, the sense of smell is so acute that newborn babies can distinguish the scent of their own mother's breast milk from that of other mothers.[2] Much of our ability to taste foods actually comes from our sense of smell. This is why foods are not as appealing when we have a stuffy nose due to a cold. Certain tastes, such as sweetness, are almost universally appealing, while others, such as the astringent taste of foods like spinach and kale, are quite individual. Because many natural poisons and spoiled foods are bitter, our distaste for bitterness is thought to be protective.[3]

Texture, or "mouth feel," is also important in food choices, as it stimulates nerve endings sensitive to touch in our mouth and on our tongue. Do you prefer mashed potatoes, thick French fries, or rippled potato chips? Even your sense of hearing can be stimulated by foods, from the fizz of cola to the crunch of peanuts to the "snap, crackle, and pop" of Rice Krispies cereal.

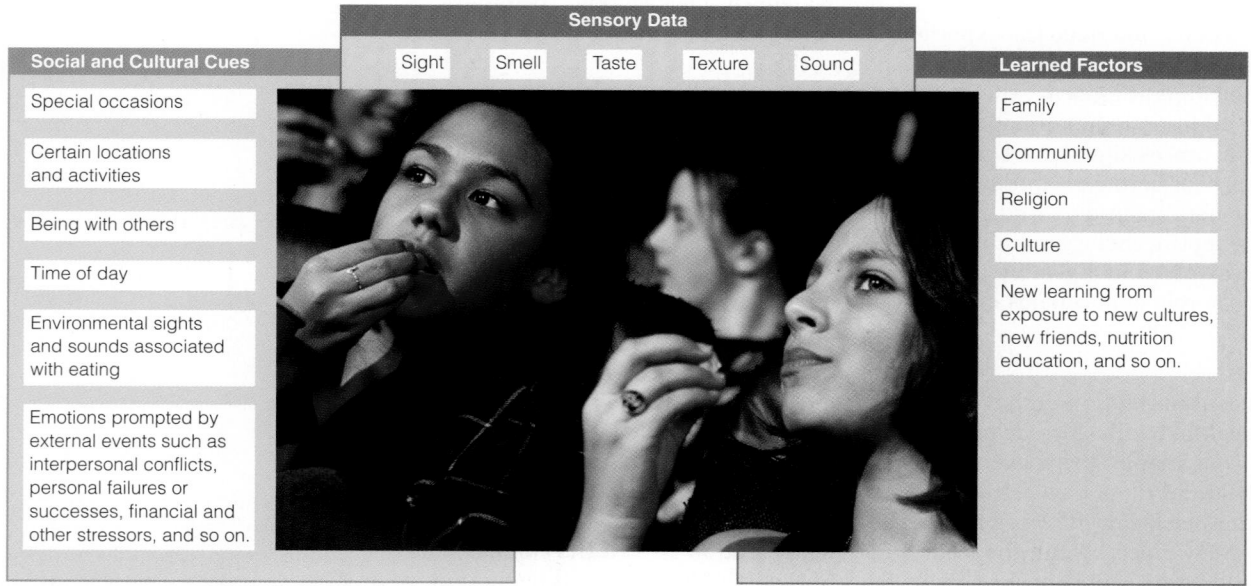

Sensory Data

| Sight | Smell | Taste | Texture | Sound |

Social and Cultural Cues

- Special occasions
- Certain locations and activities
- Being with others
- Time of day
- Environmental sights and sounds associated with eating
- Emotions prompted by external events such as interpersonal conflicts, personal failures or successes, financial and other stressors, and so on.

Learned Factors

- Family
- Community
- Religion
- Culture
- New learning from exposure to new cultures, new friends, nutrition education, and so on.

FIGURE 3.2   Appetite is a drive to consume specific foods, such as popcorn at the movies. It is aroused by social and cultural cues and sensory data and influenced by learning.

The Role of Social and Cultural Cues

In addition to sensory cues, our brain's association with certain social events like birthday parties or holiday gatherings can stimulate our appetite. At these times, our culture gives us permission to eat more than usual or to eat "forbidden" foods. Even when we feel full, these cues can motivate us to accept a second helping.

For some people, being in a certain location, such as at a baseball game or a movie theatre, can trigger appetite. Others may be triggered by certain activities such as watching television or studying, or at certain times of day associated with mealtimes. Many people feel an increase or decrease in appetite according to whom they are with; for example, they may eat more when at home with family members and less when out on a date. Even visual cues and sounds in the environment can trigger appetite. Do you start thinking about food every time you pass your refrigerator? When the bell sounds at the end of a class period, how many of your classmates head for the vending machines?

In some people, appetite masks an emotional response to an external event. For example, a person might experience a desire for food rather than a desire for emotional comfort after receiving a failing grade or arguing with a close friend. Many people crave food when they're frustrated, worried, or bored, or when they are at a party or other gathering where they feel anxious or awkward. Others subconsciously seek food as a "reward." For example, have you ever found yourself heading out for a burger and fries after handing in a term paper?

The Role of Learning

Pigs' feet, anyone? What about blood sausage, stewed octopus, or tripe? These are delicacies in various European cultures, whereas the meat of dogs, monkeys, and snakes is enjoyed in different regions of Asia. Would you eat grasshoppers? If you'd grown up in certain parts of Africa or Central America you probably would. That's because your preference for particular foods is largely a learned response. The family, community, religion, and/or culture in which you are raised teach you what plant and animal products are appropriate to eat. If your parents fed you cubes of plain tofu throughout your toddlerhood, then you are probably still eating tofu now.

That said, early introduction to foods is not essential: we can learn to enjoy new foods at any point in our lives. Immigrants from developing nations settling in the United States or Canada often adopt a typical Western diet, especially when their traditional foods are not readily available. This happens temporarily when we travel: the last time you were away from home, you probably enjoyed sampling a variety of dishes that are not normally part of your diet.

Food preferences also change when people learn what foods are most healthful in terms of nutrient density and prevention of chronic diseases. Since reading Chapter 1, has your diet changed at all? Chances are as you learn more about the health benefits of specific types of carbohydrates, fats, and proteins, you'll quite naturally start incorporating more of these foods in your diet.

We can also "learn" to dislike foods we once enjoyed. For example, if we experience an episode of food poisoning after eating undercooked scrambled eggs, we might develop a strong distaste for all types of cooked eggs. Many adults who become vegetarians do so after learning about the treatment of animals in slaughterhouses: they might have eaten meat daily when young but no longer have any appetite for it.

Now that you understand the differences between appetite and hunger, as well as the influence of learning on food choices, you might be curious to investigate your own reasons for eating what and when you do. If so, check out the accompanying Highlight: Do You Eat in Response to External or Internal Cues?

Food preferences are influenced by the family and culture you are raised in.

> RECAP: *In contrast to hunger, appetite is a psychological desire to consume specific foods. It is triggered when external stimuli arouse our senses, and often occurs in combination with social and cultural cues. Our preference for certain foods is largely learned from the culture in which we were raised, but our food choices can change with exposure to new foods or with new learning experiences.*

HIGHLIGHT

HIGHLIGHT HIGHLIGHT HIGHLIGHT HIGHLIGHT HIGHLIGHT

Do You Eat in Response to External or Internal Cues?

Whether you're trying to lose weight, gain weight, or maintain your current healthful weight, you'll probably find it intriguing to keep a log of the reasons behind your decisions about what, when, where, and why you eat. Are you eating in response to internal sensations telling you that your body needs food, or in response to your emotions, situation, or a prescribed diet? Keeping a "cues" log for 1 full week would give you the most accurate picture of your eating habits, but even logging 2 days of meals and snacks should increase your cue awareness.

Each day, every time you eat a meal, snack, or beverage other than water, make a quick note of:

- **when you eat**. Many people eat at certain times (for example, 6 PM) whether they are hungry or not.
- **what you eat, and how much**. A cup of yogurt and a handful of nuts? An apple? A 20-oz cola?
- **where you eat.** At home at the dining room table, watching television, driving in the car, and so on.
- **with whom you eat.** Are you alone or with others? If with others, are they eating as well? Have they offered you food?
- **your emotions.** Many people overeat when they are happy, especially when celebrating with others. Some people eat excessively when they are anxious, depressed, bored, or frustrated. Still others eat as a way of denying feelings because they don't want to identify and deal with them. For some, food becomes a substitute for emotional fulfillment.
- **your sensations: what you see, hear, or smell.** Are you eating because you walked past the kitchen and spied that batch of homemade cookies, or smelled coffee roasting?
- **any diet restrictions.** Are you choosing a particular food because it is allowed on your current diet plan? Or are you hungry, but drinking a diet soda to stay within a certain allowance of calories? Are you restricting yourself because you feel guilty about having eaten too much at another time?
- **your physiologic hunger.** Rate your hunger on a scale from 1 to 5 as follows:
  1 = you feel full or even stuffed
  2 = you feel satisfied but not uncomfortably full
  3 = neutral; you feel no discernible satiation nor hunger
  4 = you feel hungry and want to eat
  5 = you feel strong physiologic sensations of hunger and need to eat.

After keeping a log for 2 or more days, you might become aware of patterns you'd like to change. For example, maybe you notice that you often eat when you are not actually hungry, but are worried about homework or personal relationships. Or maybe you notice that you can't walk past the snack bar without going in. This self-awareness may prompt you to take positive steps to change those patterns. For instance, instead of stifling your worries with food, sit down with a pen and paper and write down exactly what you are worried about, including steps you can take to address your concerns. And the next time you approach the snack bar, before going in, check with your gut: are you truly hungry? If so, then purchase a healthful snack, maybe a yogurt, a piece of fruit, or a bag of peanuts. If you're not really hungry, then take a moment to acknowledge the strength of this visual cue—and then walk on by.

Apricots are an example of a healthful snack.

NUTRI-CASE JUDY

"Ever since I was diagnosed with type 2 diabetes, I've felt as if there's a "food cop" spying on me. Sometimes I feel like I have to look over my shoulder when I pull into the Dunkin' Donuts parking lot. My doctor says I'm supposed to eat fresh fruits and vegetables, fish, brown bread, brown rice . . . I didn't bother telling him I don't like that stuff and I don't have the money to buy it or the time to cook it even if I did. Besides, that kind of diet is for movie stars. All the real people I know eat the same way I do."

According to what you learned in Chapter 2, is the diet Judy's doctor described really just for "movie stars"? Of the many factors influencing why we eat what we eat, identify at least two that might be affecting Judy's food choices. If you learned that Judy had not finished high school, would that fact have any bearing on your answer? If so, in what way?

Are We Really What We Eat?

You've no doubt heard over and over again the saying that "you are what you eat." Is this scientifically true? To answer that question, and to better understand how we digest and process foods, we'll need to look at how our body is organized (FIGURE 3.3).

Atoms Bond to Form Molecules

Like all substances on earth, our bodies are made up of atoms. Atoms are tiny units of matter that cannot be broken down by natural means. Atoms almost constantly bind to each other in nature. When they do, they form groups called molecules. For example, a molecule of water is composed of two atoms of hydrogen and an atom of oxygen, which is abbreviated H_2O.

Food Is Composed of Molecules

Every particle of food we eat is composed of molecules. During digestion, we chew our food, moisten it with saliva, churn it around in the stomach, and mix it with digestive chemicals in the small intestine. These actions break down food into molecules small enough to be easily absorbed through the gastrointestinal wall and transported in the bloodstream to our body's cells. Our cells can then use these molecules to help build the structures of the body and to provide the energy we need to live.

Molecules Join to Form Cells

Cells are the smallest units of life. That is, cells can grow, reproduce, and perform certain basic functions, such as taking in nutrients, transmitting impulses, producing chemicals, and excreting wastes. The human body is composed of billions of cells that are constantly replacing themselves, destroying worn or damaged cells, and manufacturing new ones. To support this constant demand for new cells, we need a ready supply of nutrient molecules, such as simple sugars, amino acids, and fatty acids, to serve as building blocks. All cells, whether of the skin, bones, or brain, are made of these same basic nutrient molecules, which are derived from the foods we eat.

cell The smallest unit of matter that exhibits the properties of living things, such as growth, reproduction, and metabolism.

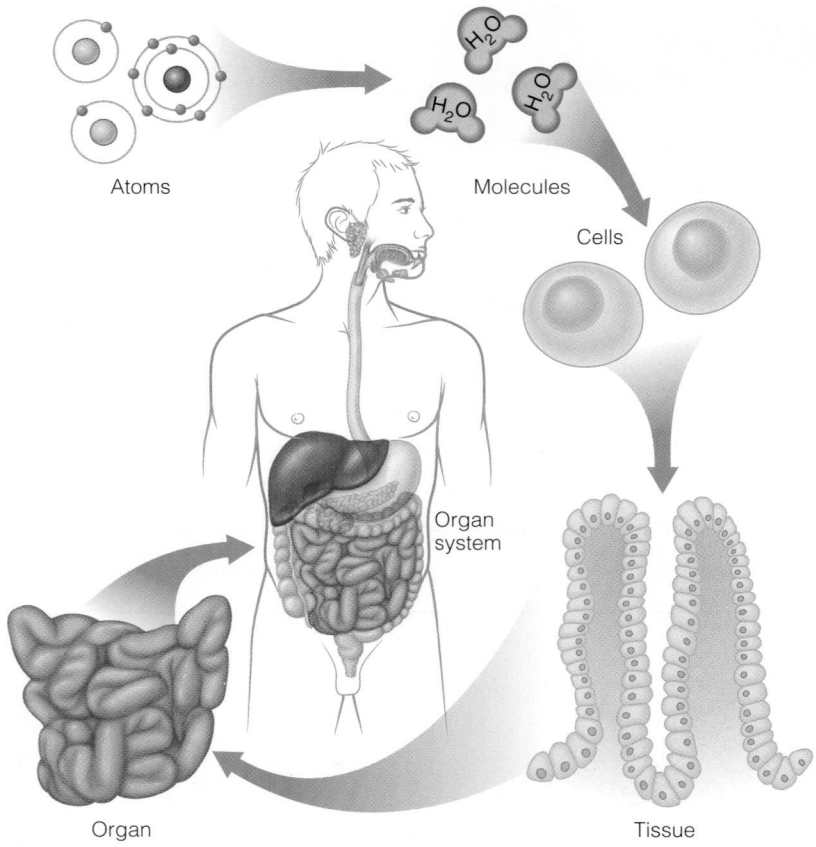

Atoms

Molecules

Cells

Organ system

Organ

Tissue

FIGURE 3.3 The organization of the human body. Atoms bind together to form molecules, and our body's cells are composed of molecules of the food we eat. Cells join to form tissues, one or more types of which form organs. Body systems, such as the gastrointestinal system, are made up of several organs, each of which performs a discrete function within that system. For example, the stomach is the primary site of chemical breakdown of food into molecules.

Cells Are Encased in a Functional Membrane

Cells are encased by a thin covering called the **cell membrane** or plasma membrane (FIGURE 3.4). This membrane defines the cell's boundaries: it encloses the cell's contents and acts as a gatekeeper, either allowing or denying the entry and exit of molecules such as nutrients and wastes.

Cell membranes are composed of two layers. Each layer is made of molecules called phospholipids, which consist of a long lipid "tail" bound to a round phosphate "head." The phosphate head interacts with water, whereas the lipid tail repels water. In the cell membrane, the lipid tails of each layer face each other, forming the membrane interior, whereas the phosphate heads contact either the extracellular fluid or the intracellular fluid. Located throughout the membrane are molecules of another lipid, cholesterol, which helps keep the membrane flexible. The membrane is also studded with various proteins, which assist in the transport of nutrients and other substances across the cell membrane and in the manufacture of certain chemicals.

Recall that the cell membrane is the gatekeeper which, along with its proteins, determines what goes into and out of the cell. This means that cell membranes are *selectively permeable*, allowing only some compounds to enter and leave the cell.

cell membrane The boundary of an animal cell that separates its internal cytoplasm and organelles from the external environment.

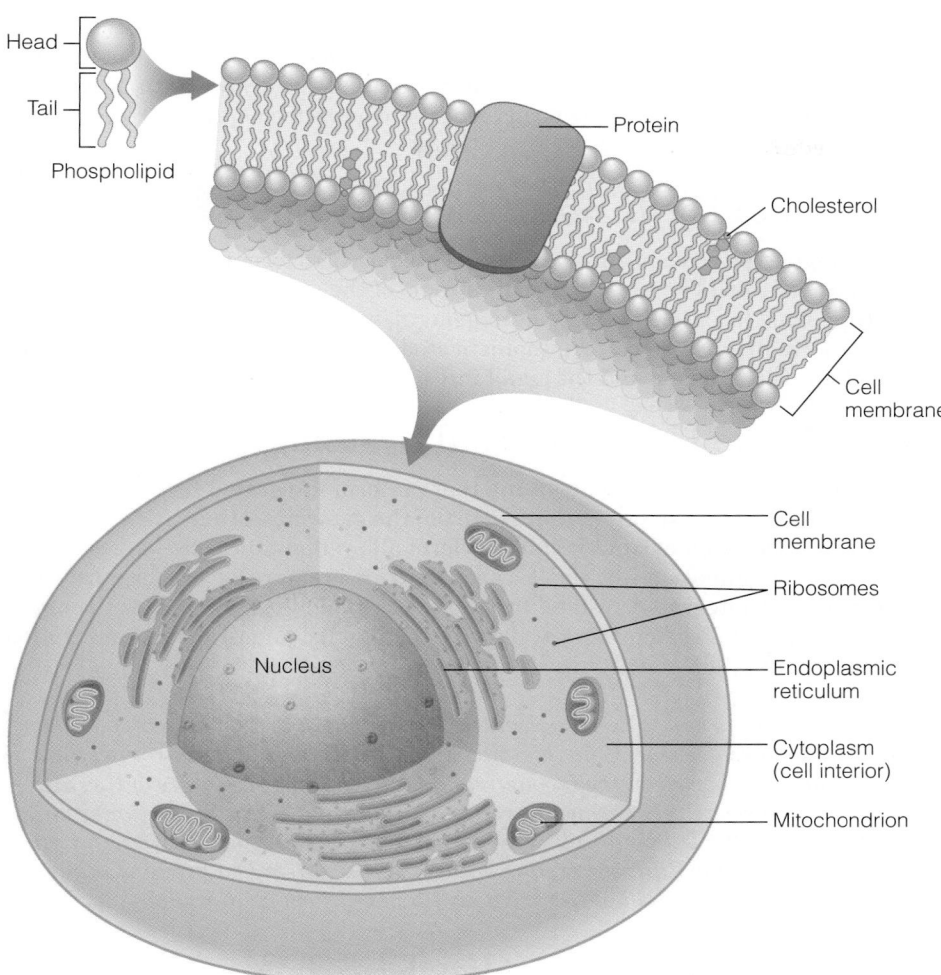

FIGURE 3.4 Representative cell of the small intestine, showing the cell membrane, cytoplasm, and a variety of organelles. The cell membrane is a double layer of phospholipid molecules, each composed of two lipid tails and a phosphate head. The two layers of the membrane align such that the lipid tails form the interior and the phosphate heads interact with the environment inside and outside the cell. Inside the cell is the cytoplasm, which includes a variety of organelles.

Cells Contain Organelles That Support Life

Enclosed within the cell membrane is the semi-liquid **cytoplasm,** which includes a variety of **organelles** (see FIGURE 3.4). These tiny structures accomplish some surprisingly sophisticated functions. A full description of all structures within the cell and their roles is beyond the scope of this book. In terms of nutrition, the most important are:

- *Nucleus.* The nucleus is where our genetic information, in the form of deoxyribonucleic acid (DNA), is located. The cell nucleus is darkly colored because DNA is a huge molecule that is tightly packed within it. A cell's DNA contains the instructions that the cell uses to make certain proteins.

- *Ribosomes.* Ribosomes use the instructions from DNA to assemble proteins.

- *Endoplasmic Reticulum (ER).* Proteins assembled on the ribosomes enter this network of channels and are further processed and packaged for transport. The ER is also responsible for the breakdown of lipids and for storage of the mineral calcium.

cytoplasm The interior of an animal cell, not including its nucleus.

organelle A tiny "organ" within a cell that performs a discrete function necessary to the cell.

- *Mitochondria.* Often called the cell's powerhouse, mitochondria produce the energy molecule ATP (adenosine triphosphate) from basic food components. ATP can be thought of as a stored form of energy that can be drawn upon as we need it. Cells that have high energy needs contain more mitochondria than cells with lower energy needs.

Cells Join to Form Tissues and Organs

Cells of a single type, such as muscle cells, join together to form functional sheets or cords of cells called **tissues.** We'll introduce some of the unique tissues of the gastrointestinal tract later in this chapter. In general, several types of tissues join together to form **organs,** which are sophisticated structures that perform a unique body function. The stomach and the small intestine are examples of organs.

Organs Make Up Functional Systems

Organs are further grouped into **systems** that perform integrated functions. The stomach, for example, is an organ that is part of the gastrointestinal system. It holds and partially digests a meal, but it can't perform all system functions—digestion, absorption, and elimination—by itself. These functions require several organs working together in an integrated system. In the next section, we describe how the organs of the gastrointestinal system work together to accomplish digestion and absorption of foods and elimination of waste products.

> RECAP: *Atoms join to form molecules. The goal of digestion is to break down food into molecules small enough to be absorbed through the gastrointestinal tract and transported in the bloodstream. Cells, the smallest units of life, are encased in a selectively permeable cell membrane and contain functional units called organelles. Different cell types give rise to different tissue types and ultimately to all of the different organs of the body. A system is a group of organs that together accomplish a discrete body function, such as digestion.*

What Happens to the Food We Eat?

When we eat, the food is digested, then the useful nutrients are absorbed, and finally, the waste products are eliminated. But what does each of these processes really entail? In the simplest terms, **digestion** is the process by which foods are broken down into their component molecules, either mechanically or chemically. **Absorption** is the process of taking these products of digestion through the wall of the intestine. **Elimination** is the process by which the undigested portions of food and waste products are removed from the body.

The processes of digestion, absorption, and elimination occur in the **gastrointestinal (GI) tract,** the organs of which work together to process foods. The GI tract is a long tube: if held out straight, an adult GI tract would be close to 30 feet in length. Food within this tube is digested; in other words, it is broken down into molecules small enough to be absorbed by the cells lining the GI tract and thereby passed into the body.

The GI tract begins at the mouth and ends at the anus (FIGURE 3.5). It is composed of several distinct organs, including the mouth, esophagus, stomach, small intestine, and large intestine. The flow of food between these organs is controlled by muscular **sphincters,** which are tight rings of muscle that open when a nerve signal indicates that food is ready to pass into the next section. Surrounding the GI tract are several accessory organs, including the salivary glands, liver, pancreas, and gallbladder, each of which has a specific role in digestion and absorption of nutrients.

Now let's take a look at the role of each of these organs in processing the food we eat. Imagine that you ate a turkey sandwich for lunch today. It contained two slices of bread spread with mayonnaise, some turkey, two lettuce leaves, and a slice of tomato. Let's travel along with the sandwich and see what happens as it enters your GI tract and is digested and absorbed into your body.

tissue A grouping of like cells that performs a function, for example, muscle tissue.

organ A body structure composed of two or more tissues and performing a specific function, for example, the esophagus.

system A group of organs that work together to perform a unique function, for example, the gastrointestinal system.

digestion The process by which foods are broken down into their component molecules, either mechanically or chemically.

absorption The physiologic process by which molecules of food are taken from the gastrointestinal tract into the circulation.

elimination The process by which the undigested portions of food and waste products are removed from the body.

gastrointestinal (GI) tract A long, muscular tube consisting of several organs: the mouth, esophagus, stomach, small intestine, and large intestine.

sphincter A tight ring of muscle separating some of the organs of the GI tract and opening in response to nerve signals indicating that food is ready to pass into the next section.

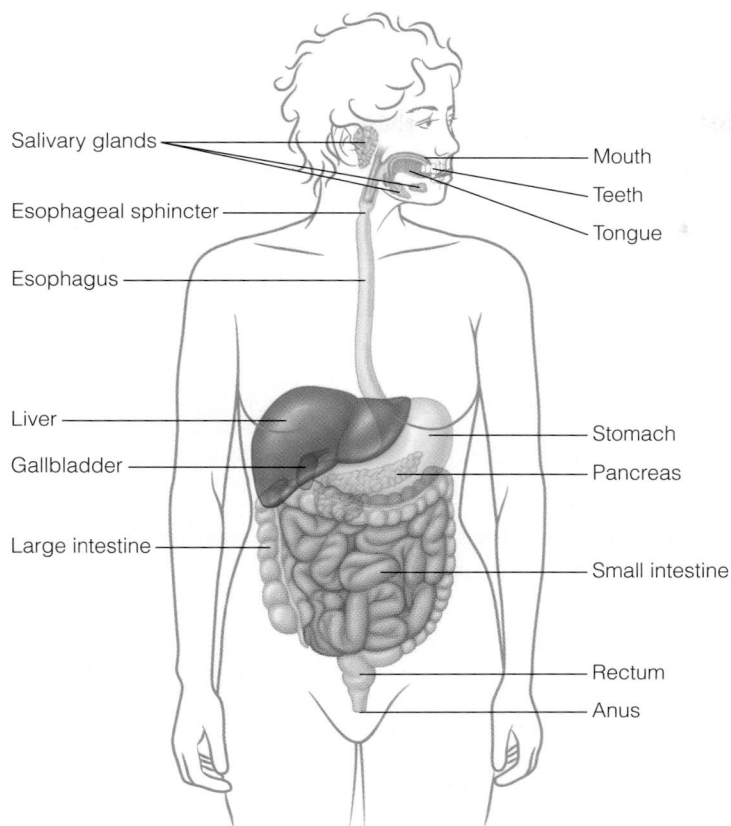

FIGURE 3.5 An overview of the gastrointestinal (GI) tract. The GI tract begins in the mouth and ends at the anus and is composed of numerous organs.

Digestion Begins in the Mouth

Believe it or not, the first step in the digestive process is not your first bite of that sandwich. It is your first thought about what you wanted for lunch and your first whiff of turkey and freshly baked bread as you stood in line at the deli. In this **cephalic phase** of digestion, hunger and appetite work together to prepare the GI tract to digest food. The nervous system stimulates the release of digestive juices in preparation for food entering the GI tract, and sometimes we experience some involuntary movement commonly called "hunger pangs."

Now let's stop smelling that sandwich and take a bite and chew! Chewing is very important because it moistens the food and mechanically breaks it down into pieces small enough to swallow **(FIGURE 3.6)**. Thus, chewing initiates the mechanical digestion of food. The tough coating or skin surrounding the lettuce fibers and tomato seeds is also broken open, facilitating digestion. This is especially important when eating foods that are high in fiber such as grains, fruits, and vegetables.

When you chew, everything in your sandwich mixes together: the protein in the turkey; the carbohydrates in the bread, lettuce, and tomato; the fat in the mayonnaise; and the vitamins and minerals in all of the foods. The presence of food initiates not only mechanical digestion via chewing, but also chemical digestion through the secretion of various substances throughout the gastrointestinal tract. As your teeth cut and grind the different foods in your sandwich, more surface area is exposed to the digestive juices in your mouth. Foremost among these is **saliva,** which you secrete from your **salivary glands.** Saliva not only moistens your food, but also begins the process of chemical breakdown. One component of saliva is *amylase*, an enzyme that starts the process of carbohydrate digestion in the mouth.

Digestion of a sandwich starts before you even take a bite.

cephalic phase Earliest phase of digestion in which the brain thinks about and prepares the digestive organs for the consumption of food.

saliva A mixture of water, mucus, enzymes, and other chemicals that moistens the mouth and food, binds food particles together, and begins the digestion of starch.

salivary glands Group of glands found under and behind the tongue and beneath the jaw that release saliva continually as well as in response to the thought, sight, smell, or presence of food.

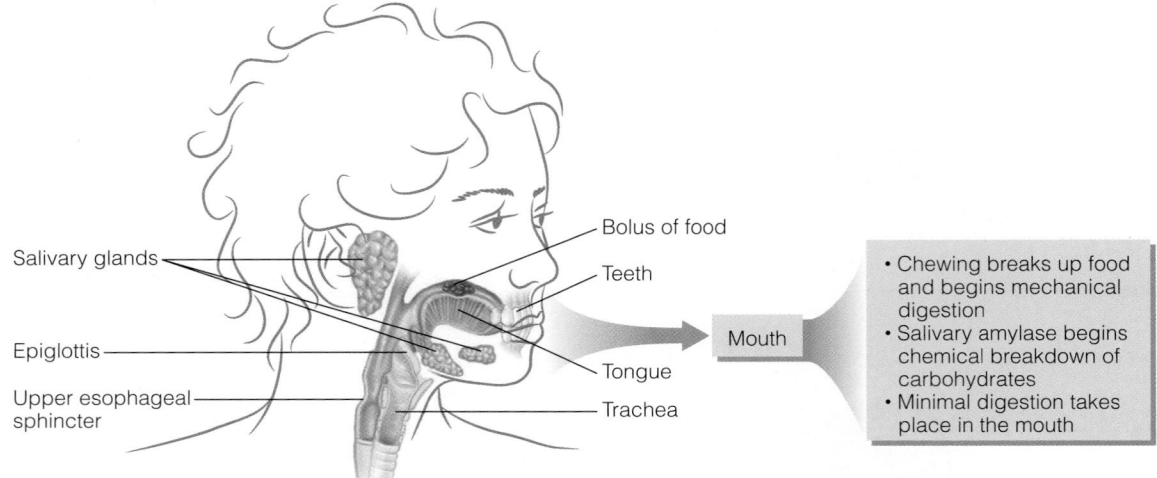

Salivary glands

Epiglottis

Upper esophageal
sphincter

Bolus of food

Teeth

Tongue

Trachea

Mouth

- Chewing breaks up food
  and begins mechanical
  digestion
- Salivary amylase begins
  chemical breakdown of
  carbohydrates
- Minimal digestion takes
  place in the mouth

FIGURE 3.6 Where your food is now: the mouth. Chewing moistens food and mechanically breaks it down into pieces small enough to swallow, while salivary amylase begins chemical digestion of carbohydrates.

Saliva also contains other components such as antibodies that protect the body from foreign bacteria entering the mouth and keep the oral cavity free from infection.

Salivary amylase is the first of many enzymes that assist the body in digesting and absorbing food. Since we will encounter enzymes throughout our journey through the GI tract, let's discuss them briefly here. **Enzymes** are complex proteins that induce chemical changes in other substances to speed up bodily processes and that may be reused since they essentially are unchanged by the chemical reactions they catalyze. Imagine them as facilitators: a chemical reaction that might take an hour to occur independently might happen in a few seconds with the help of one or more enzymes. The action of enzymes can result in the production of new substances or can assist in breaking substances apart. Our bodies make hundreds of enzymes, and the process of digestion—as well as many other biochemical processes that go on in our bodies—could not happen without them. By the way, enzyme names typically end in *–ase* (as in amylase), so they are easy to recognize as we go through the digestive process.

In reality, very little digestion occurs in the mouth. This is because we do not hold food in the mouth for very long and because all of the enzymes needed to break down food are not present in saliva. Salivary amylase starts the digestion of carbohydrates in the mouth, and this digestion continues until food reaches the stomach. Once in the stomach, salivary amylase is no longer active because it is destroyed by the acidic environment of the stomach.

RECAP: *Digestion, absorption, and elimination take place in the gastrointestinal (GI) tract. The cephalic phase of digestion involves hunger and appetite working together to prepare your GI tract for digestion and absorption. Chewing initiates mechanical digestion by breaking the food mass apart and mixing it together. Release of saliva moistens food and starts the process of chemical digestion of carbohydrates through the action of the enzyme salivary amylase.*

enzymes Small chemicals, usually proteins, that act on other chemicals to speed up body processes but are not apparently changed during those processes.

bolus The mass of food that has been chewed and moistened in the mouth.

The Esophagus Propels Food into the Stomach

The mass of food that has been chewed and moistened in the mouth is referred to as a **bolus.** This bolus is swallowed (FIGURE 3.7) and propelled to the stomach through the esophagus. Most of us take swallowing for granted. However, it is a very complex process involving voluntary and involuntary motion. A tiny flap of tissue called the *epiglottis* acts like a trapdoor covering the entrance to the trachea (or windpipe). The epiglottis is normally open, allowing us to breathe freely even while chewing (FIGURE 3.7a). As a food bolus moves to the very back of the mouth, the brain is sent a signal to temporarily raise the soft palate and close the openings to the nasal passages, preventing aspiration of food or liquid into the sinuses (FIGURE 3.7b). The brain also signals the epiglottis to close during swallowing so food and liquid cannot enter the trachea.

Sometimes this protective mechanism goes awry, for instance, when we try to eat and talk at the same time. When this happens, food or liquid enters the trachea. This causes us to experience the sensation of choking and typically to cough involuntarily and repeatedly until the offending food or liquid is expelled.

As the trachea closes, the **esophagus** opens. This muscular tube connects and transports food from the mouth to the stomach (FIGURE 3.8). It does this by contracting

esophagus Muscular tube of the GI tract connecting the back of the mouth to the stomach.

Soft palate

Bolus of food

Epiglottis (open)

Esophagus (closed)

Trachea

(a) Chewing

Epiglottis is open; esophagus is closed

Soft palate rises to close opening to nasal passages

Epiglottis (closed)

Esophagus (open)

Epiglottis bends to close off trachea and open esophagus

(b) Swallowing

FIGURE 3.7 Chewing and swallowing are complex processes. **(a)** During the process of chewing, the epiglottis is open and the esophagus is closed so that we can continue to breathe as we chew. **(b)** During swallowing, the epiglottis closes so that food does not enter the trachea and obstruct our breathing. The soft palate also rises to seal off our nasal passages to prevent aspiration of food or liquid into the sinuses.

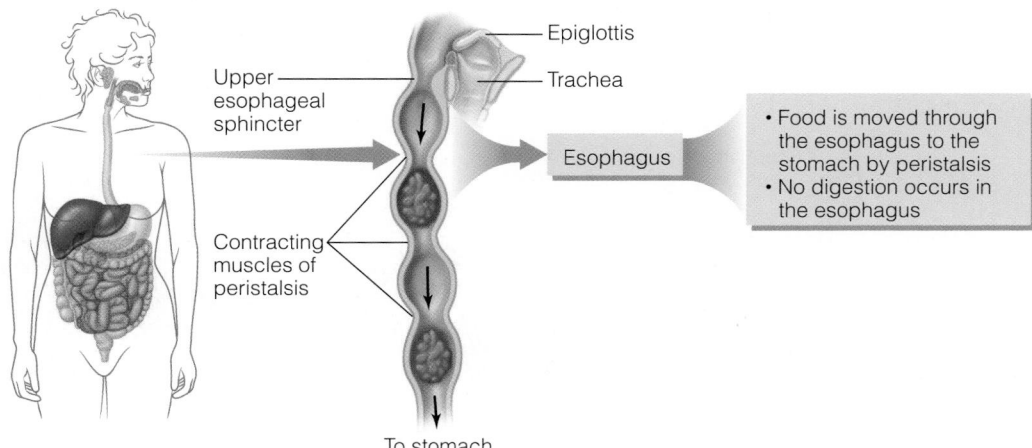

Epiglottis

Trachea

Upper esophageal sphincter

Esophagus

Contracting muscles of peristalsis

- Food is moved through the esophagus to the stomach by peristalsis
- No digestion occurs in the esophagus

To stomach

FIGURE 3.8 Where your food is now: the esophagus. Peristalsis, the rhythmic contraction and relaxation of both circular and longitudinal muscles in the esophagus, propels food toward the stomach. Peristalsis occurs throughout the GI tract.

two sets of muscles: inner sheets of circular muscle squeeze the food, while outer sheets of longitudinal muscle push food along the length of the tube. Together, these rhythmic waves of squeezing and pushing are called **peristalsis.** We will see later in this chapter that peristalsis occurs throughout the GI tract.

Gravity also helps transport food down the esophagus, which is one reason why it is wise to sit or stand upright while eating. Together, peristalsis and gravity can transport a bite of food from our mouth to the opening of the stomach in 5 to 8 seconds. At the end of the esophagus is a sphincter muscle, the *gastroesophageal sphincter* (*gastro-* indicates the stomach), which is normally tightly closed. When food reaches the end of the esophagus, this sphincter relaxes to allow the passage of food into the stomach. In some people, this sphincter is continually somewhat relaxed. Later in the chapter, we'll discuss this disorder and the unpleasant symptoms caused when this sphincter does not function properly.

The Stomach Mixes, Digests, and Stores Food

The **stomach** is a J-shaped organ. Its size is fairly individual; in general, its volume is about 6 fl. oz (or ¾ cup) when it is empty. When the stomach is full, it can expand to hold about 32 fl. oz, or about 4 cups. Before any food reaches the stomach, the brain sends signals telling it to be ready for the food to arrive. This causes an increased secretion of **gastric juice,** which contains several important compounds:

- *Hydrochloric acid (HCl)* keeps the stomach interior very acidic—more so than many citrus juices. This acid is extremely important for digestion because it starts to **denature** proteins, which means it destroys the bonds that maintain their structure. HCl also converts *pepsinogen*, an inactive substance, into the active enzyme *pepsin*, which assists in protein digestion. HCl performs another important function: it kills many bacteria and/or germs that may have entered your body with your sandwich.

- *Pepsin* begins to digest proteins into smaller components. Recall that salivary amylase begins to digest carbohydrates in the mouth. In contrast, proteins and fats enter the stomach largely unchanged. Pepsin begins the digestion of protein and activates many other GI enzymes needed to digest your meal.

- *Gastric lipase* is an enzyme responsible for fat digestion. Thus, it begins to break apart the fat in the turkey and the mayonnaise in your sandwich. Only minimal digestion of fat occurs in the stomach.

- Your stomach also secretes *mucus* that protects its lining from being digested by the HCl and pepsin.

With these gastric juices already present, chemical digestion of proteins and fats begins as soon as food enters your stomach (FIGURE 3.9). In this *gastric phase* of diges-

peristalsis Wave of squeezing and pushing contractions that move food in one direction through the length of the GI tract.

stomach A J-shaped organ where food is partially digested, churned, and stored until released into the small intestine.

gastric juice Acidic liquid secreted within the stomach; it contains hydrochloric acid, pepsin, and other compounds.

denature Term used to describe the action of unfolding proteins. Proteins must be denatured before they can be digested.

- Mechanical digestion occurs when peristaltic waves mix contents of stomach
- Gastric juice is secreted by stomach
- Pepsin initiates protein digestion
- Gastric lipase intiates fat digestion
- Small amounts of water, some minerals, drugs, and alcohol are absorbed

Esophagus

Lower esophageal sphincter

Pyloric sphincter

Stomach

Contracting muscles

FIGURE 3.9 Where your food is now: the stomach. In the stomach, the protein and fat in your sandwich begin to be digested. Your meal is churned into chyme and stored until released into the small intestine.

tion, the hormone *gastrin* is secreted. This hormone acts to increase the secretions of the gastric cells, making the gastric juices even more acidic. It also stimulates stomach contractions, which begin to mix and churn the food until it becomes a liquid called **chyme.** This physical mixing and churning of food is another example of mechanical digestion that takes place in the gastrointestinal tract. Enzymes can access the liquid chyme more readily than solid forms of food. This access facilitates chemical digestion.

Although most absorption occurs in the small intestine, the stomach lining does begin absorbing a few substances. These include water, some medium-chain fatty acids (components of certain types of lipids), some minerals, and some drugs, including aspirin and alcohol.[4]

Another of your stomach's jobs is to store your sandwich (or what's left of it!) while the next part of the digestive tract, the small intestine, gets ready for the next wave of food. Remember that the stomach can hold about 4 cups of food. If this amount suddenly moved into the small intestine all at once, it would overwhelm it. Instead, chyme stays in your stomach about 2 to 4 hours: liquids pass more quickly, whereas a high-fat meal may remain for up to 6 hours before being released periodically in spurts into the duodenum, which is the first part of the small intestine. Regulating this release is the *pyloric sphincter* (see FIGURE 3.9).

> RECAP: *The esophagus is a muscular tube that transports food from the mouth to the stomach via waves of peristalsis. The stomach prepares itself for digestion by secreting gastric juice, which contains hydrochloric acid and the enzymes pepsin and gastric lipase. The stomach also secretes mucus to protect its lining. As the hormone gastrin causes the stomach to churn food into a liquid called chyme, digestion of proteins and fats begins. The stomach stores chyme and releases it periodically into the small intestine through the pyloric sphincter.*

Most Digestion and Absorption Occurs in the Small Intestine

The **small intestine** is the longest portion of the GI tract, accounting for about two-thirds of its length. However, at only an inch in diameter, it is comparatively narrow.

The small intestine is composed of three sections (FIGURE 3.10). The *duodenum* is the section of the small intestine that is connected via the pyloric sphincter to the stomach. The *jejunum* is the middle portion, and the last portion is the *ileum*. It connects to the large intestine at another sphincter, called the *ileocecal valve*.

Most digestion and absorption take place in the small intestine. Here, food is broken down into its smallest components, molecules that the body can then absorb into its internal environment. In this next section we identify a variety of accessory organs, enzymes, and unique anatomical features of the small intestine that permit maximal absorption of most nutrients.

The Gallbladder and Pancreas Aid in Digestion

We left your sandwich as chyme, being released periodically into the small intestine. As the chyme enters the duodenum, a hormone-like substance called cholecystokinin (or CCK) is released in response to the presence of protein and fat from the turkey and mayonnaise. CCK signals an accessory organ, the **gallbladder,** to contract. The gallbladder is located beneath the liver (see FIGURE 3.5), and stores a greenish fluid, **bile,** produced by the liver. Contraction of the gallbladder sends bile through the *common bile duct* into the duodenum. Bile then *emulsifies* the fat; that is, it reduces the fat into smaller globules and disperses them so they are more accessible to digestive enzymes. If you've ever noticed how a drop of liquid detergent breaks up a film of fat floating at the top of a basin of greasy dishes, you understand the function of bile.

The **pancreas,** another accessory organ, manufactures, holds, and secretes different digestive enzymes. It is located behind the stomach (see FIGURE 3.5). Enzymes secreted by the pancreas include *pancreatic amylase*, which continues the digestion of carbohydrates, and *pancreatic lipase*, which continues the digestion of fats.

chyme Semifluid mass consisting of partially digested food, water, and gastric juices.

small intestine The longest portion of the GI tract where most digestion and absorption takes place.

gallbladder A tissue sac beneath the liver that stores bile and secretes it into the small intestine.

bile Fluid produced by the liver and stored in the gallbladder; it emulsifies fats in the small intestine.

pancreas Gland located behind the stomach; it secretes digestive enzymes.

- Bile from the gallbladder emulsifies fat to aid digestion
- Pancreatic lipase digests fats
- Pancreatic amylase digests carbohydrates
- Proteases digest protein
- Bicarbonate secreted by the pancreas neutralizes acidic chyme coming from the stomach into the small intestine

FIGURE 3.10 Where your food is now: the small intestine. Here, most digestion and absorption of the nutrients in your sandwich take place.

Proteases secreted in pancreatic juice digest proteins. The pancreas is also responsible for manufacturing hormones that are important in metabolism. Earlier we mentioned insulin and glucagon, two pancreatic hormones that help regulate the amount of glucose in the blood.

Another essential role of the pancreas is to secrete bicarbonate into the duodenum. Bicarbonate is a base and, like all bases, is capable of neutralizing acids. Recall that chyme leaving the stomach is very acidic. The pancreatic bicarbonate neutralizes this acidic chyme. This action helps the pancreatic enzymes work more effectively. It also ensures that the lining of the duodenum is not eroded.

Now the protein, carbohydrate, and fat in your sandwich have been processed into a liquid that contains molecules of nutrients small enough for absorption. This molecular "soup" continues to move along the small intestine via peristalsis, encountering the absorptive cells of the intestinal lining all along the way.

A Specialized Lining Enables the Small Intestine to Absorb Food

The lining of the GI tract is especially well suited for absorption. If you looked at the inside of the lining, which is also referred to as the mucosal membrane, you would notice that it is heavily folded (FIGURE 3.11). This feature increases the surface area of the small intestine and allows it to absorb more nutrients than if it were smooth. Within these larger folds, you would notice even smaller finger-like projections called *villi*, whose constant movement helps them to encounter and trap nutrient molecules. Inside each villus are *capillaries*, or tiny blood vessels, and a **lacteal**, which is a small lymph vessel. (The role of the lymphatic system is presented on page 98.) These vessels take up the final products of digestion. Water-soluble nutrients are absorbed directly into the bloodstream, while fat-soluble nutrients are absorbed into lymph.

Covering the villi are specialized cells covered with hairlike structures called *microvilli*. The microvilli look like tiny brushes and are sometimes referred to as the **brush border.** These intricate folds multiply the surface area of the small intestine more than 500 times, which tremendously increases its absorptive capacity.

lacteal A small lymph vessel located inside of the villi of the small intestine.

brush border Term that describes the microvilli of the small intestine's lining. These microvilli tremendously increase the small intestine's absorptive capacity.

FIGURE 3.11 Absorption of nutrients occurs via the specialized lining of the small intestine. The lining of the small intestine is heavily folded and has thousands of finger-like projections called *villi*. The cells covering the villi end in hairlike projections called *microvilli* that together form the brush border. These features significantly increase the absorptive capacity of the small intestine.

Intestinal Cells Readily Absorb Vitamins, Minerals, and Water

The turkey sandwich you ate contained several vitamins and minerals in addition to protein, carbohydrate, and fat. For instance, the bread contained B-complex vitamins and iron, and the tomato contained vitamin C. If you had a glass of milk with your sandwich, you also consumed the mineral calcium as well as vitamin D. The turkey contained some of the mineral zinc. Most of the sandwich also contained small amounts of sodium, potassium, and chloride.

Vitamins and minerals are not really "digested" in the same way that macronutrients are. These compounds do not have to be broken down because they are small enough to be readily absorbed by the small intestine. For example, fat-soluble vitamins such as vitamins A, D, E, and K are soluble in lipids and are absorbed into the intestinal cells along with the fats in our foods. Water-soluble vitamins such as the B vitamins and vitamin C typically use some type of transport process to cross the intestinal lining.

Minerals are absorbed all along the small intestine, and in some cases in the large intestine as well, by a wide variety of mechanisms. For example, the absorption of sodium, potassium, and chloride is regulated by nerves and hormones working together to maintain water and salt balance (see Chapter 7). These minerals are

Water is readily absorbed along the entire length of the GI tract.

absorbed in both the small and large intestines. Iron absorption increases or decreases according to the body's needs. One way the body regulates the amount of iron absorbed is by holding iron in the mucosal cells until needed. The cells turn over every 24 to 72 hours, so any excess iron will be lost as the cell is sloughed off. There is also a specialized protein in the membrane of intestinal cells that can transport needed iron into the body (see Chapter 10). Zinc, copper, and manganese can each be absorbed with the help of a carrier protein, but they can also pass through the intestinal cells unassisted.

Finally, a large component of food is water, and of course you also drink lots of water throughout the day. Water is readily absorbed along the entire length of the GI tract because it is a small molecule that can easily pass through the cell membrane. However, as we will see shortly, a significant percentage of water is absorbed in the large intestine.

Blood and Lymph Transport Nutrients and Fluids

Two fluids are primarily responsible for transporting nutrients and waste products throughout the body: blood and lymph. Blood travels through the cardiovascular system, and lymph travels through the lymphatic system (FIGURE 3.12).

The oxygen we inhale into our lungs is absorbed by our red blood cells. This oxygen-rich blood then travels to the heart, where it is pumped out to the rest of the body. Blood

FIGURE 3.12 Blood travels through the cardiovascular system to transport nutrients and fluids and pick up waste products. Lymph travels through the lymphatic system and transports most fats and fat-soluble vitamins.

travels to all of our tissues to deliver nutrients and other materials and pick up waste products. As blood travels through the GI tract, it picks up most nutrients, including water, that are absorbed through the mucosal membrane of the small intestine.

The lymphatic vessels pick up most fats, fat-soluble vitamins, and fluids that have escaped from the cardiovascular system and transport them in the lymph. This lymph eventually returns to the bloodstream in an area near the heart where the lymphatic and blood vessels join together.

As the blood leaves the GI system, it is transported to the liver. The role of the liver in digestion is described in the following section. The waste products picked up by the blood as it circulates around the body are filtered and excreted by the kidneys. In addition, much of the carbon dioxide remaining in the blood once it reaches the lungs is exhaled into the outside air, making room for oxygen to attach to the red blood cells and repeat this cycle of circulation again.

The Liver Regulates Blood Nutrients

Once nutrients are absorbed from the small intestine, most enter the *portal vein*, which carries them to the **liver.** The liver is a triangular wedge-shaped organ weighing about 3 pounds and resting almost entirely within the protection of the rib cage on the right side of the body (see FIGURE 3.5). It is not only the largest digestive organ, but also one of the most important organs in the body, performing more than 500 discrete functions.

One function of the liver is to receive the products of digestion and then release into the bloodstream those nutrients needed throughout the body. The liver also processes and stores monosaccharides, triglycerides (fats), and amino acids and plays a major role in regulating these energy nutrients. For instance, after we eat a meal, the liver picks up excess glucose from the blood and stores it as glycogen, releasing it into the bloodstream when we need energy later in the day. It also stores certain vitamins. But the liver is more than a nutrient warehouse: it also manufactures blood proteins and can even make glucose when necessary to keep our blood glucose levels constant. Thus, the liver plays a major role in regulating the level and type of energy nutrients circulating in the blood.

Have you ever wondered why people who abuse alcohol are at risk for liver damage? It's because another of the liver's functions is to filter the blood, removing wastes and toxins like alcohol, medications, and other drugs. When you drink, your liver works hard to replace the cells poisoned with alcohol, but, over time, scar tissue forms. The scar tissue blocks the free flow of blood through the liver, so that any further toxins accumulate in the blood, causing confusion, coma, and ultimately, death.

Another important job of the liver is to synthesize many of the chemicals used by the body in carrying out metabolic processes. For example, the liver synthesizes bile, which, as we just discussed, is then stored in the gallbladder until needed to emulsify fats.

> RECAP: *Most digestion occurs in the small intestine. Its three sections are the duodenum, the jejunum, and the ileum. The gallbladder stores bile, which emulsifies fats, and the pancreas synthesizes and secretes digestive enzymes that break down carbohydrates, fats, and proteins. The lining of the small intestine is heavily folded, with the surface area expanded by villi and microvilli. Nutrients are absorbed across the mucosal membrane. Vitamins and minerals can be absorbed directly into lymph or the bloodstream. The liver processes all nutrients absorbed from the small intestine and stores and regulates monosaccharides, triglycerides, and amino acids.*

The Large Intestine Stores Food Waste Until It Is Excreted

The **large intestine** is a thick tubelike structure that frames the small intestine on three-and-a-half sides (FIGURE 3.13). It begins with a tissue sac called the *cecum*, which explains the name of the sphincter—the *ileocecal valve*—which connects it to

liver The largest auxiliary organ of the GI tract and one of the most important organs of the body. Its functions include production of bile and processing of nutrient-rich blood from the small intestine.

large intestine Final organ of the GI tract consisting of the cecum, colon, rectum, and anal canal, and in which most water is absorbed and feces are formed.

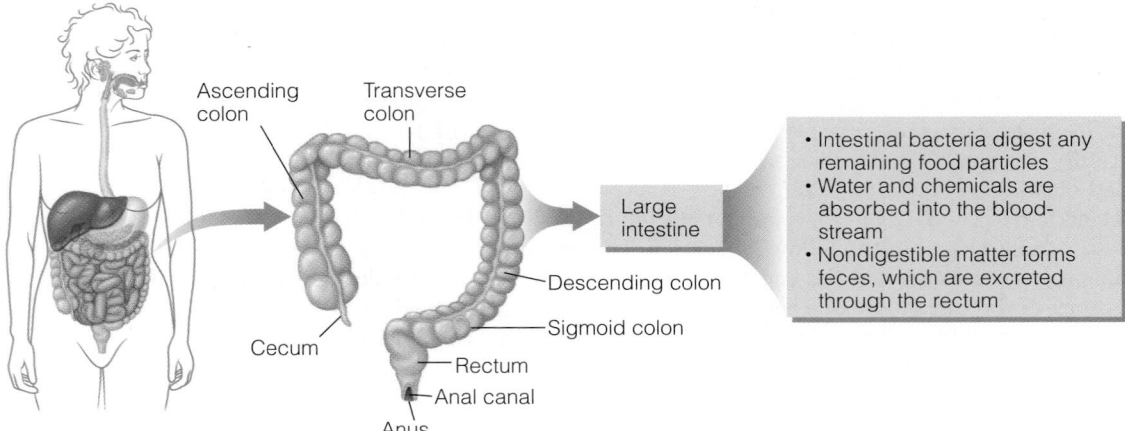

FIGURE 3.13 Where your food is now: the large intestine. Most water absorption occurs here, as does the formation of food wastes into semisolid feces. Peristalsis propels the feces to the body exterior.

The large intestine is a thick tube-like structure that stores the undigested mass leaving the small intestine and absorbs any remaining nutrients and water.

the ileum of the small intestine. From the cecum, the large intestine continues up along the left side of the small intestine as the *ascending colon*. The *transverse colon* runs across the top of the small intestine, and then the *descending colon* comes down on the right. The *sigmoid colon* is the last segment of the colon; it extends from the bottom right corner to the *rectum*. The last segment of the large intestine is the *anal canal*, which is about an inch and a half long.

What has happened to our turkey sandwich? The undigested food components in the chyme finally reach the large intestine. By this time, the digestive mass entering the large intestine does not resemble the chyme that left the stomach several hours before. This is because a majority of the nutrients have been absorbed, leaving mostly nondigestible food material such as fiber, bacteria, and water. As in the stomach, cells lining the large intestine secrete mucus, which helps protect it from the abrasive materials passing through it.

Bacteria colonizing the large intestine are normal and helpful residents, since they finish digesting some of the nutrients from your sandwich. The by-products of this digestion, such as short-chain fatty acids, are reabsorbed into the body where they return to the liver and are either stored or used as needed. Intestinal bacteria, called *intestinal flora*, also help synthesize certain vitamins and are thought to promote intestinal motility. In fact, the types of bacteria that thrive in our large intestine are so helpful that many people consume them deliberately! They are found in foods such as yogurt and supplements called probiotics. These and other "functional foods" are discussed *In Depth* on pages 350–359.

No other digestion occurs in the large intestine. Instead, its main functions are to store the digestive mass for 12 to 24 hours, and during that time to absorb nutrients and water from it, leaving a semisolid mass called *feces*. Peristalsis occurs weakly to move the feces through the colon, except for one or more stronger waves of peristalsis each day that force the feces more powerfully toward the rectum for elimination.

> RECAP: *The large intestine is composed of six sections: the cecum, ascending colon, descending colon, sigmoid colon, rectum, and anal canal. Small amounts of undigested and indigestible food material, bacteria, and water enter the large intestine. Intestinal bacteria accomplish final digestion of any remaining digestible food products. No other digestion occurs here. The main functions of the large intestine are to store the digestive mass and absorb any remaining nutrients and water. A semisolid mass called feces is then eliminated from the body.*

How Does the Body Coordinate and Regulate Digestion?

To complete your picture of the gastrointestinal system, it might help to think of your body as a manufacturing plant with the GI tract as its assembly line. Here, all the raw, unprocessed materials (foods) needed by the manufacturing plant to synthesize new products arrive. These raw materials are broken down into usable parts, which are then sent to other departments to be reassembled into new products. Wastes are excreted at the end of the assembly line. Now that you can identify the organs involved and the jobs they perform, you might be wondering—who's the boss? In other words, what organ or system directs and coordinates all of these interrelated processes? The answer is the neuromuscular system. Each of its two components, the nervous and muscular systems, is an essential partner in coordinating and regulating the digestion, absorption, and elimination of food.

The Muscles of the Gastrointestinal Tract Mix and Move Food

The purpose of the muscles of the GI tract is to mix food and move it in one direction, that is, from the mouth toward the anus. When food is present, nerves respond to the stretching of the tract walls and send signals to its muscles, stimulating peristalsis. As with the assembly line, the entire GI tract functions together so that materials are moved in one direction in a coordinated manner and wastes are removed as needed.

   In order to process the large amount of food we consume daily, we use both voluntary and involuntary muscles. Muscles in the mouth are primarily voluntary; that is, they are under our conscious control. Once we swallow, involuntary muscles largely take over to propel food through the rest of the GI tract. This enables us to continue digesting and absorbing our food while we're working, exercising, and even sleeping. Let's now reveal the master controller behind these involuntary muscular actions.

When we eat, both voluntary and involuntary muscles help us digest the food.

The Enteric Nerves Coordinate and Regulate Digestive Activities

The nervous system in your body is like the communications system in a manufacturing plant. Within this communications system, the central nervous system (CNS), composed of the brain and spinal cord, is like the main control desk. For example, as discussed earlier in this chapter, the hypothalamus of the brain plays an important role in control of hunger and satiation.

   There is also an intricate system of nerves branching out from the CNS; this system is called the peripheral nervous system. The nerves of the GI tract are found within the peripheral nervous system and are collectively known as the **enteric nervous system.**

   Enteric nerves work both independently of and in collaboration with the CNS. For example, they can respond independently to signals produced within the GI tract without first relaying them to the CNS for interpretation or assistance. On the other hand, many jobs require the involvement of the CNS. For instance, as we discussed earlier, special nerves in the GI tract pick up mechanical signals indicating how far the tract wall is stretched, that is, how full it is. These receptors signal the brain that your digestive tract is full, and then your brain sends out messages that prompt you to stop eating. Another type of enteric nerve picks up chemical signals about how acidic the digestive environment is or if there is protein or fat present. The CNS receives and responds to these signals, sending out a message to the pancreas to secrete enzymes for fat and protein digestion, for example.

   All along the GI tract are a series of glands that secrete digestive juice, mucus, and water. The actions of these glands are also controlled by the nervous system. When food

enteric nervous system The nerves of the GI tract.

digestion products reach various locations within the GI tract, these glands are stimulated to release digestive enzymes, mucus, or water and electrolytes. For example, as chyme moves from the stomach into the small intestine, neural signals are sent to stimulate the pancreas, gallbladder, and mucosal cells lining the intestinal tract. These signals cause these glands and cells to secrete digestive enzymes, bile, bicarbonate, and water, secretions necessary to continue digestion in the small intestine.

> RECAP: *The coordination and regulation of digestion are directed by the neuromuscular system. Voluntary muscles assist us with chewing and swallowing. Once food is swallowed, the involuntary muscles along the entire length of the GI tract function together so that materials are moved in one direction in a coordinated manner and wastes are removed as needed. The enteric nerves of the GI tract work with the central nervous system to achieve digestion, absorption, and elimination of food.*

What Disorders Are Related to Digestion, Absorption, and Elimination?

Considering the complexity of digestion, absorption, and elimination, it's no wonder that sometimes things go wrong. Clinical disorders can disturb gastrointestinal functioning, as can merely consuming the wrong types or amounts of food for our unique needs. Whenever there is a problem with the GI tract, absorption of nutrients can be affected. If absorption of a nutrient is less than optimal for a long period of time, malnutrition can result. Let's look more closely at some GI tract disorders and what you might be able to do if they affect you.

Heartburn Is Caused by Reflux of Stomach Acid

heartburn The painful sensation that occurs over the sternum when hydrochloric acid backs up into the lower esophagus.

gastroesophageal reflux disease (GERD) A painful type of heartburn that occurs more than twice per week.

When you eat food, your stomach secretes hydrochloric acid to start the digestive process. In many people, the amount of HCl secreted is occasionally excessive, or the gastroesophageal sphincter opens too soon. In either case, the result is that HCl seeps back up into the esophagus (FIGURE 3.14). Although the stomach is protected from HCl by a thick coat of mucus, the esophagus does not have this mucus coating. Thus, the HCl burns it. When this happens, a person experiences a painful sensation in the region of his or her chest above the sternum (breastbone). This condition is commonly called **heartburn.** People often take over-the-counter antacids to neutralize the HCl, thereby relieving the heartburn. A non-drug approach is to repeatedly swallow: this action causes any acid within the esophagus to be swept down into the stomach, eventually relieving the symptoms.

Gastroesophageal reflux disease (GERD) is a more painful type of heartburn that occurs more than twice per week. GERD affects about 19 million Americans and, like heartburn, occurs when HCl flows back into the esophagus. Although people who experience occasional heartburn usually have no structural abnormalities, many people with GERD have an overly relaxed or damaged esophageal sphincter or damage to the esophagus itself. Symptoms of GERD include persistent heartburn and acid regurgitation. Some people have GERD without heartburn and instead experience chest pain, trouble swallowing, burning in the mouth, the feeling that food is stuck in the throat, or hoarseness in the morning.[5]

The exact causes of GERD are unknown. However, there are a number of factors that may contribute, including the following:[5]

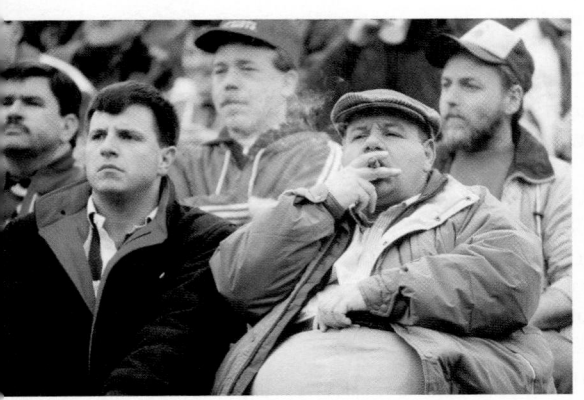

Although the exact causes of gastroesophageal reflux disease (GERD) are unknown, smoking and being overweight may be contributing factors.

- A *hiatal hernia*, which occurs when the upper part of the stomach lies above the diaphragm muscle. Normally, the horizontal diaphragm muscle separates the stomach from the chest and helps keep acid from coming into the esophagus. Stomach acid can more easily enter the esophagus in people with a hiatal hernia.

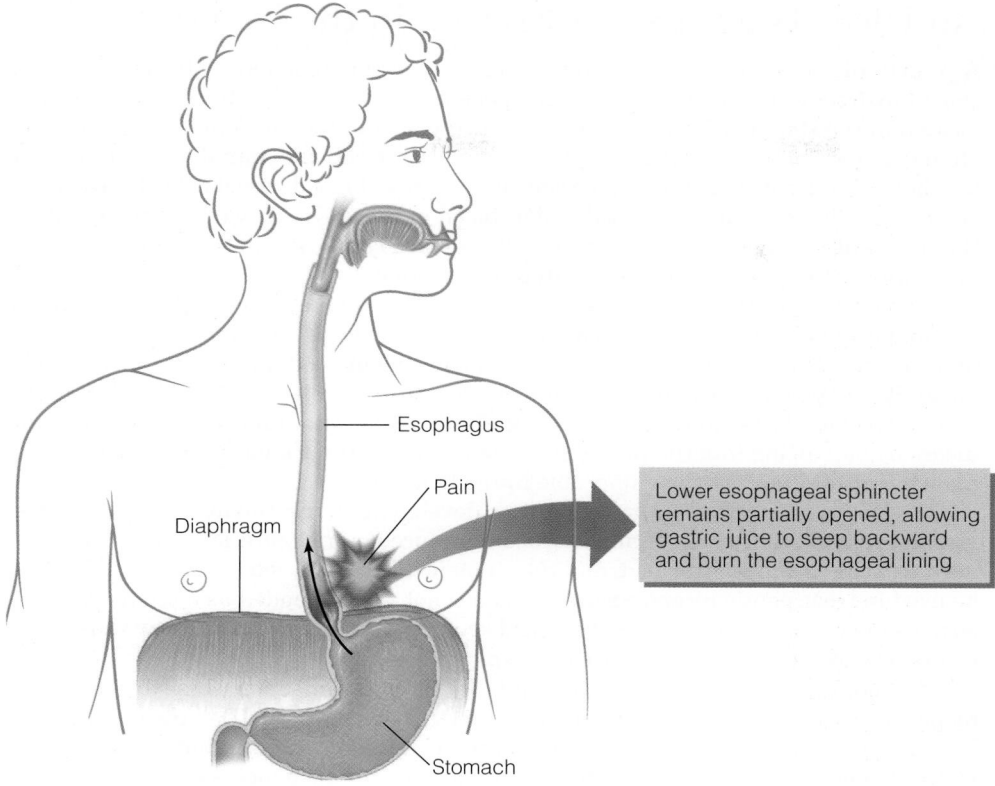

Lower esophageal sphincter remains partially opened, allowing gastric juice to seep backward and burn the esophageal lining

FIGURE 3.14 The mechanism of heartburn and gastroesophageal reflux disease is the same: acidic gastric juices seep backward through an open or relaxed sphincter into the lower portion of the esophagus, burning its lining. The pain is felt above the sternum, over the heart.

- Cigarette smoking.
- Alcohol use.
- Overweight.
- Pregnancy.
- Foods such as citrus fruits, chocolate, caffeinated drinks, fried foods, garlic and onions, spicy foods, and tomato-based foods such as chili, pizza, and spaghetti sauce.
- Large, high-fat meals. These meals stay in the stomach longer and increase stomach pressure, making it more likely that acid will be pushed up into the esophagus.
- Lying down soon after a meal. This is almost certain to bring on symptoms, since it positions the body so it is easier for the stomach acid to back up into the esophagus.

There are ways to reduce the symptoms of GERD. One way is to identify the types of foods or situations that trigger episodes, and then avoid them. Eating smaller meals also helps. After a meal, waiting at least 3 hours before lying down is recommended. Some people relieve their nighttime symptoms by elevating the head of the bed 4 to 6 inches, for instance, by placing a wedge between the mattress and the box spring. This keeps the chest area elevated and minimizes the amount of acid that can back up into the esophagus. People with GERD who smoke should stop, and if they are overweight, they should lose weight. Taking an antacid before a meal can help prevent symptoms if a person accidentally eats an offending food, and there are also many other medications now prescribed to treat GERD.

It is important to treat GERD, as it can cause serious health problems. GERD can lead to bleeding and ulcers in the esophagus. Scar tissue can develop in the esophagus, making swallowing very difficult. Some people can also develop a condition called Barrett's esophagus, which can lead to cancer. Asthma can also be aggravated or even caused by GERD.

An Ulcer Is an Area of Erosion in the GI Tract

A **peptic ulcer** is an area of the GI tract that has been eroded away by a combination of hydrochloric acid and the enzyme pepsin (FIGURE 3.15). In almost all cases, it is located in the stomach area (*gastric ulcer*) or the part of the duodenum closest to the stomach (*duodenal ulcer*). It causes a burning pain in the abdominal area, typically 1 to 3 hours after eating a meal. In serious cases, eroded blood vessels bleed into the GI tract, causing vomiting of blood and/or blood in the stools, as well as anemia. If the ulcer entirely perforates the tract wall, stomach contents can leak into the abdominal cavity, causing a life-threatening infection.

The bacterium *Helicobacter pylori* (*H. pylori*) plays a key role in the development of a majority of peptic ulcers, which include both gastric and duodenal ulcers.[6] It appears that *H. pylori* infects about 20% of people younger than 40 years of age and about 50% of people older than 60 years of age.[6] Most people with *H. pylori* infection do not develop ulcers, however, and the reason for this is not known. *H. pylori* causes ulcers by burrowing into the protective mucus coating the stomach and duodenum, allowing acid to contact the vulnerable lining beneath.

Because of the role of *H. pylori* in ulcer development, treatment usually involves antibiotics and other types of medications to reduce gastric secretions. Antacids are used to weaken the gastric acid, and the same medications used to treat GERD can be used to treat peptic ulcers. Special diets are not recommended as often as they once were because they do not reduce acid secretion. In fact, we now know that ulcers are not caused by stress or eating spicy foods.

Although most peptic ulcers are caused by *H. pylori* infection, some are caused by prolonged use of nonsteroidal anti-inflammatory drugs (NSAIDs); these drugs include pain relievers such as aspirin, ibuprofen, and naproxen sodium. Acetaminophen use does not cause ulcers. The NSAIDs appear to cause ulcers by preventing the stomach from protecting itself from acidic gastric juices. Ulcers caused by NSAID use generally heal once a person stops taking the medication.[7]

FIGURE 3.15 A peptic ulcer.

> RECAP: *Heartburn is caused by the seepage of gastric juices into the esophagus. Gastroesophageal reflux disease (or GERD) is a painful type of heartburn that occurs more than twice per week. It can cause serious health consequences such as esophageal bleeding, ulcers, and cancer. Peptic ulcers are caused by erosion of the GI tract by hydrochloric acid and pepsin. The main culprit is infection with a bacterium called* Helicobacter pylori. *Ulcers are painful and can cause internal bleeding, anemia, and potentially fatal infections.*

Some People Experience Disorders Related to Specific Foods

You check out the ingredients list on your energy bar, and you notice that it says, "Produced in a facility that processes peanuts." The package on your microwave dinner cautions: "Contains wheat, milk, and soy." Why all the warnings about these healthful foods? The reason is that, to some people, consuming these normally healthful foods can be dangerous, even life-threatening. To learn more about product labeling for potential food offenders, see the Nutrition Label Activity.

Disorders related to specific foods can be clustered into three main groupings: food intolerances, food allergies, and a genetic disorder called celiac disease. We discuss these separately.

Food Intolerance

A **food intolerance** is a cluster of GI symptoms (often gas, pain, and diarrhea) that occur following consumption of a particular food. The immune system plays no role in intolerance, and although episodes are unpleasant, they are usually transient, resolving after the offending food has been eliminated from the body. An example is lactose intolerance. It occurs in people whose bodies do not produce sufficient quantities of the enzyme lactase, which is needed for the breakdown of the milk sugar lactose. (Lactose intolerance is discussed in more detail in Chapter 4.) People can also

peptic ulcer Area of the GI tract that has been eroded away by the acidic gastric juice of the stomach. The two main causes of peptic ulcers are an *H. pylori* infection or chronic use of nonsteroidal anti-inflammatory drugs.

food intolerance Gastrointestinal discomfort caused by certain foods that is not a result of an immune system reaction.

have an intolerance to wheat, soy, and other foods, but as with lactose intolerance, the symptoms pass once the offending food is out of the person's system.

Food Allergy

A **food allergy** is a hypersensitivity reaction of the immune system to a particular component (usually a protein) in a food. This reaction causes the immune cells to release chemicals that cause either limited or systemic (whole-body) inflammation. About 5% of infants and young children and 2% of adults experience food allergies.[8] Although this makes them much less common than food intolerances, food allergies can be far more serious. Approximately 30,000 consumers require emergency room treatment and 150 Americans die each year because of allergic reactions to foods.[8]

You may have heard stories of people being allergic to foods as common as peanuts. This is the case for Liz. She was out to dinner with her parents, celebrating her birthday, when the dessert cart came around. The caramel custard looked heavenly and was probably a safe choice, but she asked the waiter just to be sure that it contained no peanuts. He checked with the chef, then returned and assured her that, no, the custard was peanut-free—but within minutes of consuming it, Liz's skin became flushed, and she struggled to breathe. As her parents were dialing 911, she lost consciousness. Fortunately, the paramedics arrived within minutes and were able to resuscitate her. It was subsequently determined that, unknown to the chef, the spoon that his prep cook had used to scoop the baked custard into serving bowls had been resting on a cutting board where he had chopped peanuts for a different dessert. Just this small exposure to peanuts was enough to cause a severe allergic reaction in Liz.

How can a food that most people consume regularly, such as peanuts, shellfish, eggs, or milk, cause another person's immune system to react so violently? In Liz's case, a trace amount of peanut stimulated immune cells throughout her body to release their inflammatory chemicals. In some people, the inflammation is localized, so the damage is limited. For instance, some people's mouth and throat itch when they eat cantaloupe, whereas others develop a rash whenever they eat eggs. What made Liz's experience so terrifyingly different was that the inflammation was widespread, affecting essentially all of her body systems and sending her into a state called *anaphylactic shock*. Left untreated, anaphylactic shock is nearly always fatal, so many people with known food allergies carry with them a kit containing an injection of a powerful stimulant called epinephrine. This drug can reduce symptoms long enough to buy the victim time to get emergency medical care.

Celiac Disease

Celiac disease, also known as *celiac sprue*, is a digestive disease that severely damages the lining of the small intestine and interferes with absorption of nutrients.[9] As in food allergy, the body's immune system causes the disorder. However, because there is a strong genetic predisposition to celiac disease, with the risk now linked to specific gene markers, it is also classified as a genetic disorder.[9]

In celiac disease, the offending food component is *gliadin*, a fraction of a protein called *gluten* that is found in wheat, rye, and barley. When people with celiac disease eat one of these grains, their immune system triggers an inflammatory response that erodes the villi of the small intestine. If the person is unaware of the disorder and continues to eat gluten, repeated immune reactions cause the villi to become greatly decreased so there is less absorptive surface area. In addition, the enzymes located at the brush border of the small intestine become reduced. As a result, the person becomes unable to absorb certain nutrients properly—a condition known as *malabsorption*. Over time malabsorption can lead to malnutrition (poor nutrient status). Deficiencies of vitamins A, D, E, and K, iron, folic acid, and calcium are common in those suffering from celiac disease, as are inadequate intakes of protein and total energy.[10]

Symptoms of celiac disease often mimic those of other intestinal disturbances like irritable bowel syndrome (discussed shortly), and so the condition is often misdiagnosed. Some of the symptoms of celiac disease include fatty stools (due to poor fat absorption); frequent stools, either watery or hard, with an odd odor; cramping;

For some people, eating a meal of grilled shrimp with peanut sauce would cause a severe allergic reaction.

food allergy An inflammatory reaction to food caused by an immune system hypersensitivity.

celiac disease A genetic disorder characterized by an inability to absorb a component of gluten called gliadin. This causes an inflammatory immune response that damages the lining of the small intestine.

For people with celiac disease, corn is a gluten-free source of carbohydrates.

anemia; pallor; weight loss; fatigue; and irritability. However, other puzzling symptoms do not appear to involve the GI tract. These include an intensely itchy rash called *dermatitis herpetiformis*, osteoporosis (poor bone density), infertility, epilepsy, anxiety, irritability, depression, and migraine headaches, among others.[10]

Diagnostic tests for celiac disease include a variety of blood tests that screen for the presence of immune proteins called antibodies, or for the genetic markers of the disease. However, the "gold standard" for diagnosis is a biopsy of the small intestine showing atrophy of the intestinal villi. Because long-term complications of undiagnosed celiac disease include an increased risk for intestinal cancer, early diagnosis can be life-saving. Unfortunately, celiac disease is currently thought to be widely underdiagnosed in the United States.[10] We'll explore some reasons for this in the Nutrition Debate on pages 114–115.

Currently there is no cure for celiac disease. Treatment is with a special diet that excludes all forms of wheat, rye, and barley. Oats are allowed, but they are often contaminated with wheat flour from processing, and even a microscopic amount of wheat can cause an immune response. The diet is especially challenging because many binding agents and other unfamiliar ingredients in processed foods are derived from gluten. Thus, nutritional counseling is essential. Fortunately, more gluten-free foods are now available, including breads made from corn, rice, tapioca, potato, arrowroot, cassava, soy, and even garbanzo bean flours.

RECAP: *Food intolerance is a condition in which a person experiences gastrointestinal discomfort following consumption of certain foods, but the symptoms are not prompted by the immune system. In contrast, both food allergies and celiac disease are caused by an immune response. Food allergies cause inflammation that results in localized problems such as skin rash or systemic problems such as life-threatening anaphylactic shock. Celiac disease is a genetic disorder that causes damage to the intestinal villi whenever an individual with the disease consumes gluten, a protein found in wheat, rye, and barley. Food allergies and celiac disease can be treated only by avoiding foods that cause the immune reactions.*

NUTRI-CASE LIZ

"I used to think of my peanut allergy as no big deal, but ever since my experience at that restaurant last year, I've been pretty obsessive about it. For months afterwards, I refused to eat anything that I hadn't prepared myself. I do eat out now, but I always insist that the chef prepare my food personally, with clean utensils, and I avoid most desserts. They're just too risky. Shopping is a lot harder too, because I have to check every label. The worst, though, is eating at my friends' houses. I have to ask them, do you keep peanuts or peanut butter in your house? Some of them are really sympathetic, but others look at me as if I'm a hypochondriac! I wish I could think of something to say to them to make them understand that this isn't something I have any control over."

What could Liz say in response to friends who don't understand the cause and seriousness of her food allergy? Do you think it would help Liz to share her fears with her doctor and to discuss possible strategies? If so, why? In addition to shopping, dining out, and eating at friends' houses, what other situations might require Liz to be cautious about her food choices?

NUTRITION LABEL ACTIVITY

Recognizing Common Allergens in Foods

Beginning on January 1, 2006, the U.S. Food and Drug Administration (FDA) required food labels to clearly identify any ingredients containing protein derived from the eight major allergenic foods.[8] Manufacturers were required to identify "in plain English" the presence of ingredients that contain protein derived from milk, eggs, fish, crustacean shellfish (crab, lobster, shrimp, and so on), tree nuts (almonds, pecans, walnuts, and so on), peanuts, wheat, soybeans

Although more than 160 foods have been identified as causing food allergies in sensitive individuals, the FDA requires labeling for only these eight foods because together they account for over 90% of all documented food allergies in the United States and represent the foods most likely to result in severe or life-threatening reactions.[11]

These eight allergenic foods must be indicated in the list of ingredients; alternatively, adjacent to the ingredients list, the label must say "Contains" followed by the name of the food. For example, the label of a product containing the milk-

derived protein casein would have to use the term "milk" in addition to the term "casein" so that those with milk allergies would clearly understand the presence of an allergen they need to avoid.[11] Any food product found to contain an undeclared allergen is subject to recall by the FDA.

Look at the ingredients list from an energy bar, shown below. How many of the FDA's eight allergenic foods does this bar contain? If you were allergic to peanuts, would you eat this bar? Would you eat it if you had celiac disease? Explain your answers.

Ingredients: Soy protein isolate, rice flour, oats, milled flaxseed, brown rice syrup, evaporated cane juice, sunflower oil, soy lecithin, cocoa, nonfat milk solids, salt.

Contains soy and dairy. May contain traces of peanuts and other nuts.

Diarrhea and Constipation

Diarrhea is the frequent passage (more than three times in 1 day) of loose, watery stools. Other symptoms may include cramping, abdominal pain, bloating, nausea, fever, and blood in the stools. Diarrhea is usually caused by an infection of the gastrointestinal tract, a chronic disease, stress, food intolerances, or reactions to medications, or a result of a bowel disorder.[12]

Acute diarrhea lasts less than 3 weeks and is usually caused by an infection from bacteria, a virus, or a parasite. Chronic diarrhea, which lasts more than 3 weeks, affects about 3% to 5% of the U.S. population and is usually caused by allergies to cow's milk, irritable bowel syndrome (discussed shortly), lactose intolerance, celiac disease, or conditions such as Crohn's disease or ulcerative colitis.

Whatever the cause, diarrhea can be harmful if it persists for a long period of time because the person can lose large quantities of water and electrolytes and become severely dehydrated. Table 3.1 reviews the signs and symptoms of dehydration, which is particularly dangerous in infants and young children. In fact, a child can die from dehydration in just a few days. Adults, particularly the elderly, can also become dangerously ill if severely dehydrated. A doctor should be seen immediately if diarrhea persists for more than 24 hours in children or more than 3 days in adults, diarrhea is bloody, fever is present, or there are signs of dehydration.

A condition referred to as *traveler's diarrhea* has become

diarrhea Condition characterized by the frequent passage of loose, watery stools.

TABLE 3.1 Signs and Symptoms of Dehydration in Adults and Children

Symptoms in Adults	Symptoms in Children
Thirst	Dry mouth and tongue
Light-headedness	No tears when crying
Less frequent urination	No wet diapers for 3 hours or more
Dark colored urine	High fever
Fatigue	Sunken abdomen, eyes, or cheeks
Dry skin	Irritable or listless
	Skin that does not flatten when pinched and released

Source: National Digestive Diseases Information Clearinghouse (NDDIC). 2001, January. Diarrhea. NIH Publication No. 01-2749. http://digestive.niddk.nih.gov/ddiseases/pubs/diarrhea/index.htm.

HIGHLIGHT

HIGHLIGHT HIGHLIGHT HIGHLIGHT HIGHLIGHT HIGHLIGHT

Traveler's Diarrhea—What Is It and How Can I Prevent It?

Diarrhea is the rapid movement of fecal matter through the large intestine, often accompanied by large volumes of water. *Traveler's diarrhea* is experienced by people traveling to countries outside of their own and is usually caused by viral or bacterial infections. Diarrhea represents the body's way of ridding itself of the invasive agent. The large intestine and even some of the small intestine become irritated by the microbes and the body's defense against them. This irritation leads to increased secretion of fluid and increased motility of the large intestine, causing watery stools and a higher than normal frequency of bowel movements.

People generally get traveler's diarrhea from consuming water or food that is contaminated with fecal matter. High-risk destinations include developing countries in Africa, Asia, Latin America, and the Middle East. Low-risk destinations include the United States, Canada, most European countries, Japan, Australia, and New Zealand. Very risky foods include any raw or undercooked fish, meats, and raw fruits and vegetables. Tap water, ice made from tap water, and unpasteurized milk and dairy products are also common sources of infection.

Traveler's diarrhea usually starts about 5 to 15 days after you arrive at your destination. Symptoms include fatigue, lack of appetite, abdominal cramps, and watery diarrhea. In some cases, you may also experience nausea, vomiting, and low-grade fever. Usually, this diarrhea passes within 4 to 6 days, and people recover completely. However, infants and toddlers, the elderly, and people with AIDS (acquired immunodeficiency syndrome), cancer, or other disorders that weaken their immune system are at greater risk for serious illness resulting from traveler's diarrhea, and these people do not recover as well. This is also true for people with digestive disorders such as celiac disease and ulcers.[13]

What can you do to prevent traveler's diarrhea? Because the primary cause is contaminated water and food,

a common health concern due to the expansion in global travel. Traveler's diarrhea is discussed in the accompanying Highlight box.

At the opposite end of the spectrum is **constipation,** which is typically defined as a condition in which no stools are passed for 2 or more days; however, it is important to recognize that some people normally experience bowel movements only every second or third day. Thus, the definition of constipation varies from one person to another. In addition to being infrequent, the stools are usually hard, small, and somewhat difficult to pass.

Constipation is frequent in people who have disorders affecting the nervous system and in which the muscles of the large bowel do not receive the appropriate neurologic signals needed for involuntary muscle movement to occur. For these individuals, drug therapy is often needed to keep the large bowel functioning.

Many people experience temporary constipation at some point in their lives in response to a variety of factors. Often people have trouble with it when they travel, when their schedule is disrupted, if they change their diet, or if they are on certain medications. Many healthcare providers suggest increasing fiber and fluid in the diet. Five to nine servings of fruits and vegetables each day and six or more servings

constipation Condition characterized by the absence of bowel movements for a period of time that is significantly longer than normal for the individual. When a bowel movement does occur, stools are usually small, hard, and difficult to pass.

HIGHLIGHT

TABLE 3.2 Foods and Beverages Linked with Traveler's Diarrhea

Foods/Beverages That Can Cause Traveler's Diarrhea	Foods/Beverages Considered Safe to Consume
Tap water	Boiled tap water
Local bottled water	Brand name bottled waters
Iced tea	Hot coffee and hot tea
Unpasteurized dairy products or juices	Wine and beer
Ice (in both alcoholic and nonalcoholic beverages)	Well-cooked foods
Undercooked or raw foods (includes meats, vegetables, and most fruits)	Fruit that can be peeled (for example, bananas and oranges)
Cooked foods that are no longer hot in temperature	
Shellfish	
Vegetables with high water content (for example, lettuce and salads)	
Food from street vendors	

Source: Stanley, S. L. 1999. Advice to travelers. In: Yamada, T., ed. *Textbook of Gastroenterology,* vol. 1, 3rd edn. Philadelphia: Lippincott Williams & Wilkins.

avoiding those identified in Table 3.2 can help reduce your risk of contracting this illness. In general, it is smart to assume that all local water and foods and beverages exposed to or cleaned with local water are contaminated and should be avoided. Brand name bottled waters, wine, beer, and beverages made with boiling water are typically safe, but beware of drinking them over ice, and wipe all bottles clean and dry before drinking from them. To render local water safe, you need to boil it; chemicals such as chlorine bleach and iodine can also be used to sterilize water, but boiling is more effective. Remember the adage "Boil it, peel it, cook it, or forget it" when making food choices. All food should be well cooked. Fruit from which the peel is removed is generally safe, but raw vegetables, including salads, should not be eaten.

If you do suffer from traveler's diarrhea, it is important to replace the fluid and nutrients lost as a result of the illness. There are specially formulated oral rehydration solutions available to help replenish vital nutrients that are lost; these solutions are available in most countries. Antibiotics may also be taken to kill bacteria. Once treatment is initiated, the diarrhea should cease within 2 to 3 days. If the diarrhea persists for more than 10 days after the initiation of treatment, or if there is blood in your stools, you should see a physician immediately to determine the cause of the diarrhea and get appropriate treatment to avoid serious medical consequences.

of whole grains is recommended. If you use breakfast cereal, make sure you buy a cereal containing at least 2 to 3 g of fiber per serving. The dietary recommendation for fiber and the role it plays in maintaining healthy elimination are discussed in detail in Chapter 4. Staying well hydrated by drinking lots of water is especially important when increasing fiber intake. Regular exercise may also help reduce the risk of constipation.

Irritable Bowel Syndrome

Irritable bowel syndrome (IBS) is a disorder that interferes with normal functions of the colon. Symptoms include abdominal cramps, bloating, and either constipation or diarrhea. It is one of the most common medical diagnoses, applied to approximately 20% of the U.S. population.[14] Three times more women than men are diagnosed with IBS, which typically first appears by early adulthood.[14]

IBS shows no sign of disease that can be observed or measured.[14] However, it appears that the colon is more sensitive to physiologic or emotional stress in people with IBS than in healthy people. Some researchers believe that the problem stems

irritable bowel syndrome A bowel disorder that interferes with normal functions of the colon. Symptoms are abdominal cramps, bloating, and constipation or diarrhea.

Consuming caffeinated drinks is one of several factors that have been linked with irritable bowel syndrome (IBS), a bowel disorder that interferes with normal functions of the colon.

from conflicting messages between the central nervous system and the enteric nervous system. The immune system may also trigger symptoms of IBS. Whatever the cause, the normal movement of the colon appears to be disrupted. In some people with IBS, food moves too quickly through the colon and fluid cannot be absorbed fast enough, which causes diarrhea. In others, the movement of the colon is too slow and too much fluid is absorbed, leading to constipation. Some of the foods thought to cause physiologic stress linked to IBS include caffeinated drinks, such as tea, coffee, and colas; foods such as chocolate, alcohol, dairy products, and wheat; and large meals.

Some women with IBS find that their symptoms worsen during their menstrual period, indicating a possible link between reproductive hormones and IBS. Certain medications may also increase the risk.

The high prevalence of the diagnosis in the United States, along with the lack of any sign of physical disease, has led to charges that IBS is overdiagnosed or misdiagnosed. Some physicians do not even agree that IBS qualifies as a disease, pointing out that the stresses of everyday life have always led to digestive problems, and probably always will.[14] Other researchers argue that U.S. physicians too often apply the diagnosis of IBS before screening for more serious disorders. In one study, 65% of patients with diarrhea-predominant IBS exhibited findings associated with celiac disease; thus, some researchers are arguing that all diarrhea-predominant IBS patients should be screened for celiac disease.[15]

If you think you have IBS, it is important to have a complete physical examination to rule out any other health problems, including celiac disease. Treatment options include certain medications to treat diarrhea or constipation, stress management, regular physical activity, eating smaller meals, avoiding foods that exacerbate symptoms, eating a higher fiber diet, and drinking at least six to eight glasses of water each day.[16] Although IBS is uncomfortable, it does not appear to endanger long-term health. However, severe IBS can be disabling and prevent people from leading normal lives; thus, accurate diagnosis and effective treatment are critical.

RECAP: *Diarrhea is the frequent passage of loose or watery stools. It should be treated quickly to avoid dehydration or even death. Constipation is failure to have a bowel movement for 2 or more days or within a time period that is normal for the individual. Irritable bowel syndrome (IBS) causes abdominal cramps, bloating, and constipation or diarrhea. The causes of IBS are unknown; however, physiologic and emotional stress is implicated.*

CHAPTER SUMMARY

- Hunger is a physiologic drive that prompts us to eat.
- In response to signals from the gastrointestinal tract and from hormones, the hypothalamus causes us to feel hungry or satiated.
- Foods that contain fiber, water, and large amounts of protein have the highest satiety value.
- Appetite is a psychological desire to consume specific foods. The most significant factors influencing our

appetite are sensory data, social and cultural cues, and learning.
- Atoms are the smallest units of matter, and they bond together to form molecules.
- The primary goal of digestion is to break food into molecules small enough to be absorbed and transported throughout the body.
- Cells are the smallest units of life. We build the billions of cells in the body from the nutrients we absorb as a result of digesting food.

- Cells are encased in a cell membrane, which acts as a gatekeeper to determine which substances go into and out of the cell.

- Cells contain a nucleus and organelles, tiny structures that perform highly sophisticated functions. Ribosomes and mitochondria are examples.

- Cells of a single type join together to form tissues. Several types of tissues join together to form organs, such as the liver.

- Organs group together to form systems that perform integrated functions. The gastrointestinal system and the central nervous system are examples.

- Digestion is the process of breaking down foods into molecules; absorption is the process of taking molecules of food into the body; and elimination is the process of removing undigested food and waste products from the body.

- Chewing starts mechanical digestion of food. Saliva contains salivary amylase, which is an enzyme that initiates the chemical digestion of carbohydrates.

- Food moves down to the stomach through the esophagus via a process called peristalsis. Peristalsis involves rhythmic waves of squeezing and pushing food through the gastrointestinal tract.

- The action of the hormone gastrin prompts the stomach to mix and churn food together with gastric juices. Hydrochloric acid and the enzyme pepsin initiate protein digestion, and a minimal amount of fat digestion begins through the action of gastric lipase.

- The stomach periodically releases the partially digested food, referred to as chyme, into the small intestine.

- Most digestion and absorption of nutrients occurs in the small intestine.

- The lining of the small intestine has thousands of folds and finger-like projections that increase the surface area over 500 times, significantly increasing its absorptive capacity.

- The gallbladder stores bile and secretes it into the small intestine to assist with the digestion of fat.

- The pancreas manufactures and secretes digestive enzymes into the small intestine. Pancreatic amylase digests carbohydrates, pancreatic lipase digests fats, and proteases digest proteins. The pancreas also synthesizes two hormones that play a critical role in carbohydrate metabolism, insulin and glucagon.

- The liver processes and stores all absorbed nutrients, alcohol, and drugs. The liver also synthesizes bile and regulates metabolism of monosaccharides, fatty acids, and amino acids.

- The large intestine digests any remaining food particles, absorbs water and chemicals, and moves feces to the rectum for elimination.

- The neuromuscular system involves coordination of the muscles, the central nervous system, and the enteric nervous system to move food along the gastrointestinal tract and to control all aspects of digestion, absorption, and elimination.

- Heartburn is caused by hydrochloric acid seeping into the esophagus and burning its lining.

- Gastroesophageal reflux disease (GERD) is a painful type of heartburn that occurs more than twice per week. GERD can cause bleeding, ulcers, and cancer of the esophagus.

- A peptic ulcer is an area in the stomach or duodenum that has been eroded by hydrochloric acid and pepsin. A bacterium, *Helicobacter pylori*, is the most common cause of peptic ulcers. Prolonged use of nonsteroidal anti-inflammatory drugs (NSAIDs) can also cause peptic ulcers.

- A food intolerance is gastrointestinal discomfort caused by foods. It is not a result of an immune system reaction. A food allergy is an inflammatory reaction to food that is caused by a hypersensitivity of the immune system.

- Celiac disease is a genetic disorder caused by an immune response to a wheat protein called gluten that damages the lining of the small intestine. Celiac disease can lead to malabsorption of nutrients and to significant malnutrition. Undiagnosed celiac disease increases the risk for certain intestinal cancers.

- Diarrhea is the frequent (more than three times per day) elimination of loose, watery stools. Diarrhea should be treated promptly to avoid dehydration.

- Constipation is a condition in which no stools are passed for 2 or more days or for a length of time considered abnormally long for the individual.

- Irritable bowel syndrome is a bowel disorder that interferes with normal functions of the colon, causing pain, diarrhea, and constipation.

TEST YOURSELF ANSWERS

1. **True.** Sometimes you may have an appetite even though you are not hungry. These feelings are referred to as "cravings" and are associated with physical or emotional cues.

2. **True.** Although there are individual variations in how we respond to food, the entire process of digestion and absorption of one meal usually takes about 24 hours.

3. **True.** Certain bacteria are normal and helpful residents of the large intestine, where they assist in digestion. They also appear to protect the tissue lining the intestinal walls and may improve immune function. Food products and supplements containing these bacteria are called *probiotics*.

4. **True.** Most ulcers result from an infection of the bacterium *Helicobacter pylori* (*H. pylori*). Contrary to popular belief, ulcers are not caused by stress or spicy food.

5. **False.** Irritable bowel syndrome is a common disorder, diagnosed in about 20% of the U.S. population. It typically appears by early adulthood.

FIND THE QUACK

Christine is heading to her favorite department store at the mall when she notices a sign at a small kiosk:

Flush Your Fat Away! New fat magnet blocks fat absorption! Lose more than a pound a day! Eat whatever you want and lose all the weight you want! Your dieting days are over!

A trim young woman in a white lab coat hands her a flyer. It says that the product is a formulation of chitosan and is made from a type of carbohydrate called chitin found in the exoskeleton of shellfish. "Chitosan," says the flyer, "will bind to fats and prevent their absorption. All the fat you eat will simply be excreted with your normal bowel movements! This will cause you to lose a lot of weight very quickly: more than a pound every day, no matter how much you eat!" The product is sold in capsules, and the daily recommended dose is five per day. A bottle of 200 capsules costs $40.

1. Do you think it is possible that four capsules of a carbohydrate substance could bind to and block the absorption of all of the fat an individual consumes throughout a day?

2. What do you think an individual would experience if all of the dietary fat eaten throughout each day were excreted in the feces?

3. Given that an individual needs to expend 3,500 more kcal than he or she consumes in order to achieve a loss of 1 pound of weight, discuss the possibility that the chitosan supplement can enable an individual to lose "more than a pound a day, no matter how much you eat."

4. How much would a consumer spend each day on the chitosan supplement if taken at the recommended dosage? Do you think the product is worth the investment? Why or why not?

Answers can be found at www.aw-bc.com/thompson.

REVIEW QUESTIONS

1. Which of the following represents the levels of organization in the human body?
   a. cells, molecules, atoms, tissues, organs, systems
   b. atoms, molecules, cells, organs, tissues, systems
   c. atoms, molecules, cells, tissues, organs, systems
   d. molecules, atoms, cells, tissues, organs, systems

2. Bile is a greenish fluid that
   a. is stored by the pancreas.
   b. is produced by the gallbladder.
   c. denatures proteins.
   d. emulsifies fats.

3. The region of brain tissue that is responsible for prompting us to seek food is the
   a. pituitary gland.
   b. cephalic phase.
   c. hypothalamus.
   d. peripheral nervous system.

4. Heartburn is caused by
   a. seepage of gastric acid into the esophagus.
   b. seepage of gastric acid into the cardiac muscle.
   c. seepage of bile into the stomach.
   d. seepage of salivary amylase into the stomach.

5. Most digestion of carbohydrates, fats, and proteins takes place in the
   a. mouth.
   b. stomach.
   c. small intestine.
   d. large intestine.

6. True or false? Hunger is more physiologic, and appetite is more psychologic.

7. True or false? The nerves of the GI tract are collectively known as the enteric nervous system.

8. True or false? Vitamins and minerals are digested in the small intestine.

9. True or false? A person with celiac disease cannot tolerate milk or milk products.

10. True or false? Atoms are the smallest units of life.

11. Explain why it is true that you are what you eat.

12. Identify the type of remedy most commonly prescribed to treat a peptic ulcer.

13. Imagine that the lining of your small intestine were smooth, like the inside of a rubber tube. Would this design be efficient in performing the main function of this organ? Why or why not?

14. Why doesn't the acidic environment of the stomach cause it to digest itself?

15. After dinner, your roommate lies down to rest for a few minutes before studying. When he gets up, he complains of a sharp, burning pain in his chest. Offer a possible explanation for his pain.

WEB LINKS

http://digestive.niddk.nih.gov
National Digestive Diseases Information Clearinghouse (NDDIC)

Explore this site to learn more about diarrhea, celiac disease, irritable bowel syndrome (IBS), heartburn, and gastroesophageal reflux disease (GERD).

www.nlm.nih.gov/medlineplus
MEDLINE Plus Health Information

Search for "food allergies" to obtain additional resources as well as the latest news about food allergies.

www.healthfinder.gov
Health Finder

Search this site to learn more about disorders related to digestion, absorption, and elimination.

www.ific.org
International Food Information Council Foundation (IFIC)

Scroll down to "Food Safety Information" and click on the link for "Food Allergies and Asthma" for additional information on food allergies.

www.foodallergy.org
The Food Allergy and Anaphylaxis Network (FAN)

Visit this site to learn more about common food allergens.

www.americanceliac.org/cd.htm
American Celiac Disease Alliance

Learn more about the diagnosis and treatment of celiac disease, ongoing research, and living with celiac disease.

www.csaceliacs.org
Celiac Sprue Association—National Celiac Disease Support Group

Get information on the Celiac Sprue Association, a national educational organization that provides information and referral services for persons with celiac disease.

www.gfmall.com
Gluten-Free Mall

Find out where you can buy gluten-free products.

www.ibsgroup.org
Irritable Bowel Syndrome Self-Help and Support Group

Visit this site for information on self-help measures and support for people diagnosed with IBS.

REFERENCES

1. Orr, J., and B. Davy. 2005. Dietary influences on peripheral hormones regulating energy intake: potential applications for weight management. *J. Am. Diet. Assoc.* 105:1115–1124.
2. Gardner, S. L., and E. Goldson. 2002. The neonate and the environment: impact on development. In: Merenstein, G. G., and S. L. Gardner, eds. *Handbook of Neonatal Intensive Care*, 5th ed., pp. 219–282. St. Louis: Mosby.
3. Marieb, E., and K. Hoehn. 2007. *Human Anatomy and Physiology*, 7th edn., p. 582. San Francisco: Benjamin Cummings.
4. Davidson, N. O. 2003. Intestinal lipid absorption. In: Yamada, T., D. H. Alpers, N. Kaplowitz, L. Laine, C. Owyang, and D. W. Powell, eds. *Textbook of Gastroenterology,* vol. 1, 4th edn. Philadelphia: Lippincott Williams & Wilkins.
5. National Digestive Diseases Information Clearinghouse (NDDIC). 2003. Heartburn, Hiatal Hernia, and Gastroesophageal Reflux Disease (GERD). NIH Publication No. 03-0882. http://digestive.niddk.nih.gov/ddiseases/pubs/gerd/index.htm. (Accessed March 2007.)
6. National Digestive Diseases Information Clearinghouse (NDDIC). 2004. *H. pylori* and Peptic Ulcer. NIH Publication No. 05-4225. http://digestive.niddk.nih.gov/ddiseases/pubs/hpylori/.
7. National Digestive Diseases Information Clearinghouse (NDDIC). 2002. NSAIDs and Peptic Ulcers. NIH Publication No. 02-4644. Available at http://digestive.niddk.nih.gov/ddiseases/pubs/nsaids/index.htm.
8. U.S. Food and Drug Administration (FDA). December 20, 2005. FDA to Require Food Manufacturers to List Food Allergens. FDA News. www.fda.gov/bbs/topics/NEWS/2005/NEW01281.html.
9. National Digestive Diseases Information Clearinghouse (NDDIC). October 2005. Celiac Disease. NIH Publication No. 06-4269. http://digestive.niddk.nih.gov.
10. National Institutes of Health. June 2004. NIH Consensus Development Conference on Celiac Disease. http://consensus.nih.gov/2004/2004CeliacDisease118html.htm.
11. U.S. Food and Drug Administration (FDA). July 18, 2006. Information for Consumers: Food Allergen Labeling and Consumer Protection Act of 2004 Questions and Answers. www.cfsan.fda.gov/~dms/alrgqa.html.
12. National Digestive Diseases Information Clearinghouse (NDDIC). 2003. Diarrhea. NIH Publication No. 04-2749. http://digestive.niddk.nih.gov/ddiseases/pubs/diarrhea/index.htm.
13. DuPont, H. L. 2006. New insights and directions in traveler's diarrhea. *Gastroenterol. Clin. N. Am.* 35(2):337–353, viii–ix.
14. Lewis, C. July–August 2001. Irritable Bowel Syndrome: A Poorly Understood Disorder. *FDA Consumer Magazine.* www.fda.gov/fdac/features/2001/401_ibs.html.
15. National Institutes of Health. March 12, 2002. Celiac Disease Meeting Summary. DDICC Meeting Minutes. http://digestive.niddk.nih.gov/federal/ddicc/minutes_3-12-02.pdf.
16. National Digestive Diseases Information Clearinghouse (NDDIC). 2003, April. Irritable Bowel Syndrome. NIH Publication No. 03-693. http://digestive.niddk.nih.gov/ddiseases/pubs/ibs/index.htm.
17. Ladewig, P., M. London, and M. Davidson. 2006. *Contemporary Maternal-Newborn Nursing Care*, 6th edn., p. 655. Upper Saddle River, NJ: Pearson Prentice Hall.
18. Early, E. 2003. Celiac Disease More Prevalent in Diabetic Children. Medical College of Wisconsin. http://healthlink.mcw.edu/article/1009402816.html.

NUTRITION DEBATE

Should All School-Age Children Be Screened for Celiac Disease?

a *screening test* is a diagnostic procedure that elicits data about the presence or absence of characteristic signs of a disorder. Every baby born in a U.S. hospital undergoes at least two screening tests within the first 48 hours of life.[17] These are for the metabolic disorder phenylketonuria, discussed in Chapter 4, and hypothyroidism, a disorder affecting the thyroid gland. Most school-age children in the United States are also screened for vision and hearing problems, learning disorders, excessive sleepiness, head lice, and other problems. With all this screening going on, should school-age children also be screened for celiac disease?

Researchers and healthcare professionals in favor of screening children for celiac disease point to several factors in support of their position. First, the prevalence in the United States is high enough to be of general concern: from 0.5% to 1% of the U.S. population, or 1 in every 100 to 200 Americans, is believed to have celiac disease. This is in line with prevalence rates in Europe, where celiac disease is the most common genetic disease.[10]

In addition, celiac disease is thought to be greatly underdiagnosed. Three reasons for this include the following: many doctors and healthcare providers in the United States are not knowledgeable about celiac disease; only a small number of U.S. laboratories are experienced and skilled in testing for celiac disease; and celiac symptoms can be attributed to other problems.[9] Although in many

people celiac disease presents as a "classic" syndrome of diarrhea, weight loss, abdominal bloating, and excessive intestinal gas, the symptoms are in reality highly variable, with some patients experiencing constipation, vomiting, or abdominal pain. In people with neurologic and other nondigestive symptoms, celiac disease may never even be considered without routine, population-wide screening. Moreover, general screening both in Europe and in limited studies in the United States reveals a significant prevalence of "silent celiac disease"; that is, the individual is not aware of having symptoms, but has a positive antibody test and upon biopsy is shown to have atrophy of the intestinal villi. Although asymptomatic, the intestinal damage in these people puts them at risk for all of the complications of untreated celiac disease, including malnutrition and GI cancers. In Italy, where the prevalence of celiac disease is about 1 in 250 people, all children are screened by age 6 so that even asymptomatic disease is caught early.[18] In addition, some U.S. researchers are recommending that all children with type 1 diabetes be screened for celiac disease, as an association between the two diseases has been recognized for some time. A recent U.S. study showed that at least 4.6% of children with type 1 diabetes also have celiac disease.[18] Many children with Down syndrome are screened; in these children the prevalence is 5–12%.[10]

Further considerations in favor of routine screening are the potentially serious consequences of a missed diagnosis. In children, short stature results when childhood celiac disease prevents nutrient absorption during the years when nutrition is critical to a child's normal growth and development.[9] Children who are diagnosed and treated before their growth period ends may be able to catch up to the growth of their peers, but after that time, the short stature is irreversible. Other possible consequences of a missed diagnosis include an increased risk of depression, anxiety, learning disorders, epilepsy, autoimmune disorders, type 1 diabetes, thyroid disease, liver disease, poor bone density, and GI cancers.[9]

Finally, a simple blood test that is highly sensitive and specific to antibodies produced in celiac disease is available. Routine screening would provide a financial incentive for laboratories to make the antibody test more widely available, benefiting all Americans.

Arguments against routine testing center on the invasiveness and questions of reliability of the available tests. Unlike the screening tests for vision, hearing, or head lice, the antibody test for celiac disease is invasive, requiring that the healthcare provider draw a small amount of

School children may have celiac disease and not know it. Undiagnosed celiac disease can lead to physical and mental disorders as children grow.

blood. Some families object to invasive medical tests for religious or other reasons. Second, although the antibody test is considered generally reliable for diagnosing celiac disease, false negatives are not uncommon. Indeed, the reliability of the test for children younger than 5 is controversial.[9] The only definitive proof of celiac disease is via a biopsy of the small intestine that shows atrophy of the villi. Since few people would argue that all children should undergo a biopsy, should routine screening wait until a reliable but noninvasive test is developed?

Another area of controversy exists over the benefit of identifying people with "latent celiac disease," that is, people who test positive with the antibody screen but do not currently have symptoms or any damage to the intestinal villi. Do these people need to go on the highly restrictive gluten-free diet? Because current data do not indicate a clear benefit of a gluten-free diet in people with latent disease, this question is the subject of debate.[10]

Finally, the concept of routine screening itself is a matter of some controversy. While few would argue against simple, low-cost screening tests such as those for vision or hearing problems, some people hesitate when tests become more costly. The United States does not currently require screening of all children for type 1 or type 2 diabetes, obesity, or many other serious health problems, so why should the public be burdened with screening for celiac disease?

In 2004, the National Institutes of Health Consensus Development Conference on Celiac Disease concluded that, at this time, there are insufficient data to recommend routine screening for celiac disease. Instead, the Conference recommended further research into the benefits and cost-effectiveness of screening in the general population. Ongoing with this research, the Conference recommends heightened awareness of the disease: education of physicians, registered dietitians, and other health-care providers is imperative.[10]

Now that you've read the arguments for and against routine screening of American children for celiac disease, do you think that all children should have the test? Why or why not? If you voted yes, who should pay for it? Parents? School districts? The public health department? Given the number of children who are homeschooled or in private schools, how could we ensure that all families were offered screening? Would you be in favor of routine screening of children for type 2 diabetes, hypertension, obesity, and other disorders? What factors seem most important to consider when deciding which diseases we screen for in American children?

A simple blood test can identify celiac disease.

CHAPTER 4

CHAPTER OBJECTIVES

After reading this chapter you will be able to:

1. Describe the difference between simple and complex carbohydrates, pp. 118–124.

2. List four functions of carbohydrates in our bodies, pp. 124–126.

3. Discuss how carbohydrates are digested and absorbed by our bodies, pp. 128–130.

4. Define the Acceptable Macronutrient Distribution Range for carbohydrates, the Adequate Intake for fiber, and the recommended intake of added sugars, pp. 134–137.

5. Identify the potential health risks associated with diets high in simple sugars, pp. 135–137.

6. List five foods that are good sources of carbohydrates, pp. 140–141.

7. Identify at least three alternative sweeteners, pp. 143–146.

8. Describe type 1 and type 2 diabetes, and discuss how diabetes differs from hypoglycemia, pp. 146–151.

TEST YOURSELF TRUE OR FALSE?

1. Type 2 diabetes is typically only seen in adults. T or F

2. Diets high in sugar cause hyperactivity in children and diabetes. T or F

3. Carbohydrates are fattening. T or F

4. Carbohydrates are the primary fuel source for our brain and body tissues. T or F

5. Alternative sweeteners, such as aspartame, are safe for us to consume. T or F

Test Yourself answers can be found after the Chapter Summary.

Carbohydrates: Plant-Derived Energy Nutrients

i t was a typical day at a large medical center in the Bronx, New York: two patients were having toes amputated, another had nerve damage, one was being treated for kidney failure, another for infection, and another was blind. Despite their variety, these problems were due to just one disease: diabetes. On an average day, nearly half of the inpatients at the medical center have diabetes. And the problem isn't limited to the Bronx. Every day in the United States, 230 people with diabetes have surgery to remove toes, a foot, or an entire leg; 120 people with diabetes enter the final stage of kidney disease; and 55 go blind. A little over a decade ago, these complications, which typically develop about 10 to 15 years after the onset of the disease, were rarely seen in people younger than age 60. But now, as more and more children are being diagnosed with diabetes, experts are predicting that the typical patient will be more like Iris, one of the patients with diabetes at the Bronx medical center this day. Iris is 26 years old.[1]

What is diabetes, and why are we discussing it in a chapter on carbohydrates? Does the consumption of carbohydrates somehow lead to diabetes—or, for that matter, to obesity or any other disorder? Several popular diets—including the Zone Diet, Sugar Busters, and Dr. Atkins' New Diet Revolution—claim that carbohydrates are bad for your health and advocate reducing carbohydrate consumption and increasing protein and fat intake.[2-4] Should we reduce our intake of carbohydrates? If you noticed that a friend regularly consumed four or five soft drinks a day, plus chips, cookies, candy, and other high-carbohydrate snacks, would you say anything? Are carbohydrates a health menace, and is one type of carbohydrate as bad as another?

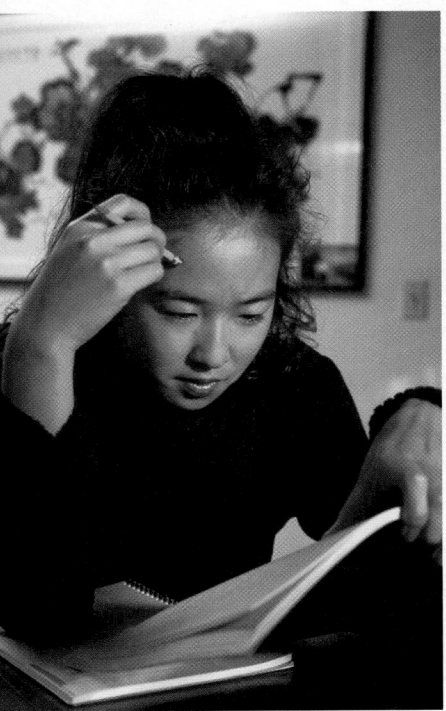

In our bodies, glucose is the preferred source of energy for the brain.

In this chapter, we explore the differences between simple and complex carbohydrates and learn why some carbohydrates are better than others. We also learn how the human body breaks down carbohydrates and uses them to maintain our health and to fuel our activity and exercise. Because carbohydrate metabolism sometimes does go wrong, we'll also discuss its relationship to some common health disorders.

What Are Carbohydrates?

As we mentioned in Chapter 1, **carbohydrates** are one of the three macronutrients. As such, they are an important energy source for the entire body and are the preferred energy source for nerve cells, including those of the brain. We will say more about their functions later in this chapter.

The term *carbohydrate* literally means "hydrated carbon." You know that water (H_2O) is made of hydrogen and oxygen, and that when something is said to be *hydrated*, it contains water. Thus, the chemical abbreviation for carbohydrate (CHO) indicates the atoms it contains: **c**arbon, **h**ydrogen, and **o**xygen.

We obtain carbohydrates predominantly from plant foods such as fruits, vegetables, and grains. Plants make the most abundant form of carbohydrate, called **glucose,** through a process called **photosynthesis.** During photosynthesis, the green pigment of plants, called *chlorophyll*, absorbs sunlight, which provides the energy needed to fuel the manufacture of glucose. As shown in FIGURE 4.1, water absorbed from the earth by the plants' roots combines with carbon dioxide present in the leaves to produce the carbohydrate glucose. Plants continually store glucose and use it to support their own growth. Then, when we eat plant foods, our bodies digest, absorb, and use the stored glucose.

> RECAP: *Carbohydrates are one of the three macronutrient types that provide energy to our bodies. Carbohydrates contain carbon, hydrogen, and oxygen. Plants make one type of carbohydrate, glucose, through the process of photosynthesis.*

What's the Difference Between Simple and Complex Carbohydrates?

Carbohydrates can be classified as *simple* or *complex*. Simple carbohydrates contain either one or two molecules, while complex carbohydrates contain hundreds to thousands of molecules.

Simple Carbohydrates Include Monosaccharides and Disaccharides

Simple carbohydrates are commonly referred to as *sugars*. Three of these sugars are called **monosaccharides** because they consist of a single sugar molecule (*mono*-meaning "one," and *saccharide* meaning "sugar"). The other three sugars are **disaccharides,** which consist of two molecules of sugar joined together (*di* meaning "two").

Glucose, Fructose, and Galactose Are Monosaccharides

Glucose, fructose, and *galactose* are the three most common monosaccharides in our diet. Each of these monosaccharides contains six carbon atoms, twelve hydrogen atoms, and six oxygen atoms (FIGURE 4.2). Very slight differences in the structure of the molecules in these three monosaccharides cause major differences in their level of sweetness.

Given what you've just learned about how plants manufacture glucose, it probably won't surprise you to discover that glucose is the most abundant sugar molecule found in our diets and in our bodies. Glucose does not generally occur by itself in foods but attaches to other sugars to form disaccharides and complex carbohydrates.

carbohydrate One of the three macronutrients, a compound made up of carbon, hydrogen, and oxygen that is derived from plants and provides energy.

glucose The most abundant sugar molecule, a monosaccharide generally found in combination with other sugars. The preferred source of energy for the brain and an important source of energy for all cells.

photosynthesis Process by which plants use sunlight to fuel a chemical reaction that combines carbon and water into glucose, which is then stored in their cells.

simple carbohydrate Commonly called *sugar;* a monosaccharide or disaccharide such as glucose.

monosaccharide The simplest of carbohydrates. Consists of one sugar molecule, the most common form of which is glucose.

disaccharide A carbohydrate compound consisting of two sugar molecules joined together.

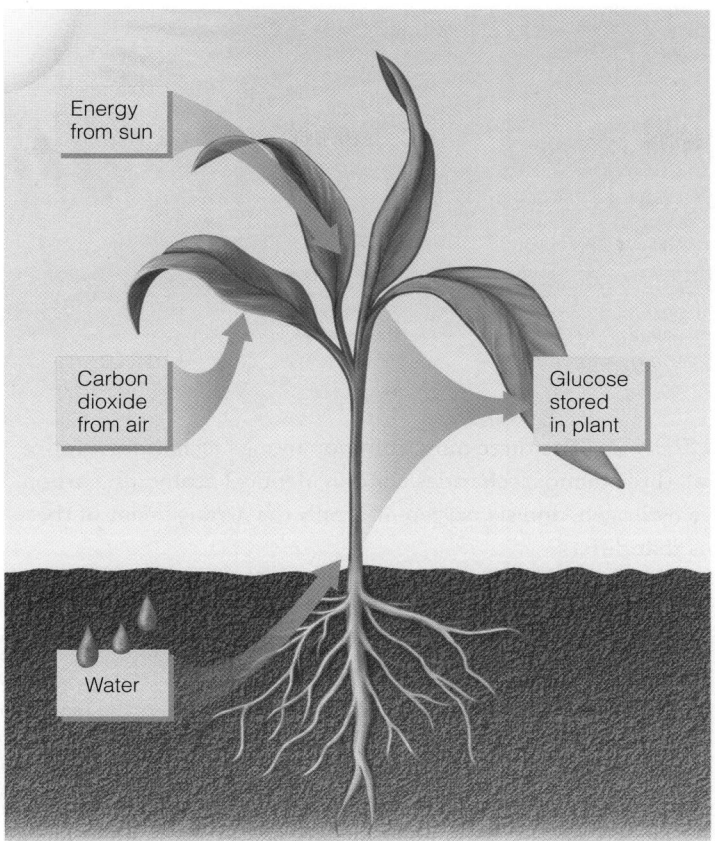

FIGURE 4.1 Plants make carbohydrates through the process of photosynthesis. Water, carbon dioxide, and energy from the sun are combined to produce glucose.

In our bodies, glucose is the preferred source of energy for the brain, and it is a very important source of energy for all cells.

Fructose, the sweetest natural sugar, is found in fruits and vegetables. Fructose is also called *levulose*, or *fruit sugar*. In many processed foods, it comes in the form of *high-fructose corn syrup*. This syrup is manufactured from corn and is used to sweeten soft drinks, desserts, candies, and jellies.

Galactose does not occur alone in foods. It joins with glucose to create lactose, one of the three most common disaccharides.

Lactose, Maltose, and Sucrose Are Disaccharides

The three most common disaccharides found in foods are *lactose*, *maltose*, and *sucrose* (FIGURE 4.3). **Lactose** (also called *milk sugar*) consists of one glucose molecule and one galactose molecule. Interestingly, human breast milk has a higher amount of lactose than cow's milk, which makes human breast milk taste sweeter.

Maltose (also called *malt sugar*) consists of two molecules of glucose. It does not generally occur by itself in foods, but rather is bound together with other molecules. As our bodies break these larger molecules down, maltose results as a by-product. Maltose is also the sugar that is fermented during the production of beer and liquor products. Contrary to popular belief, very little maltose remains in alcoholic beverages after the fermentation process is complete; thus, alcoholic beverages are not good sources of carbohydrate.

Sucrose is composed of one glucose molecule and one fructose molecule. Because sucrose contains fructose, it is sweeter than lactose or maltose. Sucrose provides much of the sweet taste found in honey, maple syrup, fruits, and vegetables. Table sugar, brown sugar, powdered sugar, and many other products are made by refining the sucrose found in sugarcane and sugar beets. You will learn more about the different forms of sucrose commonly used in foods later in this chapter. Are naturally

fructose The sweetest natural sugar; a monosaccharide that occurs in fruits and vegetables. Also called *levulose,* or *fruit sugar.*

galactose A monosaccharide that joins with glucose to create lactose, one of the three most common disaccharides.

lactose Also called *milk sugar,* a disaccharide consisting of one glucose molecule and one galactose molecule. Found in milk, including human breast milk.

maltose A disaccharide consisting of two molecules of glucose. Does not generally occur independently in foods but results as a by-product of digestion. Also called *malt sugar.*

sucrose A disaccharide composed of one glucose molecule and one fructose molecule. Sweeter than lactose or maltose.

FIGURE 4.2 The three most common monosaccharides. Notice that all three monosaccharides contain identical atoms: six carbon, twelve hydrogen, and six oxygen. It is only the arrangement of these atoms that differs.

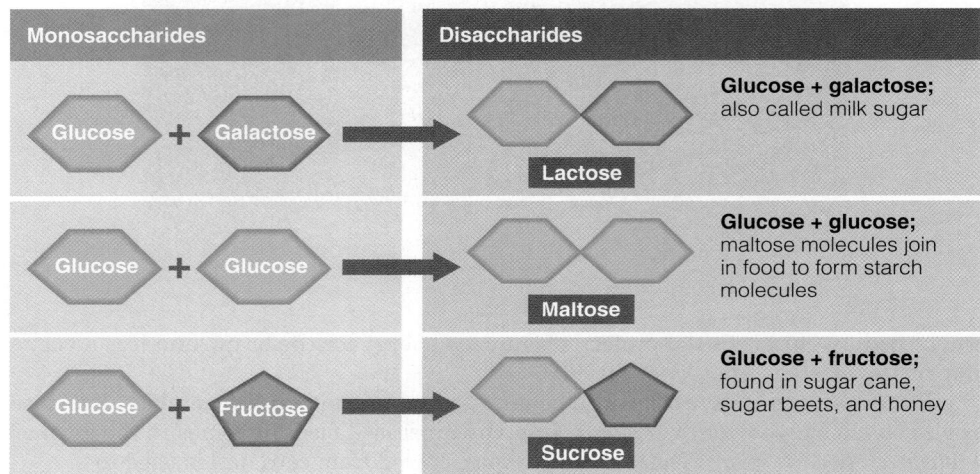

FIGURE 4.3 Galactose, glucose, and fructose join together to make the disaccharides lactose, maltose, and sucrose.

occurring forms of sucrose more healthful than manufactured forms? The Nutrition Myth or Fact? box on page 122 investigates the common belief that honey is more nutritious than table sugar.

RECAP: *Simple carbohydrates include monosaccharides and disaccharides. Glucose, fructose, and galactose are monosaccharides; lactose, maltose, and sucrose are disaccharides.*

complex carbohydrate A nutrient compound consisting of long chains of glucose molecules, such as starch, glycogen, and fiber.

polysaccharide A complex carbohydrate consisting of long chains of glucose.

All Complex Carbohydrates Are Polysaccharides

Complex carbohydrates, the second major type of carbohydrate, generally consist of long chains of glucose molecules. The technical name for complex carbohydrates is **polysaccharides** (*poly* meaning "many"). They include starch, glycogen, and most fibers (FIGURE 4.4).

FIGURE 4.4 Polysaccharides, also referred to as complex carbohydrates, include starch, glycogen, and fiber.

Tubers, such as these sweet potatoes, are excellent food sources of starch.

Starch Is a Polysaccharide Stored in Plants

Plants store glucose not as single molecules, but as polysaccharides in the form of **starch.** Excellent food sources of starch include grains (wheat, rice, corn, oats, and barley), legumes (peas, beans, and lentils), and tubers (potatoes and yams). Our cells cannot use the complex starch molecules exactly as they occur in plants. Instead, our bodies must break them down into the monosaccharide glucose, from which we can then fuel our energy needs.

Our bodies easily digest most starches; however, some starch in plants is not digestible and is called *resistant*. When our intestinal bacteria try to digest resistant starch, a fatty acid called *butyrate* is produced. Consuming resistant starch may be beneficial because some research suggests that butyrate consumption reduces the risk of cancer.[5] Legumes contain more resistant starch than do grains, fruits, or vegetables. This quality, plus their high protein and fiber content, makes legumes a healthful food.

Glycogen Is a Polysaccharide Stored by Animals

Glycogen is the storage form of glucose for animals, including humans. Very little glycogen exists in food; thus, glycogen is not a dietary source of carbohydrate. We can break down glycogen very quickly into glucose when we need it for energy. We store glycogen in our muscles and liver; the storage and use of glycogen are discussed in more detail on page 129.

Fiber Is a Polysaccharide That Gives Plants Their Structure

Like starch, fiber is composed of long polysaccharide chains; however, the body does not easily break down the bonds that connect fiber molecules. This means that most fibers pass through the digestive system without being digested and absorbed, so they contribute no energy to our diet. However, fiber offers many other health benefits, as we will see shortly (page 127).

There are currently a number of definitions of fiber. Recently, the Food and Nutrition Board of the Institute of Medicine has proposed three distinctions: *dietary fiber, functional fiber*, and *total fiber*.[6] **Dietary fiber** is the nondigestible parts of plants that form the support structures of leaves, stems, and seeds (see FIGURE 4.4). In a sense, you can think of dietary fiber as the plant's "skeleton." **Functional fiber** consists of nondigestible forms of carbohydrates that are extracted from plants or

starch A polysaccharide stored in plants; the storage form of glucose in plants.

glycogen A polysaccharide stored in animals; the storage form of glucose in animals.

dietary fiber The nondigestible carbohydrate parts of plants that form the support structures of leaves, stems, and seeds.

functional fiber The nondigestible forms of carbohydrate that are extracted from plants or manufactured in the laboratory and have known health benefits.

NUTRITION MYTH OR FACT?

Is Honey More Nutritious Than Table Sugar?

Liz's friend Tiffany is dedicated to eating healthful foods. She advises Liz to avoid sucrose and to eat foods that contain honey, molasses, or raw sugar. Like many people, Tiffany believes these sweeteners are more natural and nutritious than refined table sugar. How can Liz sort sugar fact from fiction?

Remember that sucrose consists of one glucose molecule and one fructose molecule joined together. From a chemical perspective, honey is almost identical to sucrose, since honey also contains glucose and fructose molecules in almost equal amounts. However, enzymes in bees' "honey stomachs" separate some of the glucose and fructose molecules, resulting in honey looking and tasting slightly different from sucrose. As you know, bees store honey in combs and fan it with their wings to reduce its moisture content. This also alters the appearance and texture of honey.

Honey does not contain any more nutrients than sucrose, so it is not a more healthful choice than sucrose. In fact, per tablespoon, honey has more calories (or energy) than table sugar. This is because the crystals in table sugar take up more space on a spoon than the liquid form of honey, so a tablespoon contains less sugar. However, some people argue that honey is sweeter, so you use less.

It is important to note that honey commonly contains bacteria that can cause fatal food poisoning in infants. The more mature digestive system of older children and adults is immune to the effects of these bacteria, but babies younger than 12 months should never be given honey.

Are raw sugar and molasses more healthful than table sugar? Actually, the "raw sugar" available in the United States is not really raw. Truly raw sugar is made up of the first crystals obtained when sugar is processed. Sugar in this form contains dirt, parts of insects, and other by-products that make it illegal to sell in the United States. The raw sugar products in American stores have actually gone through more than half of the same steps in the refining process used to make table sugar. Raw sugar has a more coarse texture than white sugar and is unbleached; in most markets it is also significantly more expensive.

Molasses is the syrup that remains when sucrose is made from sugarcane. It is reddish brown in color with a distinctive taste that is less sweet than table sugar. It does contain some iron, but this iron does not occur naturally. It is a contaminant from the machines that process the sugarcane! Incidentally, blackstrap molasses is the residue of a third boiling of the syrup. It contains less sugar than light or dark molasses but more minerals.

Table 4.1 compares the nutrient content of white sugar, honey, blackstrap molasses, and raw sugar. As you can see, none of them contain many nutrients that are important for health. This is why highly sweetened products are referred to as "empty calories."

---

manufactured in a laboratory and have known health benefits. Functional fiber is added to foods during processing and is the form used in fiber supplements. **Total fiber** is the sum of dietary fiber and functional fiber.

Fiber can also be classified according to its chemical and physical properties as soluble or insoluble. **Soluble fibers** dissolve in water. They are also **viscous,** forming a gel when wet, and they are fermentable; that is, they are easily digested by bacteria in the colon. Soluble fibers are typically found in citrus fruits, berries, oat products, and beans.

Research suggests that regular consumption of soluble fibers reduces the risks for cardiovascular disease and type 2 diabetes by lowering blood cholesterol and blood glucose levels. The exact mechanism by which soluble fibers decrease blood cholesterol is not known. They may reduce the absorption of dietary cholesterol from the intestine, which would directly lower blood cholesterol. They may also reduce the

total fiber The sum of dietary fiber and functional fiber.

soluble fibers Fibers that dissolve in water.

viscous Term referring to a gel-like consistency; viscous fibers form a gel when dissolved in water.

TABLE 4.1 Nutrient Comparison of Four Different Sugars

	Table Sugar	Raw Sugar	Honey	Molasses
Energy (kcal)	49	48.8	64	58
Carbohydrate (g)	12.60	12.6	17.3	14.95
Fat (g)	0	0	0	0.02
Protein (g)	0	0	0.06	0
Fiber (grams)	0	0	0	0
Vitamin C (mg)	0	0	0.1	0
Vitamin A (IU)	0	0	0	0
Thiamin (mg)	0	0	0	0.008
Riboflavin (mg)	0.002	0.003	0.008	0
Folate (µg)	0	0	0	0
Calcium (mg)	0	0.042	1	41
Iron (mg)	0	0	0.09	0.94
Sodium (mg)	0	0	1	7
Potassium (mg)	0	0.25	11	293

Source: U.S. Department of Agriculture, Agricultural Research Service. 2006. USDA National Nutrient Database for Standard Reference, Release 19. Nutrient Data Laboratory Home Page, http://www.ars.usda.gov/ba/bhnrc/ndl.
Note: Nutrient values are identified for one tablespoon of each product.

absorption of bile acids from the intestine, which would force the liver to synthesize more cholesterol to meet the need for bile acids. Increased synthesis would require the removal of more cholesterol from the blood and thereby indirectly reduce blood cholesterol levels. Soluble fibers are known to decrease the absorption of dietary fat and carbohydrate, which could decrease blood lipid concentrations in general and also decrease blood glucose levels.

Examples of soluble fibers include the following:

- *Pectins* contain chains of galacturonic acid and other monosaccharides. Pectins are found in the cell walls and intracellular tissues of many fruits and berries. They can be isolated and used to thicken foods such as jams and yogurts.

- *Gums* contain galactose, glucuronic acid, and other monosaccharides. Gums are a diverse group of polysaccharides that are viscous. They are typically isolated from seeds and are used as thickening, gelling, and stabilizing agents. Guar gum and gum arabic are common gums used as food additives.

- *Mucilages* are similar to gums and contain galactose, mannose, and other mono-saccharides. Two examples include psyllium and carrageenan. Psyllium is the husk of psyllium seeds, which are also known as plantago or flea seeds. Carrageenan comes from seaweed. Mucilages are used as food stabilizers.

Insoluble fibers are those that do not typically dissolve in water. These fibers are usually nonviscous and typically cannot be fermented by bacteria in the colon. Insoluble fibers are generally found in whole grains such as wheat, rye, and brown rice and are also found in many vegetables. These fibers are not associated with reducing cholesterol levels but are known for promoting regular bowel movements,

Dissolvable laxatives can be examples of soluble fibers.

insoluble fibers Fibers that do not dissolve in water.

alleviating constipation, and reducing the risk for diverticulosis (discussed later in this chapter). Examples of insoluble fibers include the following:

- *Lignins* are noncarbohydrate forms of fiber. Lignins are found in the woody parts of plant cell walls and are also in carrots and in the seeds of fruits and berries. Lignins are also found in brans (or the outer husk of grains such as wheat, oats, and rye) and other whole grains.

- *Cellulose* is the main structural component of plant cell walls. Cellulose is a chain of glucose units similar to amylose, but unlike amylose, cellulose contains bonds that are nondigestible by humans. Cellulose is found in whole grains, fruits, vegetables, and legumes. It can also be extracted from wood pulp or cotton, and it is added to foods as an agent for anticaking, thickening, and texturizing of foods.

- *Hemicelluloses* contain glucose, mannose, galacturonic acid, and other monosaccharides. Hemicelluloses are found in plant cell walls and they surround cellulose. They are the primary component of cereal fibers and are found in whole grains and vegetables. Although many hemicelluloses are insoluble, some are also classified as soluble.

As you can see from these definitions of fiber, good food sources include oat and wheat brans, oats, wheat, rye, barley, brown rice, seeds, legumes, fruits, and vegetables. Examples of functional fiber sources you might see on nutrition labels include cellulose, guar gum, pectin, and psyllium.

> RECAP: *All complex carbohydrates are polysaccharides. They include starch, glycogen, and fiber. Starch is the storage form of glucose in plants, while glycogen is the storage form of glucose in animals. Fiber forms the support structures of plants; soluble fibers dissolve in water, are viscous, and can be digested by bacteria in the colon, whereas insoluble fibers do not dissolve in water, are not viscous, and cannot be digested.*

Our red blood cells can utilize only glucose and other monosaccharides, and our brain and other nervous tissues primarily rely on glucose. This is why you get tired, irritable, and shaky when you have not eaten for a prolonged period of time.

Why Do We Need Carbohydrates?

We have seen that carbohydrates are an important energy source for our bodies. Let's now learn more about this and discuss other functions of carbohydrates.

Carbohydrates Provide Energy

Carbohydrates, an excellent source of energy for all our cells, provide 4 kilocalories (kcal) of energy per gram. Some of our cells can also use fat and even protein for energy if necessary. However, our red blood cells can utilize only glucose, and our brain and other nervous tissues primarily rely on glucose. This is why you get tired, irritable, and shaky when you have not eaten any carbohydrate for a prolonged period of time.

Carbohydrates Fuel Daily Activity

Many popular diets—such as Dr. Atkins' New Revolution Diet and the Sugar Busters plan—are based on the idea that our bodies actually "prefer" to use fat and/or protein for energy. They claim that current carbohydrate recommendations are much higher than we really need.

In reality, the body relies mostly on both carbohydrates and fat for energy. In fact, as shown in FIGURE 4.5, our bodies always use some combination of carbohydrates and fat to fuel daily activities. Fat is the predominant energy source used by our bodies at rest and during low-intensity activities such as sitting, standing, and walking. Even during rest, however, our brain cells and red blood cells still rely on glucose.

Carbohydrates Fuel Exercise

When we exercise, whether running, briskly walking, bicycling, or performing any other activity that causes us to breathe harder and sweat, we begin to use more glu-

Exercise intensity	Percent (%) contribution of total energy
Light	12.5% Carbohydrate / 87.5% Fat
Moderate	45% Carbohydrate / 55% Fat
Intense	67% Carbohydrate / 33% Fat

FIGURE 4.5 Amounts of carbohydrate and fat used during light, moderate, and intense exercise. (Adapted from Romijn, J. A., E. F. Coyle, L. S. Sidossis, A. Gastaldelli, J. F. Horowitz, E. Endert, and R. R. Wolfe. 1993. Regulation of endogenous fat and carbohydrate metabolism in relation to exercise intensity and duration. *Am. J. Physiol.* 265 (*Endocrinol. Metab.* 28): E380–E391.)

cose than fat. While fat breakdown is a slow process and requires oxygen, we can break down glucose very quickly either with or without oxygen. Even during very intense exercise, when less oxygen is available, we can still break down glucose very quickly for energy. That's why when you are exercising at maximal effort, carbohydrates are providing almost 100% of the energy your body requires.

If you are physically active, it is important to eat enough carbohydrates to provide energy for your brain, red blood cells, and muscles. In Chapter 13, we discuss in more detail the carbohydrate recommendations for active people. In general, if you do not eat enough carbohydrate to support regular exercise, your body will have to rely upon fat and protein as alternative energy sources. When your carbohydrate intake is insufficient, body protein is used for energy (the consequences of which are discussed beginning on page 126). In addition, you will have to reduce the amount and intensity of your exercise so that you can rely more on fat for energy. One advantage of becoming highly trained for endurance-type events such as marathons and triathlons is that our muscles are able to store more glycogen, which provides us with additional glucose we can use during exercise. (See Chapter 13 for more information on how exercise improves our use and storage of carbohydrates.)

If you are trying to lose weight, you may be wondering whether you should exercise at a lower intensity so you will use more fat for energy. This is a question that researchers are still trying to answer. Weight loss studies show that, to lose weight and keep it off, it is important to exercise daily. A lower-intensity activity such as walking is generally recommended because it is easy to do and we know that fat provides much of the energy we need for walking. However, a study of highly trained athletes found that they actually lost more body fat when they performed very high-intensity exercise![7]

Based on the evidence currently available, there is no magic formula for weight loss. It is likely that people who combine aerobic-type exercises, such as walking, jogging, or bicycling, with strength-building exercises will be more successful in losing weight and keeping it off. It is important to find activities we can do every day. The current recommendations for health suggest that people perform at least 30 minutes

When we exercise or perform any other activity that causes us to breathe harder and sweat, we begin to use more glucose than fat.

of activity daily, but for weight loss, it is more effective to exercise for at least 1 hour each day. We can help our bodies stay active and healthy by eating the proper balance of carbohydrate, fat, and protein. (For more information on weight loss, see Chapter 11.)

Low Carbohydrate Intake Can Lead to Ketoacidosis

When we do not eat enough carbohydrate, the body seeks an alternative source of fuel for the brain and begins to break down stored fat. This process, called **ketosis,** produces an alternative fuel called **ketones.**

Ketosis is an important mechanism for providing energy to the brain during situations of fasting, low carbohydrate intake, or vigorous exercise.[8] However, ketones also suppress appetite and cause dehydration and acetone breath (the breath smells like nail polish remover). If inadequate carbohydrate intake continues for an extended period of time, the body will produce excessive amounts of ketones. Because many ketones are acids, high ketone levels cause the blood to become very acidic, leading to a condition called **ketoacidosis.** The high acidity of the blood interferes with basic body functions, causes the loss of lean body mass, and damages many body tissues. People with untreated diabetes are at high risk for ketoacidosis, which can lead to coma and even death. (See pages 146–150 for further details about diabetes.)

Carbohydrates Spare Protein

Most cells can use fat for energy, but some cells require glucose. If the diet does not provide enough carbohydrate, the body will make its own glucose from protein. This involves breaking down the proteins in blood and tissues into amino acids, then converting them to glucose. This process is called **gluconeogenesis** (or "generating new glucose").

When our body uses proteins for energy, the amino acids from these proteins cannot be used to make new cells, repair tissue damage, support our immune system, or perform any of their other functions. During periods of starvation or when eating a diet that is very low in carbohydrate, our body will take amino acids from the blood first, and then from other tissues like muscles, heart, liver, and kidneys. Using amino acids in this manner over a prolonged period of time can cause serious, possibly irreversible, damage to these organs. (See Chapter 6 for more details on using protein for energy.)

> RECAP: *Carbohydrates are an excellent energy source at rest and during exercise, and provide 4 kcal of energy per gram. Carbohydrates are necessary in the diet to spare body protein and prevent ketosis.*

Complex Carbohydrates Have Health Benefits

The relationship between carbohydrates, heart disease, and obesity is the subject of considerable controversy. Proponents of low-carbohydrate diets claim that eating carbohydrates, not fat, makes you overweight. However, anyone who consumes extra calories, whether in the form of sugar, complex carbohydrates, protein, or fat, may eventually become obese. Studies indicate that overweight people tend to eat higher amounts of energy, including both sugar and fat, and they are not physically active enough to expend this extra energy. Thus, weight gain occurs.

Fat is more energy dense than carbohydrate: it contains 9 kcal per gram, while carbohydrate contains only 4 kcal per gram. Thus, gram for gram, fat is twice as "fattening" as carbohydrate. In fact, eating complex carbohydrates that are high in fiber and other nutrients has been shown to reduce the overall risk for obesity, heart disease, and diabetes. Thus, all carbohydrates are not bad, and a small amount of simple carbohydrate can be included in a healthful diet. People who are very active and need more calories can eat more simple carbohydrate, while those who are older, less active, or overweight should limit their consumption of simple carbohydrate and focus on complex carbohydrates.

---

ketosis The process by which the breakdown of fat during fasting states results in the production of ketones.

ketones Substances produced during the breakdown of fat when carbohydrate intake is insufficient to meet energy needs. Provide an alternative energy source for the brain when glucose levels are low.

ketoacidosis A condition in which excessive ketones are present in the blood, causing the blood to become very acidic, which alters basic body functions and damages tissues. Untreated ketoacidosis can be fatal. This condition is found in individuals with untreated diabetes mellitus.

gluconeogenesis The generation of glucose from the breakdown of proteins into amino acids.

Fiber Helps Us Stay Healthy

Although we cannot digest fiber, it is still an important substance in our diet. Research indicates that it helps us stay healthy and may prevent many digestive and chronic diseases. The potential benefits of fiber consumption include the following:

- May reduce the risk of colon cancer. While there is some controversy surrounding this issue, many researchers believe that fiber binds cancer-causing substances and speeds their elimination from the colon. However, recent studies of colon cancer and fiber have shown that the relationship between them is not as strong as previously thought.

- Helps prevent hemorrhoids, constipation, and other intestinal problems by keeping our stools moist and soft. Fiber gives gut muscles "something to push on" and makes it easier to eliminate stools.

- Reduces the risk of *diverticulosis*, a condition that is caused in part by trying to eliminate small, hard stools. A great deal of pressure must be generated in the large intestine to pass hard stools. This increased pressure weakens intestinal walls, causing them to bulge outward and form pockets (FIGURE 4.6). Feces and fibrous materials can get trapped in these pockets, which become infected and inflamed. This is a painful condition that must be treated with antibiotics or surgery.

- May reduce the risk of heart disease by delaying or blocking the absorption of dietary cholesterol into the bloodstream (FIGURE 4.7). Fiber also contributes small fatty acids that may lower the amount of low-density lipoprotein (or LDL) to healthful levels in our bodies.

- May enhance weight loss, as eating a high-fiber diet causes a person to feel more full. Fiber absorbs water, expands in our intestine, and slows the movement of food through the upper part of the digestive tract. People who eat a fiber-rich diet tend to eat fewer fatty and sugary foods.

- May lower the risk of type 2 diabetes. In slowing digestion, fiber also slows the release of glucose into the blood. It thereby improves the body's regulation of insulin production and blood glucose levels.

> RECAP: *Complex carbohydrates contain fiber and other nutrients that can reduce the risk for obesity, heart disease, and diabetes. Fiber helps prevent hemorrhoids, constipation, and diverticulosis; may reduce risk of colon cancer and heart disease; and may assist with weight loss.*

Brown rice is a good food source of dietary fiber.

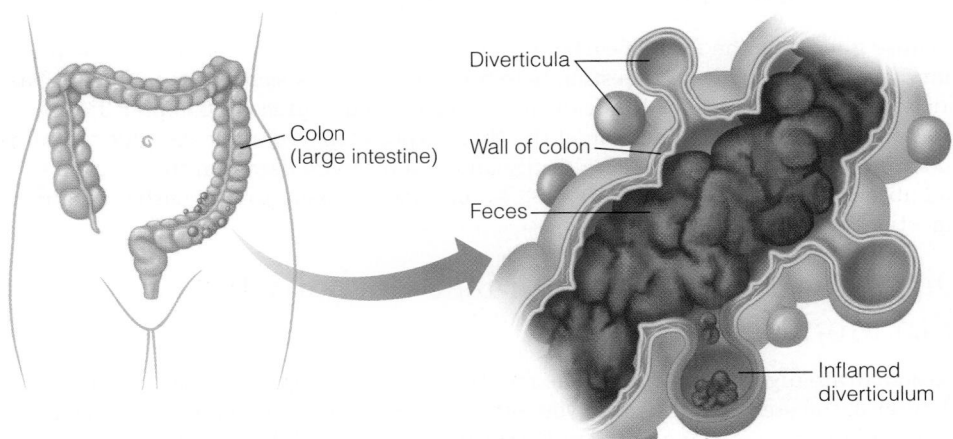

FIGURE 4.6 Diverticulosis occurs when bulging pockets form in the wall of the colon. These pockets become infected and inflamed, demanding proper treatment.

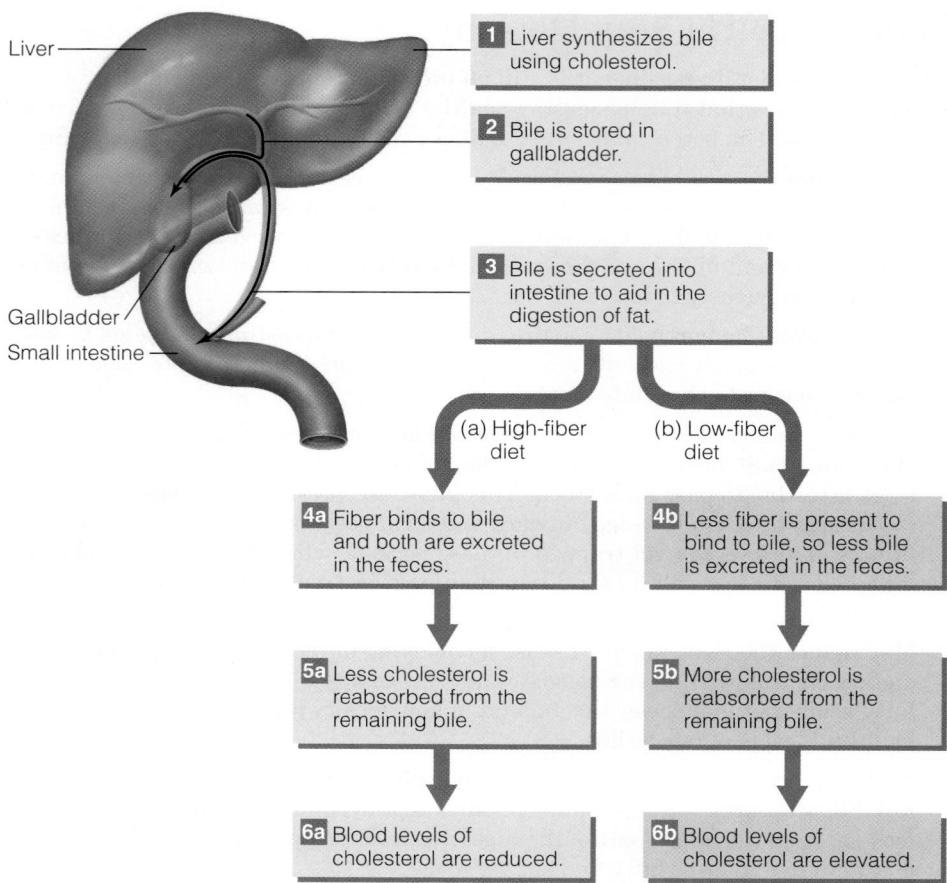

Liver

1 Liver synthesizes bile using cholesterol.

2 Bile is stored in gallbladder.

3 Bile is secreted into intestine to aid in the digestion of fat.

Gallbladder

Small intestine

(a) High-fiber diet

(b) Low-fiber diet

4a Fiber binds to bile and both are excreted in the feces.

4b Less fiber is present to bind to bile, so less bile is excreted in the feces.

5a Less cholesterol is reabsorbed from the remaining bile.

5b More cholesterol is reabsorbed from the remaining bile.

6a Blood levels of cholesterol are reduced.

6b Blood levels of cholesterol are elevated.

FIGURE 4.7 How fiber might help decrease blood cholesterol levels. **(a)** When eating a high-fiber diet, fiber binds to the bile that is produced from cholesterol, resulting in relatively more cholesterol being excreted in the feces. **(b)** When a lower fiber diet is consumed, less bile (and thus cholesterol) is bound to bile and excreted in the feces.

How Do Our Bodies Break Down Carbohydrates?

Because glucose is the form of carbohydrate that our bodies use for energy, the primary goal of carbohydrate digestion is to break down polysaccharides and disaccharides into monosaccharides that can then be converted to glucose. Chapter 3 provided an overview of digestion of the three types of macronutrients, plus vitamins and minerals. Here, we focus specifically and in a bit more detail on the digestion and absorption of carbohydrates. FIGURE 4.8 provides a visual tour of carbohydrate digestion.

Digestion Breaks Down Most Carbohydrates into Monosaccharides

Carbohydrate digestion begins in the mouth (FIGURE 4.8, step 1). As you saw in Chapter 3, the starch in the foods you eat mixes with your saliva during chewing. Saliva contains an enzyme called **salivary amylase,** which breaks starch into smaller particles and eventually into the disaccharide maltose. The next time you eat a piece of bread, notice that you can actually taste it becoming sweeter; this indicates the breakdown of starch into maltose. Disaccharides are not digested in the mouth.

salivary amylase An enzyme in saliva that breaks starch into smaller particles and eventually into the disaccharide maltose.

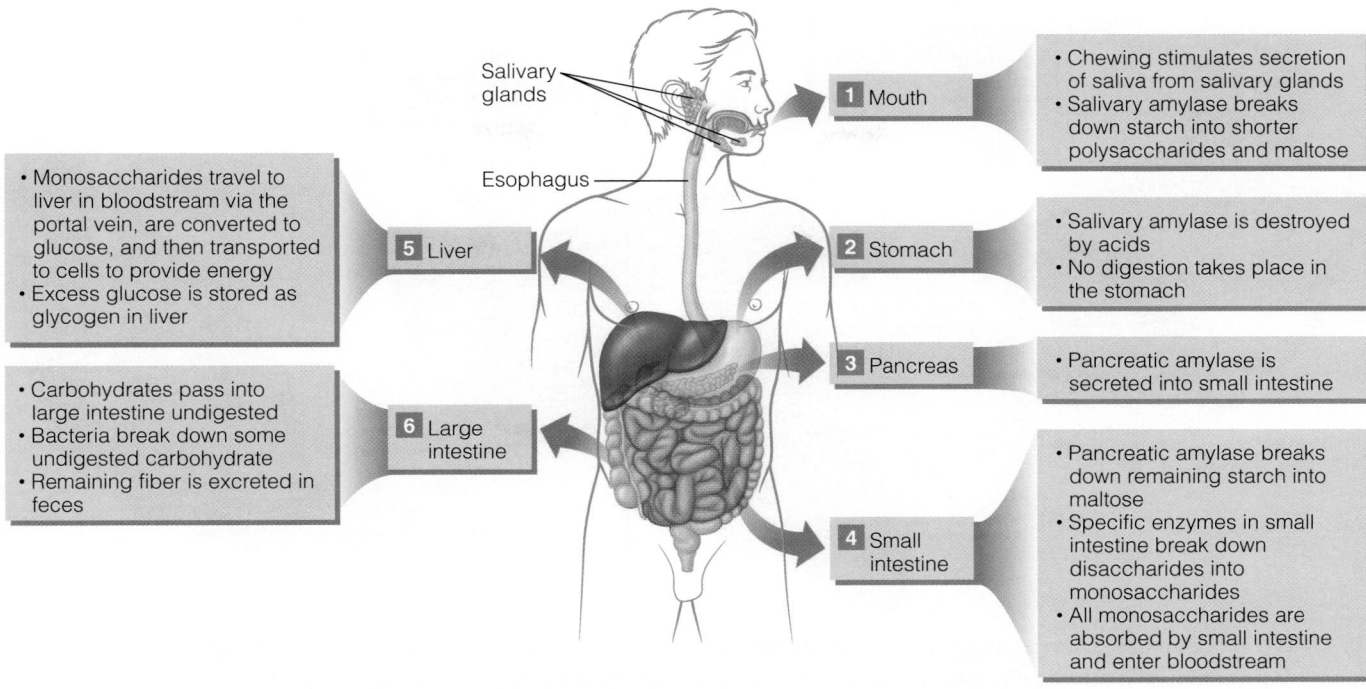

Salivary glands

Esophagus

1 Mouth
- Chewing stimulates secretion of saliva from salivary glands
- Salivary amylase breaks down starch into shorter polysaccharides and maltose

2 Stomach
- Salivary amylase is destroyed by acids
- No digestion takes place in the stomach

3 Pancreas
- Pancreatic amylase is secreted into small intestine

4 Small intestine
- Pancreatic amylase breaks down remaining starch into maltose
- Specific enzymes in small intestine break down disaccharides into monosaccharides
- All monosaccharides are absorbed by small intestine and enter bloodstream

5 Liver
- Monosaccharides travel to liver in bloodstream via the portal vein, are converted to glucose, and then transported to cells to provide energy
- Excess glucose is stored as glycogen in liver

6 Large intestine
- Carbohydrates pass into large intestine undigested
- Bacteria break down some undigested carbohydrate
- Remaining fiber is excreted in feces

FIGURE 4.8 A review of carbohydrate digestion and absorption.

As the bolus of food leaves the mouth and enters the stomach, all digestion of carbohydrates ceases. This is because the acid in the stomach inactivates most of the salivary amylase enzyme (FIGURE 4.8, step 2).

The majority of carbohydrate digestion occurs in the small intestine. As the contents of the stomach enter the small intestine, an enzyme called *pancreatic amylase* is secreted by the pancreas into the small intestine (FIGURE 4.8, step 3). **Pancreatic amylase** continues to digest any remaining starch into maltose. Additional enzymes found in the microvilli of the mucosal cells that line the intestinal tract work to break down disaccharides into monosaccharides. Maltose is broken down into glucose by the enzyme **maltase.** Sucrose is broken down into glucose and fructose by the enzyme **sucrase.** The enzyme **lactase** breaks lactose into glucose and galactose (FIGURE 4.8, step 4). Notice that enzyme names are identifiable by the *–ase* suffix. All monosaccharides are then absorbed into the mucosal cells lining the small intestine, where they pass through and enter into the bloodstream.

The Liver Converts All Monosaccharides into Glucose

Once the monosaccharides enter the bloodstream, they travel to the liver. There, fructose and galactose are converted to glucose (FIGURE 4.8, step 5). If needed immediately for energy, the liver releases glucose into the bloodstream where it can travel to the cells to provide energy. If there is no immediate demand by the body for glucose, it is stored as glycogen in our liver and muscles. Enzymes in liver and muscle cells combine glucose molecules to form glycogen (an anabolic, or building, process) and break glycogen into glucose (a catabolic, or destructive, process), depending on our bodily needs. Our liver can store 70 g (or 280 kcal) of glycogen, and our muscles can normally store about 120 g (or 480 kcal) of glycogen. Between meals, our bodies draw on liver glycogen reserves to maintain blood glucose levels and support the needs of our cells, including those of our brain, spinal cord, and red blood cells (FIGURE 4.9).

The glycogen stored in our muscles provides energy to the muscles during intense exercise. Endurance athletes can increase their storage of muscle glycogen from two to four times the normal amount through a process called *glycogen, or carbohydrate,*

pancreatic amylase An enzyme secreted by the pancreas into the small intestine that digests any remaining starch into maltose.

maltase A digestive enzyme that breaks maltose into glucose.

sucrase A digestive enzyme that breaks sucrose into glucose and fructose.

lactase A digestive enzyme that breaks lactose into glucose and galactose.

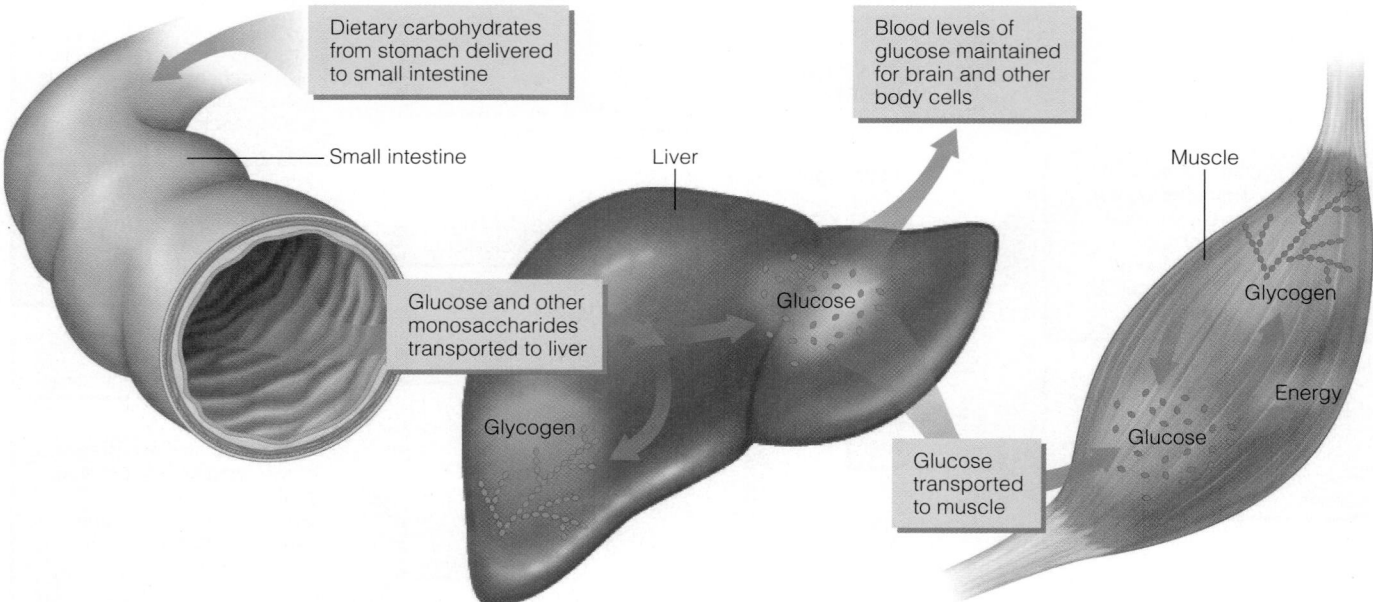

FIGURE 4.9 Glucose is stored as glycogen in both liver and muscle. The glycogen stored in the liver maintains blood glucose between meals; muscle glycogen provides immediate energy to the muscle during exercise.

loading (see Chapter 13). Any excess glucose is stored as glycogen in the liver and muscles and saved for such future energy needs as exercise.

Fiber Is Excreted from the Large Intestine

We do not possess enzymes that can break down fiber. Thus, fiber passes through the small intestine undigested and enters the large intestine, or colon. Once in the large intestine, bacteria break down some previously undigested carbohydrates, causing the production of gas and a few fatty acids. The cells of the large intestine use these fatty acids for energy. The fiber remaining in the colon adds bulk to our stools and is excreted (FIGURE 4.8, step 6) in feces. In this way, fiber assists in maintaining bowel regularity.

> RECAP: *Carbohydrate digestion starts in the mouth and continues in the small intestine. Glucose and other monosaccharides are absorbed into the bloodstream and travel to the liver, where non-glucose sugars are converted to glucose. Glucose either is used by the cells for energy or is converted to glycogen and stored in the liver and muscle for later use.*

Insulin and Glucagon Regulate the Level of Glucose in Our Blood

Our bodies regulate blood glucose levels within a fairly narrow range to provide adequate glucose to the brain and other cells. Two hormones, insulin and glucagon, assist the body with maintaining blood glucose. Specialized cells in the pancreas synthesize, store, and secrete both hormones.

When we eat a meal, our blood glucose level rises. But glucose in our blood cannot help the nerves, muscles, and other tissues function unless it can cross into them. Glucose molecules are too large to cross the cell membranes of our tissues independently. To get in, glucose needs assistance from the hormone **insulin,** which is secreted by the beta cells of the pancreas (FIGURE 4.10A). Insulin is transported in the blood to the cells of tissues throughout the body, where it stimulates special molecules located in the cell membrane to transport glucose into the cell. Insulin can be thought of as a key that

insulin Hormone secreted by the beta cells of the pancreas in response to increased blood levels of glucose. Facilitates uptake of glucose by body cells.

opens the gates of the cell membrane and carries the glucose into the cell interior, where it can be used for energy. Insulin also stimulates the liver and muscles to take up glucose and store it as glycogen.

When you have not eaten for some period of time, your blood glucose levels decline. This decrease in blood glucose stimulates the alpha cells of the pancreas to secrete another hormone, **glucagon** (FIGURE 4.10B). Glucagon acts in an opposite way to insulin: it causes the liver to convert its stored glycogen into glucose, which is then secreted into the bloodstream and transported to the cells for energy. Glucagon also assists in the breakdown of body proteins to amino acids so the liver can stimulate *gluconeogenesis*, or the production of new glucose from amino acids.

glucagon Hormone secreted by the alpha cells of the pancreas in response to decreased blood levels of glucose. Causes breakdown of liver stores of glycogen into glucose.

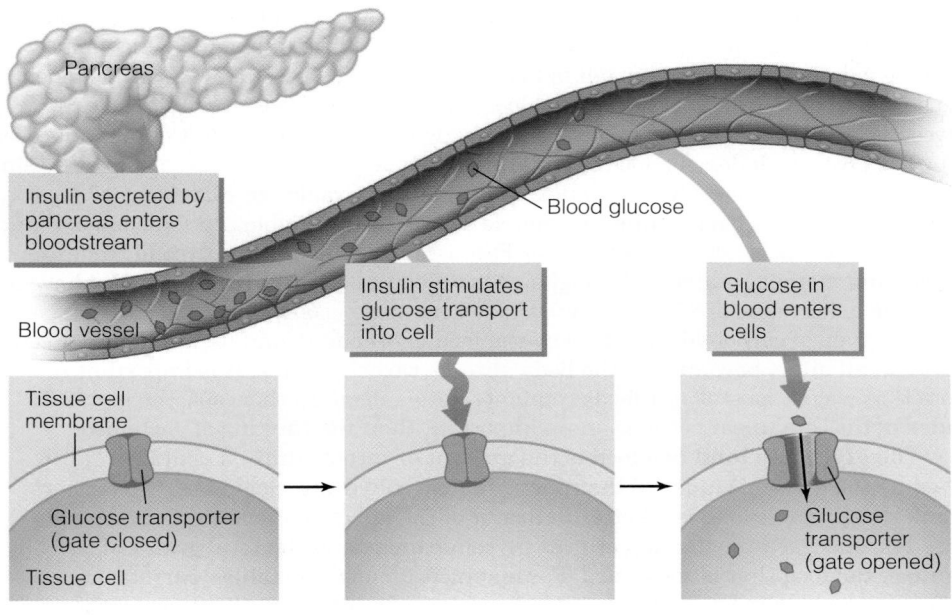

(a)

FIGURE 4.10 Regulation of blood glucose by the hormones insulin and glucagon. **(a)** When blood glucose levels increase after a meal, the pancreas secretes insulin. Insulin opens gates in the cell membrane to allow the passage of glucose into the cell. **(b)** When blood glucose levels are low, the pancreas secretes glucagon. Glucagon enters the cell, where it stimulates the breakdown of stored glycogen into glucose. This glucose is then released into the bloodstream.

(b)

Normally the effects of insulin and glucagon balance each other to maintain blood glucose within a healthy range. An alteration in this balance can lead to health conditions such as diabetes (pages 146–150) or hypoglycemia (page 151).

> RECAP: *Two hormones, insulin and glucagon, are involved in regulating blood glucose. Insulin lowers blood glucose levels by facilitating the entry of glucose into cells. Glucagon raises blood glucose levels by stimulating gluconeogenesis and the breakdown of glycogen stored in the liver.*

The Glycemic Index Shows How Foods Affect Our Blood Glucose Levels

The **glycemic index** refers to the potential of foods to raise blood glucose levels. Consumption of foods with a high glycemic index causes a sudden large increase in blood glucose. This surge in blood glucose in turn triggers a surge in insulin, which may then be followed by a dramatic fall in blood glucose. Foods with a low glycemic index cause low to moderate fluctuations in blood glucose. When foods are assigned a glycemic index value, they are often compared with the glycemic effect of pure glucose.

The glycemic index of a food is not always easy to predict. FIGURE 4.11 ranks certain foods according to their glycemic index. Do any of these rankings surprise you? Most people assume that foods containing simple sugars have a higher glycemic index than starches, but this is not always the case. For instance, compare the glycemic index for apples and instant potatoes. Although instant potatoes are a starchy food, they have a glycemic index value of 85, while the value for an apple is only 38!

The type of carbohydrate, the way the food is prepared, and its fat and fiber content can all affect how quickly the body absorbs carbohydrates. It is important to note that we eat most of our foods combined into a meal. In this case, the glycemic index of the total meal becomes more important than the ranking of each food.

The **glycemic load** of a food is the amount of carbohydrate it contains multiplied by the glycemic index of that particular carbohydrate. Some nutrition experts think the glycemic load is a better indicator of the effect of a food on a person's glucose response, as it factors in both the glycemic index and the total grams of carbohydrate of the food that is consumed. For instance, among vegetables, carrots are recognized as having a relatively high glycemic index of about 68; however, the glycemic load of carrots is only 3.[9] This is because there is very little total carbohydrate in a serving of carrots. The low glycemic load of carrots means that it is unlikely to cause a significant rise in glucose and insulin.

Why do we care about the glycemic index and glycemic load? Foods or meals with a lower glycemic load are a better choice for someone with diabetes, for instance, because they will not trigger dramatic fluctuations in blood glucose. They may also reduce the risk of heart disease and colon cancer because they generally contain more fiber, and it is known that fiber helps decrease fat levels in the blood.

glycemic index Rating of the potential of foods to raise blood glucose and insulin levels.

glycemic load The amount of carbohydrate in a food multiplied by the glycemic index of the carbohydrate.

An apple (36) has a much lower glycemic index than a serving of white rice (56).

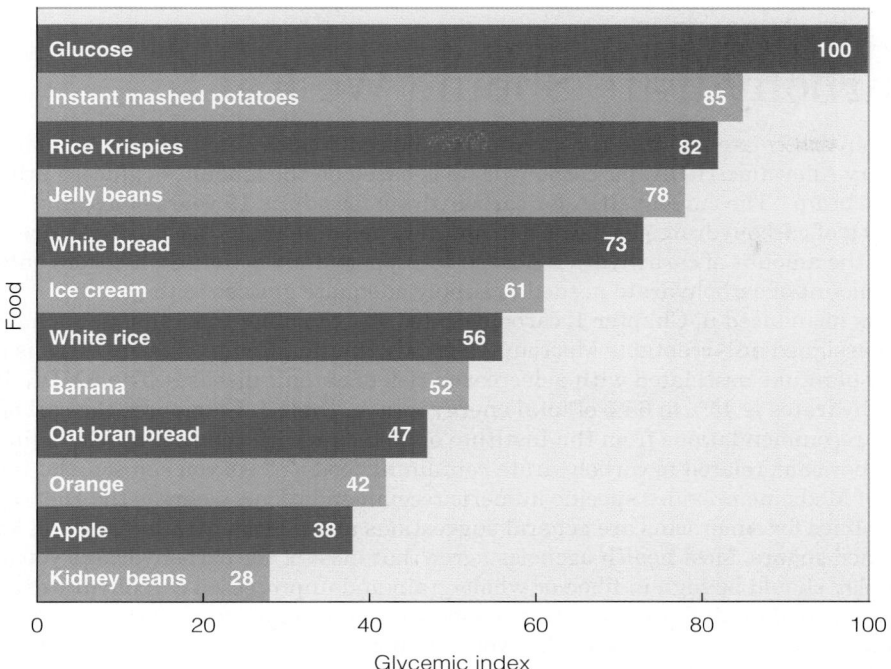

FIGURE 4.11 Glycemic index values for various foods as compared to pure glucose. (Values derived from K. Foster-Powell, S. H. A. Holt, and J. C. Brand-Miller. 2002. International table of glycemic index and glycemic load values. *Am. J. Clin. Nutr.* 76:5–56.)

Recent studies have shown that people who eat lower glycemic index diets have higher levels of high-density lipoprotein, or HDL (a healthful blood lipid), and lower levels of LDL (a blood lipid associated with increased risk for heart disease), and their blood glucose values are more likely to be normal.[10–12] Diets with a low glycemic index and low glycemic load are also associated with a reduced risk for prostate cancer.[13] The easiest way to eat lower glycemic index and glycemic load foods and meals without having to look up their values is to consume foods such as beans and lentils, fresh vegetables, and whole-wheat bread.

Despite some encouraging research findings, the glycemic index and glycemic load remain controversial. Many nutrition researchers feel that the evidence supporting their health benefits is weak and that we do not know enough about the impact of low glycemic index/load foods on long-term health. In addition, many believe the concepts of the glycemic index/load are too complex for people to apply to their daily lives. Other researchers insist that helping people to choose foods with a lower glycemic index/load is critical to the prevention and treatment of many chronic diseases. Until this controversy is resolved, people are encouraged to eat a variety of fiber-rich and less processed carbohydrates because we know these forms of carbohydrates are lower in glycemic load and they also contain a multitude of important nutrients.

RECAP: *The glycemic index is a value that indicates the potential of foods to raise blood glucose and insulin levels. The glycemic load is the amount of carbohydrate in a food multiplied by the glycemic index of the carbohydrate in that food. Foods with a high glycemic index/load cause sudden large increases in blood glucose and insulin, whereas foods with a low glycemic index/load cause low to moderate fluctuations in blood glucose. Diets with a low glycemic index/load are associated with a reduced risk for chronic diseases such as cardiovascular disease, type 2 diabetes, and prostate cancer.*

How Much Carbohydrate Should We Eat?

Carbohydrates are an important part of a balanced, healthy diet. The Recommended Dietary Allowance (RDA) for carbohydrate is based on the amount of glucose utilized by the brain.[6] The current RDA for carbohydrate for adults 19 years of age and older is 130 g of carbohydrate per day. It is important to emphasize that this RDA does not cover the amount of carbohydrate needed to support daily activities; it covers only the amount of carbohydrate needed to supply adequate glucose to the brain.

As introduced in Chapter 1, carbohydrates and the other macronutrients have been assigned an Acceptable Macronutrient Distribution Range (AMDR). This is the range of intake associated with a decreased risk of chronic diseases. The AMDR for carbohydrates is 45% to 65% of total energy intake. Table 4.2 compares the carbohydrate recommendations from the Institute of Medicine with the Dietary Guidelines for Americans related to carbohydrate-containing foods.[6, 14] As you can see, the Institute of Medicine provides specific numeric recommendations, whereas the Dietary Guidelines for Americans are general suggestions about foods high in fiber and low in added sugars. Most health agencies agree that most of the carbohydrates you eat each day should be high in fiber, or whole-grain and unprocessed carbohydrates. As recommended in MyPyramid, eating a wide variety of whole grains and fruits and vegetables each day will ensure that you get enough fiber and other complex carbohydrates in your diet. Keep in mind that fruits are predominantly composed of simple sugar and contain little or no starch. They are healthful food choices, however, as they are good sources of vitamins, some minerals, and fiber.

> RECAP: *The RDA for carbohydrate is 130 g per day; this amount is only sufficient to supply adequate glucose to the brain. The AMDR for carbohydrate is 45% to 65% of total energy intake.*

Most Americans Eat Too Much Simple Carbohydrate

The average carbohydrate intake in the United States is approximately 50%. For some people, almost half of this amount consists of simple sugars. Where does all this

TABLE 4.2 Dietary Recommendations for Carbohydrates

Institute of Medicine Recommendations*	Dietary Guidelines for Americans†
Recommended Dietary Allowance (RDA) for adults 19 years of age and older is 130 g of carbohydrate per day.	Choose fiber-rich fruits, vegetables, and whole grains often.
The Acceptable Macronutrient Distribution Range (AMDR) for carbohydrate is 45–65% of total daily energy intake.	Choose and prepare foods and beverages with little added sugars or caloric sweeteners, such as amounts suggested by the USDA Food Guide and the DASH eating plan.
Added sugar intake should be 25% or less of total energy intake each day.	Reduce the incidence of dental caries by practicing good oral hygiene and consuming sugar- and starch-containing foods and beverages less frequently.

*From "Dietary Reference Intakes for Energy, Carbohydrates, Fiber, Fat, Fatty Acids, Cholesterol, Protein, and Amino Acids (Macronutrients)," © 2002 by the National Academy of Sciences, courtesy of the National Academies Press, Washington, DC. Used by permission.
† U.S. Department of Health and Human Services (USDHHS) and U.S. Department of Agriculture (USDA). 2005. *Dietary Guidelines for Americans, 2005.* 6th edn. Washington, DC: U.S. Government Printing Office, www.healthierus.gov/dietaryguidelines.

sugar come from? Some sugar comes from healthful food sources, such as fruit and milk. However, much of our simple sugar intake comes from *added sugars*. **Added sugars** are defined as sugars and syrups that are added to foods during processing or preparation.[6] The most common source of added sugars in the U.S. diet is sweetened soft drinks; we drink an average of 40 gallons per person each year. Consider that one 12-oz sugared cola contains 38.5 g of sugar, or almost 10 tsp. If you drink the average amount, you are consuming more than 16,420 g of sugar (about 267 cups) each year! Other common sources of added sugars include cookies, cakes, pies, fruit drinks, fruit punches, and candy.

Added sugars are not chemically different from naturally occurring sugars. However, foods and beverages with added sugars have lower levels of vitamins and minerals than foods that naturally contain simple sugars. Due to these nutrient limitations, it is recommended that we choose and prepare foods and beverages with little added sugars. People who are very physically active are able to consume relatively more added sugars, while smaller or less active people should consume relatively less. The Nutrition Facts Panel includes a listing of total sugars, but a distinction is not generally made between added sugars and naturally occurring sugars. You need to check the ingredients list for added sugars (refer to Highlight: Forms of Added Sugars Commonly Used in Foods on page 136 for a list of terms indicating added sugars). To limit foods that are high in added sugars, a good strategy is to limit foods in which some form of added sugar is listed as one of the first few ingredients on the label.[15]

Foods with added sugars, like candy, have lower levels of vitamins and minerals than foods that naturally contain simple sugars.

Simple Carbohydrates Are Blamed for Many Health Problems

Why do simple carbohydrates have such a bad reputation? First, they are known to cause tooth decay. Second, many people believe they cause hyperactivity in children. Third, eating a lot of simple carbohydrates could increase the levels of unhealthful lipids, or fats, in our blood, increasing our risk for heart disease. High intakes of simple carbohydrates have also been blamed for causing diabetes and obesity. Let's now learn the truth about these accusations related to simple carbohydrates.

Sugar Causes Tooth Decay

Simple carbohydrates do play a role in dental problems because the bacteria that cause tooth decay thrive on them. These bacteria produce acids that eat away at tooth enamel and can eventually cause cavities and gum disease (FIGURE 4.12). Eating sticky foods that adhere to teeth—such as caramels, crackers, sugary cereals, and licorice—and sipping sweetened beverages over a period of time are two behaviors that increase the risk of tooth decay. This means that people shouldn't suck on hard candies or caramels, slowly sip soda or juice, or put babies to bed with a bottle unless it contains water. As we have seen, even breast milk contains sugar, which can slowly drip onto the baby's gums. As a result, infants should not routinely be allowed to fall asleep at the breast.

To reduce your risk for tooth decay, brush your teeth after each meal and especially after drinking sugary drinks and eating candy. Drinking fluoridated water and using a fluoride toothpaste also will help protect your teeth.

There Is No Link Between Sugar and Hyperactivity in Children

Although many people believe that eating sugar causes hyperactivity and other behavioral problems in children, there is little scientific evidence to support this claim. Some children actually become less active shortly after a high-sugar meal! However, it is important to emphasize that most studies of sugar and children's behavior have only looked at the effects of sugar a few hours after ingestion. We know very little about the long-term effects of sugar intake on the behavior of children. Behavioral and learning problems are complex issues, most likely caused by a multitude of factors. Because of this complexity, the Institute of Medicine has stated that overall, there currently does not appear to be enough evidence to state that eating too much sugar causes hyperactivity or other behavioral problems in children.[6] Thus, they have not set a Tolerable Upper Intake Level for sugar.

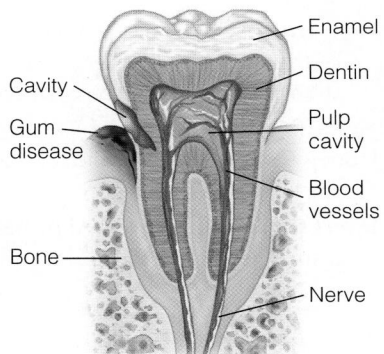

FIGURE 4.12 Eating simple carbohydrates can cause an increase in cavities and gum disease. This is because bacteria in the mouth consume simple carbohydrates present on the teeth and gums and produce acids, which eat away at these tissues.

added sugars Sugars and syrups that are added to food during processing or preparation.

HIGHLIGHT

Forms of Added Sugars Commonly Used in Foods

Brown sugar A highly refined sweetener made up of approximately 99% sucrose and produced by adding to white table sugar either molasses or burnt table sugar for coloring and flavor.

Concentrated fruit juice sweetener A form of sweetener made with concentrated fruit juice, commonly pear juice.

Confectioner's sugar A highly refined, finely ground white sugar with added cornstarch to reduce clumping; also referred to as powdered sugar.

Corn sweeteners A general term for any sweetener made with cornstarch.

Corn syrup A syrup produced by the partial hydrolysis of cornstarch.

Dextrose An alternative term for glucose.

Fructose A monosaccharide that occurs in fruits and vegetables. Also called levulose, or fruit sugar.

Glucose The most abundant monosaccharide; it is the preferred source of energy for the brain and an important source of energy for all cells.

Granulated sugar Another term for white sugar, or table sugar.

High-fructose corn syrup A type of corn syrup in which part of the sucrose is converted to fructose, making it sweeter than sucrose or regular corn syrup; most high-fructose corn syrup contains 42% to 55% fructose.

Honey A sweet, sticky liquid sweetener made by bees from the nectar of flowers; contains glucose and fructose.

Invert sugar A sugar created by heating a sucrose syrup with a small amount of acid. Inverting sucrose results in its breakdown into glucose and fructose, which reduces the size of the sugar crystals. Its smooth texture makes it ideal for use in making candies such as fondant and some syrups.

Lactose A disaccharide formed by one molecule of glucose and one molecule of galactose. Occurs naturally in milk and other dairy products.

Levulose Another term for fructose, or fruit sugar.

Maltose A disaccharide consisting of two molecules of glucose. Does not generally occur independently in foods but is a by-product of digestion. Also called malt sugar.

Mannitol A type of sugar alcohol.

Maple sugar A sugar made by boiling maple syrup.

Molasses A thick brown syrup that is separated from raw sugar during manufacturing. It is considered the least refined form of sucrose.

Natural sweeteners A general term used for any naturally occurring sweeteners such as sucrose, honey, and raw sugar.

Raw sugar The sugar that results from the processing of sugar beets or sugarcane. It is approximately 96% to 98% sucrose. True raw sugar contains impurities and is not stable in storage; the raw sugar available to consumers has been purified to yield an edible sugar.

Sorbitol A type of sugar alcohol.

Turbinado sugar The form of raw sugar that is purified and safe for human consumption. Sold as "Sugar in the Raw" in the United States.

White sugar Another name for sucrose, or table sugar.

Xylitol A type of sugar alcohol.

High Sugar Intake Can Lead to Unhealthful Levels of Blood Lipids

Research evidence suggests that consuming a diet high in simple sugars, particularly fructose, can lead to unhealthful changes in blood lipids. You will learn more about blood lipids (including cholesterol and lipoproteins) in Chapter 5. In brief, higher intakes of simple sugars are associated with increases in triglycerides (lipids in our blood) and LDLs, which are commonly referred to as "bad cholesterol." At the same time, high simple sugar intake appears to *decrease* our HDLs, which are protective and are often referred to as "good cholesterol."[6,16] These changes are of concern, as increased levels of triglycerides and LDL and decreased levels of HDL are known risk factors for heart disease. However, there is not enough scientific evidence at the present time to state with confidence that eating a diet high in simple sugars causes heart disease. Based on our current knowledge, it is prudent for a person at risk for heart disease to eat a diet low in simple sugars.

High Sugar Intake Does Not Cause Diabetes but May Contribute to Obesity

There is no scientific evidence that eating a diet high in sugar causes diabetes. In fact, studies examining the relationship between sugar intake and type 2 diabetes report either no association between sugar intake and diabetes or a decreased risk of diabetes with increased sugar intake.[17,18] However, people who have diabetes need to moderate their intake of sugar and closely monitor their blood glucose levels.

To date, there is no evidence to convincingly prove that sugar intake causes obesity; however, a recent study found that overweight children consumed more sugared soft drinks than did children of normal weight.[19] Another study found that for every extra sugared soft drink consumed by a child per day, the risk of obesity increases by 60%.[20] We do know that if you consume more energy than you expend, you will gain weight. It makes intuitive sense that people who consume extra energy from high-sugar foods are at risk for obesity, just as people who consume extra energy from fat gain weight. In addition to the increased potential for obesity, another major concern about high-sugar diets is that they are inadequate in nutrients critical to maintain our health. Although we cannot state with certainty that consuming a high-sugar diet causes obesity, it is important to optimize your intake of nutrient-dense foods and limit added sugars. The relationship between sugared soft drinks and obesity is highly controversial and is discussed in more detail in the Nutrition Debate on pages 157–159.

RECAP: *Added sugars are sugars and syrups added to foods during processing or preparation. Sugar causes tooth decay but does not appear to cause hyperactivity in children. High intakes of simple sugars are associated with increases in triglycerides and lipoproteins or "bad cholesterol." Diets high in sugar cause unhealthful changes in blood sugar but do not cause diabetes. The relationship between added sugars and obesity is controversial.*

Most Americans Eat Too Little Complex Carbohydrate

Do you get enough complex carbohydrates each day? If you are like most people in the United States, you eat only about 2 servings of fruits or vegetables each day; this is far below the 5 to 9 recommended servings. Do you eat whole grains and legumes every day? Many people eat plenty of breads, pastas, and cereals, but most do not consistently choose whole-grain products. As we explained earlier, whole-grain foods have a lower glycemic index than simple carbohydrates; thus, they prompt a more gradual release of insulin and result in less severe fluctuations in both insulin and glucose. Whole-grain foods also provide more nutrients and fiber than foods made with enriched flour (FIGURE 4.13).

Table 4.3 defines terms commonly used on nutrition labels for breads and cereals. Read the label for the breads you eat—does it list *whole-wheat flour* or just *wheat flour?* Although most labels for breads and cereals list wheat flour as the first ingredient, this term actually refers to enriched white flour, which is made when wheat flour is processed. Don't be fooled—becoming an educated consumer will help you select whole grains instead of processed foods.

We Need at Least 25 Grams of Fiber Daily

How much fiber do we need? The Adequate Intake for fiber is 25 g per day for women and 38 g per day for men, or 14 g of fiber for every 1,000 kcal per day that a person eats.[6] Most people in the United States eat only 12 to 18 g of fiber each day, getting only half of the fiber they need. Although fiber supplements are available, it is best to get fiber from food because foods contain additional nutrients such as vitamins and minerals.

Eating the amounts of whole grains, vegetables, fruits, nuts, and legumes recommended in MyPyramid will ensure that you eat adequate fiber. FIGURE 4.14 shows

Whole-grain foods provide more nutrients and fiber than foods made with enriched flour.

FIGURE 4.13 Nutrients in whole-grain, enriched white, and unenriched white breads. The percentages of each nutrient reported for enriched white bread and unenriched white bread indicate the amount they contain as compared to the amount contained in whole-grain bread.

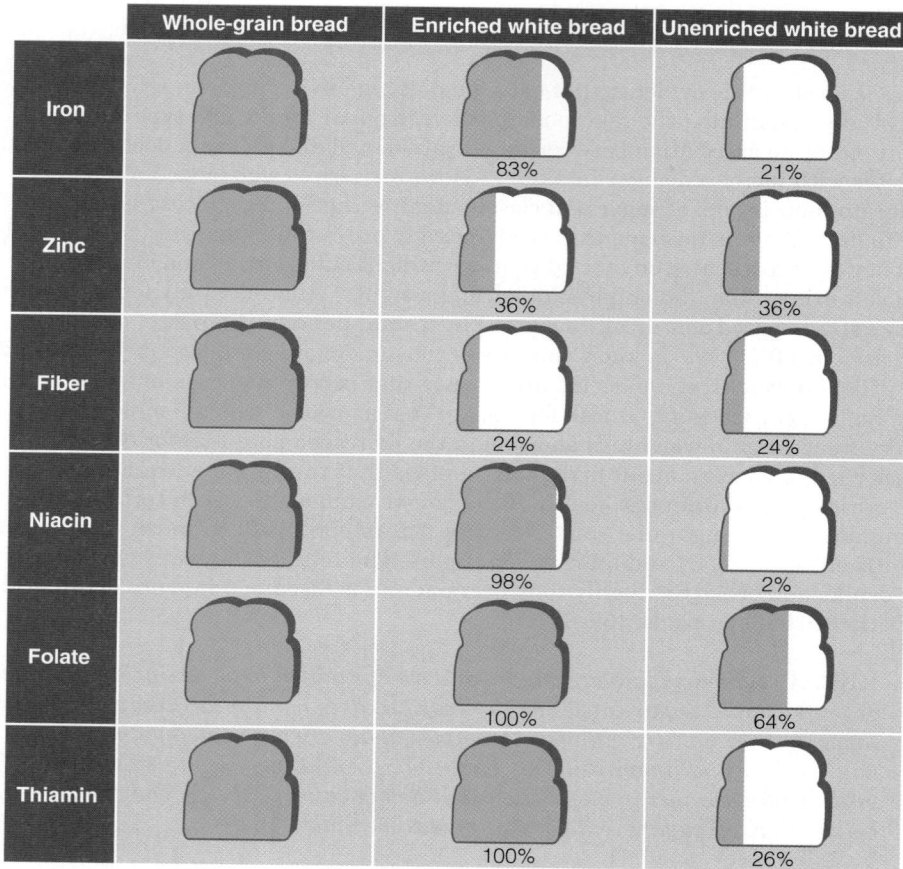

	Whole-grain bread	Enriched white bread	Unenriched white bread
Iron		83%	21%
Zinc		36%	36%
Fiber		24%	24%
Niacin		98%	2%
Folate		100%	64%
Thiamin		100%	26%

TABLE 4.3 Terms Used to Describe Grains and Cereals on Nutrition Labels

Term	Definition
Brown bread	Bread that may or may not be made using whole-grain flour. Many brown breads are made with white flour with brown (caramel) coloring added.
Enriched (or fortified) flour or grain	Enriching or fortifying grains involves adding nutrients back to refined foods. In order to use this term in the United States, a minimum amount of iron, folate, niacin, thiamin, and riboflavin must be added. Other nutrients can also be added.
Refined flour or grain	Refining involves removing the coarse parts of food products; refined wheat flour is flour in which all but the internal part of the kernel has been removed. Refined sugar is made by removing the outer portions of sugar beets or sugarcane.
Stone ground	Refers to a milling process in which limestone is used to grind any grain. Stone ground does not mean that bread is made with whole grain, as refined flour can be stone ground.
Unbleached flour	Flour that has been refined but not bleached; it is very similar to refined white flour in texture and nutritional value.
Wheat flour	Any flour made from wheat; includes white flour, unbleached flour, and whole-wheat flour.
White flour	Flour that has been bleached and refined. All-purpose flour, cake flour, and enriched baking flour are all types of white flour.
Whole-grain flour	A grain that is not refined; whole grains are milled in their complete form, with only the husk removed.
Whole-wheat flour	An unrefined, whole-grain flour made from whole-wheat kernels.

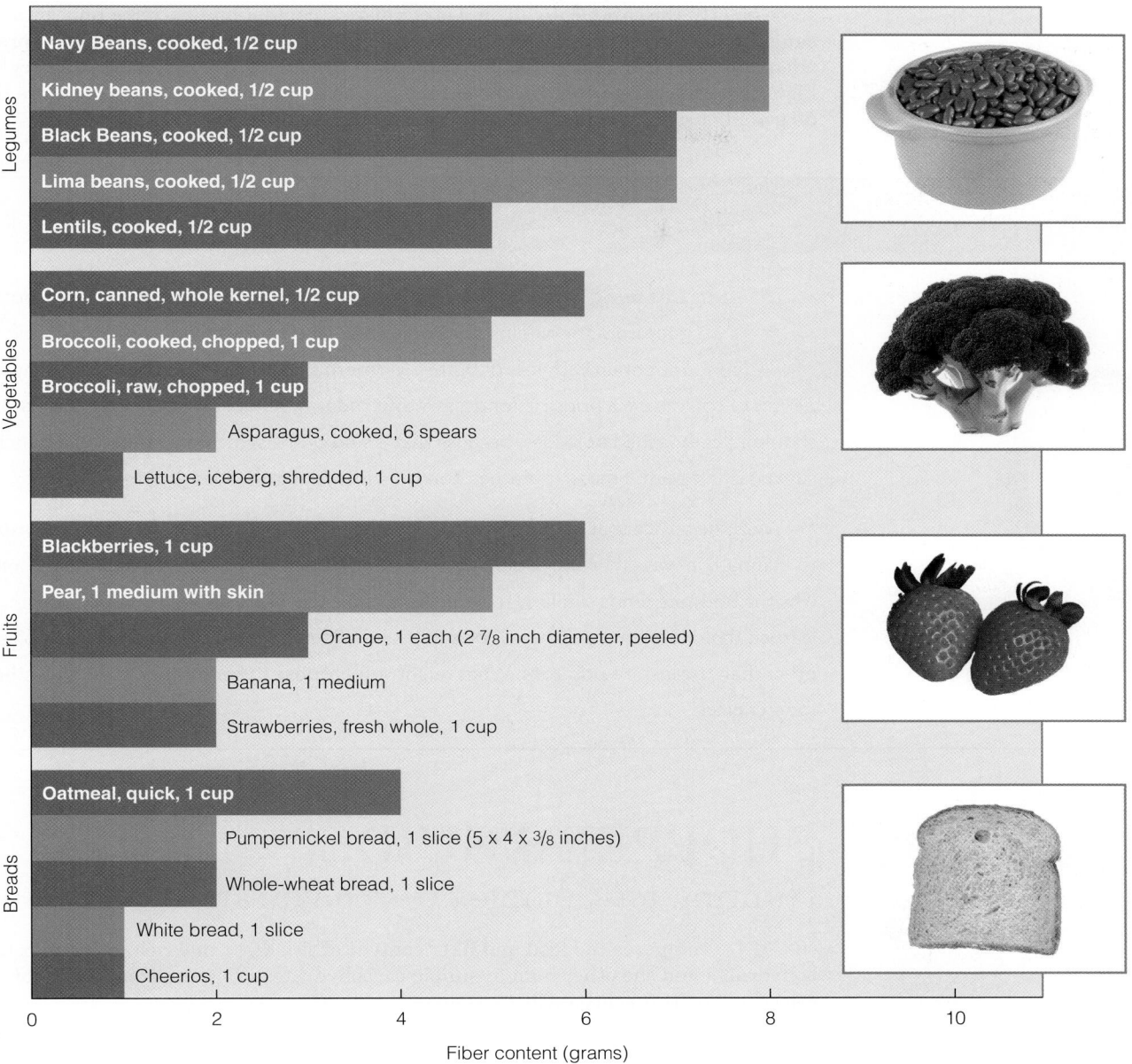

Legumes

- Navy Beans, cooked, 1/2 cup
- Kidney beans, cooked, 1/2 cup
- Black Beans, cooked, 1/2 cup
- Lima beans, cooked, 1/2 cup
- Lentils, cooked, 1/2 cup

Vegetables

- Corn, canned, whole kernel, 1/2 cup
- Broccoli, cooked, chopped, 1 cup
- Broccoli, raw, chopped, 1 cup
- Asparagus, cooked, 6 spears
- Lettuce, iceberg, shredded, 1 cup

Fruits

- Blackberries, 1 cup
- Pear, 1 medium with skin
- Orange, 1 each (2 7/8 inch diameter, peeled)
- Banana, 1 medium
- Strawberries, fresh whole, 1 cup

Breads

- Oatmeal, quick, 1 cup
- Pumpernickel bread, 1 slice (5 x 4 x 3/8 inches)
- Whole-wheat bread, 1 slice
- White bread, 1 slice
- Cheerios, 1 cup

Fiber content (grams)
0   2   4   6   8   10

FIGURE 4.14   Fiber content of common foods. *Note:* The Adequate Intake for fiber is 25 g per day for women and 38 g per day for men. (*Source:* U.S. Department of Agriculture, Agricultural Research Service. 2006. USDA National Nutrient Database for Standard Reference, Release 19. Nutrient Data Laboratory Home Page, http://www.ars.usda.gov/ba/bhnrc/ndl.)

some common foods and their fiber content. Think about how you can design your own diet to include high-fiber foods.

It is also important to drink more water as you increase your fiber intake, since fiber binds with water to soften stools. Inadequate water intake with a high-fiber diet can actually result in hard, dry stools that are difficult to pass through the colon.

Can you eat too much fiber? Excessive fiber consumption can lead to problems such as intestinal gas, bloating, and constipation. Because fiber binds with water, it causes the body to eliminate more water, so a very high-fiber diet could result in dehydration. Since fiber binds many vitamins and minerals, a high-fiber diet can reduce our absorption of important nutrients such as iron, zinc, and calcium. In children, some elderly, the chronically ill, and other at-risk populations, extreme fiber intake can even lead to malnutrition—they feel full before they have eaten enough to provide adequate energy and nutrients. So while some societies are accustomed to a very high-fiber diet, most people in the United States find it difficult to tolerate more than 50 g of fiber per day and may end up consuming too little.

NUTRI-CASE HANNAH

"Last night, my mom made sausages and she let me make the mashed potatoes from the Mr. Instant Potato box. They're my favorite, and I ate a big mountain with lots of butter. My mom said I did such a good job on my supper that I could have a popsicle for dessert. But today in school my science teacher said we shouldn't eat mashed potatoes, because that's kind of the same thing as eating a bunch of sugar. I don't get it. I mean, potatoes don't taste anything like sugar!"

Was the advice that Hannah's science teacher gave her sound? How would you explain to Hannah, in ways that she could understand, what happens to the foods she eats, and why the body responds similarly to some foods that seem very different? Suppose you learned that Hannah drank a glass of apple juice with her dinner and had no vegetables other than the instant potatoes. What might you propose to her mother, Judy, about her food choices?

SHOPPER'S GUIDE:
Hunting for Complex Carbohydrates

FIGURE 4.15 compares the food and fiber content of two diets, one rich in complex carbohydrates and the other high in simple carbohydrates. Here are some hints for selecting healthful carbohydrate sources:

√ Select breads and cereals that are made with whole grains such as wheat, oats, barley, and rye (make sure the label says "whole" before the word grain).

√ Choose foods that have at least 2 or 3 g of fiber per serving.

√ Buy fresh fruits and vegetables whenever possible. When appropriate, eat them with the skin left on.

√ Buy frozen vegetables and fruits when fresh produce is not available. Check frozen selections to make sure there is no extra sugar or salt added.

√ Be careful when buying canned fruits and vegetables, as many are high in sodium and added sugar. Foods that are packed in their own juice are more healthful than those packed in syrup.

√ Buy plenty of legumes, and eat some every day if possible. Add them to soups, casseroles, and other recipes. If you are trying to consume less sodium, rinse canned beans to remove extra salt or choose low-sodium alternatives.

High Complex Carbohydrate Diet

Breakfast:
1½ cups Cheerios
1 cup skim milk
2 slices whole-wheat toast
  with 1 tbsp. light margarine
1 medium banana
8 fl. oz fresh orange juice

Lunch:
8 fl. oz low-fat blueberry
  yogurt
Tuna sandwich (2 slices
  whole-wheat bread; ¼ cup
  tuna packed in water,
  drained; 1 tsp. Dijon mustard;
  2 tsp. low-calorie
  mayonnaise)
2 carrots, raw, with peel
1 cup raw cauliflower
1 tbsp. peppercorn ranch
  salad dressing
  (for dipping vegetables)

Snack:
3 cups non-fat popcorn

Dinner:
½ chicken breast roasted
1 cup brown rice, cooked
1 cup cooked broccoli
Spinach salad
(1 cup chopped spinach,
  1 whole egg white, 2 slices
  turkey bacon, 3 cherry
  tomatoes, and 2 tbsp. creamy
  bacon salad dressing)
2 baked apples (no added
  sugar)

(No Snack)

Nutrient Analysis:
2150 kcal
60% of energy from carbohydrates
22% of energy from fat
18% of energy from protein
38 grams of dietary fiber

High Simple Carbohydrate Diet

Breakfast:
1½ cups Fruit Loops cereal
1 cup skim milk
2 slices white bread toasted,
  with 1 tbsp. light margarine
8 fl. oz fresh orange juice

Lunch:
McDonald's Quarter Pounder—
  1 sandwich
1 large order French fries
16 fl. oz cola beverage
30 jelly beans

Snack:
1 cinnamon raisin bagel (3½-
  inch diameter)
2 tbsp. cream cheese
8 fl. oz low-fat strawberry
  yogurt

Dinner:
1 whole chicken breast,
  roasted
2 cups mixed green salad
2 tbsp. ranch salad dressing
1 serving macaroni and
  cheese
12 fl. oz cola beverage
Cheesecake (⅑ of cake)

Late Night Snack:
2 cups gelatin dessert
  (cherry flavored)
3 raspberry oatmeal no-fat
  cookies

Nutrient Analysis:
4012 kcal
60% of energy from carbohydrates
25% of energy from fat
15% of energy from protein
18.5 grams of dietary fiber

FIGURE 4.15 Comparison of two high-carbohydrate diets.
Note: Diets were analyzed using Food Processor Version 7.21 (ESHA Research, Salem, OR).

Nutrition Facts

Serving Size: 3/4 cup (30g)
Servings Per Package: About 14

Amount Per Serving	Cereal	Cereal With 1/2 Cup Skim Milk
Calories	120	160
Calories from Fat	15	15
	% Daily Value**	
Total Fat 1.5g*	2%	2%
Saturated Fat 0g	0%	0%
Trans Fat 0g		
Polyunsaturated Fat 0g		
Monounsaturated Fat 0.5g		
Cholesterol 0mg	0%	1%
Sodium 220mg	9%	12%
Potassium 40mg	1%	7%
Total Carbohydrate 26g	9%	11%
Dietary Fiber 1g	3%	3%
Sugars 13g		
Other Carbohydrate 12g		
Protein 1g		
Vitamin A	0%	4%
Vitamin C	0%	2%
Calcium	0%	15%
Iron	25%	25%
Thiamin	25%	25%
Riboflavin	25%	35%
Niacin	25%	25%
Vitamin B6	25%	25%
Folate	25%	25%
Zinc	25%	25%

* Amount in cereal. One-half cup skim milk contributes an additional 65mg sodium, 6g total carbohydrate (6g sugars), and 4g protein.

** Percent Daily Values are based on a 2,000 calorie diet. Your daily values may be higher or lower depending on your calorie needs:

	Calories	2,000	2,500
Total Fat	Less than	65g	80g
Sat. Fat	Less than	20g	25g
Cholesterol	Less than	300mg	300mg
Sodium	Less than	2,400mg	2,400mg
Potassium		3,500mg	3,500mg
Total Carbohydrate		300g	375g
Dietary fiber		25g	30g

Calories per gram:		2,500
Fat 9 • Carbohydrate 4 •		Protein 4

INGREDIENTS: Corn Flour, Sugar, Brown Sugar, Partially Hydrogenated Vegetable Oil (Soybean and Cottonseed), Oat Flour, Salt, Sodium Citrate (a flavoring agent), Flavor added [Natural & Artificial Flavor, Strawberry Juice Concentrate, Malic Acid (a flavoring agent)], Niacinamide (Niacin), Zinc Oxide, Reduced Iron, Red 40, Yellow 5, Red 3, Yellow 6, Pyridoxine Hydrochloride (Vitamin B6), Riboflavin (Vitamin B2), Thiamin Mononitrate (Vitamin B1), Folic Acid (Folate) and Blue 1.

(a)

Nutrition Facts

Serving Size: 1/2 cup dry (40g)
Servings Per Container: 13

Amount Per Serving	
Calories	150
Calories from Fat	25
	% Daily Value*
Total Fat 3g	5%
Saturated Fat 0.5g	2%
Trans Fat 0g	
Polyunsaturated Fat 1g	
Monounsaturated Fat 1g	
Cholesterol 0mg	0%
Sodium 0mg	0%
Total Carbohydrate 27g	9%
Dietary Fiber 4g	15%
Soluble Fiber 2g	
Insoluble Fiber 2g	
Sugars 1g	
Protein 5g	
Vitamin A	0%
Vitamin C	0%
Calcium	0%
Iron	10%

* Percent Daily Values are based on a 2,000 calorie diet. Your daily values may be higher or lower depending on your calorie needs:

	Calories	2,000	2,500
Total Fat	Less than	65g	80g
Sat. Fat	Less than	20g	25g
Cholesterol	Less than	300mg	300mg
Sodium	Less than	2,400mg	2,400mg
Total Carbohydrate		300g	375g
Dietary fiber		25g	30g

INGREDIENTS: 100% Natural Whole Grain Rolled Oats.

(b)

FIGURE 4.16 Labels for two breakfast cereals. **(a)** Sweetened cereal. **(b)** Whole-grain cereal.

NUTRITION LABEL ACTIVITY

Recognizing Carbohydrates on the Label

Figure 4.16 shows labels for two breakfast cereals. The cereal on the left (a) is processed and sweetened, while the one on the right (b) is a whole-grain product with no added sugar.

- Check the center of each label to locate the amount of total carbohydrate. For the sweetened cereal, the total carbohydrate is 26 g. For the whole-grain cereal, the total carbohydrate is almost the same, 27 g for a smaller serving size.

- Look at the information listed as subgroups under total carbohydrate. The label for the sweetened cereal lists all types of carbohydrates in the cereal—dietary fiber, sugars, and other carbohydrate (which refers to starches). Notice that this cereal contains 13 g of sugar—half of its total carbohydrates—but only 1 g of dietary fiber.

- The label for the whole-grain cereal lists dietary fibers by type and sugars. In contrast to the sweetened cereal, this product contains 4 g of fiber and only 1 g of sugar! Notice that on this label there is no amount listed for starches (or other carbohydrates). In this case, the amount of starch is the difference between the total carbohydrate and the sum of dietary fiber and sugars, or 27 g – 5 g = 22 g of starch.

- Now look at the percent values listed to the right of the total carbohydrate section. For both cereals (without milk), their percent contribution to daily carbohydrate is 9%. This does not mean that 9% of the calories in these cereals come from carbohydrates. Instead, this percentage refers to the Daily Values listed at the bottom of each label. For a person who eats 2,000 kcal, the recommended amount of carbohydrate each day is 300 g. One serving of each cereal contains 26–27 g, which is about 9% of 300 g.

- To calculate the percent of calories that comes from carbohydrate, do the following:

  a. Calculate the *calories* in the cereal that come from carbohydrate. Multiply the total grams of carbohydrate per serving by the energy value of carbohydrate:

     26 g of carbohydrate × 4 kcal/g = 104 kcal from carbohydrate

  b. Calculate the *percent of calories* in the cereal that come from carbohydrate. Divide the calories from carbohydrate by the total calories for each serving and multiply by 100:

     (104 kcal ÷ 120 kcal) × 100 = 87% calories from carbohydrate

Which cereal should you choose? Check the ingredients for the sweetened cereal. Remember that the ingredients are listed in the order from highest to lowest amount. The second and third ingredients listed are sugar and brown sugar, and the corn and oat flours are not whole-grain flours. Now look at the ingredients for the other cereal—it contains whole-grain oats. Although the sweetened product is enriched with more B vitamins, iron, and zinc, the whole-grain cereal packs 4 g of fiber per serving and contains no added sugars. Overall, it is a more healthful choice.

Try the Nutrition Label Activity to learn how to recognize various carbohydrates on food labels. Armed with this knowledge, you are now ready to make more healthful food choices.

> RECAP: *The Adequate Intake for fiber is 25 g per day for women and 38 g per day for men. Most Americans only eat half of the fiber they need each day. Foods high in fiber and complex carbohydrates include whole grains and cereals, fruits, and vegetables. The more processed the food, the fewer complex carbohydrates it contains.*

What's the Story on Alternative Sweeteners?

Most of us love sweets but want to avoid the extra calories and tooth decay that go along with eating simple sugars. Remember that all carbohydrates, including simple and complex, contain 4 kcal of energy per gram. Because sweeteners such as sucrose, fructose, honey, and brown sugar contribute calories (or energy), they are called **nutritive sweeteners.**

Other nutritive sweeteners include the *sugar alcohols* such as mannitol, sorbitol, isomalt, and xylitol. Popular in sugar-free gums and mints, sugar alcohols are less sweet than sucrose (FIGURE 4.17). One major advantage is that they do not promote dental problems because they do not support the bacteria that cause tooth decay. However, eating large amounts of sugar alcohols can cause diarrhea, and, because they provide 2 to 4 kcal of energy per gram, they are not calorie-free.

Alternative Sweeteners Are Non-Nutritive

A number of other products have been developed to sweeten foods without promoting tooth decay and weight gain. As these products provide little or no energy, they are called **non-nutritive,** or *alternative,* **sweeteners.**

Limited Use of Alternative Sweeteners Is Not Harmful

Contrary to popular belief, alternative sweeteners have been determined safe for adults, children, and individuals with diabetes to consume. Women who are pregnant should discuss the use of alternative sweeteners with their healthcare provider. In general, it appears safe for pregnant women, including pregnant women who have diabetes, to consume alternative sweeteners in amounts within the Food and Drug Administration (FDA) guidelines.[21] The **acceptable daily intake (ADI)** is an estimate made by the FDA of the amount of a sweetener that someone can consume each day over a lifetime without adverse effects. The estimates are based on studies

nutritive sweeteners Sweeteners such as sucrose, fructose, honey, and brown sugar that contribute calories (or energy).

non-nutritive sweeteners Also called *alternative sweeteners;* manufactured sweeteners that provide little or no energy.

acceptable daily intake (ADI) An estimate made by the Food and Drug Administration of the amount of a non-nutritive sweetener that someone can consume each day over a lifetime without adverse effects.

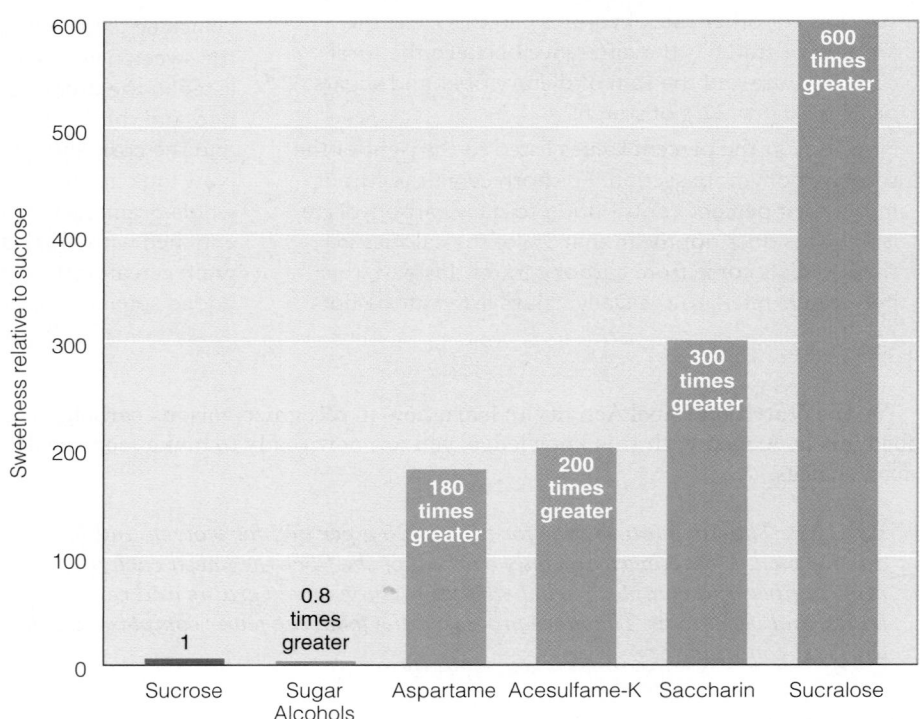

Sucrose versus alternative sweeteners

FIGURE 4.17 Relative sweetness of alternative sweeteners as compared to sucrose. (Values derived from Kroger M., K. Meister, and R. Kava. 2006. Low-calorie sweeteners and other sugar substitutes: a review of the safety issues. *Comp. Rev. Food Sci. Food Safety* 5:35–47.)

conducted on laboratory animals, and they include a 100-fold safety factor. While no ADI has been set for saccharin, the ADI for sucralose, acesulfame-K, and aspartame is 5, 15, and 50 mg per kg body weight per day, respectively. For example, the acceptable daily intake of sucralose in an adult weighing 150 pounds (or 68 kg) would be 340 mg. It is important to emphasize that actual intake by humans is typically well below the ADI.

The major alternative sweeteners available on the market today are saccharin, acesulfame-K, aspartame, and sucralose.

Saccharin

Discovered in the late 1800s, *saccharin* is about 300 times sweeter than sucrose (see FIGURE 4.17). Evidence to suggest that saccharin may cause bladder tumors in rats surfaced in the 1970s. While subsequent research with humans did not support this finding, the FDA felt it was prudent to ban the sweetener. The saccharin ban met with tremendous pressure from consumers and the food industry, so the U.S. government placed a moratorium on the ban. This moratorium has kept saccharin available for public consumption. More than 20 years of scientific research have shown that saccharin is not related to bladder cancer in humans. Based on this evidence, in May of 2000 the National Toxicology Program of the U.S. government removed saccharin from its list of products that may cause cancer. Saccharin is used in foods and beverages and sold as a tabletop sweetener. Saccharin is sold as Sweet 'N Low in the United States.

Acesulfame-K

Acesulfame-K (or acesulfame potassium) is marketed under the names Sunette and Sweet One. It is a calorie-free sweetener that is 200 times sweeter than sugar. It is used to sweeten gums, candies, beverages, instant tea, coffee, gelatins, and puddings. The taste of acesulfame-K does not change when it is heated, so it can be used in cooking. The body does not metabolize acesulfame-K, so it is excreted unchanged by the kidneys.

Aspartame

Aspartame, also called Equal and NutraSweet, is one of the most popular alternative sweeteners currently found in foods and beverages. Aspartame is composed of two amino acids, phenylalanine and aspartic acid. When these amino acids are separate, one is bitter and the other has no flavor—but joined together, they make a substance that is 180 times sweeter than sucrose. Although aspartame contains 4 kcal of energy per gram, it is so sweet that only small amounts are necessary; thus, it ends up contributing little or no energy. Because aspartame is made from amino acids, its taste is destroyed with heat (see Chapter 6); thus, it cannot be used in cooking.

A significant amount of research has been done to test the safety of aspartame. While a number of false claims have been published, especially on the Internet, there is no scientific evidence to support the claim that aspartame causes brain tumors, Alzheimer's disease, or nerve disorders.

Table 4.4 shows how many servings of aspartame-sweetened foods have to be consumed to exceed the ADI. Although eating less than the ADI is considered safe, note that children who consume many powdered drinks, diet sodas, and other aspartame-flavored products could potentially exceed this amount. Drinks sweetened with aspartame are extremely popular among children and teenagers, but they are very low in nutritional value and should not replace healthful beverages such as milk, water, and fruit juice.

There are some people who should not consume aspartame at all: those with the disease *phenylketonuria (PKU)*. This is a genetic disorder that prevents the breakdown of the amino acid phenylalanine. Because the person with PKU cannot metabolize phenylalanine, it builds up in the tissues of the body and causes irreversible brain damage. In the United States, all newborn babies are tested for PKU; those who have it are placed on a phenylalanine-limited diet. Some foods that are important sources of protein and other nutrients for growing children, such as meats and

Contrary to recent reports claiming severe health consequences related to consumption of alternative sweeteners, major health agencies have determined that these products are safe for us to consume.

TABLE 4.4   The Amount of Food that a 50-Pound Child and a 150-Pound Adult Would Have to Consume Each Day to Exceed the ADI for Aspartame

Food	50-Pound Child	150-Pound Adult
12 fl. oz carbonated soft drink	7	20
8 fl. oz powdered soft drink	11	34
4 fl. oz gelatin dessert	14	42
Packets of tabletop sweetener	32	97

Source: Adapted from International Food Information Council. 2001. *Food Safety and Nutrition Information. Sweeteners. Everything You Need to Know about Aspartame.* http://ific.org/publications/factsheets/lcsfs.cfm.

milk, contain phenylalanine. Thus, it is critical that children with PKU not waste what little phenylalanine they can consume on nutrient-poor products sweetened with aspartame.

Sucralose

The FDA has recently approved the use of *sucralose* as an alternative sweetener. It is marketed under the brand name Splenda. It is made from sucrose, but chlorine atoms are substituted for the hydrogen and oxygen normally found in sucrose, and it passes through the digestive tract unchanged, without contributing any energy. It is 600 times sweeter than sucrose and is stable when heated, so it can be used in cooking. It has been approved for use in many foods, including chewing gum, salad dressings, beverages, gelatin and pudding products, canned fruits, frozen dairy desserts, and baked goods. Safety studies have not shown sucralose to cause cancer or to have other adverse health effects.

Other Alternative Sweeteners

Two additional alternative sweeteners that are awaiting FDA approval in the United States are *alitame* and *D-tagatose*. Alitame is composed of two amino acids, but unlike aspartame it remains stable when heated. D-tagatose is made from lactose. Its sweetness is equal to that of sucrose, but it contributes only half the energy.

> RECAP: *Alternative sweeteners can be used in place of sugar to sweeten foods. Most of these products do not promote tooth decay and contribute little or no energy. The alternative sweeteners approved for use in the United States are considered safe when eaten in amounts less than the acceptable daily intake.*

What Disorders Are Related to Carbohydrate Metabolism?

Health conditions that affect the body's ability to absorb and/or use carbohydrates include diabetes, hypoglycemia, and lactose intolerance.

Diabetes: Impaired Regulation of Glucose

Diabetes is a chronic disease in which the body can no longer regulate glucose within normal limits, and blood glucose levels become dangerously high or fall dangerously low. It is imperative to detect and treat the disease as soon as possible because excessive fluctuations in glucose injure tissues throughout the body. If not controlled, diabetes can lead to blindness, seizures, kidney failure, nerve disease, amputations, stroke, and heart disease. In severe cases, it is fatal.

diabetes   A chronic disease in which the body can no longer regulate glucose.

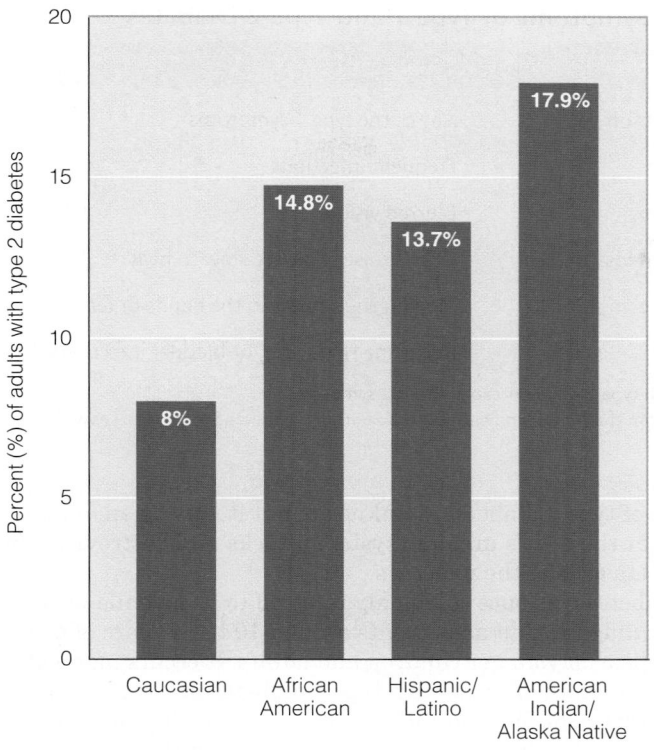

FIGURE 4.18 The percent of adults from various ethnic and racial groups with type 2 diabetes. (Values derived from the National Diabetes Information Clearinghouse (NDIC). 2005. National Diabetes Statistics. National Institutes of Health (NIH) Publication No. 06-3892. http://diabetes.niddk.nih.gov/dm/pubs/statistics/index.htm.)

Approximately 16 million people in the United States—6% of the total population including adults and children—are diagnosed with diabetes. It is speculated that another 5 million people have diabetes but do not know it.

FIGURE 4.18 shows the percentage of adults with diabetes from various ethnic groups in the United States.[22] As you can see, diabetes is more common in African Americans, Hispanic/Latino Americans, and American Indians and Alaska Natives than in Caucasians.

There are two main forms of diabetes, type 1 and type 2. Some women develop a third form, *gestational diabetes*, during pregnancy; we will discuss this in more detail in Chapter 19.

In Type 1 Diabetes, the Body Does Not Produce Enough Insulin

Approximately 10% of people with diabetes have **type 1 diabetes,** in which the body cannot produce enough insulin. When they eat a meal and their blood glucose rises, the pancreas is unable to secrete insulin in response. Glucose cannot therefore be transported into the cells, and blood glucose levels soar. The body tries to expel the excess glucose by excreting it in the urine. In fact, the medical term for the disease is *diabetes mellitus* (from the Greek *diabainein*, "to pass through," and Latin *mellitus,* "sweetened with honey"), and frequent urination is one of its warning signs (see Table 4.5 for other symptoms). If blood glucose levels are not controlled, a person with type 1 diabetes will become confused and lethargic and have trouble breathing. This is because the brain cells are not getting enough glucose to properly function. As discussed earlier, uncontrolled diabetes can lead to ketoacidosis; left untreated, the ultimate result is coma and death.

type 1 diabetes Disorder in which the body cannot produce enough insulin.

TABLE 4.5 Symptoms of Type 1 and Type 2 Diabetes

Type 1 Diabetes	Type 2 Diabetes*
Frequent urination	Any of the type 1 symptoms
Unusual thirst	Frequent infections
Extreme hunger	Blurred vision
Unusual weight loss	Cuts/bruises that are slow to heal
Extreme fatigue	Tingling/numbness in the hands or feet
Irritability	Recurring skin, gum, or bladder infections

*Some people with type 2 diabetes experience no symptoms.
Source: Adapted from the American Diabetes Association, Diabetes Symptoms. www.diabetes.org.

FIGURE 4.19 Monitoring blood glucose requires pricking the fingers each day and measuring the blood using a glucometer.

type 2 diabetes Progressive disorder in which body cells become less responsive to insulin.

impaired fasting glucose Fasting blood glucose levels that are higher than normal but not high enough to lead to a diagnosis of type 2 diabetes.

The cause of type 1 diabetes is unknown, but it may be an *autoimmune disease*. This means that the body's immune system attacks and destroys its own tissues, in this case the beta cells of the pancreas.

Type 1 diabetes was once commonly referred to as juvenile-onset diabetes, and most cases are diagnosed in adolescents around 10 to 14 years of age. However, the disease can appear in younger children and adults. It occurs more often in families, so siblings and children of those with type 1 diabetes are at greater risk.

The only treatment for type 1 diabetes is daily insulin injections. Insulin is a hormone made up of protein, so it would be digested in the intestine if taken as a pill. Individuals with type 1 diabetes must monitor their blood glucose levels closely, using a *glucometer*, and administer injections of insulin several times a day to maintain their blood glucose levels in a healthful range (FIGURE 4.19). The accompanying Highlight box describes how one young man with type 1 diabetes stays healthy.

In Type 2 Diabetes, Cells Become Less Responsive to Insulin

In **type 2 diabetes,** body cells become resistant, or less responsive to insulin. This type of diabetes develops progressively, meaning that the biological changes resulting in the disease occur over a long period of time.

In most cases, obesity is the trigger for a cascade of changes that eventually result in the disorder. Specifically, the cells of many obese people are less responsive to insulin, exhibiting a condition called *insulin insensitivity* (or insulin resistance). The pancreas attempts to compensate for this insensitivity by secreting more insulin. At first, the increased secretion of insulin is sufficient to maintain normal blood glucose levels. However, over time a person who is insulin insensitive will have to circulate very high levels of insulin to utilize glucose for energy, and eventually this excessive production is not sufficient to prevent a rise in fasting blood glucose. The resulting condition is referred to as **impaired fasting glucose,** meaning glucose levels are higher than normal but not high enough to lead to a diagnosis of type 2 diabetes. Some health professionals refer to this condition as *pre-diabetes*, as people with impaired fasting glucose are more likely to get type 2 diabetes than people with normal fasting blood glucose levels. Eventually the pancreas becomes incapable of secreting these excessive amounts of insulin, and the beta cells stop producing the hormone altogether. Thus, blood glucose levels may be elevated in a person with type 2 diabetes 1) because of insulin insensitivity, 2) because the pancreas can no longer secrete enough insulin, or 3) because the pancreas has entirely stopped insulin production.

Many factors can cause type 2 diabetes. Genetics plays a role, so relatives of people with type 2 diabetes are at increased risk (see the Highlight: Calculate Your Risk for Type 2 Diabetes on page 150). Obesity and physical inactivity also increase the risk. Indeed, diabetes is thought to have become an epidemic in the United States because of a combination of our poor eating habits, sedentary lifestyles, increased obesity, and an aging population. Most cases of type 2 diabetes develop after age 45, and almost 20% of Americans 65 years and older have diabetes. Once commonly known as *adult-*

HIGHLIGHT

Living with Type 1 Diabetes

Vincent was diagnosed with type 1 diabetes when he was 10 years old. At first, Vincent and his family were frightened by the disease and found it difficult to adapt their lifestyles to provide a safe and health-promoting environment for Vincent. For example, Vincent's mother felt frustrated because her son could no longer eat the cakes, pies, and other sweets she had always enjoyed baking for her family, and Vincent's siblings found themselves watching over their brother's meals and snacks, running to their parents whenever they feared that he was about to eat something that would harm him. Within a few months, though, Vincent's mother learned to adapt her recipes and cooking techniques to produce a variety of foods that Vincent could enjoy, and his siblings learned to allow Vincent the responsibility for his food choices and his health.

Vincent is now a college sophomore and has been living with diabetes for 9 years, but what he still hates most about the disease is that food is always a major issue. Vincent is smart and a good student, but if his blood glucose declines, he has trouble concentrating. He has to eat three nutritious meals a day on a regular schedule, and he can't snack unless his blood sugar is low. When his friends eat candy, chips, or other snacks, he can't join them. In general he knows these dietary changes are very healthy, but sometimes he wishes he could eat like all of his friends. On the other hand, he cannot skip a meal, even if he isn't hungry. It is also important for Vincent to stay on a regular schedule for exercise and sleep.

Vincent must test his blood sugar many times each day. He has to prick his fingers to do this, and they get tender and develop calluses. During his first few years with diabetes, he had to give himself two to four shots of insulin each day. He learned to measure the insulin into a syringe, and to change the injection site with each insulin shot to avoid damaging his skin and underlying tissue. Technological advances now offer easier alternatives than a needle and syringe. Vincent uses an insulin infusion pump, which looks like a small pager and delivers insulin into the body through a long, thin tube in very small amounts throughout the day. One of Vincent's friends also has type 1 diabetes but can't use a pump; instead, he uses an insulin pen, which includes a needle and a cartridge of insulin. Now that Vincent uses the insulin pump, he can choose to eat more of the foods he loves and deliver his insulin accordingly.

Insulin pumps can help those with diabetes eat a wider range of foods.

Although diabetes is challenging, it does not prevent Vincent from playing soccer and basketball almost every day. In fact, he knows that people with diabetes should be active. As long as he takes his insulin regularly, keeps an eye on his blood sugar, drinks plenty of water, and eats when he should, he knows that he can play sports and do most of the things he wants to do. There are numerous professional and Olympic athletes and other famous people who have diabetes, showing that this disease should not prevent Vincent from leading a healthful life and realizing his dreams.

Presently there is no cure for type 1 diabetes. However, there are many new treatments and potential cures being researched. The FDA has approved several devices that measure blood glucose without pricking the finger. Some of them can read glucose levels through the skin, and others take readings from a small needle implanted in the body to monitor glucose continually. Tests are also being conducted on insulin nasal sprays and inhalers. Advances in genetic engineering may soon make it possible to transplant healthy beta cells into the pancreas of virtually anyone with type 1 diabetes, so that the normal cells will secrete insulin. Vincent looks forward to seeing major changes in the treatment of diabetes in the next few years.

onset diabetes, type 2 diabetes in children was virtually unheard of until recently. Unfortunately, the disease is increasing dramatically among children and adolescents, posing serious health consequences for them and their future children.[22]

Type 2 diabetes can be treated in a variety of ways. Weight loss, healthful eating patterns, and regular exercise can control symptoms in some people. More severe cases may require oral medications. These drugs work in either of two ways: they improve body cells' sensitivity to insulin or reduce the amount of glucose the liver produces. If a person with type 2 diabetes can no longer secrete enough insulin, the patient must take daily injections of insulin just like a person with type 1 diabetes.

HIGHLIGHT

Calculate Your Risk for Type 2 Diabetes

To calculate your risk for developing type 2 diabetes, answer the following questions:

I am overweight.	yes	no
I am sedentary (I exercise fewer than three times a week).	yes	no
I have a close family member with type 2 diabetes.	yes	no
I am a member of one of the following groups:	yes	no

African American
Hispanic American (Latino)
Native American
Pacific Islander

I have had gestational diabetes, or I gave birth to at least one baby weighing more than 9 pounds.	yes	no
My blood pressure is 140/90 or higher, or I have been told that I have high blood pressure.	yes	no
My cholesterol levels are not normal. (See the discussion of cholesterol in Chapter 5.)	yes	no

The more "yes" responses you give, the higher your risk of developing type 2 diabetes. You cannot change your ethnicity or your family members' health, but you can take steps to maintain a healthful weight and increase your physical activity. For tips, see Chapters 13 and 15.

Data from the National Diabetes Information Clearinghouse (NDIC). Available at http://diabetes.niddk.nih.gov/dm/pubs/riskfortype2/.

Jerry Garcia, a member of the Grateful Dead, had type 2 diabetes.

Lifestyle Choices Can Help Control or Prevent Diabetes

In general, people with diabetes should follow many of the same dietary guidelines recommended for those without diabetes. One difference is that people with diabetes may need to eat less carbohydrate and slightly more fat or protein to help regulate their blood glucose levels. Carbohydrates are still an important part of the diet, but their intake may need to be reduced. Precise nutritional recommendations vary according to each individual's responses to foods. In addition, people with diabetes should avoid alcoholic beverages, which can cause hypoglycemia. The symptoms of alcohol intoxication and hypoglycemia are very similar. The person with diabetes and his or her companions may confuse these conditions; this can result in a potentially life-threatening situation.

While there is no cure for type 2 diabetes, many cases could be prevented or onset delayed. We cannot control our family history, but we can eat a balanced diet, exercise regularly, and maintain an appropriate body weight. Studies show that losing only 10 to 30 pounds can reduce or eliminate the symptoms of type 2 diabetes.[23] In addition, moderate daily exercise may prevent the onset of type 2 diabetes more effectively than dietary changes alone.[24] By selecting plenty of whole grains, fruits, legumes, and vegetables and by staying active and maintaining a healthful body weight, our risk for diabetes should remain low.

RECAP: *Diabetes is a disease that results in dangerously high levels of blood glucose. Type 1 diabetes typically appears at a young age; the pancreas cannot secrete sufficient insulin so insulin injections are required. Type 2 diabetes develops over time and may be triggered by obesity: body cells are no longer sensitive to the effects of insulin or the pancreas no longer secretes sufficient insulin for bodily needs. Supplemental insulin may or may not be needed to treat type 2 diabetes. Diabetes increases the risk of dangerous complications such as heart disease, blindness, kidney disease, and amputations. Many cases of type 2 diabetes could be prevented or delayed with a balanced diet, regular exercise, and achieving and/or maintaining a healthful body weight.*

NUTRI-CASE JUDY

" My daughter, Hannah, is overweight and the school nurse wants me to have her tested for type 2 diabetes. I'm against it. Even though I was just recently told I have type 2 diabetes, I think she's got enough to handle with her school work, peer pressure, and all of the changes of adolescence coming on. I think a wait-and-see approach is best for now. The last thing she needs is this scary disease!"

Do you think Judy should have Hannah tested for type 2 diabetes? What are Hannah's risk factors? Can you think of any benefits of early diagnosis, and do you think they would outweigh the possible stress of knowing she had the disease?

Hypoglycemia: Low Blood Glucose

In **hypoglycemia,** blood sugar falls to lower-than-normal levels (FIGURE 4.20). One cause of hypoglycemia is excessive production of insulin, which lowers blood glucose too far. People with diabetes can develop hypoglycemia if they inject too much insulin or when they exercise and fail to eat enough carbohydrates. Two types of hypoglycemia can develop in people who do not have diabetes: reactive and fasting.

Reactive hypoglycemia occurs when the pancreas secretes too much insulin after a high-carbohydrate meal. The symptoms of reactive hypoglycemia usually appear about 1 to 4 hours after the meal and include nervousness, shakiness, anxiety, sweating, irritability, headache, weakness, and rapid or irregular heartbeat. Although many people experience these symptoms from time to time, they are rarely caused by true hypoglycemia. A person diagnosed with reactive hypoglycemia must eat smaller meals more frequently to level out blood insulin and glucose levels.

Fasting hypoglycemia occurs when the body continues to produce too much insulin, even when someone has not eaten. This condition is usually caused by another medical condition such as cancer, liver infection, alcohol-induced liver disease, or a tumor in the pancreas. Its symptoms are similar to those of reactive hypoglycemia, but occur more than 4 hours after a meal.

hypoglycemia A condition marked by blood glucose levels that are below normal fasting levels.

FIGURE 4.20 Changes in blood glucose after a meal for people with hypoglycemia and without hypoglycemia (normal).

> RECAP: *Hypoglycemia refers to lower-than-normal blood glucose levels. Reactive hypoglycemia occurs when the pancreas secretes too much insulin after a high-carbohydrate meal. Fasting hypoglycemia occurs when the body continues to produce too much insulin even when someone has not eaten.*

Lactose Intolerance: Inability to Digest Lactose

Sometimes our bodies do not produce enough of the enzymes necessary to break down carbohydrates before they reach the colon. A common example is **lactose intolerance,** in which the body does not produce sufficient amounts of the enzyme lactase in the small intestine and therefore cannot digest foods containing lactose. Lactose intolerance should not be confused with a milk allergy. People who are allergic to milk experience an immune reaction to the proteins found in cow's milk. Symptoms of milk allergy include skin reactions such as hives and rashes; intestinal distress such as nausea, vomiting, cramping, and diarrhea; and respiratory symptoms such as wheezing, runny nose, and itchy and watery eyes. In severe cases, anaphylactic shock can occur.

Symptoms of lactose intolerance include intestinal gas, bloating, cramping, nausea, diarrhea, and discomfort. While some infants are born with lactose intolerance, it is more common to see lactase enzyme activity decrease after 2 years of age. In fact, it is estimated that up to 70% of the world's adult population lose some ability to digest lactose as they age. In the United States, lactose intolerance is more common in Native American, Asian, Hispanic, and African-American adults than in Caucasians.

Not everyone experiences lactose intolerance to the same extent. Some people can digest small amounts of dairy products, while others cannot tolerate any. Suarez et al.[25] found that many people who reported being lactose intolerant were able to consume multiple small servings of dairy products without symptoms, which enabled them to meet their calcium requirements. Thus, it is not necessary for them to avoid all dairy products; they may simply need to eat smaller amounts and experiment to find foods that do not cause intestinal distress.

It is important that people with lactose intolerance, regardless of age, find foods that can supply enough calcium for normal growth, development, and maintenance of bones. Many can tolerate specially formulated milk products that are low in lactose, while others take pills or use drops that contain the lactase enzyme when they eat dairy products. Calcium-fortified soy milk and orange juice are excellent substitutes for cow's milk. Many lactose-intolerant people can also digest yogurt and aged cheese, as the bacteria or molds used to ferment these products break down the lactose during processing.

How can you tell if you are lactose intolerant? Many people discover that they have problems digesting dairy products by trial and error. Because intestinal gas, bloating, and diarrhea may indicate other health problems too, you should consult a physician to determine the cause.

Tests for lactose intolerance include drinking a lactose-rich liquid and testing blood glucose levels over a 2-hour period. If you do not produce the normal amount of glucose, you are unable to digest the lactose present. Another test involves measuring hydrogen levels in the breath, as lactose-intolerant people breathe out more hydrogen when they drink a beverage that contains lactose.

> RECAP: *Lactose intolerance results from the inability to digest lactose due to insufficient amounts of lactase. Symptoms include intestinal gas, bloating, cramping, diarrhea, and nausea. Lactose intolerance commonly occurs in non-Caucasian populations. The extent of lactose intolerance varies from mild to severe.*

Milk products, such as ice cream, are hard to digest for people who are lactose intolerant.

lactose intolerance A disorder in which the body does not produce sufficient lactase enzyme and therefore cannot digest foods that contain lactose, such as cow's milk.

CHAPTER SUMMARY

- Carbohydrates contain carbon, hydrogen, and oxygen. Plants make the carbohydrate glucose during photosynthesis.

- Simple sugars include mono- and disaccharides. The three primary monosaccharides are glucose, fructose, and galactose.

- Two monosaccharides joined together are called disaccharides. Glucose and fructose join to make sucrose, glucose and glucose join to make maltose, and glucose and galactose join to make lactose.

- Starches are polysaccharides, and they are the storage form of glucose in plants.

- Glycogen is the storage form of glucose in humans. Glycogen is stored in the liver and in muscles. Liver glycogen provides glucose to help us maintain blood sugar levels, while muscle glycogen is used for energy during exercise.

- Dietary fiber is the nondigestible parts of plants, while functional fiber is nondigestible forms of carbohydrate extracted from plants or manufactured in the laboratory. Fiber may reduce the risk of many diseases and digestive illnesses.

- All cells can use glucose for energy. The red blood cells, brain, and central nervous system prefer to use glucose exclusively for energy.

- Using glucose for energy helps spare body proteins, and glucose is an important fuel for the body during exercise. Exercising regularly trains our muscles to become more efficient at using both glucose and fat for energy.

- Fiber helps us maintain the healthy elimination of waste products. Eating adequate fiber may reduce the risk of colon cancer, type 2 diabetes, obesity, heart disease, hemorrhoids, and diverticulosis.

- Carbohydrate digestion starts in the mouth, where chewing and an enzyme called salivary amylase start breaking down the carbohydrates in food.

- Digestion continues in the small intestine. Specific enzymes are secreted to break starches into smaller mono- and disaccharides. As disaccharides pass through the intestinal cells, they are digested into monosaccharides.

- Glucose and other monosaccharides are absorbed into the bloodstream and travel to the liver, where all molecules are converted to glucose.

- Glucose is transported in the bloodstream to the cells, where it is either used for energy or stored in the liver or muscle as glycogen.

- Insulin and glucagon are hormones secreted by the pancreas in response to changes in blood glucose.

- Insulin is secreted when blood glucose increases sufficiently, and it assists with the transport of glucose into cells.

- Glucagon is secreted when blood glucose levels are low, and it assists with the conversion of glycogen to glucose and with gluconeogenesis.

- The glycemic index and glycemic load are values that indicate how much a food increases glucose levels. High glycemic foods can trigger detrimental increases in blood glucose for people with diabetes. The usefulness of the glycemic index and glycemic load for making dietary recommendations is controversial.

- The Acceptable Macronutrient Distribution Range for carbohydrate is 45% to 65% of total energy intake.

- High added sugar intake can cause tooth decay, elevate levels of harmful blood lipids, and contribute to obesity, but it does not appear to cause hyperactivity in children.

- The Adequate Intake for fiber is 25 g per day for women and 38 g per day for men, or 14 g of fiber for every 1,000 kcal of energy consumed.

- Foods high in complex carbohydrates include whole grains and cereals, fruits, and vegetables. Eating 6 to 11 servings of breads/grains and 5 to 9 servings of fruits and vegetables helps ensure that you meet your complex carbohydrate goals.

- Alternative sweeteners are added to some foods because they sweeten foods without promoting tooth decay and add little or no calories to foods.

- Sugar alcohols, saccharin, acesulfame-K, aspartame, and sucralose are examples of alternative sweeteners used in foods and beverages.

- All alternative sweeteners approved for use in the United States are felt to be safe when eaten at levels at or below the acceptable daily intake levels defined by the FDA.

- Diabetes is caused by insufficient insulin or by the cells becoming resistant or insensitive to insulin. Diabetes causes dangerously high blood glucose levels. There are two primary types of diabetes, type 1 and type 2.

- Lower than normal blood glucose levels is defined as hypoglycemia. There are two types, reactive and fasting. Reactive occurs when too much insulin is secreted after a high-carbohydrate meal; fasting occurs when blood glucose drops even though no food has been eaten.

- Lactose intolerance results from an insufficient amount of the lactase enzyme. Symptoms include intestinal gas, bloating, cramping, diarrhea, and discomfort.

TEST YOURSELF ANSWERS

1. **False.** Although specific estimates are not yet available, significantly higher rates of type 2 diabetes are now being reported in children and adolescents; these higher rates are attributed to increasing obesity rates in young people.

2. **False.** There is no evidence that diets high in sugar cause hyperactivity in children or diabetes.

3. **False.** At 4 kcal/g, carbohydrates have less than half the energy of a gram of fat. Eating a high-carbohydrate diet will not cause people to gain body fat unless their total diet contains more energy (or kcal) than they expend. In fact, eating a diet high in complex, fiber-rich carbohydrates is associated with a lower risk for obesity.

4. **True.** Our brains rely almost exclusively on glucose for energy, and our body tissues utilize glucose for energy both at rest and during exercise.

5. **True.** Contrary to recent reports claiming harmful consequences related to consumption of alternative sweeteners, major health agencies have determined that these products are safe for most of us to consume in limited quantities.

FIND THE QUACK

Christina is surfing the Internet looking for information for a report on carbohydrates for her nutrition class when she spots something that intrigues her: Cure Diseases with Sugar! She wonders what it's all about and clicks to bring up the site (www.glycotech.net/index.html). Glyconutrients! the homepage proclaims. There are promises listed of reversing aging, increasing sporting performance, and achieving optimal health. Beside a photo of a slender, tanned couple walking along a beach are statements claiming that:

- Processed foods are devoid of nourishment and have no nutritional value. They are also toxic. We both starve and poison ourselves by consuming these foods. This is why every degenerative disease condition is on the rise.

- Pharmaceuticals (prescription and over-the-counter medications) do not work.

- Glyconutrients are plant monosaccharides that are essential plant sugars that have recently been shown to be essential to human life. We must consume glyconutrient supplements to protect our health. Without them, our cells will lose the ability to communicate with one another and perform the functions they were designed to do. We will then develop chronic diseases such as cancer and diabetes.

- A total of 96 patents have been filed on a range of glyconutrient products.

- Just about every respected scientific journal has now published documents and articles on glycobiology and glyconutrients.

- Your doctor will not know about glyconutrients because the topic is only just now beginning to be taught in medical schools.

1. In Chapter 2, you learned how to spot false nutrition claims (pages 43–47). Discuss the validity of the Web site's statement about processed foods.

2. Comment on the Web site's definition of glyconutrients as plant monosaccharides that are essential for human life.

3. Are you impressed with the statement that "96 patents have been filed on a range of glyconutrient products"? Why or why not?

4. What motive do you think might lurk behind the assertion that your doctor will not know about glyconutrients because the topic "is only 'just' being taught in medical schools"?

Answers can be found at www.aw-bc.com/thompson.

REVIEW QUESTIONS

1. The glycemic index rates
   a. the acceptable amount of alternative sweeteners to consume in 1 day.
   b. the potential of foods to raise blood glucose and insulin levels.
   c. the risk of a given food for causing diabetes.
   d. the ratio of soluble to insoluble fiber in a complex carbohydrate.

2. Carbohydrates contain
   a. carbon, nitrogen, and water.
   b. carbonic acid and a sugar alcohol.
   c. hydrated sugar.
   d. carbon, hydrogen, and oxygen.

3. The most common source of added sugar in the American diet is
   a. table sugar.
   b. white flour.
   c. alcohol.
   d. sweetened soft drinks.

4. Glucose, fructose, and galactose are
   a. monosaccharides.
   b. disaccharides.
   c. polysaccharides.
   d. complex carbohydrates.

5. Aspartame should not be consumed by people who have
   a. phenylketonuria.
   b. type 1 diabetes.
   c. lactose intolerance.
   d. diverticulosis.

6. True or false? Sugar alcohols are non-nutritive sweeteners.

7. True or false? Insulin and glucagon are both pancreatic hormones.

8. True or false? A person with lactose intolerance is allergic to milk.

9. True or false? Plants store glucose as fiber.

10. True or false? Salivary amylase breaks down starches into galactose.

11. Describe the role of insulin in regulating blood glucose levels.

12. Identify at least four ways in which fiber helps us maintain a healthy digestive system.

13. Defend the statement that obesity can trigger type 2 diabetes.

14. Create a table listing molecular composition and food sources of each of the following carbohydrates: glucose, fructose, lactose, and sucrose.

15. A few weeks after your grandfather was diagnosed with type 2 diabetes, you share a holiday meal with your family. As your grandfather is adding whipped cream to the pecan pie on his plate, your grandmother shouts, "Stu! How could you! You know you're not supposed to eat sweets anymore!" Is your grandmother correct? Why or why not?

WEB LINKS

www.eatright.org
American Dietetic Association

Visit this Web site to learn more about diabetes, low- and high-carbohydrate diets, and general healthful eating habits.

www.ific.org
International Food Information Council Foundation (IFIC)

Search this site to find out more about sugars and low-calorie sweeteners.

www.ada.org
American Dental Association

Go to this site to learn more about tooth decay as well as other oral health topics.

www.nidcr.nih.gov
National Institute of Dental and Craniofacial Research (NIDCR)

Find out more about recent oral and dental health discoveries, and obtain statistics and data on the status of dental health in the United States.

www.diabetes.org
American Diabetes Association

Find out more about the nutritional needs of people living with diabetes.

www.niddk.nih.gov
National Institute of Diabetes and Digestive and Kidney Diseases (NIDDK)

Learn more about diabetes including treatment, complications, U.S. statistics, clinical trials, and recent research.

REFERENCES

1. Kleinfield, N. R. 2006. Diabetes and its awful toll quietly emerge as a crisis. *The New York Times*. January 9, 2006. http://www.nytimes.com/2006/01/09/nyregion/nyregionspecial5/09diabetes.html. (Accessed March 2007.)
2. Sears, B. 1995. *The Zone. A Dietary Road Map*. New York: HarperCollins Publishers.

3. Steward, H. L., M. C. Bethea, S. S. Andrews, and L. A. Balart. 1995. *Sugar Busters! Cut Sugar to Trim Fat.* New York: Ballantine Books.

4. Atkins, R. C. 1992. *Dr. Atkins' New Diet Revolution.* New York: M. Evans & Company, Inc.

5. Topping, D. L., and P. M. Clifton. 2001. Short-chain fatty acids and human colonic function: roles of resistant starch and nonstarch polysaccharides. *Physiol. Rev.* 81:1031–1064.

6. Institute of Medicine, Food and Nutrition Board. 2002. *Dietary Reference Intakes for Energy, Carbohydrates, Fiber, Fat, Protein and Amino Acids (Macronutrients).* Washington, DC: The National Academy of Sciences.

7. Tremblay, A., J. A. Simoneau, and C. Bouchard. 1994. Impact of exercise intensity on body fatness and skeletal muscle metabolism. *Metabolism* 43:814–818.

8. Pan, J. W., D. L. Rothman, K. L. Behar, D. T. Stein, and H. P. Hetherington. 2000. Human brain β-hydroxybutyrate and lactate increase in fasting-induced ketosis. *J. Cerebral Blood Flow Metabol.* 20:1502–1507.

9. Foster-Powell, K., S. H. A. Holt, and J. C. Brand-Miller. 2002. International table of glycemic index and glycemic load values: 2002. *Am. J. Clin. Nutr.* 76:5–56.

10. Liu, S., J. E. Manson, M. J. Stampfer, M. D. Holmes, F. B. Hu, S. E. Hankinson, and W. C. Willett. 2001. Dietary glycemic load assessed by food-frequency questionnaire in relation to plasma high-density-lipoprotein cholesterol and fasting plasma triacylglycerols in postmenopausal women. *Am. J. Clin. Nutr.* 73:560–566.

11. Sloth, B., I. Krog-Mikkelsen, A. Flint, I. Tetens, I. Björck, S. Vinoy, H. Elmståhl, A. Astrup, V. Lang, and A. Raben. 2004. No difference in body weight decrease between a low-glycemic-index and a high-glycemic-index diet but reduced LDL cholesterol after 10-wk ad libitum intake of the low-glycemic-index diet. *Am. J. Clin. Nutr.* 80:337–347.

12. Buyken, A. E., M. Toeller, G. Heitkamp, G. Karamanos, B. Rottiers, R. Muggeo, and M. Fuller. 2001. Glycemic index in the diet of European outpatients with type 1 diabetes: relations to glycated hemoglobin and serum lipids. *Am. J. Clin. Nutr.* 73:574–581.

13. Augustin, L. S. A., C. Galeone, L. Dal Maso, C. Pelucchi, V. Ramazzotti, D. J. A. Jenkins, M. Montella, R. Talamini, E. Negri, S. Franceschi, and C. La Vecchia. 2004. Glycemic index, glycemic load and risk of prostate cancer. *Int. J. Cancer* 112: 446–450.

14. U.S. Department of Health and Human Services (USDHHS) and U.S. Department of Agriculture (USDA). 2005. *Dietary Guidelines for Americans, 2005,* 6th edn. Washington, DC: U.S. Government Printing Office. www.healthierus.gov/dietaryguidelines. (Accessed March 2007.)

15. U.S. Department of Health and Human Services (USDHHS) and U.S. Department of Agriculture (USDA). 2006. Eating healthier and feeling better using the Nutrition Facts Label. http://www.cfsan.fda.gov/~acrobat/nutfacts.pdf. (Accessed March 2007.)

16. Howard, B. V., and J. Wylie-Rosett. 2002. Sugar and cardiovascular disease. A statement for healthcare professionals from the Committee on Nutrition of the Council on Nutrition, Physical Activity, and Metabolism of the American Heart Association. *Circulation* 106:523–527.

17. Meyer, K. A., L. H. Kushi, D. R. Jacobs, J. Slavin, T. A. Sellers, and A. R. Folsom. 2000. Carbohydrates, dietary fiber, and incident type 2 diabetes in older women. *Am. J. Clin. Nutr.* 71:921–930.

18. Colditz, G. A., J. E. Manson, M. J. Stampfer, B. Rosner, W. C. Willett, and F. E. Speizer. 1992. Diet and risk of clinical diabetes in women. *Am. J. Clin. Nutr.* 55:1018–1023.

19. Troiano, R. P., R. R. Briefel, M. D. Carroll, and K. Bialostosky. 2000. Energy and fat intakes of children and adolescents in the United States: Data from the National Health and Nutrition Examination Surveys. *Am. J. Clin. Nutr.* 72:1343S–1353S.

20. Ludwig, D. S., K. E. Peterson, and S. L. Gortmaker. 2001. Relation between consumption of sugar-sweetened drinks and childhood obesity: a prospective, observational analysis. *Lancet* 357:505–508.

21. International Food Information Council Foundation. 2004. Gestational Diabetes and Low-Calorie Sweeteners: Answers to Common Questions. http://www.ific.org/publications/brochures/upload/gestationaldiabetes.pdf. (Accessed March 2007.)

22. National Diabetes Information Clearinghouse (NDIC). 2005. National Diabetes Statistics. National Institutes of Health Publication No. 06–3892. http://diabetes.niddk.nih.gov/dm/pubs/statistics/index.htm. (Accessed March 2007.)

23. American College of Sports Medicine (ACSM). 2000. Position stand: Exercise and type 2 diabetes. *Med. Sci. Sports Exerc.* 32:1345–1360.

24. Pan, X.-P., G.-W. Li, Y.-H. Hu, J. X. Wang, W. Y. Yang, Z. X. An, Z. X. Hu, J. Lin, J. Z. Xiao, H. B. Cao, P. A. Liu, X. G. Jiang, Y. Y. Jiang, J. P. Wang., H. Zheng, H. Zhang, P. H. Bennett, and B. V. Howard. 1997. Effects of diet and exercise in preventing NIDDM in people with impaired glucose tolerance. *Diabetes Care* 20:537–544.

25. Suarez, F. L., J. Adshead, J. K. Furne, and M. D. Levitt. 1998. Lactose maldigestion is not an impediment to the intake of 1500 mg calcium daily as dairy products. *Am. J. Clin. Nutr.* 68:1118–1122.

26. Ogden, C. L., M. D. Carroll, L. R. Curtin, M. A. McDowell, C. J. Tabak, and K. M. Flegal. 2006. Prevalence of overweight and obesity in the United States, 1999–2004. *JAMA* 295(13):1549–1555.

27. Elliott, S. S., N. L. Keim, J. S. Stern, K. Teff, and P. J. Havel. 2002. Fructose, weight gain, and the insulin resistance syndrome. *Am. J. Clin. Nutr.* 76:911–922.

28. Bray, G. A., S. J. Nielsen, and B. M. Popkin. 2004. Consumption of high-fructose corn syrup in beverages may play a role in the epidemic of obesity. *Am. J. Clin. Nutr.* 79:537–543.

29. Wilkinson Enns, C., S. J. Mickle, and J. D. Goldman. 2002. Trends in food and nutrient intakes by children in the United States. *Family Econ. Nutr. Rev.* 14:56–68.

30. Harnack, L., J. Stang, and M. Story. 1999. Soft drink consumption among U.S. children and adolescents: nutritional consequences. *J. Am. Diet. Assoc.* 99:436–441.

31. Ebbeling, C. B., H. A. Feldman, S. K. Osganian, S. H. Ellenbogen, and D. S. Ludwig. 2006. Effects of decreasing sugar-sweetened beverage consumption on body weight in adolescents: a randomized, controlled pilot study. *Pediatrics* 117:673–680.

32. Jacobson, M. F. 2004. Letter to the editor. High-fructose corn syrup and the obesity epidemic. *Am. J. Clin. Nutr.* 80:1081–1090.

33. Lê, K.-A., D. Faeh, R. Stettler, M. Ith, R. Kreis, P. Vermathen, C. Boesch, E. Ravussin, and L. Tappy. 2006. A 4-wk high-fructose diet alters lipid metabolism without affecting insulin sensitivity or ectopic lipids in healthy humans. *Am. J. Clin. Nutr.* 84:1374–1379.

NUTRITION DEBATE

Is High-Fructose Corn Syrup the Cause of the Obesity Epidemic?

almost every day in the news we see headlines about obesity: "More Americans Overweight!", "The Fattening of America," "Obesity is a National Epidemic!" These headlines accurately reflect the state of weight in the United States. Over the past 30 years, obesity rates have increased dramatically for both adults and children. Obesity has become public health enemy number one, as many chronic diseases such as type 2 diabetes, heart disease, high blood pressure, and arthritis go hand in hand with obesity.

Of particular concern are the rising obesity rates in children. Although national health statistics do not distinguish between obesity and overweight in children, it is estimated that the prevalence of overweight in young children aged 2 to 5 years has doubled since the 1970s, while the rate of overweight in school-aged children (6 to 19 years of age) has tripled over this same time period.[26] Why should we concern ourselves with fighting obesity in children? First, it is well established that the treatment of existing obesity is extremely challenging, and our greatest hope of combating this disease is through prevention. Most agree that prevention should start with children at a very early age. Second, approximately 30% of children who are obese will remain obese as adults, suffering all of the health problems that accompany this disease. Young children are now experiencing type 2 diabetes, high blood pressure, and high cholesterol at increasingly younger ages, only compounding the devastating effects of these illnesses as they get older. We have reached the point where serious action must be taken immediately to curb the already growing crisis.

How can we prevent obesity? This is a difficult question to answer. One way is to better understand the factors that contribute to obesity, and then take actions to alter these factors. We know of many factors that contribute to overweight and obesity. These include genetic influences, lack of adequate physical activity, and eating foods that are high in fat, added sugar, and energy. While it is easy to blame our genetics, they cannot be held entirely responsible for the rapid rise in obesity that has occurred over the past 30 years. Our genetic makeup takes thousands of years to change; thus, humans who lived 50 or 100 years ago have essentially the same genetic makeup as humans who live now. The fact that obesity rates have risen so dramatically in recent years illustrates that we need to look more closely at how our

lifestyle changes over this same period have contributed to obesity.

One factor that has recently come to the forefront of nutrition research and policy making is the contribution of added sugars, particularly in the form of high-fructose corn syrup (HFCS), to overweight and obesity. As discussed earlier in this chapter, there is disagreement about whether added sugar does cause, and how much it might contribute to, obesity. Many nutrition researchers are beginning to draw attention to the potential role of HFCS in rising obesity rates. Before we discuss why these researchers are pointing to HFCS as a major cause of the obesity epidemic, it is important to understand what HFCS is and how it is metabolized in our bodies.

HFCS is made by first converting the starch in corn to glucose, and then converting some of the glucose to fructose through a process referred to as *enzymatic isomerization*. The result is an inexpensive corn-based syrup that has been used to replace sucrose and other simple sugars as a sweetener in foods and beverages. Fructose is sweeter than glucose. It is also metabolized differently from glucose, as it is absorbed further down in the small intestine and, unlike glucose, it does not stimulate insulin release from the pancreas. It also enters the cell by a transport protein that does not require the presence of

It is estimated that the rate of overweight in children has increased 100% since the mid-1970s.

insulin. Interestingly, brain cells do not have this transport protein; thus, unlike glucose, fructose cannot enter brain cells and stimulate satiety signals. In addition, consumption of fructose increases the production of triglycerides (a form of fat) in the blood significantly more than glucose, and in animals can lead to excessive insulin production, resistance to insulin, and impaired glucose regulation—all factors that can lead to type 2 diabetes.[27]

How might the consumption of HFCS contribute to obesity? Bray et al.[28] speculate that HFCS could lead to increased obesity because of its effect on appetite regulation and its contribution to excessive energy intake. Both insulin and the hormone leptin inhibit food intake in humans, and as previously stated fructose does not stimulate insulin release. As insulin increases the release of leptin, it is possible that consuming fructose results in lower

circulating levels of both insulin and leptin, which results in an increase in appetite and food intake. At the same time, consuming foods high in HFCS could contribute to obesity because people consume significant amounts of excess energy in the form of sweetened soft drinks. Bray et al.[28] emphasize that HFCS could be a major culprit in the obesity epidemic because it is the sole caloric sweetener in sugared soft drinks and represents more than 40% of caloric sweeteners added to other foods and beverages in the United States. These researchers have linked the increased use and consumption of HFCS in beverages and foods with the rising rates of obesity since the 1970s, when HFCS was first developed and marketed (see the graph below).

The potential contribution of sweetened soft drink consumption to rising rates of obesity in children and adolescents has received a great deal of attention in recent years. Studies of soft drink consumption in children show that girls and boys ages 6 to 11 years drank about twice as many soft drinks in 1998 as compared to 1977, and consumption of milk over this same time period dropped by about 30%.[29] Equally alarming is the finding that one-fourth of a group of adolescents studied were heavy consumers of sugared soft drinks, drinking at least 26 oz of soft drinks each day. This intake is equivalent to almost 400 extra calories each day, and these individuals consumed more energy from all foods than other adolescents and drank less nutritious beverages such as milk and fruit juice.[30] One report found that for each extra sugared soft drink that children drink each day, the risk of obesity increases by 60%.[20] A recent pilot intervention study found that replacing sweetened soft drinks with noncaloric beverages in 13- to 18-year-old adolescents

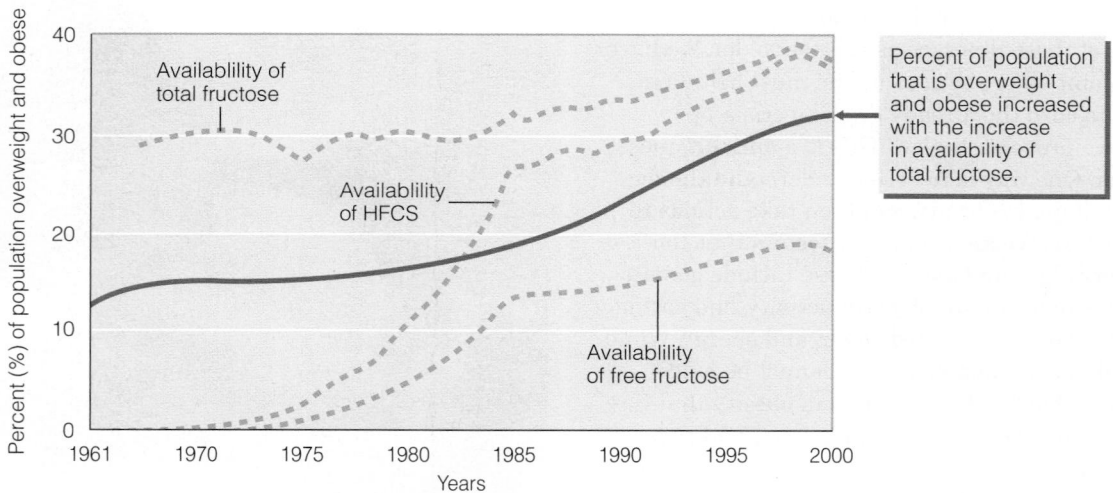

Availability of total fructose, high-fructose corn syrup (HFCS), and free fructose in relation to obesity prevalence in the United States. (*Source:* Bray, G. A., S. J. Nielsen, and B. M. Popkin. 2004. Consumption of high fructose corn syrup in beverages may play a role in the epidemic of obesity. *Am. J. Clin. Nutr.* 79:537–543. Used with permission.)

resulted in a significant decrease in body mass index in the adolescents who were the most overweight when starting the study.[31] In addition to providing significant quantities of nutritionally empty calories, soft drinks may also have a detrimental effect on bone density: soft drinks typically displace milk in the diet, and the phosphorus available in some sodas, whether sugared or diet, binds with calcium, causing it to be drawn out of the bones. This is especially harmful during childhood and adolescence, when bones are still growing.

All of this alarming information has led to dramatic changes in soft drink availability in schools and at school-sponsored events. As of 2006, the soft drink industry has agreed to a voluntary ban on sales of all sweetened soft drinks in elementary and high schools, to take effect by the start of the 2009–2010 school year. Despite these positive changes in schools, there is still ample availability of foods and beverages containing HFCS in the marketplace.

Although the evidence pinpointing HFCS as a major contributor to the obesity epidemic may appear strong, other nutrition professionals disagree with these speculations about HFCS. It has been proposed that soft drinks would have contributed to the obesity epidemic no matter whether the sweetener was sucrose or fructose and that their contribution to obesity is due to increased consumption resulting from massive increases in advertising, substantial increases in serving sizes of soft drinks, and virtually unlimited access to soft drinks throughout our everyday lives.[32] A recent study has also indicated that, although 4 weeks of increased fructose consumption in humans does cause an increased production of triglycerides as previously stated, it does not cause weight gain or increased resistance to insulin.[33] Thus, it may be that animals respond differently than humans to diets high in fructose. It is entirely possible that the obesity epidemic has resulted from increased consumption of energy (predominantly in the form of sweetened soft drinks and other high-energy foods) and a reduction in physical activity levels, and HFCS has nothing to do with this epidemic. Evidence to support this supposition stems from the fact that obesity rates are rising around the world, and many of the countries experiencing this epidemic do not use HFCS as a sweetener.

Aggressive marketing and easy availability of soft drinks make them a tempting choice for children and adults, adding HFCS and calories to their diets.

This issue is extremely complex, and it has been suggested that more research needs to be done in humans before we can fully understand how fructose contributes to our diet and our health.[27] How do you feel about this issue? Do you feel HFCS is unhealthful and a major contributor to the obesity epidemic? Should HFCS be banned from our food supply? Should soft drink companies be encouraged to replace HFCS with sucrose or some other form of caloric sweetener? Should reducing soft drink consumption be up to individuals, or should it be mandatory for those at high risk for obesity? Should families, schools, and our government play a central role in controlling the types of foods and beverages offered to young people throughout their day? As this controversy grows, it is more likely that average citizens will be asked to take a stand on this issue.

Alcohol

WANT TO FIND OUT. . .

- what "moderate drinking" really means? p. 161
- how many young Americans die in alcohol-related incidents each year? 166
- if you should be concerned about your alcohol intake? p. 166
- how to talk to someone who might have a drinking problem? pp. 166–168

READ ON.

no one should have to spend his 21st birthday in an emergency room, but that's what happened to Todd the night he turned 21. His friends took him off campus to celebrate, and, with their encouragement, he attempted to drink 21 shots before the bar closed at 2:00 AM. Fortunately for Todd, when he passed out and couldn't be roused, his best friend noticed his cold, clammy skin and erratic breathing and drove him to the local emergency room. There, his stomach was pumped and he was treated for alcohol poisoning. He regained consciousness, but felt sick and shaky for several more hours. Not everyone is so lucky. Some people with alcohol poisoning never wake up.

What makes excessive alcohol intake so dangerous, and why is moderate alcohol consumption often considered healthful? How can you tell if someone is struggling with alcohol addiction, and what can you do to help? What if that someone is you? We explore these questions *In Depth* here.

Alcohols are chemical compounds structurally similar to carbohydrates, with one or more hydroxyl (OH) groups. **Ethanol** is the specific type of alcohol found in beer, wine, and distilled spirits such as whiskey and vodka. Throughout this discussion the common term *alcohol* will be used to represent the specific compound *ethanol*.

What Are the Health Benefits and Concerns of Moderate Alcohol Intake?

Alcohol intake is usually described as "drinks per day." A **drink** is defined as the amount of a beverage that provides ½ fluid ounce of pure alcohol. For example, 12 oz of beer, 10 oz of a wine cooler, 4–5 oz of wine, and 1½ oz of 80 **proof** whiskey, scotch, gin, or vodka are each equivalent to one drink (FIGURE 1).

The 2005 Dietary Guidelines for Americans advise, "Those who choose to drink alcoholic beverages should do so sensibly and in moderation—defined as the consumption of up to one drink per day for women and up to two drinks per day for men." Notice that this definition of moderate drinking is based on a maximal daily intake; a person who does not drink any alcohol on weekdays but downs a six-pack of beer most Saturday nights would NOT be classified as a "moderate drinker"! The 2005 Dietary Guidelines for Americans also identify groups of individuals who should not consume alcohol at all, including women who are or may become pregnant and women who are breastfeeding. In addition, people with a history of alcoholism and those taking medications that interact with alcohol should not drink at all, nor should individuals driving, operating machinery, or engaged in other tasks that require attention and coordination.

As we discuss here, there are both health benefits and concerns related to moderate alcohol intake. When deciding if or how much alcohol to drink, you need to weigh the pros and cons of alcohol consumption as related to your own personal health history.

Benefits of Moderate Alcohol Intake

In most people, moderate alcohol intake offers some psychological benefits; it can reduce stress and anxiety while improving self-confidence. It can also have nutritional benefits: in the elderly, moderate use of alcohol can improve appetite and dietary intake.[1]

FIGURE 1 What does one drink look like? A drink is equivalent to 1½ oz of distilled spirits, 4–5 oz of wine, 10 oz of wine cooler, or 12 oz of beer.

In addition, moderate alcohol consumption has been linked to lower rates of heart disease. Alcohol increases levels of the "good" type of cholesterol (HDL) while lowering the concentration of "bad" cholesterol (LDL); it also reduces the risk of abnormal clot formation in the blood vessels.[2] Recently, there has been a lot of interest in **resveratrol**, which is a powerful antioxidant found in red wines and foods such as grapes and nuts. Some researchers, based on experiments with mice, are proposing that resveratrol may be able to lower our risk for certain chronic diseases such as diabetes, heart disease, and liver disease. However, if resveratrol is found to be effective in promoting human health, the amount needed would be so high that it would have to be given as a purified supplement, not in the form of red wine.

alcohol Chemically, a compound characterized by the presence of a hydroxyl group; in common usage, a beverage made from fermented fruits, vegetables, or grains and containing ethanol.

ethanol A specific alcohol compound (C_2H_5OH) formed from the fermentation of dietary carbohydrates and used in a variety of alcoholic beverages.

drink The amount of an alcoholic beverage that provides approximately 0.5 fl. oz of pure ethanol.

proof A measure of the alcohol content of a liquid; 100 proof liquor is 50% alcohol by volume, 80 proof liquor is 40% alcohol by volume, and so on.

resveratrol A potent phenolic antioxidant found in red wine as well as grapes and nuts.

161

Concerns of Moderate Alcohol Intake

Not everyone responds to alcohol in the same manner. A person's age, genetic makeup, state of health, and use of medications can influence both immediate and long-term responses to alcohol intake, even at moderate levels. For example, some women appear to be at increased risk for breast cancer when consuming low to moderate amounts of alcohol. As few as two drinks per day can increase the risk of hypertension (high blood pressure) in some people, especially if the alcohol is consumed in the absence of food.[3] Moderate use of alcohol has also been linked to a higher rate of bleeding in the brain, resulting in what is termed *hemorrhagic stroke*.[4]

Alcohol has a relatively high caloric content (7 kcal/g) and provides virtually no nutritional value. Only fat (9 kcal/g) has more calories per gram. If you are watching your weight, it makes sense to strictly limit your consumption of alcohol to stay within your daily energy needs. Alcohol intake may also increase your *total* energy intake, increasing your risk of overweight or obesity. That's because alcoholic beverages, unlike solid foods and most nonalcoholic drinks, fail to trigger the satiety or "fullness" response, leading some people to overeat.[5]

The potential for drug–alcohol interactions is well known; many medications carry a warning label advising consumers to avoid alcohol while taking the drug. Alcohol

Alcohol can interfere with and increase the risks of using various over-the-counter and prescription medications.

magnifies the effect of certain painkillers, sleeping pills, antidepressants, and antianxiety medications and can lead to loss of consciousness. It also increases the risk of aspirin- and ibuprofen-associated gastrointestinal bleeding. In diabetics using insulin or oral medications to lower blood glucose, alcohol can exaggerate the drug's effect, leading to an inappropriately low level of blood glucose.

As you can see, there are both benefits and risks to moderate alcohol consumption. Experts agree that people who are currently consuming alcohol in moderation and who have low or no risk of alcohol addiction or medication interaction can safely continue their current level of use. Adults who abstain from alcohol, however, should not start drinking just for the possible health benefits. Individuals who have a personal or family history of alcoholism or fall into any other risk category should consider abstaining from alcohol use, even at a moderate level.

How Is Alcohol Metabolized?

Alcohol is absorbed directly from both the stomach and the small intestine; it does not require digestion prior to absorption. Consuming foods with some fat, protein, and fiber slows the absorption of alcohol and can reduce *blood alcohol concentration* (*BAC*) by as much as 50% compared to peak BAC when drinking on an empty stomach. Carbonated alcoholic beverages are absorbed very rapidly, which explains why champagne and sparkling wines are so quick to generate an alcoholic "buzz." As explained below, women often absorb 30–35% more of a given alcohol intake compared to men of the same size, which may explain why females often show a greater response to alcohol compared to males.

While most alcohol is oxidized, or broken down, in the liver, a small amount is metabolized in the stomach before it has even been absorbed. The enzyme *alcohol dehydrognase* (ADH) triggers the first step in alcohol degradation, while *aldehyde dehydrogenase* (ALDH) takes the breakdown process one step further (FIGURE 2). In women, ADH activity in the stomach is less active than in men; thus, women do not oxidize as much alcohol in their stomach, leaving up to 30–35% more intact alcohol to be absorbed.

Once absorbed, the alcohol moves through the bloodstream to the liver, where it is broken down at a fairly steady rate. On average, a healthy adult metabolizes the equivalent of one drink per hour. If someone drinks more than that, such as two or three alcoholic drinks in an hour, the excess alcohol is released back into the bloodstream where it elevates BAC and triggers a variety of behavioral and metabolic reactions. Through the blood,

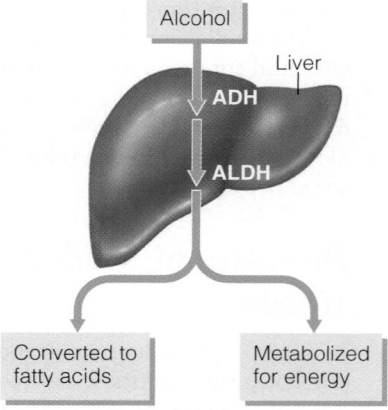

FIGURE 2   Metabolism of alcohol.

alcohol is readily distributed throughout all body fluids and tissues, including the brain. Any time you consume more than one alcoholic beverage per hour, you are exposing every tissue in your body to the toxic effects of alcohol.

Despite what you may have heard, there is no effective intervention to speed up the breakdown of alcohol (Table 1). The key to keeping your BAC below the legal limit is to drink alcoholic beverages while eating a meal or large snack, to drink very slowly, no more than one drink per hour, and to limit your total consumption of alcohol on any one occasion.

A person who steadily increases his or her alcohol consumption over time becomes more tolerant of a given intake of alcohol. Chronic drinkers experience *metabolic tolerance*, a condition in which the liver becomes more efficient in its breakdown of alcohol. This means that the person's BAC rises more slowly after consuming a certain number of drinks. In addition, chronic drinkers develop what is called *functional tolerance*, meaning they show few if any signs of impairment or intoxication even at high BACs. As a result, these individuals may need to consume twice as much alcohol as when they first started drinking in order to reach the same state of euphoria.

TABLE 1   Myths About Alcohol Metabolism

The Claim	The Reality
Physical activity, such as walking around, will speed up the breakdown of alcohol.	Muscles don't metabolize alcohol; the liver does.
Drinking a lot of coffee will keep you from getting drunk.	Coffee does not cause alcohol to be excreted in the urine.
Using a sauna or steam room will force the alcohol out of your body.	Very little alcohol is lost in the sweat; the alcohol will remain in your bloodstream.
Herbal and nutritional products are available that speed up the breakdown of alcohol.	There is no scientific evidence that commercial supplements will increase the rate of alcohol metabolism; they will not lower blood alcohol levels.

NUTRI-CASE THEO

"I was driving home from a post-game party last night when I was pulled over by the police. The officer said I seemed to be driving "erratically" and asked me how many drinks I'd had. I told him I'd only had three beers, and explained that I was pretty tired from the game. Then, just to prove I was fine, I offered to count backwards from a hundred, but I must have sounded sober, because he didn't make me do it. I can't believe he thought I was driving drunk! Still, maybe three beers after a game really is too much."

Do you think it is physiologically possible that Theo's driving might have been impaired even though he had consumed only three beers? Before you answer, consider both Theo's body weight (see page 547) and the effect of playing a long basketball game. What other factors that influence rate of alcohol absorption or breakdown could have affected Theo's BAC? How could all of these factors influence a decision about whether or not "three beers after a game really is too much"?

Effects of Excessive Alcohol Intake on Personal Health

Alcohol is a drug. It exerts a narcotic effect on virtually every part of the brain, acting as a sedative and depressant. Excessive intake of this drug can take several forms, including binge drinking, alcohol poisoning, and alcoholism.

Binge drinking or excessive drinking can lead to a number of negative consequences.

Binge drinking, the consumption of five or more alcoholic drinks on one occasion (within a 3- to 5-hour span, for example), occurs in about 15% of U.S. adults and in youth as young as 12 years of age. Young males between the ages of 18 and 25 have the highest rate of binge drinking.[6,7] Binge drinking by college students and other young adults (or even underage adolescents) increases the risk of potentially fatal falls, drownings, and automobile accidents. Acts of physical violence, including vandalism and physical and sexual assault, are also associated with binge drinking. The consequences also carry over beyond the actual binge: hangovers, which are discussed shortly, are practically inevitable given the amount of alcohol consumed.

Alcohol poisoning is a metabolic state that occurs in response to binge drinking. At high BACs, the respiratory center of the brain is depressed. This reduces the level of oxygen reaching the brain and increases the individual's risk of death by respiratory or cardiac failure. Like Todd in our opening story, many binge drinkers lose consciousness before alcohol poisoning becomes fatal, but emergency care is often essential.

Alcoholism (also called *chronic alcohol dependence*) is characterized by:

- *Craving*: a strong need or urge to drink alcoholic beverages
- *Loss of control*: the inability to stop once drinking has begun
- *Physical dependence*: the presence of nausea, sweating, shakiness, and other signs of withdrawal after stopping alcohol intake
- *Tolerance*: the need to drink larger and larger amounts of alcohol to get the same "high" or pleasurable sensations associated with alcohol intake

The Effects of Alcohol Hangovers

Alcohol hangover is a frequent and extremely unpleasant consequence of drinking too much alcohol. It lasts up to 24 hours, and its symptoms include headache, fatigue, dizziness, muscle aches, nausea and vomiting, sensitivity to light and sound, and extreme thirst. Some people also experience depression, anxiety, irritability, and other mood disturbances. While some of the aftereffects of a binge may be due to nonalcoholic compounds known as congeners (found in red wines, brandy, and whiskey, for example), most of the consequences are directly related to the alcohol itself.

Some of the symptoms occur because of alcohol's effect as a *diuretic*, a compound that increases urine output. Alcohol inhibits the release of hormones that normally regulate urine production, elevating the loss of fluid and electrolytes and contributing to dizziness and lightheadedness. Alcohol irritates the lining of the stomach and increases gastric acid production, which may account for the abdominal pain, nausea, and vomiting seen in most hangovers. Alcohol also disrupts normal body metabolism, leading to low levels of blood glucose and elevated levels of lactic acid. These disturbances contribute to the characteristic fatigue, weakness, and mood changes seen after excessive alcohol intake. Finally, alcohol disrupts various biological rhythms, such as sleep patterns and cycles of hormone secretion, leading to a jet lag type effect.

While many folk remedies, including various herbal products, are claimed to prevent or reduce hangover effects, few have been proven effective. Drinking water or other nonalcoholic beverages will minimize the risk of dehydration, while consumption of toast or dry cereal will bring blood glucose levels back to normal. Getting adequate sleep can counteract the fatigue, and use of antacids may reduce nausea and abdominal pain. While aspirin and ibuprofen might be useful for headaches, they may worsen stomach pain, increase risk of GI bleeding and, over time, may increase risk of liver damage.

---

binge drinking The consumption of five or more alcoholic drinks on one occasion.

alcohol poisoning A potentially fatal condition in which an overdose of alcohol results in cardiac and/or respiratory failure.

alcoholism A disease state characterized by chronic dependence on alcohol.

alcohol hangover A consequence of drinking too much alcohol; symptoms include headache, fatigue, dizziness, muscle aches, nausea and vomiting, sensitivity to light and sound, extreme thirst, and mood disturbances.

Reduced Brain Function

Alcohol is well known for its ability to alter behavior, mainly through its effects on the brain. Even at low intakes, alcohol impairs reasoning and judgment (Table 2). Alcohol also interferes with normal sleep patterns, alters sight and speech, and leads to loss of fine and gross motor skills such as handwriting, hand–eye coordination, and balance. Many people who drink experience unexpected mood swings, intense anger, or unreasonable irritation. Others react in the opposite direction, becoming sad, withdrawn, and lethargic. When teens or young adults chronically consume excessive amounts of alcohol, they may permanently damage brain structure and function.[8] Intellectual functioning and memory can be lost. In addition, early exposure to alcohol increases risk of future alcohol addiction and may contribute to lifelong deficits in memory, motor skills, and muscle coordination.[9,10]

At very high intakes of alcohol, a person is at risk for alcohol poisoning, defined earlier. When the brain is deprived of oxygen, the areas of the brain that regulate breathing and cardiac function shut down, leading to loss of consciousness, respiratory and cardiac failure, and death. If someone passes out after a night of hard drinking, he or she should never be left alone to "sleep it off." Instead, the person should be placed on his or her side to prevent aspiration if vomiting occurs. The person should also be watched carefully for cold and clammy skin, a bluish tint to the skin, or slow, irregular breathing. If any of these signs become evident, or there is any reason to believe he or she has alcohol poisoning, seek emergency healthcare immediately.

TABLE 2 Effects of Blood Alcohol Concentration (BAC) on Brain Activity

Blood Alcohol Concentration	Typical Response
0.02–0.05%	Feeling of relaxation, euphoria, relief
0.06–0.10%	Impaired judgment, fine motor control, and coordination; loss of normal emotional control; legally drunk in many states (at the upper end of the range)
0.11–0.15%	Impaired reflexes and gross motor control; staggered gait; legally drunk in all states; slurred speech
0.16–0.20%	Impaired vision; unpredictable behavior; further loss of muscle control
0.21–0.35%	Total loss of coordination; in a stupor
0.40% and above	Loss of consciousness; coma; suppression of respiratory response; death

(a) (b)

FIGURE 3 Cirrhosis of the liver, caused by chronic alcohol abuse. **(a)** A healthy liver. **(b)** A liver damaged by cirrhosis.

Reduced Liver Function

In addition to its effects on the brain, alcohol can damage the liver, which is the main site of alcohol metabolism. Liver cells are damaged or destroyed during periods of excessive alcohol intake; the longer the alcohol abuse continues, the greater the damage to the liver. **Fatty liver**, a condition in which abnormal amounts of fat build up in the liver, is an early yet reversible sign of liver damage linked to alcohol abuse. **Alcoholic hepatitis** causes loss of appetite, nausea and vomiting, abdominal pain, and jaundice (a yellowing of the skin and eyes, reflecting loss of liver function). **Cirrhosis of the liver** is often the result of long-term alcohol abuse; liver cells are scarred, blood flow through the liver is impaired, and liver function declines (FIGURE 3).

Increased Risk of Chronic Disease

Heavy drinking has been associated with a number of chronic diseases including osteoporosis, diabetes and pancreatic injury, and certain types of cancer. Alcohol negatively impacts bone health in several ways: there is an increased loss of calcium in the urine, vitamin D activation is impaired, and the production of testosterone and estrogen (hormones that enhance bone formation) decreases in alcoholic men and women.[11] Alcohol damages the pancreas, which produces insulin, and decreases the body's ability to properly respond to insulin. The

fatty liver An early and reversible stage of liver disease often found in people who abuse alcohol and characterized by the abnormal accumulation of fat within liver cells; also called alcoholic steatosis.

alcoholic hepatitis Inflammation of the liver caused by alcohol; other forms of hepatitis can be caused by a virus or toxin.

cirrhosis of the liver Endstage liver disease characterized by significant abnormalities in liver structure and function; may lead to complete liver failure.

Excessive alcohol intake greatly increases the risks for car accidents and other traumatic injuries.

result is chronically elevated blood glucose levels and an increased risk of diabetes. Research has most strongly linked alcohol intake to increased risk of cancer of the mouth and throat, esophagus, stomach, liver, colon, and female breast.[12] A recent study estimated that as many as 13% of cancers in a group of Japanese men were due to heavy drinking, complicated by smoking.[13] So, while moderate drinking may provide some health benefits, it is clear that chronically high intakes of alcohol damage a number of body organs and systems, increasing a person's risk of chronic disease and death.

Malnutrition

As alcohol intake increases to 30% or more of total energy intake, appetite is lost and intake of healthful foods declines. Over time, the diet becomes deficient in protein, fats, carbohydrates, vitamins A and C, and minerals such as iron, zinc, and calcium. Even if food intake is maintained, the toxic effects of alcohol damage many digestive organs including the stomach, small intestine, pancreas, and liver. The digestion of foods and absorption of nutrients such as the fat-soluble vitamins (A, D, E, and K), vitamin B_6, folate, and zinc become inadequate, leading to malnutrition and inappropriate weight loss.

Increased Risk of Traumatic Injury

Excessive alcohol intake is the leading cause of death for Americans under the age of 21. It is also the third leading cause of all U.S. deaths.[14] It has been estimated that as many as 6,000 young Americans die each year from alcohol-

---

related motor vehicle accidents, suicides, and homicides. As previously noted, rates of physical and sexual assaults, vandalism, accidental falls, and drownings also increase when people are under the influence of alcohol.

Fetal and Infant Health Problems

There is no known safe level of alcohol consumption for pregnant women. Women who are or think they may be pregnant should abstain from all alcoholic beverages. As discussed in the accompanying Highlight box, fetal alcohol syndrome, which is caused by alcohol intake in a childbearing woman, is a critical problem in the United States.

Women who are breastfeeding should also abstain from alcohol since it easily passes into the breast milk at levels equal to blood alcohol concentrations. If consumed by the infant, the alcohol in breast milk can slow motor development, depress the central nervous system, and increase sleepiness in the child. Alcohol also reduces the mother's ability to produce milk, putting the infant at risk for malnutrition.

Should You Be Concerned About Your Alcohol Intake?

Even people who are not dependent on alcohol can have a problem called **alcohol abuse** if they engage in binge drinking or drink at inappropriate times (while pregnant, before or while driving a car, to deal with negative emotions, or while at work/school). If you answer "yes" to one or more of the following questions, provided by the National Institute on Alcohol Abuse and Alcoholism, you may have a problem with alcohol abuse.

- Have you ever felt you should cut down on your drinking?
- Have people annoyed you by criticizing your drinking?
- Have you ever felt bad or guilty about your drinking?
- Do you drink alone when you feel angry or sad?
- Has your drinking ever made you late for school or work?
- Have you ever had a drink first thing in the morning to steady your nerves or get rid of a hangover?
- Do you ever drink after promising yourself you won't?

If you think you have an alcohol problem, it is important for you to speak with a trusted friend, counselor, or healthcare provider. There are many effective support groups that can help you plan a course of action to cut down or eliminate alcohol intake. Taking control of your alcohol intake will allow you to take control of your life.

Talking to Someone About Alcohol Addiction

You may suspect that a close friend or relative might be one of the nearly 14 million Americans who abuse alcohol or are dependent on alcohol.[15] If you notice that your

---

alcohol abuse The act of engaging in inappropriate or dangerous drinking behaviors.

HIGHLIGHT

Fetal Alcohol Syndrome

The March of Dimes estimates that more than 40,000 babies are born each year with some type of alcohol-related defect.[16] Alcohol is a known **teratogen** (a substance that causes fetal harm) that readily crosses the placenta into the fetal bloodstream. Since the immature fetal liver can not effectively break down the alcohol, it accumulates in the fetal blood and tissues, increasing the risk for various birth defects. The effects of maternal alcohol intake are dose related: the more the mother drinks, the greater the potential harm to the fetus. In addition to the amount of alcohol consumed during pregnancy, the timing of the mother's alcohol intake influences the risk of fetal complications. Binge or frequent drinking during the first trimester of pregnancy is more likely to result in birth defects and other permanent abnormalities, while alcohol consumption in the third trimester typically results in low birth weight and growth retardation.

Fetal alcohol syndrome (FAS) is a condition characterized by malformations of the face, limbs, heart, and nervous system. The characteristic facial features persist throughout the child's life (Figure 4). Exposure to alcohol while in the womb impairs fetal growth; FAS babies are often underweight at birth and rarely normalize their growth after birth. Newborn and infant death rates are abnormally high, and those who do survive suffer from emotional, behavioral,

social, learning, and developmental problems throughout life. FAS is one of the most common causes of mental retardation in the United States and the only one that is completely preventable.

Fetal alcohol effects (FAE) are a more subtle set of consequences related to maternal alcohol intake. While usually not identified at birth, this condition often becomes evident when the child enters preschool or kindergarten. The child may exhibit hyperactivity, attention deficit disorder, or impaired learning abilities. It is estimated that the incidence of FAE is ten times greater than that of FAS.

Can a pregnant woman safely consume any amount of alcohol? Although some pregnant women do have an occasional alcoholic drink with no apparent ill effects, there is no amount of alcohol known to be safe. In one recent study, researchers identified a number of subtle but long-term negative consequences of light to moderate alcohol consumption during pregnancy: children of women who had as little as one alcoholic drink a week during their pregnancy were more aggressive and more likely to engage in delinquent behaviors compared to children who had no fetal exposure to alcohol. The best advice regarding alcohol intake during pregnancy is to abstain if there is any chance of becoming pregnant, as well as throughout the pregnancy.

FIGURE 4 A child with fetal alcohol syndrome (FAS). The facial features typical of children with FAS include a short nose with a low, wide bridge; drooping eyes with an extra skinfold; and a flat, thin upper lip. These external traits are typically accompanied by behavioral problems and learning disorders. The effects of FAS are irreversible.

teratogen A compound known to cause fetal harm or danger.

fetal alcohol syndrome (FAS) A set of serious, irreversible alcohol-related birth defects characterized by certain physical and mental abnormalities.

fetal alcohol effects (FAE) A set of subtle consequences of maternal intake of alcohol, such as impaired learning and behavioral problems.

friend or relative uses alcohol as the primary way to calm down, cheer up, or relax, that may be a sign of alcohol dependency or addiction. The appearance of tremors or other signs of withdrawal as well as the initiation of secretive behaviors when consuming alcohol are other indications that alcohol has become a serious problem.

Many people become defensive or hostile when asked about their use of alcohol; denial is very common. The single hardest step toward sobriety is often the first: accepting the fact that help is needed. Some people respond well when confronted by a single person, while others benefit more from a group intervention. There should be no blaming or shaming; alcohol addiction and dependency are medical conditions with a strong genetic component. The National Institute on Alcoholism and Alcohol Abuse suggests the following approaches when trying to get a friend or relative into treatment:

Stop covering up and making excuses. Many times, family and friends will make excuses to others to protect the person from the results of his or her drinking. It is important, however, to stop covering for that person so he or she can experience the full consequences of inappropriate alcohol consumption.

Intervene at a vulnerable time. The best time to talk to someone about problem drinking is shortly after an alcohol-related incident such as a DUI arrest, an alcohol-related traffic accident, or a public scene. Wait until the person is sober and everyone is relatively calm.

Be specific. Tell the person exactly why you are concerned; use examples of specific problems associated with their drinking habits (poor school or work performance; legal problems; inappropriate behaviors). Explain what will happen if the person chooses not to get help, for example, no longer going out with the person if alcohol will be available, no longer riding with him or her in motor vehicles, moving out of a shared home, and so on.

Get help. Professional help is available from community agencies, healthcare providers, online sites, school or worksite wellness centers, and some religious organizations. Several contacts and Web sites are listed at the end of this *In Depth*. If the person indicates a willingness to get help, call immediately for an appointment and/or immediately bring him or her to a treatment center. The longer the delay, the more likely it is that the person will experience a change of heart.

Enlist the support of others. Whether or not the person agrees to get help, calling upon other friends and relatives can often be effective, especially if one has had alcohol-related problems of his or her own. Formal support groups such as Al-Anon and Alateen can provide additional information and guidance.

Treatment for alcohol-related problems works for many, but not all, individuals. "Success" is measured in small steps, and relapses are common. Most scientists agree that people who abuse alcohol cannot just "cut down." Complete avoidance of all alcoholic beverages is the only way for most people who abuse alcohol to achieve full and ongoing recovery.

WEB LINKS

www.aa.org
Alcoholics Anonymous, Inc.

This site provides links to local AA groups and provides information on the AA program.

www.al-anon.alateen.org
Al-Anon Family Group Headquarters, Inc.

This site provides links to local Al-Anon and Alateen groups, which provide support for spouses, children, and other loved ones of people addicted to alcohol.

www.ncadd.org
National Council on Alcoholism and Drug Dependence, Inc.

Educational materials and information on alcoholism can be obtained from this site.

www.niaaa.nih.gov
National Institute on Alcohol Abuse and Alcoholism

Visit this Web site for information on the prevelance, consequences, and treatments of alcohol-related disorders. Information for healthcare providers, people struggling with alcohol abuse, and family members is available free of charge.

www.collegedrinkingprevention.gov
College Drinking: Changing the Culture

The NIAAA developed this Web site specifically for college students seeking information and advice on the subject of college drinking. Services include self-assessment questionnaires, answers to frequently asked questions, news articles, research, and links to support groups.

www.madd.org
Mothers Against Drunk Driving

Links to local chapters, statistics related to drunk driving, and prevention strategies are easily accessed from this site.

www.marchofdimes.com
March of Dimes

Information on fetal alcohol syndrome and fetal alcohol effects.

REFERENCES

1. Dufour, M. C., L. Archer, and E. Gordis. 1992. Alcohol and the elderly. *Clin. Geriatr. Med.* 8:127–141.
2. Gunzerath, L., V. Faden, S. Zakhari, and K. Warren. 2004. National Institute on Alcohol Abuse and Alcoholism Report on moderate drinking. *Alcohol. Clin. Exp. Res.* 28L:829–847.
3. Stranges, S., T. Wu, J. M. Born., et al. 2004. Relationship of alcohol drinking pattern to risk of hypertension. *Hypertension* 44:813–819.
4. Meister, K. A., E. M. Whelan, and R. Kava. 2000. The health effects of moderate alcohol intake in humans: an epidemiologic review. *Crit. Rev. Clin. Lab. Sci.* 37:261–296.

5. Caton, S. J., M. Ball, A. Ahern, et al. 2004. Dose-dependent effects of alcohol on appetite and food intake. *Physiol. Behav.* 81:51–58.

6. Nelson, D. E., T. S. Naimi, R. D. Brewer, J. Bolen, and H. E. Wells. 2004. Metropolitan-area estimates of binge drinking in the United States. *Am. J. Pub. Health* 94:663–671.

7. Naimi, T. S., R. D. Brewer, A. Mokdad, C. Denny, and M. K. Serdula. 2003. Binge drinking among US adults. *JAMA* 289:70–79.

8. Oscar-Berman, M., and K. Marinkovic. 2003. Alcoholism and the brain: an overview. *Alc. Res. Health* 27:161–173.

9. Brown, S. A., S. F. Tapert, E. Granholm, and D. C. Delis. 2000. Neurocognitive functioning of adolescents: effects of protracted alcohol use. *Alc. Clin. Exp. Res.* 24:164–171.

10. National Institute on Alcohol Abuse and Alcoholism (NIAAA). 2006. Young Adult Drinking. *Alcohol Alert*, No. 68, April 2006.

11. National Institute of Arthritis and Musculoskeletal and Skin Diseases (NIAMS). 2005. What People Recovering from Alcoholism Need to Know About Osteoporosis. www.niams.nih.gov/bone/hi/osteoporosis_alcohol.htm. (Accessed March 2007.)

12. Bagnardi, V., M. Blangiardo, C. La Vecchia, and G. Corrao. 2001. Alcohol consumption and the risk of cancer: a meta-analysis. *Alc. Res. Health* 25:263–270.

13. Inoue, M., and S. Tsugane for the JPHC Study Group. 2004. Impact of alcohol drinking on total cancer risk: data from a large-scale population-based cohort study in Japan. *Brit. J. Cancer* 92:182–187.

14. National Institute on Alcohol Abuse and Alcoholism (NIAAA). 2005. A Snapshot of High-Risk College Drinking Consequences. www.collegedrinkingprevention.gov/facts/snapshot.aspx. (Accessed March 2007.)

15. National Institute on Alcohol Abuse and Alcoholism (NIAAA). 2005. Alcohol: How to Cut Down on Your Drinking. www.collegedrinkingprevention.gov/facts/cutdrinking.aspx. (Accessed March 2007.)

16. Sokol, R. J., et al. 2003. Fetal alcohol spectrum disorder. *JAMA* 290:2996–2999.

CHAPTER 5

CHAPTER OBJECTIVES

After reading this chapter you will be able to:

1. List and describe the three types of lipids found in foods, pp. 172–181.

2. Discuss how the level of saturation of a fatty acid affects its shape and the form it takes, pp. 173–174.

3. Explain the primary difference between a *cis* fatty acid and a *trans* fatty acid and how the change from *cis* to *trans* can negatively affect our health, pp. 175–178.

4. List three functions of fat in our bodies, pp. 181–184.

5. Identify the beneficial functions of the essential fatty acids, pp. 178–180.

6. Describe the steps involved in fat digestion, pp. 185–186.

7. Define the recommended dietary intakes for total fat, saturated fat, and the two essential fatty acids, pp. 187–188.

8. Identify at least three common food sources of beneficial fats, pp. 191–192.

9. Describe the role of dietary fat in the development of cardiovascular disease, pp. 198–201.

TEST YOURSELF TRUE OR FALSE?

1. Fat is unhealthful, and we should eat as little as possible in our diets. **T or F**

2. Fat is an important fuel source during rest and exercise. **T or F**

3. Fried foods are relatively nutritious as long as vegetable shortening is used to fry the foods. **T or F**

4. Certain fats protect against heart disease. **T or F**

5. High-fat diets cause cancer. **T or F**

Test Yourself answers can be found after the Chapter Summary.

Fats: Essential Energy-Supplying Nutrients

Only couch potatoes develop heart disease . . . or so we like to think. That's why the world was stunned in the fall of 1995 when 28-year-old skater Sergei Grinkov, a two-time Olympic gold medalist, collapsed and died of a fatal heart attack while training in Lake Placid, New York. An autopsy revealed that Grinkov's coronary arteries were as severely clogged as those of a 70-year-old with established heart disease. Although his widow reported that he had never complained of chest pain or shortness of breath, his family history revealed one very important clue: his father had died of a heart attack at age 52. In one recent study, a survey of U.S. public health records revealed that, from 1985 through 1995, 134 deaths of young athletes were due to heart disease.

Sergei Grinkov, here skating with his partner and wife Ekaterina Gordeeva, died of a heart attack at the age of 28.

What causes a heart attack, and how can you calculate your risk? Can a high-fat diet cause heart disease, and can a low-fat diet prevent it? When was the last time you heard anything good about dietary fat? If your best friend's father had died of a heart attack at age 44 and you noticed your friend regularly eating high-fat meals, would you say anything about it? If so, what would you say?

Some fats, such as olive oil, are liquid at room temperature.

lipids A diverse group of organic substances that are insoluble in water; lipids include triglycerides, phospholipids, and sterols.

triglyceride A molecule consisting of three fatty acids attached to a three-carbon glycerol backbone.

fatty acids Long chains of carbon atoms bound to each other as well as to hydrogen atoms.

glycerol An alcohol composed of three carbon atoms; it is the backbone of a triglyceride molecule.

Although some people think of dietary fat as something to be avoided, a certain amount of fat is absolutely essential for good health. In this chapter, we'll discuss the function of fat in the human body and help you distinguish between beneficial and harmful types of dietary fat. You'll also assess how much fat you need in your diet and learn about the role of dietary fat in the development of heart disease and other disorders.

What Are Fats?

Fats are just one form of a much larger and more diverse group of substances called **lipids** that are distinguished by the fact that they are insoluble in water. Think of a salad dressing made with vinegar, which is mostly water, and olive oil, which is a lipid. Shaking the bottle *disperses* the oil but doesn't *dissolve* it: that's why it separates back out again so quickly. Lipids are found in all sorts of living things, from bacteria to plants to human beings. In fact, their presence on your skin explains why you can't clean your face with water alone: you need some type of soap to break down the insoluble lipids before you can wash them away. In this chapter, we focus on the small group of lipids that are found in foods.

Fats and oils are two different types of lipids found in foods. Fats like butter are solid at room temperature, while oils such as olive oil are liquid at room temperature. Because most people are more comfortable with the term *fats* instead of *lipids,* we will use that term generically throughout this book, including when we are referring to oils. Three types of fats are commonly found in foods. These are triglycerides, phospholipids, and sterols. Let's take a look at each.

Most of the Fats We Eat Are in the Form of Triglycerides

Most of the fat we eat (95%) is in the form of triglycerides (also called triacylglycerols), which is the same form in which most of the fat in our body is stored. As reflected in the prefix *tri-,* a **triglyceride** is a molecule consisting of *three* fatty acids attached to a *three*-carbon glycerol backbone. **Fatty acids** are long chains of carbon atoms bound to each other as well as to hydrogen atoms. They are acids because they contain an acid group (carboxyl group) at one end of their chain. **Glycerol,** the backbone of a triglyceride molecule, is an alcohol composed of three carbon atoms. One fatty acid attaches to each of these three carbons to make the triglyceride (FIGURE 5.1).

FIGURE 5.1   A triglyceride consists of three fatty acids attached to a three-carbon glycerol backbone.

To understand why we want more of some fats than others, we need to know more about their properties and how they work in our body. In general, triglycerides can be classified by their chain length (number of carbons in each fatty acid), their level of saturation (how much hydrogen, H, is attached to each carbon atom in the fatty acid chain), and their shape, which is determined in some cases by how they are commercially processed. All of these factors influence how we use the triglyceride within our bodies.

Chain Length Affects Triglyceride Function

The fatty acids attached to the glycerol backbone can vary in the number of carbons they contain, referred to as their *chain length*.

- **Short-chain fatty acids** are usually fewer than six carbon atoms in length.
- **Medium-chain fatty acids** are six to twelve carbons in length.
- **Long-chain fatty acids** are fourteen or more carbons in length.

Fatty acid chain length is important because it determines the method of fat digestion and absorption and affects how fats function within the body. For example, short- and medium-chain fatty acids are digested and transported more quickly than long-chain fatty acids. We will discuss digestion and absorption of fats in more detail shortly. In addition, chain length can also determine saturation, as discussed in the next section.

Saturated Fats Contain the Maximum Amount of Hydrogen

Triglycerides can also vary by the types of bonds found in the fatty acids. If a fatty acid has no carbons bonded together with a double bond, they are referred to as **saturated fatty acids (SFA)** (FIGURES 5.2A and 5.3A). This is because every carbon atom in the chain is *saturated* with hydrogen: each has the maximum amount of hydrogen bound to it. Some foods that are high in saturated fatty acids are coconut oil, palm kernel oil, butter, cream, whole milk, and beef. Much of the fat in these foods is in the form of short- and medium-chain fatty acids that are always saturated.

Unsaturated Fats Contain Less Hydrogen

If, within the chain of carbon atoms, two are bound to each other with a double bond, then this double carbon bond excludes hydrogen. This lack of hydrogen at *one* part of the molecule results in a fat that is referred to as *monounsaturated* (recall from Chapter 4 that the prefix *mono-* means one). A monounsaturated molecule is shown in FIGURE 5.2B and FIGURE 5.3C. **Monounsaturated fatty acids (MUFA)** are usually liquid at room temperature. Foods that are high in monounsaturated fatty acids are olive oil, canola oil, and cashew nuts.

If the fat molecules have *more than one* double bond, they contain even less hydrogen and are referred to as **polyunsaturated fatty acids (PUFA)**. Polyunsaturated fatty acids are also liquid at room temperature and include cottonseed, canola, corn, and safflower oils.

Foods vary in the types of fatty acids they contain. For example, animal fats provide approximately 40–60% of their energy from saturated fats, while plant fats provide 80–90% of their energy from monounsaturated and polyunsaturated fats (FIGURE 5.4). You will notice that canola oil is listed as being high in both MUFA and PUFA. Most oils are a combination of fats, making them a good source of more than one type of fat. Diets higher in plant foods will usually be lower in saturated fats than diets high in animal products. The impact that various types of fatty acids have on health will be discussed later in this chapter (beginning on page 177).

short-chain fatty acids Fatty acids fewer than six carbon atoms in length.

medium-chain fatty acids Fatty acids that are six to twelve carbon atoms in length.

long-chain fatty acids Fatty acids that are fourteen or more carbon atoms in length.

saturated fatty acids (SFAs) Fatty acids that have no carbons joined together with a double bond; these types of fatty acids are generally solid at room temperature.

FIGURE 5.2 An atom of carbon has four attachment sites. In fatty acid chains, two of these sites are filled by adjacent carbon atoms. **(a)** In saturated fatty acids, the other two sites are always filled by two hydrogen atoms. **(b)** In unsaturated fatty acids, at one or more points along the chain, a double bond to an adjacent carbon atom takes up one of the attachment sites that would otherwise be filled by hydrogen.

FIGURE 5.3 Level of saturation affects the shape of the fatty acids. **(a)** In saturated fats, each carbon atom in the fatty acid chain is singly bonded to two other carbon atoms and two hydrogen atoms. **(b)** Saturated fats have straight fatty acid chains packed tightly together and are solid at room temperature. **(c)** In monounsaturated fats, somewhere along the fatty acid chain, two carbon atoms are doubly bonded to each other. This double carbon bond excludes hydrogen at this area of the molecule and produces one kink in the chain. Polyunsaturated fats have two or more such kinks in their fatty acid chain. **(d)** The kinks in the fatty acid chains of monounsaturated and polyunsaturated fats prevent them from packing tightly together; they are liquid at room temperature.

Carbon Bonding Affects Shape

monounsaturated fatty acids (MUFAs) Fatty acids that have two carbons in the chain bound to each other with one double bond; these types of fatty acids are generally liquid at room temperature.

polyunsaturated fatty acids (PUFAs) Fatty acids that have more than one double bond in the chain; these types of fatty acids are generally liquid at room temperature.

Have you ever noticed how many toothpicks are packed into a small box? A hundred or more! But if you were to break a bunch of toothpicks into V shapes anywhere along their length, how many could you then fit into the same box? It would be very few because the bent toothpicks would jumble together, taking up much more space. Molecules of saturated fat are like straight toothpicks: they have no double carbon bonds and always form straight, rigid chains. As they have no kinks, these chains can pack together tightly (FIGURE 5.3B). That is why saturated fats, such as the fat in meats, are solid at room temperature.

In contrast, each double carbon bond of unsaturated fats gives them a kink along their length (FIGURE 5.3D). This means that they are unable to pack together tightly—for example, to form a stick of butter—and instead are liquid at room temperature. In our body, unsaturated fatty acids are part of our cell membranes. They help keep the cell membranes flexible, allowing substances to move in and out of the cells.

	SFA	MUFA	PUFA
Butter	65	31	4
Milk, whole	63	33	4
Beef, ground	45	51	4
Egg	37	46	16
Chicken, breast	32	44	24
Turkey	32	25	35
Tuna, water packed	32	22	46
Salmon, Chinook	25	48	24
Cashews	20	59	17
Olive oil	14	74	10
Sesame oil	14	41	42
Corn oil	13	25	60
Walnuts	10	23	64
Safflower oil	9	12	74
Canola oil	7	59	30

Percentage (%) of total fat kcals

Key:
SFA
MUFA
PUFA

FIGURE 5.4   Major sources of dietary fat.

Unsaturated fatty acids can occur in either a *cis* or a *trans* shape. The prefix *cis* means things are located on the same side or near each other, while *trans* is a prefix that denotes across or opposite. These terms describe the positioning of the hydrogen atoms around the double carbon bond as follows:

- The prefix *cis* means "on the same side." A *cis fatty acid* has both hydrogen atoms located on the same side of the double bond (FIGURE 5.5A). This positioning gives the *cis* molecule a pronounced kink at the double carbon bond. We typically find the *cis* fatty acids in nature, and thus in foods like olive oil.

- In contrast, *trans* means "on the opposite side." In a *trans fatty acid*, the hydrogen atoms are attached on diagonally opposite sides of the double carbon bond (FIGURE 5.5B). This positioning makes *trans* fatty acid fats straighter and more rigid, just like saturated fats. Thus, "*trans* fats" is a collective term used to define fats with *trans* double bonds. Although a limited amount of natural *trans* fatty acids are found in cow's milk and meat, the majority of *trans* fatty acids are produced by manipulating the fatty acid during food processing.

Walnuts and cashews are high in monounsaturated fatty acids.

(a) *cis* polyunsaturated fatty acid

(b) *trans* polyunsaturated fatty acid

FIGURE 5.5 Structure of **(a)** a *cis* and **(b)** a *trans* polyunsaturated fatty acid. Notice that *cis* fatty acids have both hydrogen atoms located on the same side of the double bond. This positioning makes the molecule kinked. In the *trans* fatty acids, the hydrogen atoms are attached on diagonally opposite sides of the double carbon bond. This positioning makes them straighter and more rigid.

This process, called **hydrogenation**, was developed in the early 1900s in order to produce a type of cheap fat that could be stored in a solid form and would resist rancidity. During hydrogenation, pressurized hydrogen molecules are added directly to unsaturated fatty acids like those found in corn and safflower oils. This causes the double bonds of the unsaturated fatty acids in the oil to be partially or totally removed. As a result, the fatty acid becomes more saturated and straighter.

The hydrogenation process can be controlled to make the oil more or less saturated: if only some of the double bonds are broken, the fat produced is called *partially hydrogenated*, a term you will see frequently on food labels. For example, corn oil margarine is a partially hydrogenated fat made from corn oil. Along with making fatty acids more saturated, the hydrogenation process produces *trans* fatty acids. Unless labeled as containing zero *trans* fatty acids, most partially hydrogenated margarines will have more *trans* fatty acids than butter.

The hardening of oil provides the food industry with some important advantages.[1] First, hydrogenation improves the stability of oils, which can become rancid when the double carbon bonds are oxidized. This improves the shelf life of the fat itself and any products made with the fat. Second, by manipulating the hydrogenation process, a manufacturer can produce a customized fat with a particular texture, function, or sensory property. Third, hydrogenation allows the use of fats for spreads that could not previously be used in the food industry because of undesirable properties such as poor taste or texture. Finally, for a period of several decades

hydrogenation The process of adding hydrogen to unsaturated fatty acids, making them more saturated and thereby more solid at room temperature.

in the 20th century, partially hydrogenated oil products were in demand. Americans were being urged to reduce their intake of saturated fats, and switched to partially hydrogenated oils, including spreadable margarines, assuming that these products were more healthful. But as we discuss next, this assumption did not turn out to be true. Partial hydrogenation of fat had also created a glut of new products full of *trans* fatty acids that had never before been consumed in abundance by the American public.

Different Forms of Triglycerides Can Damage or Preserve Our Health

As we will discuss throughout the rest of this chapter, the types of fats we choose to eat can have a greater effect on our health than the amount of fat in our diet.

Both Saturated Fats and *Trans* Fats Are Harmful to Our Health

Research over the last two decades has shown that diets high in saturated fatty acids negatively impact blood lipid levels, increasing our risk of heart disease. We now know that *trans* fatty acids appear to function much like saturated fatty acids in our diet: both *trans* and saturated fatty acids lower "good" cholesterol and raise "bad" cholesterol, change cell membrane function, and alter the way cholesterol is removed from the blood. For these reasons, researchers believe that diets high in saturated and *trans* fatty acids can increase the risk of cardiovascular disease.

Many health professionals feel that diets high in *trans* fatty acids increase the risk of heart disease even more than diets high in saturated fat.[2] To understand why, let's look at some numbers. Currently the average consumption of industrially produced *trans* fatty acids is only about 2–3% of total energy intake, with the majority of these fats coming from deep-fried fast or frozen foods, bakery products, packaged snacks, margarines, and other packaged foods such as crackers, tortillas, and pancake.[2] (See Table 5.1 for examples of the amount of *trans* fatty acids in various foods prepared or fried in partially hydrogenated fats.) Although *trans* fatty acids make up only a small amount of the fat in the average American diet, their negative effect on our health appears to be dramatic. A research review that involved over 140,000 individuals showed that for every 2% increase in energy intake from *trans* fatty acids there was a 23% increase in incidence of heart disease.[2] Researchers have concluded that the scientific evidence showing that *trans* fatty acids negatively affect health is so strong that it is unethical to do any additional long-term human research trials comparing the health effects of *trans* fatty acids to other types of fatty acids.

Because of the evidence linking *trans* fatty acid consumption to heart disease, the U.S. Food and Drug Administration (FDA) has required manufacturers to list the amount of *trans* fatty acids per serving on the Nutrition Facts Panel. The requirement for the labeling of *trans* fatty acids took effect in January 2006 for all products sold with a food label. In addition, many cities are considering total bans on *trans* fatty acids in restaurants. For example, the New York City Department of Health and Mental Hygiene approved an amendment to their health code to phase out all artificial *trans* fats in New York City restaurants and other food establishments by July 2008.[3]

Unfortunately, no such requirement exists for most food establishments in the United States. Until all food establishments are required to identify or eliminate *trans* fatty acids from their foods, avoid ordering fried foods and baked goods such as cakes, cookies, and pies to limit your intake. Currently, legislators and food policy organizations around the United States and the world are lobbying for the labeling of *trans* fatty acids on menus and/or the elimination of artificial *trans* fatty acids from restaurant foods and other ready-to-eat foods. If we are to achieve our goals for public health, we need to make sure that, in eliminating *trans* fatty

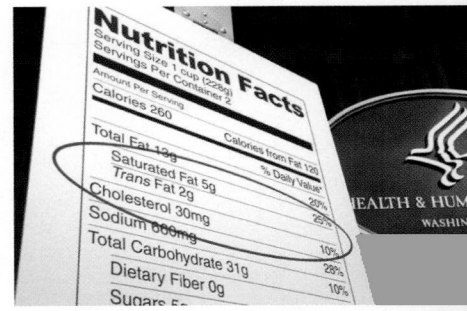

The U.S. FDA ruled that as of 2006, *trans* fatty acids, or *trans* fat, must be listed as a separate line item on Nutrition Facts Panels for conventional foods and some dietary supplements.

TABLE 5.1 *Trans* Fatty Acid Content of Common Foods*

Type of Food	*Trans* Fatty Acid Content (grams per typical serving)
Fast or Frozen Food	
French fries	4.7–6.1
Breaded fish burger	5.6
Breaded chicken nuggets	5.0
French fries, frozen	2.8
Enchilada	2.1
Burrito	1.1
Pizza	1.1
Packaged Snacks	
Tortilla corn chips	1.6
Popcorn, microwave	1.2
Granola bar	1.0
Bakery Products	
Pie	3.9
Danish or sweet roll	3.3
Cookies	1.8
Cake	1.7
Margarines	
Vegetable shortening	2.7
Hard stick margarine	0.9–2.5
Soft tub margarine	0.3–1.4

*The foods in this list typically are either produced or prepared with partially hydrogenated vegetable oils in the United States.
Source: Mozaffarian, D., M. B. Katan, A. Ascherio, M. J. Stampher, and W. C. Willet. 2006. Trans fatty acids and cardiovascular disease. *N. Engl. J. Med.* 354(15):1603–1613.

acids from foods, we don't simply substitute saturated fats. Food establishments and food manufacturers need to switch to unsaturated fats to reduce Americans' risk for heart disease.

Essential Fatty Acids Protect Our Health

Although many people think that all dietary fats should be avoided, some fats are required by the body. These **essential fatty acids (EFA)** are incorporated into the many phospholipids in our body (described shortly) and are needed to make a number of important biological compounds called *eicosanoids*. In the body, eicosanoids help regulate key physiological functions, including gastrointestinal tract motility, blood clotting, the expanding and contracting of our blood vessels to regulate blood pressure, the permeability of our blood vessels to fluid and large molecules, and the regulation of inflammation, just to name a few. Since they play an important role in "regulating" biological processes, we need a balance of the various eicosanoids and thus a balance of EFAs. For example, we need just the right amount of blood clotting at the right time—too much and we get excessive blood clotting, and too little and we get excessive bleeding.

EFAs are called "essential" because they must be consumed in the diet and cannot be made in our bodies. (Information on the EFA content of various foods is given in FIGURE 5.4, page 175.) The two EFAs required in our diet are linoleic acid and alpha-linolenic acid (FIGURE 5.6).

essential fatty acids (EFAs) Fatty acids that must be consumed in the diet because they cannot be made by our bodies. The two essential fatty acids are linoleic acid and alpha-linolenic acid.

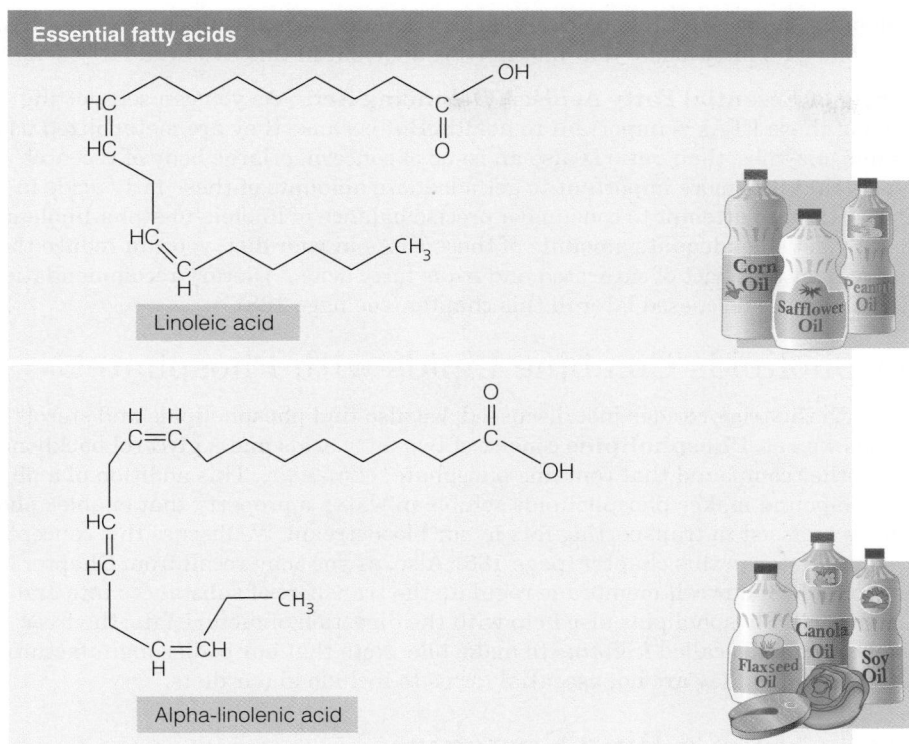

Essential fatty acids

Linoleic acid

Alpha-linolenic acid

FIGURE 5.6   The two essential fatty acids: linoleic acid (omega-6 fatty acid) and alpha-linolenic acid (omega-3 fatty acid).

Linoleic Acid: Omega-6 Fatty Acid.   **Linoleic acid,** also known as *omega-6 fatty acid*, was identified as an essential EFA more than 75 years ago, with deficiency symptoms that include poor growth and scaly skin lesions. This EFA is found in vegetable and nut oils such as sunflower, safflower, corn, soy, and peanut oil. If you eat lots of vegetables, or use vegetable oil–based margarines or vegetable oils, you are probably getting adequate amounts of this essential fatty acid in your diet. Linoleic acid is needed for cell membrane structure and is required for lipoproteins that transport fats in our blood. This EFA is also metabolized in the body to arachidonic acid, which contributes to many body functions, such as blood clotting and blood pressure.

Alpha-Linolenic Acid: Omega-3 Fatty Acid.   The second essential fatty acid is **alpha-linolenic acid,** an *omega-3 fatty acid* that was not recognized as essential until about 20 years ago, when its role in visual and neurological development in infants was identified.[4] Today, we are still learning about the biological functions of this EFA. Alpha-linolenic acid and its metabolic products are important in reducing heart disease more by altering cardiac function than by altering blood lipids. In this capacity, alpha-linolenic acid appears to reduce cardiac arrhythmia, inflammation associated with heart disease, and the development of blood clots.[5]

Alpha-linolenic acid is found primarily in leafy green vegetables, flaxseeds and flaxseed oil, soy oil and foods, canola oil, walnuts and walnut oil, and fish products. You may have read news reports of the health benefits of the omega-3 fatty acids found in many fish and fish oils. Two of these fatty acids, **eicosapentaenoic acid (EPA)** and **docosahexaenoic acid (DHA),** are metabolic derivatives of alpha-linolenic acid and are necessary for the synthesis of a number of regulatory compounds in the body. Research indicates that diets high in EPA and DHA may be protective against heart disease.[5] These fatty acids play a role in improving vascular function and reduce inflammatory responses, blood clotting, blood pressure, cardiac arrhythmias, and plasma triglycerides, all of which are associated with a reduction

linoleic acid An essential fatty acid found in vegetable and nut oils; also known as omega-6 fatty acid.

alpha-linolenic acid An essential fatty acid found in leafy green vegetables, flaxseed oil, soy oil, fish oil, and fish products; an omega-3 fatty acid.

eicosapentaenoic acid (EPA) A metabolic derivative of alpha-linolenic acid.

docosahexaenoic acid (DHA) Another metabolic derivative of alpha-linolenic acid; together with EPA, it appears to reduce our risk of a heart attack.

Salmon is high in omega-3 fatty acid content.

in risk of heart disease.[6] If you do not eat fish and do not make an effort to use oils high in omega-3 fatty acids, your diet may be deficient in this essential fatty acid.

Benefits of Essential Fatty Acids: A Balancing Act. As you can see, getting enough of these EFAs is important to health. But because they are metabolized using the same enzymes, their ratio is also an issue of concern. A large body of research suggests that it is more important to get adequate amounts of these fatty acids in your diet than to attempt to consume a precise balance of linoleic-to-alpha-linolenic acids.[5] By getting adequate amounts of these EFAs in your diet, you can reduce the negative health impact of saturated and *trans* fatty acids.[5] Dietary recommendations for the EFAs are discussed later in this chapter (see page 188).

Phospholipids Combine Lipids with Phosphate

Along with the triglycerides just discussed, we also find phospholipids and sterols in the foods we eat. **Phospholipids** consist of two fatty acids and a glycerol backbone with another compound that contains phosphate (FIGURE 5.7). This addition of a phosphate compound makes phospholipids soluble in water, a property that enables phospholipids to assist in transporting fats in our bloodstream. We discuss this concept in more detail later in this chapter (page 186). Also, as you may recall from Chapter 3, phospholipids in our cell membrane regulate the transport of substances into and out of the cell. Phospholipids also help with the digestion of dietary fats: the liver uses phospholipids called *lecithins* to make bile. Note that our bodies manufacture phospholipids, so they are not essential for us to include in our diets.

Sterols Have a Ring Structure

phospholipids A type of lipid in which a fatty acid is combined with another compound that contains phosphate; unlike other lipids, phospholipids are soluble in water.

sterols A type of lipid found in foods and the body that has a ring structure; cholesterol is the most common sterol that occurs in our diets.

Sterols are also a type of lipid found in foods and in the body, but their multiple-ring structure is quite different from that of triglycerides (FIGURE 5.8A). Sterols are found in both plant and animal foods and are produced in the body. Plants contain some sterols, but these sterols are not very well absorbed and appear to block the absorption of dietary cholesterol, the most commonly occurring sterol in the diet (FIGURE 5.8B). Cholesterol is found only in the fatty part of animal products such as butter, egg yolks, whole milk, meats, and poultry. Low- or reduced-fat animal products such as lean meats and skim milk have little cholesterol.

We don't need to consume cholesterol in our diet because our body continually synthesizes it, mostly in the liver and intestines. This continuous production is essential because cholesterol is part of every cell membrane, where it works in conjunction with fatty acids to help maintain cell membrane integrity. It is particularly plentiful in the neural cells that make up our brain, spinal cord, and nerves. The body also uses cholesterol to synthesize several important compounds including sex

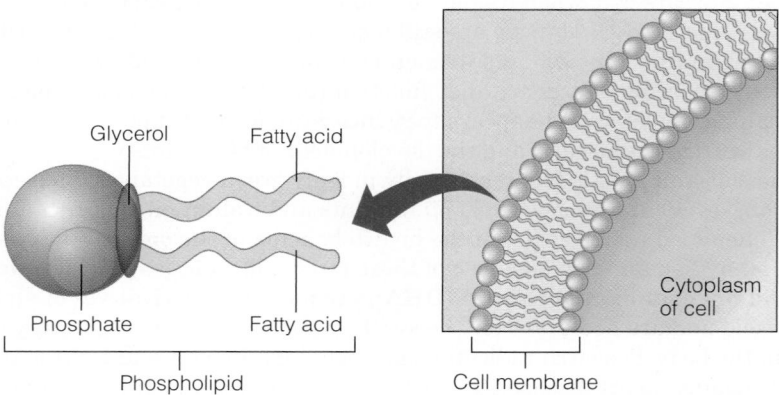

FIGURE 5.7 Structure of a phospholipid. Phospholipids consist of a glycerol backbone with two fatty acids and a compound that contains phosphate.

(a) Sterol ring structure

(b) Cholesterol

FIGURE 5.8 Sterol structure. **(a)** Sterols are lipids that contain multiple ring structures. **(b)** Cholesterol is the most commonly occurring sterol in the diet.

hormones (estrogen, androgen, and progesterone), bile acids, adrenal hormones, and vitamin D. Thus, despite cholesterol's bad reputation, it is absolutely essential to human health.

> RECAP: *Fat is essential for health. Three types of fat are found in foods: triglycerides, phospholipids, and sterols. Triglycerides are the most common. A triglyceride is made up of glycerol and three fatty acids. These fatty acids can be classified based on chain length, level of saturation, and shape. Saturated and* trans *fatty acids increase our risk for cardiovascular disease, whereas unsaturated and essential fatty acids are protective. Phospholipids combine two fatty acids and a glycerol backbone with a phosphate-containing compound, making them soluble in water. Sterols have a multiple ring structure; cholesterol is the most commonly occurring sterol in our diets.*

Why Do We Need Fats?

Dietary fat provides energy and helps our bodies perform some essential physiologic functions.

Fats Provide Energy

Dietary fat is a primary source of energy because fat has more than twice the energy per gram of carbohydrate or protein. Fat provides 9 kilocalories (kcal) per gram, while carbohydrate and protein provide only 4 kilocalories (kcal) per gram. This means that fat is much more energy dense. For example, 1 tbsp. of butter or oil contains approximately 100 kcal, while it takes 2.5 cups of steamed broccoli or 1 slice of whole-wheat bread to provide 100 kcal.

Fats Are a Major Fuel Source When We Are at Rest

At rest, we are able to deliver plenty of oxygen to our cells so that metabolic functions can occur. Just as a candle needs oxygen for the flame to burn the tallow, our cells need oxygen to burn fat for energy. Thus, approximately 30–70% of the energy used at rest by the muscles and organs comes from fat.[7] The exact percentage varies according to how much fat you are eating in your diet, how physically active you are, and whether you are gaining or losing weight. If you are dieting, more fat will be used for energy than if you are gaining weight. During times of weight gain, more of the fat consumed in the diet is stored in the adipose tissue, and the body uses more dietary protein and carbohydrate as fuel sources at rest.

Fats Fuel Physical Activity

Fat is a major energy source during physical activity, and one of the best ways to lose body fat is to exercise. During exercise, fat can be mobilized from any of the following sources: muscle tissue, adipose tissue, blood lipoproteins, and/or any

Dietary fat provides energy.

The longer you exercise, the more fat you use for energy. Cyclists in long-distance races use fat stores for energy.

dietary fat consumed during exercise. A number of hormonal changes signal the body to break down stored energy to fuel the working muscles. The hormonal responses, and the amount and source of the fat used, depend on your level of fitness; the type, intensity, and duration of the exercise; and how well-fed you are before you exercise.

For example, adrenaline strongly stimulates the breakdown of stored fat. Blood levels of adrenaline rise dramatically within seconds of beginning exercise, and this action activates additional hormones within the fat cell to begin breaking down fat. Adrenaline also signals the pancreas to *decrease* insulin production. This is important, because insulin inhibits fat breakdown. Thus, when the need for fat as an energy source is high, blood insulin levels are typically low. As you might guess, blood insulin levels are high when we are eating, because during this time our need for getting energy from stored fat is low and the need for fat storage is high.

Once fatty acids are released from the adipose cell, they travel in the blood attached to a protein, *albumin,* to the muscles, where they enter the mitochondria and use oxygen to produce ATP, which is the cell's energy source. Becoming more physically fit means you can deliver more oxygen to the muscle to use the fat that is delivered there. In addition, you can exercise longer when you are fit. Since the body has only a limited supply of stored carbohydrate as glycogen in muscle tissue, the longer you exercise, the more fat you use for energy. This point is illustrated in FIGURE 5.9. In this example, an individual is running for 4 hours at a moderate intensity. The longer the individual runs, the more depleted the muscle glycogen levels become and the more fat from adipose tissue is used as a fuel source for exercise.

Body Fat Stores Energy for Later Use

Our body stores extra energy in the form of body fat, which then can be used for energy at rest, during exercise, or during periods of low energy intake. Having a readily available energy source in the form of fat allows the body to always have

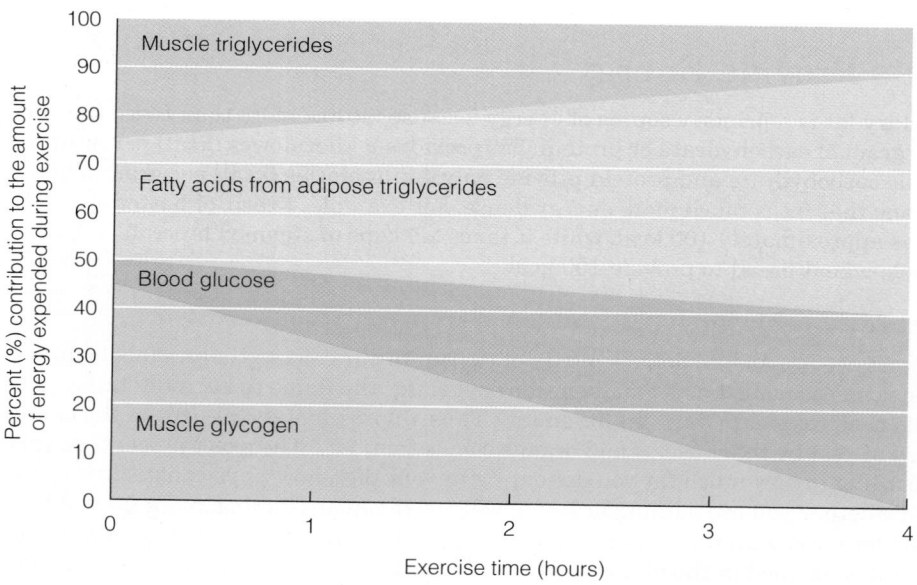

FIGURE 5.9 Various sources of energy used during exercise. As a person exercises for a prolonged period of time, fatty acids from adipose cells contribute relatively more energy than do carbohydrates stored in the muscle or circulating in our blood. (Adapted with permission by the *American Journal of Clinical Nutrition.* © American Journal of Clinical Nutrition. American Society for Clinical Nutrition.)

access to energy even when we choose not to eat (or are unable to eat), when we are exercising, and while we are sleeping. Our bodies have little stored carbohydrate—only enough to last about 1 to 2 days—and there is no place where our body can store extra protein. We cannot consider our muscles and organs as a place where "extra" protein is stored! For these reasons, the fat stored in our adipose and muscle tissues is necessary to keep the body going. Although we do not want too much stored adipose tissue, some fat storage is essential to good health.

Fats Enable the Transport of Fat-Soluble Vitamins

Dietary fat enables the transport of the fat-soluble vitamins (A, D, E, and K) needed by our body for many essential metabolic functions. For example, vitamin A is especially important for normal vision and gives you the ability to see at night. Vitamin D is important for regulating blood calcium and phosphorus concentrations within normal ranges, which indirectly helps maintain bone health. If vitamin D is low, blood calcium levels will drop below normal, and the body will draw calcium from the bones to maintain blood levels. Vitamin E functions primarily as an antioxidant in our body and keeps cell membranes healthy by preventing oxidation of body fats. Finally, vitamin K is important for proteins involved in blood clotting and bone health. We discuss these vitamins in detail in Chapters 8 and 9.

Fats Help Maintain Cell Function

Fats are a critical part of every cell membrane. The types of fats in cell membranes help to maintain membrane integrity, determine what substances are transported in and out of the cell, and regulate what substances can bind to the cell; thus, fats strongly influence the function of the cell. In addition, fats help maintain cell fluidity and other physical properties of the cell membrane. For example, wild salmon live in very cold water and have high levels of omega-3 fatty acids in their cell membranes. These fats stay fluid and flexible even in very cold environments, which allow the fish to swim in extremely cold water. In the same way, fats help our membranes stay fluid and flexible. For example, we want our red blood cells to be flexible enough to bend and move through the smallest capillaries in our body, delivering oxygen to all our cells. Fats help the red blood cells to maintain this ability.

Fats, especially PUFAs, are also primary components of the tissues of the brain and spinal cord, where they facilitate the transmission of information from one cell to another. We also need fats for the development, growth, and maintenance of these tissues.

Adipose tissue pads our body and protects our organs when we fall or are bruised.

Stored Fat Provides Protection to the Body

Stored body fat also plays an important role in our body. Besides being the primary site of stored energy, adipose tissue pads our body and protects our organs, such as the kidneys and liver, when we fall or are bruised. The fat under our skin acts as insulation to help us retain body heat. Although we often think of body fat as "bad," it does play an important role in keeping our body healthy and functioning properly.

Fats Contribute to the Flavor and Texture of Foods

Dietary fat plays an important role in making food taste good because it adds texture and flavor to foods. Fat makes salad dressings smooth and ice cream "creamy," and it gives cakes and cookies their moist, tender texture. Frying foods in melted butter, lard, or oils gives them a crisp, flavorful coating; however, eating fried foods regularly is unhealthful because these foods are high in saturated and *trans* fatty acids.

Fat adds texture and flavor to foods.

Fats Help Us to Feel Satiated

Fats in foods help us feel satiated after a meal. Two factors probably contribute to this effect: first, fat has a much higher energy density than carbohydrate or protein. For example, a pat of butter weighing 5 g will contain 35 kcal; 5 g of an apple contain only 3 kcal. For every gram of fat you consume, you get 2.25 times the amount of energy that you get with the same number of grams consumed in protein or carbohydrate.

Second, fat takes longer to digest than protein or carbohydrate because more steps are involved in the digestion process, which may make you feel fuller for a longer period of time because energy is slowly being released into your body.

On the other hand, you can eat more fat in a meal without feeling overfull because fat is generally compact in its size. Going back to our apple and butter example, one medium apple weighs 117 g (approximately 4 oz) and has 70 kcal, but the same number of calories of butter—two pats—would hardly make you feel full! Looked at another way, an amount of butter weighing the same number of grams as a medium apple would contain 840 kcal!

RECAP: *Dietary fats provide more than twice the energy of protein and carbohydrate, at 9 calories per gram, and provide the majority of energy required at rest. Fats are also a major fuel source during exercise, especially endurance exercise. Dietary fats help transport the fat-soluble vitamins into the body and help regulate cell function and maintain membrane integrity. Stored body fat in the adipose tissue helps protect vital organs and pad the body. Fats contribute to the flavor and texture of foods and the satiety we feel after a meal.*

When Are Fats Harmful?

Like many things, a little can be good, but a lot can be harmful. We have just discussed why fats are an essential part of a good diet and necessary for health, but too much fat, regardless of the type, can be damaging to our bodies.

Eating Too Much of Certain Fats Can Lead to Disease

As mentioned earlier, diets high in saturated and *trans* fatty acids increase our risk of cardiovascular disease. Conversely, diets too high in omega-3 fatty acids can increase your risk of stroke, although these types of diets are rare. It is also well documented that diets that are high in fat, regardless of the type of fat, are high in calories and can contribute to weight gain and obesity. Thus, our goal is to select the right amount and types of fats to include in our diet.

Fats Limit the Shelf Life of Foods

Fats are susceptible to oxidation and become rancid quickly if they are not stored appropriately. This means that foods high in fat such as cookies, doughnuts, crackers, chips, and breads quickly become stale on the grocery store shelf. Manufacturers add preservatives to reduce the rancidity of the fats in the products and increase their shelf life because high-fat products made without preservatives spoil quickly. For example, freshly baked muffins without preservatives will become stale and moldy more quickly than muffins made with preservatives. The consumer has to make a decision when buying products with added fat: do I want a longer shelf life or fewer preservatives? It is important to note that not all preservatives added to increase the shelf life of high-fat products are bad. For example, vitamin E, an antioxidant, is frequently added to margarines to increase their shelf life.

RECAP: *The fats we eat can either contribute to health or increase our risk of disease. Selecting the right amount and type of fats in your diet is important for improving health. Because fats added to foods can be oxidized and become rancid, foods high in fat can quickly spoil. Manufacturers add preservatives to foods high in fat to increase their shelf life.*

How Does Our Body Process Fats?

Because fats are not soluble in water, they cannot enter our bloodstream easily from the digestive tract. Thus, fats must be digested, absorbed, and transported within the body differently from carbohydrates and proteins, which are water-soluble substances.

The digestion and absorption of fat were discussed in detail in Chapter 3, but we briefly review the process here (FIGURE 5.10). Dietary fats usually come mixed with other foods. Salivary enzymes released during chewing have a limited role in the breakdown of fats, and so fat reaches the stomach intact (FIGURE 5.10, step 1). The primary role of the stomach in fat digestion is to mix and break up the fat into small droplets. Because they are not soluble in water, these fat droplets typically float on top of the watery digestive juices in the stomach until they are passed into the small intestine (FIGURE 5.10, step 2).

The Gallbladder, Liver, and Pancreas Assist in Fat Digestion

Because fat is not soluble in water, its digestion requires the help of digestive enzymes from the pancreas and mixing compounds from the gallbladder. Recall from Chapter 3 that the gallbladder is a sac attached to the underside of the liver and the pancreas is an oblong-shaped organ sitting below the stomach. Both have a duct connecting them to the small intestine. As fat enters the small intestine from the stomach, the gallbladder contracts and releases a substance called bile (FIGURE 5.10, step 3). Bile is produced in the liver from cholesterol and is stored in the gallbladder until needed. You can think of bile acting much like soap, breaking up the fat into smaller and smaller droplets. At the same time, lipid-digesting enzymes produced in the pancreas travel through the pancreatic duct into the small intestine. Once bile has broken the fat into small droplets, these pancreatic enzymes take over, breaking the fatty acids away from their glycerol backbones. Each triglyceride molecule is broken down into two free fatty acids and one *monoglyceride,* a glycerol molecule with one fatty acid still attached.

Fats and oils do not dissolve readily in water.

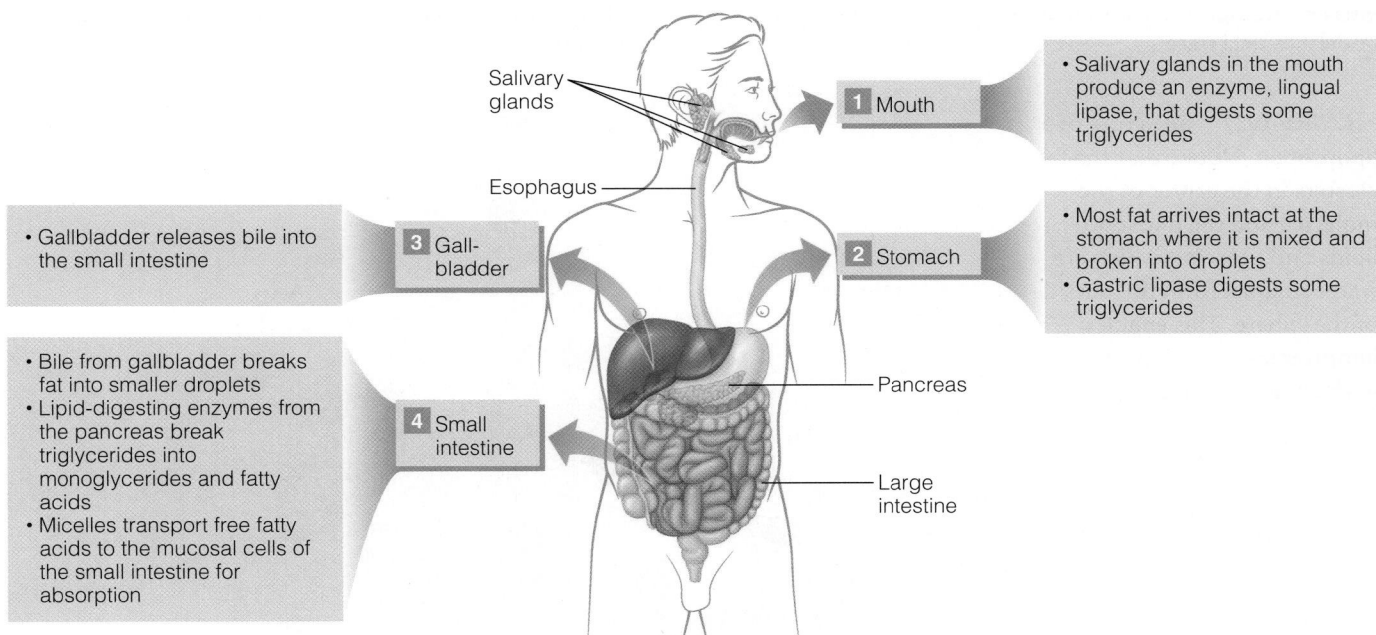

FIGURE 5.10   The process of fat digestion.

Absorption of Fat Occurs Primarily in the Small Intestine

The majority of fat absorption occurs in the mucosal lining of the small intestine with the help of a micelle (FIGURE 5.10, step 4). A *micelle* is a spherical compound made up of bile and phospholipids that can trap the free fatty acids and the monoglycerides and transport them to the mucosal cells for absorption.

How does the absorbed fat get into the bloodstream? Because fats do not mix with water, most fats cannot be transported freely in the bloodstream. To solve this problem, the fatty acids are reformulated back into triglycerides and then packaged into lipoproteins before being released into the bloodstream. A **lipoprotein** is a spherical compound in which the fat clusters in the center and phospholipids and proteins form the outside of the sphere (FIGURE 5.11). The specific lipoprotein produced in the mucosal cell to transport fat from a meal is called a **chylomicron.** This unique compound is now soluble in water because phospholipids and proteins are water soluble. Once chylomicrons are formed, they are transported from the intestinal lining to the lymphatic system and then into the blood. In this way, dietary fat finally arrives in your blood.

As mentioned earlier, short- and medium-chain fatty acids (those fewer than fourteen carbons in length) can be transported in the body more readily than the long-chain fatty acids. When short- and medium-chain fatty acids are digested and transported to the mucosal cell of the small intestine, they do not have to be reformed into triglycerides and incorporated into chylomicrons. Instead, they can travel in the bloodstream bound to either a transport protein or a phospholipid. For this reason, shorter-chain fatty acids can get into the system more quickly than long-chain fatty acids.

Fat Is Stored in Adipose Tissues for Later Use

The chylomicrons, which are filled with the dietary fat you just ate, now begin to circulate through the blood looking for a place to deliver their load. There are three primary fates of this dietary fat:

1. It can immediately be taken up and used as a source of energy for the cells.
2. It can be used to make lipid-containing compounds in the body.
3. It can be stored in the muscle or adipose tissue as a triglyceride for later use. (FIGURE 5.12 shows an adipose cell.)

lipoprotein A spherical compound in which fat clusters in the center and phospholipids and proteins form the outside of the sphere.

chylomicron A lipoprotein produced in the mucosal cell of the intestine; transports dietary fat out of the intestinal tract.

FIGURE 5.11 Structure of a lipoprotein. Notice that the fat clusters in the center of the molecule and the phospholipids and proteins, which are water soluble, form the outside of the sphere. This enables lipoproteins to transport fats in the bloodstream.

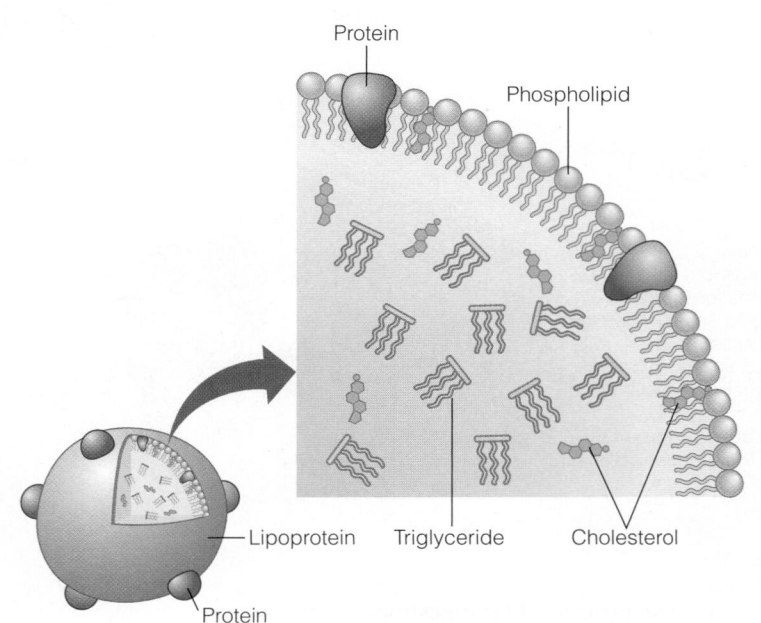

Protein

Phospholipid

Lipoprotein   Triglyceride   Cholesterol

Protein

How does the fat get out of the chylomicrons and into the cell? This process occurs with the help of an enzyme called **lipoprotein lipase,** or LPL, which sits outside of our adipose cells. LPL comes in contact with the chylomicrons when they touch the surface of the adipose cell. As a result of this contact, LPL breaks apart the triglycerides in the core of the chylomicrons. This process results in the movement of individual fatty acids from within the core of the chylomicrons and out into the adipose cell. If the cell needs the fat for energy, these fatty acids will be quickly transported into the mitochondria and used as fuel. If the body doesn't need the fatty acids for immediate energy, the cell can re-create the triglycerides and store them for later use.

The primary storage site for this extra energy is the adipose cell. However, if you are physically active, your body will preferentially store this extra fat in the muscle tissue first, so the next time you work out, the fat is readily available to the cell for energy. Thus, people who engage in physical activity are more likely to have extra fat stored in the muscle tissue and to have less body fat—something many of us would prefer. Of course, fat stored in the adipose tissue can also be used for energy during exercise, but it must be broken down first and then transported to the muscle cells.

> RECAP: *Fat digestion begins when fats are broken into droplets by bile. Pancreatic enzymes subsequently digest the triglycerides into two free fatty acids and one monoglyceride. These are transported into the intestinal mucosal cells with the help of micelles. Once inside the mucosal cells, triglycerides are re-formed and packaged into lipoproteins called chylomicrons. Dietary fat is transported by the chylomicrons to cells within the body that need energy. Fat stored in the muscle tissue is used as a source of energy during physical activity. Excess fat is stored in the adipose tissue and can be used whenever the body needs energy.*

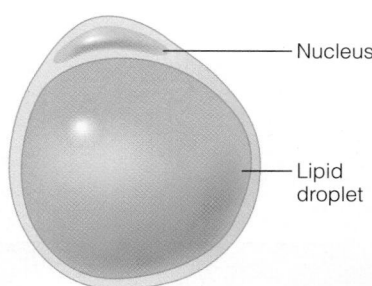

FIGURE 5.12 Diagram of an adipose cell.

How Much Fat Should We Eat?

Without a doubt, Americans think dietary fat is bad! How many people have you heard say they are trying to dramatically reduce the level of fat in their diet? Yet, because fat plays such an important role in keeping our bodies healthy, we must eat diets providing a moderate amount of energy from fat. But what, exactly, is a moderate amount? And what foods contain the most healthful fats? We'll explore these questions here.

Dietary Reference Intake for Total Fat

The Acceptable Macronutrient Distribution Range (AMDR) for fat is 20–35% of total energy.[8] This recommendation is based on evidence indicating that higher intakes of fat increase the risk of obesity and its complications, especially heart disease, but that diets too low in fat and too high in carbohydrate can also increase the risk of heart disease if they cause blood triglycerides to increase.[8] Within this range of fat intake, it is also recommended that we minimize our intake of saturated and *trans* fatty acids as much as possible; these changes will lower our risk of heart disease.

Because carbohydrate is essential in replenishing glycogen, athletes and other physically active people are advised to consume less fat and more carbohydrate than sedentary people. Specifically, it is recommended that athletes consume 20–25% of their total energy from fat, 55–60% of energy from carbohydrate, and 12–15% of energy from protein.[9] This level of fat intake represents approximately 45 to 55 g of fat per day for an athlete consuming 2,000 kcal per day, and 78 to 97 g of fat per day for an athlete consuming 3,500 kcal per day.

Although many people trying to lose weight consume less than 20% of their energy from fat, this practice may do more harm than good, especially if they are also limiting energy intake (eating fewer than 1,500 kcal per day). Research suggests that very-low-fat diets, or those with less than 15% of energy from fat, do not provide additional health or performance benefits over moderate-fat diets and are usually very difficult to follow.[10] In fact, most people find they feel better, are more successful in weight maintenance, and are less preoccupied with food if they keep their fat

lipoprotein lipase An enzyme that sits on the outside of cells and breaks apart triglycerides so that their fatty acids can be removed and taken up by the cell.

intakes at 20–25% of energy intake. Additionally, people attempting to reduce their dietary fat frequently eliminate food groups, such as meat, dairy, eggs, and nuts. Unfortunately, eliminating these food groups also eliminates potential sources of protein and many essential vitamins and minerals important for good health and maintaining an active lifestyle. Diets extremely low in fat may also be deficient in essential fatty acids.

NUTRI-CASE LIZ

"Lately I'm hungry all the time. I read on a Web site last night that if I limit my total fat intake to no more than 10% of my total calories, I can eat all the carbohydrate and protein that I want, and I won't gain weight. So I went right out to the yogurt shop down the street and ordered a large sundae with non-fat vanilla yogurt and fat-free chocolate syrup. I have to admit, though, that an hour or so after I ate it, I was hungry again. Maybe it's stress. . . ."

What do you think of Liz's approach to her persistent hunger? What have you learned in this chapter about the role of fats that might be important information to share with her?

Dietary Reference Intakes for Essential Fatty Acids

Dietary Reference Intakes (DRIs) for the two essential fatty acids were set for the first time in 2002.[8] The Adequate Intake (AI) for linoleic acid is 14 to 17 g per day for adult men and 11 to 12 g per day for women 19 years and older, whereas the AI for alpha-linolenic acid is 1.6 g per day for adult men and 1.1 g per day for adult women. Using the typical energy intakes for adult men and women, this translates into an AMDR of 5–10% of energy for linoleic acid and 0.6–1.2% for alpha-linolenic acid. These recommendations translate into a 6:1 ratio for linoleic acid to alpha-linolenic acid.

Most Americans Eat Within the Recommended Amount of Fat but Eat the Wrong Types

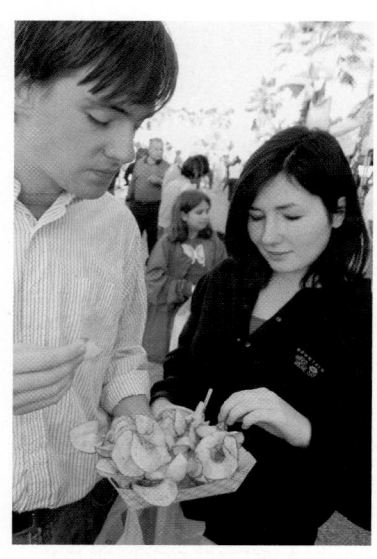

In the United States, we eat too many saturated and *trans* fats.

Nutritionists have been recommending the reduction of dietary fat for a decade. According to the most recent data, relative fat intake has decreased from 45% of total energy intake in 1965 to 34% of energy intake in 1995 for both men and women.[11] However, this reduction in the percentage of fat consumed is misleading because Americans are consuming 15% more calories overall. As shown in Table 5.2, these additional calories have come mostly in the form of carbohydrates and proteins, and less in fats, but the end result is that daily fat consumption has not decreased; instead, it has *increased* slightly.[12] The most recent dietary intake data available, collected in 1999–2000, show the same trends.[13]

Of the dietary fat we eat, saturated and *trans* fats are most highly correlated with an increased risk of heart disease because they negatively affect blood lipids by altering lipoprotein synthesis, uptake, and removal. Thus, the recommended intake of saturated fat is less than 7–10% of our total energy; unfortunately, our average intake of saturated fats is between 11% and 12% of energy.[14] The Institute of Medicine also recommends that we keep our intake of *trans* fatty acids to an absolute minimum.[8] The determination of the actual amount of *trans* fatty acids consumed in America has been hindered by the lack of an accurate and comprehensive database of foods containing *trans* fatty acids. At the present time, a best guess as to the amount of *trans* fatty acid

TABLE 5.2   Trends in Energy Availability in the United States from 1970 to 1994

Nutrient	Year						Percentage Change from 1970 to 1994
	1970	*1975*	*1980*	*1985*	*1990*	*1994*	
Food energy available (kcal/day)	3298	3203	3298	3489	3609	3800	+15.2
Protein (g/day)	95	93	96	101	105	110	+15.8
Carbohydrate (g/day)	386	385	406	420	458	491	+27.2
Total fat (g/day)	154	146	153	163	156	159	+3.2
Percentage (%) of total energy from fat	42	41	42	42	39	38	−9.5

Source: Adapted from Harnack, L. J., R. W. Jeffery, and K. N. Boutelle. 2000. Temporal trends in energy intake in the United States: an ecologic perspective. *Am. J. Clin. Nutr.* 71:1478–1484. Copyright © 2000 American Society for Nutrition. Used with permission.

consumed in the United States comes from a national survey,[15] which estimated our intake at 2.6% of our total fat intake.

> RECAP: *The Acceptable Macronutrient Distribution Range (AMDR) for total fat is 20–35% of total energy. The Adequate Intake (AI) for linoleic acid is 14 to 17 g per day for adult men and 11 to 12 g per day for adult women. The AI for alpha-linolenic acid is 1.6 g per day for adult men and 1.1 g per day for adult women. Because saturated and* trans *fatty acids can increase the risk of heart disease, health professionals recommend that we reduce our intake of saturated fat to less than 7% of our total energy intake and reduce our intake of* trans *fatty acids to an absolute minimum.*

Food Sources of Fats

The last time you popped a frozen dinner into the microwave, did you stop and read the Nutrition Facts Panel on the box? If you had, you might have been shocked to learn how much saturated fat was in the meal. As we discuss here, many processed foods are hidden sources of fat, especially saturated fat. In contrast, many whole foods, such as oils and nuts, are rich sources of the healthful fats our bodies need.

Watch Out for Invisible Fats

Americans not only eat lots of high-fat foods, but also commonly add fat to foods to improve their taste. Added fats, such as oils, butter, cream, shortening, margarine, or dressings (such as mayonnaise and salad dressings), are called **visible fats** because we can easily see that we are adding them to our food.

When we add fat to foods ourselves, we know how much we are adding and what kind. When fat is added in the preparation of a casserole or a fast-food burger and fries, we are less aware of how much or what type of fat is actually there. In fact, unless we read food labels carefully, we might not be aware that a food contains any fat at all. We call fats in prepared and processed foods **invisible fats** because they are hidden within the food. In fact, their invisibility often tricks us into choosing them over more healthful foods. For example, a slice of

visible fats Fat we can see in our foods or see added to foods, such as butter, margarine, cream, shortening, salad dressings, chicken skin, and untrimmed fat on meat.

invisible fats Fats that are hidden in foods, such as the fats found in baked goods, regular-fat dairy products, marbling in meat, and fried foods.

Baked goods are often high in invisible fats and may contain *trans* fats.

HIGHLIGHT

HIGHLIGHT HIGHLIGHT HIGHLIGHT HIGHLIGHT HIGHLIGHT

Low-Fat, Reduced-Fat, Nonfat . . . What's the Difference?

Although most people love high-fat foods, we also know that eating too much fat isn't good for our health or our waistlines. Because of this concern, food manufacturers have produced a host of modified-fat foods—so you can have your cake and eat it too! In fact, it is now estimated that there are more than 5,000 different fat-modified foods on the market.[16,17] This means that we have similar foods that come in a wide range of fat contents. For example, you can purchase full-fat, low-fat, or fat-free milk, ice cream, sour cream, cheese, and yogurt.

In Table 5.3, we list a number of full-fat foods with their lower-fat alternatives. These products, if incorporated in the diet on a regular basis, can significantly reduce the amount of fat consumed but may or may not reduce the amount of energy consumed. For example, drinking nonfat milk (86 kcal and 0.5 g of fat per serving) instead of whole milk (150 kcal and 8.2 g of fat per serving) will dramatically reduce both fat and energy intake. However, eating fat-free Fig Newton cookies (3 cookies have 204 kcal and 0 g of fat) instead of regular Fig Newton cookies (3 cookies have 210 kcal and 4.5 g of fat) will not reduce your energy intake, even though it will reduce your fat intake by 4.5 g per serving.

Thus, if you think that eating fat-free foods means you're not getting any calories and can eat all you want without gaining weight, you're mistaken. The reduced fat is often replaced with added carbohydrate, resulting in a very similar total energy intake. Thus, if you want to reduce both the amount of fat and the number of calories you consume, you must read the labels of modified-fat foods carefully before you buy.[16]

The FDA and the USDA have set specific regulations on allowable product descriptions for reduced-fat products. The following claims are defined for one serving:

- Fat-free = less than 0.5 g of fat
- Low-fat = 3 g or less of fat
- Reduced or less fat: at least 25% less fat as compared to a standard serving
- Light: one-third fewer calories or 50% less fat as compared with a standard serving size

yellow cake is much higher in fat (40% of total energy) than a slice of angel food cake (1% of total energy). Yet many consumers just assume the fat content of these foods are the same, since they are both cake. For most of us, the majority of the fat in our diets comes from invisible fat. Foods that can be high in invisible fats are baked goods, regular-fat dairy products, processed meats or meats that are not trimmed, and most convenience and fast foods, such as hamburgers, hot dogs, chips, ice cream, French fries, and other fried foods. When purchasing packaged foods, read the Nutrition Facts Panel and find out whether or not the product is high in invisible fats!

Because high-fat diets have been associated with obesity, many Americans have tried to reduce their total fat intake. Food manufacturers have been more than happy to provide consumers with low-fat alternatives to their favorite foods. However, these lower-fat foods may not always have fewer calories. Read the Highlight box above and Table 5.3 to learn how to be a better consumer of reduced-fat foods.

TABLE 5.3 Comparison of Full-Fat, Reduced-Fat, and Low-Fat Foods

Product and Serving Size	Version	Energy (kcal)	Protein (g)	Carbohydrate (g)	Fat (g)
Milk, 8 oz	Whole, 3.3% fat	150	8.0	11.4	8.2
	2% fat	121	8.1	11.7	4.7
	1% fat	102	8.0	11.7	2.6
	Skim (nonfat)	86	8.4	11.9	0.5
Cheese, cheddar, 1 oz	Regular	111	7.1	0.5	9.1
	Low-fat	81	9.1	0.0	5.1
	Nonfat	41	6.8	4.0	0.0
Mayonnaise, 1 tbsp.	Regular	100	0.0	0.0	11.0
	Light	50	0.0	1.0	5.0
	Fat-free	10	0.0	2.0	0.0
Margarine, corn oil, 1 tbsp.	Regular	100	0.0	0.0	11.0
	Reduced-fat	60	0.0	0.0	7.0
Peanut butter, 1 tbsp.	Regular	95	4.1	3.1	8.2
	Reduced-fat	81	4.4	5.2	5.4
Cream cheese, 1 tbsp.	Soft regular	50	1.0	0.5	5.0
	Soft light	35	1.5	1.0	2.5
	Soft nonfat	15	2.5	1.0	0.0
Wheat Thins, 18 crackers	Regular	158	2.3	21.4	6.8
	Reduced-fat	120	2.0	21.0	4.0
Cookies, Oreo, 3 cookies	Regular	160	2.0	23.0	7.0
	Reduced-fat	130	2.0	25.0	3.5
Cookies, Fig Newton, 3 cookies	Regular	210	3.0	30.0	4.5
	Fat-free	204	2.4	26.8	0.0
Breakfast bars, 1 bar	Regular	140	2.0	27.0	2.8
	Fat-free	110	2.0	26.0	0.0

Data Source: Food Processor-SQL, Version 9.9, ESHA Research, Salem, OR.
The Food and Drug Administration and the U.S. Department of Agriculture have set specific regulations on allowable product descriptions for reduced-fat products. The following claims are defined for 1 serving: **Fat-free**: less than 0.5 g of fat; **low-fat**: 3 g or less of fat; **reduced or less fat**: at least 25% less fat as compared to a standard serving; **light**: one-third fewer calories or 50% less fat as compared with a standard serving size.

Increase Your Consumption of Beneficial Fats

Americans appear to get adequate amounts of omega-6 fatty acids, probably because of the large amount of salad dressings, vegetable oils, margarine, and mayonnaise we eat; however, our consumption of omega-3 fatty acids is more variable and can be low in the diets of people who do not eat leafy green vegetables, fish, or walnuts; drink soy milk; or use soybean, canola, or flax oil. Table 5.4 identifies the omega-3 fatty acid content of various foods.

In general, it's best to switch to healthful sources of fats without increasing total fat intake. For example, use olive and canola oil in place of butter and margarine, and select fish more frequently instead of high-fat meat sources (hot dogs, hamburgers, sausage). Dairy products can be high in saturated fats, so select low- and reduced-fat dairy products when possible and reduce the intake of hard cheeses and cheese spreads. Read the Nutrition Label Activity on page 196 to learn how to calculate the amount of fat in the foods you buy.

TABLE 5.4   Omega-3 Fatty Acid Content of Selected Foods

Food Item	Omega-3 Fatty Acid (grams per serving)
Flaxseed oil, 1 tbsp.	7.25
Salmon oil (fish oil), 1 tbsp.	4.39
Sardine oil, 1 tbsp.	3.01
Flaxseed, whole, 1 tbsp.	2.50
Herring, Atlantic, broiled, 3 oz	1.83
Herring oil, 1 tbsp.	1.53
Canola oil, 1 tbsp.	1.30
Sardines, Atlantic, w/ bones and oil, 3 oz	1.26
Shrimp, broiled, 3 oz	1.11
Trout, rainbow fillet, baked, 3 oz	1.00
Walnuts, English, 1 tbsp.	0.68
Salmon, smoked Chinook, 3 oz	0.50
Halibut, fillet, baked, 3 oz	0.47
Tuna, white, in oil, 3 oz	0.38
Crab, Dungeness, steamed, 3 oz	0.34
Scallops, broiled, 3 oz	0.26
Tuna, light, in water, 3 oz	0.23

Source: Data from Food Processor SQL, Version 9.9, ESHA Research, Salem, OR.

Avoid Consumption of Contaminated Fish

It is important to recognize that there can be some risk associated with eating large amounts of certain fish on a regular basis. Some species of fish contain high levels of poisons such as mercury, polychlorinated biphenyls (PCBs), and other environmental contaminants. These poisons can accumulate in the bodies of individuals who regularly consume contaminated fish. Women who are pregnant or breastfeeding, women who may become pregnant, and small children are at particularly high risk for toxicity from these contaminants. It is generally considered safe for pregnant women or women who become pregnant to consume up to 12 oz of a variety of fish each week.

Not all fish are contaminated; sport-caught fish and predator fish such as shark, swordfish, and king mackerel tend to have higher levels of contaminants. Types of fish that are currently considered safe to consume include salmon (except from the Great Lakes region), farmed trout, flounder, sole, mahi-mahi, and cooked shellfish. For more information on seafood contamination, see Chapter 18.

Fat Replacers

One way to lower the fat content of foods such as chips, muffins, cakes, and cookies is by replacing the fat in a food with a *fat replacer*. Snack foods have been the primary target for fat replacers since it is more difficult to eliminate the fat from these types of products without dramatically changing the taste. In the mid-1990s, the food industry and nutritionists thought that fat replacers would be the answer to our growing obesity problem. If we could replace some of the traditional fats in snack and fast foods with these products, we might be able to reduce both energy and fat intake and help Americans manage their weight better.

Products such as olestra (brand name Olean) hit the market in 1996 with a lot of fanfare, but the hype was short-lived. Initially, foods containing olestra had to bear a label warning of potential gastrointestinal side effects. In 2003, the FDA announced that this warning was no longer necessary, as research showed that olestra causes only mild, infrequent discomfort. However, even with the new labeling, only limited foods in the marketplace contain olestra. It is also evident from our growing obesity problem that fat replacers such as olestra did not help Americans lose weight or even maintain their current weight.

Snack foods have been the primary target for fat replacers, such as Olean, since it is more difficult to eliminate the fat from these types of foods without dramatically changing the taste.

RECAP: *Visible fats are those foods that can be easily recognized as containing fat. Invisible fats are those fats added to our food during the manufacturing or cooking process so we are not aware of how much fat was added. Fat replacers are substances used to replace the typical fats found in foods. By making simple substitutions when shopping, cooking, and eating out, you can reduce the quantity of saturated and* trans *fatty acids in your diet and increase your intake of healthful fats.*

SHOPPER'S GUIDE

Improving the Type and Quantity of Fat in Your Diet

So how do you actually begin applying the recommendations related to fat intake to your daily diet? Begin by becoming a better shopper. Next, make wise choices when cooking at home with fat. Finally, make better selections while eating out. Below are some simple ways to begin improving the quality and quantity of fat in your diet. If you follow a few of these suggestions every day, you'll achieve a more healthful diet and reduce your risk for heart disease.

Shopping Tips

√ Select liquid or tub margarine/butters over hard stick forms. Fats that are solid at room temperature are usually high in trans or saturated fatty acids. Also, select margarines made from healthful fats such as canola oil.

√ Use naturally occurring oils such as olive and canola oil. These types of oils have not been hydrogenated and contain healthful unsaturated fatty acids and no trans fatty acids.

√ Read food labels. Look for foods with zero trans fatty acids and low amounts of saturated fats per serving.

√ Select reduced-fat baked products such as crackers, chips, cookies, and muffins over full-fat versions. If you are watching your weight, choose products with fewer calories per serving as well.

√ Select reduced-fat salad dressing and mayonnaise or select those made with healthful fats such as olive oil and vinegar. If you select the full-fat versions, remember that a tablespoon of oil or full-fat mayonnaise contains 100 kcal.

√ Add fish, especially those high in omega-3 fatty acids, to your shopping list. For example, select salmon, line-caught tuna, herring, and sardines. Many specialty markets now carry line-caught canned tuna, which is low in mercury. These tuna are smaller, usually less than 20 pounds, and have had less exposure to mercury in their lifetime.

√ For other healthful sources of protein, select lean cuts of meat and skinless poultry, meat substitutes made with soy, or beans or lentils.

√ Select low-fat or non-fat dairy products such as milk, cottage cheese, yogurt, sour cream, and cottage cheese.

√ Add small amounts of healthful nuts, such as walnuts or almonds, to your diet. You can do this by adding a tablespoon of nuts to breakfast cereal, yogurt, salads, sautéed vegetables, or meats. Because nuts are high in calories, add them to your diet in moderation.

Cooking Tips

√ Use naturally occurring oils in sautéing and cooking. Measure the amount used if you want to control the fat and calories you are adding to your food

√ When baking, replace butter with reduced-fat, trans fat–free tub margarines or oils to decrease the saturated fat in your recipe. You can also replace a portion of the butter with ground flaxseed. To keep baked products moist with less fat, try adding applesauce or other fruits to the product.

√ Use a cooking oil spray to coat pans for baking or sautéing. This will reduce the amount of fat added to the product. These products are typically very low in calories and fat.

(continued)

√ Experiment by adding more herbs and spices to vegetables and meats, which adds flavor when less fat is used in the cooking process.

√ Use cooking techniques that use less fat such as steaming, baking, roasting, sautéing, and grilling instead of frying.

√ Trim fats from meats and cook without adding additional fats.

√ Use low-fat spreads on your sandwiches, such as mustards or chutneys, over full-fat mayonnaise or butter.

Tips for Eating Out

√ Select restaurants or eating establishments that allow you a choice when selecting from the menu. If you like burgers, look for a restaurant that offers grilled burgers and a salad instead of fried burgers and French fries.

√ Select menu items that use cooking methods that add little or no additional fat such as grilling, steaming, or sautéing. Be alert to menu descriptions such as fried, crispy, creamed, in cream, cheese, or butter sauce, au gratin, escalloped, parmesan, hollandaise, pot pie, or pastry crust. All of these types of food preparation typically add more fat to a meal.

√ Select lower-fat menu items such as reduced-fat dairy, lean meats, fish, vegetables, salads, and whole grains.

√ Ask for visible fats, such as butter, salad dressings, sauces, sour cream, and cheese, to be served on the side instead of added in the kitchen.

√ Ask about the types of fats used in salad dressing, baked goods, and cooking processes. Many restaurants and fast-food establishments are working to eliminate trans fatty acids from their products and incorporating healthful fats into their other menu items. For example, Wendy's eliminated trans fatty acids in 2006. McDonald's and KFC have promised to do the same. McGraths lists non-trans fat items on their menu. If you have a favorite restaurant that you visit frequently, make sure you know the kinds of fats they use in their products.

√ Select broth-based soups, which are lower in fat and calories than cream-based soups, which are typically made with cream, cheese, and/or butter.

√ Select healthful appetizers, such as salads, broth-based soups, vegetables, or fruit, over high-fat chips and dip or fried foods such as chicken wings.

√ Substitute a salad or fruit for the chips or French fries that come with the meal.

√ Select lower-fat desserts, such as sorbet or a small cookie, over full-fat ice cream or a brownie. Alternatively, share a full-fat dessert with friends or family members, which will reduce both the calories and fat you consume.

√ Select your favorite coffee, chocolate, or tea drink with non-fat or reduced-fat milk and eliminate the whipped cream. For example, a Starbucks Tall Caffe Latte (12 oz) made with whole milk contains 200 kcal and 11 g of fat (7 g from saturated fat). The same drink made with non-fat milk contains 120 kcal and no fat. Thus, it is easy to see how quickly we can add both fat and calories in a liquid beverage. Also, by asking for your beverage without whipped cream, you can save 80–130 kcal and 8–12 g of fat.

√ Select lower-fat options to accompany your coffee drink. For example, choose a bagel or small cookie (biscotti or gingersnap) instead of a croissant, scone, muffin, coffee cake, or large cookie.

NUTRI-CASE HANNAH

" Friday is my favorite day at school, because it's pizza day! Today I had two slices of pepperoni pizza, a carton of milk to drink, and banana pudding for dessert. I wish it could be pizza day every day!"

What important nutrients did Hannah consume in her lunch today? What nutrients were lacking? If Hannah has this type of lunch just once a week, do you think it presents a problem? What additional information about Hannah and her mom's diet would help you to answer this question?

What Role Do Fats Play in Cardiovascular Disease and Cancer?

There appears to be a generally held assumption that if you eat fat-free or low-fat foods you will lose weight and prevent chronic diseases. Certainly, we know that high-fat diets, especially those high in saturated and *trans* fatty acids, can contribute to chronic diseases, including heart disease and cancer; however, as we have explored in this chapter, unsaturated fatty acids do not have this negative effect and are essential to good health. Thus, a sensible health goal would be to eat the appropriate amounts and types of fat.

cardiovascular disease A general term that refers to abnormal conditions involving dysfunction of the heart and blood vessels; cardiovascular disease can result in heart attack or stroke.

Fats Can Protect Against or Promote Cardiovascular Disease

Cardiovascular disease is a general term used to refer to any abnormal condition involving dysfunction of the heart and blood vessels. A common form of this disease occurs when blood vessels supplying the heart (the *coronary arteries*) become blocked or constricted; such blockage reduces blood flow to the heart and can result in a heart attack. Blockage of one of the blood vessels supplying the brain (the *cerebral arteries*) can cause a stroke. According to the Centers for Disease Control and Prevention, heart disease is the leading cause of death in the United States across racial and ethnic groups and is a major cause of permanent disability (FIGURE 5.13).[18] It accounts for more than 30% of all deaths. Stroke is the third leading cause of death and accounts for about 10% of all deaths. Overall, about 61 million Americans of all ages suffer from cardiovascular diseases, and it is estimated that in 2001 the cost of this disease was $300 billion.

Risk Factors for Cardiovascular Disease

Over the last two decades, researchers have identified a number of factors that contribute to an increased risk for cardiovascular disease. Some of

FIGURE 5.13 Cardiovascular disease, which includes heart disease, is the leading cause of death in the United States. (National Center for Chronic Disease Prevention and Health Promotion (NCCDPHP). 2002. Chronic Disease Prevention. Chronic Disease Overview. www.cdc.gov/nccdphp/overview.htm.)

NUTRITION LABEL ACTIVITY

How Much Fat Is in This Food?

How do you know how much fat is in a food you buy? One simple way to determine the amount of fat in the food you eat is to read the Nutrition Facts Panel on the label. By becoming a better label reader, you can make more healthful food selections. Two cracker labels are shown in Figure 5.14; one cracker is higher in fat than the other.

Let's review how you can read the label so you know what percentage of energy is coming from fat from each product. These calculations are relatively simple.

1. Divide the total calories from fat by the total calories per serving, and multiply the answer by 100.
   - For the regular wheat crackers: 50 calories/150 calories = 0.33 × 100 = 33%

   Thus, for the regular crackers, the total energy coming from fat is 33%.
   - For the reduced-fat wheat crackers: 35 calories/130 calories = 0.269 × 100 = 27%

   Thus, for the reduced-fat crackers, the total energy coming from fat is 27%.

   You can see that, although the total amount of energy per serving is not very different between these two crackers, the amount of fat is quite different.

2. If the total calories per serving from fat are not given on the label, you can quickly calculate this value by multiplying the grams of total fat per serving by 9 (as there are 9 calories per gram of fat).
   - For the regular wheat crackers: 6 g fat × 9 calories/gram = 54 calories of fat
   - To calculate percentage of calories from fat: 54 calories/150 calories = 0.36 × 100 = 36%

   You can see that this value is not exactly the same as the 50 calories reported on the label or the 33% of calories from fat calculated in example 1. The values on food labels are rounded off, so your estimations may not be identical when you do this second calculation. Refer to Table 5.3, which gives a list of regular, reduced-fat, and fat-free foods. You can quickly calculate the percentage of fat per serving for these foods by following the same series of steps: first, multiply the grams of fat per serving by 9 calories per gram; then divide this number by the total calories per serving; and finally, multiply by 100.

these risk factors are nonmodifiable, such as age, gender, and family history, whereas others can be modified through lifestyle changes, such as body weight, level of physical activity, and smoking. Following is a brief description of each of these major risk factors, many of which have a dietary component.[19,20]

- Overweight—Being overweight is associated with higher rates of death from cardiovascular disease. The risk is due primarily to a greater occurrence of high blood pressure, abnormal blood lipids (discussed in more detail on page 198), and higher rates of type 2 diabetes in people who are overweight. In general, an overweight condition develops from an energy imbalance from eating too much and exercising too little (see Chapter 11).

- Physical inactivity—Numerous research studies have shown that physical activity can reduce your risk of cardiovascular disease by improving several risk factors associated with the disease, including improved blood lipid levels, lower resting blood pressure, lower body fat and weight, and improved blood glucose levels both at rest and after eating.

- Smoking—There is strong evidence that smoking increases your risk for cardiovascular disease. Research indicates that smokers have a 70% greater chance of developing cardiovascular disease than nonsmokers. Without question, smoking cessation or never starting initially is one of the best ways to reduce your risk of cardiovascular disease. People who stop smoking live

Wheat Crackers

• **No Cholesterol**

Nutrition Facts

Serving Size: 16 Crackers (31g)
Servings Per Container: About 9

Amount Per Serving	
Calories	150
Calories from Fat	50

	% Daily Value*
Total Fat 6g	9%
Saturated Fat 1g	6%
Polyunsaturated Fat 0g	
Monounsaturated Fat 2g	
Trans Fat 0g	
Cholesterol 0mg	0%
Sodium 270mg	11%
Total Carbohydrate 21g	7%
Dietary Fiber 1g	4%
Sugars 3g	
Protein 2g	

Vitamin A	0%
Vitamin C	0%
Calcium	2%
Iron	6%

* Percent Daily Values are based on a 2,000 calorie diet. Your daily values may be higher or lower depending on your calorie needs:

	Calories	2,000	2,500
Total Fat	Less than	65g	80g
Sat. Fat	Less than	20g	25g
Cholesterol	Less than	300mg	300mg
Sodium	Less than	2,400mg	2,400mg
Total Carbohydrate		300g	375g
Dietary Fiber		25g	30g

INGREDIENTS: Enriched Flour (Wheat Flour, Niacin, Reduced Iron, Thiamine Mononitrate (Vitamin B1), Riboflavin (Vitamin B2), Folic Acid), Partially Hydrogenated Soybean Oil, Defatted Wheat Germ, Sugar, Cornstarch, High Fructose Corn Syrup, Corn Syrup, Salt, Malt Syrup, Leavening (Calcium Phosphate, Baking Soda), Vegetable Colors (Annatto Extract, Turmeric Oleoresin), Malted Barley Flour.

(a)

Reduced-Fat Wheat Crackers

• **No Cholesterol**
• **Low Saturated Fat**
Contains 4g Fat Per Serving

Nutrition Facts

Serving Size: 16 Crackers (29g)
Servings Per Container: About 9

Amount Per Serving	
Calories	130
Calories from Fat	35

	% Daily Value*
Total Fat 4g	6%
Saturated Fat 1g	4%
Polyunsaturated Fat 0g	
Monounsaturated Fat 1.5g	
Trans Fat 0g	
Cholesterol 0mg	0%
Sodium 260 mg	11%
Total Carbohydrate 21g	7%
Dietary Fiber 1g	4%
Sugars 3g	
Protein 2g	

Vitamin A	0%
Vitamin C	0%
Calcium	2%
Iron	6%

* Percent Daily Values are based on a 2,000 calorie diet. Your daily values may be higher or lower depending on your calorie needs:

	Calories	2,000	2,500
Total Fat	Less than	65g	80g
Sat. Fat	Less than	20g	25g
Cholesterol	Less than	300mg	300mg
Sodium	Less than	2,400mg	2,400mg
Total Carbohydrate		300g	375g
Dietary Fiber		25g	30g

Reduced Fat Wheat Crackers have 4 grams of fat per serving compared to 6 grams in Original Wheat Crackers.

INGREDIENTS: Enriched Flour (Wheat Flour, Niacin, Reduced Iron, Thiamine Mononitrate (Vitamin B1), Riboflavin (Vitamin B2), Folic Acid), Partially Hydrogenated Soybean Oil, Defatted Wheat Germ, Sugar, Cornstarch, High Fructose Corn Syrup, Corn Syrup, Salt, Malt Syrup, Leavening (Calcium Phosphate, Baking Soda), Vegetable Colors (Annatto Extract and Turmeric Oleoresin), Malted Barley Flour.

(b)

FIGURE 5.14 Labels for two types of wheat crackers. **(a)** Regular wheat crackers. **(b)** Reduced-fat wheat crackers.

longer than those who continue to smoke, and a 15-year cessation period will reduce your risk factors for cardiovascular disease to those of a nonsmoker.

- High blood pressure—High blood pressure stresses the heart and increases the chance that blockage or rupture of a blood vessel will occur. Elevated blood pressure is associated with a number of factors, including dietary factors (for example, high sodium intake, low calcium intake, high caffeine intake), elevated blood lipid levels, obesity, smoking, diabetes mellitus, and physical inactivity.

- Type 2 diabetes mellitus—As discussed in Chapter 4, in many individuals with type 2 diabetes, the condition is directly related to being overweight or obese, which is also associated with abnormal blood lipids and high blood pressure. The risk for cardiovascular disease is two to eight times higher in individuals with diabetes compared to individuals without diabetes.

- High blood cholesterol—As discussed below, high blood cholesterol, especially high LDL-cholesterol, is associated with an increased risk of cardiovascular disease. Making lifestyle changes, such as lowering saturated fat intake, increasing physical activity, and achieving a healthy body weight, can help lower LDL-cholesterol. These same lifestyle changes will also help to raise HDL-cholesterol, which also helps reduce the risk of cardiovascular disease.

Calculating Your Risk for Cardiovascular Disease

You can estimate your risk of developing cardiovascular disease if you know your blood pressure and blood lipid levels. Your blood lipid levels are a measurement of the fat in your blood and include the measurement of total blood cholesterol and some of the lipoproteins in the blood that carry fats to and from your cells. The significance of your blood lipid levels, as well as the types of lipoproteins typically measured, is discussed below. If you do not know this information about yourself, the next time you visit the doctor, ask to have your blood pressure taken and your blood lipids measured. It is especially important to do this if you have a family history of heart disease. The first step is to calculate the number of points for each risk factor in FIGURE 5.15, and then compare your total points to the points in the 10-year risk column. You can also do this quick assessment on family members or friends to help them become more aware of their risk factors for cardiovascular disease. There is also an online version of this risk calculator at http://hin.nhlbi.nih.gov/atpiii/calculator.asp?usertype=prof.

The Role of Dietary Fats in Cardiovascular Disease

As you recall from our discussion of fat metabolism, fats are transported in the blood by lipoproteins made up of a lipid center and a protein outer coat. These lipoproteins are soluble in our blood, and so they are commonly called *blood lipids*. At various times, whether eating or fasting, our blood contains a different mix of various types of these blood lipids. Research indicates that high intakes of saturated and *trans* fatty acids negatively alter the blood lipid assessment measures associated with heart disease. These blood lipid assessment measures are total blood cholesterol and the cholesterol found in very-low-density lipoproteins (VLDLs) and low-density lipoproteins (LDLs). Conversely, omega-3 fatty acids decrease our risk of heart disease in a number of ways, one of which is by increasing high-density lipoproteins (HDLs).[21] We will talk about each of these blood lipid assessment measures or lipoproteins and explain how they are linked to heart disease risk.

We have already said that high blood cholesterol increases the risk of heart disease. The question is—how? Much of this blood cholesterol is packaged in the LDLs that circulate in the blood. Normally, cells that need the cholesterol take up these lipoproteins; however, diets high in saturated fat *decrease* the removal of these lipoproteins by the cells. Failure to remove the LDLs from the blood results in their

Because foods fried in hydrogenated vegetable oils, such as French fries, are high in *trans* fatty acids, these types of foods should be limited in our diet.

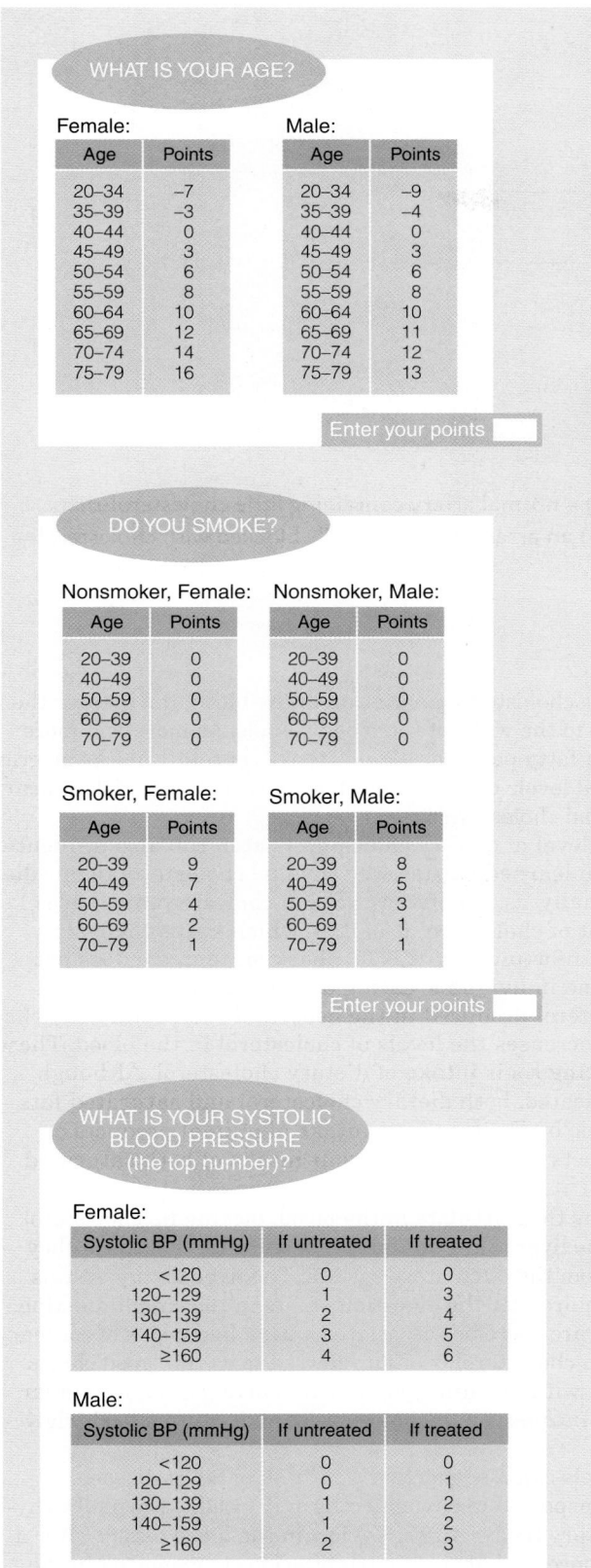

WHAT IS YOUR AGE?

Female:

Age	Points
20–34	–7
35–39	–3
40–44	0
45–49	3
50–54	6
55–59	8
60–64	10
65–69	12
70–74	14
75–79	16

Male:

Age	Points
20–34	–9
35–39	–4
40–44	0
45–49	3
50–54	6
55–59	8
60–64	10
65–69	11
70–74	12
75–79	13

Enter your points ____

WHAT IS YOUR TOTAL CHOLESTEROL NUMBER?

Female:

Age	Total Cholesterol				
	<160	160–199	200–239	240–279	≥280
20–39	0	4	8	11	13
40–49	0	3	6	8	10
50–59	0	2	4	5	7
60–69	0	1	2	3	4
70–79	0	1	1	2	2

(Points)

Male:

Age	Total Cholesterol				
	<160	160–199	200–239	240–279	≥280
20–39	0	4	7	9	11
40–49	0	3	5	6	8
50–59	0	2	3	4	5
60–69	0	1	1	2	3
70–79	0	0	0	1	1

(Points)

Enter your points ____

DO YOU SMOKE?

Nonsmoker, Female:

Age	Points
20–39	0
40–49	0
50–59	0
60–69	0
70–79	0

Nonsmoker, Male:

Age	Points
20–39	0
40–49	0
50–59	0
60–69	0
70–79	0

Smoker, Female:

Age	Points
20–39	9
40–49	7
50–59	4
60–69	2
70–79	1

Smoker, Male:

Age	Points
20–39	8
40–49	5
50–59	3
60–69	1
70–79	1

Enter your points ____

WHAT IS YOUR HIGH-DENSITY LIPOPROTEIN NUMBER (HDL)?

Female:

HDL (mg/dL)	Points
≥60	–1
50–59	0
40–49	1
<40	2

Male:

HDL (mg/dL)	Points
≥60	–1
50–59	0
40–49	1
<40	2

Enter your points ____

WHAT IS YOUR SYSTOLIC BLOOD PRESSURE (the top number)?

Female:

Systolic BP (mmHg)	If untreated	If treated
<120	0	0
120–129	1	3
130–139	2	4
140–159	3	5
≥160	4	6

Male:

Systolic BP (mmHg)	If untreated	If treated
<120	0	0
120–129	0	1
130–139	1	2
140–159	1	2
≥160	2	3

Enter your points ____

WHAT IS YOUR TOTAL NUMBER OF POINTS (what is your 10-year risk)?

Female:

Point total	10-Year risk %
<9	<1
9	1
10	1
11	1
12	1
13	2
14	2
15	3
16	4
17	5
18	6
19	8
20	11
21	14
22	17
23	22
24	27
≥25	≥30

Male:

Point total	10-Year risk %
<0	<1
0	1
1	1
2	1
3	1
4	1
5	2
6	2
7	3
8	4
9	5
10	6
11	8
12	10
13	12
14	16
15	20
16	25
≥17	≥30

Enter your 10-year risk percentage ____

FIGURE 5.15 Calculation matrix to estimate the 10-year risk for cardiovascular disease for men and women. (From National Institutes of Health, *Third Report of the National Cholesterol Education Program: Detection, Evaluation and Treatment of High Blood Cholesterol in Adults (ATP: III)*. Bethesda, MD: National Cholesterol Education Program, National Heart, Lung, and Blood Institute, NIH, May 2001. www.nhlbi.nih.gov/guideline/cholesterol/atp3xsum.pdf.)

(a)   (b)

FIGURE 5.16   These light micrographs show a cross section of **(a)** a normal artery containing little cholesterol-rich plaque and allowing adequate blood flow through the heart, and **(b)** an artery that is partially blocked with cholesterol-rich plaque, which can lead to a heart attack.

continued circulation. The more cholesterol circulating in the blood, the greater the risk that some of it will adhere to the walls of the blood vessels. As more and more cholesterol builds up, it forms a fatty patch, or *plaque,* that eventually blocks arteries (FIGURE 5.16). Because high blood levels of LDL-cholesterol increase your risk of heart disease, it is often called the "bad cholesterol."

For some individuals, the level of dietary cholesterol eaten can also influence blood cholesterol levels. As you learned earlier, we consume cholesterol in our diet and make it in our body. Normally, as the dietary level of cholesterol increases, the body decreases the amount of cholesterol it makes, which keeps the body's level of cholesterol constant. Unfortunately, this feedback mechanism does not work well in everyone. For some individuals, eating dietary cholesterol doesn't decrease the amount of cholesterol produced in the body, and their total body cholesterol levels rise. This also increases the levels of cholesterol in the blood. These individuals benefit from reducing their intake of dietary cholesterol. Although this appears somewhat complicated, both dietary cholesterol and saturated fats are found in animal foods; thus, by limiting your intake of animal products or selecting low-fat animal products you will reduce your intake of both saturated fat and cholesterol.

HDLs are small lipoproteins that circulate in the blood, picking up cholesterol and returning it to the liver. The liver takes up the HDLs and the cholesterol they carry, effectively removing it from the circulatory system. The liver then uses this cholesterol to make the bile required for the digestion of fats in the small intestine. High levels of HDL-cholesterol are therefore associated with a lower risk of coronary artery disease. That's why HDL-cholesterol is often referred to as the "good cholesterol." Replacing saturated fats with unsaturated fats and participating in regular physical exercise can modestly *increase* HDL-cholesterol and decrease blood triglyceride levels.[22]

High blood triglyceride levels can also increase your risk of heart disease. Triglycerides are primarily transported in chylomicrons and VLDLs. Normally, chylomicrons, which transport dietary triglycerides, are low in the blood except after a meal. Therefore, we are most concerned about the triglycerides transported in the VLDLs, which are made primarily in the liver and intestines and are filled with endogenous triglycerides (triglycerides made in the body). Diets high in fat, simple sugars, and extra calories can increase the production of endogenous VLDLs, while diets high in omega-3 fatty acids can help reduce the production of endogenous triglycerides and VLDLs. In addition, exercise can reduce VLDLs because the fat produced in the body is quickly used for energy instead of remaining to circulate in the blood.

HIGHLIGHT

Blood Lipid Levels: Know Your Numbers!

One of the most important steps you can take to reduce your risk of heart disease is to know your "numbers"—that is, your blood lipid values. The next time you go to a physician, ask to have your blood lipid levels measured. Record these numbers and have them checked every 1 to 2 years, or each time you visit your physician for a checkup. Many college and university health clinics, as well as community health fairs, offer a screening for total cholesterol as well. Based on your total cholesterol values, you can go to your physician to have a more complete testing of all your blood lipids. In this way you can know your own blood lipid levels and keep track of your risk for heart disease.

How are your blood lipids actually measured? First, a blood sample is taken, and the lipoproteins in your blood are extracted. Total cholesterol is determined by breaking apart all the lipoproteins and measuring their combined cholesterol content. You can see from Figure 5.17 that each of the lipoproteins contains some cholesterol and some triglycerides. This same process is used to determine your total blood triglycerides level. The next step is to measure the amount of cholesterol in the LDLs and HDLs, since these two lipoproteins can either raise or lower your risk of heart disease. These lipoproteins are separated, and the amount of cholesterol in each one is determined to give you an LDL-cholesterol and an HDL-cholesterol value. Once you have these values, you can compare them to the "target" level and see how you measure up.

Let's look at the blood lipid profile for Liz. Notice that each of the blood lipids discussed in this chapter is listed here, along with the normal, or target, values. How does Liz measure up? (Remember, Liz is a dancer and watches everything she eats!) We've also included space for you to write in and evaluate your own blood lipid values.

Liz's Blood Lipid Profile: How Does She Measure Up?

Blood Lipid Parameter	Liz's Target Values*	Liz's Values	How Does She Measure Up?	Your Values	How Do You Measure Up?
Total blood cholesterol	<200 mg/dl	151 mg/dl			
HDL-cholesterol	>40 mg/dl	56 mg/dl			
LDL-cholesterol	<100 mg/dl	88 mg/dl			
Triglycerides	<150 mg/dl	42 mg/dl			

*Values from the National Institutes of Health, *Third Report of the National Cholesterol Education Program: Detection, Evaluation and Treatment of High Blood Cholesterol in Adults (ATP: III)*. Bethesda, MD. National Cholesterol Education Program, National Heart, Lung, and Blood Institute, NIH, May 2001. http://www.nhlbi.nih.gov/guidelines/cholesterol/atp3xsum.pdf.

FIGURE 5.17 contains a brief description and overview of the functions of the various blood lipoproteins. Refer to the Highlight box to gain more insight into understanding your blood lipid levels.

We have known for a long time that saturated fats increase our blood levels of total cholesterol and LDL-cholesterol and increase our risk of heart disease. Because saturated fat is found primarily in the fats of animal products, we can easily reduce our intake of saturated fats by eating low-fat dairy and meat products. As mentioned earlier, recent research indicates that *trans* fatty acids can raise blood LDL-cholesterol levels as much as saturated fat.[23,24] Thus, we should also avoid eating products made with partially hydrogenated oils.

Lifestyle Changes Can Prevent or Reduce Cardiovascular Disease

Diet and exercise interventions aimed at reducing the risk of cardiovascular disease center on reducing high levels of triglycerides and LDL-cholesterol while raising HDL-cholesterol. The Centers for Disease Control and Prevention (CDC) and the

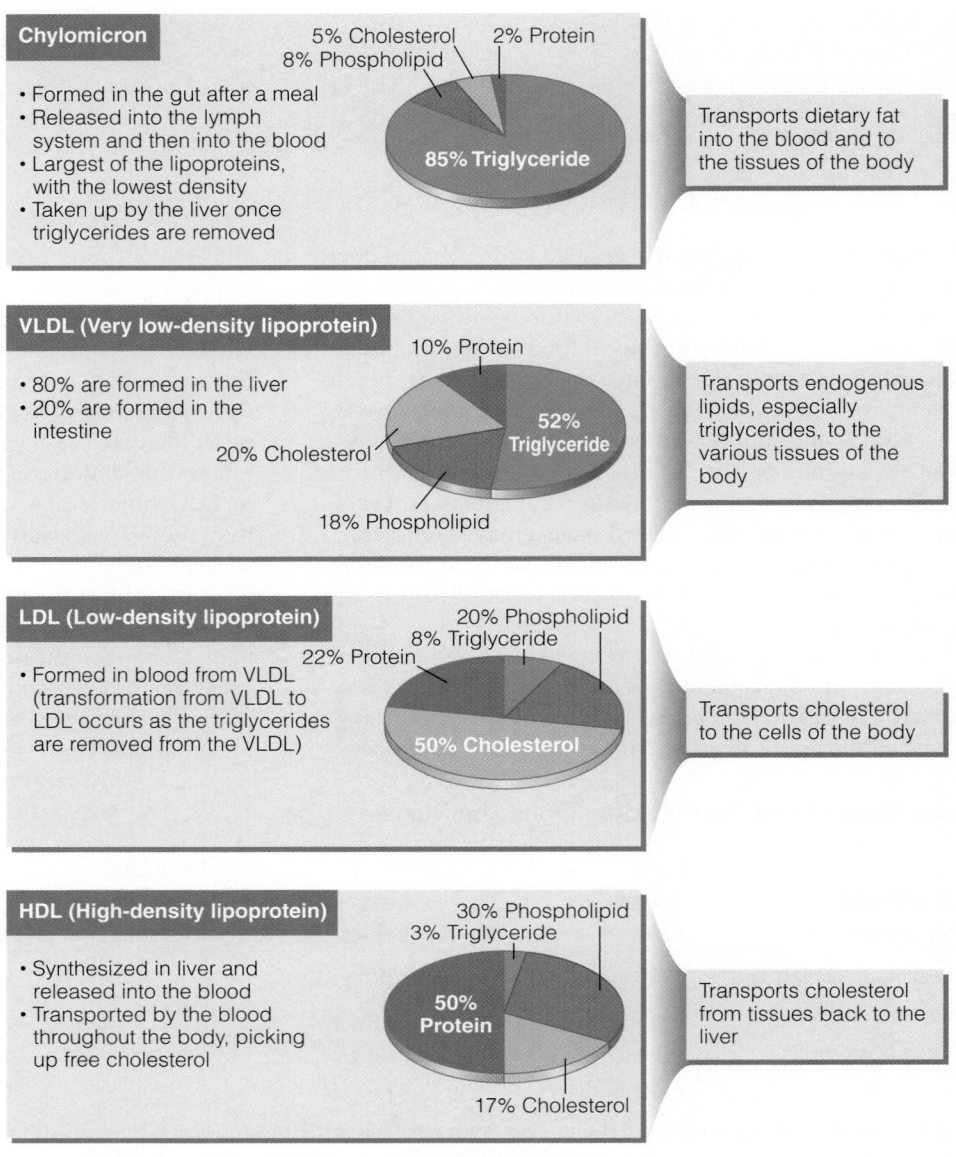

Chylomicron

- Formed in the gut after a meal
- Released into the lymph system and then into the blood
- Largest of the lipoproteins, with the lowest density
- Taken up by the liver once triglycerides are removed

5% Cholesterol 2% Protein
8% Phospholipid
85% Triglyceride

Transports dietary fat into the blood and to the tissues of the body

VLDL (Very low-density lipoprotein)

- 80% are formed in the liver
- 20% are formed in the intestine

10% Protein
52% Triglyceride
20% Cholesterol
18% Phospholipid

Transports endogenous lipids, especially triglycerides, to the various tissues of the body

LDL (Low-density lipoprotein)

- Formed in blood from VLDL (transformation from VLDL to LDL occurs as the triglycerides are removed from the VLDL)

20% Phospholipid
8% Triglyceride
22% Protein
50% Cholesterol

Transports cholesterol to the cells of the body

HDL (High-density lipoprotein)

- Synthesized in liver and released into the blood
- Transported by the blood throughout the body, picking up free cholesterol

30% Phospholipid
3% Triglyceride
50% Protein
17% Cholesterol

Transports cholesterol from tissues back to the liver

FIGURE 5.17   The chemical components of various lipoproteins. Notice that chylomicrons contain the highest proportion of triglycerides, making them the least dense, while high-density lipoproteins (HDLs) have the highest proportion of protein, making them the most dense.

Expert Panel on Detection, Evaluation, and Treatment of High Blood Cholesterol in Adults (APT: III) have made the following dietary and lifestyle recommendations to improve blood lipid levels and reduce the risk of cardiovascular disease:[14, 19]

- Maintain total fat intake to within 20–35% of energy.[8] Polyunsaturated fats (for example, soy and canola oil) can comprise up to 10% of total energy intake, while monounsaturated fats (for example, olive oil) can comprise up to 20% of total energy intake. For some people, a lower fat intake may help to maintain a healthful body weight.

- Decrease dietary saturated fat to less than 7% of total energy intake. Decrease cholesterol intake to less than 300 mg per day, and keep *trans* fatty acid intake as low as possible. Lowering the intakes of these fats will lower your LDL-cholesterol level. Replace saturated fat (for example, butter, margarine, vegetable shortening, or lard) with more healthful cooking oils, such as olive or canola oil.

- Increase dietary intakes of whole grains, fruits, and vegetables so that total dietary fiber is 20 to 30 g per day, with 10 to 25 g per day coming from fiber sources such as oat bran, beans, and fruits. Foods high in fiber decrease blood LDL-cholesterol levels.

- Maintain blood glucose and insulin concentrations within normal ranges. High blood glucose levels are associated with high blood triglycerides. Consume foods whole (such as whole-wheat breads and cereals, whole fruits and vegetables, and beans and legumes), and select low-saturated-fat meats and dairy products, while limiting your intake of high-sugar and high-fat foods (for example, cookies, high-sugar drinks and snacks, candy, fried foods, and convenience and fast foods).

- Eat throughout the day (for example, smaller meals and snacks) instead of eating most of your calories in the evening before bed.

- Maintain an active lifestyle. Exercise most days of the week for 30 to 60 minutes if possible. Exercise will increase HDL-cholesterol while lowering blood triglyceride levels. Exercise also helps maintain a healthy body weight and a lower blood pressure and reduces your risk for type 2 diabetes.

- Maintain a healthy body weight. Blood lipids and glucose levels typically improve when obese individuals lose weight and engage in regular physical activity.

Whole fruits and vegetables can reduce your risk for cardiovascular disease.

The impact of diet on reducing the risk of cardiovascular disease was clearly demonstrated in the Dietary Approaches to Stop Hypertension (DASH) study, which is discussed in Chapter 2. Although this study focused on dietary interventions to reduce hypertension (high blood pressure), the results of the study showed that eating the DASH way could dramatically improve blood lipids and lower blood pressure. The DASH diet includes high intakes of fruits, vegetables, whole grains, low-fat dairy products, poultry, fish, and nuts and low intake of fats, red meat, sweets, and sugar-containing beverages. Combining the DASH dietary approach with an active lifestyle significantly reduces the risk of cardiovascular disease.

Does a High-Fat Diet Cause Cancer?

Cancer develops as a result of a poorly understood interaction between the environment and genetic factors. In addition, most cancers take years to develop, so examining the impact of diet on cancer development can be a long and difficult process. Nevertheless, research does suggest that diet and lifestyle are two important environmental factors that influence the development of cancer.[25]

Of several dietary factors that have been studied, the influence of dietary fat intake on the development of cancer has been extensively researched. There appears to be a weak relationship between type and amount of fat consumed and increased risk for breast cancer.[26] Early research suggested an association between intake of meats and increased risk for colon cancer, but more recent research indicates that the association involves factors other than fat that are found in red meat. Because we now know that physical activity can reduce the risk of colon cancer, earlier diet and colon cancer studies that did not control for this factor are now being questioned. The strongest association between dietary fat intake and cancer is for prostate cancer. Research shows that there is a consistent link between prostate cancer risk and consumption of meats and high-fat dairy products, but not plant oils. The exact mechanism by which animal fats may contribute to prostate cancer has not yet been identified.

RECAP: *The types of fats we eat can significantly affect our health and risk of disease. Saturated and* trans *fatty acids increase our risk of heart disease, while omega-3 fatty acids can reduce our risk. Other risk factors for heart disease include being overweight, being physically inactive, smoking, having high blood pressure, and having diabetes mellitus. High levels of LDL-cholesterol and low levels of HDL-cholesterol increase your risk of heart disease. Selecting appropriate types of fat in the diet may also reduce your risk of some cancers, especially prostate cancer.*

CHAPTER SUMMARY

- Fats and oils are forms of a larger and more diverse group of substances called lipids; most lipids are insoluble in water.

- The three types of lipids commonly found in foods are triglycerides, phospholipids, and sterols.

- Most of the fat we eat is in the form of triglycerides; a triglyceride is a molecule that contains three fatty acids attached to a glycerol backbone.

- The various fatty acids in triglycerides are classified based on chain length, level of saturation, and shape.

- Saturated fatty acids have no carbons attached together with a double bond, which means that every carbon atom in the fatty acid chain is saturated with hydrogen.

- Monounsaturated fatty acids contain one double bond between two carbon atoms; polyunsaturated fatty acids contain more than one double bond between carbon atoms.

- Saturated fats are straight in shape, allowing the fatty acid chains to pack tightly together and making them solid at room temperature.

- Unsaturated fats (those with one or more double bonds in their fatty acid chains) have a kink along their length, which prevents them from packing tightly together and results in their being liquid at room temperature.

- A *cis* fatty acid has hydrogen atoms located on the same side of the double bond in an unsaturated fatty acid. This *cis* positioning produces a kink in the unsaturated fatty acid and is the shape found in naturally occurring fatty acids.

- A *trans* fatty acid has hydrogen atoms located on opposite sides of the double carbon bond. This positioning causes *trans* fatty acids to be straighter and more rigid, like saturated fats. This *trans* positioning results when oils are partially hydrogenated during food processing.

- The essential fatty acids, linoleic acid and alpha-linolenic acid, cannot be synthesized by the body and must be consumed in our diet.

- Phospholipids consist of a glycerol backbone and two fatty acids with a phosphate group; phospholipids are soluble in water and assist with transporting fats in our bloodstream.

- Sterols have a ring structure; cholesterol is the most common sterol in our diets.

- Fats are a primary energy source during rest and exercise, are our major source of stored energy, enable the transport of fat-soluble vitamins, help maintain cell function, provide protection for body organs, contribute to the texture and flavor of foods, and help us feel satiated after a meal.

- The majority of fat digestion and absorption occurs in the small intestine. Fat is broken down into smaller components by bile, which is produced by the liver and stored in the gallbladder.

- Because fats are not soluble in water, triglycerides are packaged into lipoproteins before being released into the bloodstream for transport to the cells.

- Dietary fat is primarily used either as an energy source for the cells or to make lipid-containing compounds in the body, or it is stored in the muscle and adipose tissue as triglyceride for later use.

- The AMDR for fat is 20–35% of total energy. Our intake of saturated fats and *trans* fatty acids should be kept to a minimum. Individuals who limit fat intake to less than 15% of energy intake need to make sure that essential fatty acid needs are met, as well as protein and energy needs.

- For the essential fatty acids, 5–10% of energy intake should be in the form of linoleic acid and 0.6% as alpha-linolenic acid.

- Visible fats are those we can easily see, such as butter, cream, shortening, oils, dressings, poultry skin, and fat on the edge of meats.

- Invisible fats are hidden in foods such as processed foods, baked goods, fried foods, and regular-fat dairy products.

- Diets high in saturated fat and *trans* fatty acids increase our risk for cardiovascular disease. Other risk factors for cardiovascular disease are overweight or obesity, physical inactivity, smoking, high blood pressure, and diabetes mellitus.

- High levels of circulating low-density lipoproteins, or LDLs, increase total blood cholesterol and the formation of plaque on arterial walls, leading to an increased risk for cardiovascular disease. This is why LDLs are sometimes called the "bad cholesterol."

- High levels of circulating high-density lipoproteins, or HDLs, reduce our blood cholesterol level and our risk for cardiovascular disease. This is why HDLs are sometimes called the "good cholesterol."

- There are some studies showing that diets high in meats and high-fat dairy products may increase our risk for prostate cancer, while the role of dietary fat in breast and colon cancer is still controversial.

TEST YOURSELF ANSWERS

1. **False.** Eating too much fat, or too much of unhealthful fats such as saturated and *trans* fatty acids, can increase our risk for diseases such as cardiovascular disease and obesity. However, fat is an important part of a nutritious diet, and we need to consume a certain minimum amount to provide adequate levels of essential fatty acids and fat-soluble vitamins.

2. **True.** Fat is our primary source of energy, both at rest and during low-intensity exercise. Fat is also an important fuel source during prolonged exercise.

3. **False.** Even foods fried in vegetable shortening can be unhealthful because they are higher in *trans* fatty acids. In addition, fried foods are high in fat and energy and can contribute to overweight and obesity.

4. **True.** Certain essential fatty acids, including EPA and DHA, reduce inflammation, blood clotting, and plasma triglycerides and thereby reduce an individual's risk of heart disease.

5. **False.** Cancer develops as a result of a poorly understood interaction between environmental and genetic factors. Some research indicates an association between high dietary fat consumption and certain cancers, but this research is inconclusive.

REVIEW QUESTIONS

1. Omega-3 fatty acids are
   a. a form of *trans* fatty acids.
   b. metabolized in the body to arachidonic acid.
   c. synthesized in the liver and small intestine.
   d. found in leafy green vegetables, flaxseeds, soy milk, and fish.

2. One of the most sensible ways to reduce body fat is to
   a. limit intake of fat to less than 15% of total energy consumed.
   b. exercise regularly.
   c. avoid all consumption of *trans* fatty acids.
   d. restrict total calories to 1,200 per day.

3. Fats in chylomicrons are taken up by cells with the help of
   a. lipoprotein lipase.
   b. micelles.
   c. sterols.
   d. pancreatic enzymes.

4. The risk of heart disease is reduced in people who have high blood levels of
   a. triglycerides.
   b. very-low-density lipoproteins.
   c. low-density lipoproteins.
   d. high-density lipoproteins.

5. Triglycerides with a double bond at one part of the molecule are referred to as
   a. monounsaturated fats.
   b. hydrogenated fats.
   c. saturated fats.
   d. sterols.

6. True or false? The Acceptable Macronutrient Distribution Range (AMDR) for fat is 20–35% of total energy.

7. True or false? During exercise, fat cannot be mobilized from adipose tissue for use as energy.

8. True or false? Triglycerides are the same as fatty acids.

9. True or false? *Trans* fatty acids are produced by food manufacturers; they do not occur in nature.

10. True or false? A serving of food labeled *reduced fat* has at least 25% less fat and 25% fewer calories than a full-fat version of the same food.

11. Explain how the saturated and *trans* fatty acids we eat affect our risk for heart disease.

12. Explain the contributions of the essential fatty acids to health.

13. You have volunteered to participate in a 20-mile walk-a-thon to raise money for a local charity. You have been training for several weeks, and the event is now 2 days away. An athlete friend of yours advises you to "load up on carbohydrates" today and tomorrow and says you should avoid eating any foods that contain fat during the day of the walk-a-thon. Do you take this advice? Why or why not?

14. Your father returns from an appointment with his doctor feeling down. He tells you that his "blood test didn't turn out so good." He then adds, "My doctor told me I can't eat any of my favorite foods anymore. He says red meat and butter have too much fat. I guess I'll have to switch to cottage cheese and margarine!" What type of blood test do you think your father had? How would you respond to his intention to switch to cottage cheese and margarine? Finally, suggest a non-dietary lifestyle choice that might improve his health.

15. Your friend Maria has determined that she needs to consume about 2,000 calories per day to maintain her healthful weight. Create a chart for Maria showing the

recommended maximum number of calories she should consume in each of the following forms: unsaturated fat, saturated fat, linoleic acid, alpha-linolenic acid, and *trans* fatty acids.

FIND THE QUACK

Yesterday, Luiz had his blood lipids checked at a campus health center and was dismayed to discover that his total cholesterol and LDL-cholesterol were high, and his HDL-cholesterol was low. On this morning's news broadcast, the health segment discusses the Dr. Dean Ornish Diet. It is supposed to be designed specifically for people with risk factors for cardiovascular disease. Luiz learns that the diet consists of the following:

- Abundant consumption of legumes, fruits, vegetables, and grains
- Moderate consumption of nonfat dairy products and nonfat or very-low-fat processed foods (such as nonfat yogurt bars, very-low-fat frozen dinners, and so on)
- Avoidance of all of the following: meats, oils, oil-containing products such as margarines and salad dressings, avocados, nuts, seeds, alcohol, sugars (including honey, molasses, and high-fructose corn syrup)
- The program also advises 30 minutes a day of moderate physical activity or three 1-hour sessions per week.

The TV health segment states that the Dr. Dean Ornish Diet has been proven in clinical studies to reduce the risk factors for cardiovascular disease.

1. Compare the Dr. Dean Ornish Diet to the Healthy Eating Pyramid illustrated in Chapter 2. What are the main similarities? What are the main differences you see?

2. Comment on the level of essential fatty acids the Dr. Dean Ornish Diet provides.

3. Based on the diet's recommendations, how much total fat do you think this diet provides?

4. Do you think the Dr. Dean Ornish Diet is a quack diet or a legitimate diet? If legitimate, do you think it is advisable for someone with unhealthful blood lipids, like Luiz? Why or why not?

Answers can be found at www.aw-bc.com/thompson.

WEB LINKS

www.americanheart.org
American Heart Association

Learn the best way to help lower your blood cholesterol level. Access the AHA's online cookbook for healthy-heart recipes and cooking methods.

www.caloriecontrol.org
Calorie Control Council

Go to this site to find out more about fat replacers.

www.nhlbi.nih.gov/chd
Live Healthier, Live Longer

Take a cholesterol quiz, and test your heart disease IQ. Create a diet using the Heart Healthy Diet or the TLC Diet online software.

www.nhlbi.nih.gov
National Heart, Lung, and Blood Institute

Learn how a healthful diet can lower your cholesterol levels. Use the online risk assessment tool to estimate your 10-year risk of having a heart attack.

www.cfsan.fda.gov/~dms/transfat.html
Consumer Information on the New *Trans* Fat Labeling Requirements

This page, created by the U.S. Food and Drug Administration, provides information about the newly required *trans* fat labeling.

www.nih.gov
The National Institutes of Health (NIH)
U.S. Department of Health and Human Services

Search this site to learn more about dietary fats and the DASH diet (Dietary Approaches to Stop Hypertension).

www.nlm.nih.gov/medlineplus
MEDLINE Plus Health Information

Search for "fats" or "lipids" to obtain additional resources and the latest news on dietary lipids, heart diseases, and cholesterol.

www.hsph.harvard.edu/nutritionsource
The Nutrition Source: Knowledge for Healthy Eating
Harvard School of Public Health

Go to this site, and click on "Fats & Cholesterol" to find out how selective fat intake can be part of a healthful diet.

www.ific.org
International Food Information Council Foundation

Access this site to find out more about fats and dietary fat replacers.

REFERENCES

1. Krover, O., and M. B. Katan. 2006. The elimination of trans fats from spreads: how science helped to turn an industry around. *Nutr. Rev.* 64(6):275–279.

2. Mozaffarian, D., M. B. Katan, A. Ascherio, M. J. Stampher, and W. C. Willet. 2006. Trans fatty acids and cardiovascular disease. *N. Engl. J. Med.* 354(15):1601–1613.

3. New York Department of Health and Mental Hygiene, Board of Health. 2006. *Notice of Adoption of an Amendment (81.08) to Article 81 of the New York City Health Code to Restrict the Service of Products Containing Artificial Trans Fats at All Food Service Establishments.* December 5, 2006. www.nyc.gov/html/ doh/downloads/pdf/public/notice-adoption-hc-art81-08.pdf. (Accessed March 2007.)

4. Heird, W. C., and A. Lapillonne. 2005. The role of essential fatty acids in development. *Annu. Rev. Nutr.* 25:549–571.

5. Wijendran, V., and K. C. Hayes. 2004. Dietary n-6 and n-3 fatty acid balance and cardiovascular health. *Annu. Rev. Nutr.* 24:597–615.

6. Din, J. N., D. E. Newby, and A. D. Flapan. 2004. Omega 3 fatty acids and cardiovascular disease—fishing for a natural treatment. *British Med. J.* 328(3):30–35.

7. Jebb, S. A., A. M. Prentice, G. R. Goldberg, P. R. Murgatroyd, A. E. Black, and W. A. Coward. 1996. Changes in macronutrient balance during over- and underfeeding assessed by 12-d continuous whole-body calorimetry. *Am. J. Clin. Nutr.* 64:259–266.

8. Institute of Medicine, Food and Nutrition Board. 2002. *Dietary Reference Intakes for Energy, Carbohydrate, Fiber, Fat, Fatty Acids, Cholesterol, Protein, and Amino Acids (Macronutrients).* Washington, DC: National Academies Press.

9. Manore, M. M., S. I. Barr, and G. E. Butterfield. 2000. Position of the American Dietetic Association, Dietitians of Canada, and the American College of Sports Medicine: nutrition and athletic performance. *J. Am. Diet. Assoc.* 100:1543–1556.

10. Lichtenstein, A. H., and L. Van Horn. 1998. Very low fat diets. *Circulation* 98:935–939.

11. U. S. Department of Agriculture (USDA), Center for Nutrition Policy and Promotion (CNPP). 1998. Is total fat consumption really decreasing? *Nutrition Insights,* vol. 5. Reprinted in *Nutr. Today* 33:171–172.

12. Harnack, L. J., R. W. Jeffery, and K. N. Boutelle. 2000. Temporal trends in energy intake in the United States: an ecologic perspective. *Am. J. Clin. Nutr.* 71:1478–1484.

13. Briefel, R. R., and C. L. Johnson. 2004. Secular trends in dietary intake in the United States. *Annu. Rev. Nutr.* 24:401–431.

14. Expert Panel on Detection, Evaluation, and Treatment of High Blood Cholesterol in Adults, National Institutes of Health. 2001. Executive summary of the Third Report of the National Cholesterol Education Program (NCEP) Expert Panel on Detection, Evaluation, and Treatment of High Blood Cholesterol in Adults (Adult Treatment Panel III). *JAMA* 285(19):2486–2509.

15. Allison, D. B., S. K. Egan, L. M. Barraj, C. Caughman, M. Infante, and J. T. Heimbach. 1999. Estimated intakes of *trans* fatty and other fatty acids in the U.S. population. *J. Am. Diet. Assoc.* 99:166–174.

16. Calloway, C. W. 1998. The role of fat-modified foods in the American diet. *Nutr. Today* 33:156–163.

17. Sigman-Grant, M. 1997. Can you have your low-fat cake and eat it too? The role of fat-modified products. *J. Am. Diet. Assoc.* 97(suppl.):S76–S81.

18. National Center for Chronic Disease Prevention and Health Promotion (NCCDPHP). 2002. *Chronic Disease Prevention. Chronic Disease Overview.* www.cdc.gov/nccdphp/overview.htm. (Accessed March 2007.)

19. Hahn, R. A., and G. W. Heath. 1998. Cardiovascular disease risk factors and preventive practices among adults—United States, 1994: a behavioral risk factor atlas. *Morbid. Mortal. Wkly. Rep.* 47(SS-5):35–69.

20. Rippe, J. M., T. J. Angelopoulos, and L. Zukley. 2007. The rationale for intervention to reduce the risk of coronary heart disease. *Am. J. Lifestyle Med.* 1(1):10–19.

21. Harris, W. S. 1997. n-3 Fatty acids and serum lipoproteins: human studies. *Am. J. Clin. Nutr.* 65(suppl.):1645S–1654S.

22. Zoeller, R. F. 2007. Physical activity and fitness in the prevention of coronary heart disease and associated risk factors. *Am. J. Lifestyle Med.* 1(1):29–33.

23. Oomen, C. M., M. C. Ocké, E. J. Feskens, M. A. van Erp-Baart, F. J. Kok, and D. Kromhout. 2001. Association between *trans* fatty acid intake and 10-year risk of coronary heart disease in the Zutphen Elderly Study: a prospective population-based study. *Lancet* 357(9258):746–751.

24. Wootan, M., B. Lieberman, and W. Rosoesky. 1996. Trans: the phantom fat. *Nutr. Action Health Lett.* 23(7):10–13.

25. Kim, Y. I. 2001. Nutrition and cancer. In: Bowman, B. A., and R. M. Russell, eds. *Present Knowledge in Nutrition*, 8th edn. Washington, DC: International Life Sciences Institute Press.

26. Willett, W. C. 1999. Diet, nutrition and the prevention of cancer. In: Shils, M. E., J. A. Olsen, M. Shike, and A. C. Ross, eds. *Modern Nutrition in Health and Disease*, 9th edn. Baltimore, MD: Williams & Wilkins.

27. Variyam, J. N. 2004. The price is right. Economics and the rise of obesity. Amber Waves. USDA Economic Research Service, Vol. 3 (Issue 1): 20-27.

28. Nestle, M., and L. B. Dixon. 2004. Taking Sides. Clashing Views on Controversial Issues in Food and Nutrition. Guilford, CA: McGraw-Hill/Dushin, pp. 24–39.

29. DHHS/USDA. 2005. Dietary Guidelines for Americans. www. health.gov/dietaryguidelines/dga2005/report/.

30. American Dietetic Association. 2002. Position of the American Dietetic Association: Total Diet Approaches to Communicating Food and Nutrition Information. *J. Am. Diet. Assoc.* 102(1):100–108.

NUTRITION DEBATE

Should Nutrition Professionals Speak Out Against "Bad" Foods?

"Bad" foods and food ingredients are in the news. As mentioned earlier in this chapter, New York City caused a furor by banning *trans* fatty acids in foods prepared in restaurants and other prepared foods. Portland, Oregon, is likely to follow suit, as will perhaps dozens of other cities across the United States. At the same time, school districts are removing sodas and high-sugar juice drinks from school vending machines, General Mills is replacing some of the refined grains in its cereals with whole grains, Safeway food stores is eliminating milk and dairy products containing a controversial artificial growth hormone (called rBGH) from its shelves, and the Hannaford food store chain is using a "star" rating system to help shoppers distinguish between foods that are healthful and foods that are not. And what about fast food, perhaps the most-vilified "bad" food of all? From lawsuits to feature films like *Super Size Me* and *Fast Food Nation*, fast food is at the center of a growing debate about when and whether nutrition professionals should speak our against "bad" foods.

Fast food is cheap, tasty, and easy, but it is often an unhealthful choice.

Look around you. How many fast-food restaurants are within walking distance of your home, place of work, or campus? These restaurants are notorious for the high-calorie meals they serve containing unhealthful levels of saturated and *trans* fats. So why do consumers choose them? Fast food has three major advantages over traditional restaurant meals and home-cooked meals: It is

quick to obtain, it tastes good to a majority of consumers, and it is relatively cheap for the number of calories it provides.[27] Many Americans view the large portions served in fast-food restaurants as evidence that they are getting good "value" for their money and may not realize how quickly eating these large portions of high-fat foods can pack on the pounds and harm their health.

The fast, high-fat, low-cost food environment in which we live prompts several questions we might ask about any food or food ingredient our culture has labeled as "bad." First, can all foods fit into a healthful diet, or are there certain foods and ingredients, such as French fries or rBGH, that we should avoid entirely? Will banning "bad" foods and ingredients make us more healthful and help curb our growing obesity problem? And finally, what type of food recommendations should nutrition professionals make to government agencies, media, clients, and friends and family members? Fundamentally, these questions all contribute to the same debate, that is, whether or not nutrition professionals should advise their clients to avoid specific foods or food ingredients.

This debate touches on the interaction between science and politics in the matter of nutrition advice. On one side of the debate, we have a growing body of scientific evidence that indicates which foods are more healthful and which are harmful. Dietitians and healthcare professionals on this side of the debate say that they have an obligation to share this information with their clients.[28] They argue that consumers have a right to information about which foods promote health and which increase the risk of disease.[28] They point out that most Americans are light-years away from meeting the 2005 Dietary Guidelines and thus need specific, straightforward advice on what to eat and what to avoid if their diets are to improve and if we are to curb the epidemic of obesity we face as a nation.[29]

On the other side of the debate are the politics of food and what sells. Every nutrition professional knows that quick, good-tasting, and low-cost food sells extremely well, even among consumers who know it does not promote their health.[28] Thus, nutrition professionals on this side of the debate attempt to work with clients' food preferences to the extent possible. Many dietitians and professional groups, including the American Dietetic Association, share the philosophy that all foods can fit into a healthful diet.[30] They believe that it is important to look at an individual's total diet and dietary patterns, including portion sizes, and not focus on just one or two "bad" foods or meals. They also argue that you cannot

Should some foods be avoided entirely?

assign "moral" qualities to foods. They believe their responsibility is to communicate positive nutrition messages that help people make better food choices.

Dietitians on this side of the debate believe that it is unrealistic to tell people to stop eating their favorite foods, and that change will be achieved by encouraging clients to eat these foods in moderation. They point out that a significant percentage of people advised to make dramatic dietary changes get discouraged and give up. Thus, in working with a client who eats fast food daily, they would not tell the client to stop eating it altogether, but rather would suggest the client eat fast food less often and make better food choices when he or she does. Their goal is to help individuals set achievable goals and make small steps toward changing their diet.

But consumers need information they can understand to help them make better food choices. For instance, New York City is also requiring food establishments to post in a public place the number of calories in a serving of each food sold. Even then, will consumers know what their ideal calorie consumption level is, and will they be able to make the necessary calculations? And even if they do realize that a sweetened coffee beverage with whipped cream provides one-fourth of their daily energy needs, will other factors cause them to purchase it anyway? And about those *trans* fats: just because your morning croissant will be *trans* fat free if you buy it in New York City, this doesn't mean it won't contain a lot of fat, including saturated fat. The bakery will probably just replace one type of fat with another, so your almond croissant will probably still contain 360 kcal, and 53% of the kcal will probably still come from fat. What's more, the calories in the croissant will still represent nearly 20% of the calories needed for most non-active adults. This is another reason that some nutritionists suggest that we stop focusing on individual foods and ingredients and start helping people think about changing the way they think about food.

What's your opinion? Should nutrition professionals be more forthright with consumers and clients about what they should and shouldn't be eating? Should they give specific advice on what foods to eliminate and what foods to include in their diet? Should professional nutrition organizations speak out against "bad" foods or support food policy changes, such as banning *trans* fatty acids in restaurants? What approach is best in helping people make positive dietary changes? Certainly more research is needed to determine what kinds of advice are most helpful in producing health-promoting dietary changes in large populations.

Prior to taking this class, how frequently did you consider the fat and energy content of the food you ordered? Did you frequently order high-fat, large-portion meals at fast-food restaurants? Did you "super size"? Now that you know more about nutrition and food, what do you think is the best approach to making positive dietary changes for most Americans? Do you agree that all foods can fit into a healthful diet, or do you think that some foods should be avoided completely? If someone were to ask you for dietary advice, what would *you* recommend?

What kind of information will help you make the best dietary choices?

CHAPTER 6

CHAPTER OBJECTIVES

After reading this chapter you will be able to:

1. Describe how proteins differ from carbohydrates and fats, p. 212.

2. Identify non-meat food combinations that are complete protein sources, p. 219.

3. Describe four functions of proteins in our bodies, pp. 220–224.

4. Discuss how proteins are digested, absorbed, and synthesized by our bodies, pp. 214–217, 224–225.

5. Calculate your recommended daily allowance for protein, p. 229.

6. Identify the potential health risks associated with high-protein diets, pp. 230–231.

7. List five foods that are good sources of protein, pp. 231–233.

8. Describe two disorders related to inadequate protein intake or genetic abnormalities, pp. 242–244.

TEST YOURSELF TRUE OR FALSE?

1. Protein is a primary source of energy for our bodies. **T or F**

2. We must consume amino acid supplements in order to build muscle tissue. **T or F**

3. Any protein eaten in excess is excreted in your urine. **T or F**

4. Vegetarian diets are inadequate in protein. **T or F**

5. Most people in the United States consume more protein than they need. **T or F**

Test Yourself answers can be found after the Chapter Summary.

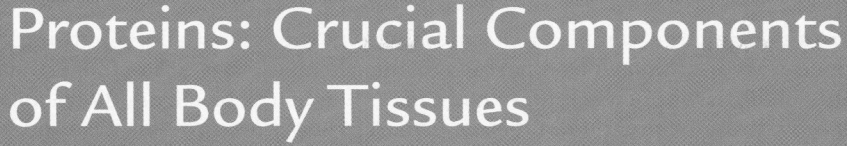

Proteins: Crucial Components of All Body Tissues

What do "Mr. Universe" Bill Pearl, Olympic figure skating champion Surya Bonaly, wrestler "Killer" Kowalski, and hundreds of other athletes have in common? They're all vegetarians! Olympic track icon Carl Lewis states: "A person does not need protein from meat to be a successful athlete . . . my best year of track competition was the first year I ate a vegan diet." Although precise statistics on the number of vegetarian American athletes aren't available, a total of 2.8% of the U.S. population—approximately 5.7 million American adults—are estimated to be vegetarians.[1]

What is a protein, and what makes it so different from carbohydrates and fats? How much protein do you really need, and do you get enough in your daily diet? What exactly is a vegetarian anyway? Do you qualify? If so, how do you plan your diet to include sufficient protein, especially if you play competitive sports? Are there real advantages to eating meat, or is plant protein just as good?

It seems as if everybody has an opinion about protein, both how much you should consume and from what sources. In this chapter, we address these and other questions to clarify the importance of protein in the diet and dispel common myths about this crucial nutrient.

Proteins are an integral part of our body tissues, including our muscle tissue.

proteins Large, complex molecules made up of amino acids and found as essential components of all living cells.

amino acids Nitrogen-containing molecules that combine to form proteins.

What Are Proteins?

Proteins are large, complex molecules found in the cells of all living things. While proteins are best known as a part of our muscle mass, they are in fact critical components of all tissues of the human body, including bones, blood, and hormones. As *enzymes,* proteins function in metabolism. As *antibodies,* proteins are fundamental to a healthy immune system. Without adequate proteins, the body cannot maintain its balance of fluids or its ratio of acids to bases. Although our bodies prefer to use carbohydrates and fats for energy, proteins do provide energy in certain circumstances. All of these functions of proteins will be discussed later in this chapter.

How Do Proteins Differ from Carbohydrates and Lipids?

As we saw in Chapter 1, proteins are one of the three macronutrients and are found in a wide variety of foods. Our bodies are able to manufacture, or synthesize, proteins, carbohydrates, and lipids. But unlike carbohydrates and lipids, our genetic material, or DNA, dictates the structure of each protein molecule. We'll explore how our body synthesizes proteins and the role that DNA plays in this process shortly.

Another key difference between proteins and the other macronutrients lies in their chemical makeup. In addition to the carbon, hydrogen, and oxygen also found in carbohydrates and lipids, proteins contain a special form of nitrogen that our bodies can readily use. This nitrogen is found in amino acids, which are the building blocks of proteins. By eating proteins found in plants and animals, we are able to break down these proteins into their respective amino acid components and utilize the nitrogen for many important body processes. Carbohydrates and lipids cannot provide this critical form of nitrogen.

The Building Blocks of Proteins Are Amino Acids

The proteins in our bodies are made from a combination of building blocks called **amino acids,** molecules composed of a central carbon atom connected to four other groups: an amine group, an acid group, a hydrogen atom, and a side chain (FIGURE 6.1A). The word *amine* means *nitrogen-containing,* and nitrogen is indeed the essential component of the amine portion of the molecule.

As shown in FIGURE 6.1B, the portion of the amino acid that makes each unique is its side chain. The amine group, acid group, and carbon and hydrogen atoms do not

(a)

(b)

FIGURE 6.1 Structure of an amino acid. **(a)** All amino acids contain five parts: a central carbon atom, an amine group around the atom that contains nitrogen, an acid group, a hydrogen atom, and a side chain. **(b)** Only the side chain differs for each of the twenty amino acids, giving each its unique properties.

TABLE 6.1 Amino Acids of the Human Body

Essential Amino Acids	Nonessential Amino Acids
These amino acids must be obtained from food.	*These amino acids can be manufactured by the body.*
Histidine	Alanine
Isoleucine	Arginine
Leucine	Asparagine
Lysine	Aspartic acid
Methionine	Cysteine
Phenylalanine	Glutamic acid
Threonine	Glutamine
Tryptophan	Glycine
Valine	Proline
	Serine
	Tyrosine

vary. Variations in the structure of the side chain give each amino acid its distinct properties. In addition to containing carbon, hydrogen, oxygen, and nitrogen, amino acid side chains may also contain sulfur.

The singular term *protein* is misleading, as there are potentially an infinite number of unique types of proteins in living organisms. Most of the proteins in our bodies are made from combinations of just twenty amino acids, identified in Table 6.1. By combining a few dozen to more than 300 copies of these twenty amino acids in various sequences, our bodies form an estimated 10,000 to 50,000 unique proteins.

We Must Obtain Essential Amino Acids from Food

Of the twenty amino acids in our bodies, nine are classified as essential. This does not mean that they are more important than the eleven nonessential amino acids. Instead, an **essential amino acid** is one that our bodies cannot produce at all or cannot produce in sufficient quantities to meet our physiological needs. Thus, we must obtain an essential amino acid from our food. Without the proper amount of essential amino acids in our bodies, we lose our ability to make the proteins and other nitrogen-containing compounds we need.

The Body Can Make Nonessential Amino Acids

Nonessential amino acids are just as important to our bodies as essential amino acids, but our bodies can make them in sufficient quantities so we do not need to consume them in our diet. We make nonessential amino acids by transferring the nitrogen-containing group from an essential amino acid to a different acid group and side chain. The process of transferring the amine group from one amino acid to another acid group and side chain is called **transamination,** and it is shown in FIGURE 6.2. The acid groups and side chains can be donated by amino acids, or they can be made from the breakdown products of carbohydrates and fats. Thus, by combining parts of different amino acids, the nonessential amino acids can be made.

Under some conditions, a nonessential amino acid can become an essential amino acid. In this case, the amino acid is called a *conditionally essential amino acid.* Consider what occurs in the disease known as phenylketonuria (PKU). As discussed in Chapter 4, someone with PKU cannot metabolize phenylalanine (an essential amino acid). Normally the body uses phenylalanine to produce the nonessential amino acid tyrosine, so the inability to metabolize phenylalanine results in failure to make tyrosine. If PKU is not diagnosed immediately after birth, it results in irreversible brain damage. In this situation, tyrosine becomes a conditionally essential amino acid that must be provided by the diet.

essential amino acids Amino acids not produced by the body that must be obtained from food.

nonessential amino acids Amino acids that can be manufactured by the body in sufficient quantities and therefore do not need to be consumed regularly in our diet.

transamination The process of transferring the amine group from one amino acid to another in order to manufacture a new amino acid.

FIGURE 6.2 Transamination. Our bodies can make nonessential amino acids by transferring the amine group from an essential amino acid to a different acid group and side chain.

> RECAP: *Proteins are critical components of all tissues of the human body. They contain carbon, hydrogen, oxygen, and nitrogen, and their structure is dictated by DNA. The building blocks of proteins are amino acids. The amine group of the amino acid contains nitrogen. The portion of the amino acid that changes, giving each amino acid its distinct identity, is the side chain. The body cannot make essential amino acids so we must obtain them from our diet. Our body can make nonessential amino acids from parts of other amino acids, carbohydrates, and fats.*

How Are Proteins Made?

As we have stated, our bodies can synthesize proteins by selecting the needed amino acids from the pool of all amino acids available at any given time. Let's look more closely at how this occurs.

Amino Acids Bond to Form a Variety of Peptides

peptide bonds Unique types of chemical bonds in which the amine group of one amino acid binds to the acid group of another in order to manufacture dipeptides and all larger peptide molecules.

FIGURE 6.3 shows that when two amino acids join together, the amine group of one binds to the acid group of another in a unique type of chemical bond called a **peptide bond.** In the process, a molecule of water is released as a by-product.

Two amino acids joined together form a *dipeptide,* and three amino acids joined together are called a *tripeptide.* The term *oligopeptide* is used to identify a string of four to nine amino acids, while a *polypeptide* is ten or more amino acids bonded

FIGURE 6.3 Amino acid bonding. Two amino acids join together to form a dipeptide. By combining multiple amino acids, proteins are made.

together. As a polypeptide chain grows longer, it begins to fold into any of a variety of complex shapes that give proteins their sophisticated structure.

Genes Regulate Amino Acid Binding

Each of us is unique because we inherited a specific genetic code from our parents. Each person's specific genes direct minute differences in amino acid sequences, which in turn lead to slight differences in our bodies' individual proteins. These differences in proteins result in the unique physical and physiological characteristics each one of us possesses.

As mentioned earlier, DNA dictates the structure of each protein our body synthesizes. FIGURE 6.4 shows how this process occurs. **Gene expression** is a term used

gene expression The process of using a gene to make a protein.

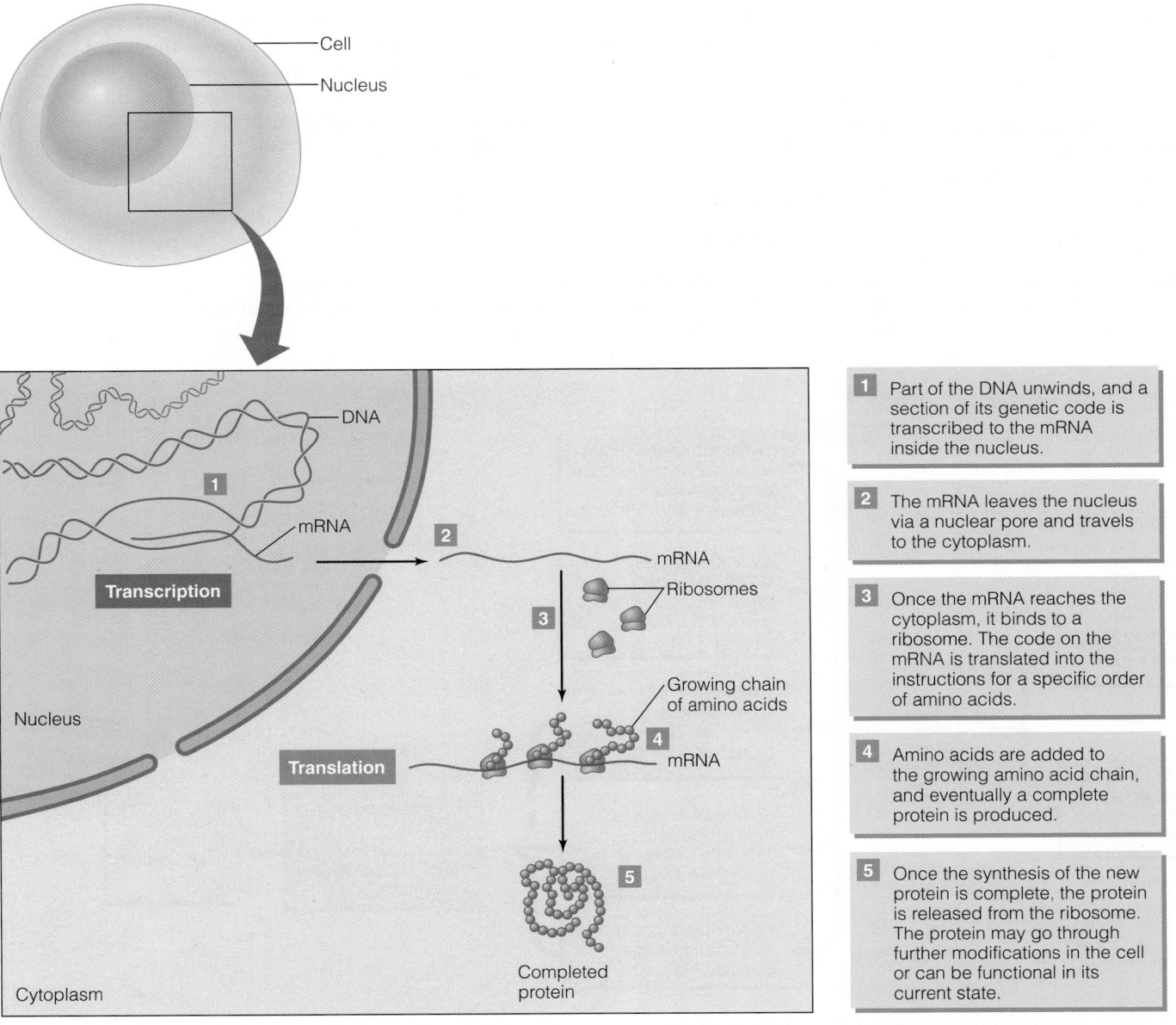

1 Part of the DNA unwinds, and a section of its genetic code is transcribed to the mRNA inside the nucleus.

2 The mRNA leaves the nucleus via a nuclear pore and travels to the cytoplasm.

3 Once the mRNA reaches the cytoplasm, it binds to a ribosome. The code on the mRNA is translated into the instructions for a specific order of amino acids.

4 Amino acids are added to the growing amino acid chain, and eventually a complete protein is produced.

5 Once the synthesis of the new protein is complete, the protein is released from the ribosome. The protein may go through further modifications in the cell or can be functional in its current state.

FIGURE 6.4 Gene expression. Messenger RNA (mRNA) transcribes the genetic information from DNA in the nucleus and carries it to the ribosomes in the cytoplasm. At the ribosome, this genetic information is translated into a chain of amino acids that eventually make a protein.

to refer to the process of using a gene in a cell to make a protein. A gene is a segment of DNA that serves as a template for the structure of a protein. As proteins are manufactured at the site of ribosomes in the cytoplasm, and DNA never leaves the nucleus, a special molecule is needed to copy, or transcribe, the information from DNA and carry it to the ribosome. This is the job of *messenger RNA* (*messenger ribonucleic acid*, or *mRNA*); during **transcription,** mRNA copies the genetic information from DNA in the nucleus and carries it to the ribosomes in the cytoplasm. Once this genetic information is at the ribosome, **translation** occurs: genetic information from the mRNA is translated into a growing chain of amino acids that are bonded together to make a specific protein.

Although the DNA for making every protein in our bodies is contained within each cell nucleus, not all genes are expressed and each cell does not make every type of protein. For example, each cell contains the DNA to manufacture the hormone insulin. However, only the cells of the pancreas express the insulin gene; that is, they are the only cells that produce insulin. Our physiological needs alter gene expression, as do various nutrients. For instance, a cut in the skin that causes bleeding leads to the production of various proteins that clot the blood. If we consume more dietary iron than we need, the gene for ferritin (a protein that stores iron) is expressed so that we can store this excess iron. Our genetic makeup and how appropriately we express our genes are important factors in our health. Gene expression is discussed in more detail in the Nutrition Debate on pages 33–35.

transcription The process through which messenger RNA copies genetic information from DNA in the nucleus.

translation The process that occurs when the genetic information carried by messenger RNA is translated into a chain of amino acids at the ribosome.

Protein Turnover Involves Synthesis and Degradation

Our bodies constantly require new proteins to function properly. *Protein turnover* involves both the synthesis of new proteins and the degradation of existing proteins to provide the building blocks for those new proteins (FIGURE 6.5). This process allows

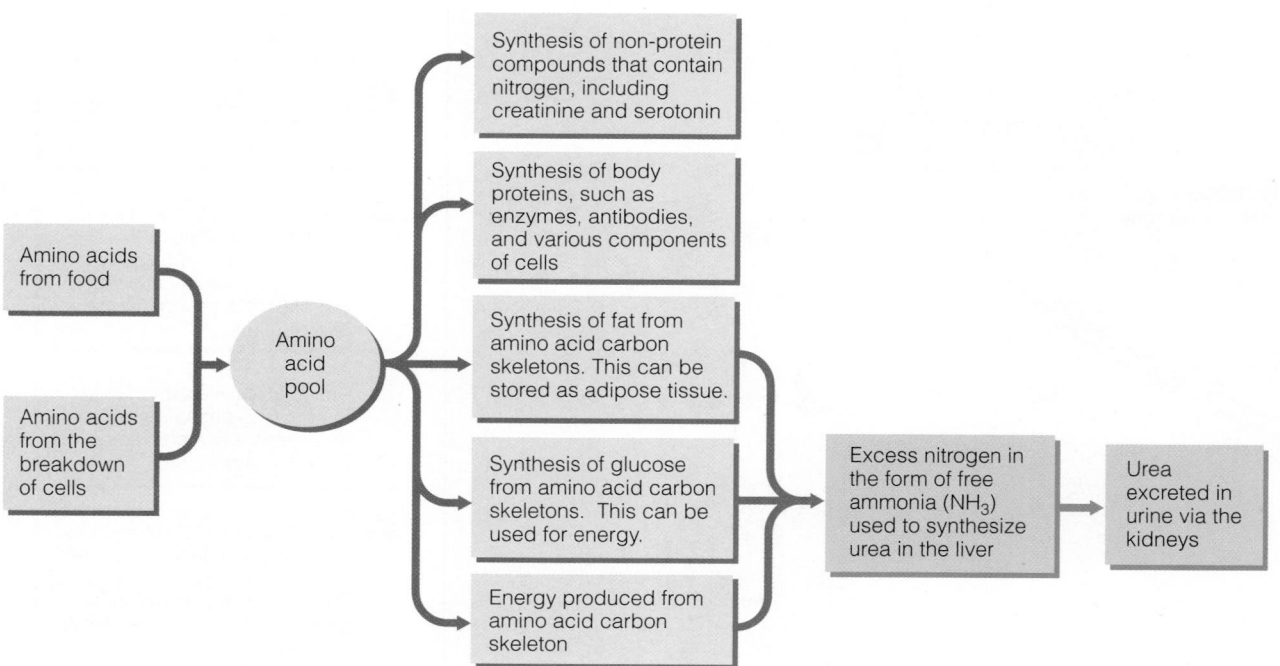

FIGURE 6.5 Protein turnover involves the synthesis of new proteins and breakdown of existing proteins to provide building blocks for new proteins. Amino acids are drawn from the body's amino acid pool and can be used to build proteins, fat, glucose, and non-protein nitrogen-containing compounds. Urea is produced as a waste product from any excess nitrogen, which is then excreted by the kidneys.

the cells to respond to the constantly changing demands of physiologic functions. For instance, skin cells live only for about 30 days and must continually be replaced. The amino acids needed to produce these new skin cells can be obtained from the body's *amino acid pool*, which includes those amino acids we consume in our diets as well as those that are released from the breakdown of other cells in our bodies. The body's pool of amino acids is used to produce not only new amino acids but also other products including glucose, fat, and urea.

Protein Organization Determines Function

Four levels of protein structure have been identified. The sequential order of the amino acids in a protein is called the *primary structure* of the protein. The different amino acids in a polypeptide chain possess unique chemical characteristics that cause the chain to twist and turn into a characteristic spiral shape referred to as the protein's *secondary structure*. The stability of the secondary structure is achieved through the bonding of hydrogen atoms (referred to as hydrogen bonds) or sulfur atoms (referred to as a *disulfide bridge*); these bonds create a bridge between two protein strands or two parts of the same strand of protein. The spiral of the secondary structure further folds into a unique three-dimensional shape referred to as the protein's *tertiary structure*; this structure is critically important because it determines each protein's function in the body. Often, two or more separate polypeptides bond to form an even larger protein with a *quaternary structure* that may be *globular* or *fibrous*. FIGURE 6.6 illustrates the four levels of protein structure.

Again, the tertiary structure of a protein determines its function in the body. For example, the proteins that form tendons are much longer than they are wide. Tendons are connective tissues that attach bone to muscle, and their long, rod-like structure provides strong, fibrous connections. In contrast, the proteins that form red blood cells are globular in shape, and they result in the red blood cells being shaped like flattened discs with depressed centers, similar to a miniature doughnut (FIGURE 6.7). This

(a) Primary structure   (b) Secondary structure   (c) Tertiary structure   (d) Quaternary structure

FIGURE 6.6 Levels of protein structure. **(a)** The primary structure of a protein is the sequential order of amino acids. **(b)** The secondary structure of a protein is the folding of the amino acid chain. **(c)** The tertiary structure is a further folding that results in the three-dimensional shape of the protein. **(d)** The quaternary structure of a protein refers to molecules containing two or more polypeptides that bond to form a larger protein such as the actin molecule illustrated here. In this figure, strands of actin molecules intertwine to form contractile elements involved in generating muscle contractions.

Polypeptide chain

Heme group with iron atom

(a)

(b)

FIGURE 6.7 Protein shape determines function. **(a)** Hemoglobin, the protein that forms red blood cells, is globular in shape. **(b)** The globular shape of hemoglobin results in red blood cells being shaped like flattened discs.

Stiffening egg whites denatures some of the proteins within them.

structure and the flexibility of the proteins in the red blood cells permit them to change shape and flow freely through even the tiniest capillaries to deliver oxygen and still return to their original shape.

Proteins can uncoil and lose their shape when they are exposed to heat, acids, bases, heavy metals, alcohol, and other damaging substances. The term used to describe this change in the shape of proteins is *denaturation*. When a protein is denatured, its function is also lost. Examples of protein denaturation that we can see are stiffening of egg whites when they are whipped, the curdling of milk when lemon juice or another acid is added, and the solidifying of eggs as they cook. Denaturation also occurs when we digest proteins.

> RECAP: *Amino acids bind together to form proteins. Genes regulate the amino acid sequence, and thus the structure, of all proteins. The shape of a protein determines its function. When a protein is denatured by damaging substances such as heat and acids, it loses its shape and its function.*

Protein Synthesis Can Be Limited by Missing Amino Acids

For protein synthesis to occur, all essential amino acids must be available to the cell. If this is not the case, the amino acid that is missing or in the smallest supply is called the **limiting amino acid.** Without the proper combination and quantity of essential amino acids, protein synthesis slows to the point at which proteins cannot be generated. For instance, the protein hemoglobin contains the essential amino acid histidine. If we do not consume enough histidine, it becomes the limiting amino acid in hemoglobin production. As no other amino acid can be substituted, our body becomes unable to make adequate hemoglobin, and we lose the ability to transport oxygen to our cells. Our cells cannot function and will eventually die if they do not receive adequate oxygen.

Inadequate energy consumption also limits protein synthesis. If there is not enough energy available from our diets, our bodies will use any accessible proteins for energy, thus preventing them from being used to build new proteins.

A protein that does not contain all of the essential amino acids in sufficient quantities to support growth and health is called an **incomplete** (or *low-quality*)

limiting amino acid The essential amino acid that is missing or in the smallest supply in the amino acid pool and is thus responsible for slowing or halting protein synthesis.

incomplete proteins Foods that do not contain all of the essential amino acids in sufficient amounts to support growth and health.

protein. Proteins that have all nine of the essential amino acids are considered **complete** (or *high-quality*) **proteins.** The most complete protein sources are from animal sources and include egg whites, ground beef, chicken, fish, and milk. Soybeans are the most complete source of vegetable protein. In general, the typical American diet is very high in complete proteins, as we eat proteins from a variety of food sources.

Protein Synthesis Can Be Enhanced by Mutual Supplementation

Many people believe that we must consume meat or dairy products to obtain complete proteins. Not true! Consider a meal of beans and rice. Beans are low in the amino acids methionine and cysteine but have adequate amounts of isoleucine and lysine. Rice is low in isoleucine and lysine but contains sufficient methionine and cysteine. By combining beans and rice, a complete protein source is created.

    Mutual supplementation is the process of combining two or more incomplete protein sources to make a complete protein. The two foods involved are called complementary foods; these foods provide **complementary proteins** (FIGURE 6.8) that, when combined, provide all nine essential amino acids. It is not necessary to eat these foods at the same meal. Recall that we maintain a free pool of amino acids in the blood; these amino acids come from food and sloughed-off cells. When we eat one complementary protein, its amino acids join those in the free amino acid pool. These free amino acids can then combine to synthesize complete proteins. However, it is wise to eat complementary-protein foods during the same day, as partially completed proteins cannot be stored and saved for a later time. Mutual supplementation is important for people eating a vegetarian diet, particularly if they consume no animal products whatsoever.

complete proteins Foods that contain all nine essential amino acids.

mutual supplementation The process of combining two or more incomplete protein sources to make a complete protein.

complementary proteins Two or more foods that together contain all nine essential amino acids necessary for a complete protein. It is not necessary to eat complementary proteins at the same meal.

Food with limiting amino acid	+	Foods high in limiting amino acid	→	Complementary food combination	
Legumes: limited in methionine and cysteine	+	**Grains, Nuts and seeds**		• Rice and lentils • Red beans and rice • Rice and black-eyed peas • Hummus (garbanzo beans and sesame seeds)	
Grains: limited in lysine	+	**Legumes**		• Peanut butter and bread • Barley and lentil soup • Corn tortilla and beans	
Vegetables: limited in lysine, methionine, and cysteine	+	**Legumes** (lysine) **Grains, Nuts and seeds** (methionine and cysteine)		• Tofu and broccoli with almonds • Spinach salad with pine nuts and kidney beans	
Nuts and seeds: limited in lysine and isoleucine	+	**Legumes**		• Sesame seeds with mixed bean salad • Lentil soup with slivered almonds	

FIGURE 6.8 Complementary food combinations.

> **RECAP:** *When a particular amino acid is limiting, protein synthesis cannot occur. A complete protein provides all nine essential amino acids. Mutual supplementation combines two complementary-protein sources to make a complete protein.*

Why Do We Need Proteins?

The functions of proteins in the body are so numerous that only a few can be described in detail in this chapter. Note that proteins function most effectively when we also consume adequate amounts of energy as carbohydrates and fat. When there is not enough energy available, the body uses proteins as an energy source, limiting their availability for the functions described below.

Proteins Contribute to Cell Growth, Repair, and Maintenance

The proteins in our body are dynamic, which means that they are constantly being broken down, repaired, and replaced. When proteins are broken down, many amino acids are recycled into new proteins. Think about all of the new proteins that are needed to allow an embryo to develop and grow. In this case, an entirely new human body is being made! In fact, a newborn baby has more than 10 trillion body cells.

Even in the mature adult, our cells are constantly turning over, meaning that old cells are broken down and parts are used to create new cells. In addition, cellular damage that occurs must be repaired in order to maintain our health. Our red blood cells live for only 3 to 4 months, then are replaced by new cells that are produced in our bone marrow. The cells lining our intestinal tract are replaced every 3 to 6 days. The "old" intestinal cells are treated just like the proteins in food; they are digested and the amino acids absorbed back into the body. The constant turnover of proteins from our diet is essential for such cell growth, repair, and maintenance.

Proteins Act as Enzymes and Hormones

enzymes Proteins that speed up chemical reactions without being changed by the chemical reaction themselves.

Enzymes are proteins that speed up chemical reactions, without being changed by the chemical reaction themselves. Enzymes can act to bind substances together or break them apart and can transform one substance into another. FIGURE 6.9 shows how an enzyme can bind two substances together.

FIGURE 6.9   Proteins act as enzymes. Enzymes facilitate chemical reactions such as joining two compounds together.

Each cell contains thousands of enzymes that facilitate specific cellular reactions. For example, the enzyme phosphofructokinase (PFK) increases carbohydrate metabolism during physical exercise. This enzyme is critical for driving the rate at which we break down glucose and use it for energy during exercise. Without PFK, we would be unable to generate energy at a fast enough rate to allow us to be physically active.

Hormones are substances that act as chemical messengers in the body. Some hormones are made from amino acids, while others are made from lipids (refer to Chapter 5). Hormones are stored in various glands in the body, which release them in response to changes in the body's environment. They then act on the body's organs and tissues to restore the body to normal conditions.

Insulin, a hormone made from amino acids, plays an important role in regulating blood concentrations of glucose (refer to Chapter 4). While glucose is an important source of energy for body cells, high blood levels can damage cells. When you digest a meal, the breakdown of the carbohydrates raises your blood glucose levels, which stimulates your pancreas to increase its production and release of insulin. Insulin acts on cell membranes to speed up the transport of glucose into the cells and return blood glucose levels to normal.

Other examples of amino acid–containing hormones are glucagon, which responds to conditions of low blood glucose, and thyroid hormone, which helps control our resting metabolic rate.

Proteins Help Maintain Fluid and Electrolyte Balance

Electrolytes are electrically charged particles that assist in maintaining fluid balance. For our bodies to function properly, fluids and electrolytes must be maintained at healthy levels inside and outside cells and within blood vessels. Proteins attract fluids, and the proteins that are in the bloodstream, in the cells, and in the spaces surrounding the cells work together to keep fluids moving across these spaces in the proper quantities to maintain fluid balance and blood pressure. When protein intake is deficient, the concentration of proteins in the bloodstream is insufficient to draw fluid from the tissues and across the blood vessel walls; fluid then collects in the tissues, causing **edema** (FIGURE 6.10). In addition to being uncomfortable, edema can lead to serious medical problems.

Sodium (Na^+) and potassium (K^+) are examples of common electrolytes. Under normal conditions, Na^+ is more concentrated outside the cell, and K^+ is more concentrated inside the cell. This proper balance of Na^+ and K^+ is accomplished by the action of **transport proteins** located within the cell membrane. FIGURE 6.11 shows how these transport proteins work to pump Na^+ outside and K^+ inside of the cell. Conduction of nerve signals and contraction of muscles depend on a proper balance of electrolytes. If protein intake is deficient, we lose our ability to maintain these functions, resulting in potentially fatal changes in the rhythm of the heart. Other consequences of chronically low protein intakes include muscle weakness and spasms, kidney failure, and, if conditions are severe enough, death.

Proteins Help Maintain Acid–Base Balance

The body's cellular processes result in the constant production of acids and bases. These substances are transported in the blood to be excreted through the kidneys and the lungs. The human body maintains very tight control over the **pH,** or the acid–base balance, of the blood. The body goes into a state called **acidosis** when the blood becomes too acidic. **Alkalosis** results if the blood becomes too basic. Both acidosis and alkalosis can be caused by respiratory or metabolic problems. Acidosis and alkalosis can cause coma and death by denaturing body proteins.

Proteins are excellent **buffers,** meaning that they help maintain proper acid–base balance. Acids contain hydrogen ions, which are positively charged. The side chains of proteins have negative charges that attract the hydrogen ions and neutralize their detrimental effects on the body. Proteins can release the hydrogen ions when the blood becomes too basic. By buffering acids and bases, proteins maintain acid–base balance and blood pH.

edema A disorder in which fluids build up in the tissue spaces of the body, causing fluid imbalances and a swollen appearance.

transport proteins Protein molecules that help to transport substances throughout the body and across cell membranes.

pH Stands for percentage of hydrogen. It is a measure of the acidity—or level of hydrogen—of any solution, including human blood.

acidosis A disorder in which the blood becomes acidic; that is, the level of hydrogen in the blood is excessive. It can be caused by respiratory or metabolic problems.

alkalosis A disorder in which the blood becomes basic; that is, the level of hydrogen in the blood is deficient. It can be caused by respiratory or metabolic problems.

buffers Proteins that help maintain proper acid–base balance by attaching to, or releasing, hydrogen ions as conditions change in the body.

(a) Normal fluid balance

(b) Edema caused by insufficient protein in blood stream

FIGURE 6.10 The role of proteins in maintaining fluid balance. The heartbeat exerts pressure that continually pushes fluids in the bloodstream through the arterial walls and out into the tissue spaces. By the time blood reaches the veins, the pressure of the heartbeat has greatly decreased. In this environment, proteins in the blood are able to draw fluids out of the tissues and back into the bloodstream. **(a)** This healthy (non-swollen) tissue suggests that body fluids in the bloodstream and in the tissue spaces are in balance. **(b)** When the level of proteins in the blood is insufficient to draw fluids out of the tissues, edema can result. This foot with edema is swollen due to fluid imbalance.

Proteins Help Maintain a Strong Immune System

Antibodies are special proteins that are critical components of the immune system. When a foreign substance attacks the body, the immune system produces antibodies to defend against it. Bacteria, viruses, toxins, and allergens (substances that cause allergic reactions) are examples of antigens that can trigger antibody production. (An *antigen* is any substance—but typically a protein—that our bodies recognize as foreign and that triggers an immune response.)

antibodies Defensive proteins of the immune system. Their production is prompted by the presence of bacteria, viruses, toxins, allergens, and so on.

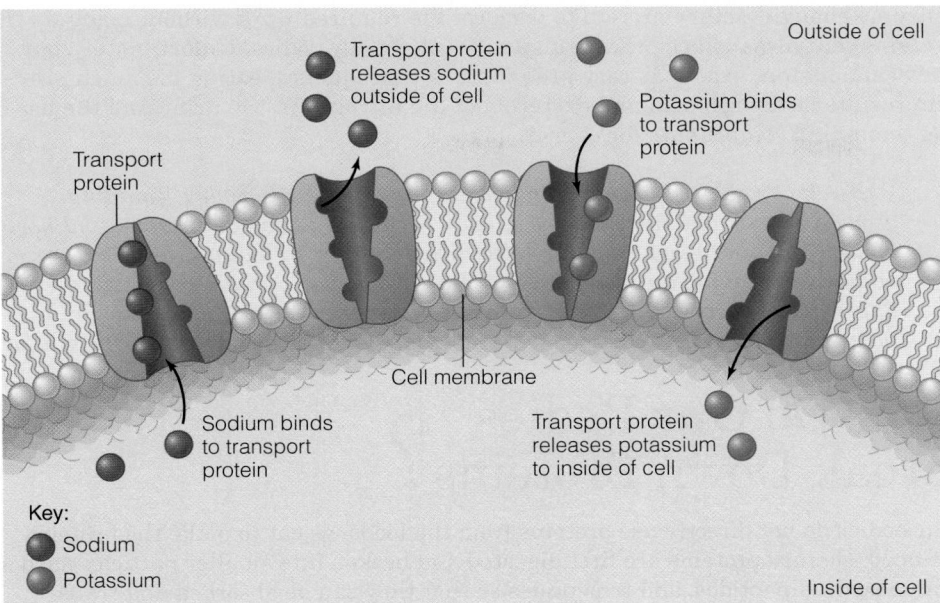

FIGURE 6.11 Transport proteins help maintain electrolyte balance. Transport proteins in the cell membrane pick up potassium and sodium and transport them across the cell membrane.

When an unfamiliar antigen invades the body, antibodies are produced that are specialized to recognize that particular antigen. These antibodies multiply and attach to the antigen, marking it for destruction. This production of a new group of antibodies is somewhat slow, which is why it takes your body some time to vanquish certain infections. But once antibodies have been made, they continue to circulate in the bloodstream and can respond quickly the next time that particular invader appears, often before we experience any symptoms of infection. *Immunity* refers to the development of the molecular memory to produce antibodies quickly upon subsequent invasions.

Adequate protein is necessary to support the production of antibodies. If we do not consume enough protein, our resistance to certain diseases is weakened. On the other hand, eating more protein than we need does not improve immune function.

Proteins Serve as an Energy Source

The body's primary energy sources are carbohydrate and fat. Remember that both carbohydrate and fat have specialized storage forms that can be used for energy—glycogen for carbohydrate and triglycerides for fat. Proteins do not have a specialized storage form for energy. This means that when proteins need to be used for energy, they are taken from the blood and body tissues such as the liver and skeletal muscle. In healthy people, proteins contribute very little to energy needs. Because we are efficient at recycling amino acids, protein needs are relatively low as compared to carbohydrate and fat needs.

To use proteins for energy, the nitrogen (or amine) group is removed from the amino acid in a process called **deamination.** The nitrogen is then transported to the kidneys, where it is excreted in the urine as *urea.* The remaining fragments of the amino acid contain carbon, hydrogen, and oxygen. The body can directly metabolize these fragments for energy or use them to build carbohydrate. Certain amino acids can be converted into glucose. This is a critical process during times of low carbohydrate intake or starvation. Fat cannot be converted into glucose, but body proteins can be broken down and converted into glucose to provide needed energy to the brain.

To protect the proteins in our body tissues, it is important that we regularly eat an adequate amount of carbohydrate and fat to provide energy. We also need to

deamination The process by which an amine group is removed from an amino acid. The nitrogen is then transported to the kidneys for excretion in the urine, while the carbon and other components are metabolized for energy or used to make other compounds.

consume enough dietary protein to perform the required work without using up the proteins that already are playing an active role in our bodies. Unfortunately, our body cannot store excess dietary protein. As a consequence, eating too much protein results in the removal and excretion of the nitrogen in the urine and the use of the remaining components for energy.

> RECAP: *Proteins serve many important functions, including 1) enabling growth, repair, and maintenance of body tissues; 2) acting as enzymes and hormones; 3) maintaining fluid and electrolyte balance; 4) maintaining acid–base balance; 5) making antibodies, which strengthen our immune system; and 6) providing energy when carbohydrate and fat intake are inadequate. Proteins function best when we also consume adequate amounts of carbohydrate and fat.*

How Do Our Bodies Break Down Proteins?

Our bodies do not directly use proteins from the foods we eat to make the proteins we need. Dietary proteins are first digested and broken into smaller particles such as amino acids, dipeptides, and tripeptides so that they can be absorbed and transported to the cells. In this section, we will review how proteins are digested and absorbed. As you read about each step in this process, refer to FIGURE 6.12 for a visual tour through the digestive system.

Stomach Acids and Enzymes Break Proteins into Short Polypeptides

Virtually no enzymatic digestion of proteins occurs in the mouth. As shown in step 1 in FIGURE 6.12, proteins in food are chewed, crushed, and moistened with saliva to ease swallowing and to increase the surface area of the protein for more efficient digestion. There is no further digestive action on proteins in the mouth.

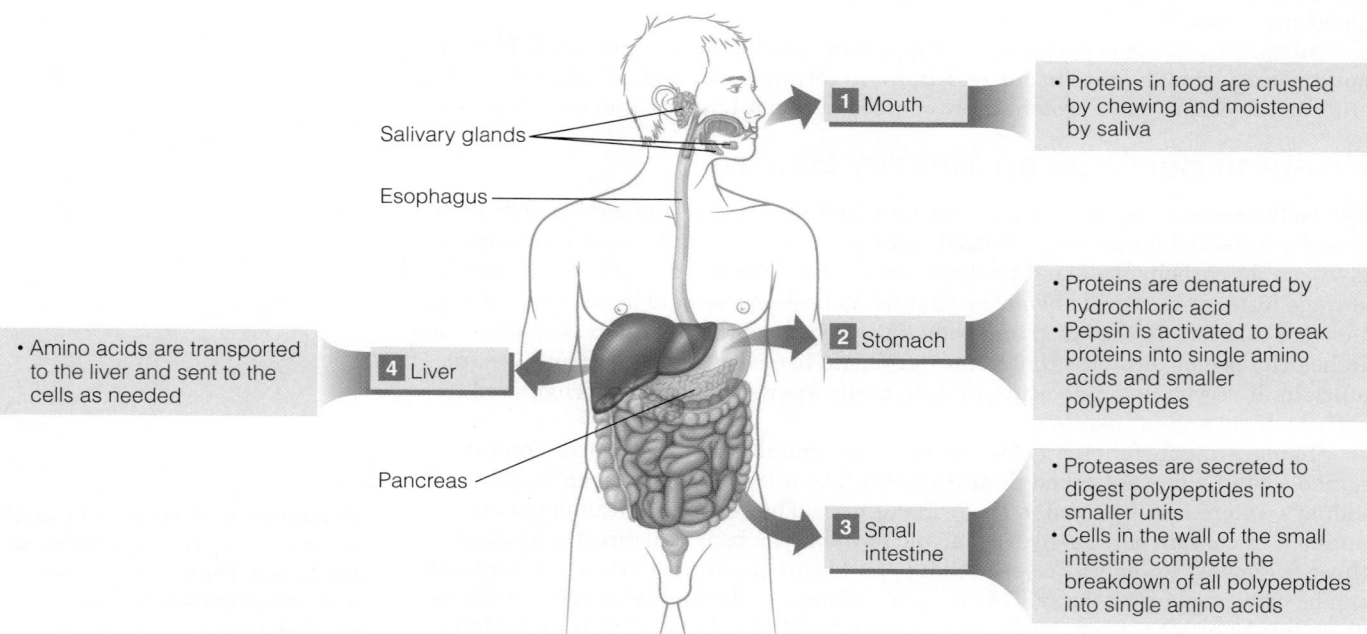

Salivary glands

Esophagus

Pancreas

1 Mouth
• Proteins in food are crushed by chewing and moistened by saliva

2 Stomach
• Proteins are denatured by hydrochloric acid
• Pepsin is activated to break proteins into single amino acids and smaller polypeptides

3 Small intestine
• Proteases are secreted to digest polypeptides into smaller units
• Cells in the wall of the small intestine complete the breakdown of all polypeptides into single amino acids

4 Liver
• Amino acids are transported to the liver and sent to the cells as needed

FIGURE 6.12 The process of protein digestion.

When proteins reach the stomach, they are broken apart by *hydrochloric acid* (FIGURE 6.12, step 2). Hydrochloric acid denatures the strands of protein and converts the inactive enzyme, *pepsinogen,* into its active form, **pepsin.** Although pepsin is a protein, it is not denatured by the acid in the stomach because it has evolved to work optimally in an acidic environment. Pepsin begins breaking proteins into single amino acids and shorter polypeptides that then travel to the small intestine for further digestion.

Enzymes in the Small Intestine Break Polypeptides into Single Amino Acids

As the polypeptides reach the small intestine, the pancreas and the small intestine secrete enzymes that digest them into oligopeptides, tripeptides, dipeptides, and single amino acids (FIGURE 6.12, step 3). The enzymes that digest proteins in the small intestine are called **proteases.**

The cells in the wall of the small intestine then absorb the single amino acids, dipeptides, and tripeptides. Enzymes in the intestinal cells break the dipeptides and tripeptides into single amino acids. The amino acids are then transported into the bloodstream to the liver and on to cells throughout the body as needed (FIGURE 6.12, step 4).

Cells of the small intestine have different sites that specialize in transporting certain types of amino acids, dipeptides, and tripeptides. When very large doses of single amino acids are taken on an empty stomach, there is the potential that similar amino acids may be competing for the same absorption sites. Thus, consumption of too much of one amino acid could, in theory, block the absorption of others. Some people believe that this is why it is not beneficial to consume individual amino acid supplements. In reality, people rarely take very large doses of single amino acids on an empty stomach. The primary reason people should not take single amino acids is that the amount taken is usually so small that they don't have any beneficial effect. For more information on amino acid supplements, refer to Chapter 13.

Protein Digestibility Affects Protein Quality

Earlier in this chapter we discussed how various foods differ in the quality of protein they contain. The quantity of essential amino acids in a protein determines its quality: foods of higher protein quality contain more essential amino acids, and foods of lower protein quality contain fewer essential amino acids.

Another factor to consider when determining protein quality is *digestibility,* or how well our bodies can digest a protein. Complete proteins are more highly digestible than incomplete proteins. Thus animal protein sources such as meat and dairy products are highly digestible, as are many soy products; we can absorb more than 90% of these proteins. Legumes are also highly digestible (about 80%). Grains and many vegetable proteins are less digestible, ranging from 60% to 90%. The **protein digestibility corrected amino acid score (PDCAAS)** uses an amino acid score and a correction factor for digestibility to calculate a value for protein quality.

Other measures of protein quality include the protein efficiency ratio and net protein utilization. The *protein efficiency ratio* assesses protein quality by comparing the weight gained by a laboratory animal consuming a test protein with the weight gained by a laboratory animal consuming a reference, or standardized, protein. *Net protein utilization* is a process that compares the amount of nitrogen retained in our bodies with the amount of nitrogen we consume in our diets. The more nitrogen we retain, the higher the quality of the protein we have consumed.

These measures of protein quality are useful when determining the quality of protein available to populations of people. However, these measures are not practical or useful for individual diet planning.

Meats are highly digestible sources of dietary protein.

pepsin An enzyme in the stomach that begins the breakdown of proteins into shorter polypeptide chains and single amino acids.

proteases Enzymes that continue the breakdown of polypeptides in the small intestine.

protein digestibility corrected amino acid score (PDCAAS) A measurement of protein quality that considers the balance of amino acids as well as the digestibility of the protein in the food.

RECAP: In the stomach, hydrochloric acid denatures proteins and converts pepsinogen to pepsin; pepsin breaks proteins into smaller polypeptides and individual amino acids. In the small intestine, proteases break polypeptides into smaller fragments and single amino acids. The cells in the wall of the small intestine break the smaller peptide fragments into single amino acids, which are then transported to the liver for distribution to our cells. Protein digestibility as well as provision of essential amino acids influences protein quality.

How Much Protein Should We Eat?

Consuming adequate protein is a major concern of many people. In fact, one of the most common concerns among active people and athletes is that their diets are deficient in protein (see the Nutrition Myth or Fact? box for a discussion of this topic). This concern about dietary protein is generally unnecessary, as we can easily consume the protein our bodies need by eating an adequate amount of various foods.

Nitrogen Balance Is a Method Used to Determine Protein Needs

A highly specialized procedure referred to as *nitrogen balance* is used to determine a person's protein needs. Nitrogen is excreted through the body's processes of recycling or using proteins; thus, the balance can be used to estimate whether protein intake is adequate to meet protein needs. Typically performed only in experimental laboratories, the nitrogen balance procedure involves measuring both nitrogen intake and nitrogen excretion over a 2-week period. A standardized diet with a set amount of protein is fed to a person, and the nitrogen content of the diet is measured and recorded. The person is required to consume all of the foods he or she is given. Because the majority of nitrogen is excreted in the urine and feces, laboratory technicians directly measure the nitrogen content of the subject's urine and fecal samples. Small amounts of nitrogen are excreted in the skin, hair, and body fluids such as mucus and semen, but because of the complexity of collecting nitrogen excreted via these routes, the measurements are estimated. Then, technicians add the estimated nitrogen losses to the nitrogen measured in the subject's urine and feces. Nitrogen balance is then calculated as the difference between nitrogen intake and nitrogen excretion.

When a person consumes more nitrogen than is excreted, this person is considered to be in positive nitrogen balance (FIGURE 6.13). This state indicates that the body is retaining, or adding, protein, and it occurs during periods of growth, pregnancy, or recovery from illness or a protein deficiency. When a person excretes more nitrogen than is consumed, this person is considered to be in negative nitrogen balance. This situation indicates that the body is losing protein, and it occurs during starvation or when people are consuming very-low-energy diets. This is because when energy intake is too low to meet energy demands over a prolonged period of time, the body metabolizes body proteins for energy and the nitrogen from these proteins is excreted in the urine and feces. Negative nitrogen balance also occurs during severe illness, infections, high fever, serious burns, or injuries that cause significant blood loss. People in these situations require increased dietary protein. A person is in nitrogen balance when nitrogen intake equals nitrogen excretion. This indicates that protein intake is sufficient to cover protein needs. Healthy adults who are not pregnant are in nitrogen balance.

Recommended Dietary Allowance (RDA) for Protein

How much protein should we eat? The RDA for sedentary people is 0.8 g per kg body weight per day. The recommended percentage of energy that should come from protein is 10–35% of total energy intake. Protein needs are higher for children, adolescents, and pregnant/lactating women because more protein is needed during times of growth and development (refer to Chapters 19 and 20 for details on protein needs

NUTRITION MYTH OR FACT?

Do Athletes Need More Protein Than Inactive People?

At one time it was believed that the Recommended Dietary Allowance (RDA) for protein, which is 0.8 g per kg body weight, was sufficient for both inactive people and athletes. Recent studies, however, show that athletes' protein needs are higher. Why do athletes need more protein? Regular exercise increases the transport of oxygen to body tissues, requiring changes in the oxygen-carrying capacity of the blood. To carry more oxygen, we need to produce more of the protein that carries oxygen in the blood (i.e., hemoglobin, which is a protein). During intense exercise, we use a small amount of protein directly for energy. We also use protein to make glucose to maintain adequate blood glucose levels and to prevent hypoglycemia (low blood sugar) during exercise. Regular exercise stimulates tissue growth and causes tissue damage, which must be repaired by additional proteins. Strength athletes (such as bodybuilders and weightlifters) need 1.8 to 2 times more protein than the current RDA, while

Some athletes who persistently diet are at risk of low protein intake.

endurance athletes (such as distance runners and triathletes) need 1.5 to 1.75 times more protein than the current RDA.[2] Later in this chapter we will calculate the protein needs for inactive and active people.

Does this mean you should add more protein to your diet? Not necessarily. Contrary to popular belief, most Americans, including inactive people *and* athletes, already consume more than twice the RDA for protein. Thus, taking amino acid and protein supplements is not necessary. In fact, eating more protein or taking individual amino acids does not cause muscles to become bigger or stronger. Only regular strength training can achieve these goals. For healthy individuals, evidence does not support eating more than two times the RDA for protein to increase strength, build muscle, or improve athletic performance. By eating a balanced diet and con-

suming a variety of foods, both inactive and active people can easily meet their protein requirements.

during these portions of the life cycle). Protein needs can also be higher for active people and for vegetarians.

Table 6.2 lists the daily recommendations for protein for a variety of lifestyles. How can we convert this recommendation into total grams of protein for the day? In the You Do the Math box on page 229, let's calculate Theo's RDA for protein.

Is it possible for Theo to eat this much protein each day? It may surprise you to discover that most Americans eat 1.5 to 2 times the RDA for protein without any effort! In the following sections, we describe the average protein intake in the United States, review foods that are good sources of protein, and give an example of calculating your daily protein intake. We will also look at potential risks of high-protein diets.

Most Americans Meet or Exceed the RDA for Protein

Surveys indicate that Americans eat 15–17% of their total daily energy intake as protein.[3–5] In these studies, women reported eating about 65 to 70 g of protein each day, while men consumed 88 to 110 g per day. Putting these values into perspective,

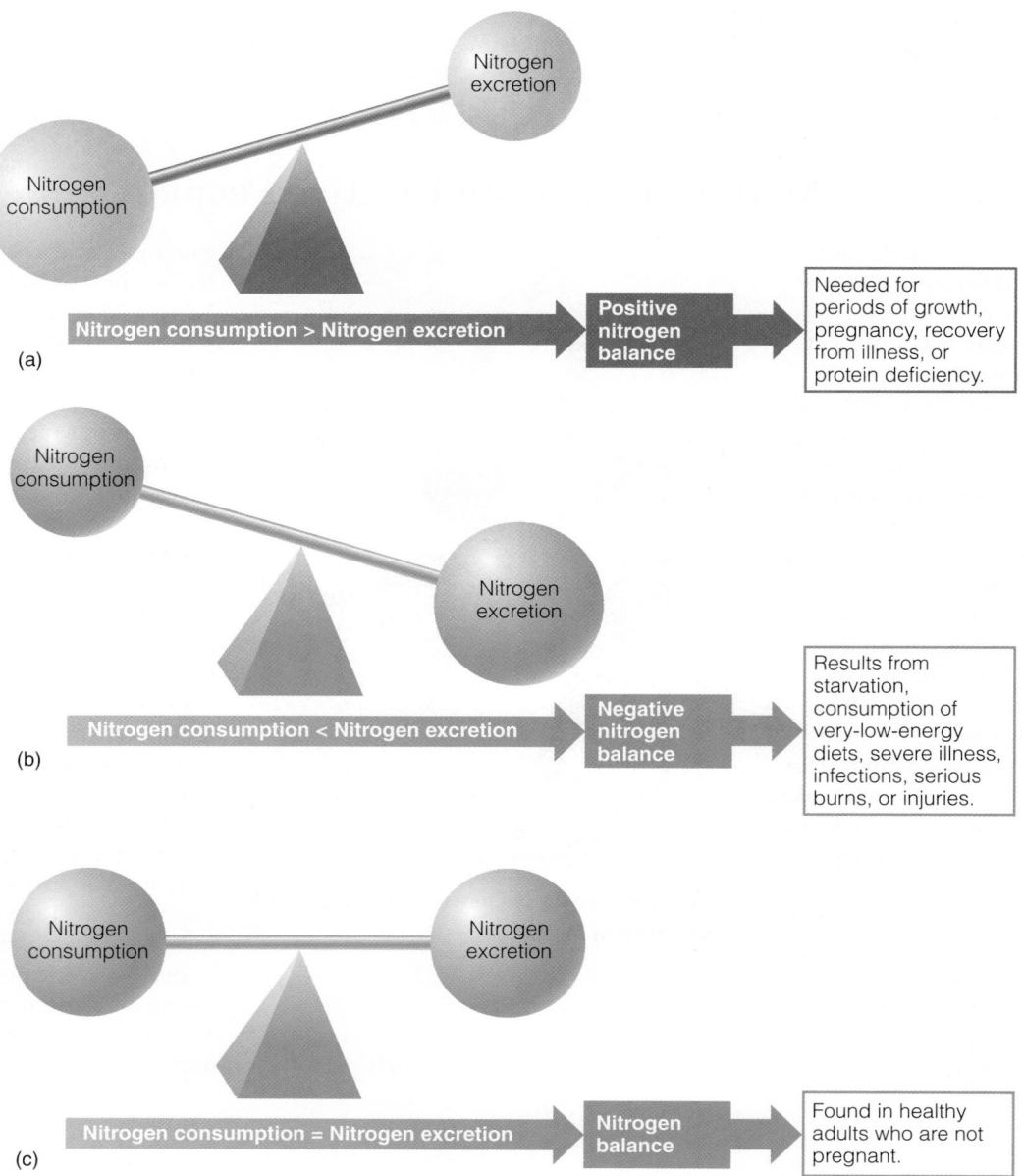

FIGURE 6.13   Nitrogen balance describes the relationship between how much nitrogen (or protein) we consume and excrete each day. **(a)** Positive nitrogen balance occurs when nitrogen consumption is greater than excretion. **(b)** Negative nitrogen balance occurs when nitrogen consumption is less than excretion. **(c)** Nitrogen balance is maintained when nitrogen consumption equals excretion.

let's assume that the average man weighs 75 kg (165 pounds) and the average woman weighs 65 kg (143 pounds). Their protein requirements (assuming they are not athletes or vegetarians) are 60 g and 52 g per day, respectively. As you can see, most adults in the United States appear to have no problems meeting their protein needs each day.

What are the typical protein intakes of active people? Table 6.3 reviews the self-reported protein intake of athletes participating in a variety of sports.[6] As you can see, the protein intake ranges from 1.1 to 3.1 g per kg body weight per day and accounts for 13–36% of the total daily energy intake in these active individuals. If you compare this to the recommended intakes in Table 6.2, you'll find that many ath-

TABLE 6.2 Recommended Protein Intakes

Group	Protein Intake (g/kg body weight/day)*
Most adults[†]	0.8
Nonvegetarian endurance athletes[‡]	1.2 to 1.4
Nonvegetarian strength athletes[‡]	1.6 to 1.7
Vegetarian endurance athletes[‡]	1.3 to 1.5
Vegetarian strength athletes[‡]	1.7 to 1.8

*To convert body weight to kilograms, divide weight in pounds by 2.2.
Weight (lb)/2.2 = Weight (kg)
Weight (kg) × protein recommendation (g/kg body weight/day) = protein intake (g/day)
Sources: [†]Food and Nutrition Board, Institute of Medicine. 2005. *Dietary Reference Intakes for Energy, Carbohydrate, Fiber, Fat, Fatty Acids, Cholesterol, Protein, and Amino Acids (Macronutrients)*, pp. 465–608. Washington, DC: National Academies Press.
[‡]American College of Sports Medicine, American Dietetic Association, and Dietitians of Canada. 2001. Joint Position Statement. Nutrition and athletic performance. *Med. Sci. Sports Exerc.* 32:2130–2145.

letes are consuming significantly more protein than they need. In contrast, athletes who consume inadequate energy and limit food choices, such as distance runners, figure skaters, female gymnasts, and wrestlers who are dieting, are all at risk for low protein intakes. Unlike people who consume adequate energy, individuals who are restricting their total energy intake (kilocalories) need to pay close attention to their protein intake.

RECAP: *The RDA for protein for most nonpregnant, nonlactating, nonvegetarian adults is 0.8 g per kg body weight. Children, pregnant women, nursing mothers, vegetarians, and active people need slightly more. Most people who eat enough kilocalories and carbohydrates have no problem meeting their RDA for protein.*

YOU DO THE MATH % = >

Calculating Your Protein Needs

Theo wants to know how much protein he needs each day. During the off-season, he works out three times a week at a gym and practices basketball with friends every Friday night. He is not a vegetarian. Although Theo exercises regularly, he does not qualify as an endurance athlete or as a strength athlete. At this level of physical activity, Theo's RDA for protein probably ranges from 0.8 to 1.0 g per kg body weight per day (see Table 6.3). To calculate the total number of grams of protein Theo should eat each day:

1. Convert Theo's weight from pounds to kilograms. Theo presently weighs 200 pounds. To convert this value to kilograms, divide by 2.2:
   200 pounds ÷ 2.2 pounds/kg = 91 kg.

2. Multiply Theo's weight in kilograms by his RDA for protein:
   91 kg × 0.8 g/kg = 72.8 grams of protein per day.
   91 kg × 1.0 g/kg = 91 grams of protein per day.

   What happens during basketball season, when Theo practices or has games 5 to 6 days a week? This will probably raise his protein needs to approximately 1.0 to 1.2 g per kg body weight per day. How much more protein should he eat?

   91 kg × 1.2 g/kg = 109.2 grams of protein per day.

   Now calculate your recommended protein intake based upon your activity level.

TABLE 6.3   Self-Reported Protein Intakes of Athletes

Sport Type	Gender	Protein Intake (g/kg body weight/day)	Protein Intake (% total kcal)
Football	M	1.5	15.0
Weightlifting	M	1.9	18.0
Soccer	M	2.2	14.4
Triathlon	M	2.0	13.0
Marathon running	M	2.0	14.5
Distance running	M	1.6	12.8
	F	1.1	14.1
Ultradistance running	M	1.4	16.7
	F	1.2	15.1
Bodybuilding	M	2.7–3.1	22.5–37.7
	F	1.9–2.7	22.6–35.8

Source: Adapted by permission from M. Manore and J. Thompson, 2000, *Sport Nutrition for Health and Performance,* page 118, Table 4.5. © 2000 by Melinda Manore and Janice Thompson. Reprinted with permission from Human Kinetics (Champaign, IL).

Too Much Dietary Protein Can Be Harmful

High protein intake may increase the risk of health problems. Three health conditions that have received particular attention are heart disease, bone loss, and kidney disease.

High Protein Intake Is Associated with High Cholesterol

High-protein diets in which the protein is derived predominantly from animal sources are associated with higher blood cholesterol levels. This is probably due to the saturated fat in animal products, which is known to increase blood cholesterol levels and the risk of heart disease. One study showed that people with heart disease improved their health when they ate a diet that was high in whole grains, fruits, and vegetables and met the RDA for protein.[7] However, some of the people in this study chose to eat a high-protein diet, and their risk factors worsened. In addition, vegetarians have been shown to have a greatly reduced risk of heart disease.[8,9]

High Protein Intake May Contribute to Bone Loss

How might a high-protein diet lead to bone loss? Until recently, nutritionists have been concerned about high-protein diets because they increase calcium excretion. This may be because animal products contain more of the sulfur amino acids (methionine and cysteine). Metabolizing these amino acids makes the blood more acidic, and calcium is pulled from the bone to buffer these acids. Although eating more protein can cause you to excrete more calcium, whether high protein intakes actually cause bone loss is very controversial. We do know that eating too little protein causes bone loss, which increases the risk of fractures and osteoporosis. Higher intakes of animal and soy protein have been shown to protect bone in middle-aged and older women.[10,11] There does not appear to be enough direct evidence at this time to show that higher protein intakes cause bone loss in healthy people.

High Protein Intake Can Increase the Risk for Kidney Disease

A third risk associated with high protein intakes is kidney disease. People with kidney problems are advised to eat a low-protein diet because a high-protein diet can increase the risk of acquiring kidney disease in people who are susceptible. People with diabetes have higher rates of kidney disease and may benefit from a lower protein diet.[12] The American Diabetes Association states that people with diabetes have a higher protein need than people without diabetes, but a protein intake of 15–20% of total energy is adequate to meet these increased protein needs.[13] This level of protein intake is deemed safe for people with diabetes who have normal renal function. There is no evidence, however, that eating more protein causes kidney disease in healthy people who are not susceptible to this condition. In fact, one study found that athletes consuming up to 2.8 g of protein per kg body weight per day experienced no unhealthy changes in kidney function.[14] Experts agree that eating no more than 2 g of protein per kg body weight each day is safe for healthy people.

It is important for people who consume a lot of protein to drink more water. This is because eating more protein increases protein metabolism and urea production. As we mentioned earlier, urea is a waste product that forms when nitrogen is removed during amino acid metabolism. Adequate fluid is needed to flush excess urea from the kidneys. This is particularly important for athletes, who need more fluid to counterbalance higher sweat losses.

NUTRI-CASE LIZ

" One of my dancer friends, Silvie, was always a little pudgy, but now she's tighter than I've ever seen her. Yesterday, even our teacher commented on how great she looks! After class, I asked her secret and she said she's been on a high-protein diet for 2 months. She said it's pretty easy to stick to—you just have to avoid starches like bread and pasta. Oh, and most sweets, too, though you can still have ice cream. She said she never feels hungry anymore, that the meat and eggs and cheese keep her feeling full. I'm thinking to myself, heck, I'm hungry all the time. So I asked her to bring me her book about the diet so I can try it for myself."

One issue that has been a major controversy for many years is the use of high-protein diets for weight loss. Popular diets such as the Atkins Diet, the Zone Diet, and the Sugar Busters Diet support the use of high-protein or low-carbohydrate meals to achieve weight loss. The Nutrition Debate at the end of the chapter (page 249) has a detailed discussion of this controversial topic. After reading it, what do you think of Liz's idea of trying the diet? Would your opinion change if you learned that Liz has high LDL-cholesterol and that her father suffered a heart attack last year at age 49? How might you advise Liz to adapt the diet for her unique health concerns?

SHOPPER'S GUIDE
Good Food Sources of Protein

Table 6.4 compares the protein content of a variety of foods. In general, good sources of protein include meats (beef, pork, poultry, seafood), dairy products (milk-based products and eggs), soy products, legumes, whole grains, and nuts. While most people are aware that meats are an excellent source of protein, many people are surprised to learn that the quality of the protein in some legumes is almost equal to that of meat.

Legumes include foods such as kidney beans, pinto beans, black beans, soybeans, garbanzo beans (or chickpeas), lentils, green peas, black-eyed peas, and lima beans.

TABLE 6.4 Protein Content of Commonly Consumed Foods

Food	Serving Size	Protein (g)	Food	Serving Size	Protein (g)
Beef:			*Beans:*		
Ground, lean, baked (16% fat)	3.0 oz	22	Refried	0.5 cup	7
Corned beef, brisket, cooked	3.0 oz	15	Kidney, red	0.5 cup	7.7
Prime rib, broiled (½-in. trim)	3.0 oz	17	Black	0.5 cup	7
Top sirloin, broiled (⅛-in. trim)	3.0 oz	23	Pork and beans, canned	0.5 cup	6.5
Poultry:			*Nuts:*		
Chicken breast, broiled, no skin	3.0 oz	28	Peanuts, dry roasted	1 oz	6.7
Chicken thigh, roasted, no skin	3.0 oz	23	Peanut butter, creamy	2 tbsp.	8
Chicken drumstick, broiled, with skin	3.0 oz	24	Almonds, blanched	1 oz	6
Turkey breast, roasted, Louis Rich	3.0 oz	14	Sunflower seeds	1 oz	5.5
Turkey dark meat, roasted, no skin	3.0 oz	26	Pecan halves	1 oz	2.6
Seafood:			*Cereals, Grains, and Breads:*		
Cod, cooked	3.0 oz	19	Barley, cooked	1 cup	3.6
Salmon, Chinook, baked	3.0 oz	22	Oatmeal, quick instant	1 cup	5.4
Shrimp, steamed	3.0 oz	18	Cheerios	1 cup	3
Oysters, steamed	3.0 oz	16	Corn Bran	1 cup	2
Tuna, in water, drained	3.0 oz	22	Grape-Nuts	0.5 cup	6
Pork:			Raisin Bran	1 cup	5
			Brown rice, cooked	1 cup	5
Pork loin chop, broiled	3 oz	25	Whole-wheat bread	1 slice	2.7
Beef ribs, roasted	3 oz	19	Rye bread	1 slice	2.7
Ham, roasted, lean	3 oz	20	Bagel, 3½-in. diameterameter	1 each	7
Dairy:			*Vegetables:*		
Whole milk (3.3% fat)	8 fl. oz	7.9	Carrots, raw (7.5 × 1⅛ in.)	1 each	0.7
1% milk	8 fl. oz	8.5	Asparagus, boiled	6 spears	2
Skim milk	8 fl. oz	8.8	Green beans, cooked	1 cup	2.4
Low-fat, plain yogurt	8 fl. oz	13	Broccoli, raw, chopped	1 cup	2.6
American cheese, processed	1 oz	6	Collards, cooked from frozen	1 cup	5
Swiss cheese	1 oz	7.6	Spinach, raw	1 cup	0.9
Cottage cheese, low-fat (2%)	1 cup	28			
Soy Products:					
Tofu	3.3 oz	7			
Tempeh, cooked	3.3 oz	18			
Soy milk beverage	1 cup	11			

Source: Values obtained from U.S. Department of Agriculture, Agricultural Research Service. 2006. USDA National Nutrient Database for Standard Reference, Release 19. Nutrient Data Laboratory Home Page, http://www.ars.usda.gov/Main/docs.htm?docid=4451

Interestingly, the quality of soybean protein is almost identical to that of meat, and the protein quality of other legumes is relatively high. In addition to being excellent sources of protein, legumes are also high in fiber, iron, calcium, and many of the B vitamins. They are also low in saturated fat and cholesterol. Legumes are not nutritionally complete, however, as they do not contain vitamins B_{12}, C, or A and are deficient in methionine, an essential amino acid. Eating legumes regularly, including foods made from soybeans, may help reduce the risk of heart disease by lowering blood cholesterol levels. Diets high in legumes and soy products are also associated with lower rates of some cancers.

Fruits and many vegetables are not particularly high in protein; however, these foods provide fiber and many vitamins and minerals and are excellent sources of carbohydrates. Thus, eating these foods can help provide the carbohydrates and energy that our body needs so that we can spare protein for use in building and maintaining our bodies rather than using it for energy. Try the Nutrition Label Activity on page 235 to determine how much protein you typically eat.

The quality of the protein in some legumes is almost equal to that of meat.

Tips for Adding Legumes to Your Daily Diet

They're high in protein and fiber, low in fat, and fill you up with fewer calories than meat sources of protein. What's more, they taste good! Maybe that's why nutrition experts consider legumes an almost perfect food. Legumes include peas, lentils, and beans, as well as products made from soybeans, such as tofu and soy burgers. From main dishes to snacks, here are some simple ways to add legumes to your daily diet.

Breakfast

√ Instead of cereal, eggs, or a muffin, microwave a frozen bean burrito for a quick, portable breakfast.

√ Make your pancakes with soy milk, or pour soy milk on your cereal.

√ If you normally have a side of bacon, ham, or sausage with your eggs, have a side of black beans instead.

Lunch and Dinner

√ Try a sandwich made with hummus (a garbanzo bean spread), cucumbers, tomato, avocado, and/or lettuce on whole-wheat bread or in a whole-wheat pocket.

√ Use deli "meats" made with soy in your sandwich. Also try soy hot dogs, burgers, and "chicken" nuggets.

√ Add garbanzo beans, kidney beans, or fresh peas to tossed salads, or make a three-bean salad with kidney beans, green beans, and garbanzo beans.

√ Make a side dish using legumes such as peas with pearl onions, or succotash (lima beans, corn, and tomatoes), or homemade chili with kidney beans and tofu instead of meat.

√ Make black bean soup, lentil soup, pea soup, minestrone soup, or a batch of dal (a type of yellow lentil used in Indian cuisine) and serve over brown rice. Top with plain yogurt, a traditional accompaniment in many Asian cuisines.

√ Use soy "crumbles" in any recipe calling for ground beef.

√ Make burritos with black or pinto beans instead of shredded meat.

√ To stir-fried vegetables, add cubes of tofu or strips of tempeh.

√ Make a "meatloaf" using cooked, mashed lentils instead of ground beef.

√ For fast food at home, keep canned beans on hand. Serve over rice with a salad for a complete and hearty meal.

Snacks

√ Instead of potato chips or pretzels, try one of the new bean chips.

√ Dip fresh vegetables in bean dip.

(continued)

√ Serve hummus on wedges of pita bread.

√ Add roasted soy "nuts" to your trail mix.

√ Keep frozen tofu desserts such as tofu ice cream in your freezer.

RECAP: *Eating too much protein may increase your risk for heart disease and kidney disease if you are already at risk for these diseases. Good sources of protein include meats, eggs, dairy products, soy products, legumes, whole grains, and nuts.*

Can a Vegetarian Diet Provide Adequate Protein?

Vegetarianism is the practice of restricting the diet to food substances of vegetable origin, including fruits, grains, and nuts. Over the last 15 years, the number of vegetarians has increased in the United States from approximately 6 million to 12 million people. Many vegetarians are college students; moving away from home and taking responsibility for one's eating habits appears to influence some young adults to try vegetarianism as a lifestyle choice.

Types of Vegetarian Diets

There are almost as many types of vegetarian diets as there are vegetarians. Some people who consider themselves vegetarians regularly eat poultry and fish. Others avoid the flesh of animals, but consume eggs, milk, and cheese liberally. Still others strictly avoid all products of animal origin, including milk and eggs, and even by-products such as candies and puddings made with gelatin.

Table 6.5 identifies the various types of vegetarian diets, ranging from the most inclusive to the most restrictive. Notice that the more restrictive the diet, the more challenging it becomes to achieve an adequate protein intake.

Soy products are a good source of dietary protein.

Why Do People Become Vegetarians?

When discussing vegetarianism, one of the most often-asked questions is why people would make this food choice. The most common responses are included here.

Religious, Ethical, and Food-Safety Reasons

Some make the choice for religious or spiritual reasons. Several religions prohibit or restrict the consumption of animal flesh; however, generalizations can be misleading. For example, while certain sects within Hinduism forbid the consumption of meat, perusing the menu at any Indian restaurant will reveal that many other Hindus regularly consume small quantities of meat, poultry, and fish. Many Buddhists are vegetarians, as are some Christians, including Seventh-Day Adventists.

Many vegetarians are guided by their personal philosophy to choose vegetarianism. These people feel that it is morally and ethically wrong to consume animals and any products from animals (such as dairy or egg products) because they view the practices in the modern animal industries as inhumane. They may consume milk and eggs but choose to purchase them only from family farms where animals are treated humanely.

vegetarianism The practice of restricting the diet to food substances of plant origin, including vegetables, fruits, grains, and nuts.

NUTRITION LABEL ACTIVITY

How Much Protein Do You Eat?

Theo wants to know if his diet contains enough protein. To calculate his protein intake, he records all foods that he eats for 3 days in a food diary. The foods Theo consumed for 1 of his 3 days are listed below on the left, and the protein content of those foods is listed on the right. Theo recorded the protein content listed on the Nutrition Facts label for those foods with labels. For products without labels, he used the nutrient analysis program that came with this book. There is also a U.S. Department of Agriculture Web site that lists the energy and nutrient content of thousands of foods (go to www.ars.usda.gov/ba/bhnrc/ndl).

Foods Consumed	Protein Content (g)
Breakfast:	
Brewed coffee (2 cups) with 2 tbsp. cream	1
1 large bagel (5-in. diameter)	10
Low-fat cream cheese (1.5 oz)	4.5
Mid-morning snack:	
Cola beverage (32 fl. oz)	0
Low-fat strawberry yogurt (1 cup)	10
Snackwells Apple Cinnamon Bars (37 g each bar; 2 bars eaten)	2
Lunch:	
Ham and cheese sandwich:	
Whole-wheat bread (2 slices)	4
Mayonnaise (1.5 tbsp.)	1
Lean ham (4 oz)	24
Swiss cheese (2 oz)	16
Iceberg lettuce (2 leaves)	0.5
Sliced tomato (3 slices)	0.5
Banana (1 large)	1

	Protein Content (g)
Triscuit crackers (20 crackers)	7
Bottled water (20 fl. oz)	0
Dinner:	
Cheeseburger:	
Broiled ground beef (½ lb cooked)	64
American cheese (1 oz)	6
Seeded bun (1 large)	6
Ketchup (2 tbsp.)	1
Mustard (1 tbsp.)	1
Shredded lettuce (½ cup)	0.5
Sliced tomato (3 slices)	0.5
French fries (2- to 3-in. strips; 30 fries)	6
Baked beans (2 cups)	28
2% low-fat milk (2 cups)	16
Evening snack:	
Chocolate chip cookies (4 3-in. diameter cookies)	3
2% low-fat milk (1 cup)	8
Total Protein Intake for the Day:	**221.5 g**

As calculated in the You Do the Math box on page 229, Theo's RDA is 72.8 to 91 g of protein. He is consuming 2.4 to 3 times that amount! You can see that he does not need to use amino acid or protein supplements, since he has more than adequate amounts of protein to build lean tissue. Now calculate your own protein intake using food labels and a diet analysis program. Do you obtain more protein from animal or non-animal sources? If you consume mostly non-animal sources, are you eating soy products and complementary foods throughout the day? If you eat animal-based products on a regular basis, notice how much protein you consume from even small servings of meat and dairy products.

There is also a great deal of concern about meat handling practices, as contaminated meat is allowed into our food supply. For example, in 1982, there was an outbreak of severe bloody diarrhea that was eventually traced to hamburgers served at a fast-food restaurant. The hamburgers were contaminated with the *Escherichia coli* O157:H7 bacteria; several people became seriously ill and one child died after eating them. The Centers for Disease Control and Prevention estimates that 73,000 cases of infection and 61 deaths occur each year in the United States due to consuming foods contaminated by this bacterial strain.[15] Although many individuals feel that avoiding meat products will prevent exposure to this deadly strain, this is not true, as alfalfa sprouts, lettuce, and unpasteurized milk and juice are also foods commonly contaminated with it.

TABLE 6.5   Terms and Definitions of a Vegetarian Diet

Type of Diet	Foods Consumed	Comments
Semivegetarian (also called partial vegetarian)	Vegetables, grains, nuts, fruits, legumes; sometimes seafood, poultry, eggs, and dairy products	Typically exclude or limit red meat; may also avoid other meats
Pescovegetarian	Similar to a semivegetarian but excludes poultry	*Pesco* means fish, the only animal source of protein in this diet
Lacto-ovo-vegetarian	Vegetables, grains, nuts, fruits, legumes, dairy products (*lacto*) and eggs (*ovo*)	Excludes animal flesh and seafood
Lactovegetarian	Similar to a lacto-ovo-vegetarian but excludes eggs	Relies on milk and cheese for animal sources of protein
Ovovegetarian	Vegetables, grains, nuts, fruits, legumes, and eggs	Excludes dairy, flesh, and seafood products
Vegan (also called strict vegetarian)	Only plant-based foods (vegetables, grains, nuts, seeds, fruits, legumes)	May not provide adequate vitamin B_{12}, zinc, iron, or calcium
Macrobiotic diet	Vegan-type of diet; becomes progressively more strict until almost all foods are eliminated. At the extreme, only brown rice and small amounts of water or herbal tea are consumed	Taken to the extreme, can cause malnutrition and death
Fruitarian	Only raw or dried fruit, seeds, nuts, honey, and vegetable oil	Very restrictive diet; deficient in protein, calcium, zinc, iron, vitamin B_{12}, riboflavin, and other nutrients

One recent concern surrounding beef that has taken Europe by storm is the epidemic of **mad cow disease.** See the Highlight box for a review of mad cow disease and its impact on the United States and other countries.

Ecological Benefits

Many people choose vegetarianism because of their concerns about the effect of meat industries on the global environment. Due to the high demand for meat in developed nations, meat production has evolved from small family farming operations to the larger system of agribusiness. Critics of agribusiness are concerned with the environmental damages that agribusiness can cause. When animals are raised on smaller farms and/or allowed to range freely, they consume grass, crop wastes, and scraps recycled from the kitchen, which is an efficient means of utilizing food sources that humans do not consume. The waste produced by these animals can be used for fertilizer and fuel.

Activists against agribusiness and meat consumption point out that animals raised in large agribusinesses consume large quantities of grain that humans could consume. Water use can also be tremendous; it is estimated that in the United

mad cow disease A fatal brain disorder prompted by consumption of food containing *prions,* which are abnormally folded infectious proteins found in the brains and other organs of infected sheep, cows, and other livestock.

HIGHLIGHT

Mad Cow Disease—What's the Beef?

Mad cow disease is a fatal brain disorder caused by a *prion*, which is an abnormally folded, infectious protein. Prions influence other proteins to take on their abnormal shape, and these abnormal proteins cause brain damage. Mad cow disease is also called *bovine spongiform encephalopathy (BSE)*. The disease eats away at a cow's brain, leaving it full of spongelike holes. Eventually the brain can no longer control vital life functions, and the cow literally "goes mad." Unfortunately, people who eat infected cattle will also be infected. This disease has killed at least 100 people, most of them in Great Britain.

Scientists are not certain how the prions are introduced to cattle. They think that cattle become infected by eating feed made with the brains and spinal cords of other infected cattle. In Great Britain and Europe, it was common practice to feed livestock with meal made from other animals. Even after exposure, it takes years for mad cow disease to manifest itself. Scientists speculate that older cattle are more infectious than younger animals. Since cattle are slaughtered at an older age in Europe, this increases the risk of passing the disease from one animal to another.

The effect of mad cow disease on the European beef market has been staggering, with beef consumption dropping 25–70% in certain countries; Great Britain, France, and Germany have been particularly affected. Even cattle that are only potentially infected must be slaughtered. To date, almost 5 million cattle have been destroyed.

Three cases of mad cow disease were found in Canada from 2003 to early 2005. To date, no person eating Canadian beef has developed symptoms suggestive of infection. However, the occurrence of this disease in Canadian cattle has prompted the United States to temporarily ban the import of Canadian beef.

In December 2003, the first case of mad cow disease was reported in the United States, shocking those who believed the food supply to be safe from this disease. This discovery prompted many countries to immediately ban importation of American beef. As a result of this discovery,

the federal government and beef industry took aggressive steps to destroy any potentially infected beef. Additional steps taken to protect beef included feeding U.S. cattle high-protein meal made from soybeans and working to ensure that the banning of the use of animal feed made with animal by-products is strictly enforced. In addition, cattle in the United States have for many years been slaughtered at an early age, reducing the likelihood of advanced infection. Finally, the United States has banned the import of all cattle, sheep, and goats from Europe. It is unclear whether, or how long, the ban on Canadian beef will continue.

Should Americans fear our beef supply? The U.S. Department of Agriculture, the FDA, the National Institutes of Health, and the Centers for Disease Control and Prevention are working together to eliminate the use of animal-based feed and to enhance technology that can track signs of the disease and act quickly if it reappears in our food supply. In addition, the U.S. beef industry is highly motivated to comply with safety regulations since reduced beef intake translates into millions of dollars in lost income.

Although it is not possible for the United States to be completely immune to mad cow disease, adherence to strict safety standards should minimize our risk and keep our beef safe for human consumption.

States, it takes 430 gallons of water to produce one pound of pork. This is in contrast to the 151 gallons of water it takes to produce one pound of wheat. Another concern is related to the waste produced from meat production. While much of the waste produced by animals in the agribusiness system is used as fertilizer, some of it can run off into surrounding bodies of water, resulting in the pollution of neighboring streams, rivers, and lakes, as well as irrigation fields for produce crops. Livestock are also blamed for the majority of methane production, which is a gas associated with increased global warming. There is also concern that to provide ample room to raise animals for human consumption, a great deal of land that could be used for plant food production is destroyed. It is speculated that millions of acres of rain forests around the world have been destroyed to provide enough grazing land for livestock and that destroying the rain forests has been a major contributor to global warming.

In response to many of these claims, meat industry organizations have published information in defense of their practices. In a recent fact sheet, the National Cattlemen's Beef Association lists several facts that contradict many of the claims made by agribusiness critics:[16]

- Virtually all of the grain consumed by livestock is unfit for human consumption.

- While it does take more water to produce a pound of beef than a pound of vegetables, the amount is much lower than that claimed by many activists and represents 11% of the total amount of water used in the United States each year.

- The waste produced by cattle is very minor. In fact, the primary source of methane emissions is landfills; only about 2% of the total methane production in the United States comes from domestic livestock.

- Much of the land used to raise livestock is not suitable for use in growing vegetable or grain crops. Interestingly, soil erosion, which is a significant problem in the United States, occurs most extensively with crops such as cotton.

- Although many countries have destroyed significant areas of rain forest to provide grazing land for domestic livestock, less than 1% of the total 2001 beef supply in the United States was imported from rain forest countries, and the largest fast-food chains have policies in place that prohibit the purchase of beef from these same countries.

This is obviously a complex, emotionally and politically charged topic. While some individuals choose vegetarianism to protect the environment, it is not practical or realistic to expect every human around the world to adopt this lifestyle. Animal products provide important nutrients for our bodies, and many people on the brink of starvation cannot survive without small amounts of milk and meat. The environmental damage caused by the raising of livestock is due not only to how animals are raised but also to the large number of animals produced. There is currently a trend toward people reducing their consumption of animal products so that the overall demand for meat is considerably lessened. In this way, many hope that it may be possible to return to the system of small family farming, which is more environmentally friendly. In addition to the environmental benefits, eating less meat may also reduce our risk for chronic diseases such as heart disease and some cancers.

Health Benefits

Still others practice vegetarianism because of its health benefits. Research over several years has consistently shown that a varied and balanced vegetarian diet can reduce the risk of many chronic diseases. Health benefits include the following:[17]

- Reduced intake of fat and total energy, which reduces the risk for obesity. This may in turn lower a person's risk of type 2 diabetes.

- Lower blood pressure, which may be due to a higher intake of fruits and vegetables. People who eat vegetarian diets tend to be nonsmokers, drink little or no alcohol, and exercise more regularly, which are also factors known to reduce blood pressure and help maintain a healthy body weight.

- Reduced risk of heart disease, which may be due to lower saturated fat intake and a higher consumption of *antioxidants* that are found in plant-based foods. Antioxidants, discussed in detail in Chapter 8, are substances that can protect our cells from damage. They are abundant in fruits and vegetables.

- Fewer digestive problems such as constipation and diverticular disease, most likely due to the higher fiber content of vegetarian diets. Diverticular disease, discussed in Chapter 4, occurs when the wall of the bowel (large intestine) pouches and becomes inflamed.

- Reduced risk of some cancers. Research shows that vegetarians may have lower rates of cancer, particularly prostate and colon and rectal cancers.[18] Many components of a vegetarian diet could contribute to reducing cancer risks, including higher fiber, fruit and vegetable, and antioxidant intakes; lower dietary fat intake; lower consumption of **carcinogens** (cancer-causing agents) that are formed when cooking meat; and higher consumption of soy protein, which may have anticancer properties, although the research related to higher soy intake and lower cancer risk is not consistent.[17]

- Reduced risk of kidney disease, kidney stones, and gallstones. The lower protein contents of vegetarian diets, plus the higher intake of legumes and vegetable proteins such as soy, may be protective against these conditions.

What Are the Challenges of a Vegetarian Diet?

While a vegetarian diet can be healthful, it also presents many challenges. By limiting consumption of flesh and dairy products, there is the potential for inadequate intakes of certain nutrients. It is important to emphasize that these nutrients are plentiful in a well-planned lacto-ovo-vegetarian diet but can be of concern in a vegan type of eating pattern. These nutrients include:

A well-balanced vegetarian diet can provide adequate protein and other nutrients.

- Iron, calcium, and zinc: Iron is most readily available from meats, poultry, and fish. Deficiency is not a big concern in vegetarian diets that include eggs, but is a significant concern in vegan diets (see Chapter 10). Calcium is a concern because of the avoidance of milk, yogurt, and cheese. Many adults cannot consume enough calcium from plant sources to meet their daily requirement, and supplementation is advised. Zinc is also commonly low in vegan diets.

- Vitamins D and B_{12}: Both vitamins are typically lower in strict vegan diets. Some cereals and soy milks are now fortified with vitamin D; however, some individuals may still need a vitamin D–containing supplement. Vitamin B_{12}, though found in many fortified breakfast cereals, is not available in any amount from plant foods and must be supplemented in vegan diets.

Table 6.6 provides an overview of the nutrients that can be deficient in a vegan diet plan and describes good non-animal sources that can provide these nutrients.

Vegetarians who consume dairy and/or egg products obtain these nutrients more easily. However, it is important for vegetarians and nonvegetarians to consume a varied and adequate diet. Research indicates that disordered eating practices are more prevalent in university women who report eating a vegetarian diet.[19,20] Instead of eating a healthy variety of non-animal foods, people with disordered eating problems may use vegetarianism as an excuse to restrict many foods from their diets.

Can a vegetarian diet provide enough protein? Since high-quality protein sources are quite easy to obtain in developed countries, a well-balanced vegetarian diet can provide adequate protein. In fact, the American Dietetic Association and Dietitians of Canada endorses an appropriately planned vegetarian diet as healthful, nutritionally adequate, and providing many benefits in reducing and preventing various diseases.[17] As you can see, the emphasis is on a *balanced* and *adequate* vegetarian diet; thus, it is important for vegetarians to consume soy products, eat complementary proteins, and obtain enough energy from other macronutrients to spare protein from being used as an energy source. Although the digestibility of a vegetarian diet is potentially lower than that of an animal-based diet, there is no separate protein recommendation for vegetarians who consume complementary plant proteins.[21]

carcinogens Cancer-causing agents, such as certain pesticides, industrial chemicals, and pollutants.

TABLE 6.6 Nutrients of Concern in a Vegan Diet

Nutrient	Functions	Non-Meat/Non-Dairy Food Sources
Vitamin B_{12}	Assists with DNA synthesis; protection and growth of nerve fibers	Vitamin B_{12}–fortified cereals, yeast, soy products, and other meat analogs; vitamin B_{12} supplements
Vitamin D	Promotes bone growth	Vitamin D-fortified cereals, margarines, and soy products; adequate exposure to sunlight; supplementation may be necessary for those who do not get adequate exposure to sunlight
Riboflavin (vitamin B_2)	Promotes release of energy; supports normal vision and skin health	Whole and enriched grains, green leafy vegetables, mushrooms, beans, nuts, and seeds
Iron	Assists with oxygen transport; involved in making amino acids and hormones	Whole-grain products, prune juice, dried fruits, beans, nuts, seeds, leafy vegetables such as spinach
Calcium	Maintains bone health; assists with muscle contraction, blood pressure, and nerve transmission	Fortified soy milk and tofu, almonds, dry beans, leafy vegetables, calcium-fortified juices, fortified breakfast cereals
Zinc	Assists with DNA and RNA synthesis, immune function, and growth	Whole-grain products, wheat germ, beans, nuts, and seeds

NUTRI-CASE THEO

"No way would I ever become a vegetarian! The only way to build up your muscles is to eat meat. I was reading in a bodybuilding magazine last week about some guy who doesn't eat anything from animals, not even milk or eggs, and he looked pretty buff—but I don't believe it. They can do anything to photos these days. Besides, after a game I just crave red meat. If I don't have it, I feel sort of like my batteries don't get recharged. It's just not practical for a competitive athlete to go without meat."

What two claims does Theo make here about the role of red meat in his diet? Do you think these claims are valid? Why or why not? Without trying to convert Theo to vegetarianism, what facts might you offer him about the nature of plant and animal proteins?

Using the Vegetarian Food Guide Pyramid to Achieve the RDA for Protein

The Vegetarian Food Guide Pyramid was introduced in Chapter 2, and it is illustrated again in **FIGURE 6.14**. Vegetarians can use this pyramid to design a healthful diet that contains all of the necessary nutrients. **FIGURE 6.14** emphasizes the importance of eating whole grains, fruits, vegetables, and legumes at every meal. Daily

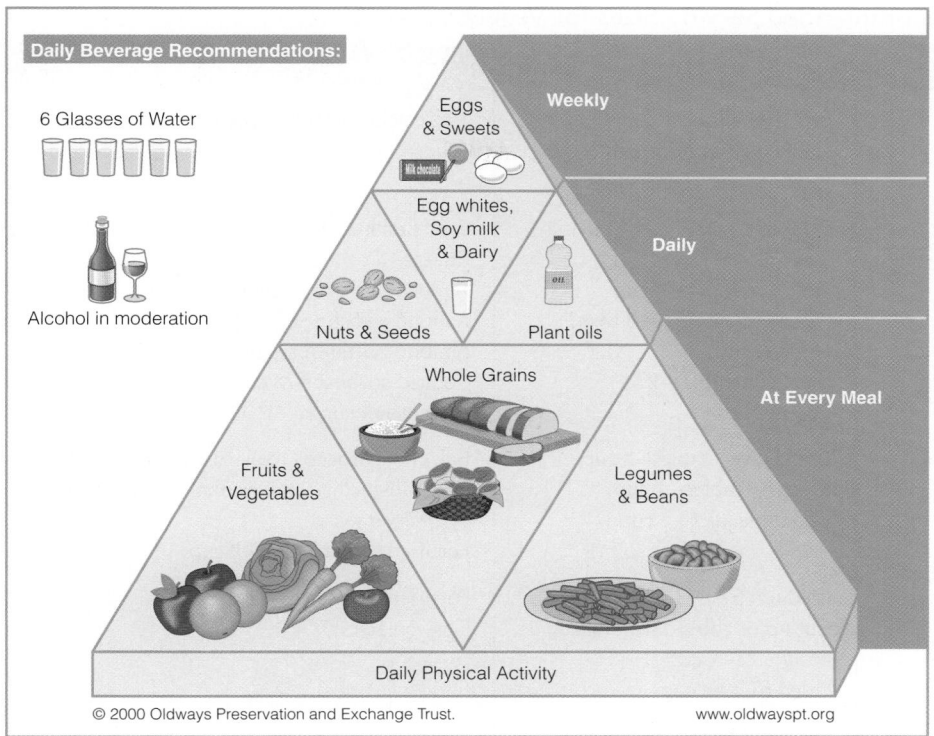

FIGURE 6.14 The Vegetarian Food Guide Pyramid. This pyramid guides general food choices at each meal, daily, and weekly.

foods include nuts and seeds, egg whites, soy milk and dairy products, and plant oils. Weekly choices include eggs and sweets. While this version provides a helpful illustration of the types of foods recommended for vegetarians, it does not give suggestions for daily number of servings.

Table 6.7 lists food groups and serving recommendations for vegetarians.[22] Notice that there is no separate listing for a group exclusive to milk, yogurt, and cheese. It is recommended that vegetarians should eat 8 or more servings each day of calcium-rich foods and that these foods can come from any of the calcium-rich foods listed in each food group. Lacto- and lacto-ovo-vegetarians can consume low-fat or nonfat dairy products, while vegans and ovovegetarians can consume calcium-fortified soy or rice products to meet their calcium needs. Another excellent source of calcium is calcium-fortified orange juice. Vegetarians should consume 5 servings daily of foods from the legumes, nuts, and other protein-rich foods group. It is also recommended that vegetarians consume at least 3 good food sources of vitamin B_{12} each day. Examples of these include 1 cup of fortified soy milk, 1 large egg, ½ cup cow's milk, ¾ cup yogurt, 1 oz of fortified breakfast cereal, and 1½ oz of a fortified meat substitute.

With careful menu planning, vegetarians can meet their nutritional needs. Vegans need to pay special attention to consuming foods high in vitamins D, B_{12}, and riboflavin (B_2) and the minerals calcium, zinc, and iron. Supplementation of these nutrients may be necessary for certain individuals if they cannot consume adequate amounts in their diet.

Vegetarians should eat 5 servings of beans, nuts, seeds, eggs, or meat substitutes daily.

> **RECAP:** *A balanced vegetarian diet may reduce the risk of obesity, type 2 diabetes, heart disease, digestive problems, some cancers, kidney disease, kidney stones, and gallstones. While varied vegetarian diets can provide enough protein, vegetarians who consume no animal products need to supplement their diet with good sources of vitamin B_{12}, vitamin D, riboflavin, iron, calcium, and zinc.*

TABLE 6.7 Food Groups and Recommended Serving Sizes for Vegetarians

Food Group	Number of Servings	Foods and Serving Sizes	Calcium-Rich Food Sources
Grains	6	Bread—1 slice Cooked grain or cereal—½ cup Ready-to-eat cereal—1 oz	1 oz calcium-fortified breakfast cereal
Legumes, nuts, and other protein-rich foods	5	Cooked beans, peas, or lentils—½ cup Tofu or tempeh—½ cup Nut or seed butter—2 tbsp. Nuts—¼ cup Meat substitute—1 oz Egg—1 each	Cow's milk or yogurt or fortified soy milk—½ cup Cheese—¾ oz Tempeh or calcium-set tofu—½ cup Almonds—¼ cup Almond butter or sesame tahini—2 tbsp. Cooked soybeans—½ cup Soy nuts—¼ cup
Vegetables	4	Cooked vegetables—½ cup Raw vegetables—1 cup Vegetable juice—½ cup	Bok choy, broccoli, collards, Chinese cabbage, kale, mustard greens, or okra—1 cup cooked or 2 cups raw Fortified tomato juice—½ cup
Fruits	2	Medium fruit—1 each Cut up or cooked fruit—½ cup Fruit juice—½ cup Dried fruit—¼ cup	Fortified fruit juice—½ cup Figs—5 each
Fats	2	Oil, mayonnaise, or soft margarine—1 tsp.	None

Source: From *Journal of the American Dietetic Association,* V 103(6), Messina et al.: "A new food guide for North American Vegetarians." © 2003 American Dietetic Association. Used by permission of Elsevier.

What Disorders Are Related to Protein Intake or Metabolism?

As we have seen, consuming inadequate protein can result in severe illness and death. Typically, this occurs when people do not consume enough total kilocalories, but a diet deficient specifically in protein can have similar effects.

Protein-Energy Malnutrition Can Lead to Debility and Death

When a person consumes too little protein and energy, the result is **protein-energy malnutrition** (also called *protein-calorie malnutrition*). Two diseases that can follow are marasmus and kwashiorkor (FIGURE 6.15).

Marasmus Results from Grossly Inadequate Energy Intake

Marasmus is a disease that results from grossly inadequate intakes of protein, energy, and other nutrients. Essentially, people with marasmus slowly starve to death. It is most common in young children (6 to 18 months of age) who are living in impoverished conditions. These children are fed diluted cereal drinks that are inadequate in energy, protein, and most nutrients. People suffering from marasmus have the look of "skin and bones" as their body fat and tissues are wasting. Consequences of marasmus include:

- Wasting and weakening of muscles, including the heart muscle
- Stunted brain development and learning impairment

protein-energy malnutrition A disorder caused by inadequate consumption of protein. It is characterized by severe wasting.

marasmus A form of protein-energy malnutrition that results from grossly inadequate intakes of protein, energy, and other nutrients.

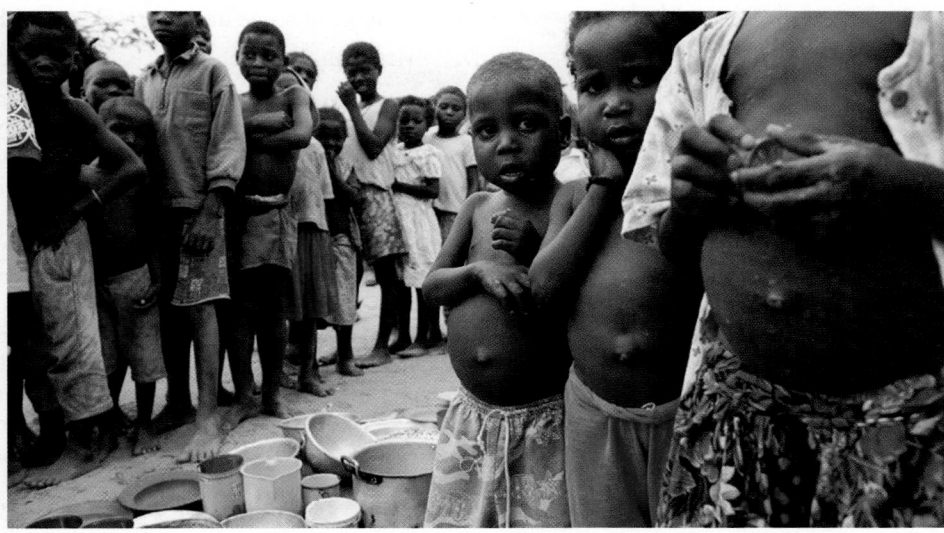

(b)

(a)

FIGURE 6.15 Two forms of protein-energy malnutrition are **(a)** marasmus and **(b)** kwashiorkor.

- Depressed metabolism and little insulation from body fat, causing a dangerously low body temperature
- Stunted physical growth and development
- Deterioration of the intestinal lining, which further inhibits absorption of nutrients
- *Anemia* (abnormally low levels of hemoglobin in the blood)
- Severely weakened immune system
- Fluid and electrolyte imbalances

If marasmus is left untreated, death from dehydration, heart failure, or infection will result. Treating marasmus involves carefully correcting fluid and electrolyte imbalances. Protein and carbohydrates are provided once the body's condition has stabilized. Fat is introduced much later, as the protein levels in the blood must improve to the point where they can carry fat so it can be safely metabolized by the body.

Kwashiorkor Results from a Low-Protein Diet

Kwashiorkor often occurs in developing countries where infants are weaned early due to the arrival of a subsequent baby. This deficiency disease is typically seen in young children (1 to 3 years of age) who no longer drink breast milk. Instead, they often are fed a low-protein, starchy cereal. Unlike marasmus, kwashiorkor often develops quickly and causes the person to look swollen, particularly in the belly. This is because the low protein content of the blood is inadequate to keep fluids from seeping into the tissue spaces. Other symptoms of kwashiorkor include:

- Some weight loss and muscle wasting, with some retention of body fat
- Retarded growth and development; less severe than that seen with marasmus
- Edema, which results in extreme distension of the belly
- Fatty degeneration of the liver
- Loss of appetite, sadness, irritability, apathy

kwashiorkor A form of protein-energy malnutrition that is typically seen in developing countries in infants and toddlers who are weaned early because of the birth of a subsequent child. Denied breast milk, they are fed a cereal diet that provides adequate energy but inadequate protein.

- Development of sores and other skin problems; skin pigmentation changes
- Dry, brittle hair that changes color, straightens, and falls out easily

Kwashiorkor can be reversed if adequate protein and energy are given in time. Because of their severely weakened immune systems, many individuals with kwashiorkor die from diseases they contract in their weakened state. Of those who are treated, many return home to the same impoverished conditions, only to develop this deficiency once again.

Many people think that only children in developing countries suffer from these diseases. However, protein-energy malnutrition occurs in all countries and affects both children and adults. In the United States, poor people living in inner cities and isolated rural areas are affected. Others at risk include the elderly, the homeless, people with eating disorders, those addicted to alcohol and drugs, and individuals with wasting diseases such as AIDS and cancer. Despite producing more than enough food, malnutrition can and does occur in the United States; more information on this topic is provided in the *In Depth* chapter on Global Nutrition on pages 778–787.

Disorders Related to Genetic Abnormalities

There are numerous disorders caused by defects in our DNA, or genetic material. A few of these disorders include phenylketonuria (or PKU), sickle cell anemia, and cystic fibrosis.

As discussed in Chapter 4, *phenylketonuria* is an inherited disease in which a person does not have the ability to break down the amino acid phenylalanine. As a result, phenylalanine and its metabolic by-products build up in the body and cause brain damage if left untreated. Individuals with PKU must eat a diet that is severely limited in phenylalanine.

Sickle cell anemia is an inherited disorder of the red blood cells in which a single amino acid present in hemoglobin is changed. As shown in FIGURE 6.7 (page 218), normal hemoglobin is globular, which results in red blood cells having a round, doughnut-like shape. The genetic alteration that occurs with sickle cell anemia causes the red blood cells to be shaped like a sickle, or a crescent (FIGURE 6.16). Sickled red blood cells are stiff and sticky and so cannot flow smoothly through small blood vessels. The cells rupture easily and become clogged in the vessels, causing reduced blood flow downstream of the area and lack of oxygen to tissues. Severe pain, respiratory distress, stroke, and organ failure can result. This disease occurs in any person who inherits the sickle cell gene from both parents.

Cystic fibrosis is an inherited disease that primarily affects the respiratory system and digestive tract. Cystic fibrosis is caused by an abnormal protein that prevents the normal passage of chloride into and out of certain cells. This alteration in chloride transport causes cells to secrete thick, sticky mucus. The linings of the lungs and pancreas are particularly affected, causing breathing difficulties, lung infections, and digestion problems that lead to nutrient deficiencies. Symptoms include wheezing, coughing, and stunted growth. The severity of this disease varies greatly among those with it; some individuals with cystic fibrosis live relatively normal lives, while others are seriously debilitated and die in childhood.

FIGURE 6.16   A sickled red blood cell.

sickle cell anemia A genetic disorder that causes red blood cells to be sickle-, or crescent-, shaped. These cells cannot travel smoothly through blood vessels, rupture easily, and cause inadequate delivery of oxygen to tissues.

cystic fibrosis A genetic disorder that causes an alteration in chloride transport, leading to the production of thick, sticky mucus that causes life-threatening respiratory and digestive problems.

RECAP: *Protein-energy malnutrition can lead to marasmus and kwashiorkor. These diseases primarily affect impoverished children in developing nations. However, residents of developed countries are also at risk, especially the elderly, the homeless, alcoholics, drug addicts, and people with AIDS, cancer, and other wasting diseases. Genetic disorders that cause protein abnormalities include phenylketonuria, sickle cell anemia, and cystic fibrosis.*

CHAPTER SUMMARY

- Proteins are large, complex molecules that are critical components of all tissues, including blood, bone, and hormones.

- Unlike carbohydrates and fat, the structure of proteins is dictated by DNA, and proteins contain nitrogen.

- Amino acids are the building blocks of proteins; they are composed of a central carbon atom, an amine group, an acid group, a hydrogen atom, and a unique side chain.

- There are twenty amino acids in our bodies: nine are essential amino acids, meaning that our bodies cannot produce them, and we must obtain them from food; eleven are nonessential, meaning that our bodies can make them so they do not need to be consumed in the diet.

- Our genetic makeup determines the sequence of amino acids in our proteins. Gene expression refers to using a gene in a cell to make a protein.

- The three-dimensional shape of proteins determines their function in the body.

- When proteins are exposed to damaging substances such as heat, acids, bases, and alcohol, they are denatured, meaning they lose their shape and function.

- A limiting amino acid is one that is missing or in limited supply, preventing the synthesis of adequate proteins.

- Mutual supplementation is the process of combining two incomplete protein sources to make a complete protein. The two foods involved in this process are called complementary proteins.

- Proteins are needed to promote cell growth, repair, and maintenance. They act as enzymes and hormones; help maintain the balance of fluids, electrolytes, acids, and bases; and support healthy immune function.

- Most digestion of proteins occurs in the small intestine.

- Protein digestibility affects its quality, with proteins that are more digestible being of higher quality. Animal sources, soy protein, and legumes are highly digestible forms of protein.

- The RDA for protein for sedentary people is 0.8 g protein per kg body weight per day; protein should comprise 10–35% of total energy intake.

- Most people in the United States routinely eat 1.5 to 2 times the RDA for protein.

- High protein intakes may be harmful and can lead to increased blood cholesterol levels, increased calcium excretion, and increased risk for kidney disease in people who are susceptible to kidney problems.

- Good sources of protein include meats, dairy products, eggs, legumes, whole grains, and nuts.

- There are many forms of vegetarianism: lacto-ovo-vegetarians eat plant foods plus eggs and dairy products; pescovegetarians consume plant foods and rely on fish as the only meat source; vegans are considered strict vegetarians and consume only plant foods.

- Consuming a well-planned vegetarian diet may reduce the risk of obesity, heart disease, type 2 diabetes, and some forms of cancer.

- Vegans may need to supplement their diet with vitamins B_{12} and D, riboflavin, iron, calcium, and zinc.

- Marasmus and kwashiorkor are two forms of protein-energy malnutrition that results from grossly inadequate energy and protein intake.

- Phenylketonuria is a genetic disease in which the person cannot break down the amino acid phenylalanine. The buildup of phenylalanine and its by-products leads to brain damage.

- Sickle cell anemia is a genetic disorder of the red blood cells. Due to an alteration of one amino acid in hemoglobin, the red blood cells become sickle shaped, rupture easily, and clog smaller blood vessels, resulting in inadequate delivery of oxygen to tissues.

- Cystic fibrosis is a genetic disease that causes an alteration in chloride transport that leads to the production of thick, sticky mucus. This mucus causes serious respiratory and digestive problems, which leads to variable levels of debilitation and, in some cases, premature death.

TEST YOURSELF ANSWERS

1. **False.** Although protein can be used for energy in certain circumstances, fats and carbohydrates are the primary sources of energy for our bodies.

2. **False.** There is no evidence that consuming amino acid supplements assists in building muscle tissue. Exercising muscles, specifically using weight training, is the stimulus needed to build muscle tissue.

3. **False.** Excess protein is broken down and its component parts are either stored as fat or used for energy or tissue building and repair. Only the nitrogen component of protein is excreted in the urine.

4. **False.** Vegetarian diets can meet and even exceed an individual's protein needs, assuming that adequate energy-yielding macronutrients, a variety of protein sources, and complementary protein sources are consumed.

5. **True.** Most people in the United States consume 1.5 to 2 times more protein than they need.

FIND THE QUACK

Colby is sensitive about his slender frame and works out at a public gym three times a week, trying to gain muscle mass. One afternoon, as he is leaving the workout room to head for the showers, he is approached by a friendly looking young man he has never seen at the gym before. Introducing himself as Russ, a new member of the gym, the man compliments Colby on his workout. Colby can't help noticing Russ's extremely muscular physique, and so when he offers to tell Colby all about how he, too, can build muscle fast, Colby agrees to talk with him. Here is what Russ tells him:

- Protein shakes are the secret to gaining muscle.

- Bodybuilding causes microscopic tears in the muscle tissue that have to be repaired with protein. This process of tearing down and rebuilding is increasing Colby's protein requirement so greatly that he cannot get the amount of protein he needs from foods alone.

- Russ asks Colby how much he weighs, and Colby tells him he is 150 pounds. Russ tells Colby that bodybuilders need to eat at least a gram of protein per pound of body weight per day. He says this means that Colby needs to eat a minimum of 150 g of protein every day, and asks him how much protein he is currently consuming. Colby answers that he has no idea, but he eats a sandwich with meat or poultry for lunch most days, and usually has meat at dinner as well. Russ raises his eyebrows. "That's all?" he asks. "You're only getting maybe 50 g of protein a day! How do you expect to build muscle on that?"

- Russ then tells Colby that he must start drinking protein shakes three times a day, first thing in the morning and as a mid-afternoon and evening snack. He also insists that, in addition to these three shakes, Colby drink a protein shake after every workout. He says that, after a workout, the muscles get totally depleted of their protein stores and need to have them replenished. Then he assures Colby that every scoop of the protein powder used for one shake will provide 25 g of pure protein with no fat and no carbohydrates.

Colby asks how much the protein powder costs, but instead of answering, Russ hands him a brochure. "Visit my Web site and register as a first-time buyer and you can order all you want for half-price! I guarantee you, it's a lot less expensive than eating five or six steaks a day, and a lot more convenient, too!"

1. Russ claims that bodybuilders need to consume at least a gram of protein per pound of body weight per day. Does this assertion sound correct to you?

2. Colby weighs 150 pounds and works out intensely with weights three times a week. Refer to the information on pages 226–230 of this chapter. How much protein does Colby actually need to consume each day? Do you think that he is only consuming about 50 g of protein a day, as Russ claims? (Hint: See the Nutrition Label Activity on page 235.)

3. Do our muscles get "totally depleted of their protein stores" after an intensive workout, as Russ claims? Explain your answer.

4. Is Colby at risk for any health problems if he begins to consume 150 g or more of protein every day as Russ suggests?

Answers can be found at www.aw-bc.com/thompson.

REVIEW QUESTIONS

1. The process of combining peanut butter and whole-wheat bread to make a complete protein is called
   a. deamination.
   b. vegetarianism.
   c. transamination.
   d. mutual supplementation.

2. Which of the following meals is typical of the vegan diet?
   a. Rice, pinto beans, acorn squash, soy butter, and almond milk
   b. Veggie dog, bun, and a banana blended with yogurt
   c. Brown rice and green tea
   d. Egg salad on whole-wheat toast, broccoli, carrot sticks, and soy milk

3. The substance that breaks down polypeptides in the small intestine is called
   a. hydrochloric acid.
   b. pepsin.
   c. protease.
   d. ketones.

4. The portion of an amino acid that contains nitrogen is called the
   a. side chain.
   b. amine group.
   c. acid group.
   d. nitrate cluster.

5. Proteins contain
   a. carbon, oxygen, and nitrogen.
   b. oxygen and hydrogen.
   c. carbon, oxygen, hydrogen, and nitrogen.
   d. carbon, oxygen, and hydrogen.

6. True or false? After leaving the small intestine, amino acids are transported to the liver for distribution throughout the body.

7. True or false? When a protein is denatured, its shape is lost but its function is retained.

8. True or false? All hormones are proteins.

9. True or false? Buffers help the body maintain its fluids in proper balance.

10. True or false? Athletes typically require about three times as much protein as nonactive people.

11. Explain the relationship between inadequate protein intake and the swollen bellies of children with kwashiorkor.

12. Explain the relationship between excessive protein intake and an increased risk for kidney disease.

13. Identify six ways in which proteins are indispensable to human functioning.

14. Katja is a 20-year-old lacto-ovo-vegetarian. She takes an aerobics class twice a week and walks 10 minutes to and from campus each day, and requires approximately 2,500 kcal/day to maintain her current body weight. She weighs 130 pounds and wants to maintain her healthful weight. Design a 1-day diet for her that provides the recommended amount of protein and is adequate in total energy.

15. Draw a sketch showing how amino acids bond to form proteins.

WEB LINKS

www.eatright.org
American Dietetic Association

Search for vegetarian diets to learn how to plan healthful meat-free meals.

www.aphis.usda.gov
Animal and Plant Health Inspection Service

Select "Hot Issues" or search for "Bovine Spongiform Encephalopathy (BSE)" to learn more about mad cow disease.

www.vrg.org
The Vegetarian Resource Group

Obtain vegetarian and vegan news, recipes, information, and additional links.

www.beef.org
National Cattlemen's Beef Association

An industry Web site providing information about beef production.

www.cdc.gov
Centers for Disease Control and Prevention

Click on "A-Z Index" to learn more about *E. coli* and mad cow disease.

www.who.int/nut/en
World Health Organization Nutrition Site

Visit this site to find out more about the worldwide magnitude of protein-energy malnutrition and the diseases that can result from inadequate intakes of protein, energy-yielding carbohydrates and fats, and various additional nutrients.

www.nlm.nih.gov/medlineplus
MEDLINE Plus Health Information

Search for "sickle cell anemia" and "cystic fibrosis" to obtain additional resources and the latest news about these inherited diseases.

REFERENCES

1. Vegetarian Resource Group. 2003. *Vegetarian Journal* 2003 Issue 1. www.vrg.org/journal/vj2003issue3/vj2003issue3poll.htm. (Accessed April 2007.)

2. Lemon, P. W. 2000. Beyond the zone: protein needs of active individuals. *J. Am. Coll. Nutr.* 19(5 suppl.):513S–521S.

3. McDowell, M. A., R. R. Briefel, K. Alaimo, A. M. Bischof, C. R. Caughman, M. D. Carroll, C. M. Lona, and C. L. Johnson. 1994. Energy and macronutrient intakes of persons ages 2 months and over in the United States: Third National Health and Nutrition Examination Survey, Phase I 1988–1991. *Adv. Data* 255:1–24.

4. Tillotson, J. L., G. E. Bartsch, D. Gorder, G. A. Grandits, and J. Stamler. 1997. Food group and nutrient intakes at baseline in the Multiple Risk Factor Intervention Trial. *Am. J. Clin. Nutr.* 65(suppl.):228S–257S.

5. Smit, E., J. Nieto, C. J. Crespo, and P. Mitchell. 1999. Estimates of animal and plant protein intake in US adults: results from the Third National Health and Nutrition Examination Survey, 1988–1991. *J. Am. Diet. Assoc.* 99:813–820.

6. Manore, M., and J. Thompson. 2000. *Sport Nutrition for Health and Performance.* Champaign, IL: Human Kinetics.

7. Fleming, R. M. 2000. The effect of high-protein diets on coronary blood flow. *Angiology* 51:817–826.

8. Leitzmann, C. 2005.Vegetarian diets: what are the advantages? *Forum Nutr.* 57:147–156.

9. Szeto, Y. T., T. C. Y. Kwok, and I. F. F. Benzie. 2004. Effects of a long-term vegetarian diet on biomarkers of antioxidant status and cardiovascular disease risk. *Nutrition* 20:863–866.

10. Munger, R. G., J. R. Cerhan, and B. C.-H. Chiu. 1999. Prospective study of dietary protein intake and risk of hip fracture in postmenopausal women. *Am. J. Clin. Nutr.* 69:147–152.

11. Alekel, D. L., A. St. Germain, C. T. Peterson, K. B. Hanson, J. W. Stewart, and T. Toda. 2000. Isoflavone-rich soy protein isolate attenuates bone loss in the lumbar spine of perimenopausal women. *Am. J. Clin. Nutr.* 72:844–852.

12. Kontessis, P., I. Bossinakou, L. Sarika, E. Iliopoulou, A. Papantoniou, R. Trevisan, D. Roussi, K. Stipsanelli, S. Grigorakis, and A. Souvatzoglou. 1995. Renal, metabolic, and hormonal responses to proteins of different origin in normotensive, nonproteinuric type 1 diabetic patients. *Diabet. Care* 18:1233–1240.

13. American Diabetes Association (ADA). 2003. Evidence-based nutrition principles and recommendations for the treatment and prevention of diabetes and related complications. *Diabet. Care* 26:S51–S61.

14. Poortmans, J. R., and O. Dellalieux. 2000. Do regular high protein diets have potential health risks on kidney function in athletes? *Int. J. Sport Nutr.* 10:28–38.

15. Centers for Disease Control and Prevention (CDC). 2004. Division of Bacterial and Mycotic Diseases. Disease Information. *Escherichia coli* O157:H7. www.cdc.gov/ncidod/dbmd/diseaseinfo/escherichiacoli_g.htm. (Accessed April 2007.)

16. National Cattlemen's Beef Association. November 2003. Beef Industry "Factoid" Fighter. www.beef.org/documents/Factoid%20Fighter%20Revisions%2011-03-03.doc. (Accessed April 2007.)

17. American Dietetic Association and Dietitians of Canada. 2003. Position of the American Dietetic Association and Dietitians of Canada: Vegetarian diets. *J. Am. Diet. Assoc.* 103(6):748–765.

18. Fraser, G. E. 1999. Associations between diet and cancer, ischemic heart disease, and all-cause mortality in non-Hispanic white California Seventh-Day Adventists. *Am. J. Clin. Nutr.* 70:532S–538S.

19. McLean, J. A., and S. I. Barr. 2003. Cognitive dietary restraint is associated with eating behaviors, lifestyle practices, personality characteristics, and menstrual irregularity in college women. *Appetite* 40(2):185–192.

20. Klopp, S. A., C. J. Heiss, and H. S. Smith. 2003. Self-reported vegetarianism may be a marker for college women at risk for disordered eating. *J. Am. Diet. Assoc.* 103(6):745–747.

21. Institute of Medicine, Food and Nutrition Board. 2002. *Dietary Reference Intakes for Energy, Carbohydrate, Fiber, Fat, Fatty Acids, Cholesterol, Protein, and Amino Acids (Macronutrients).* Washington, DC: National Academies Press.

22. Messina, V., V. Melina, and A. Reed Mangels. 2003. A new food guide for North American vegetarians. *J. Am. Diet. Assoc.* 103(6):771–775.

23. Taubes, G. 2002. What if fat doesn't make you fat? *The New York Times Magazine,* July 7, section 6.

24. Liebman, B. 2002. Big fat lies: the truth about the Atkins Diet. *Center Sci. Public Interest Nutr. Action Health Letter* 29(9): 1–7.

25. Stern, L., N. Iqbal, P. Seshadri, K. L. Chicano, D. A. Daily, J. McGrory, M. Williams, E. J. Gracely, and F. F. Samaha. 2004. The effects of low-carbohydrate versus conventional weight loss diets in severely obese adults: one-year follow-up of a randomized trial. *Ann. Intern. Med.* 140:778–785.

26. Samaha, F. F., N. Iqbal, P. Seshadri, K. L. Chicano, D. A. Daily, J. McGrory, T. Williams, M. Williams, E. J. Gracely, and L. Stern. 2003. A low-carbohydrate as compared with a low-fat diet in severe obesity. *N. Engl. J. Med.* 348:2074–2081.

27. Foster, G. D., H. R. Wyatt, J. O. Hill, B. G. McGuckin, C. Brill, B. S. Mohammed, P. O. Szapary, D. J. Rader, J. S. Edman, and S. Klein. 2003. A randomized trial of a low-carbohydrate diet for obesity. *N. Engl. J. Med.* 348:2082–2090.

28. Boden, G., K. Sargrad, C. Homko, M. Mozzoli, and T. P. Stein. 2005. Effect of a low-carbohydrate diet on appetite, blood glucose levels, and insulin resistance in obese patients with type 2 diabetes. *Ann. Intern. Med.* 142:403–411.

29. Bravata, D. M., L. Sanders, J. Huang, H. M. Krumholz, I. Olkin, C. D. Gardner, and D. M. Bravata. 2003. Efficacy and safety of low carbohydrate diets. A systematic review. *JAMA* 289:1837–1850.

NUTRITION DEBATE

High-Protein Diets—Are They the Key to Weight Loss?

High-protein diets have been popular over the last 40 years. Very-low-energy, high-protein programs (200 to 400 kcal per day, 1.5 g of protein per kg body weight) were very popular in the 1970s. Many of these diets consisted of low-quality protein, however, and at least fifty-eight people died from heart problems while following them. As a result of these deaths, we now know that these extreme diets are only appropriate for severely obese people and must include high-quality protein sources. Supervision by a qualified physician is critical when following this type of diet plan.

Proponents of high-protein diets claim that you can eat all your favorite foods and still lose weight. Is this possible? Chapter 11 provides a detailed explanation of weight loss. However, the key to weight loss is eating less energy than you expend. If you eat more energy than you expend, you can gain weight. Thus, any type of diet, even high-protein diets, must contain fewer kilocalories than a person expends to result in weight loss.

It is important to recognize that high-protein diets are synonymous with low-carbohydrate diets, since high-protein foods typically replace those high in carbohydrates. In addition, many high-protein diets are also high in fat. It is well established that reducing carbohydrate intake causes the body to break down its stored carbohydrate (or glycogen) in the liver and muscle; this is necessary to maintain blood glucose levels and provide energy to the brain. As water is stored along with glycogen, using stored carbohydrate for energy results in the loss of water from the body, which registers on the scale as rapid weight loss.

There are many supporters of high-protein diets, particularly people supporting the Atkins Diet. A highly controversial article in support of the Atkins Diet was published in the *New York Times Magazine*.[23] In this article, the Atkins Diet is touted as the most effective program for weight loss. Supporters of this diet emphasize that eating a high-carbohydrate diet (including potatoes, white bread, pasta, and refined sugars) has caused obesity in the United States. Supporters emphasize that not

High-protein diets are a multimillion-dollar industry.

only does the Atkins Diet result in substantial weight loss, but also it does not cause unhealthy changes in blood cholesterol despite its high saturated fat content.

Detractors of the Atkins Diet tell a different story. According to many nutrition and obesity experts, the U.S. population is substantially overweight because we eat too many calories, not because of eating too much carbohydrate or fat per se. There are a number of potential health risks associated with eating a low-carbohydrate (and high-fat) diet, and these risk factors have prevented many nutrition experts from endorsing the Atkins Diet as a healthy weight loss plan. Some of these health risks include the following:

- Low blood glucose levels, or hypoglycemia, leading to low energy levels, diminished cognitive functioning, and elevated ketones. As high-protein diets are low in carbohydrate, the body does not receive enough glucose to maintain brain function. This could lead to low energy levels (which could prevent some people from exercising regularly) and detrimental changes in memory and cognitive function. Because blood glucose levels are not sufficient to support brain function, the body produces ketones from body fat, as ketones are an alternative energy source for the brain and central nervous system when carbohydrate is not available. High ketone levels in the blood can be toxic, as they increase blood acidity. This state is called *ketoacidosis*, and it can be dangerous if maintained over a prolonged period of time. Left untreated, increased blood acidity causes disorientation, eventual loss of consciousness, coma, and even death. Despite this concern, there is no evidence that following the Atkins Diet has resulted in any serious disability or death due to ketoacidosis.

- Increased risk of heart disease caused by eating foods high in saturated fat. The Atkins Diet promotes the consumption of foods that are high in protein and saturated fat. For instance, daily intakes of cheese, whole-fat dairy products, and fatty meats such as bacon, sausage, and regular ground beef are encouraged. It is well established that eating a diet high in saturated fat increases a person's LDL-cholesterol, which in turn increases the risk for heart disease.

- Increased risk of some forms of cancer due to eating a diet that is high in fat and low in fiber. As the Atkins Diet recommends few, if any, foods that contain fiber and antioxidants, many nutrition experts are concerned that eating this type of a diet over many years will increase a person's risk for some forms of cancer.

It appears that the Atkins Diet will continue to be controversial for many years. After the publication of the article in the *New York Times Magazine*, the Center for Science in the Public Interest (CSPI) published a response that claimed irresponsible and inaccurate reporting.[24] CSPI interviewed many of the experts quoted in the article as supporting the Atkins Diet. These experts state they were misquoted or quoted out of context and that the information they shared that was contrary to supporting the Atkins Diet was ignored.

Are there any research studies to support the contention that the Atkins Diet is effective for weight loss? Until recently, most reports of substantial weight loss on this diet were anecdotal, meaning they came from individuals who were not participants in a controlled, scientific study. However, a few randomized controlled trials conducted over 1 year have recently shed light on the effects low-carbohydrate diets have on weight loss in obese individuals. Stern and colleagues placed participants on either the Atkins Diet or a low-fat diet plan recommended by the American Heart Association.[25] Participants consuming the Atkins Diet lost significantly more weight than those on the low-fat diet during the first 6 months, but weight loss between the two groups was no longer different after 1 year.[26] People consuming the Atkins Diet had lower triglyceride levels and had less of a decrease in HDL-cholesterol (the "good" cholesterol) as compared with people eating the low-fat diet. In another study conducted over a 1-year period using similar diet plans, the results were quite similar.[27]

Few of these trials have included participants with type 2 diabetes, which is a group that could benefit from both weight loss and a decreased intake of refined carbohydrate foods. Boden and colleagues studied how ten peo-

Many people will try any diet to lose weight, but is it worth it in the long run?

ple with type 2 diabetes responded after following the Atkins diet for 2 weeks.[28] Unlike the relatively larger randomized controlled trials done previously, the researchers in this study controlled food intake by having the participants select approved foods through a modified hospital diet. All foods consumed were weighed and recorded daily. Participants were found to lose an average of 1.65 kg (or 3.63 lb) of body weight during the 2-week study period. Surprisingly, this rapid loss of body weight was not exclusively due to the loss of body water in all participants. In fact, six participants lost body water, three participants gained body water, and one had no change in body water during the diet period. Positive changes in the health of these individuals included normalization of blood glucose levels, an increase in insulin sensitivity, and significant decreases in blood triglyceride and cholesterol levels. The participants were able to lose weight because they spontaneously reduced their energy intake by 1,000 kcal per day. It is important to emphasize that this study is of a very short duration and included only ten people. The researchers concluded that this diet was beneficial in the short term, but they recognized that we cannot speculate about the long-term implications of this type of diet.

A recent review of all of the published studies of low-carbohydrate diets resulted in the conclusion that there are not enough data to currently make recommendations for or against the use of low-carbohydrate diets.[29] The authors of this review state that the weight loss that occurs with low-carbohydrate diets appears to be associated with a decreased energy intake and longer diet duration and is not necessarily due to the reduced carbohydrate content of the diet per se. Thus, at this time, it is not possible to state with any certainty that the Atkins Diet is better than other diet plans recommending higher carbohydrate intakes. The long-term health implications of this type of a diet are also unknown at this time, and more research must be conducted in this area.

Should you adopt a high-protein diet? This is not an easy question to answer. Each of us must decide on the type of diet to consume based on our own needs, preferences, health risks, and lifestyle. At the present time,

there is not enough evidence to prove that the Atkins Diet or other high-protein diets are better or worse alternatives to higher carbohydrate, lower fat diets. Based on what we currently know, the healthiest weight loss plans are those that are moderately reduced in energy intake and contain ample fruits, vegetables, and whole grains; adequate carbohydrate and protein; moderate amounts of total fat; and relatively low amounts of saturated fat. It is also important to choose a food plan that you can follow throughout your lifetime. By researching the benefits and risks of various diet plans, you can make an educated decision about the type of diet that will work best to maintain a healthful weight and muscle mass and provide enough energy and nutrients to maintain your lifestyle and your long-term health.

Vitamins and Minerals: Micronutrients with Macro Powers

WANT TO FIND OUT. . .

- how a few fortunate accidents led to the discovery of micronutrients? p. 253

- where vitamins and minerals come from?
  pp. 253–257

- why large doses of certain micronutrients could kill you—and which ones?   p. 262

- whether micronutrient supplements have the same health benefits as nutrients in whole foods?
  pp. 262–263

READ ON.

have you heard the one about the college student on the junk-food diet who developed scurvy, a disease caused by inadequate intake of vitamin C? This "urban legend" seems to circulate on most college campuses every year, but that might be because there's some truth behind it. Away from their families, many college students do adopt diets that are deficient in one or more micronutrients. For instance, some students adopt a vegan diet with insufficient iron, whereas others stop choosing foods rich in calcium and vitamin D. Why is it important to consume adequate levels of the micronutrients, and exactly what constitutes a micronutrient anyway? This *In Depth* explores the discovery of micronutrients, their classification and naming, and their impact on our health.

Discovering the "Hidden" Nutrients

As you recall from Chapter 1, there are three general classes of nutrients. Fluids provide water, which is essential for our survival and helps regulate many body functions. Macronutrients, which include carbohydrates, fats, and proteins, provide energy; thus, we need to consume them in relatively large amounts. **Micronutrients,** which include vitamins and minerals, are needed in much smaller amounts. They assist body functions like energy metabolism and the formation and maintenance of healthy cells and tissues.

Much of our knowledge of vitamins and minerals comes from accidental observations of animals and humans. For instance, in the 1890s, a Dutch physician by the name of C. Eijkman noticed that chickens fed polished rice developed paralysis, which could be reversed by feeding them whole-grain rice. Noting the high incidence of beriberi, which results in extensive nerve damage, among hospital patients fed polished rice, he hypothesized that a highly refined diet was the main cause of beriberi. We now know that whole-grain rice, with its nutrient-rich bran layer, contains the vitamin thiamin and that thiamin deficiency results in beriberi. Similarly, in the early 1900s, it was observed that Japanese children living in fishing villages rarely developed a type of blindness common among Japanese children who did not eat fish. Experiments soon showed that cod liver oil, chicken liver, and eel fat prevented the disorder. We now know that each of these foods contains vitamin A, which is essential for healthy vision.

Such observations were followed by years of laboratory research before nutritionists came to fully accept the idea that very small amounts of substances present in food were critical to good health. In 1906, the term *accessory factors* was coined by the English scientist F. G. Hopkins; we now categorize these accessory factors as vitamins and minerals.

How Are Vitamins Classified?

Vitamins are carbon-containing compounds that regulate a wide range of body processes. Of the thirteen vitamins recognized as essential, humans can synthesize only small amounts of

Fruits contain many vitamins.

vitamins D and K, so we must consume virtually all the vitamins in our diets. Almost everyone who eats a varied and healthful diet can readily meet their vitamin needs from foods alone. The exceptions to this will be discussed shortly.

Fat-Soluble Vitamins

Vitamins A, D, E, and K are **fat-soluble vitamins** (Table 1). They are found in the fatty portions of foods (butterfat, cod liver oil, corn oil, etc.) and are absorbed along with dietary fat. Fat-containing meats, dairy products, nuts, seeds, vegetable oils, and avocados are all sources of one or more fat-soluble vitamins.

In general, the fat-soluble vitamins are readily stored in the body's adipose tissue; thus, we don't need to consume them every single day. While this may simplify day-to-day menu planning, there is

Avocados are a source of fat-soluble vitamins.

micronutrients Nutrients that are needed in the daily diet in relatively small amounts; vitamins and minerals are micronutrients.

vitamins Organic compounds that assist in regulating body processes.

fat-soluble vitamins Vitamins that are not soluble in water but are soluble in fat, including vitamins A, D, E, and K.

TABLE 1 Fat-Soluble Vitamins

Vitamin Name	Primary Functions	Recommended Intake*	Reliable Food Sources	Toxicity/Deficiency Symptoms
A (retinol, retinal, retinoic acid)	Required for ability of eyes to adjust to changes in light Protects color vision Assists cell differentiation Required for sperm production in men and fertilization in women Contributes to healthy bone Contributes to healthy immune system	RDA: Men = 900 µg Women = 700 µg UL = 3,000 µg/day	Preformed retinol: Beef and chicken liver, egg yolks, milk Carotenoid precursors: Spinach, carrots, mango, apricots, cantaloupe, pumpkin, yams	*Toxicity:* Fatigue; bone and joint pain; spontaneous abortion and birth defects of fetuses in pregnant women; nausea and diarrhea; liver damage; nervous system damage; blurred vision; hair loss; skin disorders *Deficiency:* Night blindness, xerophthalmia; impaired growth, immunity, and reproductive function
D (cholecalciferol)	Regulates blood calcium levels Maintains bone health Assists cell differentiation	AI (assumes that person does not get adequate sun exposure): Adult aged 19 to 50 = 5 µg/day Adult aged 50 to 70 = 10 µg/day Adult aged >70 = 15 µg/day UL = 50 µg/day	Canned salmon and mackerel, milk, fortified cereals	*Toxicity:* Hypercalcemia *Deficiency:* Rickets in children; osteomalacia and/or osteoporosis in adults
E (tocopherol)	As a powerful antioxidant, protects cell membranes, polyunsaturated fatty acids, and vitamin A from oxidation Protects red blood cells Enhances immune function Improves absorption of vitamin A	RDA: Men = 15 mg/day Women = 15 mg/day UL = 1,000 mg/day	Sunflower seeds, almonds, vegetable oils, fortified cereals	*Toxicity:* Rare *Deficiency:* Hemolytic anemia; impairment of nerve, muscle, and immune function
K (phylloquinone, menaquinone, menadione)	Serves as a coenzyme during production of specific proteins that assist in blood coagulation and bone metabolism	AI: Men = 120 µg/day Women = 90 µg/day	Kale, spinach, turnip greens, brussels sprouts	*Toxicity:* None known *Deficiency:* Impaired blood clotting; possible effect on bone health

*Abbreviations: RDA, Recommended Dietary Allowance; UL, upper limit; AI, Adequate Intake.

also a disadvantage to our ability to store these nutrients. When we consume more of them than we can use, they build up in the adipose tissue, liver, and other tissues and can reach toxic levels. Symptoms of fat-soluble vitamin toxicity, described in Table 1, include damage to our hair, skin, bones, eyes, and nervous system. Overconsumption of vitamin supplements is the most common cause of vitamin toxicity in the United States; rarely do our dietary choices lead to toxicity. Of the four fat-soluble vitamins, vitamins A and D are the most toxic; **megadosing** with ten or more times the recommended intake of either can result in irreversible organ damage and even death.

Even though we can store the fat-soluble vitamins, deficiencies can occur, especially in people who have a disorder that reduces their ability to absorb dietary fat. In addition, people who are "fat phobic," or eat very small amounts of dietary fat, are at risk for a deficiency. The consequences of fat-soluble vitamin deficiencies, described in Table 1, include osteoporosis, the loss of night vision, and even death in the most severe cases.

Water-Soluble Vitamins

Vitamin C (ascorbic acid) and the B-complex vitamins (thiamin, riboflavin, niacin, vitamin B_6, vitamin B_{12}, folate, pantothenic acid, and biotin) are all **water-soluble vitamins** (Table 2). They are found in a wide variety of foods, including whole grains, fruits, vegetables, meats, and dairy products. They are easily absorbed through the intestinal tract directly into the bloodstream, where they then travel to target cells.

Water-soluble vitamins can be found in a variety of foods.

With the exception of vitamin B_{12}, we do not store large amounts of water-soluble vitamins. Instead, our kidneys filter from our bloodstream any excess amounts, and they are excreted in urine. Because we do not store large amounts of these vitamins in our tissues, toxicity is rare. When it does occur, however, it is often from overuse of high-potency vitamin supplements. Toxicity can cause nerve damage and skin lesions.

Since most water-soluble vitamins are not stored in large amounts, they need to be consumed on a daily or weekly basis. Deficiency symptoms, including diseases or syndromes, can arise fairly quickly, especially during fetal development and in growing infants and children. The signs of water-soluble vitamin deficiency vary widely and are identified in Table 2.

Same Vitamin, Different Names and Forms

Food and supplement labels, magazine articles, and even nutrition textbooks such as this often use simplified alphabetic (A, D, E, K) names for the fat-soluble vitamins. The letters reflect their order of discovery: Vitamin A was discovered in 1916, whereas vitamin K was not isolated until 1939. These lay terms, however, are more appropriately viewed as "umbrellas" that unify a small cluster of chemically related compounds. For example, the term *vitamin A* refers to the specific compounds retinol, retinal, and retinoic acid. There are eight naturally occurring forms of *vitamin E*, known as tocopherols, the primary form of which is alpha-tocopherol. Compounds with *vitamin D* activity include cholecalciferol and ergocalciferol, and the *vitamin K* "umbrella" includes phylloquinone and menaquinone. As you can see, most of the individual compounds making up a fat-soluble vitamin cluster have similar chemical designations (tocopherols, calciferols, etc.). Table 1 lists both the alphabetic and chemical terms for the fat-soluble vitamins.

Similarly, there are both alphabetic and chemical designations for water-soluble vitamins. In some cases, such as *vitamin C* and *ascorbic acid*, you may be familiar with both terms. But few people would recognize *cobalamin* as designating the same micronutrient as *vitamin B_{12}*. Some of the water-soluble vitamins, such as niacin and vitamin B_6, mimic the "umbrella" clustering seen with vitamins A, E, D, and K: the term *vitamin B_6* includes pyridoxal, pyridoxine, and pyridoxamine. If you read any of these three terms on a supplement label, you'll know it refers to vitamin B_6.

Some vitamins exist in only one form. For example, thiamin is the only chemical compound known as *vitamin B_1*. There are no other related chemical compounds. Table 2 lists both the alphabetic and chemical terms for the water-soluble vitamins.

How Are Minerals Classified?

Minerals are inorganic (non-carbon-containing) elements such as calcium, iron, and zinc. As elements, they are already in the simplest chemical form possible and

megadoses Nutrient intakes that are ten or more times the recommended amount.

water-soluble vitamins Vitamins that are soluble in water, including vitamin C and the B-complex vitamins.

minerals Inorganic substances that are not broken down during digestion or absorption; they assist in regulating body processes.

TABLE 2 Water-Soluble Vitamins

Vitamin Name	Primary Functions	Recommended Intake*	Reliable Food Sources	Toxicity/Deficiency Symptoms
Thiamin (vitamin B_1)	Required as enzyme cofactor for carbohydrate and amino acid metabolism	RDA: Men = 1.2 mg/day Women = 1.1 mg/day	Pork, fortified cereals, enriched rice and pasta, peas, tuna, legumes	*Toxicity:* None known *Deficiency:* Beriberi; fatigue, apathy, decreased memory, confusion, irritability, muscle weakness
Riboflavin (vitamin B_2)	Required as enzyme cofactor for carbohydrate and fat metabolism	RDA: Men = 1.3 mg/day Women = 1.1 mg/day	Beef liver, shrimp, milk and dairy foods, fortified cereals, enriched breads and grains	*Toxicity:* None known *Deficiency:* Ariboflavinosis; swollen mouth and throat; seborrheic dermatitis; anemia
Niacin, nicotinamide, nicotinic acid	Required for carbohydrate and fat metabolism Plays role in DNA replication and repair and cell differentiation	RDA: Men = 16 mg/day Women = 14 mg/day UL = 35 mg/day	Beef liver, most cuts of meat/fish/poultry, fortified cereals, enriched breads and grains, canned tomato products	*Toxicity:* Flushing, liver damage, glucose intolerance, blurred vision *Deficiency:* Pellagra; vomiting, constipation, or diarrhea; apathy
Pyridoxine, pyridoxal, pyridoxamine (vitamin B_6)	Required as enzyme cofactor for carbohydrate and amino acid metabolism Assists synthesis of blood cells	RDA: Men and women aged 19 to 50 = 1.3 mg/day Men aged >50 = 1.7 mg/day Women aged >50 = 1.5 mg/day UL = 100 mg/day	Chickpeas (garbanzo beans), most cuts of meat/fish/poultry, fortified cereals, white potatoes	*Toxicity:* Nerve damage, skin lesions *Deficiency:* Anemia; seborrheic dermatitis; depression, confusion, and convulsions
Folate (folic acid)	Required as enzyme cofactor for amino acid metabolism Required for DNA synthesis Involved in metabolism of homocysteine	RDA: Men = 400 µg/day Women = 400 µg/day UL = 1,000 µg/day	Fortified cereals, enriched breads and grains, spinach, legumes (lentils, chickpeas, pinto beans), greens (spinach, romaine lettuce), liver	*Toxicity:* Masks symptoms of vitamin B_{12} deficiency, specifically signs of nerve damage *Deficiency:* Macrocytic anemia; neural tube defects in a developing fetus; elevated homocysteine levels
Cobalamin (vitamin B_{12})	Assists with formation of blood Required for healthy nervous system function Involved as enzyme cofactor in metabolism of homocysteine	RDA: Men = 2.4 µg/day Women = 2.4 µg/day	Shellfish, all cuts of meat/fish/poultry, milk and dairy foods, fortified cereals	*Toxicity:* None known *Deficiency:* Pernicious anemia; tingling and numbness of extremities; nerve damage; memory loss, disorientation, and dementia
Pantothenic acid	Assists with fat metabolism	AI: Men = 5 mg/day Women = 5 mg/day	Meat/fish/poultry, shiitake mushrooms, fortified cereals, egg yolk	*Toxicity:* None known *Deficiency:* Rare

*Abbreviations: RDA, Recommended Dietary Allowance; UL, upper limit; AI, Adequate Intake.

TABLE 2   Water-Soluble Vitamins, *continued*

Vitamin Name	Primary Functions	Recommended Intake*	Reliable Food Sources	Toxicity/Deficiency Symptoms
Biotin	Involved as enzyme cofactor in carbohydrate, fat, and protein metabolism	RDA: Men = 30 μg/day Women = 30 μg/day	Nuts, egg yolk	*Toxicity:* None known *Deficiency:* Rare
Ascorbic acid (vitamin C)	Antioxidant in extracellular fluid and lungs Regenerates oxidized vitamin E Assists with collagen synthesis Enhances immune function Assists in synthesis of hormones, neurotransmitters, and DNA Enhances iron absorption	RDA: Men = 90 mg/day Women = 75 mg/day Smokers = 35 mg more per day than RDA UL = 2,000 mg	Sweet peppers, citrus fruits and juices, broccoli, strawberries, kiwi	*Toxicity:* Nausea and diarrhea, nosebleeds, increased oxidative damage, increased formation of kidney stones in people with kidney disease *Deficiency:* Scurvy; bone pain and fractures, depression, and anemia

*Abbreviations: RDA, Recommended Dietary Allowance; UL, upper limit; AI, Adequate Intake.

Plants absorb minerals from soil and water.

are not digested or broken down prior to absorption. Unlike vitamins, they cannot be synthesized in the laboratory or by any plant or animal, including humans. The minerals in our foods ultimately come from the environment; for example, the selenium in soil and water is taken up into plants and then incorporated into the animals that eat the plants. Whether humans eat the plant foods directly or eat the animal products, all of the minerals in our food supply originate from Mother Earth!

Major Minerals

Major minerals are those that are required in amounts of at least 100 mg per day. In addition, these minerals are found in the human body in amounts of 5 g (5,000 mg) or higher. There are seven major minerals: sodium, potassium, phosphorus, chloride, calcium, magnesium, and sulfur. Table 3 summarizes the primary functions, recommended intakes, food sources, and toxicity/deficiency symptoms of these minerals.

Trace Minerals

Trace minerals are those we need to consume in amounts of less than 100 mg per day. They are found in the human body in amounts of less than 5 g (5,000 mg). Currently, the Dietary Reference Intake (DRI) Committee recognizes eight trace minerals as essential for human health: selenium, fluoride, iodine, chromium, manganese, iron, zinc, and copper.[1] Table 4 identifies the primary functions, recommended intakes, food sources, and toxicity, and deficiency symptoms of these minerals.

Minerals help maintain healthy skin and nails.

major minerals Minerals that must be consumed in amounts of 100 mg/day or more and that are present in the body at the level of 5 g or more.

trace minerals Minerals that must be consumed in amounts of less than 100 mg/day and that are present in the body at the level of less than 5 g.

TABLE 3   Major Minerals

Mineral Name	Primary Functions	Recommended Intake*	Reliable Food Sources	Toxicity/Deficiency Symptoms
Sodium	Fluid balance Acid–base balance Transmission of nerve impulses Muscle contraction	AI: Adults = 1.5 g/day (1,500 mg/day)	Table salt, pickles, most canned soups, snack foods, cured luncheon meats, canned tomato products	*Toxicity:* Water retention, high blood pressure, loss of calcium *Deficiency:* Muscle cramps, dizziness, fatigue, nausea, vomiting, mental confusion
Potassium	Fluid balance Transmission of nerve impulses Muscle contraction	AI: Adults = 4.7 g/day (4,700 mg/day)	Most fresh fruits and vegetables: potatoes, bananas, tomato juice, orange juice, melons	*Toxicity:* Muscle weakness, vomiting, irregular heartbeat *Deficiency:* Muscle weakness, paralysis, mental confusion, irregular heartbeat
Phosphorus	Fluid balance Bone formation Component of ATP, which provides energy for our bodies	RDA: Adults = 700 mg/day	Milk/cheese/yogurt, soy milk and tofu, legumes (lentils, black beans), nuts (almonds, peanuts and peanut butter), poultry	*Toxicity:* Muscle spasms, convulsions, low blood calcium *Deficiency:* Muscle weakness, muscle damage, bone pain, dizziness
Chloride	Fluid balance Transmission of nerve impulses Component of stomach acid (HCl) Antibacterial	AI: Adults = 2.3 g/day (2,300 mg/day)	Table salt	*Toxicity:* None known *Deficiency:* Dangerous blood acid–base imbalances, irregular heartbeat
Calcium	Primary component of bone Acid–base balance Transmission of nerve impulses Muscle contraction	AI: Adults aged 19 to 50 = 1,000 mg/day Adults aged >50 = 1,200 mg/day UL = 2,500 mg/day	Milk/yogurt/cheese (best absorbed form of calcium), sardines, collard greens and spinach, calcium-fortified juices	*Toxicity:* Mineral imbalances, shock, kidney failure, fatigue, mental confusion *Deficiency:* Osteoporosis, convulsions, heart failure
Magnesium	Component of bone Muscle contraction Assists more than 300 enzyme systems	RDA: Men aged 19 to 30 = 400 mg/day Men aged >30 = 420 mg/day Women aged 19 to 30 = 310 mg/day Women aged >30 = 320 mg/day UL = 350 mg/day (supplements)	Greens (spinach, kale, collards), whole grains, seeds, nuts, legumes (navy and black beans)	*Toxicity:* None known *Deficiency:* Low blood calcium, muscle spasms or seizures, nausea, weakness, increased risk of chronic diseases such as heart disease, hypertension, osteoporosis, and type 2 diabetes
Sulfur	Component of certain B-vitamins and amino acids Acid–base balance Detoxification in liver	No DRI	Protein-rich foods	*Toxicity:* None known *Deficiency:* None known

*Abbreviations: RDA, Recommended Dietary Allowance; UL, upper limit; AI, Adequate Intake; DRI, Dietary Reference Intake.

TABLE 4 Trace Minerals

Mineral Name	Primary Functions	Recommended Intake*	Reliable Food Sources	Toxicity/Deficiency Symptoms
Selenium	Required for carbohydrate and fat metabolism	RDA: Adults = 55 mg/day UL = 400 μg/day	Nuts, shellfish, meat/fish/poultry, whole grains	*Toxicity:* Brittle hair and nails, skin rashes, nausea and vomiting, weakness, liver disease *Deficiency:* Specific forms of heart disease and arthritis, impaired immune function, muscle pain and wasting
Fluoride	Development and maintenance of healthy teeth and bones	RDA: Men = 4 mg/day Women = 3 mg/day UL: 2.2 mg/day for children aged 4 to 8; children aged >8 = 10 mg/day		*Toxicity:* Fluorosis of teeth and bones *Deficiency:* Dental caries, low bone density
Iodine	Synthesis of thyroid hormones Temperature regulation Reproduction and growth	RDA: Adults = 150 μg/day UL = 1,100 μg/day		*Toxicity:* Goiter *Deficiency:* Goiter, hypothyroidism, cretinism in infant of mother who is iodine deficient
Chromium	Glucose transport Metabolism of DNA and RNA Immune function and growth	AI: Men aged 19 to 50 = 35 μg/day Men aged >50 = 30 μg/day Women aged 19 to 50 = 25 μg/day Women aged >50 = 20 μg/day		*Toxicity:* None known *Deficiency:* Elevated blood glucose and blood lipids, damage to brain and nervous system
Manganese	Assists many enzyme systems Synthesis of protein found in bone and cartilage	AI: Men = 2.3 mg/day Women = 1.8 mg/day UL = 11 mg/day for adults		*Toxicity:* Impairment of neuromuscular system *Deficiency:* Impaired growth and reproductive function, reduced bone density, impaired glucose and lipid metabolism, skin rash
Iron	Component of hemoglobin in blood cells Component of myoglobin in muscle cells Assists many enzyme systems	RDA: Adult men = 8 mg/day Women aged 19 to 50 = 18 mg/day Women aged >50 = 8 mg/day	Meat/fish/poultry (best absorbed form of iron), fortified cereals, legumes, spinach	*Toxicity:* Nausea, vomiting, and diarrhea; dizziness, confusion; rapid heartbeat, organ damage, death *Deficiency:* Iron-deficiency microcytic (small red blood cells), hypochromic anemia

*Abbreviations: RDA, Recommended Dietary Allowance; UL, upper limit; AI, Adequate Intake; DRI, Dietary Reference Intake.

(continued)

TABLE 4   Trace Minerals, *continued*

Mineral Name	Primary Functions	Recommended Intake*	Reliable Food Sources	Toxicity/Deficiency Symptoms
Zinc	Assists more than 100 enzyme systems Immune system function Growth and sexual maturation Gene regulation	RDA: Men = 11 mg/day Women = 8 mg/day UL = 40 mg/day	Meat/fish/poultry (best absorbed form of zinc), fortified cereals, legumes	*Toxicity:* Nausea, vomiting, and diarrhea; headaches, depressed immune function, reduced absorption of copper *Deficiency:* Growth retardation, delayed sexual maturation, eye and skin lesions, hair loss, increased incidence of illness and infection
Copper	Assists many enzyme systems Iron transport	RDA: Adults = 900 μg/day UL = 10 mg/day	Shellfish, organ meats, nuts, legumes	*Toxicity:* Nausea, vomiting, and diarrhea; liver damage *Deficiency:* Anemia, reduced levels of white blood cells, osteoporosis in infants and growing children

*Abbreviations: RDA, Recommended Dietary Allowance; UL, upper limit; AI, Adequate Intake.

Same Mineral, Different Forms

Unlike most vitamins, which can be identified by either alphabetic designations or the more complicated chemical terms, minerals are known by one name only. Iron, calcium, sodium, and all other minerals are simply referred to by their chemical name. That said, minerals do often exist within different chemical compounds; for example, a supplement label might identify calcium as calcium lactate, calcium gluconate, or calcium citrate. As we will discuss shortly, these different chemical compounds, while all containing the same elemental mineral, may differ in their ability to be absorbed by the body.

How Do Our Bodies Use Micronutrients?

In Chapter 3, we investigated the truth behind the claim that "You are what you eat." We found out that the body has to change food in order to use it. This is also true for foods containing vitamins and minerals, because the micronutrients found in foods and supplements are not always in a chemical form that can be used by our cells. This discussion will highlight some of the ways in which our bodies modify the food forms of vitamins and minerals in order to maximize their absorption and utilization.

What We Eat Differs from What We Absorb

The most healthful diet is of no value to our bodies unless the nutrients can be absorbed and transported to the cells that need them. Unlike carbohydrates, fats, and proteins, which are efficiently absorbed (85–99% of what is eaten makes it into the blood), some micronutrients are so poorly absorbed that only 3–10% of what is eaten ever arrives in the bloodstream.

The absorption of many vitamins and minerals depends on their chemical form. Dietary iron, for exam-

heme iron Iron that is part of the proteins hemoglobin and myoglobin; found only in animal-based foods such as meat, fish, and poultry.

non-heme iron Iron that is not a part of hemoglobin or myoglobin; found in both animal-based and plant-based foods.

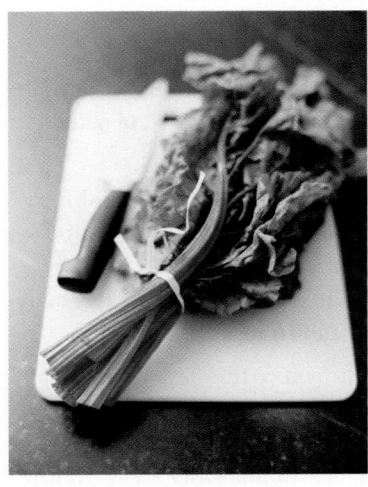

Foods high in oxalic acid, like rhubarb, can decrease zinc and iron absorption.

ple, can be in the form of **heme iron** (found only in meats, fish, and poultry) or **non-heme iron** (found in plant and animal foods as well as iron-fortified foods and supplements). Healthy adults absorb about 25% of heme iron but as little as 3–5% of non-heme iron.

In addition, the presence of other factors within the same food influences mineral absorption. For example, approximately 30–45% of the calcium found in milk and dairy products is absorbed, but the calcium in spinach, Swiss chard, seeds, and nuts is absorbed at a much lower rate because factors in these foods bind the calcium and prevent its absorption. Non-heme iron, zinc, vitamin E, and vitamin B_6 are other micronutrients whose absorption can be reduced by various binding factors in foods.

The absorption of many vitamins and minerals is also influenced by other foods within the meal. For example, the fat-soluble vitamins are much better absorbed when the meal contains some dietary fat. Calcium absorption is increased by the presence of lactose, found in milk, and non-heme iron absorption can be dou-

bled if the meal includes vitamin C–rich foods such as red peppers, oranges, or tomatoes. On the other hand, high-fiber foods such as whole grains and foods high in oxalic acid such as tea, spinach, and rhubarb can decrease the absorption of zinc and iron. It may seem an impossible task to correctly balance your food choices to optimize micronutrient absorption, but the best approach, as always, is to eat a variety of healthful foods every day.

What We Eat Differs from What Our Cells Use

Many vitamins undergo one or more chemical transformations after they are eaten and absorbed into our bodies. For example, before they can go to work for our bodies, the B-complex vitamins must combine with other substances. For many, such as thiamin and vitamin B_6, a phosphate group is added. Vitamin D is another example: before cells can use it, the food form of vitamin D must have two hydroxyl (—OH) groups added to its structure. These combinations activate the vitamin: because they don't occur randomly, but only when the compound is needed, they help the body maintain control over its metabolic pathways.

While the basic nature of minerals does not, of course, change, they can undergo minor modifications that change their atomic structure. Iron (Fe) may alternate between Fe^{2+} (ferrous) and Fe^{3+} (ferric); copper (Cu) may exist as Cu^{1+} or Cu^{2+}. These are just two examples of how micronutrients can be modified from one form to another to help the body make the best use of dietary nutrients.

NUTRI-CASE LIZ

" I used to have dinner in the dorm cafeteria, but not anymore. It's too tempting to see everybody eating all that fattening food and then topping it off with a big dessert. . . . My weight would double in a week if I ate like that! So instead I stay in my dorm room and have a bowl of cereal with skim milk. The cereal box says it provides a full day's supply of all the vitamins and minerals, so I know it's nutritious. And when I eat cereal for dinner, it doesn't matter if I didn't eat all the right things earlier in the day!"

What do you think of Liz's "cereal suppers"? If the cereal provides 100% of the DRI for all vitamins and minerals, then is Liz correct that it doesn't matter what else she eats during the day? If not, why not? What factors besides the percentage of DRI does Liz need to consider?

Controversies in Micronutrient Metabolism

Our current understanding of vitamins and minerals will no doubt change over the next several years or decades. While some people interpret the term *controversy* as negative, nutrition controversies are exciting developments, proof of new information and a sign of continued growth in the field.

Are Supplements Healthful Sources of Micronutrients?

For millions of years, humans relied solely on natural foodstuffs as their source of nutrients. It is only within the past 60 years or so that a second option became available: nutrient supplements, including those added to fortified foods. Are the micronutrients in supplements any better or worse than those in foods? Do our bodies use the nutrients from these two sources any differently?

Thousands of supplements are marketed to consumers.

As previously noted, the availability or "usefulness" of micronutrients in foods depends in part on the food itself. The iron and calcium in spinach are poorly absorbed, whereas the iron in beef and the calcium in milk are absorbed efficiently. Because of these and other differences in the availability of micronutrients from different sources, it is difficult to generalize about the usefulness of supplements. Nevertheless, we can say a few things about this issue:

- In general, it is much easier to develop a toxic overload of nutrients from supplements than it is from foods. It is very difficult, if not impossible, to develop a vitamin or mineral toxicity through diet (food) alone.

- Some micronutrients consumed as supplements appear to be harmful to the health of certain subgroups of consumers. For example, recent research has shown that use of antioxidant supplements such as vitamins A, C, and E may actually increase rates of death.[2] Earlier, it had been shown that high-potency beta-carotene supplements increased death rates among male smokers. There is also some evidence that high intake of vitamin A, including supplement use, increases risk of osteoporosis and hip fracture in older women.[3]

- Most minerals are better absorbed from animal food sources than they are from supplements. The one exception might be calcium citrate-malate, used in calcium-fortified juices. This form is used by the body as effectively as the calcium from milk or yogurt.

- Enriching a low-nutrient food with a few vitamins and/or minerals does not turn it into a healthful food. For example, soda that has been fortified with selected micronutrients is still basically soda whether it is diet or regular, caffeine-free or caffeinated.

- Eating a variety of healthful foods provides you with many more nutrients, phytochemicals, and other dietary factors than supplements alone. Nutritionists are not even sure they have identified all essential nutrients; it is possible that the list of essential micronutrients may, in the future, expand. Supplements provide only those nutrients that the manufacturer puts in; foods provide nutrients that have been identified as well as yet-unknown factors.

- Foods often provide a balance of micronutrients and other factors that work in concert with one another. The whole food is more healthful than its individual nutrients, providing benefits not always seen with purified supplements or highly refined, highly enriched food products. As one science reporter recently suggested, "Don't eat anything your great-great-grandmother wouldn't recognize as food."[4]

- A healthful diet, built from a wide variety of foods, offers social, emotional, and other benefits that are absent from supplements. Humans eat food, not nutrients.

This is not to say that nutrient supplements do not play an important role in promoting good health. Certain subgroups are likely to benefit from vitamin/mineral supplements. These include pregnant women, children with poor eating habits, and people with certain illnesses. The relative benefits of supplements versus whole foods are discussed further in the Nutrition Debate in Chapter 8 (pages 344–348).

Can Micronutrients Really Prevent or Treat Disease?

Nutritionists and other healthcare professionals clearly accept the role that dietary fat plays in the prevention and treatment of coronary heart disease. The relationship between total carbohydrate intake and the management of diabetes is also firmly established. Less clear, however,

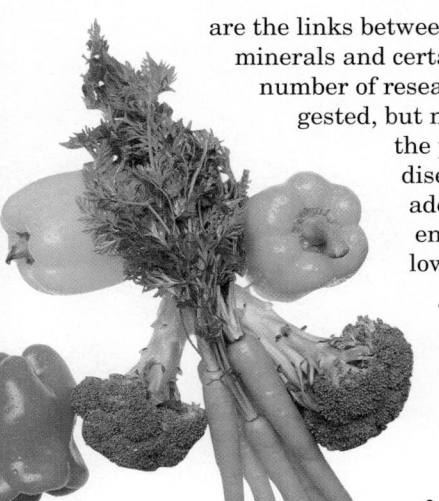

are the links between individual vitamins and minerals and certain chronic diseases. A number of research studies have suggested, but not proven, links between the protective nutrients and disease states. In each case, adequate intake of the nutrient has been associated with lower disease risk.

- Vitamin C and cataracts
- Vitamin D and colon cancer
- Vitamin E and complications of diabetes
- Vitamin K and osteoporosis
  - Calcium and high blood pressure (hypertension)
- Chromium and type 2 diabetes in older adults
- Magnesium and muscle wasting in older adults
- Selenium and certain types of cancer

As consumers, it is important to critically evaluate any claim that might be made regarding the protective or disease-preventing ability of a specific vitamin or mineral. Megadoses of micronutrients are potentially harmful, and vitamin/mineral therapies should never replace more traditional, proven methods of disease treatment. Current, reputable information can provide updates as the research into micronutrients continues.

Do More Essential Micronutrients Exist?

Nutrition researchers continue to explore the potential of a variety of substances to qualify as essential micronutrients. Vitamin-like factors such as carnitine and trace minerals such as boron, nickel, and silicon seem to have beneficial roles in human health, yet additional information is needed in order to fully define their metabolic roles. Until more research is done, we cannot classify such substances as essential micronutrients.

Another subject of controversy is the question, "What is the appropriate intake of each micronutrient?" Contemporary research suggests that the answer to this question is to be found in each individual's genetic profile. As you learned in the Nutrition Debate in Chapter 1, the science of *nutrigenomics* blends the study of human nutrition with that of genetics. It is becoming clear that some individuals, for example, require much higher intakes of folate in order to

achieve optimal health. Researchers have identified a specific genetic variation in a subset of the population that increases their need for dietary folate.[5] Future studies may identify other examples of how a person's genetic profile influences his or her individual need for vitamins and minerals.

As explained in Chapter 1, the DRI Committees rely on Adequate Intake (AI) guidelines to suggest appropriate nutrient intake levels when research has not clearly defined an Estimated Average Requirement (EAR). As the science of nutrition continues to evolve, the next 50 years will be an exciting time for micronutrient research. Who knows? Within a few decades, we all might have personalized micronutrient prescriptions matched to our gender, age, and DNA!

WEB LINKS

www.fda.gov
U.S. Food and Drug Administration

Select "Dietary Supplements" on the menu for information on how to evaluate dietary supplements.

www.ars.usda.gov/ba/bhnrc/ndl
Nutrient Data Laboratory Home Page

Click on "Reports for Single Nutrients" to find information on food sources of selected vitamins and minerals.

http://dietary-supplements.info.nih.gov
Office of Dietary Supplements

This site provides summaries of current research results and helpful information about use of dietary supplements.

http://lpi.oregonstate.edu
Linus Pauling Institute of Oregon State University

This site provides up-to-date information on vitamins and minerals that promote health and lower disease risk. You can search for individual nutrients (vitamin C) as well as types of nutrients (antioxidants).

REFERENCES

1. Institute of Medicine, Food and Nutrition Board. 2001. *Dietary Reference Intakes for Vitamin A, Vitamin K, Arsenic, Boron, Chromium, Copper, Iodine, Iron, Manganese, Molybdenum, Nickel, Silicon, Vanadium, and Zinc.* Washington, DC: National Academies Press.
2. Bjelakovic, G., D. Nikolova, L. L. Gluud, R. G. Simonetti, and C. Gluud. 2007. Mortality in randomized trials of antioxidant supplements for primary and secondary prevention. *J. Am. Med. Assoc.* 297:842–857.
3. Feskanich, D., V. Singh, W. C. Willett, and G. A. Colditz. 2002. Vitamin A intake and hip fractures among postmenopausal women. *J. Am. Med. Assoc.* 287:47–54.
4. Pollan, M. 2007. The age of nutritionism. *The New York Times Magazine,* January 28.
5. Stover, P. J. 2006. Influence of human genetic variation on nutritional requirements. *Am. J. Clin. Nutr.* 83:436S–443S.

CHAPTER 7

CHAPTER OBJECTIVES

After reading this chapter you will be able to:

1. Identify four nutrients that function as electrolytes in our bodies, p. 268.

2. List three functions of water in our bodies, pp. 269–270.

3. Describe how electrolytes assist in the regulation of healthful fluid balance, pp. 270–272.

4. Discuss the physical changes that occur to trigger our thirst mechanism, p. 273.

5. Describe the avenues of fluid intake and excretion in our bodies, pp. 274–275.

6. Define hyponatremia and identify factors that can cause this condition, pp. 283–284.

7. Identify four symptoms of dehydration, p. 290.

8. Define hypertension and list three ways we can change our lifestyle to reduce hypertension, pp. 291–293.

TEST YOURSELF TRUE OR FALSE?

1. About 50–70% of our body weight is made up of water. T or F

2. Sodium is an unhealthful nutrient, and we should avoid consuming it in our diets. T or F

3. Drinking until we are no longer thirsty always ensures that we are properly hydrated. T or F

4. Alcohol is a diuretic, causing the body to lose excessive fluid. T or F

5. Eating a high-sodium diet causes high blood pressure. T or F

Test Yourself answers can be found after the Chapter Summary.

Nutrients Involved in Fluid and Electrolyte Balance

i n April of 2002, Cynthia Lucero, a healthy 28-year-old woman who had just completed her doctoral dissertation, was running the Boston Marathon. Although not a professional athlete, Cynthia was running in her second marathon, and, in the words of her coach, she had been "diligent" in her training. While her parents, who had traveled from Ecuador, waited at the finish line, friends in the crowd watched as Cynthia steadily completed mile after mile, drinking large amounts of fluid as she progressed through the course. They described her as looking strong as she jogged up Heartbreak Hill, about 6 miles from the finish. But then she began to falter. One of her friends ran to her side and asked if she was okay. Cynthia replied that she felt dehydrated and rubber-legged, then she fell to the pavement. She was rushed to nearby Brigham and Women's Hospital, but by the time she got there, she was in an irreversible coma. The official cause of her death was hyponatremia, commonly called "low blood sodium." According to a study involving the 488 runners in that 2002 Boston Marathon, 13% had hyponatremia by the end of the race.[1] Hyponatremia continues to cause illness and death in runners, triathletes, and even hikers today.

What is hyponatremia, and are you at risk? Even if you don't run marathons, do you or any of your friends play sports, exercise, or work a physically demanding job in hot weather? If so, do you drink sports drinks or just plain water? If at the start of football practice on a hot, humid afternoon, a friend confided to you that he had been on a drinking binge the night before, would you know how to advise him? Should you tell his coach, and why?

In this chapter, we explore the role of fluids and electrolytes in keeping our bodies properly hydrated and maintaining the functions of our nerves and muscles. We also discuss how we maintain blood pressure and take a look at some disorders that occur when our fluids and electrolytes are out of balance.

What Are Fluids and Electrolytes, and What Are Their Functions?

Of course you know that orange juice, blood, and shampoo are all fluids, but what makes them so? A **fluid** is characterized by its ability to move freely, adapting to the shape of the container that holds it. This might not seem very important, but as you'll learn in this chapter, the fluid composition of your cells and tissues is critical to your body's ability to function.

Body Fluid Is the Liquid Portion of Our Cells and Tissues

Between 50% and 70%, or approximately 42 liters, of a healthy adult's body weight is fluid. When we cut a finger, we can see some of this fluid dripping out as blood, but that can't account for such a large percentage. So where is all this fluid hiding?

About two-thirds, or 28 liters, of an adult's body fluid is held within the walls of cells and is therefore called **intracellular fluid** (FIGURE 7.1A). Every cell in our body contains fluid. When our cells lose their fluid, they quickly shrink and die. On the other hand, when cells take in too much fluid, they swell and can burst apart. This is why appropriate fluid balance—which we'll discuss throughout this chapter—is so critical to life.

The remaining third, or approximately 14 liters, of an adult's body fluid is referred to as extracellular fluid because it flows outside of our cells (see FIGURE 7.1A). There are two types of extracellular fluid:

1. *Tissue fluid* (sometimes called *interstitial fluid*) flows between the cells that make up a particular tissue or organ, such as muscle fibers or the liver (FIGURE 7.1B). Other extracellular fluids such as cerebrospinal fluid, mucus, and synovial fluid within joints are also considered tissue fluid.

2. *Intravascular fluid* is extracellular fluid. Plasma is the liquid portion of blood, and it carries the red blood cells through our blood vessels. Plasma also contains

fluid A substance composed of molecules that move past one another freely. Fluids are characterized by their ability to conform to the shape of whatever container holds them.

intracellular fluid The fluid held at any given time within the walls of the body's cells.

extracellular fluid The fluid outside of the body's cells, either in the body's tissues or as the liquid portion of blood, called *plasma*.

As we age, our body water content decreases: Approximately 75% of an infant's body weight is composed of water while an elderly adult's body weight is only 50% water (or less).

Cell

Intracellular fluid
(inside of cell)

Extracellular fluid
(outside of cell)

(a)

Liver

Intracellular fluid

Extracellular fluid
(tissue fluid, or
interstitial fluid)

(b)

Capillary
network

Extracellular fluid
(plasma)

Intracellular fluid

Blood cell
inside capillary

Extracellular fluid
(tissue fluid)

(c)

FIGURE 7.1 The components of body fluid. **(a)** Intracellular fluid is contained inside the cells that make up our body tissues. **(b)** Extracellular fluid is external to cells. Tissue fluid is external to tissue cells. **(c)** Another form of extracellular fluid is intravascular fluid, that is, fluid contained within vessels. Plasma is the fluid in blood vessels and is external to blood cells.

proteins that are too large to leak out of blood vessels into the surrounding tissue fluid. As you learned in Chapter 6, protein concentration plays a major role in regulating the movement of fluids in and out of the bloodstream (FIGURE 7.1C).

Not every tissue in our body contains the same amount of fluid. Lean tissues, such as muscle, are more than 70% fluid, whereas fat tissue is only between 10% and 20% fluid. This is not surprising considering the hydrophobic nature of lipid cells, which we discussed in Chapter 5.

Body fluid also varies according to gender and age. FIGURE 7.2 compares the body composition of a 160-pound adult male and a 135-pound adult female. As you can see, males have more lean tissue and thus more body fluid than females. Our total

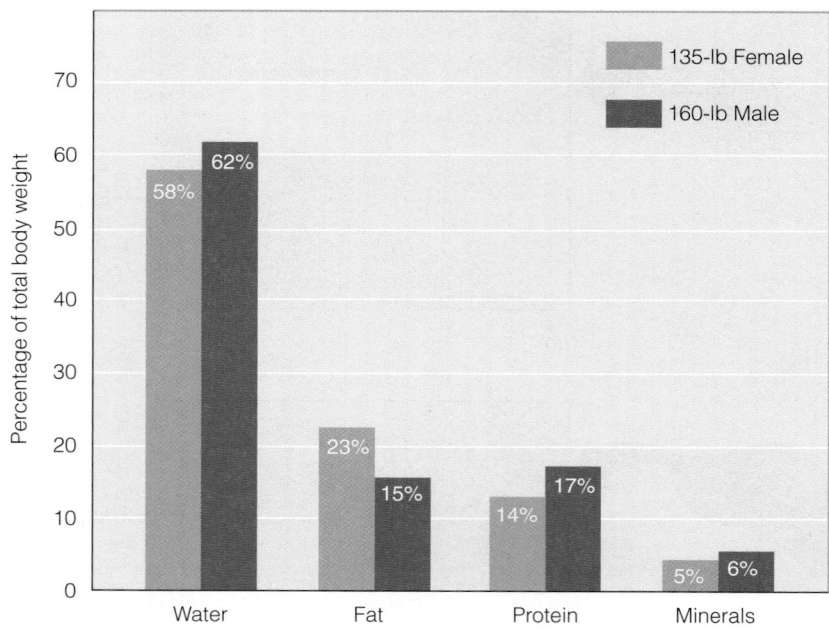

FIGURE 7.2   Body composition of an average adult male and female.

amount of body fluid decreases as we age. About 75% of an infant's body weight is water, whereas the total body water of an elderly person is generally less than 50% of body weight. This decrease in total body water is a result of the loss of lean tissue that occurs as we age.

Body Fluid Is Composed of Water and Dissolved Substances Called Electrolytes

Pure water is made up of molecules consisting of two hydrogen atoms bound to one oxygen atom (H_2O). You might think that such pure water would be healthful, but if our cell and tissue fluids contained only pure water, we would quickly die. Instead, within our body fluids are a variety of dissolved substances (called *solutes*) critical to life. These include four major minerals: sodium, potassium, chloride, and phosphorus. We consume these minerals in compounds called *salts,* especially table salt, which is made of sodium and chloride.

These mineral salts are called **electrolytes,** because when they dissolve in water, the two component minerals separate and form particles called **ions,** which are capable of carrying an electrical current. The electrical charge is the "spark" that stimulates nerves and causes muscles to contract, so electrolytes are critical to body functioning.

If you've ever jump-started a car, you know that electrical charges can be either positive or negative. Of the four major minerals just mentioned, sodium (Na^+) and potassium (K^+) are positively charged, whereas chloride (Cl^{2-}) and phosphorus (in the form of hydrogen phosphate, or HPO_4^{2-}) are negatively charged. In the intracellular fluid, potassium and phosphate are the predominant electrolytes. In contrast, in the extracellular fluid, sodium and chloride predominate. There is a slight difference in electrical charge on either side of the cell's membrane that is needed in order for the cell to perform its normal functions.

Fluids Serve Many Critical Functions

Water not only quenches our thirst, but also performs a number of functions that are critical to support life.

electrolyte A substance that disassociates in solution into positively and negatively charged ions and is thus capable of carrying an electrical current.

ion Any electrically charged particle, either positively or negatively charged.

Fluids Dissolve and Transport Substances

Water is involved in almost all chemical reactions in our bodies because it is an excellent **solvent.** This means it is capable of dissolving (i.e., mixing with and breaking apart) a wide variety of substances. Since blood plasma and the interior of blood cells are mostly water, blood is an excellent vehicle for transporting these dissolved substances, or solutes, throughout our body. All water-soluble substances—such as amino acids, glucose, vitamins, minerals, and medications—are readily transported via the bloodstream. In contrast, fats do not dissolve in water. To overcome this chemical incompatibility, fatty substances such as cholesterol and fat-soluble vitamins are either attached to or surrounded by water-soluble proteins so they too can be transported in the blood to the cells.

Fluids Account for Blood Volume

Blood volume is the amount of fluid in blood. As you might expect, appropriate fluid levels are essential to maintaining healthful blood volume. When blood volume rises, blood pressure increases; when blood volume decreases, blood pressure decreases. High blood pressure is an important risk factor for heart disease and stroke, whereas low blood pressure can cause us to feel tired, lethargic, confused, or dizzy, or even to faint. The heart, blood vessels, certain blood proteins, and kidneys work together to regulate blood volume and blood pressure in a fairly complex process that we will not describe here. We discuss high blood pressure (called *hypertension*) in the disorders section at the end of this chapter.

Fluids Help Maintain Body Temperature

Just as overheating or freezing is disastrous to a car engine, too high or low an internal temperature can cause our bodies to stop functioning. Fluids are vital to our ability to maintain our body temperature within a safe range. Two factors account for the ability of fluids to keep us cool. First, water has a relatively high heat capacity. In other words, it takes a lot of external energy to raise its temperature. For example, consider a newly filled swimming pool. Would you be willing to dive right in? If so, you'd be in for a shock because the large amount of water in the pool would not have had a chance to warm up. Because of water's high heat capacity, it will take days for the pool heater, plus the warmth of the sun, to bring the water to a suitable temperature. Likewise, once the water is warm it will take a long time for it to cool off. Since our bodies contain a lot of water, it takes sustained high heat to increase our body temperature and sustained cold temperatures to cool it down. Thus, the water content of our bodies protects us from extreme swings in temperature.

Second, body fluids are our primary coolant. When we need to release heat from the body, we increase the flow of blood from our warm body core to the vessels lying just under the skin. This action transports the heat from the core of the body out to the periphery where it can be released from the skin. When we are hot, the sweat glands secrete more sweat from the skin. As this sweat evaporates off of the skin's surface, heat is released and the skin and underlying blood are cooled (FIGURE 7.3). This cooler blood flows back to the body's core and reduces internal body temperature.

Fluids Protect and Lubricate Our Tissues

Water is a major part of the fluids that protect our organs and tissues from injury. The cerebrospinal fluid that surrounds our brain and spinal column protects these vital tissues from damage, and a fetus in a mother's womb is protected by amniotic fluid. Body fluids also act as lubricants. Synovial fluid secreted by membranes surrounding our joints acts as a lubricant for smooth joint motion, and tears cleanse and lubricate our eyes. Our saliva moistens the food we eat, which helps us to effectively swallow and transport it to the stomach. The fluid-filled mucus lining the walls of our stomach and intestines facilitates the smooth movement of food and nutrients through our digestive tract, and the pleural fluid covering our lungs allows their friction-free expansion and retraction behind our chest wall.

A hiker must consume adequate amounts of water to prevent heat illness in hot and dry environments.

solvent A substance that is capable of mixing with and breaking apart a variety of compounds. Water is an excellent solvent.

blood volume The amount of fluid in blood.

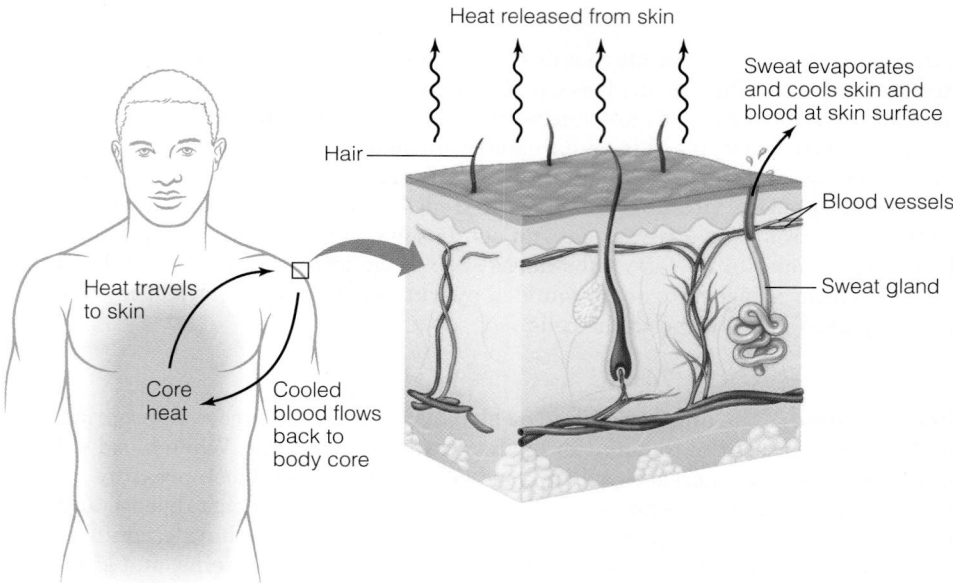

FIGURE 7.3 Evaporative cooling occurs when heat is transported from the body core through the bloodstream to the surface of the skin. The water evaporates into the air and carries away heat. This cools the blood, which circulates back to the body core, reducing body temperature.

> RECAP: *Our body fluid consists of water plus a variety of dissolved substances, including electrically charged minerals called electrolytes. Water serves many important functions in our bodies, including dissolving and transporting substances, accounting for blood volume, regulating body temperature, and cushioning and lubricating body tissues.*

Electrolytes Support Many Body Functions

Now that you know why fluid is so essential to our bodies' functioning, we're ready to explore the critical role of the minerals within it.

Electrolytes Help Regulate Fluid Balance

Our cell membranes are *permeable* to water. This means that water flows easily through them. Our cells cannot voluntarily regulate this flow of water and thus have no active control over the balance of fluid between the intracellular and extracellular compartments. In contrast, our cell membranes are *not* freely permeable to electrolytes. Sodium, potassium, and the other electrolytes (as well as proteins) stay where they are, either inside or outside of a cell, unless they are actively transported elsewhere by special transport proteins within the cell membrane. So how do electrolytes help our cells maintain their fluid balance? Answering this question requires an understanding of a process called **osmosis.**

    Imagine that you have a special filter that has the same properties as our cell membranes; in other words, this filter is freely permeable to water but not permeable to electrolytes. Now imagine that you insert this filter into a glass of pure distilled water to divide the glass into two separate chambers (FIGURE 7.4A). The level of water on either side of the filter would of course be identical, since it is freely permeable to water. Now imagine that you add a teaspoon of salt (which contains the electrolytes sodium and chloride) to the water on one side of the filter only (FIGURE 7.4B). You would see the water on the "pure water" side of the glass suddenly begin to flow through the filter to the "salt water" side of the glass (FIGURE 7.4C). This mysterious

osmosis The movement of water (or any solvent) through a semipermeable membrane from an area where solutes are less concentrated to areas where they are highly concentrated.

(a) (b) (c)

FIGURE 7.4   Osmosis. **(a)** A filter that is freely permeable to water is placed in a glass of pure water. **(b)** Salt is added to only one side of the glass. **(c)** Drawn by the high concentration of electrolytes, pure water flows to the "salt water" side of the filter. This flow of water into the concentrated solution will continue until the concentration of electrolytes on both sides of the membrane is equal.

movement of water obeys the principle of osmosis, which states that water always moves from areas where solutes such as sodium and chloride are low in concentration to areas where they are high in concentration. To put it another way, electrolytes *draw* water toward areas where they are more concentrated. This movement of water toward solutes continues until the concentration of solutes is equal on both sides of the cell membrane.

Water follows the movement of electrolytes; this action provides a means to control movement of fluid into and out of the cells. Our cells can regulate the balance of fluids between their internal and extracellular environments by using special transport proteins to actively pump electrolytes across their membranes. An example of how transport proteins pump sodium and potassium across the cell membrane was illustrated in Chapter 6 (FIGURE 6.11). By maintaining the appropriate movement of electrolytes into and out of the cell, the proper balance of fluid and electrolytes is maintained between the intracellular and extracellular compartments (FIGURE 7.5A). If the concentration of electrolytes is much higher inside of the cells as compared to outside, water will flow into the cells in such large amounts that the cells can burst (FIGURE 7.5B). On the other hand, if the extracellular environment contains too high a concentration of electrolytes, water flows out of the cells, and they can dry up (FIGURE 7.5C).

Certain illnesses can threaten this delicate balance of fluid inside and outside of the cells. You may have heard of someone being hospitalized because of excessive diarrhea and vomiting. When this happens, the body loses a great deal of fluid from the intestinal tract and extracellular compartment. This heavy fluid loss causes the extracellular electrolyte concentration to become very high. In response, a great deal of intracellular fluid leaves the cells to try to dilute this concentration of electrolytes. This imbalance in fluid and electrolytes changes the flow of electrical impulses through the heart, causing an irregular heart rate that can eventually lead to death if left untreated. Food poisoning and eating disorders involving repeated vomiting and diarrhea can also result in death due to these life-threatening fluid and electrolyte imbalances.

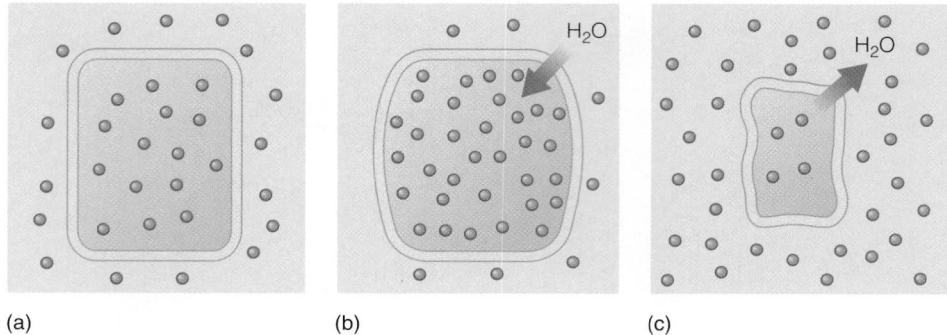

(a) (b) (c)

FIGURE 7.5 The health of our body's cells depends on maintaining the proper balance of fluids and electrolytes on either side of the cell membrane. **(a)** The concentration of electrolytes is the same on either side of the cell membrane. **(b)** The concentration of electrolytes is much greater inside the cell, drawing water into the cell and making it swell. **(c)** The concentration of electrolytes is much greater outside the cell, drawing water out of the cell and making it shrink.

Electrolytes Enable Our Nerves to Respond to Stimuli

In addition to their role in maintaining fluid balance, electrolytes are critical in enabling our nerves to respond to stimuli. Nerve impulses are initiated at the membrane of a nerve cell in response to a stimulus, for example, the touch of a hand or the clanging of a bell. Stimuli prompt changes to occur that allow an influx of sodium into the cell, causing the cell to become slightly less negatively charged. This is called *depolarization*. If enough sodium enters the cell, the change in electrical charge triggers an *action potential*, an electrical impulse that is propagated along the cell and transmitted to neighboring cells (FIGURE 7.6). Once this signal is complete, the cells return to their normal electrical state through the release of potassium to the outside of the cell. This return of the cell to its initial electrical state is termed *repolarization*. Thus, both sodium and potassium play critical roles in ensuring that nerve impulses are generated in response to a variety of stimuli.

Electrolytes Signal Our Muscles to Contract

Our muscles' ability to contract is due to a series of complex physiological changes that we will not describe in detail here. Simply stated, our muscles are stimulated to contract in response to stimulation of nerve cells. As described above, sodium and potassium play a key role in the generation of nerve impulses, or electrical signals. When a muscle cell is stimulated by an electrical signal, changes occur in the cell membrane that lead to an increased flow of calcium into the muscle from the extracellular space. This release of calcium into the muscle provides the stimulus for muscle contraction. Our muscles can relax after a contraction once the electrical signal is complete and calcium has been pumped out of the muscle cell.

[RECAP: *Electrolytes help regulate fluid balance by controlling the movement of fluid into and out of cells. Electrolytes, specifically sodium and potassium, play a key role in generating nerve impulses in response to stimuli. Calcium is an electrolyte that stimulates muscle contraction.*

How Do Our Bodies Maintain Fluid Balance?

We maintain the proper balance of fluid in our bodies by a series of mechanisms that prompt us to drink and retain fluid when we are dehydrated and to excrete fluid as urine when we consume more than we need.

(a) Resting state   (b) Depolarization   (c) Repolarization

FIGURE 7.6 The role of electrolytes in conduction of a nerve impulse. **(a)** In the resting state, the intracellular fluid has slightly more electrolytes with a negative charge. **(b)** A stimulus causes changes to occur that prompt the influx of sodium into the interior of the cell. Sodium has a positive charge, so when this happens, the charge inside the cell becomes slightly positive. This is called depolarization. If enough sodium enters the cell, an action potential is transmitted to adjacent regions of the cell membrane. **(c)** Release of potassium to the exterior of the cell allows the first portion of the membrane almost immediately to return to the resting state. This is called repolarization.

Our Thirst Mechanism Prompts Us to Drink Fluids

Imagine that, at lunch, you ate a ham sandwich and a bag of salted potato chips. Now it's almost time for your afternoon seminar to end, and suddenly you are very thirsty. The last 5 minutes of class are a torment, and when the instructor ends the session you dash to the nearest drinking fountain. What happened here? What prompted you suddenly to feel so thirsty?

Our body's command center for fluid intake is a cluster of nerve cells in a part of the brain called the *hypothalamus*. It is this group of cells, collectively referred to as the **thirst mechanism,** that causes you to consciously desire fluids. Our thirst mechanism prompts us to feel thirsty when it is stimulated by the following:

- Increased concentration of salt and other dissolved substances in our blood. Remember that ham sandwich and those potato chips? Both these foods are salty, and eating them causes the release of high concentrations of sodium into the blood.

- A reduction in blood volume and blood pressure. This can occur when fluids are lost because of profuse sweating, blood loss, vomiting, or diarrhea, or simply when fluid intake is too low. Remember that plasma is an extracellular fluid; therefore, when you sweat or lose fluid through vomiting or other means, your blood volume will decrease.

- Dryness in the tissues of the mouth and throat. Tissue dryness reflects a lower amount of fluid in the bloodstream, which causes a reduced production of saliva.

Once the hypothalamus detects such changes, it stimulates the release of a hormone that signals the kidneys to reduce urine flow and return more water to the bloodstream. The kidneys also secrete an enzyme that triggers blood vessels throughout our body to constrict. This helps us to retain water. Water is drawn out of the salivary glands in our mouths in an attempt to further dilute the concentration of substances in our blood; this causes our mouth and throat to become even drier. Together, these mechanisms allow us to prevent a further loss of body fluid and help avoid dehydration.

Although our thirst mechanism can trigger us to drink more water, this mechanism alone is not always sufficient: we tend to drink until we are no longer thirsty,

thirst mechanism A cluster of nerve cells in the hypothalamus that stimulate our conscious desire to drink fluids in response to an increase in the concentration of salt in our blood or a decrease in blood pressure and blood volume.

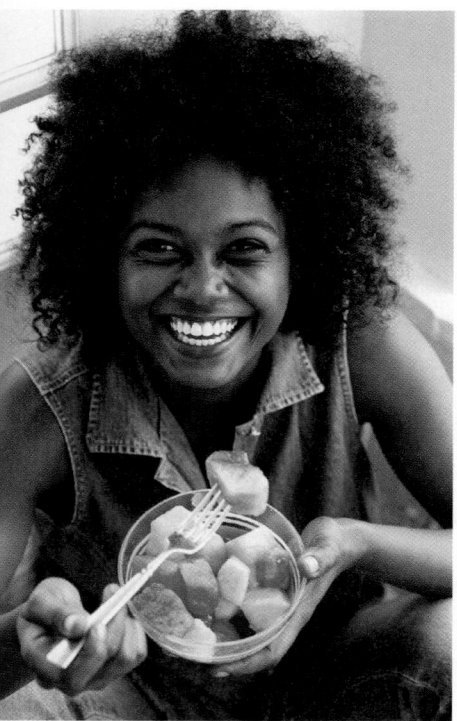

Fruits and vegetables are delicious sources of water.

metabolic water The water formed as a by-product of our body's metabolic reactions.

sensible water loss Water loss that is noticed by a person, such as through urine output and visible sweating.

but the amount of fluid we consume may not be enough to achieve fluid balance. This is particularly true when we lose body water rapidly, such as during intense exercise in the heat. Because our thirst mechanism has some limitations, it is important that you drink regularly throughout the day and not wait to drink until you become thirsty, especially if you are active.

Because our thirst mechanism becomes less sensitive as we age, elderly people can fail to drink adequate amounts of fluid and thus are at increased risk for dehydration. For this reason, elderly people should be careful to drink fluids on a regular basis throughout the day. Infants are also at increased risk for dehydration. A large proportion of an infant's body weight is water, so they need to drink a relatively large amount of fluid for their body size. For the same reason, fluid loss from diarrhea and vomiting are also more serious in this age group.

We Gain Fluids by Consuming Beverages and Foods and Through Metabolism

We obtain the fluid we need each day from three primary sources: beverages, foods, and the production of metabolic water by our bodies. Of course you know that beverages are mostly water, but it isn't as easy to see the water content in the foods we eat. For example, iceberg lettuce is almost 99% water, and even nuts such as pecans contain a small amount of water. FIGURE 7.7 shows the water content of a few commonly consumed foods.

Metabolic water is the water formed from our body's metabolic reactions. In the breakdown of fat, carbohydrate, and protein, ATP—the cell's basic energy source—and water are produced. The water that is formed during metabolic reactions contributes about 10–14% of the water we need each day.

We Lose Fluids Through Urine, Sweat, Evaporation, Exhalation, and Feces

Water loss that is noticeable, such as through urine output and sweating, is referred to as **sensible water loss.** Most water we consume is excreted through the kidneys in the form of urine. When we consume more water than we need, the kidneys process and excrete it in the form of dilute urine.

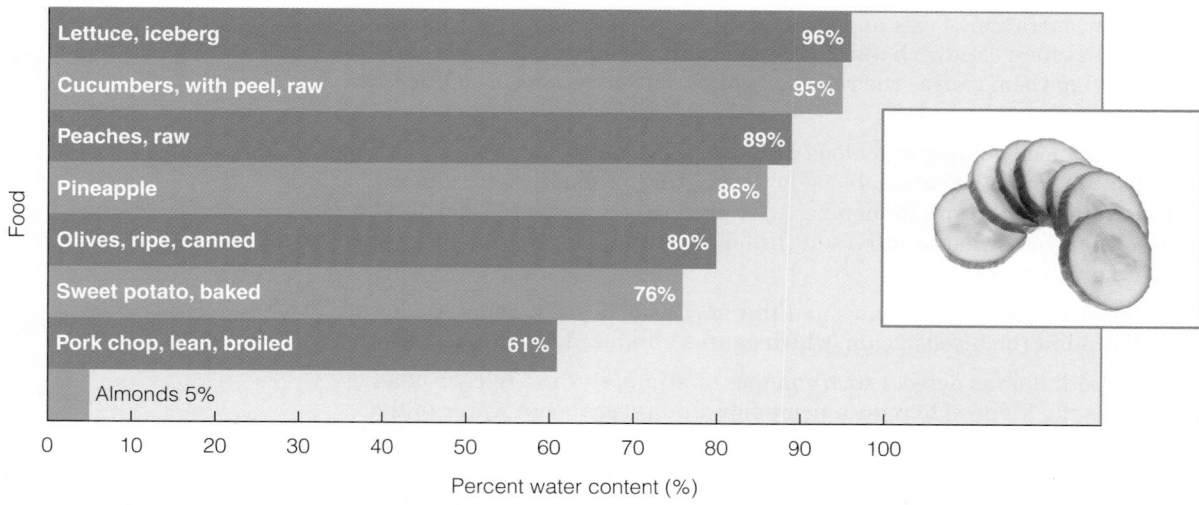

FIGURE 7.7 Water content of different foods. Much of your daily water intake comes from the foods you eat. (Data from U.S. Department of Agriculture, Agricultural Research Service. 2006. USDA Nutrient Database for Standard Reference, Release 19. Nutrient Data Laboratory Home Page. www.ars.usda.gov/ba/bhnrc/ndl.)

During times when we need to conserve body water, the sodium concentration of our extracellular fluid increases. Special cells in the hypothalamus of the brain sense this increase in sodium levels and cause hormones to be secreted that signal the kidneys to reabsorb water instead of excreting it. When we don't consume enough fluid, urine becomes concentrated.

Our kidneys also respond to massive changes in fluid balance and blood pressure such as those that occur when someone suffers a large loss of blood. Major blood loss causes a significant drop in blood pressure. This drop in blood pressure signals the kidneys to retain more water and reduce urine output, thus helping to maintain extracellular fluid levels. In addition, the kidneys excrete certain enzymes and hormones that cause constriction of blood vessels and also allow for the retention of water and sodium. Since water follows sodium, retaining sodium in the kidneys also helps retain water. The sodium and water can then be absorbed back into the bloodstream and cause an increase in blood volume and blood pressure.

The second type of sensible water loss is via sweat. Our sweat glands produce more sweat during exercise or when we are in a hot environment. The evaporation of sweat from our skin releases heat, which cools our skin and reduces our core temperature.

Water is continuously evaporated from our skin even when we are not visibly sweating, and water is also continuously exhaled from our lungs during breathing. Water loss through these mechanisms is referred to as **insensible water loss,** as we do not perceive this loss. Under normal resting conditions, our insensible water loss is less than 1 liter of fluid each day; during heavy exercise or in hot weather, we can lose up to 2 liters of water per hour due to insensible water loss.

We excrete a relatively small amount of water in our feces. Under normal conditions, we lose only about 150 to 200 ml of water each day in our feces. Our gastrointestinal tract typically reabsorbs much of the large amounts of fluids that pass through it each day. However, when someone suffers from extreme diarrhea due to illness or from consuming excess laxatives, water loss via the feces can be as high as several liters per day.

In addition to these avenues of regular fluid loss, certain situations can cause a significant loss of fluid from our bodies:

Drinking beverages that contain alcohol causes an increase in water loss, because alcohol is a diuretic.

- Illnesses that involve fever, coughing, vomiting, diarrhea, and a runny nose significantly increase fluid loss. This is why doctors advise people to drink plenty of fluids when they are ill.

- Traumatic injury, internal hemorrhaging, blood donation, and surgery also increase loss of fluid because of the blood loss involved.

- Exercise increases fluid loss via sweat and respiration: although urine production typically decreases during exercise, fluid losses increase through the skin and lungs.

- Environmental conditions that increase fluid loss include high altitudes, cold and hot temperatures, and low humidity such as in a desert or flying in an airplane. The water content of the environment is much lower at high altitude, in an airplane, and in the desert. Thus, water from our body more easily evaporates into the dry environment. We also breathe faster at higher altitudes due to the lower oxygen pressure, which results in greater fluid loss via the lungs. We sweat more in the heat, thus losing more water. Cold temperatures can trigger hormonal changes that result in an increased fluid loss.

- Pregnancy increases fluid loss to the mother because fluids are continually diverted to the fetus and amniotic fluid.

- Breastfeeding requires a tremendous increase in fluid intake to make up for the loss of fluid.

- Consumption of **diuretics**—substances that increase fluid loss via the urine— can result in dangerously excessive fluid loss. Diuretics include certain prescription medications, alcohol, and many over-the-counter weight-loss remedies.

insensible water loss The loss of water not noticeable by a person, such as through evaporation from the skin and exhalation from the lungs during breathing.

diuretic A substance that increases fluid loss via the urine. Common diuretics include alcohol, some prescription medications, and many over-the-counter weight-loss pills.

> [**RECAP:** *We maintain healthy fluid levels in our body by balancing intake with excretion. Primary sources of fluids include water and other beverages, foods, and the production of metabolic water in the body. Fluid losses occur through urination, sweating, our feces, and evaporation from our lungs.*

A Profile of Nutrients Involved in Hydration and Neuromuscular Function

Nutrients that assist us in maintaining hydration and neuromuscular function include water and the minerals sodium, potassium, chloride, and phosphorus. As discussed in Chapter 1, these minerals are classified as *major minerals,* as the body needs more than 100 mg of each per day. Table 7.1 reviews the primary functions of these minerals. As you can see, they play many roles in the body.

TABLE 7.1   Functions, Recommended Intakes, and Toxicity and Deficiency Symptoms of Primary Electrolytes

Nutrient	Primary Functions	Recommended Intake	Toxicity Symptoms	Deficiency Symptoms
Sodium	Major positively charged electrolyte in extracellular fluid Maintains proper acid–base balance Assists with transmission of nerve signals Aids muscle contraction Assists in the absorption of glucose and other nutrients	AI: 1.5 g/day UL: 2.3 g/day	Water retention High blood pressure May increase loss of calcium in urine	Muscle cramps Loss of appetite Dizziness Fatigue Nausea Vomiting Mental confusion
Potassium	Major positively charged electrolyte in intracellular fluid Regulates contraction of muscles Regulates transmission of nerve impulses Assists in maintaining healthy blood pressure levels	AI: 4.7 g/day UL: none established	Muscle weakness Vomiting Irregular heartbeat	Muscle weakness Muscle paralysis Mental confusion
Chloride	Assists with maintaining fluid balance Aids in preparing food for digestion (as HCl) Helps kill bacteria Assists in the transmission of nerve impulses	AI: 2.3 g/day UL: 3.6 g/day	Vomiting	Dangerous changes in pH Irregular heartbeat
Phosphorus	Major negatively charged electrolyte in intracellular fluid Maintains proper fluid balance Plays critical role in bone formation Component of ATP, which provides energy for our bodies Helps regulate biochemical reactions Major part of genetic materials (DNA, RNA) A component in cell membranes, LDL	RDA: 700 mg/day UL: 4 g/day	Muscle spasms Convulsions Low blood calcium levels	Muscle weakness Bone pain Dizziness

Calcium and magnesium also function as electrolytes and influence our body's fluid balance and neuromuscular function. However, because of their critical importance to bone health, they are discussed in Chapter 9.

Water

Water is essential for life. Although we can live weeks without food, we can only survive 1 to 2 days without water, depending on environmental temperature. We do not have the capacity to store water, so we must continuously replace the water we lose each day.

How Much Water Should We Drink?

Our need for water varies greatly depending upon our age, body size, health status, physical activity level, and exposure to environmental conditions. It is important to pay attention to how much our need for water changes under various conditions so that we can avoid dehydration.

Vigorous exercise causes significant water loss that must be replenished to optimize performance and health.

Recommended Intake Fluid requirements are very individualized. For example, a highly active male athlete training in a hot environment may require up to 10 liters of fluid per day to maintain healthy fluid balance, while an inactive, petite woman who lives in a mild climate and works in a temperature-controlled office building may only require about 3 liters of fluid per day.

The DRI for adult men aged 19 to 50 years is 3.7 liters of total water per day. This includes approximately 3.0 liters (or 13 cups) as beverages, including water.[2] The DRI for adult women aged 19 to 50 is 2.7 liters of total water per day. This includes about 2.2 liters (or 9 cups) as beverages.[2]

FIGURE 7.8 shows the amount and sources of water intake and output for a woman expending 2,500 kcal/day. Based on current recommendations, this woman needs about 2,700 ml (or a little over 2 liters) of fluid per day. As you can see:

• Water from metabolism provides 300 to 400 ml of water.

• The foods she eats provides her with an additional 1,000 ml or 1 liter of water each day.

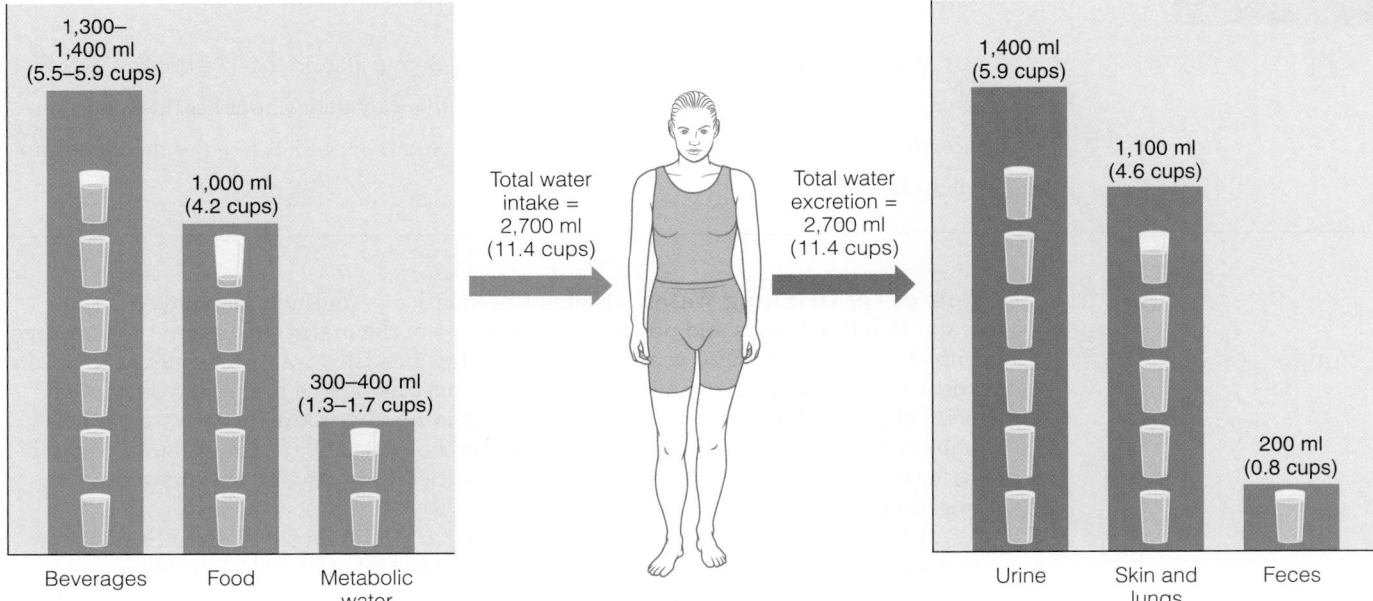

FIGURE 7.8 Amount and sources of water intake and output for a woman expending 2,500 kcal/day.

- The beverages she drinks provide the remainder of water needed, which is equal to 1,300 to 1,400 ml, or approximately a liter and a half of fluid.

An 8-oz glass of water is equal to 240 ml. In this example, the woman would need to drink 5 to 6 glasses of fluid to meet her needs. You can now see why drinking 8 glasses of fluid each day is recommended for most people; however, this recommendation is a general guideline. You may need to drink a different amount to meet your fluid needs.

Athletes or people who are active, especially those working in very hot environments, may require more fluid than the current recommendations. The amount of sweat lost during exercise is very individualized and depends on body size, exercise intensity, environmental temperature, and humidity. We do know that some people can lose as much as 4 pounds of fluid (or 1.8 kg) per hour as sweat![3] Thus, these individuals need to drink more to replace the fluid they lose. One liter of sweat contains about 1 g of sodium; we also lose some potassium and small amounts of minerals such as iron and calcium in sweat.[4]

Because of these fluid and electrolyte losses during exercise, some athletes drink sports beverages instead of plain water to help them maintain fluid balance. Recently, sports beverages have also become popular with recreationally active people and non-athletes. Is it really necessary for people to consume these beverages? See the Nutrition Debate on sports beverages at the end of this chapter to learn whether they are right for you.

NUTRI-CASE LIZ

"My dance teacher says we should be drinking at least 80 oz (or 10 cups) of fluid a day. That sounds like an awful lot, but yesterday, I kept track of how much I drank all day, and I'm pretty close: I drank a 10-oz cup of coffee with breakfast, a 16-oz bottle of spring water during dance class, and a 12-oz diet cola at lunch. After classes, I treated myself to a skim milk latté, the 12-oz size, and then I had another bottle of water during rehearsal. I had half a glass of cranberry juice with dinner, probably about 4 oz, and then I had an 8-oz cup of green tea just before bed. So I'm on target. The only problem is, I have to go to the bathroom all the time!"

What do you think of Liz's dance teacher's recommendation that she drink 80 oz of fluid a day? How is Liz doing toward that goal? Is there anything about her fluid consumption that you would advise her to change? Why do you think Liz has to go to the bathroom all the time?

Sources of Drinking Water. Millions of Americans routinely consume the tap water found in homes and public places. But one of the major changes in the beverage industry over the past 20 years is the marketing of bottled water. The meteoric rise in bottled water production and consumption is most likely due to the convenience of drinking bottled water, the health messages related to drinking more water, and the public's fears related to the safety of tap water. Is bottled water safer than tap water? Refer to the Nutrition Myth or Fact? box on bottled water to find the answer to this question.

There are so many types of bottled water available in the United States; how can we distinguish among them? If we prefer to drink water with bubbles—carbonation—we can choose carbonated water. This type of water contains carbon

NUTRITION MYTH OR FACT?

Is Bottled Water Safer Than Tap Water?

Bottled water has become increasingly popular over the past 20 years. One industry source estimated that Americans drink approximately 7.5 billion gallons of bottled water each year, and that number continues to grow.[5] Many people prefer the taste, and feel that bottled water is safer than tap water. Is this true?

The water we drink in the United States generally comes from two sources: surface water and ground water. *Surface water* comes from lakes, rivers, and reservoirs. Common contaminants of surface water include runoff from highways, pesticides, animal wastes, and industrial wastes. Many of the cities across the United States obtain their water from surface water sources. *Ground water* comes from underground rock formations called *aquifers*. People who live in rural areas generally pump ground water from a well as their water source. Hazardous substances leaking from waste sites, dumps, landfills, and oil and gas pipelines can contaminate ground water.

The most common chemical used to treat and purify our water is *chlorine*. Chlorine is effective in killing many contaminants in our water supply. Water treatment plants also routinely check our water supplies for hazardous chemicals, minerals, and other contaminants. Because of these efforts, the United States has one of the safest water systems in the world.

The Environmental Protection Agency (EPA) sets and monitors the standards for our city water systems. The EPA does not monitor water from private wells, but it publishes recommendations for well owners to help them maintain a safe water supply. Local water regulatory agencies must provide an annual report on specific water contaminants to all households served by that agency.

In contrast, the Food and Drug Administration (FDA) regulates bottled water. As with tap water, bottled water is taken from either surface water or ground water sources. Bottled water is often treated and filtered differently than tap water, which changes its taste and appearance.

Although bottled water may taste better than tap water, there is no evidence that it is safer to drink. Look closely at the label of your favorite bottled water. It may come directly from the tap! Some types of bottled water may contain more minerals than tap water, but there are no other additional nutritional benefits of drinking bottled water. As discussed in the Nutrition Label Activity, bottling plants use a variety of other treatments to disinfect water instead of chlorine, and many people feel these processes leave the water tasting better than water treated with chlorine.

Should you spend money on bottled water? The answer depends on personal preference and your source of drinking water. For instance, many supermarkets have a water filtration machine in the front of the store where you can purchase and fill your own bottles of water. These machines may not be cleaned and the filters not changed on a regular basis, making this water less safe than tap water. Some people may not have access to safe drinking water where they live, making bottled water the safest alternative water source. If you choose to drink bottled water, look for brands that carry the trademark of the International Bottled Water Association (IBWA). This association follows the regulations of the FDA. If you get your water from a water cooler, make sure the cooler is cleaned once per month by running half a gallon of white vinegar through it, then rinsing thoroughly with about 5 gallons of clean water. If you use a special filtration system at home, be familiar with the contaminants it filters from your water and make sure that you change the filters regularly as recommended by the manufacturer.

Be cautious of companies that may test your water and publish false claims about impurities in your tap water. Verify any tests conducted by a private company with your local water agency. It could save you hundreds or thousands of dollars on an unnecessary or ineffective home purifying system.

For more information on drinking water safety, go to the EPA Web site at www.epa.gov. For information on bottled water go to www.bottledwater.org.

dioxide gas that either occurs naturally or is added to the water. Mineral water is another beverage option. Mineral waters contain 250 to 500 parts per million (ppm) of minerals. While many people prefer the unique taste of mineral water, a number of brands contain high amounts of sodium so should be avoided by people who are trying to reduce their sodium intake. See the Nutrition Label Activity on page 281 for information on how to determine the source of your water, how it is treated, and its nutrient content.

Numerous varieties of drinking water are available to consumers.

What Happens If We Drink Too Much Water?

Drinking too much water and becoming overhydrated is very rare, but it can occur. Some individuals suffering from certain forms of mental illness have an uncontrollable urge to consume large quantities of water. If these individuals have healthy kidneys, this condition generally does not lead to major health problems because their kidneys are able to process this excess water. Certain illnesses can cause increases in levels of a hormone that stimulates reabsorption of water by the kidneys. When this occurs, overhydration and dilution of sodium result. As we saw in the chapter-opening story, dilution of sodium, also called *hyponatremia,* causes headaches, confusion, seizures, and coma. Hyponatremia is discussed in more detail in the next section.

What Happens If We Don't Drink Enough Water?

Dehydration results when we do not drink enough water. Fluid loss is one of the leading causes of death around the world, with infants and elderly individuals being particularly affected. Dehydration is generally due to some form of illness or gastrointestinal infection that causes diarrhea and vomiting. When these occur over a prolonged period of time, fluid loss is excessive and dehydration results, leading to impaired physical and mental function and even death if not treated quickly. The impact of dehydration on our health is discussed in detail on page 289.

Sodium

Over the last 20 years, researchers have linked high sodium intake to an increased risk for high blood pressure. Because of this link, many people have come to believe that sodium is harmful to the body. This simply is not true: in reality, sodium is an essential nutrient that our body needs to function optimally.

Functions of Sodium

Sodium has a variety of functions. As discussed earlier in this chapter, it is the major positively charged electrolyte in the extracellular fluid. Its exchange with potassium across cell membranes allows cells to maintain proper fluid balance, blood pressure, and acid–base balance.

Sodium also assists with the transmission of nerve signals and aids in muscle contraction. To review, the release of sodium from inside to outside the cell stimu-

Many popular snack foods are high in sodium.

NUTRITION LABEL ACTIVITY

How Pure Is Your Favorite Bottled Water?

The next time you reach for a bottle of water, check the label. First, find out where it comes from. Many brands of bottled water contain municipal water that has simply been purified in the plant. If no location is provided, even a bottle labeled "spring water" may actually contain tap water with minerals added to improve the taste. What you're looking for are the words "Bottled at the source." Water that comes from a protected ground water source is less likely to have contaminants such as disease-causing microbes. If the label doesn't identify the water's source, it should at least provide contact information such as a phone number or Web site of the bottled water company so that you can track down that information. Check out the labels of the two bottled waters in the accompanying photo. What is the source of the water in each? Can you tell?

Next, find out how the water in the bottle has been treated. There are several ways of treating water:

- *Distillation* is a process whereby water is boiled and then condensed back into water. This process removes salts, metals, minerals, and other organic compounds, creating a purer form of the water.
- *Micron filtration* is a process whereby water is filtered through screens with various-sized microscopic holes.

High-quality micron filtration can eliminate most chemical contaminants and microbes.

- *Reverse osmosis* is a process often referred to as *ultrafiltration* because it uses a membrane with microscopic openings that allow water to pass through but not larger compounds. Reverse osmosis membranes also utilize electrical charges to reject harmful chemicals.
- *Ozonation* is a process that exposes water to ozone (a form of oxygen), which kills most microbes.
- *Ultraviolet light (UV) exposure* is a process that also kills most microbes; however, the success varies according to how long the water is exposed to the UV light.

Of these, the following methods have been proven to be effective against the most common waterborne disease-causing microorganisms: distillation, micron filtration through a filter with holes sized 1 micron or smaller, and reverse osmosis.

If the label on your bottle of water says that the water was purified using any of the following methods, you might want to consider switching brands. That's because the following methods have not been proven to be effective against the most common waterborne disease-causing microorganisms: filtration, carbon filtration, particle filtration, ozonation or ozone treatment, ultraviolet light exposure, ion exchange, and deionization. How was the water in the two brands shown here treated? If the process is not identified on the label, how could you determine this information?

Finally, check the nutrient content on the label. Ideally, water should be high in magnesium (at least 90 mg/liter) and calcium, but low in sodium (less than 10 mg/liter).

Finally, avoid bottled waters sweetened with high-fructose corn syrup and other sweeteners, as their "empty calories" can contribute significantly to your energy intake. These products are often promoted as healthful beverage choices, but they are essentially "liquid candy." Check the Nutrition Facts Panel and don't be fooled!

Can you tell where the water in each bottle comes from?

lates the spread of nerve signals to nervous tissue and muscles. The stimulation of muscles by nerve impulses provides the impetus for muscle contraction.

How Much Sodium Should We Consume?

Many people are concerned with consuming too much sodium in the diet, as they believe it causes high blood pressure and bloating. Although this concern is warranted for certain individuals, sodium is an important nutrient that is necessary for maintaining health.

Recommended Dietary Intake for Sodium   The AI for sodium is listed in Table 7.1. Most people in the United States consume two to four times the AI daily.

SHOPPER'S GUIDE
Sources of Sodium

Sodium is found naturally in many everyday foods, and many processed foods contain large amounts of added sodium. Because sodium is so abundant, it is easy for us to consume excess amounts in our daily diet. Try to guess which of the following foods contains the most sodium: 1 cup of tomato juice, 1 oz of potato chips, or 4 saltine crackers? Now look at Table 7.2 to find the answer. This table shows foods that are high in sodium and gives lower-sodium alternatives. Are you surprised to find out that of all of these food items, the tomato juice has the most sodium? Below are some tips for lowering your sodium intake. Following them might help reduce your risk for hypertension.

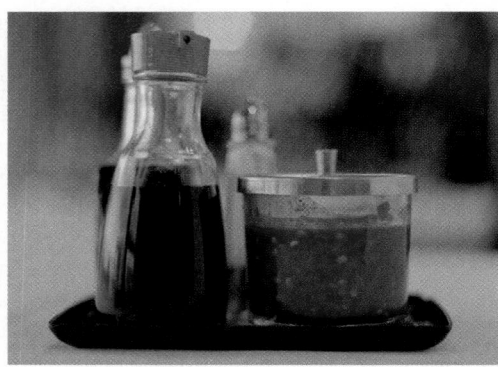

Condiments can add sodium to your diet.

Tips for Reducing the Sodium in Your Diet[6]

√ Follow the DASH diet plan (see Table 2.4, page 68).

√ Look for the words low sodium when buying processed foods. These foods should contain 5% or less of the daily value.

√ Foods can vary greatly in their sodium content, so compare labels of various name brands of the same food.

√ Choose fresh or frozen vegetables, as they are usually much lower in sodium than those found in canned or mixed processed foods like soups and stews.

TABLE 7.2   High-Sodium Foods and Lower-Sodium Alternatives

High-Sodium Food	Sodium (mg)	Lower-Sodium Food	Sodium (mg)
Dill pickle (1 large, 4 in.)	1,731	Low-sodium dill pickle (1 large, 4 in.)	23
Ham, cured, roasted (3 oz)	1,023	Pork, loin roast (3 oz)	54
Chipped beef (3 oz)	913	Beef chuck roast, cooked (3 oz)	53
Tomato juice, regular (1 cup)	877	Tomato juice, lower sodium (1 cup)	24
Tomato sauce, canned (½ cup)	741	Fresh tomato (1 medium)	11
Creamed corn, canned (1 cup)	730	Cooked corn, fresh (1 cup)	28
Tomato soup, canned (1 cup)	695	Lower-sodium tomato soup, canned (1 cup)	480
Potato chips, salted (1 oz)	168	Baked potato, unsalted (1 medium)	14
Saltine crackers (4 crackers)	156	Saltine crackers, unsalted (4 crackers)	100

Source: U.S. Department of Agriculture. 1999. USDA Nutrient Database for Standard Reference, Release 13. Nutrient Data Laboratory Home Page. http://www.ars.usda.gov/ba/bhnrc/ndl.

√ Use other spices instead of salt to flavor your food. Spices that end in the word salt such as garlic salt or celery salt are high in sodium.

√ Reduce the amount of condiment you use. Condiments such as ketchup, mustard, pickle relish, and soy sauce can add a considerable amount of sodium to your foods. Again, check the label of these items.

√ Stay away from stews and pasta sauces that are high in sodium.

√ Snack on fruits and vegetables instead of salty snack foods.

√ Look for hidden salt content on food labels; for example, both monosodium glutamate and sodium benzoate are forms of sodium.

√ Check the label on your medications. Many medications, including aspirin, are high in sodium.

√ If you drink alcoholic beverages, be aware that both beer and wine have a significant amount of sodium.

What Happens If We Consume Too Much Sodium?

High blood pressure is more common in people who consume high-sodium diets. This strong relationship between high-sodium diets and high blood pressure has prompted many health organizations to recommend low- sodium intakes. Whether high-sodium diets actually cause high blood pressure is unclear and controversial; this controversy is discussed on page 293. In addition, there are other, less controversial reasons to consume no more than the recommended amount of sodium each day. Eating excess sodium can cause an increased excretion of calcium in some people, which in turn may increase the risk for bone loss; however, the extent to which excess sodium intake affects bone health is also the subject of controversy.[7] Consuming excess sodium also causes bloating, as water is pulled from inside the cells into the extracellular space in an attempt to dilute the excess sodium.

Hypernatremia refers to an abnormally high blood sodium concentration (clinically defined as greater than 145 milliequivalents per liter of blood). It is usually caused by a rapid intake of high amounts of sodium, such as when a shipwrecked sailor drinks seawater. Eating too much sodium does not usually cause hypernatremia in a healthy person, as the kidneys are able to excrete excess sodium and avoid hypernatremia. But people with congestive heart failure or kidney disease are not able to excrete sodium effectively, making them more prone to the condition. Hypernatremia is dangerous because it causes an abnormally high blood volume, again, by pulling water from the intracellular environment to dilute the sodium in the extracellular tissue spaces and vessels. This leads to edema (swelling) of our tissues and raises blood pressure to unhealthy levels.

What Happens If We Don't Consume Enough Sodium?

Because the dietary intake of sodium is so high among Americans, deficiencies are extremely rare, except in individuals who sweat heavily or consume little or no sodium in the diet. Nevertheless, certain conditions can cause dangerously low blood sodium levels.

Hyponatremia, or low blood sodium levels (clinically defined as less than 136 milliequivalents per liter of blood), can occur in people engaged in strenuous physical activity who drink large volumes of water and fail to replace sodium. This was the case with Cynthia Lucero in our chapter-opening story, and it is discussed further in the accompanying Highlight box on page 284. Severe diarrhea, vomiting, or excessive prolonged sweating can also cause hyponatremia. Symptoms include

hypernatremia A condition in which blood sodium levels are dangerously high.

hyponatremia A condition in which blood sodium levels are dangerously low.

HIGHLIGHT

Can Water Be Too Much of a Good Thing?
Hyponatremia in Marathon Runners

At the beginning of this chapter, we described the death of marathon runner Cynthia Lucero. Her case is only one of several that have gained attention in recent years. How can seemingly healthy, highly fit individuals competing in marathons collapse and even die during or shortly after a race? One common issue faced by these athletes is maintaining a proper balance of fluid and electrolytes during the race.

It is well known that people participating in distance events such as marathons (26.2 miles) need to drink enough fluid to ensure proper fluid balance. Surprisingly, recent research has shown that some runners, especially novice runners, drink too much water and develop hyponatremia, or abnormally low blood sodium levels.

A recent study examined marathon runners who were treated for hyponatremia after a race.[8] The major contributing factors appeared to be longer race time and drinking large amounts of water during the race. Specifically, the researchers speculate that less experienced athletes run more slowly, increasing the total time that they are competing; at the same time, they consume very large amounts of water to avoid potential dehydration. The longer these individuals run, the more water they drink and the more diluted their blood sodium levels become. About half of the hyponatremic runners in these studies had to be hospitalized.

A study of long-distance triathletes (competing in swimming, cycling, and running) found that about 18% of these athletes also suffered from hyponatremia.[9] Thus, other individuals competing in long-distance events or activities are also at risk for this disorder. Hyponatremia is a dangerous and potentially fatal condition. Drinking sports beverages, which contain electrolytes, and moderating fluid intake during marathons and other long-distance activities can help prevent it.

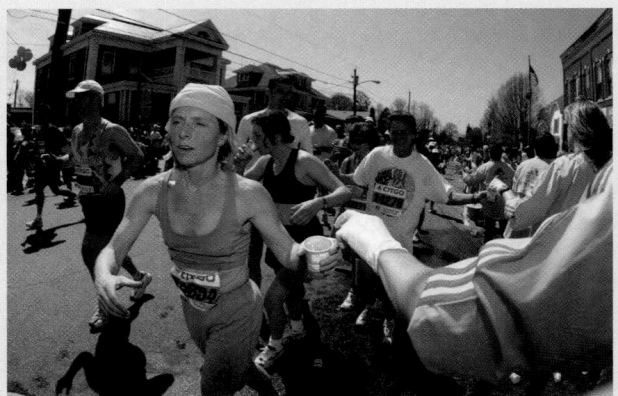

Consuming too much water can deplete blood sodium levels.

headaches, dizziness, fatigue, nausea, vomiting, and muscle cramps. If hyponatremia is left untreated it can lead to seizures, coma, and death. Treatment for hyponatremia includes replacement of the lost minerals by consuming liquids and foods high in sodium and other minerals. It may be necessary to administer electrolyte-rich solutions intravenously if the person has lost consciousness or is not able to consume beverages and foods by mouth.

> RECAP: *Sodium is the primary positively charged electrolyte in the extracellular fluid. It works to maintain fluid balance and blood pressure, assists in acid–base balance and transmission of nerve signals, aids muscle contraction, and assists in the absorption of some nutrients. Sodium deficiencies are rare, since the typical American diet is high in sodium. Excessive sodium intake has been related to high blood pressure, bloating, and loss of bone density in some studies. Low blood sodium, called hyponatremia, can cause seizures, coma, and death.*

Potassium

As we discussed previously, potassium is the major positively charged electrolyte in the intracellular fluid. It is a major constituent of all living cells and is found in both plants and animals.

Functions of Potassium

Potassium and sodium work together to maintain proper fluid balance. In addition, potassium plays a major role in regulating the contraction of muscles and transmission of nerve impulses, and it assists in maintaining blood pressure. Recent research also indicates that higher levels of potassium may benefit our bones and kidneys in part by helping the body maintain acid–base balance. Excessive acid causes the body to leach calcium from bones. This not only reduces bone density but also can contribute to the formation of calcium-containing kidney stones. In contrast to a high-sodium diet, eating a diet high in potassium actually helps to reduce the risk of high blood pressure and stroke.

How Much Potassium Should We Consume?

Potassium is found in abundance in many fresh foods. We can reduce our risk for high blood pressure by consuming adequate potassium in our diet.

Recommended Dietary Intake for Potassium   The AI for potassium is listed in Table 7.1. According to a recent survey by the Institute of Medicine, Americans typically consume less than half the amount of potassium they need daily.[10]

SHOPPER'S GUIDE

Good Food Sources of Potassium

Processing foods generally increases their sodium content and decreases their potassium content. Many researchers think that this sodium–potassium imbalance is a major factor contributing to the increased incidence of hypertension in the United States. Thus, the best sources of potassium include fresh foods, particularly fresh fruits and vegetables. FIGURE 7.9 identifies foods that are high in potassium. Below are some specific tips for increasing your potassium intake.

Tomato juice is an excellent source of potassium.

Tips for Increasing Your Potassium Intake

√ Avoid processed foods that are high in sodium and low in potassium. Check the Nutrition Facts Panel!

√ For breakfast, look for cereals containing bran and/or wheat germ.

√ Sprinkle wheat germ on yogurt and top with banana slices.

√ Add wheat germ to baked goods such as homemade pancakes and muffins.

√ Drink milk! If you don't like milk, try one of the new drinkable yogurts. Many brands of soy milk are also good sources of potassium.

√ Make a smoothie by blending ice cubes and low-fat vanilla ice cream with a banana.

(continued)

√ Pack a can of low-sodium vegetable or tomato juice in your lunch in place of a soft drink.

√ Serve avocado or bean dip with veggie slices.

√ Replace the meat in your sandwich with thin slices of avocado or marinated tofu.

√ Replace the meat in tacos and burritos with black or pinto beans.

√ For a healthful alternative to French fries, toss slices of sweet potato in olive oil, place on a cookie sheet, and oven bake at 400° for 10–15 minutes.

√ Toss a banana, some dried apricots, or a bag of sunflower seeds into your lunch bag.

√ Make a fruit salad with apricots, bananas, cantaloupe, honeydew melon, mango, or papaya.

√ Bake a pumpkin pie!

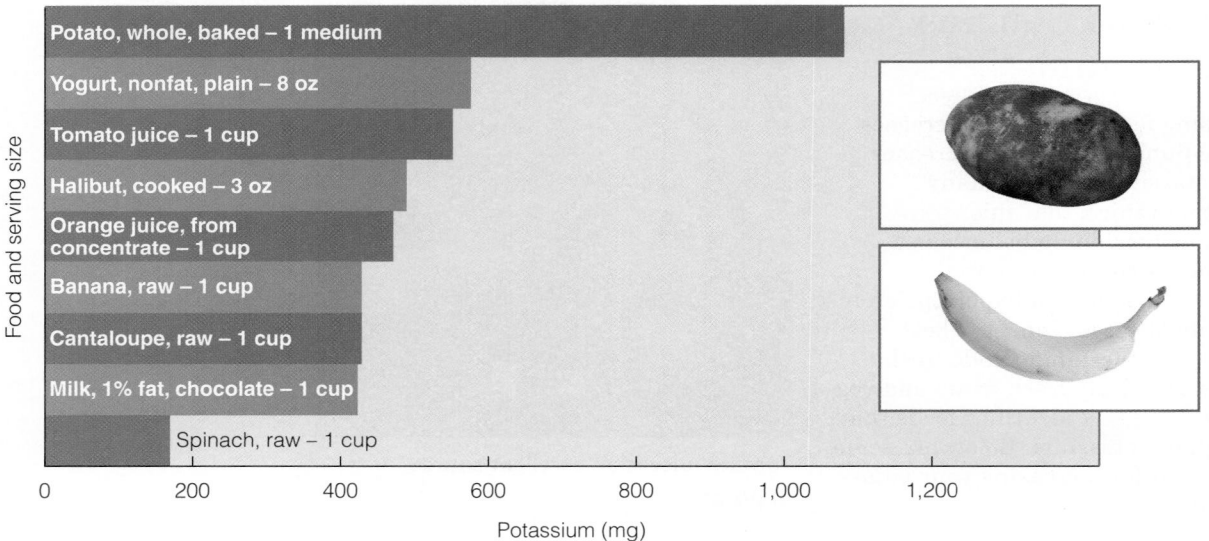

FIGURE 7.9 Common food sources of potassium. The AI for potassium is 4.7 g/day. (Data from U.S. Department of Agriculture, Agricultural Research Service. 2006. USDA Nutrient Database for Standard Reference, Release 19. Nutrient Data Laboratory Home Page. www.ars.usda.gov/ba/bhnrc/ndl.)

What Happens If We Consume Too Much Potassium?

People with healthy kidneys are able to excrete excess potassium effectively. However, people with kidney disease are not able to regulate their blood potassium levels. **Hyperkalemia,** or high blood potassium levels (clinically defined as greater than 5 milliequivalents per liter of blood), occurs when potassium is not excreted efficiently from the body. Because of potassium's role in cardiac muscle contraction, severe hyperkalemia can alter the normal rhythm of the heart, resulting in heart attack and death. People with kidney failure must monitor their potassium intake very carefully to prevent complications from hyperkalemia. Individuals at risk for hyperkalemia should avoid consuming salt substitutes, as these products are high in potassium.

hyperkalemia A condition in which blood potassium levels are dangerously high.

What Happens If We Don't Consume Enough Potassium?

Because potassium is widespread in many foods, a dietary potassium deficiency is rare. However, potassium deficiency is not uncommon among people who have serious medical disorders. Kidney disease, diabetic acidosis, and other illnesses can lead to potassium deficiency.

In addition, people with high blood pressure who are prescribed diuretic medications to treat their disease are at risk for potassium deficiency. As we noted earlier, diuretics promote the excretion of fluid as urine through the kidneys. Some diuretics also increase the body's excretion of potassium. People who are taking diuretic medications should have their blood potassium monitored regularly and should eat foods that are high in potassium to prevent **hypokalemia,** or low blood potassium levels (clinically defined as less than 3.8 milliequivalents per liter of blood). This is not a universal recommendation, however, because some diuretics are specially formulated to spare potassium, and, therefore, people taking this class of diuretic should not increase their dietary potassium above recommended levels.

Extreme dehydration, vomiting, and diarrhea can also cause hypokalemia. People who abuse alcohol or laxatives can also suffer from hypokalemia. Symptoms include confusion, loss of appetite, and muscle weakness. Severe cases of hypokalemia result in fatal changes in heart rate; many deaths attributed to extreme dehydration or an eating disorder are caused by abnormal heart rhythms due to hypokalemia.

> RECAP: *Potassium is the major positively charged electrolyte inside of the cell. It regulates fluid and acid–base balance, blood pressure, and muscle contraction, and it helps in the transmission of nerve impulses. Potassium is found in abundance in fresh foods, particularly fruits, vegetables, and meats. Potassium levels have been found to be below normal in most Americans because of the consumption of processed foods. Both hyperkalemia, or excessive blood potassium, and hypokalemia, or low blood potassium, can result in heart failure and death.*

Chloride

Chloride should not be confused with *chlorine,* which is a poisonous gas used to kill bacteria and other germs in our water supply. Chloride is a negatively charged ion that we obtain almost exclusively in our diets from consuming sodium chloride, or table salt.

Functions of Chloride

Coupled with sodium in the extracellular fluid, chloride assists with the maintenance of fluid balance. Chloride is also a part of hydrochloric acid (HCl) in the stomach, which aids in preparing food for further digestion (see Chapter 3). Chloride works with the white blood cells of our body during an immune response to help kill bacteria, and it assists in the transmission of nerve impulses.

How Much Chloride Should We Consume?

The AI for chloride is listed in Table 7.1. As chloride is coupled with sodium to form table salt, our primary dietary source of chloride is salt in our foods. Chloride is also found in some fruits and vegetables.

What Happens If We Consume Too Much Chloride?

As we consume virtually all of our dietary chloride in the form of sodium chloride, consuming excess amounts of this mineral over a prolonged period leads to hypertension in salt-sensitive individuals. There is no other known toxicity symptom for chloride.[11]

What Happens If We Don't Consume Enough Chloride?

Because of our relatively high dietary salt intake in the United States, most people consume more than enough chloride. Even when a person consumes a low-sodium

Almost all chloride is consumed through table salt.

hypokalemia A condition in which blood potassium levels are dangerously low.

diet, chloride intake is usually adequate. A chloride deficiency can occur, however, during conditions of severe dehydration and frequent vomiting. For example, it can develop in people with eating disorders who regularly vomit to rid their bodies of unwanted calories.

> **RECAP:** *Chloride is the major negatively charged electrolyte outside of the cell. It assists with maintaining fluid balance and aids digestion of food. It also helps our immune system fight infection and assists in the transmission of nerve impulses. Our main dietary source is table salt, excessive consumption of which can lead to hypertension in salt-sensitive individuals. Chloride deficiencies are rare but can occur during severe dehydration and frequent vomiting.*

Phosphorus

Phosphorus is the major intracellular negatively charged electrolyte. In our bodies, phosphorus is most commonly found combined with oxygen in the form of phosphate, PO_4^{2-}. Phosphorus is an essential constituent of all cells and is found in both plants and animals.

Functions of Phosphorus

Phosphorus works with potassium inside of the cell to maintain proper fluid balance. It also plays a critical role in bone formation, as it is a part of the mineral complex of bone (see Chapter 9). Indeed, about 85% of our body's phosphorus is stored in our bones.

As a primary component of adenosine triphosphate (ATP), phosphorus plays a key role in creating energy for our bodies. It also helps regulate many biochemical reactions by activating and deactivating enzymes. Phosphorus is a part of our genetic materials including deoxyribonucleic acid (DNA) and ribonucleic acid (RNA), and it is a component in cell membranes (as phospholipids) and lipoproteins.

How Much Phosphorus Should We Consume?

The RDA for phosphorus is listed in Table 7.1. The average U.S. adult consumes about twice this amount each day; thus, phosphorus deficiencies are rare. Phosphorus is widespread in many foods and is found in high amounts in foods that contain protein. Milk, meats, and eggs are good sources. FIGURE 7.10 shows the phosphorus content of various foods.

It is important to note that we absorb the phosphorus from animal sources more readily than that from plant sources. The phosphorus in plant foods such as beans, cereals, and nuts is found in the form of **phytic acid,** a plant storage form of phosphorus. Our bodies do not produce enzymes that can break down phytic acid, but we are still able to absorb up to 50% of the phosphorus found in plant foods because other foods and the bacteria in our large intestines can break down phytic acid. Soft drinks are another common source of phosphorus in our diet; refer to Chapter 9 to learn how heavy consumption of soft drinks may be detrimental to bone health.

What Happens If We Consume Too Much Phosphorus?

People suffering from kidney disease and people taking too many vitamin D supplements or too many phosphorus-containing antacids can suffer from high blood phosphorus levels. Severely high levels of blood phosphorus cause muscle spasms and convulsions.

What Happens If We Don't Consume Enough Phosphorus?

As mentioned previously, deficiencies of phosphorus are rare. People who may suffer from low phosphorus levels include premature infants, elderly people with poor diets, and people who abuse alcohol. People with vitamin D deficiency, those with hyperparathyroidism (oversecretion of parathyroid hormone), and those who overuse antacids that bind with phosphorus may also have low blood phosphorus levels.

Milk is a good source of phosphorus.

phytic acid The form of phosphorus stored in plants.

dehydration Depletion of body fluid that results when fluid excretion exceeds fluid intake.

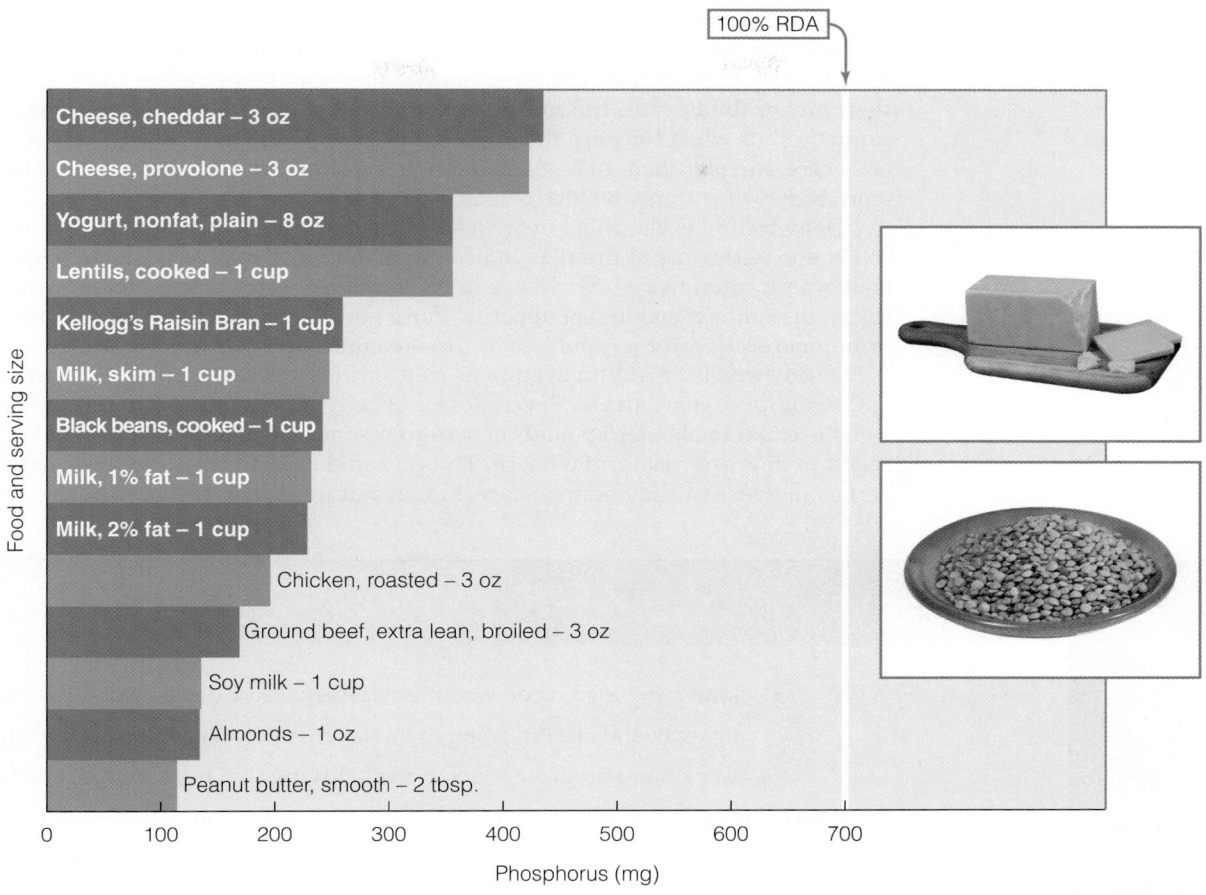

FIGURE 7.10 Common food sources of phosphorus. The RDA for phosphorus is 700 mg/day. (Data from U.S. Department of Agriculture, Agricultural Research Service. 2006. USDA Nutrient Database for Standard Reference, Release 19. Nutrient Data Laboratory Home Page. www.ars.usda.gov/ba/bhnrc/ndl.)

> RECAP: *Phosphorus is the major negatively charged electrolyte inside of the cell. It helps maintain fluid balance and bone health. It also assists us in making energy available and in regulating chemical reactions, and it is a primary component of our genetic materials. The RDA for phosphorus is 700 mg/day, and it is commonly found in high-protein foods. Excess phosphorus can lead to muscle spasms and convulsion, while phosphorus deficiencies are rare.*

What Disorders Are Related to Fluid and Electrolyte Imbalances?

There are a number of serious, and potentially fatal, disorders resulting from the imbalance of fluid and electrolytes in our bodies. Let's review some of these now.

Dehydration

Dehydration is a serious health problem that results when fluid excretion exceeds fluid intake. It commonly occurs as a result of heavy exercise or exposure to high environmental temperatures, when the body loses significant amounts of water through increased sweating and breathing. However, elderly people and infants can get dehydrated even when inactive, as their risk for dehydration is much higher than

Dehydration occurs when fluid excretion exceeds fluid intake.

that of healthy young and middle-aged adults. The elderly are at increased risk because they have a lower total amount of body water and their thirst mechanism is less effective than that of a younger person; they are therefore less likely to meet their higher fluid needs. Infants, on the other hand, excrete urine at a higher rate, cannot tell us when they are thirsty, and have a greater ratio of body surface area to body core, causing them to respond more dramatically to heat and cold and to lose more body water than an older person.

Dehydration is classified in terms of the percentage of weight loss that is exclusively due to the loss of fluid. As indicated in Table 7.3, relatively small losses in body water, equal to a 1–2% change in body weight, result in symptoms such as thirst, discomfort, and loss of appetite. For a person weighing 160 pounds, these symptoms occur after a rapid loss of 1 to 4 pounds. More severe water losses, equal to 3–5% body weight, result in symptoms that include sleepiness, nausea, flushed skin, and inability to concentrate. Severe losses of body water, greater than 8% of body weight (equal to about 13 pounds of water for someone weighing 160 pounds), can result in delirium, coma, and death. Thus, a rapid loss of body fluid leads to a dangerous increase in body temperature, kidney failure, and eventual death.

NUTRI-CASE GUSTAVO

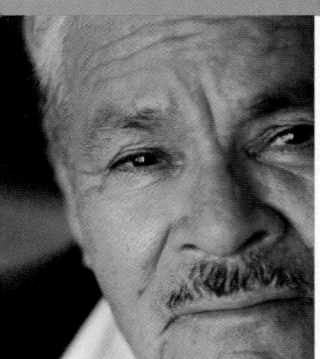

"Something is going on with me this week. Every day, at work, I've been feeling weak and like I'm going to be sick to my stomach. It's been really hot, over a hundred degrees out in the fields, but I'm used to that, and besides, I've been drinking lots of water. It's probably just my high blood pressure acting up again."

What do you think might be wrong with Gustavo? If you learned that he was following a low-sodium diet prescribed to manage his high blood pressure, would this information argue for or against your theory, and why? What would you advise Gustavo to do differently at work tomorrow?

We discussed earlier the importance of fluid replacement when you are exercising. How can you tell whether you are drinking enough fluid before, during, and after

TABLE 7.3 Percentages of Body Fluid Loss Correlated with Weight Loss and Symptoms

Body Water Loss (%)	Weight Lost If You Weigh 160 lbs	Weight Lost If You Weigh 130 lbs	Symptoms
1–2	1.6–3.2 lbs	1.3–2.6 lbs	Strong thirst, loss of appetite, feeling uncomfortable
3–5	4.8–8.0 lbs	3.9–6.5 lbs	Dry mouth, reduced urine output, greater difficulty working and concentrating, flushed skin, tingling extremities, impatience, sleepiness, nausea, emotional instability
6–8	9.6–12.8 lbs	7.8–10.4 lbs	Increased body temperature that doesn't decrease, increased heart rate and breathing rate, dizzy, difficulty breathing, slurred speech, mental confusion, muscle weakness, blue lips
9–11	14.4–17.6 lbs	11.7–14.3 lbs	Muscle spasms, delirium, swollen tongue, poor balance and circulation, kidney failure, decreased blood volume and blood pressure

Source: Based on pp. 107–125 in *Nutrition and Aerobic Exercise,* edited by D. K. Layman. © 1986 American Chemical Society.

your exercise sessions? First, you can measure your body weight before and after each session. If you weighed in at 160 pounds before basketball practice, and immediately afterward you weigh 158 pounds, then you have lost 2 pounds of body weight. This is equal to 1.3% of your body weight prior to practice. As you can see in Table 7.3, you are most likely feeling strong thirst and diminished appetite, and you may even feel generally uncomfortable. Your goal is to consume enough water and other fluids to bring your body weight back to 160 pounds prior to your next exercise session.

A simpler method of monitoring your fluid levels is to observe the color of your urine (FIGURE 7.11). If you are properly hydrated, your urine should be clear to pale yellow in color, similar to diluted lemonade. Urine that is medium to dark yellow in color, similar to apple juice, indicates an inadequate fluid intake. Very dark or brown colored urine, such as the color of a cola beverage, is a sign of severe dehydration and indicates potential muscle breakdown and kidney damage. People should strive to maintain a urine color that is clear or pale yellow.

Warning: clear urine is not a reliable indicator of adequate hydration if you have been drinking alcohol. A hormone called antidiuretic hormone helps to regulate fluid balance by triggering the body to retain water when internal conditions suggest the body is becoming dehydrated. Alcohol inhibits this hormone. When people drink alcohol, its diuretic affect causes copious amounts of fluid to be excreted. As a result, the body should begin retaining water, but because alcohol inhibits antidiuretic hormone, the body continues to lose water and the urine is clear. This mechanism explains why alcohol is often a factor in dehydration.

Heat Stroke

Athletes who work out in hot weather are particularly vulnerable to dangerous fluid loss. In August 2001, 27-year-old National Football League all-star player Korey Stringer died of complications from **heat stroke** after working out in a hot and humid environment. Heat stroke is a potentially fatal heat illness characterized by failure of the body's heat-regulating mechanisms. Symptoms include rapid pulse; hot, dry skin; high temperature; and loss of consciousness. As illustrated in the Korey Stringer case, heat stroke can also be fatal. Despite having access to ample fluid and excellent medical assistance, Stringer's body core temperature rose to 108°F. It appears that a combination of dehydration, heat, humidity, protective clothing and headgear, and Stringer's large body size (6'4", 330 pounds) contributed to his death. Although there were suspicions that ephedra, a stimulant used by many athletes, contributed to his death, no evidence was found to support this. Our ability to sweat is extremely limited in a humid environment, and large individuals with a great deal of muscle mass produce a lot of body heat. In addition, people who have excess body fat have an extra layer of insulation that makes it even more difficult to dissipate body heat at rest and during exercise.

Similar deaths of collegiate and high school football players have occurred in the past. These deaths have prompted national attention and resulted in strict guidelines encouraging regular fluid breaks and cancellation of events or changing the time of the event to avoid high heat and humidity. In addition, people who are active in a hot environment should stop exercising if they feel dizzy, light-headed, disoriented, or nauseated. Injury and death due to heat illnesses can be avoided by maintaining a healthy fluid balance before, during, and after exercise.

Water Intoxication

Is it possible to drink too much water? **Overhydration,** or *water intoxication,* can occur but it is rare. It generally only occurs in people with health problems that cause the kidneys to retain too much water, causing overhydration and hyponatremia, which were discussed earlier.

Hypertension

One of the major chronic diseases in the United States is high blood pressure, which health care professionals refer to as **hypertension.** A person with hypertension is

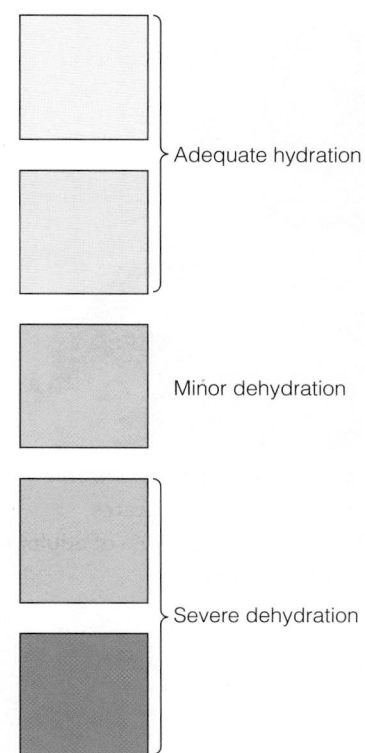

Adequate hydration

Minor dehydration

Severe dehydration

FIGURE 7.11 Urine color chart. Color variations indicate levels of hydration.

heat stroke A potentially fatal response to high temperature characterized by failure of the body's heat-regulating mechanisms. Symptoms include rapid pulse; reduced sweating; hot, dry skin; high temperature; headache; weakness; and sudden loss of consciousness. Commonly called *sunstroke* or *heatstroke*.

overhydration Dilution of body fluid. It results when water intake or retention is excessive.

hypertension A chronic condition characterized by above-average blood pressure readings, specifically, systolic blood pressure over 140 mm Hg or diastolic blood pressure over 90 mm Hg.

Hypertension is a major chronic disease in the United States, affecting more than 50% of adults over 65 years old.

unable to maintain blood pressure in a healthy range. This disease affects over 25% of all adults in the United States and more than 50% of people over the age of 65 (see FIGURE 7.12).[12] Although hypertension itself is often without symptoms, it increases a person's risk for many other serious conditions including heart disease, stroke, and kidney disease; it can also reduce brain function, impair physical mobility, and cause death.

We measure blood pressure in two phases, systolic and diastolic. *Systolic blood pressure* represents the pressure exerted in our arteries at the moment that the heart contracts, sending blood into our blood vessels. *Diastolic blood pressure* represents the pressure in our arteries between contractions, when our heart is relaxed. You can also think of diastolic blood pressure as the resistance in our arteries that our heart must pump against every time it beats.

Blood pressure measurements are recorded in millimeters of mercury (mm Hg). Optimal systolic blood pressure is *less than* 120 mm Hg, while optimal diastolic blood pressure is *less than* 80 mm Hg. Prehypertension is defined as a systolic blood pressure between 120 and 139 mm Hg, or a diastolic blood pressure between 80 and 89 mm Hg. You would be diagnosed with hypertension if your systolic blood pressure were greater than or equal to 140 mm Hg or your diastolic blood pressure were greater than or equal to 90 mm Hg.

What Causes Hypertension?

What causes hypertension? For about 95% of people who have it, the causes are unknown. This type is referred to as *primary* or *essential hypertension*. For the other 5% of people with hypertension, causes may include kidney disease, sleep apnea (a sleep disorder that affects breathing), and sensitivity to salt.

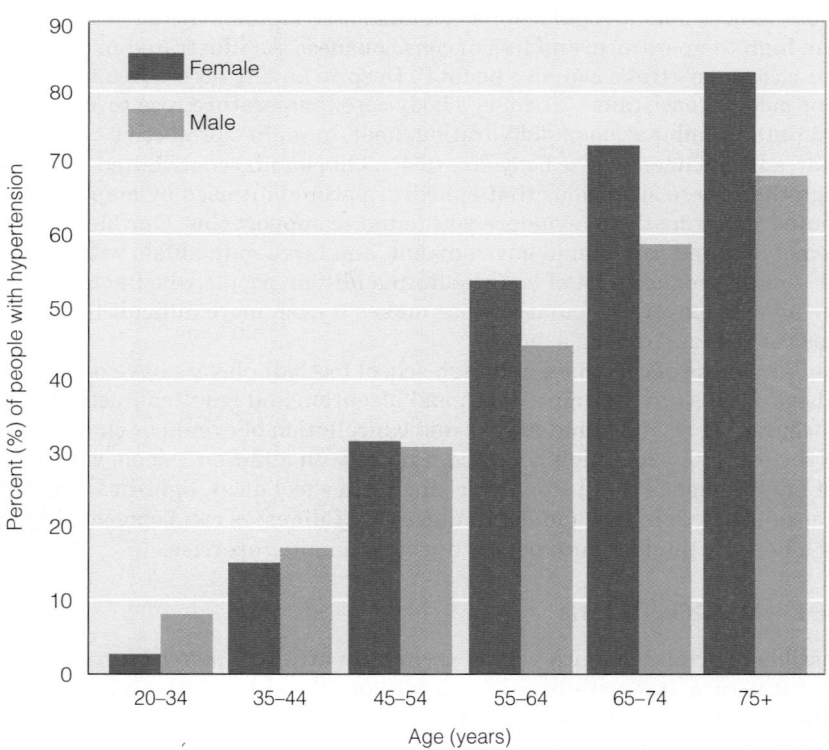

FIGURE 7.12 Hypertension is one of the major chronic diseases in the United States. (From Centers for Disease Control and Prevention, National Center for Health Statistics, Division of Health Examination Statistics. Hypertension. www.cdc.gov/nchs/fastats/hyprtens.htm.)

What Can Be Done to Reduce Hypertension?

Although we do not know what causes most cases of hypertension, there are five primary lifestyle changes that can help reduce it. These changes include the following:

- Losing weight. Blood pressure values have been shown to decrease six to seven points in people who have lost less than 20 pounds of body weight.[13]

- Increasing physical activity. The amount and intensity of exercise needed to improve blood pressure are easily achievable for most people. Light-intensity exercise lasting 30 to 60 minutes can reduce blood pressure, as can more intense exercise lasting 20 to 30 minutes.[14]

- Reducing alcohol intake. Because heavy alcohol consumption can worsen high blood pressure, it is suggested that people with this disease abstain from drinking alcohol or drink no more than two drinks per day for males and one drink per day for females.

- Reducing sodium intake in salt-sensitive individuals (people whose blood pressure increases when they eat high-sodium foods); some people who are not salt sensitive also benefit from eating lower-sodium diets.

- Eating more whole grains, fruits, vegetables, and low-fat protein sources.

Losing weight and increasing physical activity can help fight hypertension.

One area of controversy is the impact that sodium intake has on our blood pressure. For years it was believed that the high sodium intakes of the typical American diet lead to hypertension. This is because people who live in countries where sodium intake is high have greater rates of hypertension than people from countries where sodium intake is low. We have recently learned, however, that not everyone with hypertension is sensitive to sodium. Unfortunately, it is impossible to know who is sensitive to sodium, as there is not an easy test for sodium sensitivity. Because lowering sodium intake does not reduce blood pressure in all people with hypertension, there is significant debate over whether everyone can benefit from eating a lower-sodium diet. Despite this debate, the leading health organizations, including the American Heart Association, the National High Blood Pressure Education Program, and the National Heart, Lung, and Blood Institute of the National Institutes of Health, continue to support a reduction in dietary sodium to 2,400 mg/day as recommended in the Dietary Guidelines for Americans.[15] Currently, the average sodium intake in the United States is about 3,300 mg/day.

In contrast to sodium, other minerals such as calcium, magnesium, and potassium have been shown to help reduce hypertension. As discussed in Chapter 2, the DASH (Dietary Approaches to Stop Hypertension) diet is an eating plan that is high in these minerals, moderately low in sodium, and low in saturated fat, and it includes 10 servings of fruits and vegetables each day. The DASH diet has been shown to significantly reduce blood pressure in people with and without hypertension, with even greater reductions occurring in a lower-sodium version of the DASH diet.[16,17] Thus, eating a healthful diet that contains plenty of fruits, vegetables, whole grains, and low-fat dairy products has been proven to reduce blood pressure levels.

For some individuals, lifestyle changes are not completely effective in normalizing hypertension. When this is the case, a variety of medications can be prescribed to bring a person's blood pressure into the normal range. Individuals taking medications to control blood pressure should also continue to practice the healthful lifestyle changes listed earlier in this section, as these changes will continue to benefit their long-term health.

Hypertension is called "the silent killer" because often there are no obvious symptoms of this disease. For this reason, it is important that people get their blood pressure checked on a regular basis. Tragically, many people with hypertension fail to take their prescribed medication because they do not feel sick. Many of these people eventually suffer the consequences of their actions by experiencing a heart attack or stroke.

Neuropsychiatric Disorders

Electrolyte imbalances can cause changes in nervous function that result in psychiatric disorders. Low levels of magnesium, hypokalemia, and chronic hyponatremia may be associated with conditions of apathy and depression. High blood levels of calcium can also cause depression. A variety of electrolyte imbalances can cause confusion, delirium, and psychosis, including hyponatremia, excessive blood calcium, and low blood calcium. Electrolyte disorders can also impair cognitive function, diminishing a person's capacity to think, concentrate, solve problems, and remember information.

Muscle Disorders

Muscle function can be altered by electrolyte imbalances because of disturbances in nervous system signaling. For example, electrolyte imbalances can prompt **seizures,** uncontrollable muscle spasms that may be localized to one area of the body, such as the face, or can violently wrack a person's entire body. Some people lose consciousness during seizures, while others may experience hallucinations, flashbacks, or emotional outbursts. Severe seizures can result in bone fractures, dislocated joints, loss of bowel and bladder function, and severe biting of the tongue.

Muscle cramps are involuntary, spasmodic, and painful muscle contractions that last for many seconds or even minutes. Hypernatremia that occurs with dehydration is known to cause cramps, as are other electrolyte imbalances. Muscle weakness and paralysis can also occur with imbalances in potassium and phosphorus.

Contribution of Fluids to Obesity

Until about 50 years ago, beverage choices were limited. But the introduction of a new, cheap sweetener derived from corn, *high-fructose corn syrup* (see the Nutrition Debate in Chapter 4), caused soda and other sweetened beverages to flood the market. Today, Americans take in approximately 21% of their calories from beverages, mostly in the form of sweetened soft drinks and fruit juices. Recently, sweetened bottled waters, bottled teas, and specialty coffee drinks have contributed to the problem: a coffee mocha at one national chain of cafes provides 400 calories, which is 20% of an average adult's total daily calorie needs.

It's not surprising, then, that researchers believe that calories from such beverages have contributed to half of the rise in caloric intake among Americans since the late 1970s. That's because beverages with a high calorie content do little to curb appetite, so most people do not compensate for the extra calories they drink by eating less.[18] In addition, sweetened sodas, teas, and other specialty beverages displace more nutritious beverages such as milk, which provides protein, calcium, vitamin D, and other nutrients important for bone health (see Chapter 9).

seizures Uncontrollable muscle spasms caused by increased nervous system excitability that can result from electrolyte imbalances.

muscle cramps Involuntary, spasmodic, and painful muscle contractions that last for many seconds or even minutes; electrolyte imbalances are often the cause of muscle cramps.

RECAP: *Dehydration, heat stroke, and even death can occur when water loss exceeds water intake. Since our thirst mechanism is not always sufficient, it is important to drink water regularly throughout the day to promote adequate fluid intake. High blood pressure is a major chronic illness in the United States; it can be controlled by losing weight, increasing physical activity, decreasing alcohol intake, and making specific dietary changes. Electrolyte imbalances can lead to neuropsychiatric disorders such as depression, delirium, and psychosis; they can also lead to muscle disorders such as seizures and muscle cramps. Intake of sugary beverages can contribute to obesity.*

CHAPTER SUMMARY

- Between approximately 50% and 70% of a healthy adult's body weight is fluid. Two-thirds of this fluid is intracellular fluid, and the remainder is extracellular fluid.

- Electrolytes are electrically charged particles found in our body fluid that assist in maintaining fluid balance and the normal functioning of our cells and nervous system.

- Water acts as a solvent in our bodies, provides protection and lubrication for our organs and tissues, and acts to maintain blood volume, body temperature, and blood pressure.

- The three primary sources of fluid intake are beverages, foods, and metabolic water produced by our bodies.

- The primary avenues of fluid excretion are sensible water loss (via urine and sweat), insensible water loss (via evaporation and exhalation), and feces.

- Conditions that significantly increase water loss from our bodies include fever, vomiting, diarrhea, hemorrhage, blood donation, heavy exercise, and exposure to heat, cold, and altitude.

- Fluid intake needs are highly variable and depend upon body size, age, physical activity, health status, and environmental conditions.

- Drinking too much water can lead to overhydration and hyponatremia, or dilution of blood sodium, whereas drinking too little water leads to dehydration, one of the leading causes of death around the world.

- Sodium assists in maintaining fluid balance, blood pressure, nervous function, and muscle contraction.

- Consuming excess sodium can cause high blood pressure or hypernatremia. Sodium deficiencies are rare, but hyponatremia can occur from excessive fluid intake not accompanied by adequate sodium intake.

- Potassium assists in maintaining fluid balance, healthy blood pressure, transmission of nerve impulses, and muscle function.

- Hyperkalemia is excess blood potassium, which occurs due to kidney disease or malfunction. Hypokalemia is low blood potassium and can occur as a result of kidney disease, diabetic acidosis, and the use of some diuretic medications.

- Chloride assists in maintaining fluid balance, normal nerve transmission, and the digestion of food via the action of HCl.

- Excessive chloride intake occurs with excessive sodium intake, leading to hypertension in salt-sensitive people. Chloride deficiency is rare but can occur with prolonged dehydration and vomiting.

- Phosphorus assists in maintaining fluid balance and transferring energy via ATP. It is also a component of bone, phospholipids, genetic material, and lipoproteins.

- High blood phosphorus levels can occur with kidney disease and when individuals consume too many vitamin D supplements or phosphorus-containing antacids. Phosphorus deficiencies are rare but can occur with vitamin D deficiency and in premature infants or people with poor diets.

- Dehydration occurs when water excretion exceeds water intake. Individuals at risk include the elderly, infants, people exercising heavily for prolonged periods in the heat, and individuals suffering from prolonged vomiting and diarrhea.

- Heat stroke occurs when the body's core temperature rises above 100°F. Heat stroke can lead to death if left untreated.

- Overhydration, or water intoxication, is caused by consuming too much water. Hyponatremia can also result from water intoxication.

- Hypertension, or high blood pressure, increases the risk for heart disease, stroke, and kidney disease. Consuming excess sodium is associated with hypertension in some people.

- Electrolyte imbalances can cause neuropsychiatric disorders such as apathy, depression, confusion, and psychosis. They can also cause seizures, muscle cramps, muscle weakness, and paralysis.

TEST YOURSELF ANSWERS

1. **True.** Between approximately 50% and 70% of our body weight consists of water.

2. **False.** Sodium is a nutrient necessary for health, but we should not consume more than recommended amounts.

3. **False.** Our thirst mechanism signals that we need to replenish fluids, but it is not sufficient to ensure we are completely hydrated.

4. **True.** Alcohol inhibits a specific hormone that signals the body to retain water. Thus, when alcohol is consumed, the body loses excess water.

5. **False.** We do not know the cause of high blood pressure in most people. A high-sodium diet can cause high blood pressure in people who are sensitive to sodium.

REVIEW QUESTIONS

1. Which of the following is a characteristic of potassium?
   a. It is the major positively charged electrolyte in the extracellular fluid.
   b. It can be found in fresh fruits and vegetables.
   c. It is a critical component of the mineral complex of bone.
   d. It is the major negatively charged electrolyte in the extracellular fluid.

2. Which of the following people probably has the greatest percentage of bodily fluid?
   a. A female adult who is slightly overweight and vomits nightly after eating dinner.
   b. An elderly male of average weight who has low blood pressure.
   c. An overweight football player who has just completed a practice session in high heat.
   d. A healthy infant of average weight.

3. Plasma is one example of
   a. extracellular fluid.
   b. intracellular fluid.
   c. tissue fluid.
   d. metabolic water.

4. Which of the following is true of the cell membrane?
   a. It is freely permeable to most solutes except fats.
   b. It is freely permeable to water and all solutes.
   c. It is freely permeable only to fats.
   d. It is freely permeable to water but impermeable to solutes.

5. In a group of people diagnosed with hypertension, which of the following lifestyle changes is most likely to reduce blood pressure?
   a. consuming a low-sodium diet
   b. losing weight
   c. getting at least 8 hours of sleep nightly
   d. consuming at least two glasses of red wine daily

6. True or false? Drinking lots of water throughout a marathon will prevent fluid imbalances.

7. True or false? A decreased concentration of electrolytes in our blood stimulates the thirst mechanism.

8. True or false? Hypernatremia commonly occurs when we are dehydrated.

9. True or false? Absence of thirst is a reliable indicator of adequate hydration.

10. True or false? Conditions that increase fluid loss include constipation, blood transfusions, and high humidity.

11. Explain why chronic diarrhea in a young child can lead to death from abnormal heart rhythms.

12. After winning a cross-country relay race, you and your teammates celebrate with a trip to the local tavern for a few beers. That evening, you feel shaky and disoriented, and you have a "pins and needles" feeling in your hands and feet. What could be going on that is contributing to these feelings?

13. For lunch today, your choices include (a) chicken soup, a ham sandwich, and a can of tomato juice or (b) potato salad, a tuna fish sandwich, and a bottle of mineral water. You have hockey practice in mid-afternoon. Which lunch should you choose, and why?

14. Your cousin, who is breastfeeding her 3-month-old daughter, confesses to you that she has resorted to taking over-the-counter weight loss pills to help her lose the weight she gained during pregnancy. What would you advise her?

15. Your mother has been diagnosed with hypertension, and her physician has prescribed medication. She tells you that she has no intention of filling the prescription because, as she puts it, "I feel great! Why should I fix something that isn't broken?" What information, if any, might you share with her regarding her decision, and why?

FIND THE QUACK

Libby is shopping for groceries with her 10-year-old daughter, Jen. When they turn into the beverage aisle, Jen exclaims over a colorful display offering a free hot-pink Frisbee with the purchase of a six-pack of a new vitamin-fortified sparkling water. The poster above the display shows a family in a park playing Frisbee together while drinking or holding a bottle of the new water. A banner above the photograph proclaims: "Part of Your Healthy Life!"

"Mom, can we get some?" Jen asks.

Libby reads the product packaging, which describes the beverage as follows:

- "Lightly carbonated delicious sparkling water!"

- "All natural flavor and color!"

- "Packed with vitamins!"

- A 12-oz serving of the water contains 10% of the DRI for vitamins E, B_6, B_{12}, and niacin.

- No other vitamins or minerals are listed.

- A serving contains 128 calories and 32 g of carbohydrate.

- The product is sweetened with high-fructose corn syrup.

- The cost is $4.99 per six-pack.

Libby can't decide whether to give in and buy the water or not. "I don't know, honey," she tells her daughter. "It looks healthy, but $4.99 seems like a lot to pay for a Frisbee and some vitamins!"

1. The product packaging claims that the beverage is "Packed with vitamins!" Evaluate this statement by checking out the label of a multivitamin supplement either at home or at a market. How many vitamins does it contain, and at what percentage of the DRI? Which provides more nutrients: the fortified water, or a glass of plain water plus a multivitamin tablet? Calculate the difference in cost per serving.

2. It's summer, and Jen plays children's soccer two mornings a week on an unshaded field. Would Libby be smarter to purchase a sports beverage such as Gatorade for her daughter to drink during her soccer matches or this new vitamin-fortified water, or should she give Jen plain water to drink? Explain. (Hint: See the Nutrition Debate at the end of this chapter.)

3. Check out the nutrition information on a carton of milk. Which contains the greater variety of nutrients, and at what cost, the fortified water or the milk?

4. The vitamin-fortified water is sweetened with high-fructose corn syrup and contains 128 calories per serving. This is about equivalent to a can of grape soda. The promoters characterize the beverage as "Part of Your Healthy Life." Do you agree or disagree? Why?

Answers can be found at www.aw-bc.com/thompson.

WEB LINKS

www.epa.gov/OW
U.S. Environmental Protection Agency: Water

Go to the EPA's water Web site for more information about drinking water quality, standards, and safety.

www.bottledwater.org
International Bottled Water Association

Find current information about bottled water from this trade association that represents the bottled water industry.

www.mayoclinic.com
MayoClinic.com

Search for "hyponatremia" to learn more about this potentially fatal condition.

www.nlm.nih.gov/medlineplus
MedlinePlus Health Information

Search for "dehydration" and "heat stroke" to obtain additional resources and the latest news about the dangers of these heat-related illnesses.

www.nhlbi.nih.gov

National Heart, Lung, and Blood Institute

Go to this site to learn more about heart and vascular diseases including how to prevent high blood pressure and hypertension.

www.americanheart.org

American Heart Association

Discover the best way to help lower your blood pressure.

www.nih.gov

The National Institutes of Health (NIH)

Search this site to learn more about the DASH (Dietary Approaches to Stop Hypertension) diet.

http://digestive.niddk.nih.gov

National Digestive Diseases Information Clearinghouse (NDDIC)

Go to this site to find out more about the causes, symptoms, and treatment of diarrhea.

www.nephrologychannel.com/electrolytes

Nephrologychannel.com: Electrolyte Imbalances

Visit this Web site to learn more about hyponatremia, hypernatremia, hypokalemia, and hyperkalemia.

www.wqa.org

Water Quality Association

A trade association for the water treatment industry, the WQA Web site lists recent news affecting municipal water supplies, home water testing, and water quality.

REFERENCES

1. Almond, C. S. D., A. Y. Shin, E. B. Fortescue, R. C. Mannix, D. Wypij, B. A. Binstadt, C. N. Duncan, D. P. Olson, A. E. Salerno, J. W. Newburger, and D. S. Greenes. 2005. Hyponatremia among runners in the Boston Marathon. *N. Engl. J. Med.* 352:1150–1156.
2. Institute of Medicine. 2004. *Dietary Reference Intakes for Water, Potassium, Sodium, Chloride, and Sulfate.* Washington, DC: National Academies Press.
3. American College of Sports Medicine (ACSM). 1996. Exercise and fluid replacement. *Med. Sci. Sports Exerc.* 28:i–vii.
4. American College of Sports Medicine (ACSM). 2000. Nutrition and athletic performance. *Med. Sci. Sports Exerc.* 32:2130–2145.
5. Beverage Marketing Corporation. Beverage Marketing's 2006 Market Report Findings. Accessed through the International Bottled Water Association (IBWA) website. http://www.bottledwater.org/public/statistics_main.htm.
6. The University of Maine Cooperative Extension. 2007. Sodium content of your food. http://www.umext.maine.edu/onlinepubs/htmpubs/4059.htm. (Accessed May 2007.)
7. Cohen, A. J., and F. J. Roe. 2000. Review of risk factors for osteoporosis with particular reference to a possible aetiological role of dietary salt. *Food Chem. Toxicol.* 38:237–253.
8. Davis, D. P., J. S. Videen, A. Marino, G. M. Vilke, J. V. Dunford, S. P. Van Camp, and L. G. Maharam. 2001. Exercise-associated hyponatremia in marathon runners: a two-year experience. *J. Emerg. Med.* 21:47–57.
9. Speedy, D. B., T. D. Noakes, I. R. Rogers, J. M. Thompson, R. G. Campbell, J. A. Kuttner, D. R. Boswell, S. Wright, and M. Hamlin. 1999. Hyponatremia in ultradistance triathletes. *Med. Sci. Sports Exerc.* 31:809–815.
10. Hendly, J. 2007. Featured nutrient: potassium. WebMD. http://www.webmd.com/food-recipes/features/featured-nutrient-potassium?print=true. (Accessed April 2007.)
11. National Research Council. Food and Nutrition Board. 1989. *Recommended Dietary Allowances,* 10th edn. Washington, DC: National Academies Press.
12. Centers for Disease Control and Prevention (CDC). 2006. Hypertension. National Center for Health Statistics, Division of Health Examination Statistics. www.cdc.gov/nchs/fastats/hyprtens.htm. (Accessed July 2007.)
13. Blumenthal, J. A., A. Sherwood, E. C. D. Gullette, M. Babyak, R. Waugh, A. Georgiades, L. W. Craighead, D. Tweedy, M. Feinglos, M. Applebaum, J. Hayano, and A. Hinderliter. 2000. Exercise and weight loss reduce blood pressure in men and women with mild hypertension. *Arch. Intern. Med.* 160:1947–1958.
14. Lesniak, K. T., and P. M. Dubbert. 2001. Exercise and hypertension. *Curr. Opin. Cardiol.* 16:356–359.
15. U.S. Department of Agriculture (USDA). U.S. Department of Health and Human Services. 2000. *Dietary Guidelines for Americans,* 5th edn. Home and Garden Bulletin No. 232.
16. Appel, L. J., T. J. Moore, E. Obarzanek, W. M. Vollmer, L. P. Svetkey, F. M. Sacks, G. A. Bray, T. M. Vogt, J. A. Cutler, M. M. Windhauser, P.-H. Lin, and N. Karanja. 1997. A clinical trial of the effects of dietary patterns on blood pressure. *New Engl. J. Med.* 336:1117–1124.
17. Sacks, F. M., L. P. Svetkey, W. M. Vollmer, L. J. Appel, G. A. Bray, D. Harsha, E. Obarzanek, P. R. Conlin, E. R. Miller III, D. G. Simons-Morton, N. Karanja, and P.-H. Lin. 2001. Effects on blood pressure of reduced dietary sodium and the Dietary Approaches to Stop Hypertension (DASH) diet. *New Engl. J. Med.* 344:3–10.
18. Brody, J. 2007. You are also what you drink. *New York Times,* Personal Health; March 27, 2007, Section F, p. 8.
19. Manore, M., and J. Thompson. 2000. *Sport Nutrition for Health and Performance.* Champaign, IL: Human Kinetics.
20. Bilzon, J. L., A. J. Allsopp, and C. Williams. 2000. Short-term recovery from prolonged constant pace running in a warm environment: the effectiveness of a carbohydrate-electrolyte solution. *Eur. J. Appl. Physiol.* 82:305–312.
21. Galloway, S. D., and R. J. Maughan. 2000. The effects of substrate and fluid provision on thermoregulatory and metabolic responses to prolonged exercise in a hot environment. *J. Sports Sci.* 18:339–351.

NUTRITION DEBATE

Sports Beverages: Help or Hype?

Once considered specialty items used exclusively by elite athletes, sports beverages have become popular everyday beverage choices for both active and nonactive people. The market for these drinks has become so lucrative that many of the large soft drink companies now produce these drinks. This surge in popularity of sports beverages leads us to ask three important questions:

Sports beverages were originally designed to meet the needs of competitive athletes.

- Do these beverages benefit highly active athletes?
- Do these beverages benefit recreationally active people?
- Do non-athletes need to consume sports beverages?

The first question is relatively easy to answer. Sports beverages were originally developed to meet the unique fluid, electrolyte, and carbohydrate needs of competitive athletes. As you learned in this chapter, highly active people need to replenish both fluids and electrolytes to avoid either dehydration or hyponatremia. Sports beverages can especially benefit athletes who exercise in the heat and are thus at an even greater risk for loss of water, electrolytes, and carbohydrates through respiration and sweat. The carbohydrates in sports beverages provide critical fuel during relatively intense (more than 60% of maximal effort) exercise bouts lasting more than 1 hour. Thus, endurance athletes are able to exercise longer, maintain a higher intensity, and improve performance times when they drink a sports beverage during

exercise.[19] Sports beverages may help athletes consume more energy than they could by eating solid foods and water alone. Some athletes, such as endurance bicyclists, train or compete for 6 to 8 hours each day on a regular basis. It is virtually impossible for these athletes to consume enough solid foods to support this intense level of exercise.

Do recreationally active people need to consume sports beverages? Most probably do not, but if they exercise for periods longer than 1 hour at more than 60% maximal effort, they can benefit from consuming the carbohydrate and electrolytes in sports beverages during exercise. In addition, recent laboratory studies found that healthy people who are active but not elite athletes are able to exercise longer in high temperatures when they consume sports beverages.[20,21] These beverages can also be beneficial when exercising in an indoor environment, because many times the temperature in indoor areas is relatively high and results in a large volume of fluid being lost during the activity.

It is not always easy to determine whether someone should consume a sports beverage. However, keep in mind that these beverages were originally formulated for people who exercise. Whether these beverages are needed depends on the duration and intensity of exercise, the environmental conditions, and the characteristics of the individual. Here are some situations in which drinking a sports beverage is appropriate:[19]

- Before exercise during which dehydration can occur, especially if someone is already dehydrated prior to exercise.
- During exercise or physical work in high heat and/or high humidity, or if someone has recently had diarrhea or vomiting; this may also be appropriate for someone who is not accustomed to activity in the heat.
- During exercise at high altitude and in cold environments; these conditions increase fluid and electrolyte losses.
- After exercise for rapid rehydration or between exercise bouts when it is difficult to consume food, such as between multiple soccer matches during a tournament.
- During long-duration exercise when blood glucose levels get low. For bouts of continuous, vigorous exercise lasting longer than 60 minutes, sports beverages may be needed to maintain energy levels and to provide the fluid necessary to prevent dehydration.

TABLE 7.4 Nutrient Content of Sports Beverages and Other Common Beverages*

Beverage	Energy (kcal)	Carbohydrate (g)	Sodium (mg)	Potassium (mg)
Cola, regular	153	39	15	4
Ginger ale	124	32	26	4
Beer, regular	146	9	18	89
Gatorade	90	22.5	144	39
All Sport	80	22.5	55.5	55.5
Beer, light	8	<1	1	5
Coffee, brewed	7.5	1.5	7.5	192
Cola, diet	4	<1	21	0
Tea, brewed	3	<1	7	88
Water, bottled	0	0	2	0
Water, tap	0	0	7	0

*Amounts compared are 12 fl. oz (1.5 cups).

- During exercise in people who may have poor glycogen stores prior to exercise or who are not well fed due to illness or inability to eat enough solid food prior to exercise.

Interestingly, sports beverages have become very popular with people who do little or no regular exercise. Are there any benefits or negative consequences for inactive or lightly active people who regularly consume these drinks? There does not appear to be any evidence that people who do not exercise derive any benefits from consuming sports beverages. Even if these individuals live in a hot environment, they should be able to replenish the fluid and electrolytes they lose during sweating by drinking water and other beverages and eating a normal diet.

Negative consequences could result when inactive people drink sports beverages. The primary consequence is weight gain, which could lead to obesity. As you can see in Table 7.4, sports beverages contain not only fluid and electrolytes, but also energy. Drinking 12 fl. oz (1.5 cups) of Gatorade adds 90 kcal to a person's daily energy

Sports and energy beverages are now marketed heavily to everyone, even people who are inactive.

intake. Many inactive people consume two to three times this amount each day, adding 180 to 270 kcal of energy to their diet. An inactive person has much lower energy needs than someone who is physically active. As with any other food, sports beverages could contribute to excess energy consumption, especially if these drinks are consumed in addition to alcoholic beverages and sugared drinks. With obesity rates at an all-time high, it is important that we attempt to consume only the foods and beverages necessary to support our health. Sports beverages are not designed to be consumed by inactive people, and they do not contribute to the overall health of inactive or lightly active people. What do you think—are there any reasons why an inactive person might benefit from drinking sports beverages? Should these drinks be used exclusively by athletes and highly active people?

CHAPTER 8

CHAPTER OBJECTIVES

After reading this chapter you will be able to:

1. Define free radicals and discuss how they can damage cells, pp. 305–307.

2. Describe how antioxidants protect cells from the oxidative damage caused by free radicals, pp. 307–308.

3. List three antioxidant enzyme systems and describe how these systems help fight oxidative damage, p. 307.

4. Identify two vitamins and one mineral that have significant antioxidant properties, pp. 308–327.

5. Identify food sources that are high in nutrients with antioxidant properties, pp. 310–311, 314–316, 318–319, 323–324, 326.

6. Identify at least four modifiable factors that increase our risk for cancer, pp. 328–333.

7. Describe the relationship between antioxidant nutrients and cancer risk, pp. 333–334.

8. Discuss how consuming nutrients with antioxidant properties can reduce our risk for cardiovascular disease, pp. 335–336.

TEST YOURSELF TRUE OR FALSE?

1. Free radicals are a normal by-product of our bodily functions. T or F

2. Taking large doses of vitamin C supplements reduces our risk of suffering from the common cold. T or F

3. Eating carrots promotes good vision. T or F

4. Smoking is the most preventable cause of death in our society. T or F

5. Consuming a diet high in antioxidant nutrients can help cure cancer. T or F

Test Yourself answers can be found after the Chapter Summary.

Nutrients Involved in Antioxidant Function

baseball greats Eric Davis and Darryl Strawberry have a special bond that goes beyond their childhood friendship and amiable rivalry in the major leagues. At the height of their careers, each began experiencing the same symptoms: extreme weight loss, debilitating fatigue, rectal bleeding, and severe abdominal pain. Davis was diagnosed in the spring of 1997, and Strawberry's diagnosis came in the fall of 1998—both had colon cancer. Both were treated successfully, and although Strawberry's cancer made a comeback in 2000, both are currently cancer-free.

Baseball star Darryl Strawberry, who fought colon cancer.

But wait a minute! Isn't cancer supposed to strike only elderly people? And isn't regular physical activity supposed to protect against it? What exactly is cancer anyway? Does any aspect of your lifestyle increase your risk? Can a poor diet cause it, and can a healthful diet prevent it? What are antioxidants, and why do some people claim they fight cancer? If your health food store were promoting an antioxidant supplement, would you buy it?

It isn't easy to sort fact from fiction when it comes to antioxidants. Fitness and health magazines, supplement companies, and even food manufacturers tout their benefits. In contrast, some researchers claim that antioxidants do not give any added protection from diseases and in some cases may even be harmful. In this chapter, you will learn what antioxidants are and how they work in our bodies. We will also profile the antioxidant nutrients and discuss their relationship to health. Finally, you'll learn about the role antioxidants may play in preventing cancer and heart disease and in slowing the aging process.

What Are Antioxidants, and How Do Our Bodies Use Them?

Antioxidants are compounds that protect our cells from the damage caused by oxidation. *Anti* means "against," and antioxidants work *against,* or *prevent,* oxidation. Before we can go further in our discussion of antioxidants, we need to learn what oxidation is and how it damages cells.

Oxidation Is a Chemical Reaction in Which Atoms Lose Electrons

A review of some basic chemistry will help us understand the process of oxidation.

Molecules Are Composed of Atoms

Think back to the illustrations we included in Chapters 4–6 of the structure of macronutrients. These figures show *molecules,* the smallest *physical units* of a substance. Some molecules, such as hydrogen gas (H_2), contain only one type of atom, in this case hydrogen. Molecules called compounds, however, contain two or more different atoms (such as water, H_2O). Our bodies are constantly breaking down compounds of food, water, and air into their component atoms, and then rearranging these freed atoms to build the different types of molecules our bodies need.

But what, really, are atoms? Simply put, an **atom** is an infinitely small but *unique* unit of matter. Elements such as hydrogen, carbon, or iron are unique because their atoms are unique. Every atom of carbon, for example, is identical to every other atom of carbon, whether it is present in coal or in cheese. All of the matter in the universe can be broken down into just ninety-two elements, each consisting of one unique type of atom. Even more surprisingly, just six elements make up 99% of the matter in our bodies.

Atoms Are Composed of Particles

During the 20th century, physicists learned how to split atoms into even smaller particles. As you can see in FIGURE 8.1, their research revealed that all atoms have a central core, called a **nucleus,** which is positively charged. Orbiting around this nucleus at close to the speed of light are one or more **electrons,** which are negatively charged. The opposite attraction between the positive nucleus and the negative electrons keeps an atom together by making the atom stable, so that its electrons remain with it and do not veer off toward other atoms.

During Metabolism, Atoms Exchange Electrons

As you recall from Chapter 1, the process by which our bodies break down and build up molecules is called *metabolism.* During metabolism, atoms may lose electrons (FIGURE 8.2A). We call this loss of electrons **oxidation,** because it is fueled by oxygen.

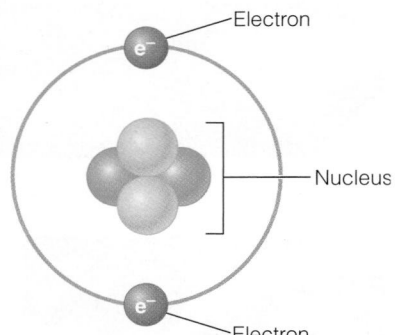

FIGURE 8.1 An atom consists of a central nucleus and orbiting electrons. The nucleus exerts a positive charge, which keeps the negatively charged electrons in its vicinity. Notice how electrons are paired with each other in their orbit around the nucleus. This pairing of electrons results in the atom being chemically stable.

Electron
Nucleus
Electron

antioxidant A compound that has the ability to prevent or repair the damage caused by oxidation.

atom A discrete, irreducible unit of matter. It is the smallest unit of an element and is identical to all other atoms of that element.

nucleus The positively charged, central core of an atom. It is made up of two types of particles—protons and neutrons—bound tightly together. The nucleus of an atom contains essentially all of its atomic mass.

electron A negatively charged particle orbiting the nucleus of an atom.

oxidation A chemical reaction in which molecules of a substance are broken down into their component atoms. During oxidation, the atoms involved lose electrons.

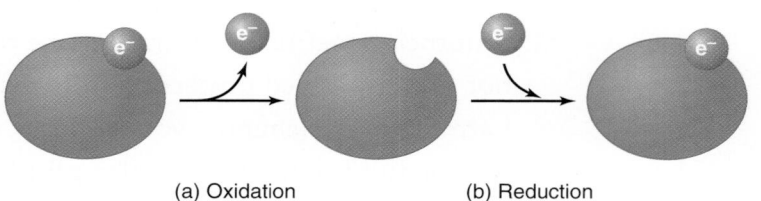

(a) Oxidation   (b) Reduction

FIGURE 8.2 The exchange reaction. Exchange reactions consist of two parts. **(a)** During oxidation, atoms *lose* electrons. **(b)** In the second part of the reaction, atoms *gain* electrons, which is called reduction.

Atoms are capable of gaining electrons during metabolism as well. We call this process *reduction* (FIGURE 8.2B). This loss and gain of electrons typically results in an even exchange of electrons. Scientists call this loss and gain of electrons an *exchange reaction*.

> RECAP: *An atom is an infinitely small and unique unit of matter having a nucleus and orbiting electrons. Atoms exist together with other atoms as molecules. During metabolism, molecules break apart and their atoms gain, lose, or exchange electrons; loss of electrons is called oxidation.*

Oxidation Sometimes Results in the Formation of Free Radicals

Stable atoms have an even number of electrons orbiting in pairs at successive distances (called *shells* or *rings*) from the nucleus. When a stable atom loses an electron during oxidation, it is left with an odd number of electrons in its outermost shell. In other words, it now has an *unpaired electron*. In most exchange reactions, unpaired electrons immediately pair up with other unpaired electrons, making newly stabilized atoms, but in some cases, atoms with unpaired electrons in their outermost shell remain unpaired. Such atoms are highly unstable and are called **free radicals.**

Energy Metabolism Involves Oxidation and Gives Rise to Free Radicals

Free radicals are formed as a by-product of many of our bodies' fundamental physiologic processes. Although some free radicals are a necessary part of our bodily functions, others cause serious damage to our cells and other body components. Let's look at the most common way they arise. As you know, our bodies use oxygen and hydrogen to generate the energy (ATP) that is needed by the body (FIGURE 8.3). We

free radical A highly unstable atom with an unpaired electron in its outermost shell.

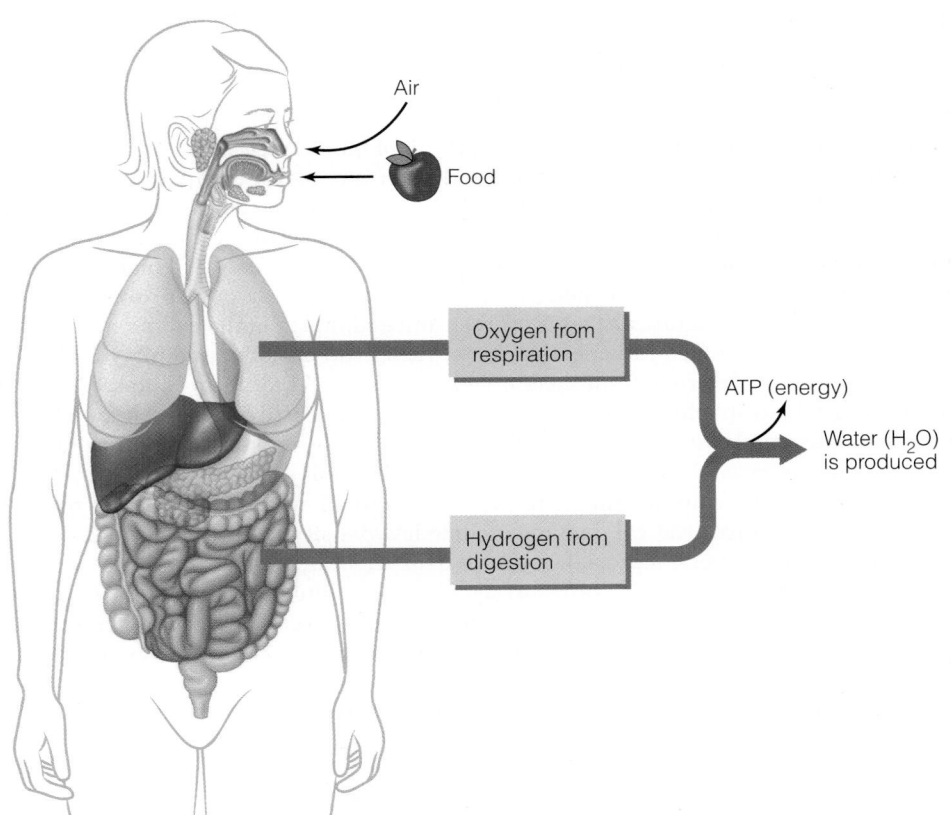

FIGURE 8.3 Oxygen (O) is consumed by inhaling air. Through the process of metabolizing food, hydrogen (H) is released. As these substances undergo exchange reactions during metabolism, electrons are freed to contribute their energy to the production of ATP, which occurs throughout the body at the cellular level. The hydrogen and oxygen then recombine to form water (H_2O).

Air

Food

Oxygen from respiration

Hydrogen from digestion

ATP (energy)

Water (H_2O) is produced

Normal oxygen · Oxygen with added electron · Free radical · Unpaired electron

FIGURE 8.4 Normally, an oxygen atom contains eight electrons. Occasionally oxygen will accept an unpaired electron during the oxidation process. This acceptance of a single electron causes oxygen to become an unstable atom called a free radical.

Exposure to pollution from car exhaust and industrial waste increases our production of free radicals.

are constantly inhaling air into our bodies, thereby providing the oxygen needed to fuel this reaction. At the same time, we generate the necessary hydrogen as a result of digesting food. As shown in FIGURE 8.4, occasionally during metabolism, oxygen accepts a single electron that was released during this process. When it does so, the newly unstable oxygen atom becomes a free radical because of the added unpaired electron.

Other Factors Can Also Cause Free Radical Formation

Free radicals are also formed from other physiologic processes, such as when the immune system produces inflammation to fight allergens or infections. Other factors that cause free radical formation include exposure to air pollution, ultraviolet (UV) rays from the sun, other types of radiation, tobacco smoke, industrial chemicals, and asbestos. Continual exposure to these factors leads to uncontrollable free radical formation, cell damage, and disease, as discussed next.

Free Radicals Can Destabilize Other Molecules and Damage Our Cells

Why are we concerned with the formation of free radicals? Simply put, it is because of their destabilizing power. If you were to think of paired electrons as a married couple, a free radical would be an extremely seductive outsider. Its unpaired electron exerts a powerful attraction toward all stable atoms and molecules around it. In an attempt to stabilize itself, a free radical will "steal" an electron from these stable neighbors, in turn generating more unstable free radicals. This is a dangerous chain reaction, since the free radicals generated can damage or destroy our cells.

One of the most significant sites of free radical damage is the cell membrane. As shown in FIGURE 8.5A, free radicals that form within the phospholipid bilayer of cell membranes steal electrons from the stable lipid heads. Recall from Chapter 5 that all lipids are hydrophobic, so when the lipid heads are destroyed, the cell membrane can no longer repel water. With the cell membrane's integrity lost, its ability to regulate the movement of fluids and nutrients into and out of the cell is also lost. This loss of cell integrity causes damage to the cell and to all systems affected by the cell.

Other sites of free radical damage include low-density lipoproteins (LDLs), cell proteins, and our genetic material (DNA, or deoxyribonucleic acid). Damage to LDLs and cell proteins disrupts the transport of substances into and out of cells and alters cell function, whereas defective DNA results in faulty protein synthesis. These changes may increase our risk for heart disease and cancer and can cause our cells to die prematurely.

Not surprisingly, many diseases are linked with free radical production, including:

* cancer
* heart disease
* diabetes

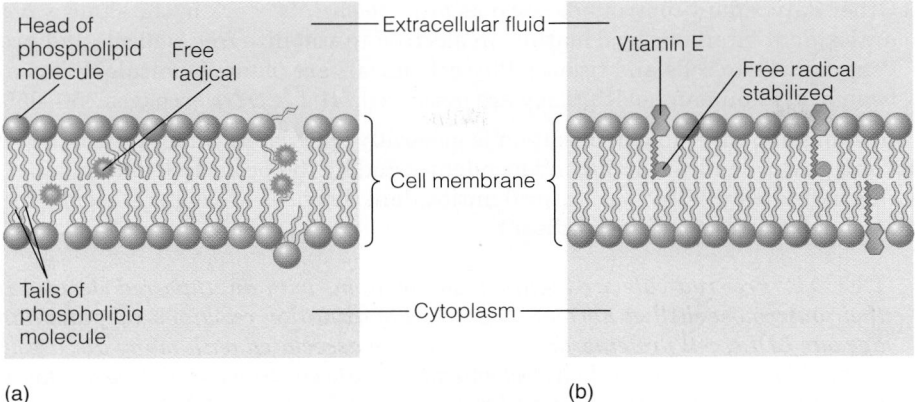

FIGURE 8.5 **(a)** The formation of free radicals in the lipid portion of our cell membranes can cause a dangerous chain reaction that damages the integrity of the membrane and can cause cell death. **(b)** Vitamin E is stored in the lipid portion of our cell membranes. By donating an electron to free radicals, it protects the lipid molecules in our cell membranes from themselves being oxidized and stops the chain reaction of oxidative damage.

- arthritis
- cataracts
- kidney disease
- Alzheimer's disease
- Parkinson's disease

Antioxidants Work by Stabilizing Free Radicals or Opposing Oxidation

How do our bodies fight free radicals and repair the damage they cause? These actions are performed by antioxidant vitamins, minerals, and phytochemicals and other compounds. These antioxidants perform their role in the following ways:

1. Antioxidant *vitamins* work independently by donating their electrons or hydrogen atoms to free radicals to stabilize them and reduce the damage caused by oxidation (FIGURE 8.5B).

2. Antioxidant *minerals* function within complex antioxidant enzyme systems that convert free radicals to less damaging substances that are excreted by our bodies. These enzymes also work to break down fatty acids that have become oxidized. In breaking down the fatty acids, they destroy the free radicals associated with them. Antioxidant enzyme systems also make more vitamin antioxidants available to fight other free radicals. Minerals typically function within enzyme systems as **cofactors,** compounds required to activate enzymes so that they can do their work. The minerals selenium, copper, iron, zinc, and manganese act as cofactors in antioxidant enzyme systems. Examples of these antioxidant enzyme systems are superoxide dismutase, catalase, and glutathione peroxidase:

   - Superoxide dismutase converts free radicals to less damaging substances, such as hydrogen peroxide.

   - Catalase removes hydrogen peroxide from our bodies by converting it to water and oxygen.

   - Glutathione peroxidase also removes hydrogen peroxide from our bodies and stops the production of free radicals in lipids.

cofactor A compound that is needed to allow enzymes to function properly.

3. Other antioxidant compounds, such as *phytochemicals,* work in the same way as antioxidant vitamins, by donating an electron to stabilize free radicals and prevent damage to cells and tissues. Phytochemicals are plant chemicals that are beneficial to human health. They are discussed ***In Depth*** on pages 350–359.

In summary, free radical formation is generally kept safely under control by vitamins and phytochemicals acting independently and by the protective antioxidant systems in our body. When our natural antioxidant defenses are not sufficient, free radical damage can be quite significant.

> RECAP: *Free radicals are highly unstable atoms with an unpaired electron in their outermost shell. A normal by-product of oxidation reactions, they can damage our LDLs, cell proteins, and DNA and are associated with many diseases. Antioxidant vitamins and phytochemicals donate electrons or hydrogen atoms to free radicals to stabilize them and reduce oxidative damage. Antioxidant minerals are part of antioxidant enzyme systems that convert free radicals to less damaging substances.*

A Profile of Nutrients That Function as Antioxidants

Our bodies cannot form antioxidants spontaneously. Instead, we must consume them in our diet. Table 8.1 reviews the antioxidant vitamins and minerals and the way they work in our bodies. Nutrients that appear to have antioxidant properties or are part of our protective antioxidant enzyme systems include vitamins E, C, and A; beta-carotene (a phytochemical that is a precursor to vitamin A); and the mineral selenium. The minerals copper, iron, zinc, and manganese play a peripheral role in fighting oxidation and are only briefly introduced in this chapter. Let's review each of these nutrients now and learn more about their functions in the body.

Vitamin E

As reviewed ***In Depth*** on pages 252–263, vitamin E is one of the fat-soluble vitamins, which means that dietary fats carry it from our intestines through the lymph system and eventually transport it to our cells. As you remember, our bodies store the fat-soluble vitamins. The liver serves as a storage site for vitamins A and D, and about 90% of the vitamin E in our bodies is stored in our adipose tissue. The remaining vitamin E is found in cell membranes.

Vitamin E is actually two separate compounds, **tocotrienol** and **tocopherol.** The tocotrienol compounds do not appear to play an active role in our bodies. The tocopherol compounds are the biologically active forms of vitamin E in our bodies. Four different tocopherol compounds have been discovered: alpha, beta, gamma, and delta. Of these, the most active, or potent, vitamin E compound found in food and supplements is *alpha-tocopherol.* The RDA for vitamin E is expressed as milligrams of alpha-tocopherol equivalents per day (mg α-tocopherol/day). Labels on foods and vitamin and mineral supplements may express vitamin E in milligrams of alpha-tocopherol equivalents (mg α-TE) or International Units (IU). For conversion purposes, 1 α-TE is equal to 1 mg of active vitamin E. In supplements, 1 IU is equal to 0.67 mg α-TE if the vitamin E in the supplement is from natural sources. If synthetic vitamin E is used in the supplement, 1 IU is equal to 0.45 mg α-TE.

Functions of Vitamin E

The primary function of vitamin E is as an antioxidant. As described earlier in this chapter, this means that vitamin E donates an electron to free radicals, stabilizing them and preventing them from destabilizing other molecules. Once vitamin E is

tocotrienol A form of vitamin E that does not play an important biological role in our bodies.

tocopherol The active form of vitamin E in our bodies.

TABLE 8.1 Functions, Recommended Intakes (RDA), Tolerable Upper Intake Levels (UL), and Toxicity and Deficiency Symptoms of Antioxidant Substances

Antioxidant	Primary Functions	Recommended Intakes	Toxicity Symptoms/ Side Effects	Deficiency Symptoms/ Side Effects
Vitamin E (fat soluble)	Protects cell membranes from oxidation Protects polyunsaturated fatty acids (PUFAs) from oxidation Protects vitamin A from oxidation Protects white blood cells and enhances immune function Improves absorption of vitamin A	RDA: Men: 5–15 mg α-tocopherol per day Women: 5–15 mg α-tocopherol per day UL: 1,000 mg α-tocopherol per day	Inhibition of blood clotting Increased risk of hemorrhagic stroke Intestinal discomfort	Red blood cell hemolysis Anemia Impairment of nerve transmission Muscle weakness and degeneration Leg cramps Difficulty walking Fibrocystic breast disease
Vitamin C (water soluble)	Antioxidant in extracellular fluid and lungs Regenerates oxidized vitamin E Reduces formation of nitrosamines in stomach Assists with collagen synthesis Enhances immune function Assists in the synthesis of hormones, neurotransmitters, and DNA Enhances absorption of iron	RDA: Men: 5–90 mg per day Women: 5–75 mg per day Smokers: 5–35 mg more per day than RDA UL: 2,000 mg/day for adults	Nausea and diarrhea Nosebleeds Abdominal cramps Increased oxidative damage Increased formation of kidney stones in those with kidney disease	Scurvy Bleeding gums and joints Loose teeth Weakness Hemorrhaging of hair follicles Poor wound healing Swollen ankles and wrists Diarrhea Bone pain and fractures Depression Anemia
Beta-carotene (fat-soluble provitamin for vitamin A)	Protects cell membranes and LDLs from oxidation Enhances immune system Protects skin from sun's ultraviolet rays Protects eyes from oxidative damage	None at this time	Carotenosis or carotenodermia (yellowing of skin)	Unknown
Vitamin A* (fat soluble)	Necessary for our ability to adjust to changes in light Protects color vision Cell differentiation Necessary for sperm production in men and fertilization in women Contributes to healthy bone growth	RDA: Men: 900 µg/day Women: 700 µg/day UL: 3,000 µg/day for adults	Spontaneous abortions and birth defects in fetus of pregnant women Loss of appetite Blurred vision Hair loss Abdominal pain, nausea, diarrhea Liver and nervous system damage	Night blindness Xerophthalmia that leads to permanent blindness Impaired immunity and increased risk of illness and infection Inability to reproduce Failure of normal growth
Selenium (trace mineral)	Part of glutathione peroxidase, an antioxidant enzyme Indirectly spares vitamin E from oxidation Assists in production of thyroid hormone Assists in maintaining immune function	RDA: Men: 55 µg/day Women: 55 µg/day UL: 400 µg/day	Brittle hair and nails Skin rashes Vomiting, nausea Weakness Cirrhosis of liver	Keshan disease: a specific form of heart disease Kashin-Beck disease: deforming arthritis Impaired immune function Increased risk of viral infections Infertility Depression, hostility Muscle pain and wasting

*Vitamin A is still under investigation as a potential antioxidant.

Vegetable oils, nuts, and seeds are good sources of vitamin E.

oxidized, it is either excreted from the body or recycled back into active vitamin E through the help of other antioxidant nutrients, such as vitamin C.

Because vitamin E is prevalent in our adipose tissues and cell membranes, its action specifically protects *polyunsaturated fatty acids* (PUFAs) and other fatty components of our cells and cell membranes from being oxidized (see FIGURE 8.5B). Vitamin E also protects our LDLs from being oxidized, which lowers our risk for heart disease. (The relationship between antioxidants and heart disease is reviewed later in this chapter.) In addition to protecting our PUFAs and LDLs, vitamin E protects the membranes of our red blood cells from oxidation and plays a critical role in protecting the cells of our lungs, which are constantly exposed to oxygen and the potentially damaging effects of oxidation.

Vitamin E serves many other roles essential to human health. It is critical for normal fetal and early childhood development of nerves and muscles, as well as for maintenance of their functions. It helps to defend our bodies against disease by protecting white blood cells and other components of our immune system. Vitamin E also improves the absorption of vitamin A if the dietary intake of vitamin A is low. A full list of the functions, recommended intake, and toxicity and deficiency symptoms associated with vitamin E is provided in Table 8.1.

How Much Vitamin E Should We Consume?

Considering the importance of vitamin E to our health, you might think that you need to consume a huge amount daily. In fact, the RDA is modest and the food sources plentiful.

Recommended Dietary Allowance for Vitamin E. The RDA for vitamin E for men and women is identified in Table 8.1. Remember that one of the primary roles of vitamin E is to protect PUFAs from oxidation. Thus, our need for vitamin E increases as we eat more oils and other foods that contain PUFAs. Fortunately these foods also contain vitamin E, so we typically consume enough vitamin E within them to protect their PUFAs from oxidation.

SHOPPER'S GUIDE
Good Food Sources of Vitamin E

Vitamin E is very widespread in the foods we eat. Much of the vitamin E that we consume comes from vegetable oils and the products made from them (FIGURE 8.6). Safflower oil, sunflower oil, canola oil, and soybean oil are good sources of vitamin E. Mayonnaise and salad dressings made from these oils also contain vitamin E. Nuts, seeds, and some vegetables also contribute vitamin E to our diet. Although no single fruit or vegetable contains very high amounts of vitamin E, eating 5 to 9 servings of fruits and vegetables along with other vitamin E–containing foods each day will help ensure adequate intake of this nutrient. Cereals are often fortified with vitamin E, and other grain products contribute modest amounts to our diet. Wheat germ and soybeans are also good sources of vitamin E. Animal and dairy products are poor sources.

Vitamin E is destroyed by exposure to oxygen, metals, ultraviolet light, and heat. Although raw (uncooked) vegetable oils contain vitamin E, heating these oils destroys vitamin E. Thus, foods that are deep-fried and processed contain little vitamin E and higher amounts of saturated and *trans* fats. This includes most fast foods and convenience foods.

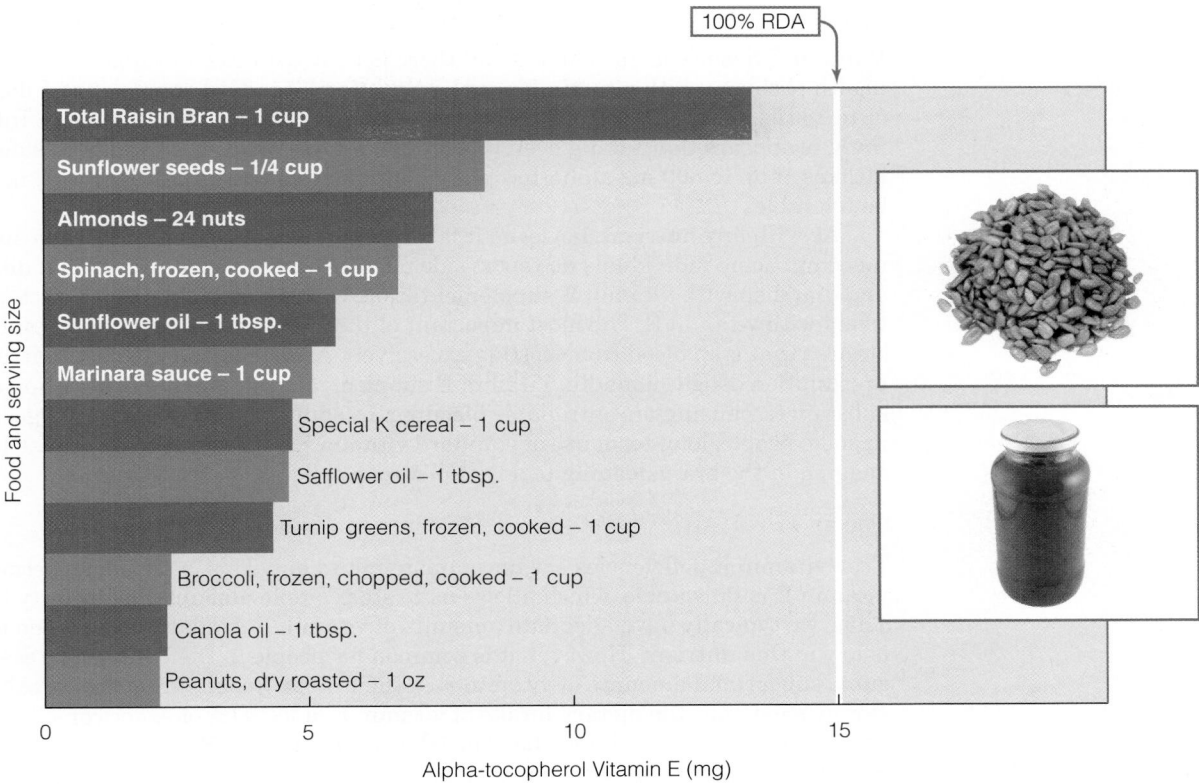

FIGURE 8.6 Common food sources of vitamin E. The RDA for vitamin E is 15 mg alpha-tocopherol per day for men and women. (Data from U.S. Department of Agriculture, Agricultural Research Service, 2006. USDA Nutrient Database for Standard Reference, Release 19. Nutrient Data Laboratory Home Page, www.ars.usda.gov/ba/ bhnrc/ndl.)

Tips for Increasing Your Vitamin E Intake

√ Eat cereals high in vitamin E for breakfast or as a snack.

√ Add sunflower seeds to salads and trail mixes; or just have them as a snack.

√ Add sliced almonds to salads, granola, and trail mixes to boost vitamin E intake.

√ Add a tablespoon of wheat germ to yogurt, cereals, or batches of homemade breads or muffins.

√ Pack a peanut butter sandwich for lunch.

√ When cooking or stir-frying, use vitamin E–rich oils, such as sunflower, safflower, corn, or canola.

√ Serve corn chips with guacamole: mash a ripe avocado with a squeeze of lime juice and a sprinkle of garlic salt.

What Happens If We Consume Too Much Vitamin E?

Vitamin E toxicity is uncommon, and there is little evidence to support significant health problems with vitamin E supplementation. Standard supplemental doses (1 to 18 times the RDA) are not associated with any adverse health effects. Interestingly, it appears that taking even much higher doses of vitamin E may be safe. Daily intakes of up to 800 mg alpha-tocopherol (or about 53 times the RDA) are known to be tolerable.

As with any nutrient, however, it is important to exercise caution when supplementing. Some individuals do report side effects such as nausea, intestinal distress, and diarrhea with vitamin E supplementation. Certain medications interact negatively with vitamin E. The most important of these are the *anticoagulants,* substances that stop blood from clotting excessively. Aspirin is an anticoagulant, as is the prescription drug Coumadin. Vitamin E supplements can augment the action of these substances, causing uncontrollable bleeding. In addition, new evidence suggests that in some people, long-term use of standard vitamin E supplements may cause hemorrhaging in the brain, leading to a type of stroke called *hemorrhagic stroke.*

What Happens If We Don't Consume Enough Vitamin E?

True vitamin E deficiencies are uncommon in humans. This is primarily because vitamin E is fat soluble, which allows us to store ample amounts in our fatty tissues. Thus, we typically have adequate amounts of vitamin E available even when our diet is low in this nutrient. However, it is common for people in the United States to consume suboptimal amounts of vitamin E in their diets. Results from the NHANES III survey show that the dietary intake of vitamin E of 27–41% of Americans is low enough that these individuals have blood levels of vitamin E putting them at increased risk for cardiovascular disease.[1]

One vitamin E deficiency symptom is *erythrocyte hemolysis,* or the rupturing (*lysis*) of red blood cells (*erythrocytes*). The rupturing of our red blood cells leads to *anemia,* a condition in which our red blood cells cannot carry and transport enough oxygen to our tissues, leading to fatigue, weakness, and a diminished ability to perform physical and mental work. We discuss anemia in more detail in Chapter 10. Premature babies can suffer from vitamin E–deficiency anemia; if born too early, the infant does not receive vitamin E from its mother, since the transfer of this vitamin from mother to baby occurs during the last few weeks of the pregnancy.

Other symptoms of vitamin E deficiency include loss of muscle coordination and reflexes, leading to impairments in vision, speech, and movement. As you might expect, vitamin E deficiency can also impair immune function. This is especially common when accompanied by low body stores of the mineral selenium.

In adults, vitamin E deficiencies are usually caused by diseases, particularly diseases that cause malabsorption of fat, such as those that affect the liver, gallbladder, pancreas, and duodenum. As reviewed in Chapter 3, the liver makes bile, which is necessary for the breakdown and absorption of fat. The gallbladder and pancreas deliver bile and pancreatic enzymes into the duodenum of the small intestine, where they facilitate digestion and absorption of fat. Thus, disease of the liver, gallbladder, pancreas, or duodenum can result in malabsorption of fat and the fat-soluble vitamins, including vitamin E, leading to their deficiency.

> RECAP: *Vitamin E protects our cell membranes from oxidation, enhances immune function, and improves our absorption of vitamin A if dietary intake is low. It is found primarily in vegetable oils and nuts. Toxicity is uncommon, but taking very high doses can cause excessive bleeding. Deficiency is rare except when disease causes malabsorption of fats, but symptoms include anemia and impaired vision, speech, and movement.*

Vitamin C

Vitamin C is a water-soluble vitamin, and any excess is excreted (primarily in our urine) rather than stored. We must therefore consume it on a regular basis. There are two active forms of vitamin C: ascorbic acid and dehydroascorbic acid. Interestingly, most animals can make their own vitamin C from glucose. Humans and guinea pigs are two groups that cannot synthesize their own vitamin C and must consume it in the diet.

Functions of Vitamin C

Vitamin C is probably most well known for its role in preventing scurvy, a disease characterized by the breakdown and bleeding of the body's tissues. Centuries ago, scurvy ravaged sailors: over half of the deaths that occurred at sea were attributable to the disease. That's because, on long voyages, the crew ate all of the fruits and vegetables early in the trip, and then had only grain and animal products available until they reached land to resupply. In 1740 in England, Dr. James Lind discovered that citrus fruits could prevent scurvy, though he had no idea that the effect was due to their high vitamin C content. Fifty years after the discovery of the link between citrus fruits and prevention of scurvy, the British Navy finally required all ships to provide daily lemon juice rations for each sailor to prevent the onset of scurvy. A century later, sailors were given lime juice rations, earning them the nickname "limeys." It wasn't until 1930 that vitamin C was discovered and identified as a nutrient. Although scurvy is not as prevalent today as it was centuries ago, people eating a "junk"-food diet consisting of burgers, crackers, chips, cookies, soda, and so on can quickly become deficient in vitamin C.

One important role of vitamin C is to assist in the synthesis of **collagen.** Collagen, a protein, is a critical component of all connective tissues in our bodies, including bone, teeth, skin, tendons, and blood vessels. Collagen assists in preventing bruises, and it ensures proper wound healing, as it is a part of scar tissue and a component of the tissue that mends broken bones. Without adequate vitamin C, our bodies cannot form collagen, and tissue *hemorrhage* (bleeding) is a major symptom of vitamin C deficiency.

Vitamin C also acts as an antioxidant. Like vitamin E, it donates electrons to free radicals, thus preventing the damage of cells and tissues. Since it is water soluble, vitamin C primarily acts as an antioxidant in the extracellular fluid. It is also an important antioxidant in the lungs, protecting us from the damage caused by ground-level ozone (O_3) and cigarette smoke. Vitamin C also regenerates vitamin E after it has been oxidized by donating an electron. This enables vitamin E to continue to protect our cell membranes and other tissues. In the stomach, vitamin C reduces the formation of *nitrosamines,* cancer-causing agents found in foods such as cured and processed meats. We discuss the role of vitamin C and other antioxidants in preventing some forms of cancer later in this chapter (page 333).

Vitamin C also enhances our immune response, protecting us from illness and infection. But contrary to popular belief, it is not a miracle cure (see the accompanying Nutrition Myth or Fact? box on vitamin C, page 314). Vitamin C also assists in the synthesis of DNA, neurotransmitters such as serotonin (which helps regulate mood), and various hormones, including *thyroxine,* a hormone produced by the thyroid gland that helps maintain basal metabolic rate and body temperature.

Vitamin C also enhances the absorption of iron. It is recommended that people with low iron stores consume vitamin C–rich foods along with iron sources to improve absorption. For people with high iron stores, this practice can be dangerous and lead to iron toxicity (discussed on page 316). Refer to Table 8.1 for a review of the functions, recommended intake, and toxicity and deficiency symptoms associated with vitamin C.

How Much Vitamin C Should We Consume?

Although popular opinion suggests our need for vitamin C is quite high, we really need only a modest amount. Indeed, a single 8-oz glass of orange juice or a few slices of sweet red pepper more than meet our daily requirements.

Recommended Dietary Allowance for Vitamin C. The RDA for vitamin C is indicated in Table 8.1. Smoking increases a person's need for vitamin C; thus the RDA for smokers is 35 mg more per day than for nonsmokers.

Many fruits, like these yellow tomatoes, are high in vitamin C.

collagen A protein found in all connective tissues in our body.

NUTRITION MYTH OR FACT?

Can Vitamin C Prevent the Common Cold?

What happens when you feel a cold coming on? If you are like many people, you will drink a lot of orange juice or take vitamin C supplements to ward it off. Do these tactics really help prevent a cold?

It is well known that vitamin C is important for a healthy immune system. A vitamin C deficiency can seriously weaken our immune cells' ability to detect and destroy invading microbes, increasing our susceptibility to many diseases and illnesses—including the common cold. Many people have taken vitamin C supplements to prevent the common cold, basing their behavior on its actions of enhancing our immune function. Interestingly, scientific studies do not support this action. A recent review of

many of the studies of vitamin C and the common cold found that people taking vitamin C experienced as many colds as people who took a placebo.[2] The amount of vitamin C taken in these studies was quite high, at least 1,000 mg/day (over ten times the RDA).

Thus, despite their popularity, vitamin C supplements do not appear to enhance our ability to fight the common cold. Consuming a healthful diet that includes excellent sources of vitamin C will assist us with maintaining a strong immune system, but vitamin C supplements do not appear to be effective in enhancing the immune system of an already well-nourished individual. So the next time you feel yourself getting a cold, you may want to think twice before taking extra vitamin C.

SHOPPER'S GUIDE
Good Food Sources of Vitamin C

As indicated in FIGURE 8.7, many fruits and vegetables are high in vitamin C. Citrus fruits (such as oranges, lemons, and limes), potatoes, strawberries, tomatoes, kiwi fruit, broccoli, spinach and other leafy greens, cabbage, green and red peppers, and cauliflower are excellent sources. Fortified beverages and cereals are also sources of vitamin C. Dairy foods, meats, and non-fortified cereals and grains provide little or no vitamin C.

Because heat and oxygen destroy vitamin C, fresh fruits and vegetables have the highest vitamin C content. Cooking foods, especially boiling them, leaches their vitamin C, which is then lost when we strain them. Forms of cooking that are least likely to compromise the vitamin C content of foods include steaming, microwaving, and stir-frying.

Fresh vegetables are good sources of vitamin C and beta-carotene.

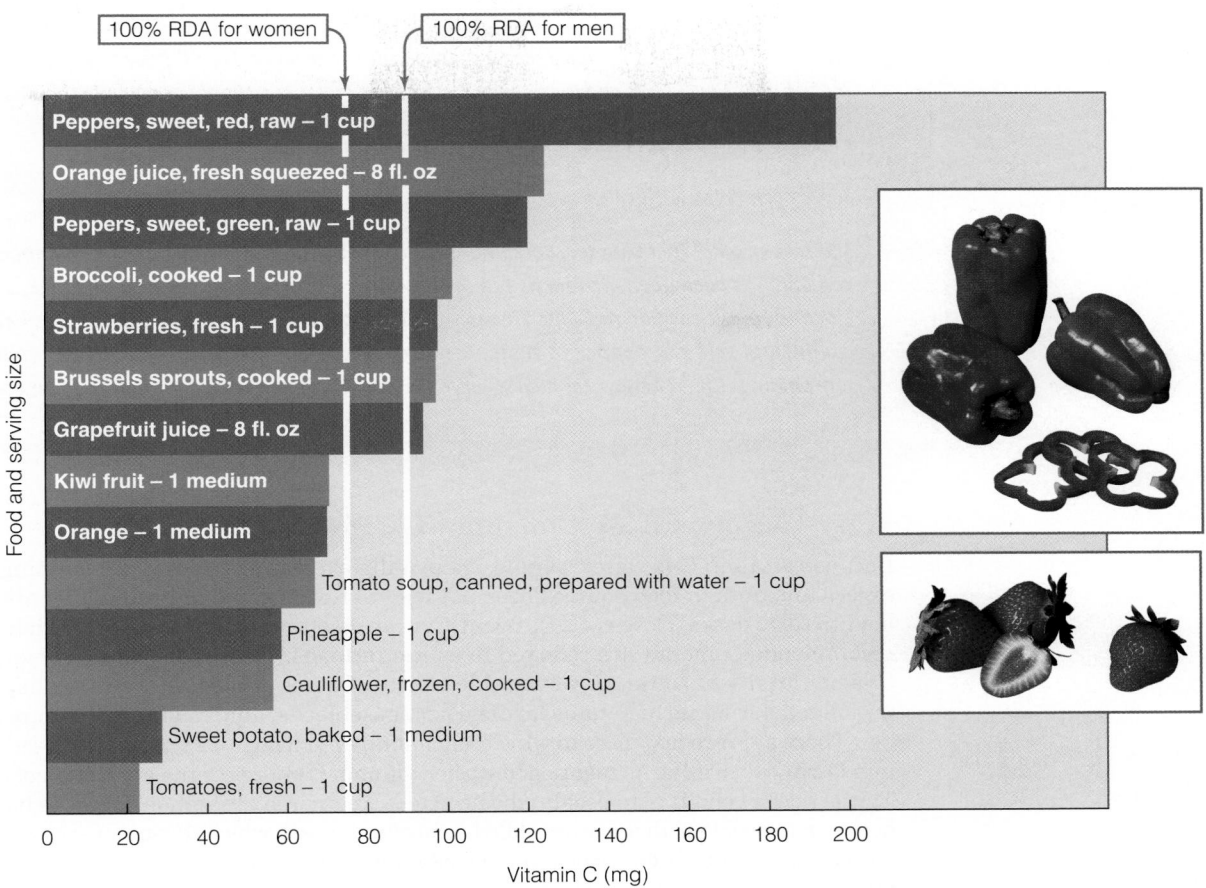

FIGURE 8.7 Common food sources of vitamin C. The RDA for vitamin C is 90 mg/day for men and 75 mg/day for women. (Data from U.S. Department of Agriculture, Agricultural Research Service, 2006. USDA Nutrient Database for Standard Reference, Release 19. Nutrient Data Laboratory Home Page, www.ars.usda.gov/ba/bhnrc/ndl.)

Healthful Tips for Eating Foods High in Vitamin C

✓ Mix strawberries, kiwi fruit, cantaloupe, and oranges for a tasty fruit salad loaded with vitamin C.

✓ Include tomatoes on salads, wraps, and sandwiches for more vitamin C.

✓ Make your own fresh-squeezed orange or grapefruit juice!

✓ Add your favorite vitamin C-rich fruits like strawberries to smoothies.

✓ Buy ready-to-eat vegetables such as baby carrots and cherry tomatoes, and toss some in a zip-lock bag to take to school or work.

✓ Put a few slices of dark-green lettuce on your sandwich.

✓ Throw a small container of orange slices, fresh pineapple chunks, or berries into your backpack for an afternoon snack.

(continued)

√ Store some juice boxes in your freezer to pack with your lunch. They'll thaw slowly, keeping the rest of your lunch cool, and many brands contain a full day's supply of vitamin C in just 6 oz.

√ Enjoy raw bell peppers with low-fat dip for a crunchy snack.

√ Serve corn chips with salsa.

√ Make gazpacho! In a blender, combine 1–3 cups tomato juice, chunks of green pepper and red onion, a cucumber with seeds removed (no need to peel), the juice of one lime, a garlic clove, a splash each of red wine vinegar and olive oil, a half teaspoon each of basil and cumin, and salt and pepper to taste. Seed and dice 2–3 fresh tomatoes and add to blended ingredients. Chill for several hours. Serve very cold, topped with a dollop of plain yogurt.

What Happens If We Consume Too Much Vitamin C?

Because vitamin C is water soluble, we usually excrete any excess. Consuming excess amounts in food sources does not lead to toxicity, and only supplements can lead to toxic doses. Doses of a nutrient that are ten or more times greater than the recommended amount are referred to as **megadoses.** Taking megadoses of vitamin C is not fatally harmful. However, side effects of doses exceeding 2,000 mg/day for a prolonged period include nausea, diarrhea, nosebleeds, and abdominal cramps.

There are rare instances in which consuming even moderately excessive doses of vitamin C can be harmful. As mentioned earlier, vitamin C enhances the absorption of iron. This action is beneficial to people who need to increase iron absorption. It can be harmful, however, to people with a disease called *hemochromatosis,* which causes an excess accumulation of iron in our bodies. Such iron toxicity can damage our tissues and lead to a heart attack. Another instance in which excessive vitamin C can be harmful is in people who have preexisting kidney disease. For these people, taking excess vitamin C can lead to the formation of kidney stones. This does not appear to occur in healthy individuals.

Critics of vitamin C supplementation claim that taking the supplemental form of the vitamin is "unbalanced" nutrition and leads vitamin C to act as a prooxidant. A **prooxidant,** as you might guess, is a nutrient that promotes oxidation. It does this by pushing the balance of exchange reactions toward oxidation, which promotes the production of free radicals. Although the results of a few studies suggested that vitamin C acts as a prooxidant, these studies were found to be flawed or irrelevant for humans. At the present time, there appears to be no strong scientific evidence that vitamin C, from either food or dietary supplements, acts as a prooxidant in humans.

megadose A dose of a nutrient that is ten or more times greater than the recommended amount.

prooxidant A nutrient that promotes oxidation and oxidative cell and tissue damage.

NUTRI-CASE JUDY

"Hannah's been fighting a lot of colds at school this winter, so I've been mixing vitamin C powder into her orange juice every morning. I guess it's helping, because she's only had to be out twice, but this morning she said her tummy hurt and she has diarrhea. I told her to stay home for the day and before I left for work I fixed her toast, a sliced banana, and her orange juice and vitamin C. So now I guess I have to worry about a stomach bug going around. I wish there was a vitamin C for that!"

Given what you've learned about the effects of vitamin C supplementation, do you think it is possible that Judy's vitamin C regimen is doing Hannah more harm than good? Explain.

What Happens If We Don't Consume Enough Vitamin C?

Vitamin C deficiencies are rare in developed countries but can occur in underdeveloped countries. Scurvy is the most common vitamin C deficiency disease. The symptoms of scurvy appear after about 1 month of a vitamin C–deficient diet. Symptoms include bleeding gums and joints, loose teeth, weakness, hemorrhages around the hair follicles of the arms and legs (FIGURE 8.8), wounds that fail to heal, swollen ankles and wrists, bone pain and fractures, diarrhea, and depression. Anemia can also result from vitamin C deficiency. People most at risk for deficiencies include those who eat few fruits and vegetables, including impoverished or home-bound individuals, and people who abuse alcohol and drugs.

> RECAP: *Vitamin C scavenges free radicals and regenerates vitamin E after it has been oxidized. Vitamin C prevents scurvy and assists in the synthesis of collagen, hormones, neurotransmitters, and DNA. Vitamin C also enhances iron absorption. Many fruits and vegetables are high in vitamin C, and our requirements are modest. Toxicity is uncommon; symptoms include nausea, diarrhea, and nosebleeds. Deficiency symptoms include scurvy, anemia, diarrhea, and depression.*

FIGURE 8.8 Bleeding gums are one symptom of scurvy, the most common vitamin C deficiency disease.

Beta-Carotene

Although beta-carotene is not considered an essential nutrient, it is a *provitamin* found in many fruits and vegetables. **Provitamins** are inactive forms of vitamins that the body cannot use until they are converted to their active form. Our bodies convert beta-carotene to the active form of vitamin A, or *retinol;* thus, beta-carotene is a precursor of retinol. It takes two units of beta-carotene to make one unit of active vitamin A. Not surprisingly, nutritionists express the units of beta-carotene in a food as Retinol Equivalents, or RE. This measurement tells us how much active vitamin A is available to the body after it has converted the beta-carotene in the food.

Beta-carotene is classified as a **carotenoid,** a class of phytochemicals (see the *In Depth* on pages 350–359). As you might guess from their name, carotenoids are a group of plant pigments that are the basis for the orange, red, and deep yellow colors of many fruits and vegetables, including carrots. (Even dark-green leafy vegetables contain plenty of carotenoids, but the green pigment, chlorophyll, masks their color!) Although there are more than 600 carotenoids found in nature, only about fifty are found in the typical human diet. The six most common carotenoids found in human blood are alpha-carotene, beta-carotene, cryptoxanthin, lutein, lycopene, and zeaxanthin. We are just beginning to learn more about how carotenoids function in our body and how they may affect our health. Most of our discussion will focus on beta-carotene, as the majority of research on carotenoids to date have focused on this substance.

Functions of Beta-Carotene

Beta-carotene and some other carotenoids are recognized to have antioxidant properties. Like vitamin E, they are fat soluble and fight the harmful effects of oxidation in the lipid portions of our cell membranes and in our LDLs; but, compared with vitamin E, beta-carotene is a relatively weak antioxidant. In fact, other carotenoids, such as lycopene and lutein, may be stronger antioxidants than beta-carotene. Research is currently being conducted to elucidate how many carotenoids are found in foods and which ones are effective antioxidants.

Carotenoids play other important roles in our bodies. Specifically:

- They enhance our immune system and boost our ability to fight illness and disease.
- They protect our skin from the damage caused by the sun's ultraviolet rays.
- They protect our eyes from damage, preventing or delaying age-related vision impairment.

provitamin An inactive form of a vitamin that the body can convert to an active form. An example is beta-carotene.

carotenoids Fat-soluble plant pigments that the body stores in the liver and adipose tissues. The body is able to convert certain carotenoids to vitamin A.

Carotenoids are also associated with a decreased risk of certain types of cancer. We discuss the influence of diet on cancer risk later in this chapter. Refer to Table 8.1 for a review of the functions and toxicity and deficiency symptoms associated with beta-carotene.

How Much Beta-Carotene Should We Consume?

Although foods rich in beta-carotene are important in a healthful diet, the question of how much beta-carotene we should consume has no easy answer.

Recommended Dietary Allowance for Beta-Carotene.   While there is evidence in the research laboratory that beta-carotene is an antioxidant, nutritionists do not consider beta-carotene and other carotenoids to be essential nutrients, as they play no known essential roles in our body and are not associated with any deficiency symptoms. Thus, no RDA for these compounds has been established. It has been suggested that consuming 6 to 10 mg of beta-carotene per day from food sources can increase the beta-carotene levels in our blood to amounts that may reduce our risks for some diseases such as cancer and heart disease.[3] Supplements containing beta-carotene have become very popular, and supplementation studies have prescribed doses of 15 to 30 mg of beta-carotene. Refer to the accompanying Nutrition Myth or Fact? box on beta-carotene, page 320, to learn more about how supplementation with this compound may affect your risk for cancer.

SHOPPER'S GUIDE
Good Food Sources of Beta-Carotene

Fruits and vegetables that are red, orange, yellow, and deep green are generally high in beta-carotene and other carotenoids such as lutein and lycopene. Tomatoes, carrots, cantaloupe, sweet potatoes, apricots, leafy greens such as kale and spinach, and pumpkin are good sources. Eating 5 to 9 fruits and vegetables each day ensures an adequate intake of beta-carotene and other carotenoids. Although beta-carotene is used as a natural coloring agent for many foods including margarine, cereal, cake mixes, gelatins, and soft drinks, these foods are not significant sources of beta-carotene. FIGURE 8.9 identifies common foods that are high in beta-carotene.

We generally absorb only between 20% and 40% of the carotenoids present in the foods we eat. In contrast to vitamins E and C, heating foods high in carotenoids improves our ability to digest and absorb these compounds. Carotenoids are bound in the cells of

Foods that are high in carotenoids are easy to recognize by their bright colors.

plants, and the process of lightly cooking these plants breaks chemical bonds and can rupture cell walls, which humans don't digest. These actions result in more of the carotenoids being released from the plant. For instance, 100 g of raw carrots contains approximately 7.3 mg of beta-carotene, while the same amount of cooked carrots contains approximately 8.0 mg.[4]

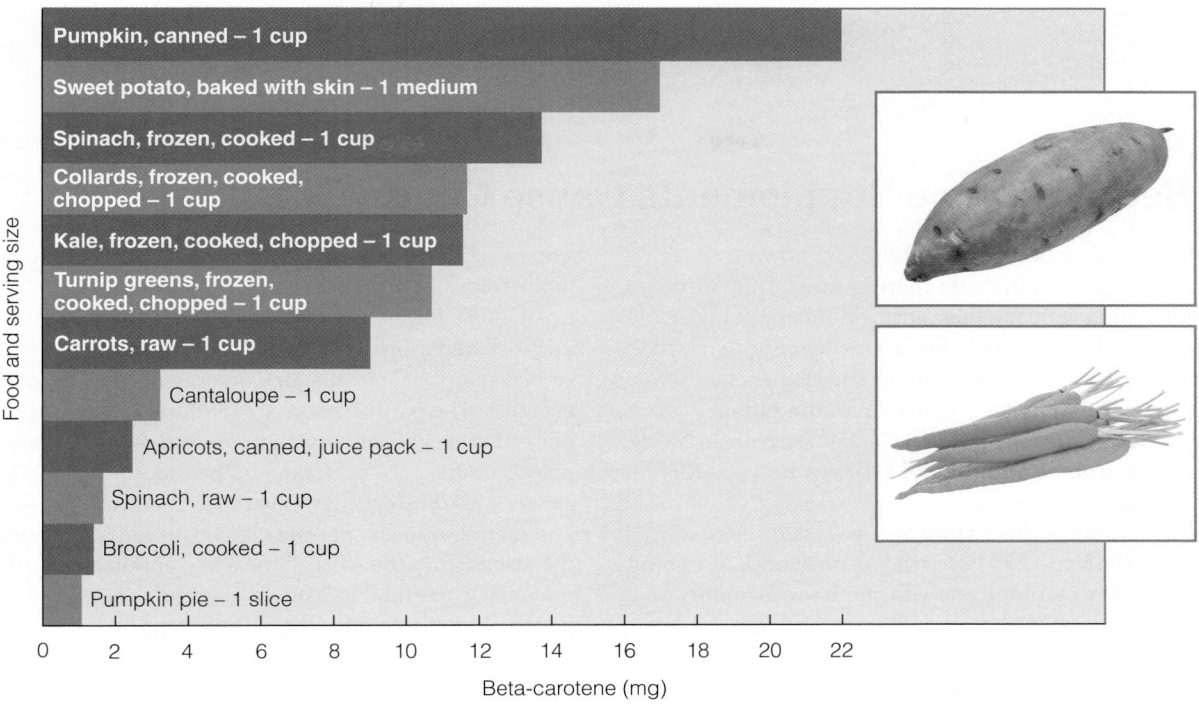

FIGURE 8.9 Common food sources of beta-carotene. There is no RDA for beta-carotene. (Data from U.S. Department of Agriculture, Agricultural Research Service. USDA—NCC Carotenoid Database for U.S. Foods, 2006. USDA Nutrient Database for Standard Reference, Release 19. Nutrient Data Laboratory Home Page, www.ars.usda.gov/ba/bhnrc/ndl.)

Tips for Increasing Your Beta-Carotene Intake

√ Start your day with oranges, grapefruits, pears, bananas, or apples, all of which are good sources of beta-carotene.

√ Pack a zip-lock bag of baby carrots or dried apricots in your lunch.

√ Instead of French fries, think orange! Slice raw sweet potatoes, toss the slices in olive or canola oil, and bake at high heat for a healthful alternative.

√ Add veggies to homemade pizza.

√ Add shredded carrots to cake and muffin batters.

√ Bringing dessert to a potluck? Make a pumpkin pie! It's easy if you use canned pumpkin and follow the recipe on the can.

√ Go green, too! The next time you have a salad, go for the dark-green leafy vegetables instead of iceberg lettuce for more beta-carotene.

√ Add raw spinach or other green leafy vegetables to wraps and sandwiches.

NUTRITION MYTH OR FACT?

Can Beta-Carotene Supplements Cause Cancer?

Beta-carotene is one of many carotenoids known to have antioxidant properties. Because there is substantial evidence that people eating foods high in antioxidants have lower rates of cancer, large-scale studies are being conducted to determine whether taking antioxidant supplements can decrease our risk for cancer. In particular, the Alpha-Tocopherol Beta-Carotene (ATBC) Cancer Prevention Study and the Beta-Carotene and Retinol Efficacy Trial (CARET) have shown surprising results.[5]

The ATBC Cancer Prevention Study was conducted in Finland from 1985 to 1993 with the purpose of determining the effects of beta-carotene and vitamin E supplements on the rates of lung cancer and other forms of cancer among male smokers between the ages of 50 and 69 years. Almost 30,000 men participated in the study for an average of 6 years. The participants were given daily a beta-carotene supplement, a vitamin E supplement, a supplement containing both beta-carotene and vitamin E, or a placebo.

Contrary to what was expected, the male smokers who took beta-carotene supplements experienced an *increased* number of deaths during the study. More men in this group died of lung cancer, heart disease, and stroke. There was also a trend in this group for higher rates of prostate and stomach cancers. This negative effect appeared to be particularly strong in men who had a higher alcohol intake.

CARET began as a pilot study in the United States in 1985 and included more than 18,000 men and women who were smokers, former smokers, or workers who were exposed to asbestos. The participants were randomly assigned to take daily supplements of beta-carotene and retinol (vitamin A) or a placebo. After a 4-year follow-up period, the incidence of lung cancer was 28% higher among those taking the beta-carotene and retinol supplement. This significant finding, in addition to the results from the ATBC Cancer Prevention Study, prompted researchers to end the CARET study early and recommend that participants discontinue the supplements.[6]

The reasons why beta-carotene increased lung cancer risk in this population are not clear. It is possible that the supplementation period was too brief to benefit these high-risk individuals, although studies of shorter duration have found beneficial effects. There may be other components besides beta-carotene in whole foods that are protective against cancer, making supplementation with an isolated nutrient ineffective. In any case, the results of this study suggest that for certain people, supplementation with beta-carotene may be harmful. There is still much to learn about how people of differing risk levels respond to antioxidant supplementation.

What Happens If We Consume Too Much Beta-Carotene?

Consuming large amounts of beta-carotene or other carotenoids in foods does not appear to cause toxic symptoms. However, your skin can turn yellow or orange if you consume large amounts of foods that are high in beta-carotene. This condition is referred to as *carotenosis* or *carotenoderma,* and it appears to be both reversible and harmless. Taking beta-carotene supplements is not generally recommended, as we can get adequate amounts of this nutrient by eating more fruits and vegetables.

What Happens If We Don't Consume Enough Beta-Carotene?

There are no known deficiency symptoms of beta-carotene or other carotenoids apart from beta-carotene's function as a precursor for vitamin A. Although studies have shown that eating foods high in carotenoids is associated with reduced risks of diseases such as heart disease and cancer, taking carotenoid supplements is not linked with any health benefits, and in some cases may be harmful, as illustrated in the Nutrition Myth or Fact? box concerning beta-carotene supplements and cancer rates.

> RECAP: *Beta-carotene is a phytochemical called a carotenoid. It is also a provitamin of vitamin A. It protects the lipid portions of our cell membranes and LDL-cholesterol from oxidative damage. It also enhances our immune function and protects our vision. There is no RDA for beta-carotene. Orange, red, and deep-green fruits and vegetables are good sources of beta-carotene. There are no known toxicity or deficiency symptoms, but yellowing of the skin can occur if too much beta-carotene is consumed.*

Vitamin A

As early as 30 AD, the Roman Aulus Cornelius Celsus described in his medical encyclopedia *De Medicina* a condition called night blindness, and recommended as a cure the consumption of liver. We now know that night blindness is due to a deficiency of vitamin A, a fat-soluble vitamin stored primarily in the liver of animals. When we consume vitamin A, we store 90% in our liver, and the remainder in our adipose tissue, kidneys, and lungs. Because fat-soluble vitamins cannot dissolve in our blood, they require proteins that can bind with and transport them through the bloodstream to target tissues and cells. *Retinol-binding protein* is one such carrier protein for vitamin A. Retinol-binding protein carries one form of vitamin A, retinol, from the liver to the cells that require it.

There are three active forms of vitamin A in our bodies: **retinol** is the alcohol form, **retinal** is the aldehyde form, and **retinoic acid** is the acid form. These three forms are collectively referred to as the *retinoids* (FIGURE 8.10). Of the three, retinol has the starring role in maintaining our bodies' physiologic functions. Remember from the previous section that beta-carotene is a precursor to vitamin A. When we eat foods with beta-carotene, it is converted to retinol in the wall of our small intestine.

The unit of expression for vitamin A is retinol activity equivalents (RAE). You may still see the expression Retinol Equivalents (RE) or International Units (IU) for vitamin A on food labels or dietary supplements. The conversions to RAE from various forms of retinol and from the units IU and RE are as follows:

- 1 RAE = 1 microgram (μg) retinol
- 1 RAE = 12 μg beta-carotene
- 1 RAE = 24 μg alpha-carotene or beta-cryptoxanthin
- 1 RAE = 1 RE
- 1 RAE = 3.3 IU

Functions of Vitamin A

The known functions of vitamin A are numerous, and researchers speculate that many are still to be discovered.

Vitamin A May Act as an Antioxidant.   Limited research indicates that vitamin A may act as an antioxidant.[7–9] For example, a recent study conducted in Sweden showed that high intakes of vitamin A and retinol from foods alone, as well as from supplements, were associated with a lower risk for gastric cancer.[7] Like vitamins E and C, vitamin A appears to scavenge free radicals and protect our LDLs from oxidation. As you might expect, adequate vitamin A levels in the blood are associated

retinol An active, alcohol form of vitamin A that plays an important role in healthy vision and immune function.

retinal An active, aldehyde form of vitamin A that plays an important role in healthy vision and immune function.

retinoic acid An active, acid form of vitamin A that plays an important role in cell growth and immune function.

FIGURE 8.10   The three active forms of vitamin A in our bodies are retinol, retinal, and retinoic acid. Retinol and retinal can be converted interchangeably; retinoic acid is formed from retinal, and this process is irreversible. Each form of vitamin A contributes to many of our bodily processes.

with lower risks of some forms of cancer and heart disease. However, the role of vitamin A as an antioxidant is not strongly established and is still under investigation.

Vitamin A Is Essential to Sight. Vitamin A's most critical role in our bodies is certainly in the maintenance of healthy vision. Specifically, vitamin A affects our sight in two ways: it enables us to react to changes in the brightness of light, and it enables us to distinguish between different wavelengths of light—in other words, to see different colors. Let's take a closer look at this process.

Light enters our eyes through the cornea, travels through the lens, and then hits the **retina,** which is a delicate membrane lining the back of the inner eyeball (see FIGURE 8.11). You might already have guessed how *retinal* got its name: it is found in—and integral to—the retina. In the retina, retinal combines with a protein called **opsin** to form **rhodopsin.** Rhodopsin is a light-sensitive pigment found in *rod cells,* which are cells that react to dim light and interpret black and white images. When light hits the retina, a reaction occurs in which rhodopsin is split into retinal and opsin. This causes the rod cells to lose their color. It also causes both retinal and opsin to change shape. These changes in turn result in the transmission of a signal to the brain that is interpreted as a black and white image. This process goes on continually, allowing our eyes to adjust moment to moment to subtle changes in our surroundings or in the level of light. Most of the retinal is recycled and combines with opsin to form rhodopsin again. However, some of the retinal is lost with each cycle and must be replaced by retinol from the bloodstream. At the same time, the *cone cells* of the retina, which are effective only in bright light, use retinal to interpret different wavelengths of light as different colors.

In summary, our abilities to adjust to dim light, recover from a bright flash of light, and see in color are all critically dependent on adequate levels of retinal in our eyes.

Vitamin A Contributes to Cell Differentiation. Another important role of vitamin A is its contribution to **cell differentiation,** the process by which

retina The delicate light-sensitive membrane lining the inner eyeball and connected to the optic nerve. It contains retinal.

opsin A protein that combines with retinal in the retina to form rhodopsin.

rhodopsin A light-sensitive pigment found in the rod cells that is formed by retinal and opsin.

cell differentiation The process by which immature, undifferentiated stem cells develop into highly specialized functional cells of discrete organs and tissues.

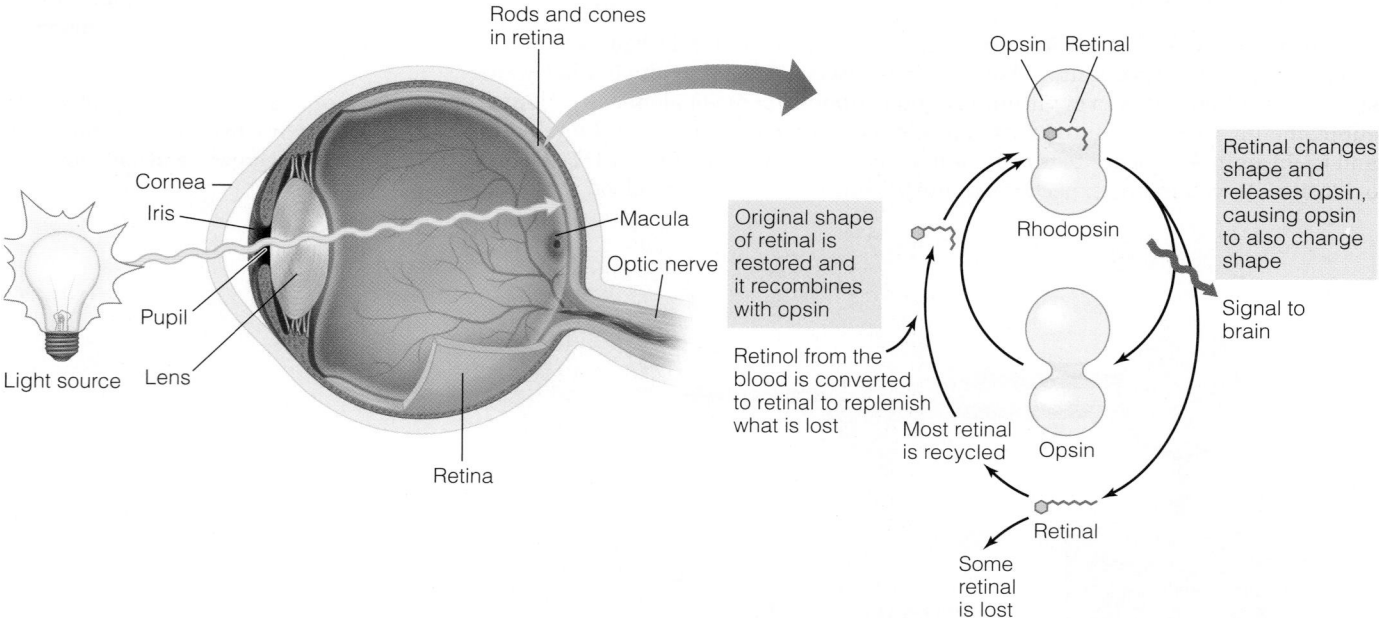

FIGURE 8.11 Vitamin A is necessary to maintain healthy vision. Light enters the eye through the cornea, travels through the lens, and hits the retina located in the back of the eye. In the rod cells of the retina, retinal is combined with opsin to form rhodopsin. As light hits the rod cells, they lose color, and the components of rhodopsin, retinal and opsin, split and change shape. These changes cause transmission of a signal to the brain that allows us to see.

immature cells develop into highly specialized cells that perform unique functions. Obviously, this process is critical to the development of healthy organs and effectively functioning body systems. As an example of cell differentiation, let's look at the development of the mucus-producing cells lining the trachea and bronchi, intestines, stomach, bladder, cornea of the eye, and other organs. The mucus that these cells produce lubricates the tissue and helps us to propel microbes, dust particles, foods, or fluids out of our body tissues (for example, when we cough up secretions or empty our bladder). When vitamin A levels are insufficient, these cells fail to differentiate appropriately, and we lose these protective mechanisms against infection and irritants. Vitamin A is also critical to the differentiation of specialized immune cells called *T-lymphocytes,* or *T-cells*, which fight infections. You can now see why vitamin A deficiency can lead to a breakdown of our immune responses and to infections and other disorders of the lungs and respiratory tract, urinary tract, vagina, and eyes.

Other Functions of Vitamin A.   Vitamin A is involved in reproduction. Although its exact role is unclear, it appears necessary for sperm production in men and for fertilization to occur in women.

Vitamin A contributes to healthy bone growth. It assists in breaking down old bone so that new, longer, and stronger bone can develop. As a result of a vitamin A deficiency, children suffer from stunted growth and wasting.

Two prescription medications for acne contain derivatives of vitamin A. Retin-A, or tretinoin, is a treatment applied to the skin. Accutane is taken orally. These medications should be used only under the supervision of a physician. Although they are relatively less toxic forms of vitamin A, they can cause birth defects in infants if used while a woman is pregnant and can lead to other toxicity problems in some individuals. It is recommended that these medications be stopped at least 2 years prior to conceiving. Interestingly, vitamin A itself has no effect on acne; thus, vitamin A supplements are not recommended in its treatment. See Table 8.1 for the functions, recommended intake, and toxicity and deficiency symptoms associated with vitamin A.

How Much Vitamin A Should We Consume?

Vitamin A toxicity can occur readily because it is a fat-soluble vitamin, so it is important to consume only the amount recommended, as shown in Table 8.1. This amount is known to be safe.

We consume vitamin A from both animal and plant sources. About half of the vitamin A in a nonvegetarian diet is the preformed vitamin A found in animal foods such as beef liver, chicken liver, eggs, and whole-fat dairy products. Vitamin A is also found in fortified reduced-fat milks, margarine, and some breakfast cereals (FIGURE 8.12).

The other half of the vitamin A we consume comes from foods high in beta-carotene and other carotenoids that can be converted to vitamin A. As discussed earlier in this chapter, dark-green, orange, and deep-yellow fruits and vegetables are good sources of beta-carotene, and thus of vitamin A. Carrots, spinach, mango, cantaloupe, and tomato juice are excellent sources of vitamin A because they contain beta-carotene.

What Happens If We Consume Too Much Vitamin A?

Vitamin A is highly toxic, and toxicity symptoms develop after consuming only three to four times the RDA. Toxicity rarely results from food sources, but vitamin A supplements are known to have caused severe illness and even death. Consuming excess vitamin A while pregnant can cause serious birth defects and spontaneous abortions. Other toxicity symptoms include loss of appetite, blurred vision, hair loss, abdominal pain, nausea, diarrhea, and damage to the liver and nervous system. If caught in time, many of these symptoms are reversible once vitamin A supplementation is stopped. However, permanent damage can occur to the liver, eyes, and other organs. Because liver contains such a high amount of vitamin A, children and pregnant women should not consume liver on a daily or weekly basis.

Liver, carrots, and cantaloupe all contain vitamin A.

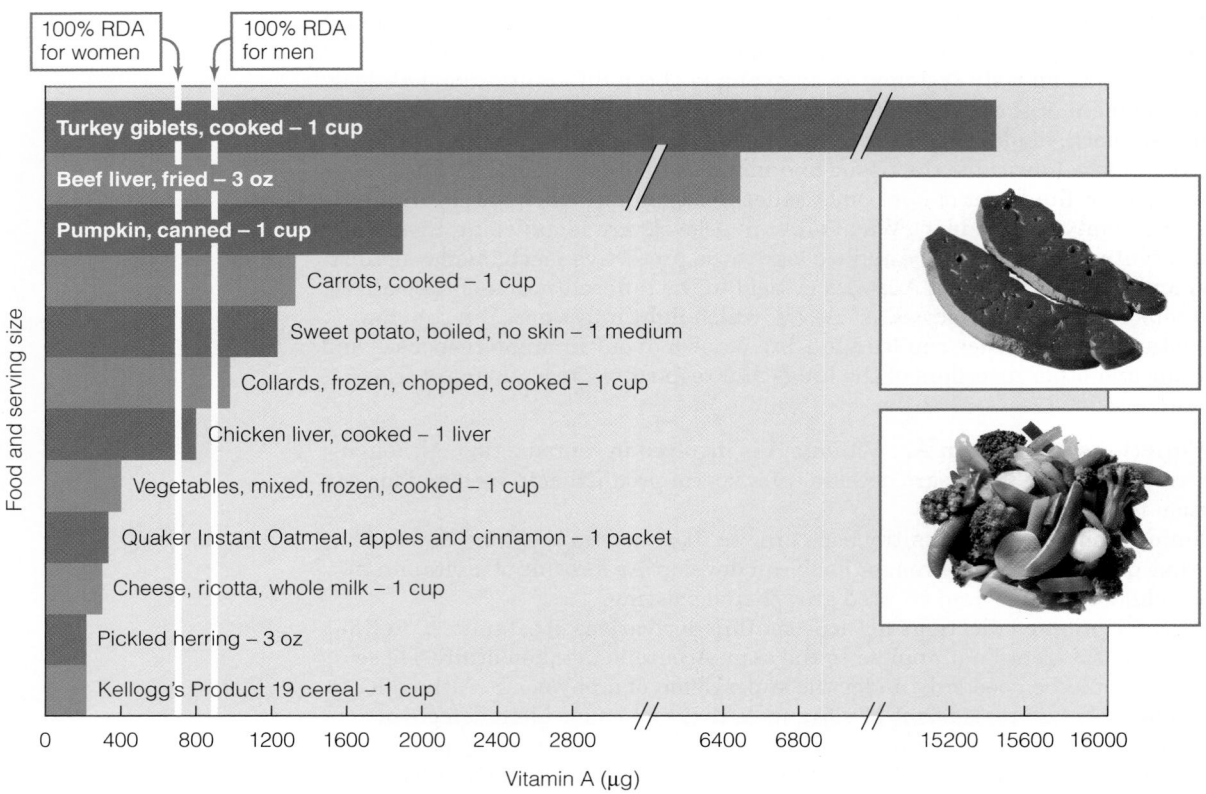

FIGURE 8.12 Common food sources of vitamin A. The RDA for vitamin A is 900 µg/day for men and 700 µg/day for women. (Data from U.S. Department of Agriculture, Agricultural Research Service, 2006. USDA Nutrient Database for Standard Reference, Release 19. Nutrient Data Laboratory Home Page, www.ars.usda.gov/ba/bhnrc/ndl.)

What Happens If We Don't Consume Enough Vitamin A?

Night blindness, the condition that results from vitamin A deficiency, is characterized by an inability to adjust to dim light as well as the failure to regain sight quickly after a bright flash of light. As we discussed earlier, since the cone cells of the retina process colors, color blindness can also result from a vitamin A deficiency.

If vitamin A deficiency progresses, it can result in irreversible blindness due to hardening of the cornea (the transparent membrane covering the front of the eye), a condition called *xerophthalmia.* The prefix of this word, *xero-,* comes from a Greek word meaning "dry." Lack of vitamin A causes the cells of the cornea to lose their ability to produce mucus, causing the eye to become very dry. This leaves the cornea susceptible to damage, infection, and hardening. Once the cornea hardens in this way, the resulting blindness is irreversible. This is why it is critical to catch vitamin A deficiency in its early stages and treat it either with the regular consumption of fruits and vegetables that contain beta-carotene or with vitamin A supplementation.

Other deficiency symptoms include impaired immunity, increased risk of illness and infections, reproductive system disorders, and failure of normal growth. Individuals who are at risk for vitamin A deficiency include anyone with a poor diet, such as people with inadequate vegetable and fruit intakes, and those who abuse alcohol or illegal drugs. Any condition that results in fat malabsorption can also lead to vitamin A deficiency. People with cystic fibrosis, celiac disease, or diseases of the liver, pancreas, or gallbladder and people who consume large amounts of the fat substitute Olestra are at risk for vitamin A deficiency.

How severe a problem is night blindness? Although uncommon among people of developed nations, vitamin A deficiency is a severe public health concern in low-income nations. Approximately 118 nations are affected, particularly African and

night blindness A vitamin A deficiency disorder that results in loss of the ability to see in dim light.

Southeast Asian countries. According to the World Health Organization, between 100 and 140 million children suffer from vitamin A deficiency.[10] Of the children affected, 250,000 to 500,000 become permanently blinded every year. At least half of these children will die within 1 year of losing their sight. Death is due to infections and illnesses, including measles and diarrhea, that are easily treated in wealthier countries.

Vitamin A deficiency is also a tragedy for pregnant women in these countries. These women suffer from night blindness, are more likely to transmit HIV to their child if HIV-positive, and run a greater risk of maternal mortality.

Programs to fight vitamin A deficiency support families in planting and maintaining home gardens with beta-carotene-rich vegetables. Other programs provide vitamin A supplements to populations at risk.

> **RECAP:** *The role of vitamin A as an antioxidant is still under investigation. Vitamin A is critical for maintaining our vision. It is also necessary for cell differentiation, reproduction, and growth. Animal livers, dairy products, and eggs are good animal sources of vitamin A; fruits and vegetables are high in beta-carotene, which is used to synthesize vitamin A. Supplementation can be dangerous, as toxicity is reached at levels of only three to four times the RDA. Toxicity symptoms include birth defects, spontaneous abortions, blurred vision, and liver damage. Deficiency symptoms include night blindness, impaired immune function, and growth failure.*

Selenium

Selenium is a trace mineral, and it is found in varying amounts in soil. As reviewed *In Depth* on pages 252–263, trace minerals are needed by our bodies in amounts less than 100 mg/day. Keep in mind that, although we need only minute amounts of trace minerals, they are just as important to our health as the major minerals.

Functions of Selenium

It is only recently that we have learned about the critical role of selenium as a nutrient in human health. In 1979, Chinese scientists reported an association between a heart disorder called **Keshan disease** and selenium deficiency. This disease occurs in children in the Keshan province of China, where the soil is depleted of selenium. The scientists found that Keshan disease can be prevented with selenium supplementation.

The selenium in our bodies is contained in proteins, or more specifically, amino acids. Two amino acid derivatives contain the majority of selenium in our bodies: *selenomethionine* is the storage form for selenium, while *selenocysteine* is the active form of selenium.

Selenium is a critical component of the glutathione peroxidase antioxidant enzyme system mentioned earlier (page 307). Thus, selenium helps spare vitamin E and prevents oxidative damage to our cell membranes.

Selenium is also needed for the production of thyroxine (thyroid hormone). By this action, selenium is involved in the maintenance of our basal metabolism and body temperature. Selenium appears to play a role in immune function, and poor selenium status is associated with higher rates of some forms of cancer. The functions, recommended intake, and toxicity and deficiency symptoms associated with selenium are listed in Table 8.1.

How Much Selenium Should We Consume?

As selenium is a trace mineral, we need only minute amounts to maintain health. (The RDA is identified in Table 8.1.) Selenium is present in both animal and plant food sources but in variable amounts. Because it is stored in the tissues of animals, selenium is found in reliably consistent amounts in animal foods. Organ meats, such as liver, kidney, pork, and seafood, are particularly good sources (see FIGURE 8.13).

Wheat is a rich source of selenium.

Keshan disease A heart disorder caused by selenium deficiency. It was first identified in children in the Keshan province of China.

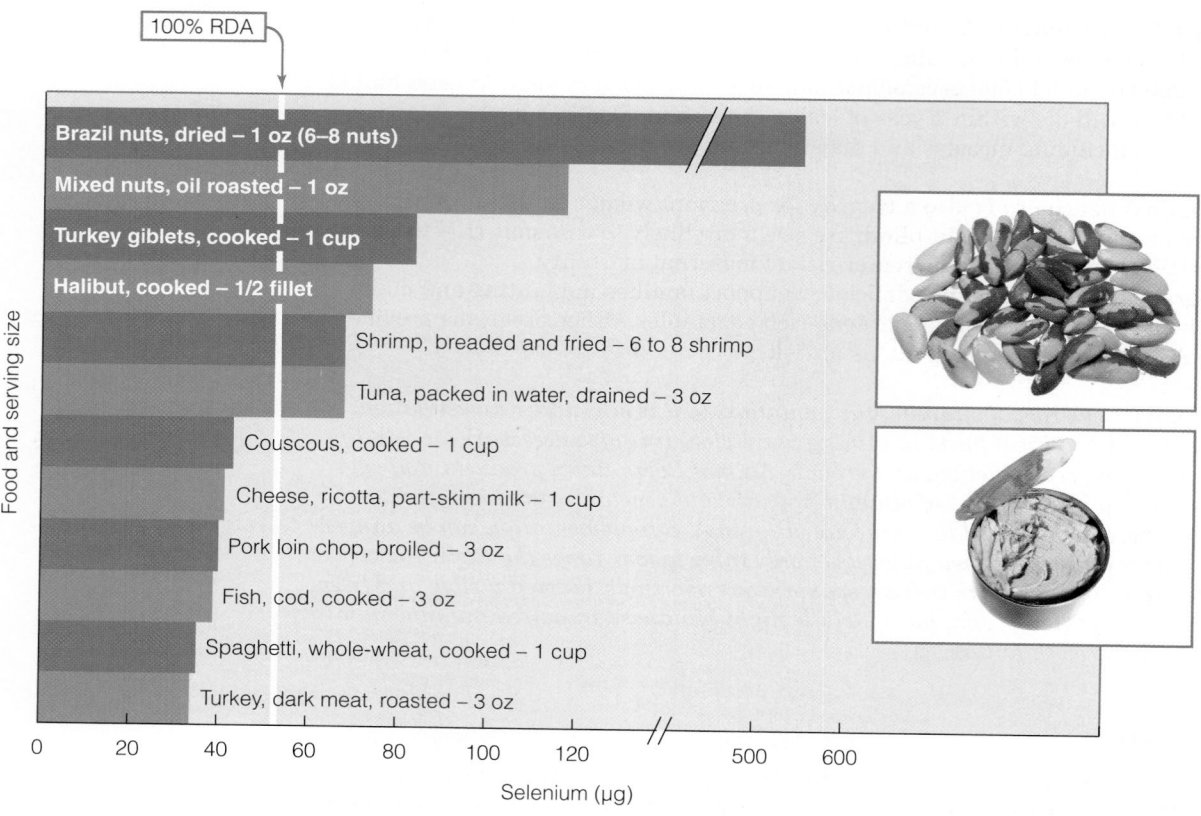

FIGURE 8.13 Common food sources of selenium. The RDA for selenium is 55 µg/day. (Data from U.S. Department of Agriculture, Agricultural Research Service, 2006. USDA Nutrient Database for Standard Reference, Release 19. Nutrient Data Laboratory Home Page, www.ars.usda.gov/ba/bhnrc/ndl.)

In contrast, the amount of selenium in plants is dependent upon the selenium content of the soil in which the plant is grown. Thus, the amount of selenium in the fruits and vegetables you eat can vary widely according to the food's origin. Many companies marketing selenium supplements warn that the agricultural soils in the United States are depleted of selenium and inform us that we need to take selenium supplements. In reality, the selenium content of soil varies greatly across North America, and because we obtain our food from a variety of geographic locations, few people in the United States suffer from selenium deficiency. This is especially true for people who eat even small quantities of meat or seafood. As indicated in FIGURE 8.13, nuts, wheat, and rice are particularly rich sources of selenium.

What Happens If We Consume Too Much Selenium?

Selenium toxicity does not result from eating foods high in selenium. However, supplementation with selenium can cause toxicity. Toxicity symptoms include brittle hair and nails that can eventually break and fall off. Other symptoms of toxicity include skin rashes, vomiting, nausea, weakness, and cirrhosis of the liver.

What Happens If We Don't Consume Enough Selenium?

As discussed previously, selenium deficiency is associated with a special form of heart disease called Keshan disease. Selenium deficiency does not cause the disease, but selenium is necessary to help the immune system effectively fight the virus that causes the disease. Another deficiency disease is *Kashin-Beck disease,* a deforming arthritis also found in selenium-depleted areas in China and in Tibet (FIGURE 8.14). Other deficiency symptoms include impaired immune responses, increased risk of viral infections, infertility, depression, hostility, impaired cognitive function, and muscle pain and wasting.

FIGURE 8.14 Selenium deficiency can lead to deforming arthritis called Kashin-Beck disease.

> RECAP: *Selenium is part of the glutathione peroxidase antioxidant enzyme system. It indirectly spares vitamin E from oxidative damage, and it assists with immune function and the production of thyroid hormone. Organ meats, pork, and seafood are good sources of selenium, as are nuts, wheat, and rice. The selenium content of plants is dependent upon the amount of selenium in the soil in which they are grown. Toxicity symptoms include brittle hair and nails, vomiting, nausea, and liver cirrhosis. Deficiency symptoms and side effects include Keshan disease, Kashin-Beck disease, impaired immune function, infertility, and muscle wasting.*

Copper, Iron, Zinc, and Manganese Assist in Antioxidant Function

As discussed earlier, there are numerous antioxidant enzyme systems in our bodies. Copper, zinc, and manganese are cofactors for the superoxide dismutase antioxidant enzyme system. Iron is a cofactor for catalase, another antioxidant enzyme system. In addition to their role in protecting our cells from oxidative damage, copper, iron, manganese, and zinc play major roles in the optimal functioning of many other enzymes in our bodies. Copper, iron, and zinc help us maintain the health of our blood, and manganese is an important cofactor in carbohydrate metabolism. The functions, requirements, food sources, and deficiency and toxicity symptoms of these nutrients are discussed in detail in Chapter 10, which focuses on the nutrients involved in energy metabolism and blood formation.

> RECAP: *Copper, zinc, and manganese are cofactors for the superoxide dismutase antioxidant enzyme system. Iron is a cofactor for the catalase antioxidant enzyme. These minerals play critical roles in blood health and energy metabolism.*

What Disorders Are Related to Free Radical Damage?

Through your experiences you may have found that there are a plethora of claims related to the functions of antioxidants. These claims include the slowing of aging and age-related diseases and the prevention of cancer and heart disease. In opposition to these claims, there is some evidence that taking antioxidant supplements may be harmful for certain people (refer back to the Nutrition Myth or Fact? box on beta-carotene, page 320). In this section, we will review what is currently known about the role of antioxidant nutrients in cancer, heart disease, and aging.

Cancer

Before we explore how antioxidants affect our risk for cancer, let's take a closer look at precisely what cancer is and how it spreads. **Cancer** is actually a group of diseases that are all characterized by cells that grow "out of control." By this we mean that cancer cells reproduce spontaneously and independently, and they are not inhibited by the boundaries of tissues and organs. Thus, they can aggressively invade tissues and organs far away from those in which they originally formed.

Most forms of cancer result in one or more **tumors,** which are newly formed masses of undifferentiated cells that are immature and have no physiologic function. Although the word "tumor" sounds frightening, it is important to note that not every tumor is *malignant,* or cancerous. Many are *benign* (not harmful to us) and are made up of cells that will not spread widely.

FIGURE 8.15 shows how changes to normal cells prompt a series of other changes that can progress into cancer.

There are three primary steps of cancer development: initiation, promotion, and progression. These steps occur as follows:

1. **Initiation**—The initiation of cancer occurs when a cell's DNA is *mutated* (or changed). This mutation causes permanent changes in the cell.

2. **Promotion**—During this phase the genetically altered cell is stimulated to repeatedly divide. The mutated DNA is locked into each new cell's genetic instructions. Since the enzymes that normally work to repair damaged cells cannot detect alterations in the DNA, the cells can continue to divide uninhibited.

3. **Progression**—During this phase, the cancerous cells grow out of control and invade surrounding tissues. These cells then *metastasize* (spread) to other sites of the body. In the early stages of progression, our immune system can sometimes detect these cancerous cells and destroy them. However, if the cells continue to grow, they develop into malignant tumors, and cancer results.

Heredity, Lifestyle Choices, and Infectious and Environmental Agents Can Increase Cancer Risk

Cancer is the second leading cause of death in the United States, and researchers estimate that about half of all men and one-third of all women will develop cancer during their lifetime. But what factors cause cancer? Are you and your loved ones at risk? The answer depends on several factors, including your heredity, your exposure to infectious and environmental agents, and various lifestyle choices.

Heredity can play a role in the development of cancer, because inherited "cancer genes," such as the BRC genes for breast cancer, increase the risk that an individual with those genes will develop cancer. However, it is important to bear in mind that a family history of cancer does not guarantee you will get cancer, too. It just means that you are at an increased risk and should take all preventive actions available to you. While some risk factors are out of your control, others are modifiable, which means that you can take positive steps to reduce that risk.

The American Cancer Society identifies five major modifiable risk factors that have been shown to have the greatest impact on an individual's chance of developing cancer: tobacco use, an unhealthful diet, infectious agents, ultraviolet radiation, and physical inactivity.[11] We discuss each of these in more detail here.

Tobacco Use. It is an established and well-known fact that smoking cigars and cigarettes and using smokeless tobacco significantly increase your risk for cancer. More than 4,000 compounds have been identified in tobacco and tobacco smoke, including tar, formaldehyde, hydrocarbons, and other chemicals. More than 40 of these compounds are **carcinogens,** or substances that can cause cancer. Using tobacco increases your risk for cancers of the lung, larynx, mouth, esophagus, bladder, and pancreas and can also cause heart disease, stroke, and emphysema (FIGURE 8.16). (See the Highlight box on disorders linked to tobacco use, page 330.) Each year more than 400,000 Americans die from cigarette smoking; this represents approximately 40 people each hour.[12]

cancer A group of diseases characterized by cells that reproduce spontaneously and independently and may invade other tissues and organs.

tumor Any newly formed mass of undifferentiated cells.

carcinogen Any substance capable of causing the cellular mutations that lead to cancer.

Carcinogen

Normal cell undergoing mutation in DNA

1 Initiation: a carcinogen causes a mutation in the DNA of a normal cell.

Rapidly dividing genetically altered cells

2 Promotion: cell with mutation in DNA divides repeatedly.

3 Progression: cancer cells invade surrounding tissues and spread to other sites in body.

Cancer cell transported in blood vessel

FIGURE 8.15 Cancer cells develop as a result of a genetic mutation in the DNA of a normal cell. The mutated cell replicates uncontrollably, eventually resulting in a tumor. If not destroyed or removed, the cancerous tumor metastasizes and spreads to other parts of the body.

The positive news is that tobacco use is a modifiable risk factor. If you smoke or use smokeless tobacco, you can reduce your risk for cancer considerably by quitting. The nicotine in tobacco is an addictive drug, so if you are trying to quit, get the professional help you need: talk with your healthcare provider about which of the various cessation methods would be right for you.

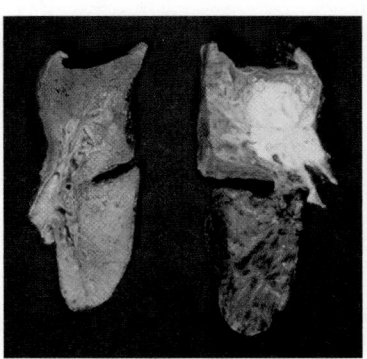

(a)   (b)

FIGURE 8.16 Cigarette smoking significantly increases our risk for lung and other types of cancer. The risk of lung cancer is 22.4 times higher in men who smoke and 12 times higher in women who smoke. **(a)** A normal, healthy lung; **(b)** the lung of a smoker. Notice the deposits of tar as well as the areas of tumor growth.

HIGHLIGHT

Disorders Linked to Tobacco Use

Many people smoke cigarettes or cigars, or use smokeless tobacco. The use of these products can lead to serious health consequences that together reduce life expectancy by more than 13 years in males and 14 years in females.[14] Tobacco use is a risk factor in development of all of the following diseases and health concerns:

1. Cancers:
   - Lung
   - Larynx
   - Mouth (Figure 8.17a)
   - Pharynx
   - Esophagus
   - Bladder
   - Pancreas
   - Uterus
   - Kidney
   - Stomach
   - Some leukemias
2. Heart disease
3. Bronchitis
4. Emphysema
5. Stroke
6. Erectile dysfunction
7. Conditions related to maternal smoking:
   - Miscarriage
   - Preterm delivery
   - Stillbirth
   - Infant death
   - Low birth weight

In addition, smoking causes a variety of other problems, such as the premature wrinkling and coarsening of the skin shown in the accompanying photo (Figure 8.17b). Smoking also causes bad breath, yellowing of the fingernails and hair, and bad-smelling clothes, hair, and living quarters. Second-hand smoke is another concern, especially for those who live or work with smokers. Nonsmokers who are exposed to secondhand smoke at home or work increase their risk of developing heart disease by 25–30% and increase their risk of developing lung cancer by 20–30%. Research indicates that there is no risk-free level of exposure to secondhand smoke.[13]

(a)

(b)

FIGURE 8.17 Effects of tobacco use. In addition to increasing your risk for lung cancer and cardiovascular disease, **(a)** using tobacco increases your risk of mouth cancer, and **(b)** smoking results in premature wrinkling of the skin, especially around the mouth.

Despite legislation banning smoking in public places, millions of Americans, including children, are exposed to secondhand smoke. Secondhand smoke has twice as much nicotine and tar as the smoke that smokers inhale. It also has five times the carbon monoxide, which decreases the amount of oxygen in the exposed person's blood. The Surgeon General reports that secondhand smoke exposure has immediate adverse effects on the cardiovascular system. Long-term inhalation of secondhand smoke causes coronary heart disease, lung cancer, and premature death.[13]

Arctic explorers wear special clothing to protect themselves from the cold as well as the high levels of ultraviolet rays from the sun.

Unhealthful Diet. Up to 30% of cancers in developed countries may be related to poor nutrition. Consumption of certain substances, including alcohol, dietary fat, and compounds found in cured and charbroiled meats, can increase our risk for cancer. See the Highlight box on page 332 for a list of nutritional factors involved in cancer risk. Nutritional factors that are protective against cancer include antioxidants, fiber, and phytochemicals (discussed *In Depth* on pages 350–359). Diets high in saturated fats and low in fruits and vegetables increase the risk of cancers of the esophagus, colon, breast, and prostate.[11] Increasing your intake of whole grains, fruits, and vegetables, decreasing your intake of red meats and fatty meats, and maintaining a healthy weight are keys to cancer prevention.

Infectious Agents. Infectious agents account for 18% of cancers worldwide. For example, infection of the female cervix with the sexually transmitted virus *Human papillomavirus* is linked to cervical cancer, and infection with the bacterium *Helicobacter pylori* is linked not only to ulcers but also to stomach cancer. As microbial research advances, it is thought that more cancers will be linked to infectious agents.

Ultraviolet Radiation. Skin cancer is the most common form of cancer in the United States and accounts for over half of all cancers diagnosed each year. Most cases of skin cancer are linked to exposure to ultraviolet (UV) rays from the sun and indoor tanning beds. UV rays damage the DNA of immature skin cells, which then reproduce uncontrollably. Research has shown that a person's risk for skin cancer doubles if he or she has had five or more sunburns; however, your risk for skin cancer still increases with UV exposure even if you do not get sunburned.[15] Exposure to tanning beds before age 35 increases by 75% your risk of developing the most invasive form of skin cancer.[16]

Skin cancer includes the nonmelanoma cancers (basal cell and squamous cell cancers), which are not typically invasive, and malignant melanoma, which is the one of the most deadly of all types of cancer (FIGURE 8.18). Skin cancer can be cured if caught early. Wearing sunscreen with at least a 15 SPF (sun protection factor) rating and protective clothing and avoiding the sun between 10 AM and 4 PM can help reduce your risk for skin cancer.

Physical Inactivity. A sedentary lifestyle increases the risk of colon cancer and may increase the risk for other forms of cancer.[11] At the same time, a recent review of

Human papillomavirus (HPV) is an infectious agent that can cause cancer.

FIGURE 8.18 A lesion associated with malignant melanoma is characterized by asymmetry, uneven or blurred borders, mixed shades of tan, brown, black, and sometimes red or blue, and a diameter larger than a pencil eraser (6 mm).

HIGHLIGHT

HIGHLIGHT HIGHLIGHT HIGHLIGHT HIGHLIGHT

Nutritional Factors That Influence Our Risk for Cancer

Nutritional factors that may increase our cancer risk include the following:

- Heterocyclic amines in cooked meat: carcinogenic chemicals formed when meat is cooked at high temperatures, such as during broiling, barbecuing, and frying.
- Nitrates in drinking water: a carcinogenic chemical found in fertilizers that is proven to increase the risk of non-Hodgkin's lymphoma. People drinking contaminated tap water in agricultural areas may be at risk.
- Nitrites and nitrates in cured meats: compounds found in some sausages, hams, bacon, and lunch meats. These compounds bind with amino acids to form nitrosamines, which are potent carcinogens.
- Obesity: appears to increase the risk of cancers of the breast, colon, prostate, endometrium (the lining of the uterus), cervix, ovary, kidney, gallbladder, liver, pancreas, rectum, and esophagus. The exact link between obesity and increased cancer risk is not clear but may be linked with hormonal changes that occur with having excess body fat.
- High saturated-fat diet: diets high in saturated fat have been associated with increased risk of many cancers, including prostate and breast. However, not all studies support this association.
- Alcohol: excessive use is linked with an increased risk of cancers of the esophagus, pharynx, and mouth. May also increase the risk for cancers of the liver, breast, colon, and rectum. Alcohol may impair cells' ability to repair damaged DNA, increasing the possibility of cancer initiation.

Factors that may protect against cancer include the following:

- Antioxidant-rich foods: includes vitamins E, C, A, beta-carotene, and other carotenoids and minerals such as selenium. Supplementation with individual antioxidants does not show consistent benefits.
- Dietary fiber: some studies show reduced risks for breast, colon, and rectal cancer with increased fiber intake, although findings are not consistent.
- Phytoestrogens: compounds found in soy-based foods and some vegetables and grains that may decrease the risk for breast, endometrial, and prostate cancers.
- Omega-3 fatty acids: includes alpha-linolenic acid, eicosapentaenoic acid (EPA), and docosahexaenoic acid (DHA). These fatty acids are found in fish and fish oils. Consuming foods high in omega-3 fatty acids is associated with reduced rates of breast, colon, and rectal cancers.

Factors falsely claimed to cause cancer include the following:

- Artificial sweeteners: there are claims that aspartame (brand name Nutrasweet) is carcinogenic. There is no evidence to support the claim that aspartame causes brain or any other form of cancer; however, these unsubstantiated claims continue to resurface on the Internet.
- Coffee: there are no studies to support the claim that drinking coffee increases the risk for cancer. Some of the chemicals used to make decaffeinated coffee are now known to be carcinogenic; most companies now use safer chemicals for this process.
- Fluoridated water: studies conducted over the past 40 years show no association between drinking fluoridated water and increased cancer risk.
- Food additives: it is estimated that more than 15,000 substances are added to our foods during growth, processing, and packaging. To date, there is no evidence that food additives contribute significantly to cancer risk.

several studies has found that higher levels of physical activity are associated with a 20–30% reduction in our overall risk for cancer.[17] A clear protective effect of exercise was found specifically for breast and colon cancers. The reduction in risk was found only for moderate or vigorous intensity activity.

At this time, we do not know how exercise reduces the overall risk for cancer or for certain types of cancers. Suggested mechanisms include 1) improved circulation; 2) increased ventilation and shortened bowel transit time, which reduces the time our lungs and bowels are exposed to potential carcinogens; 3) maintenance of healthier weight; 4) improved immune function; 5) modulation of sex hormones such as estrogen and testosterone, which could reduce the risk of breast, endometrial, ovarian, testicular, and prostate cancers; and 6) enhanced repair of damaged DNA. None of these mechanisms have been sufficiently studied to allow us to draw any firm conclusions about how physical activity may be protective against cancer. However, these findings have prompted the American Cancer Society and the National Cancer Institute to promote increased physical activity as a way to reduce our risk for cancer.

Other Factors Influencing Cancer Risk. Environmental pollution and occupational exposures also increase our cancer risk. These include such things as secondhand cigarette and cigar smoke, chemicals in our food and water supply, and radiation and chemicals found in the workplace. Proven carcinogens found in various worksites include benzene, asbestos, vinyl chloride, arsenic, coal tars, radon, wood dust, and aflatoxins (produced by molds in agricultural products such as peanuts).

Other risk factors identified by the American Cancer Society include aging, reproductive factors such as childbearing, suppressed immunity, and medicinal drugs.[11] For example, some hormonal drugs can increase the risk, and in rare cases, anti-cancer drugs can prompt another cancer years later. Finally, the risk of many types of cancer varies between racial and ethnic populations. Some of these differences are attributable to genetics, but most are due to differences in lifestyle and exposures to carcinogens.

Antioxidants Play a Role in Preventing Cancer

There is a large and growing body of evidence that antioxidants play an important role in cancer prevention. How do antioxidants work to reduce our risk for cancer? Some proposed mechanisms include the following:

- Enhancing our immune system, which assists in the destruction and removal of precancerous cells from our bodies.

- Inhibiting the growth of cancer cells and tumors.

- Preventing oxidative damage to our cells' DNA by scavenging free radicals and stopping the formation and subsequent chain reaction of oxidized molecules.

While very few studies show benefits of supplements containing individual antioxidant nutrients such as vitamins E and C, beta-carotene, and selenium, eating whole foods that are high in these nutrients—especially fruits, vegetables, and whole grains—is consistently shown to be associated with decreased cancer risk.[18] Additional studies show that populations eating diets low in antioxidant nutrients have a higher risk for cancer. These studies show a strong association between eating whole foods high in antioxidants and lower cancer risk, but they do not prove cause and effect. Nutrition experts agree that there are important interactions between antioxidant nutrients and other substances in foods, such as fiber and phytochemicals, which work together to reduce the risk for many types of cancers. Studies are now being conducted to determine whether eating foods high in antioxidants directly causes lower rates of cancer.

The link between taking antioxidant supplements and reducing cancer risk is not very clear. Laboratory animal and test tube studies show that the individual nutrients reviewed in this chapter act as antioxidants in various situations. However, supplementation studies in humans do not consistently show benefits of taking antioxidant supplements in the prevention of cancer and other diseases. For example, in the Alpha-Tocopherol Beta-Carotene Cancer Prevention Study discussed earlier, supplementation with vitamin E resulted in a lower risk for cancers of the prostate, colon, and rectum but was related to more cancers of the stomach.[5] In this same study, beta-carotene supplements increased risk for cancers of the lung, prostate, and stomach in current and former smokers.[19] In the Nutritional Prevention of Cancer Trial, selenium supplementation was found to reduce the risk of prostate, colon, and lung cancers, but it did not reduce the risk of nonmelanoma skin cancers.[20] In the Larsson study mentioned earlier, high intakes of vitamin A and retinol from foods alone, as well as from supplements, were associated with a lower risk for gastric cancer.[7] The Linxian intervention trials, named for the region of China where the studies were conducted, found that a supplement containing beta-carotene, vitamin E, and selenium reduced mortality from overall cancer, specifically reducing the risk for cancers of the esophagus and stomach.[21]

Eating more fruits and vegetables has been shown to reduce the risk of several cancers.

Why do antioxidant supplements appear to work in some studies and for some cancers but not in others? The human body is very complex, as is the development and progression of the numerous forms of cancer. People differ substantially in their susceptibility for cancer and in their response to protective factors and to cancer-causing agents. These complexities cloud the relationship between nutrition and cancer. It is impossible to control all factors that may increase our risk for cancer in any research study. Thus, there are many unknown factors that can affect study outcomes. It has also been speculated that antioxidants taken in supplemental form may act as prooxidants in some situations, but consuming antioxidants in the form of food may provide these nutrients in a more balanced state. There are many studies currently being conducted to determine the impact of whole foods and antioxidant supplements on our risk for various forms of cancers. The results of these studies will provide important insights into the link between whole foods, individual nutrients, and cancer. Refer to the Nutrition Debate box at the end of the chapter to gain a better understanding of situations that may warrant vitamin and mineral supplementation.

NUTRI-CASE GUSTAVO

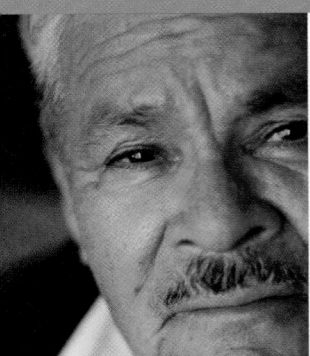

" Last night, there was an actress on TV talking about having colon cancer and saying everybody over age 50 should get tested. It brought back all the memories of my father's cancer, how thin and weak he got before he went to the doctor, so that by the time they found the cancer it had already spread too far. But I don't think I'm at risk. I only eat red meat two or three times a week, and I eat a piece of fruit or a vegetable at every meal. I don't smoke, and I get plenty of exercise, sunshine, and fresh air working in the vineyard."

What factors reduce Gustavo's risk for cancer? What factors increase his risk? Would you recommend he increase his consumption of fruits and vegetables? Why or why not? If Gustavo were your father, would you ask him to have the screening test for colon cancer that the actress on television recommended?

> RECAP: *Cancer is a group of diseases in which genetically mutated cells grow out of control. Tobacco use, an unhealthful diet, infectious agents, exposure to UV radiation, and physical inactivity are related to a higher risk for some cancers. Genetics, aging, and ethnicity/race are nonmodifiable risk factors. Eating foods high in antioxidants is associated with lower rates of cancer, but studies of antioxidant supplements and cancer are equivocal.*

Cardiovascular Disease

The details of *cardiovascular disease (CVD)* and its relationship to cholesterol and lipoproteins were presented in Chapter 5. A brief review of CVD is presented in this section, and an explanation of how antioxidants may reduce our risk is provided.

CVD is the leading cause of death for adults in the United States. CVD encompasses all diseases of the heart and blood vessels, including coronary heart disease, hypertension (or high blood pressure), and atherosclerosis (or hardening of the arteries). The two primary manifestations of CVD are heart attack and stroke. Almost 1 million people die each year from CVD, and about 61 million people (or 25% of the U.S. population) live with this disease. It is estimated that CVD costs our country $298 billion in healthcare costs and lost work revenue.[22]

Remember that the major risks for CVD are the following:

- smoking

- hypertension (high blood pressure)

- high blood levels of LDL-cholesterol

- obesity

- sedentary lifestyle

Other risk factors include a low level of high-density lipoprotein (HDL)-cholesterol, impaired glucose tolerance or diabetes, family history (CVD in males younger than 55 years of age and females younger than 65 years of age), being a male older than 45 years of age, and menopause in women. While we cannot alter our gender, family history, or age, we can change our nutrition and physical activity habits to reduce our risk for CVD.

Research has recently identified a risk factor for CVD that may be even more important than elevated cholesterol levels. This risk factor is a condition called *low-grade inflammation*.[23] This condition weakens the plaque in the blood vessels, making it more fragile. You may remember from Chapter 5 that plaque is the fatty material that builds on the inside of our arteries and causes hardening of the arteries. As the plaque becomes more fragile, it is more likely to burst and break away from the sides of our arteries. It may then form a blood clot that closes off the vessels of the heart or brain, leading to a heart attack or stroke, respectively. The marker in our bodies that indicates the degree of inflammation is C-reactive protein. Having higher levels of C-reactive protein increases our risk for a heart attack even if we do not have elevated cholesterol levels. For people with high levels of C-reactive protein and cholesterol, the risk of a heart attack is almost nine times higher than that of someone with normal cholesterol and C-reactive protein levels. These findings have prompted the medical community to develop standards for measuring C-reactive protein along with cholesterol as a test for CVD risk.

How can antioxidants decrease our risk for CVD? There is growing evidence that certain antioxidants, specifically vitamin E and lycopene, work in a variety of ways that reduce the damage to our vessels, which in turn reduces our risk of a heart attack or stroke. Some of the ways these nutrients decrease our risk for CVD include the following:

- **Scavenging free radicals**—This action prevents oxidative damage to the LDLs. Remember from Chapter 5 that oxidized LDL particles stimulate the buildup of plaque in the blood vessel walls.

- **Reducing low-grade inflammation**—This action can prevent the rupture of plaque in the blood vessels, thus preventing the release of clots that can cause a heart attack or stroke.

- **Reducing blood coagulation and the formation of clots**—Vitamin E has known anticoagulant properties. This means that it acts to prevent excessive thickening and clotting of the blood, preventing the formation of clots that can block blood vessels.

As with the research conducted on cancer, the studies of antioxidants and CVD show inconsistent results. Two large-scale surveys conducted in the United States show that men and women who eat more fruits and vegetables have a significantly reduced risk of CVD.[24,25] However, few intervention studies have been conducted to determine the effect of antioxidant supplements on risk for CVD. Vitamin E was found to lower the number of heart disease deaths in smokers in the Alpha-Tocopherol Beta-Carotene Cancer Prevention Study but had no overall effect on the risk of stroke. In the HOPE study, vitamin E had no impact on the risk for CVD in people who are at high risk for heart attack and stroke.[26, 27] Results from a more recent trial, the Women's Health Study, indicated that vitamin E supplementation provided no overall benefit for CVD or cancer among nearly 40,000 healthy women.[28] Additional studies are currently being conducted, and their results should provide more information on whether or not antioxidant supplements can reduce our risk for CVD.

The flavonoids in black tea might reduce the risk of CVD.

Aging is a natural and inevitable process of life.

macular degeneration A vision disorder caused by deterioration of the central portion of the retina and marked by loss or distortion of the central field of vision.

It is important to note that other compounds (besides antioxidants) found in fruits, vegetables, and whole grains can reduce our risk for CVD. For instance, dietary fiber in general has been shown to reduce blood pressure, lower total cholesterol levels, and improve blood glucose and insulin levels. More specifically, soluble fiber, the type found in legumes, oats, fruits, and vegetables, has been shown to reduce elevated LDL-cholesterol and total cholesterol. The most successful effects have been found in people eating oatmeal and oat bran cereals. Folate, a B-vitamin, is found in fortified cereals, green leafy vegetables, bananas, legumes, and orange juice. Folate is known to reduce homocysteine levels in the blood, and a high concentration of homocysteine in the blood is a known risk factor for CVD. A recent study from the Netherlands showed that individuals who drank more than 3 cups of black tea (which is high in flavonoids) had a lower rate of heart attacks than non-tea drinkers.[29] Thus, it appears that there are a plethora of nutrients and other components in fruits, vegetables, and whole-grain foods that may be protective against CVD. We discuss the claims and research into phytochemicals *In Depth* on pages 350–359.

RECAP: *Cardiovascular disease (CVD) is the leading cause of death in the United States. Risk factors for CVD include smoking, hypertension, high LDL-cholesterol, obesity, and a sedentary lifestyle. Antioxidants may help reduce our risk for heart disease by preventing oxidative damage to LDL-cholesterol, reducing inflammation in our vessels, and reducing the formation of blood clots.*

Vision Impairment and Other Results of Aging

In most Eastern and nonindustrialized cultures, aging is viewed as a natural and desirable process that begins with conception and ends with death. The aged are respected and valued for their wisdom and experience and are often the decision makers in their communities. In contrast, for centuries, many people in Western countries have searched to find an elixir of eternal youth. Today, in the United States and Europe, researchers continue this search, developing skin creams, supplements, botulism toxin injections, and new techniques of plastic surgery to conceal or fight the effects of aging. Despite these efforts, aging is inevitable.

Antioxidant supplements have gotten a great deal of attention as potential substances to reverse the effects of aging. This is because the process of aging is associated with increased oxidative damage and reduced activity of antioxidant enzymes in most body tissues. Despite this link between antioxidants and aging, there is no scientific evidence to support the contention that taking antioxidant supplements can prolong our lives.

However, we know that our ability to digest, absorb, and metabolize many nutrients is impaired as we age (refer to Chapter 20 for more detailed information on aging). These nutritional limitations have prompted some experts to suggest that specific RDAs be increased for adults according to new, narrower age brackets, such as 51 to 60 years, 61 to 70 years, 71 to 80 years, and 81 to 90 years. Currently, the RDAs are defined for adults 51 to 70 years and 71 years and older. A great deal more will be learned about optimal nutrition for older adults over the next decade as people live longer and we learn more about how our nutritional needs change as we age.

Some diseases associated with aging may be preventable by consuming antioxidants. Two of these diseases are macular degeneration and cataracts, both of which impair vision in older adults. Recall from earlier in the chapter that adequate intakes of beta-carotene and vitamin A are necessary for healthy vision. In addition, in some studies, vitamins C and E have shown some protective effects against these vision impairments.

Macular degeneration is the leading cause of blindness of adults 55 years and older in the United States. The macula is the central part of the retina (FIGURE 8.19A), and it is responsible for our central vision and our ability to see details. When a person has macular degeneration, he or she loses the ability to see details, such as small print, small objects, and facial features. Objects seem to fade or disappear, straight lines or edges appear wavy, and the ability to read standard

Blood vessels   Macula   Optic disk

(a)   (b)

FIGURE 8.19   Macular degeneration is the leading cause of blindness in adults ages 55 years and older. **(a)** The macula is the central part of the retina that allows us to see details and small print. **(b)** This simulation of the vision loss typical in patients with macular degeneration illustrates the loss of central vision. (*Source:* National Eye Institute, National Institutes of Health. November 2003. Photos, Images, and Videos. Ref # EDS05. www.nei.nih.gov/photo/search/ref_num.asp?ref=EDS05=&Submit=Go.)

print type is lost (FIGURE 8.19B). Macular degeneration does not affect our peripheral vision.

There is no known cure for macular degeneration. The causes of this disease are unknown, but proposed causes include the following:

- Lack of nutrients to the retina, including antioxidant nutrients like beta-carotene and vitamin A

- Poor circulation in the retina

- Untreated health problems that cause undue pressure to the eye, such as high blood pressure; other health problems such as high cholesterol and diabetes may degenerate the macula over time

- Excessive exposure to UV rays

- Genetic susceptibility

A **cataract** is a damaged portion of the eye's lens, the portion of the eye through which we focus entering light. Cataracts cause cloudiness in the lens that impairs vision (FIGURE 8.20). People with cataracts have a very difficult time seeing in bright light; for instance, they see halos around lights, glare, and scattering of light. Having cataracts also impairs a person's ability to adjust from dark to bright light. It is estimated that over one-half of all people over the age of 65 years in the United States have some cataract development.

Cataracts can be treated with surgery. As with macular degeneration, the causes of cataracts are unknown. However, some possible causes of cataracts include the following:

- Free radical damage caused by exposure to oxygen, UV light, and x-rays

- Inflammation caused by some eye diseases

- Use of certain drugs such as corticosteroids

- Complications of diabetes

Current research findings are showing some promise of reducing the risk for macular degeneration and cataracts through the use of antioxidant supplements. A recent study conducted with individuals who had early signs of macular degeneration found

cataract A damaged portion of the eye's lens, which causes cloudiness that impairs vision.

FIGURE 8.20 Cataracts can impair vision across the entire visual field. (*Source:* National Eye Institute, National Institutes of Health. November 2003. Photos, Images, and Videos. Ref # EDS03. www.nei.nih.gov/photo/search/ref_num.asp?ref=EDS03&Submit=Go.)

that consuming an antioxidant supplement containing vitamins C and E, beta-carotene, and zinc reduced the progression of this disease.[30] Earlier studies have also shown that higher blood levels of antioxidants and consuming more antioxidants in the diet are associated with a lower risk of macular degeneration.[31,32] The effects of antioxidant supplements and cataracts are mixed. Some studies show a reduced rate of cataract development in people taking antioxidant supplements containing vitamins C and E and beta-carotene or having higher blood levels of antioxidants, but other studies show no benefit of antioxidant supplements for cataracts.[33–35]

At this time, it is not possible to reach a conclusion regarding the effectiveness of antioxidant supplements to prevent these two diseases of aging. However, there is enough evidence that consuming a healthful diet that includes fruits, vegetables, and whole grains is associated with improved quality of life as we age.

RECAP: *There is no evidence that antioxidants can reverse or prevent aging or significantly prolong our lives. Macular degeneration and cataracts are two diseases of vision that are associated with aging. Antioxidant nutrients have been found to reduce the risk of these diseases in some studies.*

CHAPTER SUMMARY

- Antioxidants are compounds that protect our cells from oxidative damage.

- Free radicals are produced under many situations, including when our body generates ATP, when our immune system fights infection, and when we are exposed to environmental toxins such as pollution, overexposure to the sun, radiation, and tobacco smoke.

- Free radicals are dangerous because they can damage the lipid portion of our cell membranes, destroying their integrity. Free radicals also damage LDLs, cell proteins, and DNA.

- Antioxidant vitamins and phytochemicals such as beta-carotene donate their electrons or hydrogen atoms to free radicals to neutralize them. Antioxidant minerals are cofactors in antioxidant enzyme systems, which convert free radicals to less damaging substances that our body excretes.

- Vitamin E is an antioxidant that protects the fatty components of cell membranes from oxidation. It also protects LDLs, vitamin A, and our lungs from oxidative damage. Other functions of vitamin E are the development of nerves and muscles, enhancement of the immune function, and improvement of the absorption of vitamin A if intake of vitamin A is low.

- Vitamin C is an antioxidant that is oxidized by free radicals and prevents the damage of cells and tissues. Vitamin C also regenerates vitamin E after it has been oxidized. Other functions of vitamin C include helping the synthesis of collagen, various hormones, neurotransmitters, and DNA; enhancing immune function; and increasing the absorption of iron.

- Beta-carotene is one of about 600 carotenoids identified to date. Beta-carotene is a provitamin, or precursor, to vitamin A, meaning it is an inactive form of vitamin A that is converted to vitamin A in the body.

- Beta-carotene protects the lipid portions of our membranes and the LDL-cholesterol from oxidative damage. Other functions of beta-carotene include enhancing our immune system, protecting our skin from sun damage, and protecting our eyes from oxidative damage. The carotenoids may help reduce our risk for some forms of cancer.

- Vitamin A is a fat-soluble vitamin. The three active forms of vitamin A are retinol, retinal, and retinoic acid. Beta-carotene is converted to vitamin A in the small intestine.

- Vitamin A is extremely important for healthy vision. It ensures our ability to adjust to changes in the brightness of light, and it also helps us maintain color vision. Vitamin A may also act as an antioxidant, as it protects LDL-cholesterol from oxidative damage. Other functions of vitamin A include assistance in cell differentiation, sexual reproduction, and proper bone growth.

- Selenium is a trace mineral that is part of the structure of glutathione peroxidases, a family of antioxidant enzymes. These enzymes break down fatty acids that have become oxidized, which indirectly spares vitamin E from oxidation and helps prevent oxidative damage to our cell membranes and fatty tissues. Other functions of selenium include assisting in the production of thyroid hormone and enhancing immune function.

- Copper, iron, zinc, and manganese are minerals that act as cofactors for antioxidant enzyme systems. Cofactors are necessary to allow enzymes to function properly. Copper, zinc, and manganese are part of the superoxide dismutase complex, while iron is part of catalase. These minerals also play critical roles in energy metabolism and blood formation.

- Cancer cells arise as a result of a genetic mutation in the DNA of normal cells. This mutation may be prompted by a chronic insult such as excessive exposure to tobacco smoke or UV radiation. Uncontrolled replication of the mutated cells results in the formation of a tumor, which can spread to other sites in the body.

- Antioxidants play a role in cancer prevention. Eating foods high in antioxidants results in lower rates of some cancers, but supplementing with antioxidants can increase cancer risk in some situations.

- Antioxidants may help reduce our risk for CVD by scavenging free radicals and preventing oxidative damage to LDL-cholesterol, reducing low-grade inflammation (which in turn prevents the rupture of plaque in blood vessels), and preventing the formation of blood clots.

- Antioxidants may help prevent two age-related diseases of vision, macular degeneration and cataracts. Macular degeneration causes loss of the ability to see details, small print, and facial features. A cataract is a damaged portion of the eye's lens. This damage leads to cloudiness and impairs the ability to adjust from dark to bright light. Antioxidant supplements have been found to reduce the risk for macular degeneration and cataracts in some studies.

TEST YOURSELF ANSWERS

1. **True.** Free radicals are highly unstable atoms that can destabilize neighboring atoms or molecules and harm our cells; however, they are produced as a normal by-product of human physiology.

2. **False.** Overall, the research on vitamin C and colds does not show strong evidence that taking vitamin C supplements reduces our risk of suffering from the common cold.

3. **True.** Carrots are an excellent source of beta-carotene, a precursor for vitamin A, which helps maintain good vision.

4. **True.** According to the American Cancer Society, smoking is the most preventable cause of death in our society. In addition, tobacco use accounts for about 30% of all cancer deaths and is the primary modifiable risk factor for cancer. Among other factors known to significantly influence cancer risk are nutrition, sun exposure, and level of physical activity.

5. **False.** Currently, there is no known dietary cure for cancer. However, eating a diet that is plentiful in fruits and vegetables and exercising regularly may help reduce our risk for some forms of cancer.

FIND THE QUACK

When Bruce and Tina got married, they assumed they'd have no problem becoming parents. But 2 years later, they're still trying. So when Tina comes home from a doctor's appointment and tells Bruce she has some bad news, he doesn't know what to expect. "Bruce," she says, "I know you're not going to like this, but the doctor says you should quit smoking. She says that smoking reduces your sperm count and could be one reason we haven't conceived. And besides, your own doctor has tried to get you to quit because of your high blood pressure." Bruce feels his spirits sink. It's true he has hypertension, and his dad died of a heart attack at age 45. But he's tried to quit smoking before, and the withdrawal symptoms have always been more than he could handle.

That evening he goes onto the Internet and searches under "smoking" and "withdrawal symptoms." He finds a Web site promoting a supplement called "Quit Calm" that sounds promising, offering relief of the anxiety, sleeplessness, and cravings of nicotine withdrawal. Here's what the site states:

- Quit Calm offers an all-natural blend of herbs that work together to decrease cravings, eliminate your anxiety, promote your sleep, heal your respiratory tissues, and purge harmful toxins from your body.

- Ingredients include licorice root, peppermint, ginger, and slippery elm in a proprietary blend that soothes the body's tissues as they recover from nicotine addiction.

- Independent studies have confirmed the beneficial effects of our patented formula.

- Take one capsule three times a day 30 minutes before meals.

- If you order now, a 30-day supply (90 capsules) costs just $29.99. Why wait? Think of all the money you'll be saving by not smoking, and order today!

1. Bruce finds the statement that "Independent studies have confirmed the beneficial effects of our patented formula" reassuring. Do you? Why or why not?

2. Look up licorice root in the "Herbs at a Glance" section of the Web site of the National Center for Complementary and Alternative Medicine (**http://nccam.nih.gov**). Would you recommend that Bruce take a supplement containing licorice root? Why or why not?

3. Comment on the advertisement's final bullet urging consumers to "think of all the money you'll be saving by not smoking, and order today!"

4. Instead of a supplements Web site, where online might Bruce have found reliable help in his quest to quit smoking? What other resources should he consult?

Answers can be found at www.aw-bc.com/thompson.

REVIEW QUESTIONS

1. Which of the following is a characteristic of vitamin E?
   a. It enhances the absorption of iron.
   b. It can be manufactured from beta-carotene.
   c. It is a critical component of the glutathione peroxidase system.
   d. It is destroyed by exposure to high heat.

2. Oxidation is best described as a process in which
   a. a carcinogen causes a mutation in a stem cell's DNA.
   b. an atom loses an electron.
   c. an element loses an atom of oxygen.
   d. a compound loses a molecule of water.

3. Which of the following disorders is linked with the production of free radicals?
   a. cardiovascular disease
   b. carotenosis
   c. ulcers
   d. malaria

4. Which of the following are known carcinogens?
   a. phytochemicals
   b. antioxidants
   c. carotenoids
   d. nitrates

5. Taking daily doses of three to four times the RDA of which of the following nutrients may cause death?
   a. vitamin A
   b. vitamin C
   c. vitamin E
   d. selenium

6. True or false? Tocopherol is the biologically active form of vitamin E in our bodies.

7. True or false? Free radical formation can occur as a result of normal cellular metabolism.

8. True or false? Vitamin C helps regenerate vitamin A.

9. True or false? Reliable food sources of selenium include beef liver, pork, and seafood.

10. True or false? Pregnant women are advised to consume plentiful quantities of beef liver.

11. Explain how free radicals damage cell membranes and lead to cell death.

12. Describe the process by which cancer occurs, beginning with initiation and ending with metastasis of the cancer to widespread body tissues.

13. Explain how vitamin E reduces our risk for cardiovascular disease.

14. Discuss the contribution of trace minerals such as selenium to the prevention of oxidation.

15. Your mother has a heart condition that requires her to take the prescription drug Coumadin, an anticoagulant. While chatting with you over lunch one day, she mentions that she has started taking an antioxidant supplement that is supposed to "boost cardiovascular health." You ask to see the supplement and note that it contains 500 mg vitamin E as alpha-tocopherol, 500 mg of vitamin C, and 100 μg of selenium. Should you be concerned? Why or why not?

WEB LINKS

www.who.int
World Health Organization (WHO)

Search for "vitamin A deficiency" to find out more about vitamin A deficiency around the world.

www.americanheart.org
American Heart Association

Discover the best way to lower your risk for cardiovascular disease.

www.cancer.org
The American Cancer Society

Get ACS recommendations for smoking cessation, nutrition, sun exposure, and physical activity for cancer prevention.

www.cancer.gov
The National Cancer Institute

Learn more about the nutritional factors that can influence your risk for cancer.

www.nei.nih.gov
National Eye Institute

Visit this site to find out more about how macular degeneration and cataracts can impair vision.

www.cfsan.fda.gov/~dms/supplmnt.html
U.S. Food and Drug Administration (FDA)

This site provides information on how to make informed decisions and evaluate information related to dietary supplements.

www.nal.usda.gov/fnic
The Food and Nutrition Information Center (FNIC)

Click on the Dietary Supplements button to obtain information on vitamin and mineral supplements, including consumer reports and industry regulations.

http://dietary-supplements.info.nih.gov
Office of Dietary Supplements

Go to this site to obtain current research results and reliable information about dietary supplements.

REFERENCES

1. Ford, E. S., and A. Sowell. 1999. Serum alpha-tocopherol status in the United States population: findings from the Third National Health and Nutrition Examination Survey. *Am. J. Epidemiol.* 150(3):290–300.

2. Hemila, H. 1997. Vitamin C intake and susceptibility to the common cold. *Br. J. Nutr.* 77:59–72.

3. Burri, B. J. 1997. Beta-carotene and human health: a review of current research. *Nutr. Res.* 17:547–580.

4. U.S. Department of Agriculture (USDA), Agricultural Research Service. 1998. USDA–NCC Carotenoid Database for U.S. Foods. Nutrient Data Laboratory Home Page. www.ars.usda.gov/ba/bhnrc/ndl. (Accessed July 2007.)

5. Albanes, D., O. P. Heinonen, J. K. Huttunen, P. R. Taylor, J. Virtamo, B. K. Edwards, J. Haapakoski, M. Rautalahti, A. M. Hartman, J. Palmgren, and P. Greenwald. 1995. Effects of alpha-tocopherol and beta-carotene supplements on cancer incidence in the Alpha-Tocopherol Beta-Carotene Cancer Prevention Study. *Am. J. Clin. Nutr.* 62(suppl.):1427S–1430S.

6. Omenn, G. S., G. E. Goodman, M. D. Thornquist, J. Balmes, M. R. Cullen, A. Glass, J. P. Keogh, F. L. Meyskens, B. Valanis, J. H. Williams, S. Barnhart, and S. Hammar. 1996. Effects of a combination of beta carotene and vitamin A on lung cancer and cardiovascular disease. *New Engl. J. Med.* 334:1150–1155.

7. Larsson, S., L. Bergkvist, I. Näslund, J. Rutegård, and A. Wolk. 2007. Vitamin A, retinol, and carotenoids and the risk of gastric cancer: a prospective cohort study. *Am. J. Clin. Nutr.* 85:497–503.

8. Livrea, M. A., L. Tesoriere, A. Bongiorno, A. M. Pintaudi, M. Ciaccio, and A. Riccio. 1995. Contribution of vitamin A to the oxidation resistance of human low density lipoproteins. *Free Radic. Biol. Med.* 18:401–409.

9. Gutteridge, J. M. C., and B. Halliwell. 1994. *Antioxidants in Nutrition, Health, and Disease.* Oxford, UK: Oxford University Press.

10. World Health Organization (WHO). 2002. Vitamin A. www.who.int/vaccines/en/vitaminamain.shtml. (Accessed July 2007.)

11. American Cancer Society. 2007. Cancer Atlas. www.cancer.org /downloads/AA/CancerAtlas02.pdf. (Accessed July 2007.)

12. Centers for Disease Control and Prevention. 2006. Cigarette smoking-related mortality fact sheet. www.cdc.gov/tobacco/ data_statistics/Factsheets/cig_smoking_mort.htm. (Accessed July 2007.)

13. U.S. Department of Health and Human Services. 2006. *The Health Consequences of Involuntary Exposure to Tobacco Smoke: A Report of the Surgeon General.* U.S. Department of Health and Human Services, Centers for Disease Control and Prevention, National Center for Chronic Disease Prevention and Health Promotion, Office on Smoking and Health.

14. American Cancer Society. 2007. ACS guide to quitting smoking. www.cancer.org/docroot/PED/content/PED_10_13X_Guide_for_ Quitting_Smoking.asp?sitearea=PED.(Accessed July 2007.)

15. Pfahlberg, A., K. F. Kolmel, and O. Gefeller. 2002. Adult vs. childhood susceptibility to melanoma. Is there a difference? *Arch. Dermatol.* 138:1234–1235.

16. Heinonen, O. P., D. Albanes, J. Virtamo, P. R. Taylor, J. K. Huttunen, A. M. Hartman, J. Haapakoski, N. Malila, M. Rautalahti, S. Ripatti, H. Maepaa, and International Agency for Research on Cancer (IARC). 2007. The association of use of sunbeds with cutaneous malignant melanoma and other skin cancers: a systematic review. *Intl. J. Cancer* 120:1116–1122.

17. Thune, I., and A. S. Furberg. 2001. Physical activity and cancer risk: dose-response and cancer, all sites and site-specific. *Med. Sci. Sports Exerc.* 33 (suppl.): S530–S550.

18. Greenwald, P., C. K. Clifford, and J. A. Milner. 2001. Diet and cancer prevention. *Eur. J. Cancer* 37:948–965.

19. Heinonen, O. P., et al. 1998. Prostate cancer and supplementation with α-tocopherol and β-carotene: incidence and mortality in a controlled trial. *J. Natl. Cancer Inst.* 90:440-446.

20. Clark, L. C., B. Dalkin, A. Krongrad, G. F. Combs Jr., B. W. Turnbull, E. H. Slate, R. Witherington, J. H. Herlong, E. Janosko, D. Carpenter, C. Borosso, S. Falk, and J. Rounder. 1998. Decreased incidence of prostate cancer with selenium supplementation: results of a double-blind cancer prevention trial. *Br. J. Urol.* 81:730–734.

21. Blot, W. J., J.-Y. Li, P. R. Taylor, W. Guo, S. M. Dawsey, and B. Li. 1995. The Linxian trials: mortality rates by vitamin-mineral intervention group. *Am. J. Clin. Nutr.* 62(suppl.):1424S–1426S.

22. National Center for Chronic Disease Prevention and Health Promotion (NCCDPHP). 2002. Chronic disease prevention. Chronic disease overview. www.cdc.gov/nccdphp/overview.htm.

23. de Ferranti, S., and N. Rifai. 2002. C-reactive protein and cardiovascular disease: a review of risk prediction and interventions. *Clinica Chimica Acta* 317:1–15.

24. Joshipura, K. J., F. B. Hu, J. E. Manson, M. J. Stampfer, E. B. Rimm, F. E. Speizer, G. Colditz, A. Ascherio, B. Rosner, D. Spiegelman, and W. C. Willett. 2001. The effect of fruit and vegetable intake on risk for coronary heart disease. *Ann. Intern. Med.* 134:1106–1114.

25. Liu, S., I.-M. Lee, U. Ajani, S. R. Cole, J. E. Buring, and J. E. Manson. 2001. Intake of vegetables rich in carotenoids and risk of coronary heart disease in men: the Physicians' Health Study. *Intl. J. Epidemiol.* 30:130–135.

26. Alpha-Tocopherol, Beta-Carotene Cancer Prevention Study Group (The ATBC Study Group). 1994. The effect of vitamin E and beta carotene on the incidence of lung cancer and other cancers in male smokers. *N. Engl. J. Med.* 330:1029–1035.

27. Heart Outcomes Prevention Evaluation Study Investigators (The HOPE Investigators). 2000. Vitamin E supplementation and cardiovascular events in high-risk patients. *N. Engl. J. Med.* 342:154–160.

28. Lee, I-M., N. Cook, M. Gaziano, D. Gordon, P. Ridker, J. Manson, C. Hennekens, and J. Buring. 2005. Vitamin E in the primary prevention of cardiovascular disease and cancer: The Women's Health Study: a randomized controlled trial. *J. Am. Med. Assoc.* 294:56–65.

29. Geleijnse, J. M., L. J. Launer, D. A. M. van der Kuip, A. Hofman, and J. C. M. Witteman. 2002. Inverse association of tea and flavonoid intakes with incident myocardial infarction: the Rotterdam Study. *Am. J. Clin. Nutr.* 75:880–886.

30. Age-Related Eye Disease Study Research Group. 2001. A randomized, placebo-controlled, clinical trial of high-dose supplementation with vitamins C and E, beta-carotene, and zinc for age-related macular degeneration and vision loss: AREDS Report No. 8. *Arch. Ophthalmol.* 119:1417–1436.

31. Delcourt, C., J. P. Cristol, F. Tessier, C. L. Léger, B. Descomps, and L. Papoz. 1999. Age-related macular degeneration and antioxidant status in the POLA study. POLA Study Group. Pathologies Oculaires Liées B l'Age. *Arch. Ophthalmol.* 117:1384–1390.

32. West, S., S. Vitale, J. Hallfrisch, B. Munoz, D. Muller, S. Bressler, and N. M. Bressler. 1994. Are antioxidants or supplements protective for age-related macular degeneration? *Arch. Ophthalmol.* 112:222–227.

33. Chylack, L. T. Jr., N. P. Brown, A. Bron, M. Hurst, W. Kopcke, U. Thien, and W. Schalch. 2002. The Roche European American Cataract Trial (REACT): a randomized clinical trial to investigate the efficacy of an oral antioxidant micronutrient mixture to slow progression of age-related cataract. *Ophthalmic Epidemiol.* 9:49–80.

34. Gale, C. R., N. F. Hall, D. I. Phillips, and C. N. Martyn. 2001. Plasma antioxidant vitamins and carotenoids and age-related cataract. *Ophthalmology* 108:1992–1998.

35. Age-Related Eye Disease Study Research Group. 2001. A randomized, placebo-controlled, clinical trial of high-dose supplementation with vitamins C and E and beta-carotene for age-related cataract and vision loss: AREDS Report No. 9. *Arch. Ophthalmol.* 119:1439–1452.

36. Nutrition Business Journal. 2006. *NBJ's Supplement Business Report 2006.* ©Penton Media, Inc.

37. Blendon, R. J., C. M. DesRoches, J. M. Benson, M. Brodie, and D. E. Altman. 2001. Americans' views on the use and regulation of dietary supplements. *Arch. Intern. Med.* 26:805–810.

38. U.S. Food and Drug Administration (FDA). Center for Food Safety and Applied Nutrition. 2001. Overview of dietary supplements. www.cfsan.fda.gov/~dms/ds-oview.html. (Accessed July 2007.)

39. U.S. Food and Drug Administration (FDA). 1998. An FDA guide to dietary supplements. *FDA Consumer Magazine.* September/October. www.fda.gov/fdac/features/1998/598_guid. html. (Accessed July 2007.)

40. Dancho, C., and M. M. Manore. 2001. Dietary supplement information on the World Wide Web. Sorting fact from fiction. *ACSM's Health and Fitness J.* 5:7–12.

41. American Dietetic Association. 2001. Position of the American Dietetic Association: food fortification and dietary supplements. *J. Am. Diet. Assoc.* 101:115–125.

Vitamin and Mineral Supplementation: Necessity or Waste?

marcus has type 2 diabetes and high blood cholesterol and is worried about his health. He attended a nutrition seminar in which the health benefits of various vitamin and mineral supplements were touted. After attending this seminar, Marcus was convinced that he needed to take a series of supplements that contain more than 200% of the RDA for many vitamins and minerals. After a few months of taking these supplements on a daily basis, Marcus started to experience headaches, nausea, diarrhea, and tingling in his hands and feet. Although Marcus was not an expert in nutrition, he suspected that he might be experiencing side effects related to nutrient toxicity. He decided to talk to his doctor about the supplements he was taking to determine whether they could be causing his symptoms.

Marcus' story is not unique. The use of dietary supplements in the United States has skyrocketed in recent years. One industry source cites annual sales of supplements in the United States at $21.3 billion.[36] A recent review of national opinion surveys found that a significant number of Americans regularly take dietary supplements, but they do not report the use of these products to their physicians because they feel their physicians have little knowledge of these products and may harbor a bias toward their use.[37] Interestingly, many supplement users stated that they would continue to use these products even if scientific studies found them to be ineffective!

Why do so many people take dietary supplements? Many people believe they cannot consume adequate nutrients in their diet, and they take a supplement as extra nutritional insurance. Others have been advised by their healthcare provider to take a supplement due to a given health condition. There are people, like Marcus, who believe that certain supplements can be used to treat illness or disease. There are also people who believe supplements are necessary to enhance their physical looks or athletic performance.

Although many people believe taking dietary supplements benefits their health, this is not always the case. Who should be taking supplements? This question is not simple. Before deciding whether you may benefit from taking dietary supplements, a review of the definition of dietary supplements and their regulation is necessary to gain a more complete understanding of how these products are marketed and regulated for safety.

Supplements can be powders, pills, or liquids.

Dietary Supplements Include Vitamins, Minerals, and Other Products

According to the U.S. Food and Drug Administration (FDA), a dietary supplement is "a product taken by mouth that contains a 'dietary ingredient' intended to supplement the diet."[38] Ingredients in supplements may include vitamins, minerals, herbs or other botanicals, amino acids, enzymes, tissues from animal organs or glands, or a concentrate, metabolite, constituent, or extract. Supplements come in many forms, including pills, capsules, liquids, and powders.

How Are Dietary Supplements Regulated?

As presented in the Dietary Supplement Health and Education Act (DSHEA) of 1994, dietary supplements are categorized within the general group of foods, not drugs. This means that the regulation of supplements is much less rigorous than the regulation of drugs. Currently, the FDA is reconsidering how it regulates food and supplements that are marketed with health claims, but no changes have been finalized at this time. As an informed consumer, you should know that:

Vita-Wow

1 Statement of identity

Multivitamin/multimineral supplement with Ginseng*

100 Tablets

4 Net quantity of contents

* "Helps promote optimal energy."
This statement has not been evaluated by the Food and Drug Administration. This product is not intended to diagnose, treat, cure, or prevent any disease.

Directions: Adults: One tablet daily, with food.

5 Directions

2 Supplement facts panel

Supplement Facts
Serving Size: One tablet

	Amount Per serving	% Daily Value
Vitamin A	2500 IU	50%
Vitamin C	60 mg	100%
Vitamin D	400 IU	100%
Vitamin E	30 IU	100%
Thiamin	1.5 mg	100%
Riboflavin	1.7 mg	100%
Niacin	10 mg	50%
Vitamin B_6	2 mg	100%
Magnesium	50 mg	12%
Iron	18 mg	100%
Zinc	15 mg	100%
American Ginseng Standardized Extract	200 mg	++

++No Daily Value established for Ginseng.

Other ingredients: Cellulose, Dextrin, Gelatin, Starch, Dextrose, FD&C Yellow #6, FD&C Blue #2

Made in U.S.A.
Distributed by:
Supervitamin Corporation
P.O. Box XYZ
Energized, CA 00000

3 Name and place of business, or manufacturer, packer, or distributor. This is the address to write for more information

6 Other ingredients in descending order of predominance and by common name of proprietary blend

A multivitamin–mineral supplement label highlighting the dietary supplement guidelines.

- Supplements do not need approval from the FDA before they are marketed.
- The company that manufactures the supplements is responsible for determining that the supplement is safe; the FDA does not test any supplement for safety prior to marketing.
- Supplement companies do not have to provide the FDA with any evidence that its supplements are safe unless the company is marketing a new dietary ingredient that was not sold in the United States prior to 1994.
- There are at present no federal guidelines on practices to ensure the purity, quality, safety, and composition of dietary supplements.
- There are no rules to limit the serving size or amount of a nutrient in any dietary supplement.
- Once a supplement is marketed, the FDA must prove it unsafe before the product will be removed from the market.

Despite these limitations in supplement regulations, supplement manufacturers are required to follow dietary supplement labeling guidelines. The figure in this box shows a label from a multivitamin and mineral supplement. As you can see, there are specific requirements for the information that must be included on the supplement label. Federal advertising regulations also require that any advertising on the label must be truthful and not misleading and that advertisers must have adequate substantiation of all product claims before disseminating the advertisement. Any products not meeting these labeling and advertising guidelines can be removed from the market.

How Can We Protect Ourselves from Fraudulent or Dangerous Supplements?

Although many of the supplement products sold today are safe, there are many products that are not. In addition, some companies are less than forthright about the true content of ingredients in their supplements. How can we avoid purchasing fraudulent or dangerous supplements? The FDA suggests that consumers can do the following to protect themselves from fraudulent or dangerous supplements:[39]

1. Look for the U.S.P. (U.S. Pharmacopoeia) symbol or notation on the label. This symbol indicates that the manufacturer followed the standards established by the U.S.P. for drugs for features such as purity, strength, quality, packaging, labeling, and acceptable length of storage.

2. Consider buying recognized brands of supplements. Although not guaranteed, products made by nationally recognized companies more likely have well-established manufacturing standards.

3. Do not assume that the word "natural" on the label means that the product is safe. Arsenic, lead, and mercury are all natural substances that can kill you if consumed in large enough quantities.

4. Do not hesitate to question a company about how it makes its products. Reputable companies have nothing to hide and are more than happy to inform their customers about the safety and quality of their products.

Always research supplements and supplement manufacturers before purchasing.

Many supplements are also sold today over the Internet. Dancho and Manore suggest six criteria that can be used to evaluate dietary supplement Web sites.[40] Keep these criteria in mind each time you consider buying a dietary supplement over the Web:

1. What is the purpose of the site? Is the Web site trying to sell a product or educate the consumer? Keep in mind that the primary purpose of supplement companies is to make money. Look for sites that provide educational information about a specific nutrient or product and don't just focus on selling the products.

2. Does the site contain accurate information? Accuracy of the information on the Web site is the most difficult thing for a consumer to determine. Testimonials (claims by athletes or other famous people) are *not* reliable and accurate; claims supported by scientific research are most desirable. If what the company claims about their product sounds too good to be true, it probably is.

3. Does the site contain reputable references? References should be from articles published in peer-reviewed scientific journals. The reference should be complete and contain author names, title of article, journal title, date, volume, and page numbers. This information allows the consumer to check original research for the validity of a company's claims about their product. Be cautious of sites that refer to claims that are proven by research studies but fail to provide a complete reference.

4. Who owns or sponsors the site? Full disclosure regarding sponsorship and possible sources of bias or conflict of interest should be included in the site's information.

5. Who wrote the information? Web sites should clearly identify the author of the article and include the credentials of the author. Recognized experts include individuals with relevant health-related credentials such as R.D., Ph.D., M.D., or M.S. Keep in mind that this person is responsible for the information posted in the article but may not be the creator of the Web site.

6. Is the information current and updated regularly? As information about supplements changes regularly, Web sites should be updated regularly, and the date should be clearly posted. All Web sites should also include contact information to allow consumers to ask questions about the information posted.

For more information on how to make informed decisions and evaluate information related to dietary supplements, go to the Dietary Supplements Web site of the U.S. FDA Center for Food Safety and Applied Nutrition at **www.cfsan.fda.gov/~dms/supplmnt.html.** Other Web sites that contain reliable information about dietary supplements include The National Institutes of Health (NIH) Office of Dietary Supplements at **http://dietary-supplements.info.nih.gov**, and The Food and Nutrition Information Council (FNIC) at **www.nal.usda.gov/fnic/**.

Dietary Supplements Can Be Both Helpful and Harmful

As mentioned earlier in this debate, it is not always easy to determine who should take dietary supplements. Our nutritional needs change throughout our life span, and some of us may need to take supplements at certain times for various conditions. For instance, some athletes can benefit from consuming foods formulated to provide carbohydrate and other nutrients necessary to support intense exercise. Women at risk for osteoporosis may benefit from taking calcium and vitamin D supplements. Dietary supplements include hundreds of thousands of

products sold for many purposes, and it is impossible to discuss here all of the various situations in which these supplements may be needed. To simplify this discussion, let's focus on describing who may or may not benefit from taking vitamin and mineral supplements.

Who Might Benefit from Taking Vitamin and Mineral Supplements?

Contrary to what some people believe, the U.S. food supply is not void of nutrients, and all people do not need to supplement all of the time. In fact, we now know that foods contain a diverse combination of compounds that are critical to our health, and vitamin and mineral supplements do not contain the same amount or variety of substances found in foods. Thus, dietary supplements are not substitutes for whole foods.

However, there are certain individuals who may benefit from taking vitamin and mineral supplements. Table 8.2

TABLE 8.2   Individuals Who May Benefit from Dietary Supplementation

Example of Individual	Specific Supplements That May Help
Newborns	Routinely given a single dose of vitamin K at birth
Infants	Depends on condition; may need iron or other nutrients
Children not drinking fluoridated water	Fluoride supplements
Children on strict vegetarian diets	Vitamin B_{12}, iron, zinc, vitamin D (if not exposed to sunlight)
Children with poor eating habits or overweight children on an energy-restricted diet	Multivitamin-mineral supplement that does not exceed the RDA for the nutrients it contains
Pregnant teenagers	Iron and folic acid; other nutrients may be necessary if diet is very poor
Women who may become pregnant	Multivitamin or multivitamin-mineral supplement that contains 0.4 mg of folic acid
Pregnant or lactating women	Multivitamin-mineral supplement that contains iron, folic acid, zinc, copper, calcium, vitamin B_6, vitamin C, vitamin D
People on prolonged weight reduction diets	Multivitamin-mineral supplement
People recovering from serious illness or surgery	Multivitamin-mineral supplement
People with HIV/AIDS or other wasting diseases; people addicted to drugs or alcohol	Multivitamin-mineral supplement or single-nutrient supplements
Women	Calcium supplements: women need to consume 1000 to 1300 mg of calcium per day through food, and supplements may also be necessary
People eating a vegan diet	Vitamin B_{12}, riboflavin, calcium, vitamin D, iron, and zinc
People who have had portions of the intestinal tract removed; people who have a malabsorptive disease	Depends upon the exact condition; may include various fat-soluble and/or water-soluble vitamins and other nutrients
People with lactose intolerance	Calcium supplements
Elderly people	Multivitamin-mineral supplement, vitamin B_{12}

lists various individuals who may benefit from supplementation. It is important to remember that analyzing your total diet is an important first step in determining whether you might need to take a vitamin and mineral supplement. It is always a good idea to check with your healthcare provider or a registered dietitian (RD) before taking any supplements, as supplements can interfere with some prescription and over-the-counter medications.

When Can Taking a Vitamin and Mineral Supplement Be Harmful?

You can see from Table 8.2 that there are many people who can benefit from taking vitamin and mineral supplements in certain situations. There are also many people who do not need to take supplements but do so anyway. Instances in which taking vitamin and mineral supplements is unnecessary or harmful include:

1. Providing fluoride supplements to children who already drink fluoridated water.

2. Taking supplements in the belief that they will cure a disease such as cancer, diabetes, or heart disease.

3. Taking supplements with certain medications. For instance, people who take the blood-thinning drug Coumadin should not take vitamin E supplements, as this can cause excessive bleeding. People who take aspirin daily should check with their physician before taking vitamin E supplements, as aspirin also thins the blood.

4. Taking nonprescribed supplements if you have liver or kidney diseases. A physician may prescribe vitamin and mineral supplements for their patients because many nutrients are lost during treatment for these diseases. However, these individuals cannot properly metabolize certain supplements and should not take any that are not prescribed by their physician because of a high risk for toxicity.

5. Taking beta-carotene supplements if you are a smoker. As already mentioned, there is evidence that beta-carotene supplementation increases the risk of lung and other cancers in smokers.

6. Taking vitamins and minerals in an attempt to improve physical appearance or athletic performance. There is no evidence that vitamin and mineral supplements enhance appearance or athletic performance in healthy adults who consume a varied diet with adequate energy.

7. Taking supplements to increase your energy level. Vitamin and mineral supplements do not provide energy, because they do not contain fat, carbohydrate, or protein (sources of calories). Although many vitamins and minerals are necessary for us to produce energy, taking dietary supplements in place of eating food will not provide us with the energy necessary to live a healthy and productive life.

8. Taking single-nutrient supplements, unless a qualified healthcare practitioner prescribes a single-nutrient supplement for a diagnosed medical condition (for example, prescribing iron supplements for someone with anemia). These products contain very high amounts of the given nutrient, and taking these types of products can quickly lead to toxicity.

As advised by the American Dietetic Association, the ideal nutritional strategy for optimizing health is to eat a healthful diet that contains a variety of foods.[41] This way, you will not need to take vitamin and mineral supplements. However, some people may still need to take supplements despite their best efforts. If you do supplement your diet, select a supplement that contains no more than 100% of the recommended levels for the nutrients it contains. Avoid taking single-nutrient supplements unless advised to do so by your healthcare practitioner. Finally, avoid taking supplements that contain substances that are known to cause illness or injuries. Some of these substances are listed in Table 8.3.

TABLE 8.3   Ingredients Found in Supplements That Are Associated with Illnesses and Injuries

Ingredient	Potential Risks
Herbal Ingredients:	
Chaparral	Liver disease
Comfrey	Obstruction of blood flow to liver, possible death
Dieter's/slimming teas	Nausea, diarrhea, vomiting, stomach cramps, constipation, fainting, possible death
Ephedra (also known as ma huang, Chinese ephedra, and epitonin)	High blood pressure, irregular heartbeat, nerve damage, insomnia, tremors, headaches, seizures, heart attack, stroke, possible death
Germander	Liver disease, possible death
Lobelia	Breathing problems, excessive sweating, rapid heartbeat, low blood pressure, coma, possible death
Magnolia-Stephania preparation	Kidney disease, can lead to permanent kidney failure
Willow bark	Reyes syndrome (a potentially fatal disease that may occur when children take aspirin), allergic reaction in adults
Wormwood	Numbness of legs and arms, loss of intellectual processing, delirium, paralysis
Vitamins and Essential Minerals:	
Vitamin A (when taking 25,000 IU or more per day)	Birth defects, bone abnormalities, severe liver disease
Vitamin B_6 (when taking more than 100 mg/day)	Loss of balance, injuries to nerves that alter our touch sensation
Niacin (when taking slow-release doses of 500 mg or more per day, or when taking immediate-release doses of 750 mg or more per day)	Stomach pain, nausea, vomiting, bloating, cramping, diarrhea, liver disease, damage to the muscles, eye, and heart
Selenium (when taking 800 to 1,000 µg/day)	Tissue damage
Other Ingredients:	
Germanium (a nonessential mineral)	Kidney damage, possible death
L-tryptophan (an amino acid)	Eosinophilia-myalgia syndrome (a potentially fatal blood disorder that causes high fever, joint and muscle pain, swelling of legs and arms, skin rash, and weakness)

Source: U.S. Food and Drug Administration. 1998. Supplements associated with illnesses and injuries. *FDA Consumer Magazine.* September/October. www.fda.gov/fdac/features/1998/dietchrt.html. (Accessed July 2007.)

Phytochemicals and Functional Foods

WANT TO FIND OUT . . .

- what's behind all the fuss about phytochemicals? pp. 351–353

- why you can't put fruits and veggies in a pill? p. 353

- whether yogurt can boost your immune system? pp. 355–356

- whether "calorie-burning" drinks could help you lose weight? pp. 357–358

READ ON.

imagine a patient seeing his physician for a minor problem: "sluggish" bowel movements. The physician asks him several questions and performs an exam. At the close of the visit, he hands the patient a prescription: *One apple, two servings of dark-green leafy vegetables, 1 cup of yogurt, and 2 cups of green tea daily.* The patient accepts the prescription gratefully, assuring his physician as he says goodbye, "I'll stop at the market on my way home!"

Sound unreal? As researchers provide more and more evidence on the link between nutrition and health, it's just possible that scenarios like this might become familiar. Here, we explore *In Depth* some of the reasons why the chemicals naturally occurring in plant foods, called *phytochemicals*, are thought to promote our health. We'll also examine the claims made for so-called *functional foods* like special yogurts, eggs, chocolate, and beverages that their manufacturers say have health benefits beyond their basic nutritional function. Who knows? When you finish reading, you might find yourself writing up your own health-promoting grocery list!

What Are Phytochemicals?

Phyto- means plant, so **phytochemicals** are literally plant chemicals. These naturally occurring compounds are believed to protect plants from a variety of injurious agents, including insects, microbes, the oxygen they produce, and the UV light they capture and transform into the nutrients we need. Although more than 5,000 different phytochemicals have already been identified, researchers believe there are thousands more.[1] Any one food can contain hundreds. FIGURE 1 shows some groups of only a few of the most common.

Phytochemicals are not considered nutrients, that is, substances necessary for sustaining life. Even for carotenoids, a well-studied class of phytochemicals, the Food and Nutrition Board of the Institute of Medicine concluded in 2000 that there was not enough evidence to establish a daily recommended intake.[2] So whereas a total lack of vitamin C or iron is incompatible with life, a total lack of lutein or allylic sulfur compounds is not known to be fatal. On the other hand, eating an abundance of phytochemical-rich foods has been shown to reduce the risk of cardiovascular disease, cancer, diabetes, Alzheimer's disease, cataracts, and age-related functional decline.[1,3]

The evidence supporting this observation of a reduced disease risk stems mainly from large epidemiologic studies in which people report their usual food intake to researchers who then look for relationships between specific dietary patterns and common diseases. These large studies often find that the reduced disease risk from high intakes of plant foods cannot be attributed solely to differences in intake of macronutrients and micronutrients. This suggests that other compounds in plant

Apricots contain carotenoids, a type of phytochemical.

foods may be reducing the risk for disease.

As we noted in Chapter 1, epidemiologic studies can only reveal *associations* between general patterns of food intake and health conditions; they cannot prove that a food or dietary pattern directly *causes* a health outcome. To better understand how phytochemicals influence health and disease, researchers have turned to biochemical, cellular, and animal studies.

How Do Phytochemicals Reduce Our Risk of Disease?

For decades, laboratory experiments have shown that, at least in the test tube, many phytochemicals have antioxidant properties. Recall from Chapter 7 that antioxidants can neutralize free radicals, those unstable, highly reactive compounds that damage proteins, lipids, and DNA in our cells. Free radicals are an unavoidable by-product of normal metabolism, but are also produced in response to x-rays, air pollution, industrial chemicals, tobacco smoke, infections, and even intense exercise. The health effects of this damage, also known as oxidative damage, typically don't arise until later in life. Many **diseases of aging**, such as cardiovascular disease, cancer, cataracts, arthritis, and certain neurological disorders, have been linked to oxidative damage that accumulates over years. It's no surprise, therefore, that antioxidant-rich foods would reduce the risk of these conditions.

Unfortunately, biology is not fully explained by a few simple chemical reactions. In fact, the latest research evidence on phytochemicals suggests that their health-promoting properties are largely unrelated to the antioxidant activity measured in the test tube.[4,5] This is in part because phytochemicals can be modified during

phytochemicals Compounds found in plants that are believed to have health-promoting effects in humans.

diseases of aging Conditions that typically occur later in life as a result of lifelong accumulated risk, such as exposure to high-fat diets, lack of physical activity, and excess sun exposure.

Phytochemical	Health Claims	Food Source	
Carotenoids: alpha-carotene, beta-carotene, lutein, lycopene, zeaxanthin, etc.	Diets with foods rich in these phytochemicals may reduce the risk of cardiovascular disease, certain cancers (e.g., prostate), and age-related eye diseases (cataracts, macular degeneration).	Red, orange, and deep-green vegetables and fruits such as carrots, cantaloupe, sweet potatoes, apricots, kale, spinach, pumpkin, and tomatoes	
Flavonoids:[1] flavones, flavonols (e.g., quercetin), catechins (e.g., epigallocatechin gallate or EGCG), anthocyanidins, isoflavonoids, etc.	Diets with foods rich in these phytochemicals are associated with lower risk of cardiovascular disease and cancer, possibly because of reduced inflammation, blood clotting, and blood pressure, and increased detoxification of carcinogens or reduction in replication of cancerous cells.	Berries, black and green tea, chocolate, purple grapes and juice, citrus fruits, olives, soybeans and soy products (soy milk, tofu, soy flour, textured vegetable protein), flaxseed, whole wheat	
Phenolic acids:[1] ellagic acid, ferulic acid, caffeic acid, curcumin, etc.	Similar benefits as flavonoids.	Coffee beans, fruits (apples, pears, berries, grapes, oranges, prunes, strawberries), potatoes, mustard, oats, soy	
Phytoestrogens:[2] genistein, diadzein, lignans	Foods rich in these phytochemicals may provide benefits to bones and reduce the risk of cardiovascular disease and cancers of reproductive tissues (e.g., breast, prostate).	Soybeans and soy products (soy milk, tofu, soy flour, textured vegetable protein), flaxseed, whole grains	
Organosulfur compounds: allylic sulfur compounds, indoles, isothiocyanates, etc.	Foods rich in these phytochemicals may protect against a wide variety of cancers.	Garlic, leeks, onions, chives, cruciferous vegetables (broccoli, cabbage, cauliflower), horseradish, mustard greens	

[1] Flavonoids, phenolic acids, and stilbenes are three groups of phytochemicals called phenolics. Resveratrol, the phytochemical discussed in the Highlight "Will a PB&J Keep the Doctor Away?" is a stilbene. Flavonoids and phenolic acids are the most abundant phenolics in our diet.
[2] Phytoestrogens include phytochemicals that have mild or anti-estrogenic action in our body. They are grouped together based on this similarity in biologic function, but they also can be classified into other phytochemical groups, such as isoflavanoids.

FIGURE 1   Health claims and food sources of phytochemicals.

digestion and also after absorption so that cells are exposed to **metabolites** that are structurally different from the phytochemicals found in foods.[5] Clearly, the test tube cannot explain what is happening inside the body.

Fortunately, researchers have also employed cellular and animal studies, which have revealed that phytochemicals have many health-promoting functions independent of their antioxidant properties. These functions of phytochemicals include the following:

- Reduce inflammation,[6] which is linked to the development of Alzheimer's disease and cardiovascular disease and is symptomatic of arthritis.

- Enhance the activity of certain enzymes throughout the body that function to detoxify carcinogens.[7]

- Protect against cancer by slowing tumor cell growth and instructing cancer cells to die.[7]

- Protect against infections indirectly by enhancing our immune function and directly by acting as antibacterial and antiviral agents.[7]

- Reduce the risk of cardiovascular disease by lowering blood lipids, blood pressure, and blood clotting.[1]

Which of these roles is most important in reducing disease risk is not yet known. Many other issues are also not well understood yet, such as which phytochemicals are needed and how much.

Is There an RDA for Phytochemicals?

Most well-controlled studies in cells, animals, or people typically research only one phytochemical or food. When the results are published, we read about them in the popular press: one day we're advised to eat tomatoes, another day blueberries, then pomegranates. But these findings are only the tip of the iceberg that must be explored before we can make precise recommendations about phytochemicals and health. As scientists begin to "map" more and more phytochemical "icebergs," they're making the following discoveries:

- Phytochemicals interact with each other in the body to produce a synergistic effect that is greater than the sum of the effects of individual phytochemicals.[1] This may explain why whole tomatoes were found to reduce prostate cancer in rats, whereas a phytochemical called lycopene that is present in tomatoes, when given alone, did not.[8]

- Phytochemicals interact with macronutrients and vitamins and minerals. For example, the anticancer effect of garlic is enhanced by vitamin A, selenium, and certain fats.[9]

- Phytochemicals can act in different ways under different circumstances in the body. For example, phytoestrogens in soy appear to reduce the incidence of breast cancer in healthy women, but they may enhance cancer development when the disease is already present.[10]

For these reasons, no RDA for phytochemicals can safely be established for any life stage group.

In addition, although epidemiological studies suggest that the more phytochemicals we consume, the better our health, this benefit appears to be limited to phytochemicals found in foods. That is, phytochemicals appear to be protective in the low doses commonly provided by foods, but may have very different effects as supplements. This may be due to their mode of action: scientists now believe that, instead of *protecting* our cells, phytochemicals might benefit our health by *stressing* our cells, causing them to rev up their internal defense systems.[4] Cells are very well equipped to deal with minor stresses, but not with excessive stress, which may explain why clinical trials with phytochemical supplements rarely show the same benefits as high intakes of plant foods.[4,11]

So are phytochemical supplements harmful? Generally speaking, taking high doses of anything is risky. A basic principle of toxicology is that any compound can be toxic if the dose is high enough. Dietary supplements are no exception to this rule. For example, clinical trials found that supplementing with 20–30 mg/day of beta-carotene for 4–6 years increased lung cancer risk by 16–28% in smokers.[12,13] Based on these and other results, experts from the U.S. Preventive Health Services Task Force recommend against beta-carotene supplementation.[14]

In short, while there is ample evidence to support the health benefits of diets rich in fruits, vegetables, legumes, whole grains, and nuts, no recommendation for precise amounts can be given, and phytochemical supplements should be avoided. The best advice for optimal health is to consume a plant-based diet consisting of as many whole foods as possible.

Avoid phytochemical supplements in favor of whole foods.

metabolites The form that nutrients take when they have been used by our body. For example, lactate is a metabolite of carbohydrate that is produced when we use carbohydrate for energy.

HIGHLIGHT

Will a PB&J Keep the Doctor Away?

Whole-grain bread, natural peanut butter, and grape jelly: how could a food that tastes so good be good for the body, too? We've known for decades about some of the healthful nutrients in peanut butter and jelly sandwiches, including the fiber and micronutrients in whole-grain bread and the plant protein, fiber, monounsaturated fat, and minerals in peanuts. But recently, research has revealed that the comforting PB&J also appears to be a good source of resveratrol, a phytochemical that is being studied in labs across the world because of its health-promoting potential.[15,16] A flavonoid found in the skins of dark grapes, it is plentiful both in the raw fruit, in dark grape juice, and in most red wines, which are fermented with the grape skins still in the vat. It is also present to a lesser extent in dark berries such as blueberries and cranberries. But fruits are not the only source: resveratrol just happens to also be plentiful in peanuts, including peanut butter.

But what does resveratrol do, and does a PB&J contain enough of the stuff to make a difference? Researchers have linked resveratrol to protective effects against cancer, heart disease, obesity, viral infections, and neurological diseases like Alzheimer's; however, so far, the effects have been demonstrated only in mice. What's more, no one yet knows what an effective "dose" of resveratrol looks like, nor whether the amounts in a peanut butter and jelly sandwich could possibly confer health benefits. More disturbingly, we don't yet know whether high doses, such as those found in supplements, could be harmful. Unfortunately, these facts have not stopped supplements manufacturers from marketing hundreds of different resveratrol supplements to humans.

If you do decide to add resveratrol to your diet, we hope you'll bypass supplements in favor of the humble PB&J. Although the jury is still out on the benefits of its resveratrol content, it still makes a highly nutritious meal or snack, doesn't need refrigeration, is inexpensive, and tastes great.

What Are Functional Foods?

A **functional food** is a food that has been manipulated in order to enhance its role in a healthful diet. Functional foods (also called *nutraceuticals*) contain nutrients and/or other substances (plant extracts, phytochemicals, bacteria) that provide a health benefit beyond what is provided by the same food in an unprocessed form.[17]

Most commonly, the health-promoting substances are added to an existing food. For example, iodine is added to salt, grains are enriched with iron and B-vitamins, orange juice is fortified with calcium, or milk is enriched with *extra* calcium. Alternatively, the health-promoting substances are caused to develop in a functional food by altering the way in which the food is produced. For example, eggs with higher levels of omega-3 fatty acids result from feeding chickens a diet rich in this nutrient. Also, tomatoes can be genetically engineered to contain higher levels of phytochemicals. These qualify as functional foods.

Are Functional Foods Safe?

The U.S. Food and Drug Administration (FDA) is responsible for ensuring

Grains enriched with iron and B-vitamins are an example of a functional food.

functional food A food that has been manipulated to provide additional health benefits.

that all foods are safe and properly labeled. Currently, the FDA has no official definition or regulatory category for functional foods: it regulates them in the same way as conventional foods. This means that in order for a food to be allowed on the market, any "functional" ingredient added to that food must be generally recognized as safe.

Recently, other federal agencies and consumer advocacy groups have petitioned the FDA to re-evaluate the way it ensures the safety of ingredients in functional foods and the truthfulness of health claims on functional food labels.[18] Their concern is twofold. First, they contend that, by making unsubstantiated health claims for their products, companies are misleading consumers into wasting billions of dollars annually. Second, they point to dozens of products currently sold as foods that contain ingredients such as herbs that are not FDA approved for use in foods. They caution that such products could have adverse health effects on vulnerable consumers, including pregnant women, children, and the frail elderly, as well as consumers with chronic disease, in whom the ingredients could exacerbate symptoms or interfere with prescription medications.

In response to these and other concerns, the FDA is currently considering a new regulatory system by which any product bearing health claims would be subject to FDA oversight. Thus, not only herbs, but even conventional food ingredients promoted for use in the treatment or prevention of disease in humans would be subject to FDA control.[19] But until such a system is in effect, consumers should remain skeptical about the safety and effectiveness of the functional foods they see on the shelves.

Are Functional Foods Effective?

Is there any research to support the claims of health benefits made by manufacturers of functional foods? That depends on the product. So if you're considering regular consumption of a functional food, do your homework. To give you some practice, let's consider a few currently on the market.

Designer Yogurts

People have been consuming yogurt and other fermented milk products for thousands of years. But interest in their health benefits began only about 100 years ago, when a Russian microbiologist named Ilya Metchnikov linked the long, healthy lives of Bulgarian peasants with their consumption of such foods. Subsequent research identified bacteria in fermented milk products as responsible for their healthful effects, and the probiotics industry was born.

Probiotics means "pro-life." Probiotics are live microorganisms found in, or added to, fermented dairy foods such as yogurt, buttermilk, sour cream, and kefir (a yogurt-style liquid beverage) and fermented vegetable foods such as sauerkraut, miso, and tempeh (fermented tofu). Probiotics are also available in supplement form.

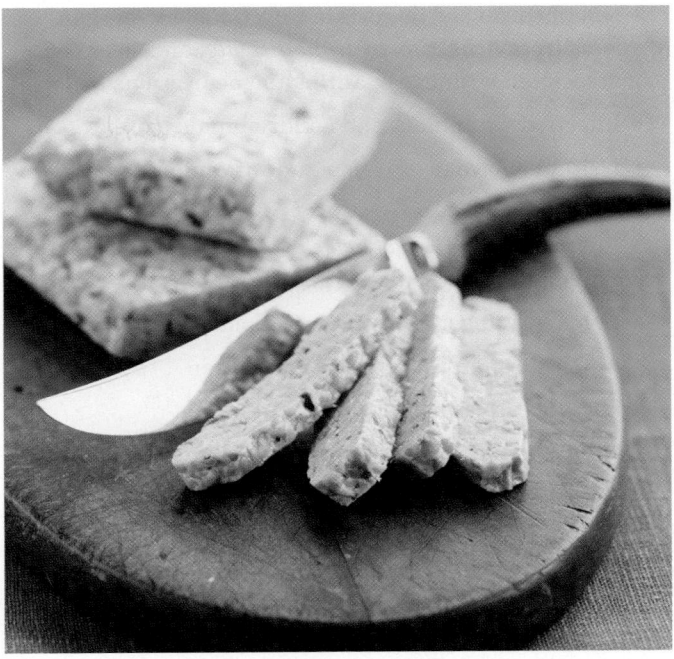

Fermented foods such as tempeh contain probiotics.

Our intestines contain an amazing number and variety of bacteria and other microorganisms. Many of these are vital to maintaining our health and supporting digestive function, but some can be harmful. The correct balance between beneficial and harmful microbes can be disturbed by medications and illness. The main symptoms of an unbalanced microbial environment are digestive, such as diarrhea or constipation, but other conditions may also be related to inadequate intestinal bacteria.

How do probiotics work? When a person consumes a product containing probiotics, these bacteria adhere to the intestinal wall for a few days. Once attached to the intestinal wall, the bacteria can exert their beneficial actions. The activity of these bacteria is short lived, and they probably need to be consumed on a daily basis to benefit human health. The exact mechanism of how probiotics work is currently being researched. It is believed that different types of bacteria provide benefits in different ways: some crowd out harmful bacterial, viral, and fungal species, some produce nutrients and other substances that influence nutrition and health, and others appear to influence our immune system.[20] Although there is still limited research on whether probiotics can really improve immune function and overall health in humans, there is promising evidence that probiotics may be beneficial in the following conditions:[20–22]

probiotics Live beneficial microorganisms in foods that can colonize the intestine and optimize the intestinal bacterial environment. There is promising research suggesting various health benefits from consuming probiotics.

- Diarrhea caused by certain infectious microorganisms (rotavirus, *Clostridium difficile*, and so on) or associated with use of antibiotic medications

- Infections in infants and children in daycare

- Irritable bowel syndrome and inflammatory bowel diseases

- Infection from *Helicobacter pylori*, the bacteria associated with peptic ulcers, gastritis, and gastric cancer

- Urinary and genital tract infections in women

- Atopic dermatitis (eczema) in children

- Lactose intolerance

- Reducing the risk of allergies in infants

It is important to remember that in order to be effective, there is a minimum number of bacteria that must be present in foods. While the exact number of bacteria is not known, it is estimated that a daily dose of at least 1 billion to 10 billion bacteria are needed to be effective.[23] Because these live cultures can survive only for a limited period of time, foods and supplements containing probiotics have a limited shelf life, and these products must be properly stored and consumed within a relatively brief period of time to receive maximal benefit.

At this time, there are no national standards for identifying the level of active bacteria in foods or supplements. In the United States, the National Yogurt Association has established a "Live Active Culture" seal, which indicates that the yogurt contains an adequate amount of active bacteria per gram.

Prebiotics are food components related to probiotics. These are types of fiber naturally found in fruits, vegetables, and whole grains that promote the growth of friendly bacteria. Inulin and oligofructose are the most widely studied. Prebiotics can be added to functional foods, typically to those that contain probiotics. For example, the yogurt manufacturer Stonyfield Farm states that the prebiotic inulin in their yogurt "increases calcium absorption . . . by as much as 20%," and their Web site lists numerous studies to support this claim.

Some food manufacturers are employing researchers to find and cultivate strains of probiotic bacteria that have specific health benefits. For example, Activia, a yogurt recently introduced by Dannon, contains a probiotic species called *Bifidus regularis*. The company states that this species promotes regular bowel movements by reducing the time

Activia yogurt.

prebiotics Types of fiber that friendly intestinal bacteria thrive on.

stool stays in the colon. As you learned in Chapter 3, the longer fecal matter remains in the colon, the more water is removed from it, so reduced transit time means softer bowel movements. Is this claim valid?

If you check out the research cited on Dannon's Web site (**http://www.activia.com**), you'll discover that four studies on Activia and *Bifidus regularis* have been published in peer-reviewed journals. The studies found that consuming 3 4-oz servings of Activia a day for 10–14 days sped up stool transit time by 10–40%. This effect was seen in men and women, and in both young (mid-twenties) and older (up to 75 years) subjects. Although benefits were seen with just 1 4-oz serving a day, the biggest benefits were seen with 2–3 daily servings. Convinced? If constipation were a problem for you, what further questions might you want to ask to determine whether or not this product would be worth purchasing?

Extraordinary Eggs

In the Nutrition Debate in Chapter 1, you learned that the diet fed to agouti mice could influence the constitution of their offspring. Similarly, the diet fed to hens can influence the nutrients present in their eggs. Feeding chickens a diet rich in omega-3 fatty acids, vitamin E, or lutein results in eggs that contain these substances. Such eggs can cost twice as much per dozen as conventional eggs. Are they worth the cost?

As you learned in Chapter 5, increased intake of omega-3 fatty acids may be important in reducing the risk of cardiovascular disease.[24–26] Typically, the positive effects are seen in clinical trials with a precisely controlled high omega-3 intake. Would the level of omega-3s in these eggs confer health benefits? We simply don't have the research to answer this question. Nevertheless, small doses of omega-3s via foods can certainly add up.

What about vitamin E? We know that diets with plenty of vitamin E–rich foods (nuts and dark-green leafy vegetables) are associated with better health, but research on vitamin E supplements has found no benefits

It is unclear whether eggs enriched with omega–3s or vitamin E are better for us, but there's no question that they are more expensive.

at all.[4,27] So there is no evidence to support recommending vitamin E–enriched eggs for disease prevention.

Lutein is a phytochemical found in many green and yellow plants. Lutein and zeaxanthin are the only carotenoids found in the retina and lens of the eye. Epidemiological studies suggest that diets rich in lutein and zeaxanthin (providing about 6 mg/day) may help slow the development of age-related macular degeneration. However, it is not known whether consuming eggs with lutein has the same effect.[5]

NUTRI-CASE GUSTAVO

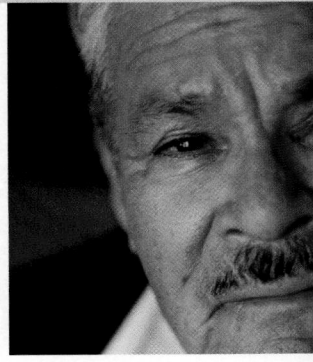

" For years, we've bought our eggs from a farm down the road, but my daughter told us yesterday that we should be buying these new so-called healthy eggs. She says they give the hens a special kind of food that makes the eggs better for us, especially as we're getting older. I asked her what they cost and she said $3.00 a dozen! That's twice what we pay at the farm, and the farm eggs are fresh! Those store-bought eggs are trucked in from miles away! I told my daughter if I want to improve my health, I'll take a vitamin."

Do you think Gustavo should switch from local eggs to the new "functional food" eggs? Why or why not? Could he get the same nutritional benefits if he were to "take a vitamin"?

Extra Dark Chocolate

You've just finished lunch when a friend offers you a piece of her extra dark chocolate bar. Should you, or shouldn't you? Recently, the results from a number of laboratory and clinical studies have suggested you *should*. Here's why.

Certain fruits, vegetables, tea, and red wine have long been associated with lower cardiovascular disease (CVD) risk. These foods are especially rich in a class of antioxidant phytochemicals called flavonoids. Cocoa has been found to have greater amounts of flavonoids per serving than teas and red wines, as well as many fruits and vegetables.[28] The darker the chocolate, the more flavonoids per serving. Thus, research interest in the potential effects of chocolate—especially dark chocolate—on CVD risk has grown.

Dozens of human feeding trials have been conducted since 2000. Most have shown that daily doses of cocoa have positive effects on one or more CVD risk factors, including improvements in blood lipids and blood pressure.[28] Several studies have shown benefits from consuming as little as 30 calories of dark chocolate daily.[29] In response, some chocolate manufacturers have produced specialty brands of "extra dark chocolate" with increased amounts of "antioxidant-rich cocoa."

So what's the hitch? One is that not all studies show the same effects. The variability in response is likely due to differences in the subjects' health and age and in the dose they consumed. And we can't ignore the fact that chocolate contains sugar and fat: some studies have fed subjects about 100 grams (3 oz) of chocolate per day, which can deliver over 400 extra calories to the diet!

Which raises a question that chocolate lovers would probably prefer to ignore: to reduce our risk of CVD, do we need to eat chocolate at all? Why not apples, for example, which contain 50% more flavonoids than a comparable serving of dark chocolate, only about 60 calories each, and no fat?[28]

For now, it seems likely that cocoa has positive health effects mediated by phytochemicals. So when debating whether or not to indulge in a small dose of extra dark chocolate, consider your diet as a whole: do you consume a wide variety of unrefined plant foods each day? If you do, then a little chocolate might be a sensible indulgence.

Calorie-Burning Beverages

Enviga is one of several so-called "calorie-burning beverages" recently brought onto the market. The manufacturers of these beverages claim that they increase the consumer's metabolic rate, causing the body to burn additional calories, and that the effect lasts for several hours after consuming the beverage. The Enviga Web site (**www.enviga.com/#Science**) states that a clinical trial

Chocolate is high in flavonoids.

Enviga claims to burn extra calories.

found that on average, participants expended 106 more calories per day after consuming 3 servings of Enviga for 3 days. The study was conducted in 2004 and has now been published in a peer-reviewed journal.[30] Although the Enviga study has not been repeated, allowing it to be reviewed suggests it is sound.

Why then does the Center for Science in the Public Interest (CSPI), a consumer advocacy group, contend in a lawsuit that the claims made for Enviga are fraudulent?[31] Here are some of the claims challenged by the CSPI: Enviga is "much smarter than fads, quick-fixes, and crash diets." It keeps "those extra calories from building up," and there is a "calorie burning effect from a single can." The CSPI is challenging these claims because not one of them was substantiated by the clinical trial.

Is it safe? Enviga contains caffeine and *epigallocatechin gallate* (*EGCG*), a phytochemical that occurs in green tea. No negative effects have been seen with EGCG. The ingredient of concern is caffeine. Three cans of Enviga provide 300 mg of caffeine, which is the caffeine equivalent of nine cans of Coke. This level of caffeine intake is generally not recommended.[32]

Is Enviga worth the cost? The Web site states that three cans would boost one's metabolism by 60–100 calories per day. At an average cost of about $1.39 per 12-oz can, drinking the effective dose of Enviga would cost about $130 a month! In comparison, you could brew coffee containing the same amount of caffeine for less than $10 a month. Even better, you could burn more calories free of charge by running 1 mile a day (about 106 calories for a 132-pound person), and you'd get all of the other health benefits of exercise to boot!

Are You Ready to Choose Functional Foods?

As these examples show, when it comes to functional foods, "Let the buyer beware." If you're considering specific products, do you know enough about their safety and effectiveness to feel confident adding them to your daily diet? Do you support the FDA proposal to more strictly regulate the health claims and safety of functional foods? How do you think food labels could be improved to assist you in identifying foods that might be beneficial for your specific health concerns? As the number of functional foods increases in the U.S. market, these are just some of the questions that consumers need to answer.

WEB LINKS

http://nccam.nih.gov/health/probiotics
National Center for Complementary and Alternative Medicine

This brochure, called "An Introduction to Probiotics," provides additional info on probiotics.

www.aicr.org
American Institute for Cancer Research

Search for "phytochemicals" to learn about the AICR's stance and recommendations about phytochemicals and their roles in cancer prevention.

http://lpi.oregonstate.edu
Linus Pauling Institute

This extensive Web site covers not only phytochemicals but also nutrients and other cutting-edge health and nutrition topics.

REFERENCES

1. Liu, R. H. 2003. Health benefits of fruit and vegetables are from additive and synergistic combinations of phytochemicals. *Am. J. Clin. Nutr.* 78(suppl.):517S–520S.
2. Panel on Dietary Antioxidants and Related Compounds. Subcommittee on Upper Reference Levels of Nutrients and Interpretation and Uses of Dietary Reference Intakes. Standing Committee on the Scientific Evaluation of Dietary Reference Intakes. Food and Nutrition Board. Institute of Medicine. 2000. *Dietary Reference Intakes for Vitamin C, Vitamin E, Selenium, and Carotenoids.* Washington, DC: National Academies Press.
3. Chun, O. K., et al. 2007. Estimated dietary flavonoid intake and major food sources of US adults. *J. Nutr.* 137:1244–1252.
4. Melton, L. 2006. The antioxidant myth: a medical fairy tale. *New Sci.* 2563:40–43.
5. Linus Pauling Institute, Oregon State University. 2005. Micronutrient information center: flavonoids. http://lpi.oregonstate.edu/infocenter/phytochemicals/flavonoids/. (Accessed July 2007.)
6. Beauchamp, G. K., R. S. Keast, D. Morel, J. Lin, J. Pika, Q. Han, C. H. Lee, A. B. Smith, and P. A. Breslin. 2005. Ibuprofen-like activity in extra virgin olive oil. *Nature* 437:45–46.
7. Liu, R. H. 2004. Potential synergy of phytochemicals in cancer prevention: mechanism of action. *J. Nutr.* 134:3479S–3485S.
8. Boileau, T. W.-M., et al. 2003. Prostate carcinogenesis in N-methyl-N-nitrosurea (NMU)-testosterone-treated rats fed tomato powder, lycopene, and energy-restricted diets. *J. Natl. Cancer Inst.* 95:1578–1586.
9. Milner, J. A. 2001. A historical perspective on garlic and cancer. *J. Nutr.* 131:1027S–1031S.

10. Rice S., and S. A. Whitehead. 2006. Phytoestrogens and breast cancer—promoters or protectors? *Endocr. Relat. Cancer* 13(4):995–1015.

11. Meyskens, F. L., and E. Szabo. 2005. Diet and cancer: the disconnect between epidemiology and randomized clinical trials. *Cancer Epidemiol. Biomarkers Prev.* 14(6):1366–1369.

12. The Alpha-Tocopherol, Beta-Carotene Cancer Prevention Study Group. 1994. The effect of vitamin E and beta carotene on the incidence of lung cancer and other cancers in male smokers. *N. Engl. J. Med.* 330(15):1029–1035.

13. Omenn, G. S., et al. 1996. Risk factors for lung cancer and for intervention effects in CARET, the Beta-Carotene and Retinol Efficacy Trial. *J. Natl. Cancer Inst.* 88(21):1550–1559.

14. U.S. Preventive Services Task Force. 2003. Routine vitamin supplementation to prevent cancer and cardiovascular disease: recommendations and rationale. *Ann. Intern. Med.* 139(1):51–55.

15. Baur, J. A., et al. 2006. Resveratrol improves health and survival of mice on a high-calorie diet. *Nature* 444:337–342.

16. Lagouge, M., et al. 2006. Resveratrol improves mitochondrial function and protects against metabolic disease by activating SIRT1 and PGC-1alpha. *Cell* 27(6):1109–1122.

17. Committee on Opportunities in the Nutrition and Food Sciences, Food and Nutrition Board, Institute of Medicine, Thomas, P. R., and R. Earl (eds.). 1994. *Opportunities in the Nutrition and Food Sciences: Research, Challenges and the Next Generation of Investigators.* Washington, DC: National Academies Press.

18. Federal Register: October 25, 2006 (Volume 71, Number 206). From the Federal Register Online via GPO Access [wais.access.gpo.gov] [DOCID:fr25oc06-12] Food and Drug Administration, HHS; 21 CFR Parts 101 and 170 [Docket No. 2002P-0122] (formerly 02P-0122). Conventional Foods Being Marketed as "Functional Foods"; Public Hearing; Request for Comments.

19. U.S. Food and Drug Administration (FDA). 2006. Docket No. 2006D-0480. Draft Guidance for Industry on Complementary and Alternative Medicine Products and Their Regulation by the Food and Drug Administration.

20. Saier, M. H., Jr., and N. M. Mansour. 2005. Probiotics and prebiotics in human health. *J. Mol. Microbiol. Biotechnol.* 10(1):22–25.

21. Doron, S., and S. L. Gorbach. 2006. Probiotics: their role in the treatment and prevention of diseases. *Expert Rev. Anti-Infect. Ther.* 4(2):261–275.

22. Ezendam, J., and H. van Loveren. 2006. Probiotics: immunomodulation and evaluation of safety and efficacy. *Nutr. Rev.* 64(1):1–14.

23. Sanders, M. E., D. C. Walker, K. M. Walker, K. Aoyama, and T. R. Klaenhammer. 1996. Performance of commercial cultures in fluid milk applications. *J. Dairy Sci.* 79:943–955.

24. American Heart Association. 2007. Fish and omega-3 fatty acids: AHA recommendation. www.americanheart.org/presenter.jhtml?identifier=4632. (Accessed July 2007.)

25. Center for Food Safety and Applied Nutrition. 2004. Questions and answers: qualified health claims for omega-3 fatty acids, eicosapentaenoic acid (EPA) and docosahexaenoic acid (DHA). CFSAN/Office of Nutritional Products, Labeling, and Dietary Supplements. www.cfsan.fda.gov/~dms/labo3qa.html. (Accessed July 2007.)

26. National Heart, Lung, and Blood Institute, NIH, DHHS. 2005. Your guide to lowering cholesterol with therapeutic lifestyle changes (TLC). www.nhlbi.nih.gov/health/public/heart/chol/chol_tlc.pdf. (Accessed July 2007.)

27. Friedrich, M. J. 2004. To "E" or not to "E," vitamin E's role in health and disease is the question. *JAMA* 292(6):671–673.

28. Ding, E. L., S. M. Hutfless, X. Ding, and S. Girotra. 2006. Chocolate and prevention of cardiovascular disease: A systematic review. *Nutr. Metab.* 3:2. www.nutritionandmetabolism.com/content/3/1/2.

29. Taubert, D., et al. 2007. Effects of low habitual cocoa intake on blood pressure and bioactive nitric oxide: a randomized controlled trial. *JAMA* 298(1):49–60.

30. Rudelle, S., et al. 2007. Effect of a thermogenic beverage on 24-hour energy metabolism in humans. *Obesity* 15(2):349–355.

31. Center for Science in the Public Interest. 2006. "Calorie burning" Enviga tea drink a fraud, group says. CSPI to sue Coke, Nestlé if weight loss claims persist. Press release: December 4, 2006. www.cspinet.org/new/200612041.html. (Accessed July 2007.)

32. McGee, W. 2005. Caffeine in the diet. Medline Plus Medical Encyclopedia. www.nlm.nih.gov/medlineplus/ency/article/002445.htm. (Accessed July 2007.)

CHAPTER 9

CHAPTER OBJECTIVES

After reading this chapter you will be able to:

1. Describe the differences between cortical bone and trabecular bone, pp. 362–363.

2. Discuss the processes of bone growth, modeling, and remodeling, pp. 363–365.

3. List two vitamins and three minerals that play important roles in maintaining bone health, p. 366.

4. Identify foods that are good sources of calcium, pp. 369–370.

5. Describe how vitamin D assists in regulating blood calcium levels, pp. 367, 375.

6. Discuss three potential reasons why consumption of soft drinks may be detrimental to bone health, pp. 383–384.

7. Define osteoporosis, and discuss how it impacts a person's health, p. 388.

8. List three factors that influence our risk for osteoporosis, pp. 388–391.

TEST YOURSELF TRUE OR FALSE?

1. Most people are unable to consume enough calcium in their diets; therefore, they must take calcium supplements. T or F

2. Osteoporosis is a disease that affects only elderly women. T or F

3. We are capable of making vitamin D within our bodies by using energy obtained from exposure to sunlight. T or F

4. Dairy products must be consumed to meet the current dietary recommendations for calcium. T or F

5. Being overweight or obese may increase a person's risk for osteoporosis. T or F

Test Yourself answers can be found after the Chapter Summary.

Nutrients Involved in Bone Health

as a young woman, Erika Goodman leapt across the stage in leading roles with the Joffrey Ballet, one of the premier dance companies in the world. Now in her mid-50s, she cannot cross a room without assistance. Goodman has a disease called *osteoporosis*, which means "porous bone." As you might suspect, the less dense the bone, the more likely it is to break; indeed, osteoporosis can cause bones to break during even minor weight-bearing activities, such as carrying groceries. In advanced cases, bones in the hip and spine fracture spontaneously, merely from the effort of holding the body erect.

If you are age 20 or older, your bones are already at or close to their peak density. But just how dense are your bones, and what changes can you make right now, no matter what your age, to keep them as strong as possible? What foods build bone? Are there foods that break it down? In this chapter, we discuss the nutrients and lifestyle factors that play a critical role in maintaining bone health.

How Does Our Body Maintain Bone Health?

Contrary to what most people think, our skeleton is not an inactive collection of bones that simply holds our body together. Bones are living organs that contain several tissues, including bone tissue, nerves, cartilage, and connective tissue. Blood vessels supply nutrients to bone to support its activities. Bones have many important functions in our bodies, some of which might surprise you (Table 9.1). For instance, did you know that most of your blood cells are formed deep within your bones? Given the importance of bones, it is critical that we maintain their health. Bone health is achieved through complex interactions between nutrients, hormones, and environmental factors. To better understand these interactions, we first need to learn about how bone structure and the constant activity of bone tissue influence bone health throughout our lifetime.

Bone Composition and Structure Provide Strength and Flexibility

We tend to think of bones as totally rigid, but if they were, how could we twist and jump our way through a basketball game or even carry an armload of books up a flight of stairs? Our bones need to be both strong and flexible so they can resist the compression, stretching, and twisting that occur throughout our daily activities. Fortunately, the composition of bone is ideally suited for its complex job: about 65% of bone tissue is made up of an assortment of minerals (mostly calcium and phosphorus) that provide hardness, but the remaining 35% is a mixture of organic substances that provide strength, durability, and flexibility. The most important of these substances is a fibrous protein called **collagen.** You might be surprised to learn that collagen fibers are actually stronger than steel fibers of similar size. Within our bones, the minerals form tiny crystals (called *hydroxyapatite*) that cluster around the collagen fibers. This design enables bones to bear our weight while responding to our demands for movement.

Bone strength and flexibility are also affected by its structure. If you examine a bone very closely, you will notice two distinct types of tissue (FIGURE 9.1): cortical bone and trabecular bone. **Cortical bone,** which is also called *compact bone,* is very dense. It comprises approximately 80% of our skeleton. The outer surface of all bones is cortical; plus many small bones of the body, such as the bones of the wrists, hands,

collagen A protein that forms strong fibers in bone and connective tissue.

cortical bone (compact bone) A dense bone tissue that makes up the outer surface of all bones as well as the entirety of most small bones of the body.

TABLE 9.1 Functions of Bone in the Human Body

Functions Related to Structure and Support	Functions Related to Metabolic Processes
Bones provide physical support for our organs and body segments.	Bone tissue acts as a storage reservoir for many minerals, including calcium, phosphorus, and fluoride. The body draws upon such deposits when these minerals are needed for various body processes; however, this can reduce bone mass.
Bones protect our vital organs; for example, the rib cage protects our lungs, the skull protects our brain, and the vertebrae in our spine protect our spinal cord.	
Bones provide support for muscles that allow movement—muscles attach to bones via tendons, and we are able to move all of our joints because of the connections between our muscles and our bones.	Most of the blood cells needed by our bodies are produced in the marrow of our bones.

and feet, are made entirely of cortical bone. Although cortical bone looks solid to the naked eye, it actually contains many microscopic openings that serve as passageways for blood vessels and nerves.

In contrast, **trabecular bone** makes up only 20% of our skeleton. It is found within the ends of the long bones (such as the bones of the arms and legs), inside the spinal vertebrae, inside the flat bones (breastbone, ribs, and most bones of the skull), and inside the bones of the pelvis. Trabecular bone is sometimes referred to as *spongy* (or *cancellous*) *bone* because to the naked eye it looks like a sponge, with no clear organization. The microscope reveals that trabecular bone is in fact aligned in a precise network of columns that protects the bone from extreme stress. You can think of trabecular bone as the scaffolding of the inside of the bone, as it supports the outer cortical bone in much the same way that the interior scaffolding of a building supports its outer walls.

Cortical and trabecular bone also differ in their rate of turnover; that is, in how quickly the bone tissue is broken down and replenished. Trabecular bone has a faster turnover rate than cortical bone, meaning that more of the trabecular bone is being broken down and replenished at any given time as compared to cortical bone. This makes trabecular bone more sensitive to changes in hormones and nutritional factors, and we can more easily detect a loss of trabecular bone than we can a loss of cortical bone. It also accounts for the much higher rate of age-related fractures in the spine and pelvis (including the hip)—all of which contain a significant amount of trabecular bone. Let's now investigate how bone turnover, or the constant activity of bone, influences our bone health.

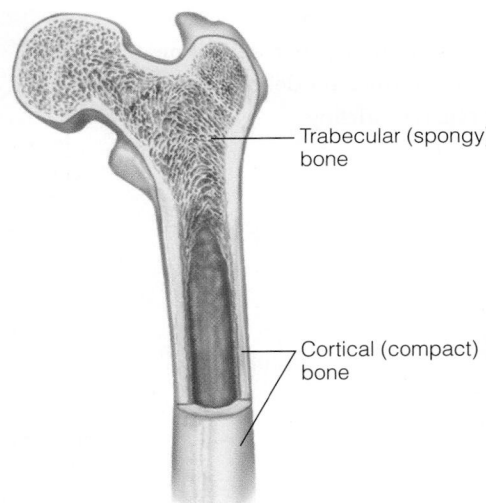

FIGURE 9.1 The structure of bone. Notice the difference in density between the trabecular (spongy) bone and the cortical (compact) bone.

> RECAP: *Bones are organs that contain metabolically active tissues composed primarily of minerals and a fibrous protein called collagen. We have two types of bone, cortical and trabecular. Cortical bone is dense and comprises about 80% of our skeleton. Trabecular bone is porous and comprises about 20% of our skeleton. Trabecular bone is more sensitive to hormonal and nutritional factors and turns over more rapidly than cortical bone.*

The Constant Activity of Bone Tissue Promotes Bone Health

Our bones develop through a series of three processes: bone growth, bone modeling, and bone remodeling (FIGURE 9.2). Bone growth and modeling begin during the early months of fetal life when our skeleton is forming and continue through infancy, childhood, and adolescence. As a result of this constant activity, the shape and size of our bones are well defined by the time we reach puberty. Bone remodeling predominates during adulthood; this process helps us to maintain a healthy skeleton as we age.

Bone Growth and Modeling Determine the Size and Shape of Our Bones

Through the process of *bone growth,* the size of our bones increases. The first period of rapid bone growth is from birth to age 2, but growth continues in spurts throughout childhood and into adolescence. Most girls reach their adult height by age 14, and boys generally reach adult height by age 17.[1] In the later decades of life, some loss in height usually occurs because of decreased bone density in the spine, as will be discussed shortly.

Bone modeling is the process by which the shape of our bones is determined, from the round "pebble" bones that make up our wrists, to the uniquely shaped bones of our face, to the long bones of our arms and legs. Although our bones stop growing in length by the time we are 18 to 21 years of age, bones can still increase in thickness if they are stressed by excessive or repetitive exercise such as weight training or if we are overweight or obese.

trabecular bone (spongy or cancellous bone) A porous bone tissue that makes up only 20% of our skeleton and is found within the ends of the long bones, inside the spinal vertebrae, inside the flat bones (breastbone, ribs, and most bones of the skull), and inside the bones of the pelvis.

FIGURE 9.2 Bone develops through three processes: bone growth, bone modeling, and bone remodeling.

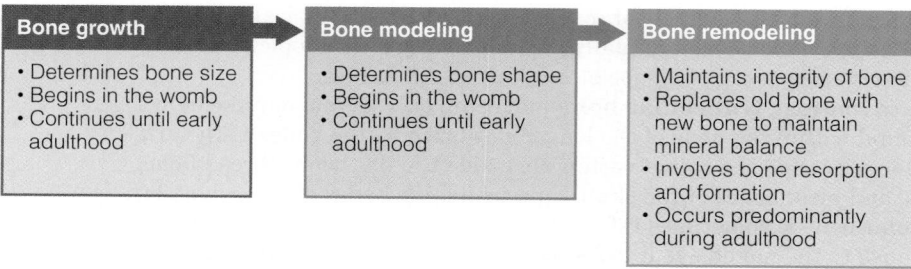

Bone Remodeling Maintains a Balance Between Breakdown and Repair

Although the shape and size of our bones do not significantly change after puberty, our **bone density,** or the strength of our bones, continues to develop into early adulthood. *Peak bone density* is the point at which our bones are strongest because they are at their highest density. Factors associated with a lower peak bone density are late pubertal age in boys and late menarchal age in girls, and inadequate calcium intakes, low body weight, and physical inactivity during the pubertal years.[2–4] About 90% of a woman's bone density is built by 17 years of age, whereas the majority of a man's bone density is built during his twenties. However, male or female, before we reach the age of 30 years, our bodies have reached peak bone mass, and we can no longer significantly add to our bone density. In our thirties, our bone density remains relatively stable, but by age 40, it begins its irreversible decline.

Although our bones cannot increase their peak density after our twenties, bone tissue still remains very active throughout adulthood. To preserve bone density to the extent possible, our bodies attempt to achieve a balance between the breakdown of older bone tissue and the formation of new bone tissue. Thus, our bone mass is regularly recycled in a process called **remodeling.** We also use remodeling to repair bone that has been broken or damaged and to strengthen bone regions that are exposed to higher physical stress. The process of remodeling involves two steps: the breakdown of existing bone and the formation of new bone.

Bone is broken down through a process referred to as **resorption** (FIGURE 9.3A). During resorption, cells called **osteoclasts** erode the bone surface by secreting enzymes and acids that dig grooves into the bone matrix. Their ruffled surface also acts much like a scrubbing brush to assist in the erosion process. But why would we ever want to break down our bones? One of the primary reasons is to release calcium into our bloodstream. As discussed in more detail later in this chapter, calcium is critical for many physiologic processes, and our bone is an important source of calcium needed to support these processes. We also want to break down bone when we fracture (or break) a bone and need to repair it. Breaking down the damaged bone at the injury site smooths the rough edges created by the break. We may also break down bone in areas away from the damaged site to obtain the minerals, or raw materials, that are needed to repair the damage caused by the break. Regardless of the reason, once bone is broken down, the resulting products of this breakdown process are transported into the bloodstream and utilized for various body functions.

New bone is formed through the action of cells called **osteoblasts,** or "bone builders" (see FIGURE 9.3B). These cells work to synthesize new bone matrix by laying down the collagen-containing organic component of bone. Within this substance, the hydroxapatite crystallizes and packs together to create new bone where it is needed.

In young healthy adults, the processes of bone resorption and formation are equal, so that just as much bone is broken down as is built, resulting in bone mass being maintained. Around 40 years of age, bone resorption begins to occur more rapidly than bone formation, and this imbalance results in an overall loss in bone density. Because this affects the vertebrae of the spine, we also tend to lose height as we age. As we will discuss shortly, achieving a high peak bone mass through proper nutrition and exercise when we are young provides us with a stronger skeleton before we begin to lose bone as we age, and it can be protective against the debilitating effects of osteoporosis.

bone density The degree of compactness of bone tissue, reflecting the strength of the bones. *Peak bone density* is the point at which a bone is strongest.

remodeling The two-step process by which bone tissue is recycled; includes the breakdown of existing bone and the formation of new bone.

resorption The process by which the surface of bone is broken down by cells called osteoclasts.

osteoclasts Cells that erode the surface of bones by secreting enzymes and acids that dig grooves into the bone matrix.

osteoblasts Cells that prompt the formation of new bone matrix by laying down the collagen-containing component of bone that is then mineralized.

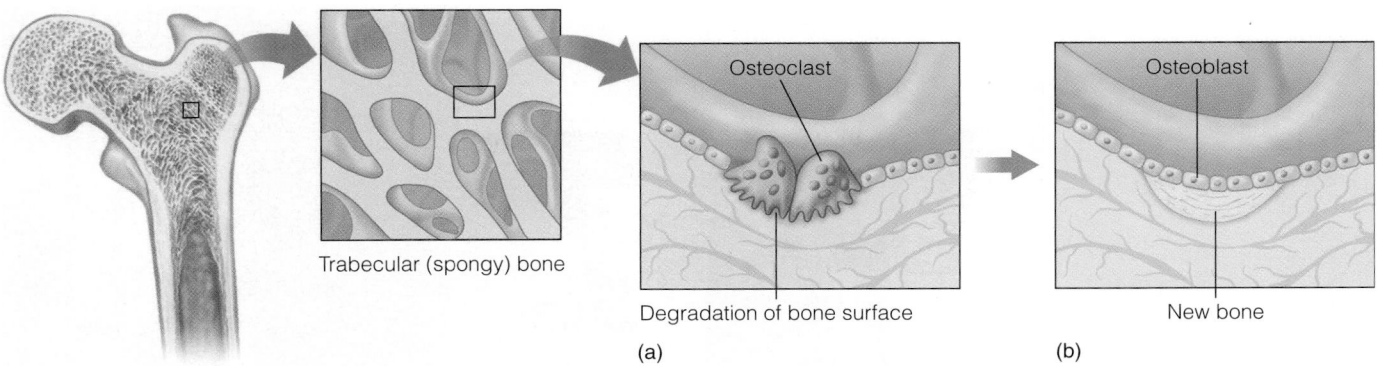

FIGURE 9.3 Bone remodeling involves resorption and formation. **(a)** Osteoclasts erode the bone surface by degrading its components, including calcium, other minerals, and collagen; these components are then transported to the bloodstream. **(b)** Osteoblasts work to build new bone by filling the pit formed by the resorption process with new bone.

> RECAP: *The three types of bone activity are growth, modeling, and remodeling. Our bones reach their peak bone mass by our late teenage years and into our twenties; bone mass begins to decline around age 40. Bone is constantly being recycled through a process called remodeling. Remodeling of bone involves the resorption of bone through the action of osteoclasts and the formation of bone through the action of osteoblasts.*

How Do We Assess Bone Health?

Until relatively recently, we had no way to measure the health of bone tissue. Over the past 30 years, however, technologic advancements have led to the development of a number of affordable methods for measuring bone health. **Dual energy x-ray absorptiometry,** also referred to as DXA (or DEXA), is considered the most accurate assessment tool for measuring bone density. This method can measure the density of the bone mass over the entire body. Special software is also available that provides an estimation of percent body fat.

The DXA procedure is simple, painless, noninvasive, and considered to be of minimal risk to humans and only takes 15 to 30 minutes to complete. The person participating in the test remains fully clothed but must remove all jewelry or other metal objects. The participant lies quietly on a table, and bone density is assessed through the use of a very low level of x-ray (FIGURE 9.4).

DXA is a very important tool to determine a person's risk for osteoporosis. Once someone's bone mineral density is determined, his or her number is compared to the average peak bone density of a 30-year-old healthy adult. Doctors use this comparison, which is known as the **T-score,** to assess the risk of fracture and determine whether or not this person has osteoporosis. A negative T-score indicates lower than normal bone mass. For instance, if the T-score is between −1 and −2.5, this person has low bone mass and is at an increased risk for fractures. If the T-score is more negative than −2.5, this person has osteoporosis. If bone density is normal, the T-score will range between +1 and −1 of the value for a 30-year-old healthy adult.

DXA tests are generally recommended for postmenopausal women because they are at highest risk for osteoporosis and fracture. Men and younger women may also be recommended for a DXA test if they have significant risk factors for osteoporosis (see page 388).

Other technologies have been developed to measure bone density. The quantitative ultrasound technique uses sound waves to measure the density of bone in the heel, shin, and kneecap. Peripheral dual energy x-ray absorptiometry, or pDXA, is a form of DXA that measures bone density in the peripheral regions of our bodies including the wrist, heel, or finger. Single energy x-ray absorptiometry is a method

dual energy x-ray absorptiometry (DXA or DEXA) Currently the most accurate tool for measuring bone density.

T-score A comparison of an individual's bone density to the average peak bone density of a 30-year-old healthy adult.

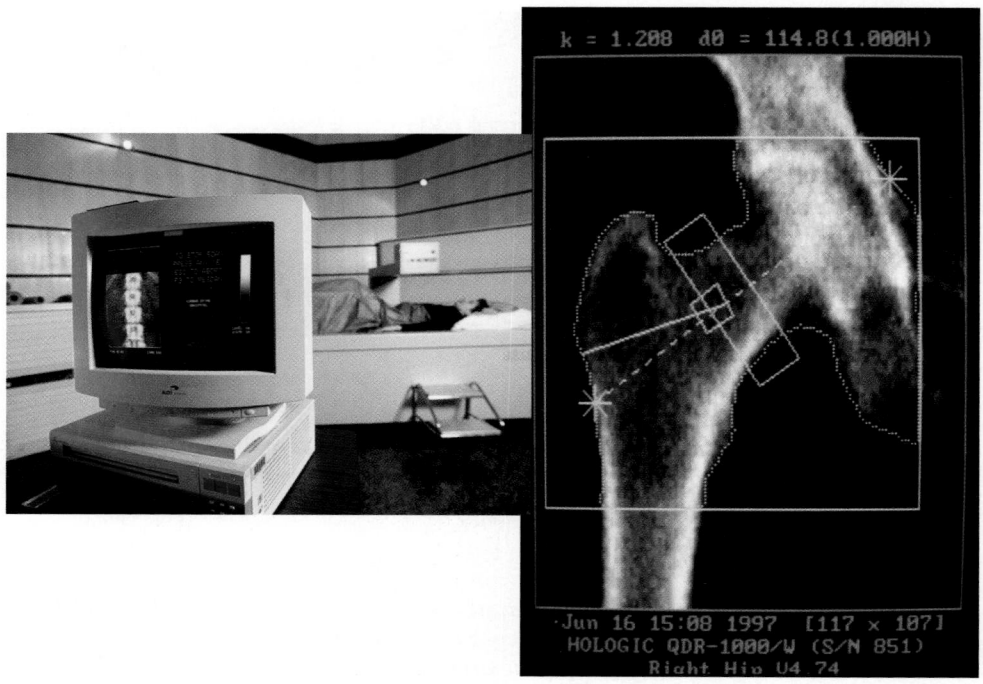

k = 1.208   d0 = 114.8(1.000H)

Jun 16 15:08 1997 [117 x 107]
HOLOGIC QDR-1000/W (S/N 851)
Right Hip U4.74

FIGURE 9.4 Dual energy x-ray absorptiometry is a simple, painless, and minimal-risk procedure that assesses bone density.

that measures bone density at the wrist or heel. These technologies are frequently used at health fairs because the machines are portable and provide scores faster than the traditional DXA.

> RECAP: *Dual energy x-ray absorptiometry (DXA or DEXA) is the gold standard measurement of bone mass. It is a simple, painless, and minimal-risk procedure. The results of a DXA include a T-score, which is a comparison of your bone density with that of a 30-year-old healthy adult. A T-score between +1 and –1 is normal; a score between –1 and –2.5 indicates poor bone density; and a score more negative than –2.5 indicates osteoporosis. Quantitative ultrasound, peripheral dual energy x-ray absorptiometry, and single energy x-ray absorptiometry are additional methods that can be used to measure bone density.*

A Profile of Nutrients That Maintain Bone Health

Calcium is the most recognized nutrient associated with bone health; however, vitamins D and K, phosphorus, magnesium, and fluoride are also essential for strong bones. Let's now learn more about these nutrients and their functions in our bodies.

Calcium

Recall from Chapter 1 that major minerals are those required in our diet in amounts greater than 100 mg per day. Calcium is by far the most abundant major mineral in our body, comprising about 2% of our entire body weight! Not surprisingly, it plays many critical roles in maintaining overall function and health.

Functions of Calcium

One of the primary roles of calcium is to provide structure to our bones and teeth. About 99% of the calcium found in our bodies is stored in our bones. As discussed

parathyroid hormone (PTH)
A hormone secreted by the parathyroid gland when blood calcium levels fall. It is also known as parathormone, and it increases blood calcium levels by stimulating the activation of vitamin D, increasing reabsorption of calcium from the kidneys, and stimulating osteoclasts to break down bone, which releases more calcium into the bloodstream.

earlier in this chapter, calcium and phosphorus crystallize to form hydroxyapatite. These crystals pack themselves tightly together and build up on the collagen foundation of bone. This combination of crystals and collagen provides both the characteristic hardness of bone and the flexibility needed to support various activities. Thus, one major role of calcium is to form and maintain bones and teeth.

The remaining 1% of calcium in our bodies is found in the blood and soft tissues. Calcium is alkaline, or basic, and because of this property it plays a critical role in helping the body maintain acid–base balance. We cannot survive for long if our blood calcium level rises above or falls below a very narrow range; therefore, our body maintains the appropriate blood calcium level at all costs.

FIGURE 9.5 illustrates how various organ systems and hormones work together to maintain blood calcium levels. When blood calcium levels fall (FIGURE 9.5A), the parathyroid gland is stimulated to produce **parathyroid hormone (PTH).** Also known as parathormone, PTH stimulates the activation of vitamin D. Together, PTH and vitamin D stimulate the kidneys to reabsorb calcium. They also stimulate osteoclasts to break down bone, releasing more calcium into the bloodstream. In addition, vitamin D increases the absorption of calcium from the intestines. Through these three mechanisms, blood calcium levels increase.

When blood calcium levels are high, the thyroid gland secretes a hormone called **calcitonin,** which inhibits the actions of vitamin D (FIGURE 9.5B). Thus, calcitonin prevents reabsorption of calcium in the kidneys, limits calcium absorption in the intestines, and inhibits the osteoclasts from breaking down bone. As just noted, the body must maintain blood calcium levels within a very narrow range. Thus, when an individual does not consume or absorb enough calcium from the diet, osteoclasts erode bone so that calcium can be released into the blood. To maintain healthy bone density, we need to consume and absorb enough calcium to balance the calcium taken from our bones.

Calcium is also critical for the normal transmission of nerve impulses. Calcium flows into nerve cells and stimulates the release of molecules called neurotransmitters,

One major role of calcium is to form and maintain bones and teeth.

calcitonin A hormone secreted by the thyroid gland when blood calcium levels are too high. Calcitonin inhibits the actions of vitamin D, preventing reabsorption of calcium in the kidneys, limiting calcium absorption in the intestines, and inhibiting the osteoclasts from breaking down bone.

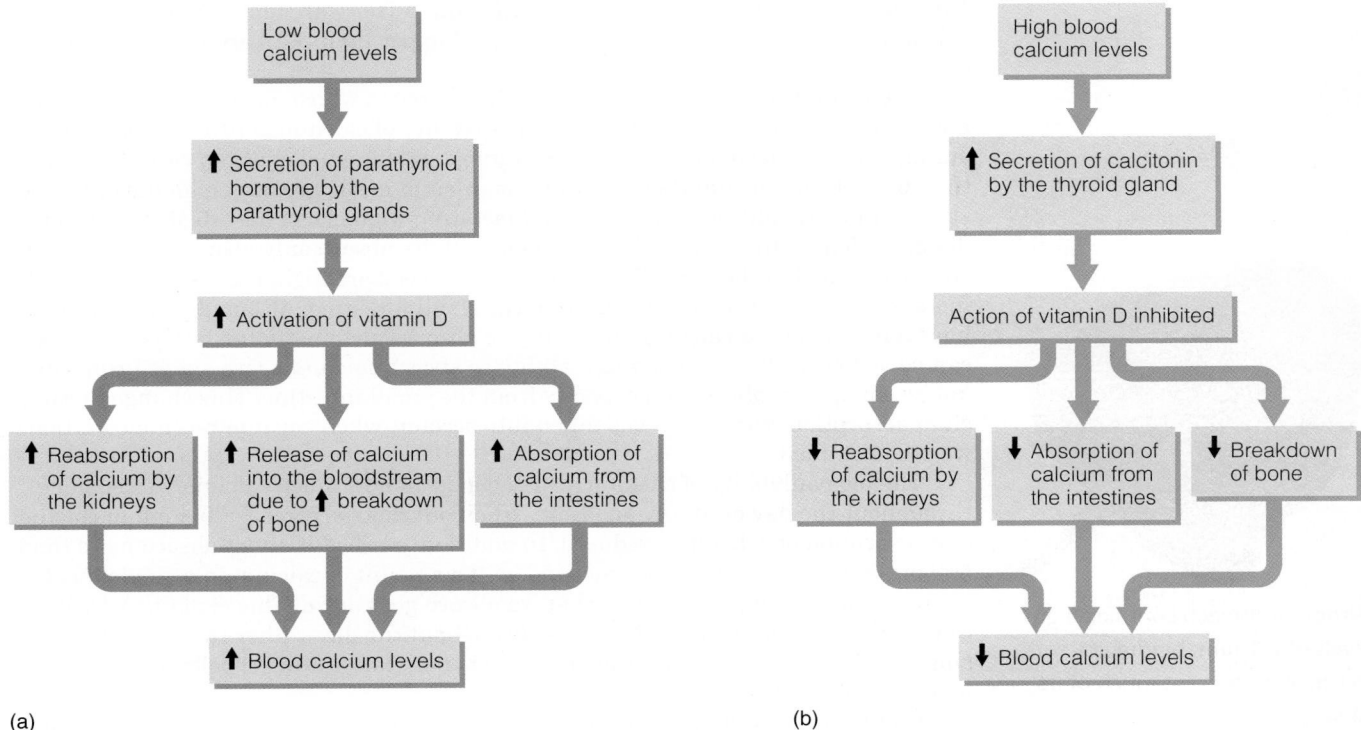

FIGURE 9.5 Regulation of blood calcium levels by various organs and hormones. **(a)** Low blood calcium levels stimulate the production of parathyroid hormone and activation of vitamin D, which in turn cause an increase in blood calcium levels. **(b)** High blood calcium levels stimulate the secretion of calcitonin, which in turn causes a decrease in blood calcium levels.

which transfer the nerve impulses from one nerve cell (neuron) to another. Without adequate calcium, our nerves' ability to transmit messages is inhibited. Not surprisingly, when blood calcium levels fall dangerously low, a person can experience convulsions.

A fourth role of calcium is to assist in muscle contraction. Our muscles are relaxed when calcium levels in the muscle are low. Contraction of our muscles is stimulated by calcium flowing into the muscle cell; conversely, our muscles relax when calcium is pumped back outside of the muscle cell. If calcium levels are inadequate, normal muscle contraction and relaxation is inhibited, and the person may suffer from twitching and spasms. This problem affects the function not only of skeletal muscles, but also of heart muscle and can cause heart failure.

A recent research study has suggested that a weight-loss diet high in calcium-rich foods may help people lose more weight than if they reduce their energy intake but do not consume enough dietary calcium.[5] This research has led to a major advertising campaign by the dairy industry, called the "3-a-Day" campaign. This campaign encourages people who want to lose weight to eat at least 3 servings of dairy foods per day, as study participants who ate calcium-rich foods experienced significantly more weight loss than those who consumed calcium supplements. Interestingly, Bowen and colleagues published a study that failed to replicate these findings.[6] Until more research is published on this topic, the question of whether dietary calcium can enhance weight loss in people who are dieting remains unanswered.

Other roles of calcium include the maintenance of healthy blood pressure, the initiation of blood clotting, and the regulation of various hormones and enzymes. A summary of the functions, recommended intakes, and toxicity and deficiency symptoms associated with calcium is provided in Table 9.3 on page 378.

How Much Calcium Should We Consume?

Much attention has recently been given to the fact that many people, particularly women, do not consume enough calcium to maintain bone health. In response to these findings, new DRI values have recently been published for calcium.[7]

Recommended Dietary Intake for Calcium. There are no RDA values for calcium. The Adequate Intake (AI) values and upper limit (UL) are listed in Table 9.3 on page 378.

The term **bioavailability** refers to the degree to which our bodies can absorb and utilize any given nutrient. The bioavailability of calcium depends in part upon our age and our need for calcium. For example, infants and children can absorb more than 60% of the calcium they consume, as calcium needs are very high during these stages of life. In addition, pregnant and lactating women can absorb about 50% of dietary calcium. In contrast, healthy young adults absorb only about 30% of the calcium consumed in the diet. When our calcium needs are high, the body can generally increase its absorption of calcium from the small intestine. Although older adults have a high need for calcium, the ability to absorb calcium diminishes as we age and can be as low as 25%. Our reduced ability to absorb calcium as we age is primarily due to changes in absorption capacity from the small intestine. This change in calcium absorption with aging was taken into account when calcium recommendations were determined.

The bioavailability of calcium also depends on how much calcium we consume throughout the day or at any one time. When our diets are generally high in calcium, our absorption of calcium is reduced. In addition, our body cannot absorb more than 500 mg of calcium at any one time, and as the amount of calcium in a single meal or supplement goes up, the fraction that we absorb goes down. This explains why it is critical to consume calcium-rich foods throughout the day, rather than relying on a single high-dose supplement. Conversely, when dietary intake of calcium is low, we increase our absorption of calcium.

Dietary factors can also affect our absorption of calcium. Binding factors such as fiber, phytates, and oxalates occur naturally in some calcium-rich seeds, nuts, grains, and vegetables such as spinach and Swiss chard. Such factors bind to the calcium in these foods and prevent their absorption from the intestine. Additionally, consuming calcium at the same time as iron, zinc, magnesium, or phosphorus has the potential

Although spinach contains high levels of calcium, binding factors in the plant prevent much of its absorption.

bioavailability The degree to which our bodies can absorb and utilize any given nutrient.

to interfere with the absorption and utilization of all of these minerals. Despite these potential interactions, the Institute of Medicine concluded that at the present time, there is not sufficient evidence to suggest that these interactions cause deficiencies of calcium or other minerals in healthy individuals.[7] However, there are people who are vulnerable to mineral deficiencies, such as elderly or people consuming very low mineral intakes, and more research needs to be done in these populations to determine the health risks associated with interactions between calcium and other minerals.

Finally, because vitamin D is necessary for the absorption of calcium, lack of vitamin D severely limits the bioavailability of calcium. We discuss this and other contributions of vitamin D to bone health shortly (pages 372–377).

SHOPPER'S GUIDE
Good Food Sources of Calcium

Dairy products are the most common sources of calcium in the United States diet. Skim milk, low-fat cheeses, and nonfat yogurt are excellent sources of calcium, and they are low in fat and calories (FIGURE 9.6). Ice cream, regular cheese, and whole milk also contain a relatively high amount of calcium, but these foods should be eaten in moderation because of their high fat and energy content. Cottage cheese is one dairy product that is a relatively poor source of calcium, as the processing of this food removes a great deal of the calcium. One cup of low-fat cottage cheese contains approximately 150 mg of calcium, while the same serving of low-fat milk contains almost 300 mg.

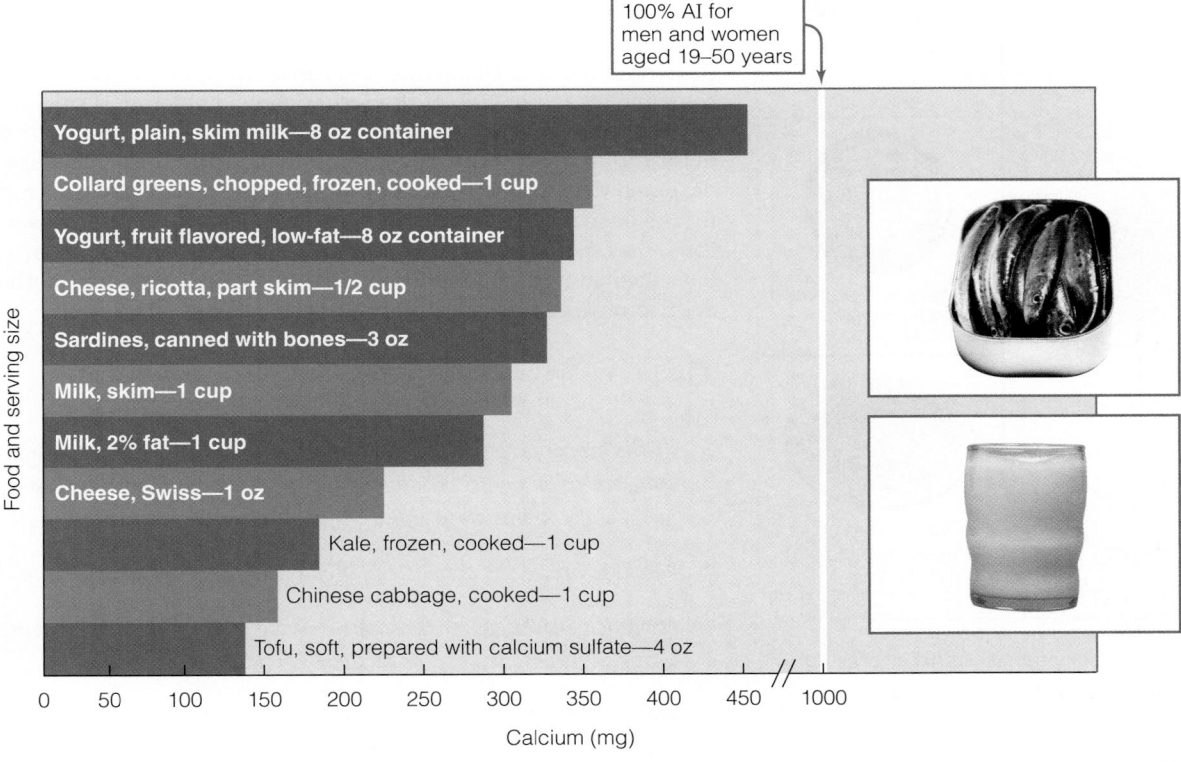

FIGURE 9.6 Common food sources of calcium. The AI for adult men and women aged 19 to 50 years is 1,000 mg of calcium per day. For men and women older than 50 years of age, the AI increases to 1,200 mg of calcium per day. (Nutrient data from U.S. Department of Agriculture, Agricultural Research Service, 2006, USDA Nutrient Database for Standard Reference, Release 19. Nutrient Data Laboratory Home Page, www.ars.usda.gov/ba/bhnrc/ndl.)

6 cups lima beans
1255 kcal

5.4 oz plain,
skim milk yogurt
86 kcal

1.4 oz Swiss cheese
151 kcal

2.8 oz canned sardines
165 kcal

9 oz tofu, soft prepared
with calcium
165 kcal

7/8 cup cooked collard
greens (from frozen)
54 kcal

8 fl. oz skim milk
306 mg Ca
83 kcal

FIGURE 9.7 Serving sizes and energy content of various foods that contain the same amount of calcium as an 8 fl. oz glass of skim milk.

Other good sources of calcium are green leafy vegetables such as kale, turnip greens, broccoli, cauliflower, green cabbage, brussels sprouts, and Chinese cabbage (bok choy). The bioavailability of the calcium in these vegetables is relatively high compared to spinach, as these vegetables contain low levels of oxalates. Many packaged foods are now available fortified with calcium. For example, you can buy calcium-fortified orange juice and soy milk, and tofu processed with calcium. Some dairies have even boosted the amount of calcium in their brand of milk! FIGURE 9.7 illustrates serving sizes of various calcium-rich foods that contain the equivalent amount of calcium as one glass (8 fl. oz) of skim milk. As you can see from this figure, a wide variety of foods can be consumed each day to contribute to adequate calcium intakes. When you are selecting foods that are good sources of calcium, it is important to remember that we do not absorb 100% of the calcium contained in our foods. For example, although a serving of milk contains approximately 300 mg of calcium, we do not actually absorb this entire amount into our bodies. To learn more about how calcium absorption rates vary for select foods, see the Nutrition Label Activity (page 373).

In general, meats and fish are not good sources of calcium. An exception is canned fish with bones (for example, sardines or salmon), providing you eat the bones. Fruits (except dried figs) and nonfortified grain products are also poor sources of calcium.

Although there are many foods in the U.S. diet that are good sources of calcium, many people in the United States do not consume adequate amounts because they consume very few dairy-based foods or other foods that are good sources of calcium. At particular risk are women and young girls. For example, a large national survey conducted by the U.S. Department of Agriculture found that teenage girls consume less than 60% of the recommended amount of calcium.[8]

There are now quick, simple tools available to assist individuals in determining their daily calcium intake. Most of these tools are designed to estimate a calcium intake score or to calculate calcium intake based on the types and amounts of calcium-rich foods a person consumes. See FIGURE 9.8 on page 372 for an example of an Internet-based calcium intake tool completed by Hannah and her mother to determine Hannah's calcium intake.

Tips for Increasing Your Calcium Intake

√ At the grocery store, stock up on calcium-fortified juice, soy milk, and rice milk. Look for single-serving portable "juice boxes" with calcium-fortified juice, milk, or chocolate milk.

√ Purchase breakfast cereals and breads that are fortified with calcium.

√ For quick snacks, purchase single-serving cups of yogurt, individually wrapped "cheese sticks," or calcium-fortified protein bars.

√ Keep on hand shredded parmesan or any hard cheese, and sprinkle it on hot soups, chili, salads, pasta, and other dishes.

√ In any recipe, replace sour cream or mayonnaise with nonfat plain yogurt.

√ Add nonfat dry milk powder to hot cereals, soups, chili, recipes for baked goods, coffee, and hot cocoa. One-third of a cup of nonfat dry milk powder provides the same amount of calcium as a whole cup of nonfat milk.

√ Make a yogurt smoothie by blending nonfat plain or flavored yogurt with fresh or frozen fruit.

√ At your favorite cafe, instead of a regular coffee or an espresso, order a skim milk latte.

√ At home, brew a strong cup of coffee, then add half a cup of warm milk for a café au lait.

√ When eating out, order milk instead of a soft drink with your meal.

√ If you do not consume enough dietary calcium, consider taking a calcium supplement. Refer to the Highlight box on page 374 to learn how to choose a calcium supplement that is right for you.

What Happens If We Consume Too Much Calcium?

In general, consuming too much calcium in the diet does not lead to significant toxicity symptoms in healthy individuals. Much of the excess calcium we consume is not absorbed from the intestine but instead is excreted in our urine and feces. However, excessive intake of calcium from supplements can lead to health problems. As mentioned earlier, one concern with consuming too much calcium is that it can lead to various mineral imbalances because calcium interferes with the absorption of other minerals, including iron, zinc, and magnesium. This interference may only be of major concern in individuals vulnerable to mineral imbalance, such as the elderly and people who consume very low amounts of minerals in their diets. In some people, the formation of kidney stones is associated with high intakes of calcium, oxalates, protein, and vegetable fiber.[9] However, more studies need to be done to determine whether high intakes of calcium actually cause kidney stones.

Various diseases and metabolic disorders can alter our ability to regulate blood calcium. **Hypercalcemia** is a condition in which our blood calcium levels reach abnormally high concentrations. Hypercalcemia can be caused by cancer and also by the overproduction of parathyroid hormone (PTH). As we noted earlier, PTH stimulates the osteoclasts to break down bone and release more calcium into the bloodstream. Symptoms of hypercalcemia include fatigue, loss of appetite, constipation, and mental confusion, and it can lead to coma and possibly death. Hypercalcemia can also result in an accumulation of calcium deposits in the soft tissues such as the liver and kidneys, causing failure of these organs.

What Happens If We Don't Consume Enough Calcium?

There are no short-term symptoms associated with consuming too little calcium. Even when we do not consume enough dietary calcium, our bodies continue to tightly regulate blood calcium levels by taking the calcium from bone. The long-term repercussion of inadequate calcium intake is osteoporosis. This disease is discussed in more detail beginning on page 388.

Hypocalcemia is a term that describes an abnormally low level of calcium in the blood. Hypocalcemia does not result from consuming too little dietary calcium, but is caused by various diseases. Some of the causes of hypocalcemia include kidney disease, vitamin D deficiency, and diseases that inhibit the production of PTH. Symptoms of hypocalcemia include muscle spasms and convulsions.

hypercalcemia A condition marked by an abnormally high concentration of calcium in the blood.

hypocalcemia A condition characterized by an abnormally low concentration of calcium in the blood.

FIGURE 9.8 This graphic illustrates the results of a calcium intake quiz that Hannah completed with her mother. As you can see, Hannah did not meet her recommended calcium intake. To try this quiz yourself, go to www.dairycouncilofca.org/Tools/CalciumQuiz/Default.aspx. (© 2005. Reprinted with permission by the Dairy Council of California.)

search _____ [Go]

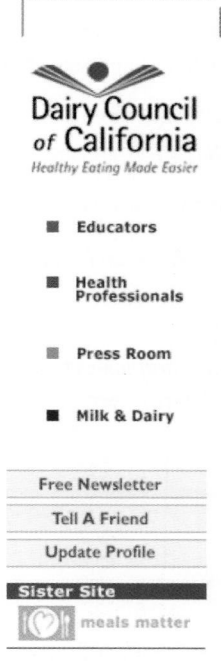

Dairy Council
of California
Healthy Eating Made Easier

- **Educators**
- **Health Professionals**
- **Press Room**
- **Milk & Dairy**

Free Newsletter
Tell A Friend
Update Profile

Sister Site
meals matter

home | about us | site map | order materials | FAQ | tools | newsletter

Learning Tools

Calcium Quiz (Ca) *what's your calcium intake?*

Name: Hannah

Gender: ○ Male ● Female

Status: ☐ Pregnant ☐ Nursing
(Check, if applicable.)

Age: 9 to 13 years ▼

Are you taking a calcium supplement daily?
○ Yes ● No

Think about **what you ate yesterday** at breakfast, lunch, dinner, and snacks. Click on each item that you ate in the List of Foods and enter the number of servings you had of that item.
Please enter servings in decimals, e.g., 1 serving or 2.5 servings.

Here is what you checked....

Item	No. of Servings	mg/Serving	Total mg
Chocolate milk (whole, low-fat or nonfat)	1.00	284	284.00
Cheese (Cheddar/ Monterey Jack types)	2.00	280	560.00
Pudding	1.00	153	153.00
Ice cream	3.00	85	255.00

Hannah, you didn't quite meet your calcium requirement yesterday.

Your Intake: ▇▇▇▇ 1,252 mg.

Recommended: ▇▇▇▇ 1,300 mg.

mg.   1,300   2500 +

To meet your calcium needs, you need 48 mg. more calcium

This is equivalent to: 0.5 more serving(s) of calcium-rich (300 mg/serving) foods every day. An easy way to make sure you are getting enough calcium is to consume at least 3 servings of dairy foods every day.

> **RECAP:** *Calcium is the most abundant mineral in the human body and a significant component of our bones. Calcium is necessary for normal nerve and muscle function, and blood calcium is maintained within a very narrow range. If dietary intake is inadequate, the body will use bone calcium to maintain normal blood calcium levels. Dairy products, canned fish with bones, and some green leafy vegetables are good sources of calcium. The most common long-term effect of inadequate calcium consumption is osteoporosis.*

Vitamin D

Vitamin D is like other fat-soluble vitamins in that we store excess amounts in the liver and adipose tissue. But vitamin D is different from other nutrients in two ways. First, vitamin D does not always need to come from the diet. This is because

NUTRITION LABEL ACTIVITY

How Much Calcium Am I Really Consuming?

As you have learned in this chapter, we do not absorb 100% of the calcium contained in our foods. This is particularly true for individuals who eat a diet predominated by foods that are high in fiber, oxalates, and phytates, such as whole grains and certain vegetables. Thus, it is important to understand how the rate of calcium absorption differs for various foods as you design an eating plan that contains adequate calcium to optimize bone health.

How do you determine the amount of calcium you are absorbing from various foods? Unfortunately, the absorption rate of calcium has not been determined for most foods. However, estimates have been established for a variety of common foods that are considered good sources of calcium. The table in the next column shows some of these foods, their calcium content per serving, the calcium absorption rate, and the estimated amount of calcium absorbed from each food.

As you can see from this table, many dairy products have a similar calcium absorption rate, just over 30%. Interestingly, many green leafy vegetables have a higher absorption rate of around 60%; however, because many times a serving of these foods contains less calcium than dairy foods, you would have to eat more vegetables to get the same calcium as you would from a standard serving of dairy foods. Note the relatively low calcium absorption rate for spinach, even though it contains a relatively high amount of calcium.

Remember that the DRIs for calcium take these differences in absorption rate into account. Thus, the 300 mg of calcium in a glass of milk counts as 300 mg toward your daily calcium goal. In general, you can trust that dairy products such as milk and yogurt (but not cottage cheese) are good, absorbable sources of calcium, as are some dark green leafy vegetables. Other good sources of calcium with good absorp-

tion rates include calcium-fortified orange juice, tofu processed with calcium, and fortified breakfast cereals such as Total and Special K.[10] Armed with this knowledge, you will be better able to select food sources that can optimize your calcium intake and support bone health.

Food	Serving Size	Calcium per Serving (mg)*	Absorption Rate (%)†	Estimated Amount of Calcium Absorbed (mg)
Yogurt, plain skim milk	8 fl. oz	488	32	156
Milk, 2%	1 cup	314	32	100
Milk, skim	1 cup	306	32	98
Kale, frozen, cooked	1 cup	179	59	106
Turnip greens, boiled	1 cup	197	52	103
Broccoli, frozen, chopped, cooked	1 cup	61	61	37
Cauliflower, boiled	1 cup	20	69	14
Spinach, frozen, cooked	1 cup	291	5	14

Sources: *U.S. Department of Agriculture, Agricultural Research Service. 2006. USDA National Nutrient Database for Standard Reference, Release 19. www.ars.usda.gov/ba/bhnrc/ndl. †Weaver, C. M., W. R. Proulx, and R. Heaney. 1999. Choices for achieving adequate dietary calcium with a vegetarian diet. *Am. J. Clin. Nutr.* 70(suppl.):543S–548S; Weaver, C. M., and K. L. Plawecki. 1994. Dietary calcium: adequacy of a vegetarian diet. *Am. J. Clin. Nutr.* 59(suppl.):1238S–1241S.

our bodies can synthesize vitamin D using energy from exposure to sunlight. However, when we do not get enough sunlight, we must consume vitamin D in our diet. Second, in addition to being a nutrient, vitamin D is considered a *hormone* because it is made in one part of the body, yet regulates various activities in other parts of the body.

FIGURE 9.9 illustrates how our body makes vitamin D by converting a cholesterol compound in our skin to the active form of vitamin D that we need to function properly. When the ultraviolet rays of the sun hit our skin, they react with 7-dehydrocholesterol. This cholesterol compound is converted into a precursor of vitamin D, cholecalciferol, which is also called provitamin D_3. This inactive form is

HIGHLIGHT

Calcium Supplements: Which Ones Are Best?

We know that calcium is a critical nutrient for bone health. Ideally, people should try to consume the recommended amount of calcium in their daily diet. Now that so many products are calcium-fortified, from cereals and energy bars to orange juice and soy milk, it is not difficult even for vegans to get sufficient calcium from the diet. Still, small or inactive people who need less energy to maintain a healthful weight may not be able to consume enough food to provide adequate calcium, and elderly people may need more calcium than they can obtain in their normal diets. In these circumstances, calcium supplements may be warranted.

An abundance of calcium supplements are available to consumers, but which ones are best? Most supplements come in the form of calcium carbonate, calcium citrate, calcium lactate, or calcium phosphate. Our bodies are able to absorb about 30% of the calcium from these various forms. Calcium citrate malate, which is the form of calcium used in fortified juices, is slightly more absorbable at 35%. Many antacids are also good sources of calcium, and it appears these are safe to take as long as you only consume enough to get the recommended level of calcium.

What is the most cost-effective form of calcium? In general, supplements that contain calcium carbonate tend to have more calcium per pill than other types. Thus, you are getting more calcium for your money when you buy this type. However, be sure to read the label of any calcium supplement you are considering taking to determine just how much calcium it contains. Some very expensive calcium supplements do not contain a lot of calcium per pill, and you could be wasting your money. Often, chelated forms of calcium supplements are touted as the best supplements available. Chelate refers to a claw-shaped protein that protects the calcium. Chelated calcium is easier to absorb, as the chelate protects the calcium from inhibitors such as phytates and oxalates that can bind with calcium in our intestine and make it harder to absorb. However, chelated calcium products are typically much more expensive and improve the absorption of calcium only by about 5–10%.

The lead content of calcium supplements is an important public health concern. Calcium supplements made from "natural" sources such as oyster shell, bone meal, and dolomite are known to be higher in lead. In fact, many of these products can contain dangerously high levels of lead and should be avoided. We have typically considered calcium supplements that include refined sources of calcium carbonate to be very low in lead. However, a recent study conducted on twenty-two calcium supplements found that eight (or 36%) of the supplements tested were unacceptably high in lead; this was true for oyster shell supplements and refined calcium carbonate.[11] Shockingly, the supplement with the highest lead content was a popular, nationally recognized brand name supplement!

How can we avoid taking supplements that contain too much lead? Unfortunately, the lead content of supplements is not reported on the label. However, there are some supplements available that claim to be lead-free; in the study by Ross et al., the supplements claiming to be lead-free were found to have no detectable levels of lead.[11] In addition, most supplements not made from oyster shell and other natural products are generally very low in lead. Look for the words "purified" on the label, and make sure the label contains the U.S.P. (U.S. Pharmacopoeia) symbol.

How should we take our supplements? Remember that our bodies cannot absorb more than 500 mg of calcium at any given time. Thus, taking a supplement that contains 1,000 mg will be no more effective than one that contains 500 mg calcium. If at all possible, try to consume calcium supplements in small doses throughout the day. In addition, we absorb calcium better with meals, as the calcium stays in our intestinal tract longer during a meal and more calcium can be absorbed. However, it is better to take one calcium supplement outside of meals than to do nothing.

By consuming foods high in calcium every day, we can minimize our need for calcium supplements. When we cannot consume enough calcium in our diets, there are many inexpensive, safe, and effective supplements available. The best supplement for you is the one that you can tolerate, is affordable, and is readily available when you need it.

FIGURE 9.9 The process of converting sunlight into vitamin D in our skin. When the ultraviolet rays of the sun hit our skin, they react with 7-dehydrocholesterol. This compound is converted to cholecalciferol, an inactive form of vitamin D also called provitamin D_3. Cholecalciferol is then converted to calcidiol in the liver. Calcidiol travels to the kidney where it is converted into calcitriol, which is considered the primary active form of vitamin D in our bodies.

then converted to calcidiol in the liver. Calcidiol travels to the kidney where it is converted into **calcitriol,** which is considered the primary active form of vitamin D in our bodies. Calcitriol then circulates to various parts of the body, performing its many functions.

Functions of Vitamin D

Vitamin D, PTH, and another hormone called *calcitonin* all work together continuously to regulate blood calcium levels, which in turn maintains bone health. They do this by regulating the absorption of calcium and phosphorus from the small intestine, causing more to be absorbed when our needs for them are higher and less when our needs are lower. They also decrease or increase blood calcium levels by signaling the kidneys to excrete more or less calcium in our urine. Finally, vitamin D works with PTH to stimulate osteoclasts to break down bone when calcium is needed elsewhere in the body.

Vitamin D is also necessary for the normal calcification of bone; this means it assists the process by which minerals such as calcium and phosphorus are crystallized. Vitamin D may also play some role in decreasing the formation of some cancerous tumors, as it can prevent certain types of cells from growing out of control. Similar to vitamin A, vitamin D appears to play a role in cell differentiation in various tissues. A review of the functions, recommended intakes, and toxicity and deficiency symptoms associated with vitamin D is provided in Table 9.3 on page 378.

How Much Vitamin D Should We Consume?

If your exposure to the sun is adequate, then you do not need to consume any vitamin D in your diet. How do you know whether or not you are getting enough sun?

Recommended Dietary Intake for Vitamin D. As with calcium, there is no RDA for vitamin D. The AI is based on the assumption that an individual does not get adequate sun exposure. Of the many factors that affect our ability to synthesize

calcitriol The primary active form of vitamin D in the body.

Vitamin D synthesis from the sun is not possible during most of the winter months for people living in high latitudes. Therefore, many people around the world, such as this couple in Russia, need to consume vitamin D in their diets, particularly during the winter.

vitamin D from sunlight, latitude and time of year are the most significant (Table 9.2). Individuals living in very sunny climates relatively close to the equator, such as the southern United States and Mexico, may synthesize enough vitamin D from the sun to meet their needs throughout the year—as long as they spend time outdoors. However, vitamin D synthesis from the sun is not possible during most of the winter months for people living in places located at a latitude of more than 40°N or more than 40°S. This is because at these latitudes the sun never rises high enough in the sky during the winter to provide the direct sunlight needed. The 40°N latitude runs like a belt across the United States from northern Pennsylvania in the east to northern California in the west (FIGURE 9.10). Thus, people living in New England, New York, the Great Lakes region, or the upper Midwestern to Pacific Northwestern states need to consume vitamin D in the winter. In addition, entire countries such as Canada and the United Kingdom are affected, as of course are countries in the far southern hemisphere. Thus, there are many people around the world who need to consume vitamin D in their diets, particularly during the winter months.

Other factors influencing vitamin D synthesis include time of day, age, level of exposure, and obesity status. More vitamin D can be synthesized during the time of day when the sun's rays are strongest, generally between 9 AM and 3 PM. Vitamin D synthesis is severely limited or may be nonexistent on overcast days. Individuals with darker skin have a more difficult time synthesizing vitamin D from the sun than do light-skinned people. In addition, it is estimated that people 65 years of age

TABLE 9.2   Factors Affecting Sunlight-Mediated Synthesis of Vitamin D in the Skin

Factors That Enhance Synthesis of Vitamin D	Factors That Inhibit Synthesis of Vitamin D
Season—Most vitamin D is produced during summer months, particularly June and July	Season—Winter months (October through February) result in little or no vitamin D production
Latitude—Locations closer to the equator get more sunlight throughout the year	Latitude—Locations that are more north of 40°N and more south than 40°S get inadequate sun
Time of day—Generally between the hours of 9 AM and 3 PM (dependent upon latitude and time of year)	Time of day—Early morning, late afternoon, and evening hours
Age—Younger age	Age—Older age, particularly elderly (due to reduced skin thickness with age)
Limited or no use of sunscreen	Use of sunscreen with SPF 8 or greater
Sunny weather	Cloudy weather
Exposed skin	Clothing or dark skin pigmentation
	Glass and plastics—Windows or other barriers made of glass or plastic (such as Plexiglas) block the sun's rays
	Obesity—May negatively impact metabolism and storage of vitamin D

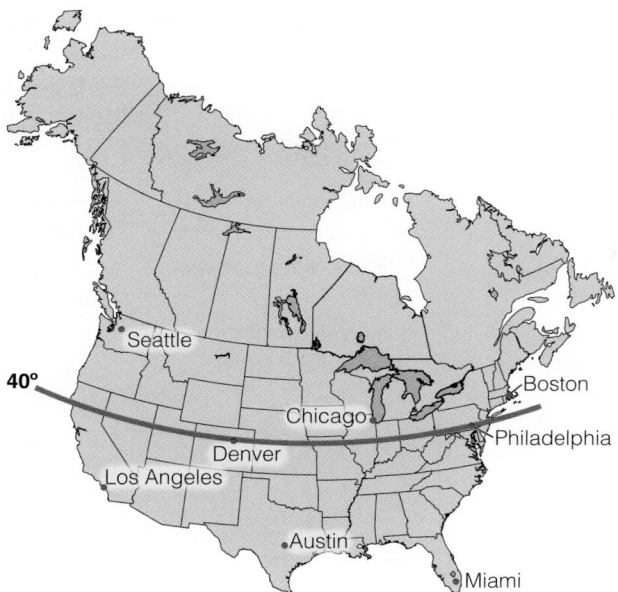

FIGURE 9.10   This map illustrates the geographical location of 40° latitude in the United States. In southern cities below 40° latitude such as Los Angeles, CA; Austin, TX; and Miami, FL, the sunlight is strong enough to allow for vitamin D synthesis throughout the year. In northern cities above 40° latitude such as Seattle, WA; Chicago, IL; and Boston, MA, the sunlight is too weak from about mid-October to mid-March to allow for adequate vitamin D synthesis.

or older experience a fourfold decrease in their capacity to synthesize vitamin D from the sun.[12,13] Obesity is associated with lower levels of circulating vitamin D, possibly due to lower bioavailability of cholecalciferol from adipose tissue, decreased exposure to sunlight due to limited mobility or time spent outdoors with skin exposed, and alterations in vitamin D metabolism in the liver.[14,15] Wearing protective clothing and sunscreen (with an SPF greater than 8) limits sun exposure, so it is suggested that we expose our hands, face, and arms to the sun two to three times per week for a period of time that is one-third to one-half of the amount needed to get sunburned.[16] This means that if you normally sunburn in 1 hour, you should expose yourself to the sun for 20 to 30 minutes two to three times per week to synthesize adequate amounts of vitamin D. Again, this guideline does not apply to people living in more northern climates during the winter months; they can only get enough vitamin D by consuming it in their diet.

Because not everyone is able to get adequate sun exposure throughout the year, an AI has been established for vitamin D (see Table 9.3). Recently, nutrition and bone health experts have called for a reevaluation of these recommendations, as much new information about vitamin D metabolism and requirements has been published since the Institute of Medicine set them in 1997.[17,18] These experts suggest that current recommendations are inadequate and that some individuals may require more than the current UL of 50 µg to maintain sufficient levels of circulating vitamin D.

When reading labels, you will see the amount of vitamin D expressed on food and supplement labels in units of either µg or IU. For conversion purposes, 1 µg of vitamin D is equal to 40 IU of vitamin D.

TABLE 9.3 Functions, Recommended Intakes (RDA), Tolerable Upper Intake Levels (UL), and Toxicity and Deficiency Symptoms of Nutrients Essential to Bone Health

Nutrient	Primary Functions	Recommended Intake	Toxicity Symptoms or Related Diseases	Deficiency Symptoms or Related Diseases
Calcium (major mineral)	Primary component of bone and teeth structure Helps maintain optimal acid–base balance Maintains normal nerve transmission Supports muscle contraction and relaxation Regulates blood pressure, blood clotting, and various hormones and enzymes	Adequate Intake (AI): Men and women 19 to 50 years = 1,000 mg/day Men and women > 50 years = 1,200 mg/day UL: 2.5 g/day	Potential mineral imbalances; calcium can interfere with absorption of iron, zinc, and magnesium; shock; kidney failure; fatigue; mental confusion	Osteoporosis: Bone fractures; convulsions and muscle spasms; heart failure; bleeder's disease
Vitamin D (fat-soluble vitamin)	Regulates blood calcium levels Maintains bone health Cell differentiation	AI*: Men and women 19 to 50 = 5 μg/day Men and women 50 to 70 = 10 μg/day Men and women > 70 = 15 μg/day UL: 50 μg/day	Hypercalcemia, including weakness, loss of appetite, diarrhea, mental confusion, vomiting, excessive urine output, extreme thirst, and formation of calcium deposits in kidney, liver, and heart Increased bone loss	Rickets (in children), leading to bone weakness and deformities Osteomalacia (in adults), leading to bone weakness and increased rate of fractures Osteoporosis, leading to increased rate of fractures
Vitamin K (fat-soluble vitamin)	Serves as a coenzyme during production of specific proteins that assist in blood coagulation and bone metabolism	AI: Men = 120 μg/day Women = 90 μg/day	No known side effects or toxicity symptoms from consuming excess vitamin K	Reduced ability to form blood clots, leading to excessive bleeding and easy bruising Effect on bone health is controversial
Phosphorus (major mineral)	Part of hydroxyapatite crystals, which are the mineral complex of bone Assists in maintaining fluid balance Primary component of ATP Helps activate and inactivate enzymes Component of DNA and RNA Component of cell membranes and lipoproteins	Recommended Dietary Allowance (RDA): Men and women = 700 mg/day UL: 4 g/day	High blood phosphorus levels, causing muscle spasms and convulsions	Low blood phosphorus levels, causing dizziness, bone pain, muscle weakness, and muscle damage

*Based on the assumption that a person does not get adequate sun exposure.

TABLE 9.3 Functions, Recommended Intakes (RDA), Tolerable Upper Intake Levels (UL), and Toxicity and Deficiency Symptoms of Nutrients Essential to Bone Health (continued)

Nutrient	Primary Functions	Recommended Intake	Toxicity Symptoms or Related Diseases	Deficiency Symptoms or Related Diseases
Magnesium (major mineral)	An essential component of bone tissue Influences formation of hydroxyapatite crystals and bone growth Cofactor for more than 300 enzyme systems, including ATP, DNA, and protein synthesis, vitamin D metabolism and action Supports muscle contraction and blood clotting	RDA: Men 19 to 30 = 400 mg/day Men > 30 = 420 mg/day Women 19 to 30 = 310 mg/day Women > 30 = 320 mg/day UL: 350 mg/day	No known toxicity symptoms of consuming excess in diet Toxicity from pharmacological use includes diarrhea, nausea, abdominal cramps; in severe cases, massive dehydration, cardiac arrest, and death can result	Hypomagnesemia, resulting in low blood calcium levels, muscle cramps, spasms or seizures, nausea, weakness, irritability, and confusion Chronic diseases such as heart disease, high blood pressure, osteoporosis, and type 2 diabetes
Fluoride (trace mineral)	Maintains health of teeth and bones Protects teeth against dental caries Stimulates new bone growth	AI: Men = 4 mg/day Women = 3 mg/day UL: 10 mg/day	Teeth fluorosis, which causes staining and pitting of teeth Skeletal fluorosis, which ranges from mild to severe; causes joint pain and stiffness, and in extreme cases can cause crippling, wasting of muscles, and osteoporosis of the extremities	High occurrence of dental caries and tooth decay Low fluoride intakes may also be associated with lower bone density

SHOPPER'S GUIDE
Good Food Sources of Vitamin D

There are many forms of vitamin D, but only two are active in our bodies. These two forms are vitamin D_2, also called **ergocalciferol,** and vitamin D_3, or **cholecalciferol.** Vitamin D_2 is found exclusively in plant foods, whereas vitamin D_3 is found in animal foods and is also the form of vitamin D we synthesize from the sun.

Most foods naturally contain very little vitamin D. Thus, our primary source of vitamin D in the diet is from fortified foods such as milk (FIGURE 9.11). In the United States, milk is fortified with 10 μg of vitamin D per quart. Because earlier studies examining the actual vitamin D content of fortified milk found that the amount of vitamin D varied widely, the USDA now monitors dairies to make sure they meet the mandated vitamin D fortification guidelines.

Fatty fish contain vitamin D.

ergocalciferol Vitamin D_2, a form of vitamin D found exclusively in plant foods.

cholecalciferol Vitamin D_3, a form of vitamin D found in animal foods and the form we synthesize from the sun.

FIGURE 9.11 Common food sources of vitamin D. For men and women aged 19 to 50 years, the AI for vitamin D is 5 µg per day. The AI for vitamin D for men and women aged 50 to 70 years is 10 µg per day, and the AI increases to 15 µg per day for adults over the age of 70 years. (Nutrient data from U.S. Department of Agriculture, Agricultural Research Service, 2006, USDA Nutrient Database for Standard Reference, Release 19. Nutrient Data Laboratory Home Page, www.ars.usda.gov/ba/bhnrc/ndl.)

Green leafy vegetables, including brussels sprouts and turnip greens, are good sources of vitamin K.

Other foods that contain high amounts of vitamin D include cod liver oil, fatty fish (such as salmon, mackerel, and sardines), and certain fortified cereals. Eggs, butter, some margarines, and liver contain small amounts of vitamin D, but we would have to eat very large amounts of these foods to consume enough vitamin D. In addition, since plants contain very little vitamin D, vegetarians who consume no dairy products need to obtain their vitamin D from sun exposure, fortified soy or cereal products, or supplements.

What Happens If We Consume Too Much Vitamin D?

We cannot get too much vitamin D from sun exposure, as our skin has the ability to limit its production, nor from food intake, since the level of vitamin D naturally found in foods is low. Thus, the only way we can consume too much vitamin D is through supplementation.

Consuming too much vitamin D causes hypercalcemia, or high blood calcium concentrations. As discussed in the section on calcium, symptoms of hypercalcemia include weakness, loss of appetite, constipation, mental confusion, vomiting, excessive urine output, and extreme thirst. Hypercalcemia also leads to the formation of calcium deposits in soft tissues such as the kidney, liver, and heart. In addition, toxic levels of vitamin D lead to increased bone loss because calcium is then pulled from the bones and excreted more readily from the kidneys.

What Happens If We Don't Consume Enough Vitamin D?

The primary deficiency associated with inadequate vitamin D is loss of bone mass. In fact, when vitamin D levels are inadequate, our intestines can only absorb 10–15% of the calcium we consume. Vitamin D deficiencies occur most often in individuals who have diseases that cause intestinal malabsorption of fat and thus the fat-soluble vitamins. People with liver disease, kidney disease, Crohn's disease, celiac disease, cystic fibrosis, or Whipple's disease commonly suffer from vitamin D deficiency and require supplements.

Vitamin D deficiency disease in children, called **rickets,** is caused by inadequate mineralization or demineralization of the skeleton. The symptoms of rickets include deformities of the skeleton such as bowed legs and knocked knees (FIGURE 9.12). Rickets is not common in the United States because of fortification of milk products with vitamin D. However, it is still a significant nutritional problem for children outside of the United States.

Vitamin D deficiency disease in adults is called **osteomalacia,** a term meaning "soft bones." With osteomalacia, bones become weak and prone to fractures. Osteoporosis, discussed in detail later in the chapter (page 388), can also result from a vitamin D deficiency.

Vitamin D deficiencies have recently been found to be more common among American adults than previously thought. This may be partly due to jobs and lifestyle choices that keep us indoors for most of the day. Not surprisingly, the population at greatest risk is older institutionalized individuals who get little or no sun exposure. Individuals who work at night and darker skinned individuals living in polluted northern cities are also at higher risk due to low sun exposure.

Various medications can also alter the metabolism and activity of vitamin D. For instance, glucocorticoids, which are medications used to reduce inflammation, can cause bone loss by inhibiting our ability to absorb calcium through the actions of vitamin D. Antiseizure medications such as phenobarbital and Dilantin alter vitamin D metabolism. Thus, people who are taking such medications may need to increase their vitamin D intake.

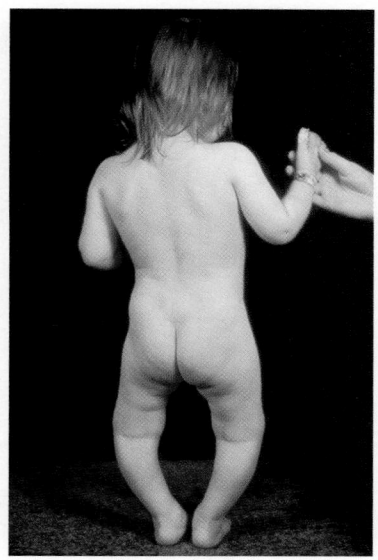

FIGURE 9.12 A vitamin D deficiency causes a bone-deforming disease in children called rickets.

RECAP: *Vitamin D is a fat-soluble vitamin and a hormone. The body can synthesize vitamin D when sunlight hits 7-dehydrocholesterol in our skin. Vitamin D regulates blood calcium levels and maintains bone health. Foods contain little vitamin D, with fortified milk being the primary source. Vitamin D toxicity causes hypercalcemia. Vitamin D deficiency causes poor bone density.*

Vitamin K

Vitamin K, a fat-soluble vitamin stored primarily in the liver, is actually a family of compounds known as quinones. **Phylloquinone** is the plant form of vitamin K, while **menaquinone** is the form of vitamin K produced by bacteria found in our large intestine.

Functions of Vitamin K

The primary function of vitamin K is to serve as a coenzyme during the production of specific proteins that play important roles in the coagulation of our blood and in bone metabolism. A **coenzyme** is an organic compound that combines with an inactive enzyme to form an active enzyme. In the case of vitamin K, it assists in the production of *prothrombin,* a protein that plays a critical role in the clotting of our blood. It also assists in the production of *osteocalcin,* a protein that is associated with bone turnover. A summary of the functions, recommended intakes, and toxicity and deficiency symptoms associated with vitamin K is provided in Table 9.3 (pages 378–379).

How Much Vitamin K Should We Consume?

We can obtain vitamin K from our diets, and we also produce vitamin K in our large intestine. These two sources of vitamin K usually provide adequate amounts of this nutrient to maintain health, and there is no RDA or UL for vitamin K. AI recommendations are listed in Table 9.3.

Only a few foods contribute substantially to our dietary intake of vitamin K. Green leafy vegetables including spinach, collard greens, turnip greens, and lettuce are good sources, as are broccoli, brussels sprouts, and cabbage. Vegetable oils, such as soybean oil and canola oil, are also good sources of vitamin K. FIGURE 9.13 identifies the amount of vitamin K in micrograms per serving for these foods.

rickets Vitamin D deficiency disease in children. Symptoms include deformities of the skeleton such as bowed legs and knocked knees.

osteomalacia Vitamin D deficiency disease in adults, in which bones become weak and prone to fractures.

phylloquinone The form of vitamin K found in plants.

menaquinone The form of vitamin K produced by bacteria in the large intestine.

coenzyme An organic compound that combines with an inactive enzyme to form an active enzyme.

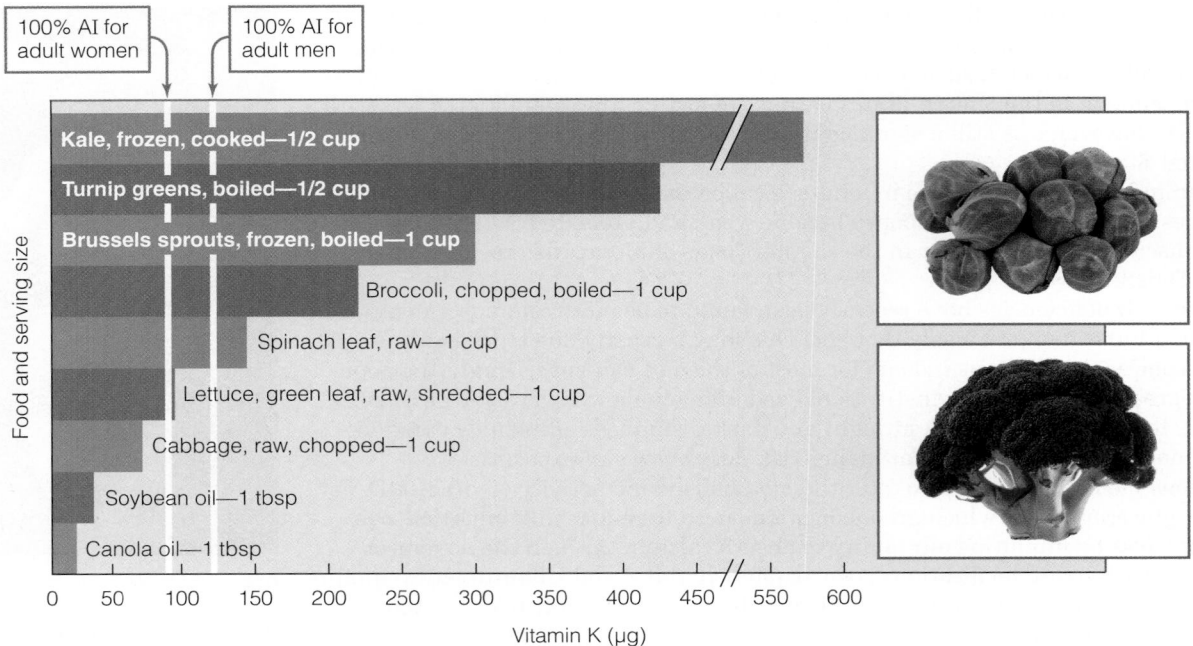

FIGURE 9.13 Common food sources of vitamin K. The AIs for adult men and adult women are 120 μg per day and 90 μg per day, respectively. (Nutrient data from U.S. Department of Agriculture, Agricultural Research Service, 2006, USDA Nutrient Database for Standard Reference, Release 19. Nutrient Data Laboratory Home Page, www.ars.usda.gov/ba/bhnrc/ndl.)

What Happens If We Consume Too Much Vitamin K?

Based on our present knowledge, for healthy individuals there appear to be no side effects associated with consuming large amounts of vitamin K.[19] This appears to be true for both supplements and food sources. In the past, a synthetic form of vitamin K was used for therapeutic purposes and was shown to cause liver damage; thus, this form is no longer used.

What Happens If We Don't Consume Enough Vitamin K?

Vitamin K deficiency is associated with a reduced ability to form blood clots, leading to excessive bleeding; however, primary vitamin K deficiency is rare in humans. People with diseases that cause malabsorption of fat, such as celiac disease, Crohn's disease, and cystic fibrosis, can suffer secondarily from a deficiency of vitamin K. Newborns are typically given an injection of vitamin K at birth, as they lack the intestinal bacteria necessary to produce this nutrient.

The impact of vitamin K deficiency on bone health is controversial. A recent study of vitamin K intake and risk of hip fractures found that women who consumed the least amount of vitamin K had a higher risk of bone fractures than women who consumed relatively more vitamin K.[20] Despite the results of this study, there is not enough scientific evidence to support the contention that vitamin K deficiency leads to osteoporosis.[19] In fact, there is no significant impact on overall bone density in people who take anticoagulant medications that result in a relative state of vitamin K deficiency.

> RECAP: *Vitamin K is a fat-soluble vitamin and coenzyme that is important for blood clotting and bone metabolism. We obtain vitamin K largely from bacteria in our large intestine. Green leafy vegetables and vegetable oils contain vitamin K. There are no known toxicity symptoms for vitamin K in healthy individuals. Vitamin K deficiency is rare and may lead to excessive bleeding.*

Phosphorus

As discussed in Chapter 7, phosphorus is the major intracellular negatively charged electrolyte. In our bodies, phosphorus is most commonly found combined with oxygen in the form of phosphate (or PO_4^{3-}). Phosphorus is an essential constituent of all cells and is found in both plants and animals.

Functions of Phosphorus

Phosphorus plays a critical role in bone formation, as it is a part of the mineral complex of bone. As discussed earlier in this chapter, calcium and phosphorus crystallize to form hydroxyapatite crystals, which provide the hardness of bone. About 85% of our body's phosphorus is stored in our bones, with the rest stored in soft tissues such as muscles and organs.

The role of phosphorus in maintaining proper fluid balance was discussed in detail in Chapter 7. Phosphorus is also a primary component of adenosine triphosphate (ATP), the energy molecule that fuels body functions. It helps activate and deactivate enzymes, is a component of the genetic material in the nuclei of our cells (including both DNA and RNA), and is a component of our cell membranes and lipoproteins. A summary of the functions, recommended intakes, and toxicity and deficiency symptoms associated with phosphorus is provided in Table 9.3 (pages 378–379).

Phosphorus, in the form of phosphoric acid, is a major component of soft drinks.

How Much Phosphorus Should We Consume?

The details of phosphorus recommendations, food sources, and deficiency and toxicity symptoms were discussed in Chapter 7 (pages 288–289). In general, phosphorus is widespread in many foods and is found in high amounts in foods that contain protein. Milk, meats, and eggs are good sources. Refer to FIGURE 7.10 (page 289) for a review of the phosphorus content of various foods.

Phosphorus is also found in many processed foods as a food additive, where it enhances smoothness, binding, and moisture retention. In the form of phosphoric acid, it is also a major component of soft drinks. Phosphoric acid is added to soft drinks to give them a sharper, or more tart, flavor and to slow the growth of molds and bacteria. Our society has increased its consumption of processed foods and soft drinks substantially over the past 20 years, resulting in an estimated 10–15% increase in phosphorus consumption.[7]

Nutrition and medical professionals have become increasingly concerned that the heavy consumption of soft drinks may be detrimental to bone health. Studies have shown that consuming soft drinks is associated with reduced bone mass or an increased risk of fractures in both youth and adults.[21–23] Researchers have proposed the following three theories to explain why consumption of soft drinks may be detrimental to bone health:

- Consuming soft drinks in place of calcium-containing beverages, such as milk, leads to a deficient intake of calcium.

- The acidic properties and high phosphorus content of soft drinks cause an increased loss of calcium because calcium is drawn from bone into the blood to neutralize the excess acid.

- The caffeine found in many soft drinks causes increased calcium loss through the urine.

A recent study of this problem tried to tease out which component of soft drinks may be detrimental to bone health.[24] Four different carbonated soft drinks were tested: two that contained phosphoric acid and two that contained citric acid. Two of these drinks also contained caffeine and two did not. Calcium loss was measured as the amount of calcium excreted in the participants' urine. Interestingly, the results showed that the contents of soft drinks had little effect on calcium status. Although the two beverages that contained caffeine caused some loss of calcium during the

5-hour testing period, this effect of caffeine on calcium tended to taper off throughout the day and night, leading to no overall impact on calcium status over a 24-hour period. The researchers concluded that the most likely explanation for the link between soft drink consumption and poor bone health is the *milk-displacement effect;* that is, soft drinks take the place of milk in our diets, depriving us of calcium and vitamin D. Additional nutritional and lifestyle factors that affect bone health are discussed later in this chapter (pages 390–391).

What Happens If We Consume Too Much Phosphorus?

As discussed in Chapter 7, people with kidney disease and those who take too many vitamin D supplements or too many phosphorus-containing antacids can suffer from high blood phosphorus levels; severely high levels of blood phosphorus can cause muscle spasms and convulsions.

What Happens If We Don't Consume Enough Phosphorus?

Phosphorus deficiencies are rare but can occur in people who abuse alcohol, in premature infants, and in elderly people with poor diets. People with vitamin D deficiency, people with hyperparathyroidism (oversecretion of parathyroid hormone), and those who overuse antacids that bind with phosphorus may also have low blood phosphorus levels.

> RECAP: *Phosphorus is the major negatively charged electrolyte inside of the cell. It helps maintain fluid balance and bone health. It also assists in regulating chemical reactions, and it is a primary component of ATP, DNA, and RNA. Phosphorus is commonly found in high-protein foods. Excess phosphorus can lead to muscle spasms and convulsions, while phosphorus deficiencies are rare.*

NUTRI-CASE HANNAH

" They only sell milk and bottled water in my school's vending machines. Some kids buy it, but not me or my friends. As soon as school's out, we go to the market across the street and buy our sodas and snacks there. Diet cola doesn't have any calories, and it tastes a whole lot better than water or milk!"

From what you know about Hannah, is her habit of drinking a diet cola after school a problem? Why or why not? Imagine that you were her nutrition teacher: what arguments could you use to try to persuade her and her friends to buy a carton of plain or chocolate milk instead of a diet cola?

Magnesium

Magnesium is a major mineral. Our total body magnesium content is approximately 25 g. About 50–60% of the body's magnesium is found in our bones, with the rest located in our soft tissues.

Functions of Magnesium

Magnesium is one of the minerals that make up the structure of bone. It is also important in the regulation of bone and mineral status. Specifically, magnesium influences the formation of hydroxyapatite crystals through its regulation of calcium balance and its interactions with vitamin D and parathyroid hormone.

Magnesium is a critical *cofactor* for more than 300 enzyme systems. A **cofactor** is a compound that is needed for an enzyme to be active. As discussed earlier in this book, a coenzyme is an organic compound that combines with an enzyme to make it active. The term *cofactor* refers to both organic compounds (coenzymes) and inorganic compounds (such as minerals) that combine with enzymes to make them active. Magnesium is necessary for the production of ATP, and it plays an important role in DNA and protein synthesis. Magnesium supports normal vitamin D metabolism and action and is necessary for normal muscle contraction and blood clotting. A review of the functions, recommended intakes, and toxicity and deficiency symptoms associated with magnesium is provided in Table 9.3 (pages 378–379).

How Much Magnesium Should We Consume?

As magnesium is found in a wide variety of foods, people who are adequately nourished generally consume adequate amounts in their diet. The RDA for magnesium is identified in Table 9.3.

Magnesium is found in green leafy vegetables such as spinach. It is also found in whole grains, seeds, and nuts. Other good food sources of magnesium include seafood, beans, and some dairy products. FIGURE 9.14 shows many foods that are good sources of magnesium. Refined and processed foods are low in magnesium.

The magnesium content of drinking water varies considerably. The "harder" the water, the higher its content of magnesium. This variability makes it impossible to estimate how much our drinking water may contribute to the magnesium content of our diets.

Trail mix with chocolate chips, nuts, and seeds is one common food source of magnesium.

cofactor Any organic or inorganic compound that combines with an enzyme to make that enzyme active.

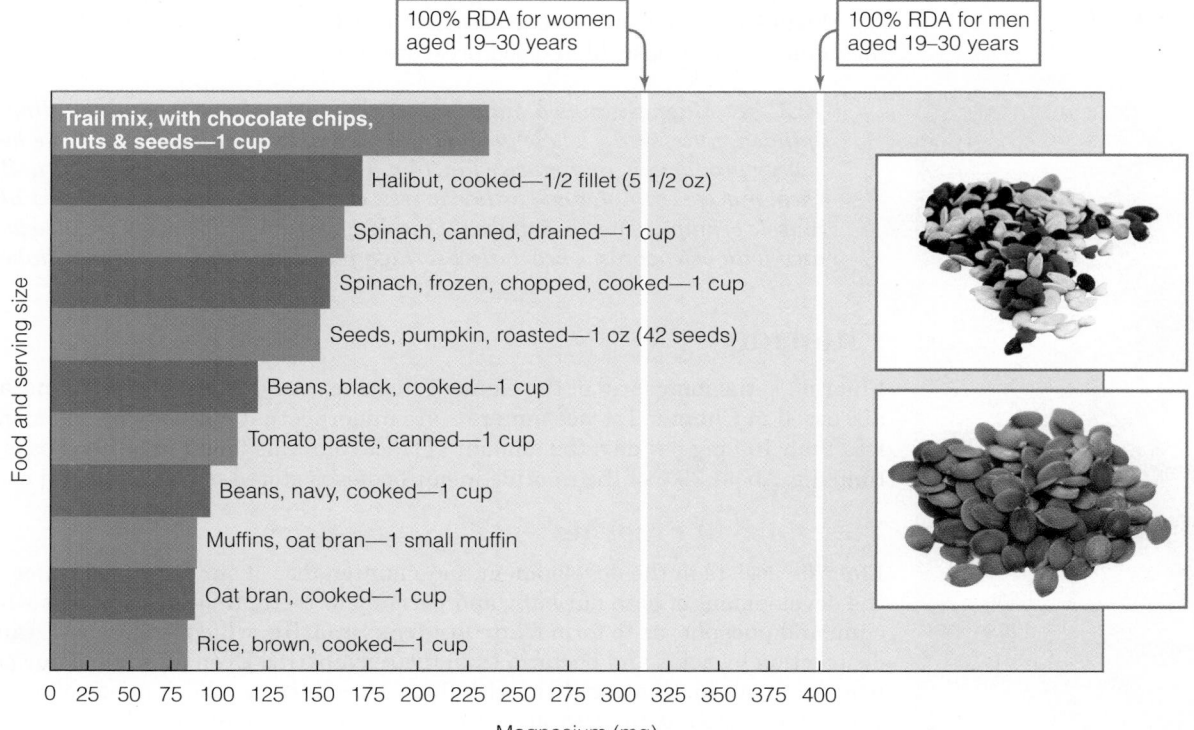

FIGURE 9.14 Common food sources of magnesium. For adult men 19 to 30 years of age, the RDA for magnesium is 400 mg per day; the RDA increases to 420 mg per day for men 31 years of age and older. For adult women 19 to 30 years of age, the RDA for magnesium is 310 mg per day; this value increases to 320 mg per day for women 31 years of age and older. (Nutrient data from U.S. Department of Agriculture, Agricultural Research Service, 2006, USDA Nutrient Database for Standard Reference, Release 19. Nutrient Data Laboratory Home Page, www.ars.usda.gov/ba/bhnrc/ndl.)

The ability of the small intestine to absorb magnesium is reduced in people who consume diets that are very high in fiber and phytates because these substances bind with magnesium. Beans, seeds, nuts, and whole grains are high in both fiber and phytates. Our absorption of magnesium should be sufficient if we consume the recommended amount of fiber each day (20 to 35 g per day). In contrast, high dietary protein intakes enhance the absorption and retention of magnesium.

What Happens If We Consume Too Much Magnesium?

There are no known toxicity symptoms related to consuming excess magnesium in the diet. The toxicity symptoms that result from pharmacological overuse of magnesium include diarrhea, nausea, and abdominal cramps. In extreme cases, large doses can result in acid–base imbalances, massive dehydration, cardiac arrest, and death. High blood magnesium levels, or **hypermagnesemia,** occur in individuals with impaired kidney function who consume large amounts of nondietary magnesium, such as antacids. Side effects include impairment of nerve, muscle, and heart function.

What Happens If We Don't Consume Enough Magnesium?

Hypomagnesemia, or low blood magnesium, results from magnesium deficiency. This condition may result from kidney disease, chronic diarrhea, or chronic alcohol abuse. Elderly people seem to be at particularly high risk of low dietary intakes of magnesium because they have a reduced appetite and blunted senses of taste and smell. In addition, the elderly face challenges related to shopping and preparing meals that contain foods high in magnesium, and their ability to absorb magnesium is reduced.

Low blood calcium levels are a side effect of hypomagnesemia. Other symptoms of magnesium deficiency include muscle cramps, spasms or seizures, nausea, weakness, irritability, and confusion. Considering magnesium's role in bone formation, it is not surprising that long-term magnesium deficiency is associated with osteoporosis. Magnesium deficiency is also associated with many other chronic diseases, including heart disease, high blood pressure, and type 2 diabetes.[7]

RECAP: *Magnesium is a major mineral found in fresh foods, including spinach, nuts, seeds, whole grains, and meats. It is important for bone health, energy production, and muscle function. Hypermagnesemia can result in diarrhea, muscle cramps, and cardiac arrest. Hypomagnesemia causes hypocalcemia, muscle cramps, spasms, and weakness. Magnesium deficiencies are also associated with osteoporosis, heart disease, high blood pressure, and type 2 diabetes.*

Fluoride

Fluoride is the ionic form of the element fluorine, and it is also a trace mineral. As discussed in Chapter 1, trace minerals are minerals that our body needs in amounts less than 100 mg per day; the amount of trace minerals found in our bodies is less than 5 g. About 99% of the fluoride in our bodies is stored in our teeth and bones.

Functions of Fluoride

Fluoride assists in the development and maintenance of our teeth and bones. During the development of both our baby and permanent teeth, fluoride combines with calcium and phosphorus to form **fluorohydroxyapatite,** which is more resistant to destruction by acids and bacteria than hydroxyapatite. Even after all of our permanent teeth are in, treating them with fluoride, whether at the dentist's office or by using fluoridated toothpaste, gives them more protection against dental caries (cavities) than teeth that have not been treated. That's because fluoride enhances tooth mineralization, decreases and reverses tooth demineralization, and inhibits the metabolism of acid-producing bacteria that cause tooth decay.

Fluoride also stimulates new bone growth, and it is currently being researched as a potential treatment for osteoporosis both alone and in combination with other

hypermagnesemia A condition marked by an abnormally high concentration of magnesium in the blood.

hypomagnesemia A condition characterized by an abnormally low concentration of magnesium in the blood.

fluorohydroxyapatite A mineral compound in human teeth that contains fluoride, calcium, and phosphorus and is more resistant to destruction by acids and bacteria than hydroxyapatite.

Fluoride is readily available in many communities in the United States through fluoridated water and dental products.

medications.[25–27] While early results are promising, more research needs to be conducted to determine if fluoride is an effective treatment for osteoporosis.[28] A review of the functions, recommended intakes, and toxicity and deficiency symptoms associated with fluoride is provided in Table 9.3 (pages 378–379).

How Much Fluoride Should We Consume?

Our need for fluoride is relatively small. Fluoride is readily available in many communities in the United States through fluoridated water and dental products. Fluoride is absorbed directly in the mouth into the teeth and gums and can also be absorbed from the gastrointestinal tract once it is ingested. In the early 1990s, there was considerable concern that our intake of fluoride was too high and could be contributing to an increased risk for cancer, bone fractures, kidney and other organ damage, infertility, and Alzheimer's disease. After reviewing the potential health hazards of fluoride, the U.S. Department of Health and Human Services found that there is no reliable scientific evidence available to indicate that fluoride increases our risk for these illnesses.[29]

Currently there are concerns that individuals whose water intake is almost exclusively from bottled water may be consuming too little fluoride and increasing their risk for dental caries, as most bottled waters do not contain fluoride. However, these individuals may still consume fluoride through other beverages that contain fluoridated water and through fluoridated dental products. Toothpastes and mouthwashes that contain fluoride are widely marketed and used by the majority of consumers in the United States, and these products can contribute as much if not more fluoride to our diets than fluoridated water. Fluoride supplements are available only by prescription, and these are generally only given to children who do not have access to fluoridated water. Incidentally, tea is a good source of fluoride: one 8-oz cup provides about 20–25% of the AI.

What Happens If We Consume Too Much Fluoride?

Consuming too much fluoride increases the protein content of tooth enamel, resulting in a condition called **fluorosis.** Because increased protein makes the enamel more porous, the teeth become stained and pitted (FIGURE 9.15). Teeth seem to be at highest risk for fluorosis during the first 8 years of life, when the permanent teeth are developing. To reduce the risk of fluorosis, children should not swallow oral care products that are meant for topical use only, and children under the age of 6 years should be supervised while using fluoride-containing products.[28] Mild fluorosis generally causes white patches on the teeth, and it has no effect on tooth function. Although moderate and severe fluorosis cause greater discoloration of the teeth, there appears to be no adverse effect on tooth function.[7]

Excess consumption of fluoride can also cause fluorosis of our skeleton. Mild skeletal fluorosis results in an increased bone mass and stiffness and pain in the joints. Moderate and severe skeletal fluorosis can be crippling, but it is extremely rare in the United States, with only five confirmed cases in the last 35 years.[7]

What Happens If We Don't Consume Enough Fluoride?

The primary result of fluoride deficiency is dental caries. Adequate fluoride intake appears necessary at an early age and throughout our adult life to reduce our risk for tooth decay. Inadequate fluoride intake may also be associated with lower bone density, but there is not enough research currently available to support the widespread use of fluoride to prevent osteoporosis. Studies are currently being done to determine the role fluoride might play in reducing our risk for osteoporosis and fractures.

> RECAP: *Fluoride is a trace mineral whose primary function is to support the health of teeth and bones. Primary sources of fluoride are fluoridated dental products and fluoridated water. Fluoride toxicity causes fluorosis of the teeth and skeleton, while fluoride deficiency causes an increase in tooth decay.*

FIGURE 9.15 Consuming too much fluoride causes fluorosis, leading to staining and pitting of the teeth.

fluorosis A condition marked by staining and pitting of the teeth; caused by an abnormally high intake of fluoride.

Osteoporosis Is a Disorder Resulting from Poor Bone Health

FIGURE 9.16 The vertebrae of a person with osteoporosis (right) are thinner and more collapsed than the vertebrae of a healthy person, in which the bone is more dense and uniform (left).

80% of Americans with osteoporosis are women.

osteoporosis A disease characterized by low bone mass and deterioration of bone tissue, leading to increased bone fragility and fracture risk.

Of the many disorders associated with poor bone health, the most prevalent in the United States is osteoporosis. **Osteoporosis** is characterized by low bone mass and deterioration of bone tissue, leading to enhanced bone fragility and increase in fracture risk. The bone tissue of a person with osteoporosis is more porous and thinner than that of a person with healthy bone. These structural changes weaken the bone, leading to a significantly reduced ability of the bone to bear weight (FIGURE 9.16).

As mentioned earlier in this chapter, the hip and the vertebrae of the spinal column are common sites of osteoporosis; thus, it is not surprising that osteoporosis is the single most important cause of fractures of the hip and spine in older adults. These fractures are extremely painful and can be debilitating, with many individuals requiring nursing home care. In addition, they cause an increased risk of infection and other related illnesses that can lead to premature death. In fact, about 20% of older adults who suffer a hip fracture die within 1 year after the fracture occurs, and death rates are higher for men than for women.[30] Osteoporosis of the spine also causes a generalized loss of height and can be disfiguring: gradual compression fractures in the vertebrae of the upper back lead to a shortening and hunching of the spine, commonly referred to as *dowager's hump.*

Unfortunately, osteoporosis is a common disease: worldwide, one in three women and one in eight men are affected,[30] and in the United States, more than 10 million people have been diagnosed.[31] Factors that influence our risk for osteoporosis include age, gender, genetics, nutrition, and physical activity (Table 9.4). Let's review these factors and discuss how we can change our lifestyle to reduce our risk for osteoporosis.

TABLE 9.4 Risk Factors for Osteoporosis

Modifiable Risk Factors	Nonmodifiable Risk Factors
Smoking	Older age (elderly)
Low body weight	Caucasian or Asian race
Low calcium intake	History of fractures as an adult
Low sun exposure	Family history of osteoporosis
Alcohol abuse	Female
History of amenorrhea (failure to menstruate) in women with inadequate nutrition	History of amenorrhea (failure to menstruate) in women with no recognizable cause
Estrogen deficiency (females)	
Testosterone deficiency (males)	
Repeated falls	
Sedentary lifestyle	

Source: Adapted from J. J. Milott et al. Osteoporosis: Evaluation and Treatment. *Comp. Ther.* 2000. 26:183–189. © 2000. Reprinted with kind permission from Springer Science and Business Media.

The Impact of Aging on Osteoporosis Risk

As discussed previously in this chapter, bone density declines as we age. Low bone mass and osteoporosis are therefore significant health concerns for both older men and women. FIGURE 9.17 illustrates how the prevalence of osteoporosis and low bone mass are predicted to increase in the United States over the next 20 years. This is primarily due to increased longevity: as the U.S. population ages, more people will live long enough to suffer from osteoporosis.

Hormonal changes that occur with aging have a significant impact on bone loss. Average bone loss approximates 0.3–0.5% per year after 30 years of age; however, during menopause in women, levels of the hormone estrogen decrease dramatically and cause bone loss to increase to about 3% per year during the first 5 years of menopause. Both estrogen and testosterone play important roles in promoting the deposition of new bone and limiting the activity of osteoclasts. Thus, men can also suffer from osteoporosis caused by age-related decreases in testosterone. In addition, reduced levels of physical activity in older people and a decreased ability to metabolize vitamin D with age exacerbate the hormone-related bone loss.

Gender and Genetics Affect Osteoporosis Risk

Osteoporosis disproportionately affects women: 80% of Americans with osteoporosis are women. There are three primary reasons for this.

- Adult women have a lower absolute bone density than men. From birth through puberty, bone mass is the same in girls as in boys. But during puberty, bone mass increases more in boys, probably because of their prolonged period of accelerated growth. Thus, when bone loss begins around age 40, women have less bone stored in their skeleton than men. Since a woman's skeleton is already less

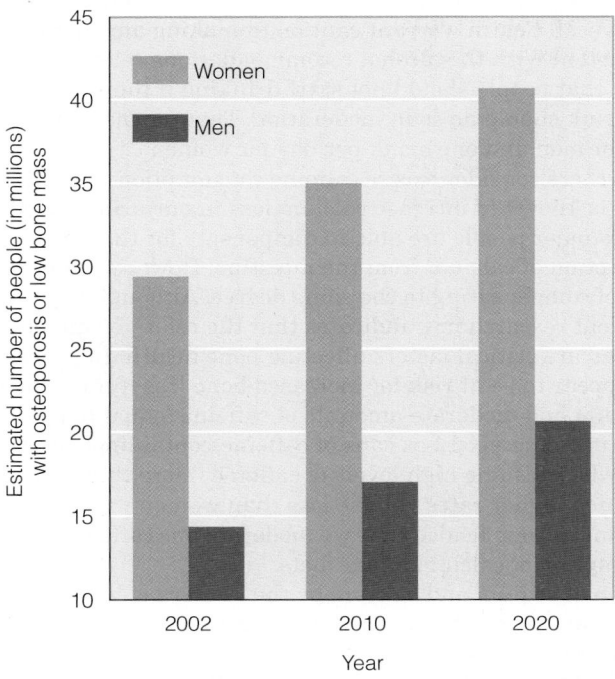

FIGURE 9.17 The prevalence of osteoporosis and low bone mass is predicted to steadily increase over the coming years in both men and women in the United States. (Adapted from National Osteoporosis Foundation, www.nof.org/advocacy/ prevalence/index.htm.)

dense, the loss of bone that occurs with aging causes osteoporosis sooner and to a greater extent in women than in men.

- As we have discussed, the hormonal changes that occur in men as they age do not have as dramatic an effect on bone density as those for women.

- Women live longer than men, and since risk increases with age, more elderly women suffer from this disease.

Secondary factors that are gender specific include social pressure on girls to be extremely thin. Extreme dieting is particularly harmful in adolescence, when bone mass is building and adequate consumption of calcium and other nutrients is critical. In many girls, weight loss causes both a loss of estrogen and reduced weight-bearing stress on the bones. In contrast, men experience pressure to "bulk up," typically by lifting weights. This puts healthful stress on the bones, resulting in increased density.

Some individuals have a family history of osteoporosis, which increases their risk for this disease. Particularly at risk are Caucasian women of low body weight who have a first degree relative (mother or sister) with osteoporosis. Asian women are also at higher risk than other non-Caucasian groups. Although we cannot change our gender or genetics, we can modify various lifestyle factors that affect our risk for osteoporosis.

Smoking and Poor Nutrition Increase Osteoporosis Risk

Cigarette smoking is known to decrease bone density because of its effects on hormones that impact bone formation and resorption; thus, cigarette smoking increases our risk for osteoporosis and resulting fractures.

Chronic alcoholism is detrimental to bone health and is associated with high rates of fractures. In contrast, numerous research studies have shown that bone density is higher in people who are *moderate* drinkers.[20,32–35] Despite the fact that moderate alcohol intake may be protective for our bone, the dangers of alcohol abuse with regard to overall health warrant caution in making any dietary recommendations. As is consistent with the alcohol recommendations related to heart disease, it is recommended that people should not start drinking if they are nondrinkers, and people who do drink should do so in moderation. That means no more than two drinks per day for men and one drink per day for women.

Some researchers consider excess caffeine consumption to be detrimental to bone health. Caffeine is known to increase calcium loss in our urine, at least over a brief period of time. Younger people are able to compensate for this calcium loss by increasing absorption of calcium from the intestine. However, older people are not always capable of compensating to the same degree. Although the findings have been inconsistent, recent research now indicates that the relative amounts of caffeine and calcium consumed are critical factors affecting bone health. In general, elderly women do not appear to be at risk for increased bone loss if they consume adequate amounts of calcium and moderate amounts of caffeine (equal to less than two cups of coffee, four cups of tea, or six 12-oz cans of caffeine-containing soft drinks per day).[36] Elderly women who consume high levels of caffeine (more than three cups of coffee per day) have much higher rates of bone loss than women with low intakes.[37] Thus, it appears important to bone health that we moderate our caffeine intake and ensure adequate consumption of calcium in our diets.

The excretion of sodium and calcium by the kidneys is linked; thus, higher intakes of sodium are known to increase the excretion of calcium in the urine. One study found an association between high urinary sodium excretion and increased bone loss from the hip in postmenopausal women.[38] However, there is no direct evidence that a high-sodium diet causes osteoporosis. The Institute of Medicine states that there is insufficient evidence to warrant different calcium recommendations based on dietary salt intake.[7]

Smoking increases our risk for osteoporosis and resulting fractures.

The effect of high dietary protein intake on bone health is controversial. While it is well established that high protein intakes increase calcium loss, protein is a critical component of bone tissue and is necessary for bone health. High protein intakes have been shown to have both a negative and a positive impact on bone health. Similar to caffeine, the key to this mystery appears to be adequate calcium intake. Elderly individuals taking calcium and vitamin D supplements and eating higher protein diets were able to significantly increase bone mass over a 3-year period, while those eating more protein and not taking supplements lost bone mass over this same time period.[39] Low protein intakes are also associated with bone loss and increased risk for osteoporosis and fractures in elderly people. Thus, there appears to be an interaction between dietary calcium and protein, in that adequate amounts of each nutrient are needed together to support bone health.

As you've learned, a multitude of nutrients play critical roles in maintaining bone health. Of these nutrients, calcium and vitamin D have received the most attention regarding their role in the prevention of osteoporosis. Research studies conducted with older individuals have shown that their risk of bone fractures is reduced by taking calcium and vitamin D supplements. We know that if people do not consume enough of these two nutrients over a prolonged period of time, their bone density is lower and they have a higher risk of bone fractures. Because our bones reach peak density when we are young, it is very important that children and adolescents consume a high-quality diet that contains the proper balance of calcium, vitamin D, protein, and other nutrients to allow for optimal bone growth. Young adults also require a proper balance of these nutrients to maintain bone mass. In older adults, diets rich in calcium and vitamin D can help minimize bone loss.

In addition to their role in reducing our risk for heart disease and cancer, diets high in fruits and vegetables are also associated with improved bone health.[40,41] This is most likely due to the fact that fruits and vegetables are good sources of nutrients that play a role in bone and collagen health, including magnesium, vitamin C, and vitamin K.

The Impact of Physical Activity on Osteoporosis Risk

Regular exercise is highly protective against bone loss and osteoporosis. Athletes are consistently shown to have more dense bones than nonathletes, and regular participation in weight-bearing exercises such as walking, jogging, tennis, and strength training can help us increase and maintain our bone mass. When we exercise, our muscles contract and pull on our bones; this stresses our bone tissue in a healthful way that stimulates increases in bone density. In addition, carrying our weight during activities such as walking and jogging stresses the bones of our legs, hips, and lower back, resulting in a healthier bone mass in these areas. It appears that people of all ages can improve and maintain bone health by consistent physical activity.

Can exercise ever be detrimental to bone health? Yes, when the body is not receiving the nutrients it needs to rebuild the hydroxyapatite and collagen broken down in response to physical activity. Thus, active people who are chronically malnourished, including people who are impoverished and those who suffer from eating disorders, are at increased fracture risk. Research has confirmed this association between nutrition, physical activity, and bone loss in the **female athlete triad,** a condition characterized by the coexistence of three (or a *triad* of) disorders in some athletic females: an eating disorder, amenorrhea, and osteoporosis. In the female athlete triad, inadequate food intake and regular strenuous exercise together result in a state of severe energy drain that causes a multitude of hormonal changes that impact menstrual function, including a reduction in estrogen production. These hormonal changes can result in the complete loss of menstrual function, called *amenorrhea*. As you have learned, estrogen is also important to maintaining healthy bone in women, so the loss of estrogen leads to osteoporosis in young women. The female athlete triad is discussed in more detail in Chapter 15.

Regular weight-bearing exercises such as jogging can help us increase and maintain our bone mass.

female athlete triad A condition characterized by the coexistence of three disorders in some athletic females: an eating disorder, amenorrhea, and osteoporosis.

NUTRI-CASE GUSTAVO

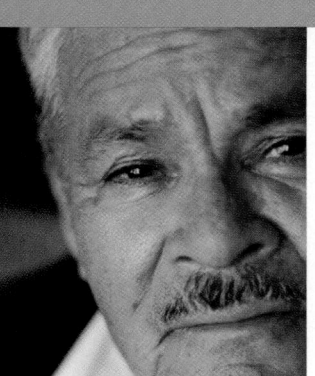

" When my wife, Antonia, fell and broke her hip, I was shocked. You see, the same thing happened to her mother, but she was an old lady by then! Antonia's only 68, and she still seems young and beautiful—at least to me! As soon as she's better, her doctor wants to do some kind of scan to see how thick her bones are. But I don't think she has that disease everyone talks about! She's always watched her weight and keeps active with our kids and grandchildren. It's true she likes her coffee and diet colas, and doesn't drink milk, but that's not enough to make a person's bones fall apart, is it?"

Study Table 9.4 (page 388). What risk factors do *not* apply to Antonia? What risk factors do? Given what Gustavo has said about his wife's nutrition and lifestyle, would you suggest he encourage her to have a DXA test? Why or why not?

Treatments for Osteoporosis

While there is no cure for osteoporosis, a variety of treatments can slow and even reverse bone loss. First, individuals with osteoporosis are encouraged to consume adequate calcium and vitamin D and to exercise regularly. Studies have shown that the most effective exercise programs include weight-bearing exercises such as jogging, stair climbing, and resistance training.[42]

In addition, several **antiresorptive** medications are available; such medications slow or stop bone resorption but do not affect bone formation. This results in an overall reduction or cessation in the rate of bone loss in people with osteoporosis. As various side effects are associated with each of these medications, patients must work closely with their physician to decide which is most appropriate.

Hormone replacement therapy (HRT) can be used for the prevention of osteoporosis in women. It combines estrogen with a hormone called progestin in brand name preparations such as Premarin and Prempro. HRT reduces bone loss, increases bone density, and reduces the risk of hip and spinal fractures. Side effects include breast tenderness, changes in mood, vaginal bleeding, and an increased risk for gallbladder disease.

Until recently, it was believed that HRT protected women against heart disease. A recent study found that one type of HRT actually increases a woman's risk for heart disease, stroke, and breast cancer. As a result, hundreds of thousands of women in the United States have recently quit taking HRT as a means to prevent or treat osteoporosis. The controversy surrounding HRT is discussed in detail in the Nutrition Debate at the end of this chapter.

Alendronate (brand name Fosamax) and risedronate (brand name Actonel) are approved for the prevention and treatment of osteoporosis. These drugs decrease bone loss, increase bone density, and reduce the risk of spinal and nonspinal fractures. Side effects are not common and include abdominal or musculoskeletal pain, nausea, diarrhea, constipation, gas, heartburn, and irritation of the esophagus. These drugs must be taken in the morning on an empty stomach, at least 30 minutes before eating, drinking, or taking any other medications, and must be taken with 8 oz of water and no other liquid. In addition, the person taking these drugs must stay upright during the 30 minutes following drug administration.

Raloxifene (brand name Evista) is a drug that was developed to mimic the beneficial effects of estrogen without the potential risks and is used for the prevention and treatment of osteoporosis. It increases bone mass and reduces the risk of spinal fractures while apparently reducing the risk of some forms of breast cancer. It may

antiresorptive Characterized by an ability to slow or stop bone resorption without affecting bone formation. Antiresorptive medications are used to reduce the rate of bone loss in people with osteoporosis.

even reduce the risk of heart disease and stroke in women who have a high risk for these diseases. Side effects are not common and include hot flashes and the formation of blood clots in the veins.

Calcitonin (brand name Miacalcin) is a hormone that occurs naturally in our bodies and assists in the regulation of calcium and in bone metabolism. When used in the treatment of osteoporosis, calcitonin slows bone loss, increases the bone density of the spine, and reduces the risk for spinal fractures. Calcitonin is a protein; thus, it cannot be taken orally or it would be digested in our intestinal tract. It therefore must be injected or inhaled through a nasal spray. Side effects of injected calcitonin include allergic reactions, flushing of the face and hands, skin rash, increased need to urinate, and nausea. Side effects of nasal calcitonin include nasal irritation, bloody nose, headaches, and backaches.

RECAP: *Osteoporosis is a major disease of concern for the elderly in the United States. Osteoporosis increases our risk for fractures and premature death from subsequent illness. Factors that increase our risk for osteoporosis include genetics, being female, being of the Caucasian or Asian race, cigarette smoking, alcohol abuse, sedentary lifestyle, and diets low in calcium and vitamin D. Medications are available for the prevention and treatment of osteoporosis.*

CHAPTER SUMMARY

- Bones are organs that are constantly active, building new bone and breaking down old bone.

- Bone develops through three processes: growth, modeling, and remodeling. Bone size is determined during growth, bone shape is determined during modeling and remodeling, and bone remodeling also affects the density of bone.

- Bone health can be assessed by measuring bone density. Dual energy x-ray absorptiometry (DXA) is the most accurate tool for measuring bone density.

- Calcium is a major mineral that is an integral component of bones and teeth. Calcium levels are maintained in our blood at all times; calcium is also necessary for normal nerve transmission, muscle contraction, healthy blood pressure, and blood clotting.

- Consuming excess calcium leads to mineral imbalance, while consuming inadequate calcium causes osteoporosis.

- Vitamin D is a fat-soluble vitamin that we can produce from the cholesterol in our skin using the energy from sunlight. Vitamin D regulates blood calcium levels, regulates absorption of calcium and phosphorus from our intestines, and helps us maintain bone health.

- Hypercalcemia results from consuming too much vitamin D, causing weakness, loss of appetite, constipation, vomiting, and formation of calcium deposits in soft tissues. Vitamin D deficiency leads to loss of bone mass, causing rickets in children or osteomalacia and osteoporosis in adults.

- Vitamin K is a fat-soluble vitamin that we obtain in the diet; it is also produced in our large intestine by normal bacteria. Vitamin K serves as a coenzyme for blood clotting and bone metabolism.

- There are no side effects of excess vitamin K intake for healthy individuals; vitamin K deficiency is rare and leads to excessive bleeding.

- Phosphorus is a major mineral that is an important part of the structure of bone; phosphorus is also a component of ATP, DNA, RNA, cell membranes, and lipoproteins.

- Consuming too much phosphorus causes high blood phosphorus levels, leading to muscle spasms and convulsions; phosphorus deficiencies are rare and cause dizziness, bone pain, and muscle damage.

- Magnesium is a major mineral that is part of the structure of bone, influences the formation of hydroxyapatite crystals and bone health through its regulation of calcium balance and the actions of vitamin D and parathyroid hormone, and is a cofactor for more than 300 enzyme systems.

- There are no known toxicity symptoms of consuming excess magnesium in the diet, though pharmacological excesses can result in such problems as diarrhea, cramping, dehydration, and cardiac arrest. Hypomagnesemia results from magnesium deficiency, resulting in low blood calcium levels, muscle cramps, seizures, confusion, and increased risk of some chronic diseases such as heart disease and type 2 diabetes.
- Fluoride is a trace mineral that strengthens our teeth and bones and reduces our risk for dental caries.
- Consuming too much fluoride causes fluorosis of the teeth and bones. Consuming too little fluoride increases our risk for dental caries and tooth decay and can weaken bones.
- Osteoporosis is a major bone disease in the United States, affecting more than 10 million Americans. About 80% of people with this disease are women.
- Osteoporosis leads to increased risk of bone fractures and premature disability and death due to subsequent illness.
- Factors that increase our risk for osteoporosis include increased age, being female, being of the Caucasian or Asian race, cigarette smoking, alcohol abuse, low calcium and vitamin D intakes, and a sedentary lifestyle.

TEST YOURSELF ANSWERS

1. **False.** By selecting foods that are good sources of calcium each day, most people can consume enough calcium in their diets to maintain bone health. People at risk for low calcium intakes include elderly people, people who do not consume enough minerals in their diets, and people who do not consume enough food to maintain a healthful weight.

2. **False.** Osteoporosis is more common among elderly women, but elderly men are also at increased risk for osteoporosis. Young women who suffer from an eating disorder and menstrual cycle irregularity may also have osteoporosis, and the combination of all three in athletic females is referred to as the female athlete triad.

3. **True.** Our bodies can convert a cholesterol compound in our skin into vitamin D.

4. **False.** There are many good sources of calcium besides dairy foods, including calcium-fortified juices and soy/rice beverages and green leafy vegetables such as kale, broccoli, and collard greens.

5. **True.** Recent studies indicate that overweight and obese people are more likely to have poorer vitamin D status than normal weight people, which could increase their risk for osteoporosis.

REVIEW QUESTIONS

1. Hydroxyapatite crystals are predominantly made up of
   a. calcium and phosphorus.
   b. hydrogen, oxygen, and titanium.
   c. calcium and vitamin D.
   d. calcium and magnesium.

2. On a DXA test, a T-score of +1.0 indicates that the patient
   a. has osteoporosis.
   b. is at greater risk of fractures than an average, healthy 30-year-old.
   c. has normal bone density as compared to an average, healthy 30-year-old.
   d. has slightly lower bone density than an average, healthy person of the same age.

3. Which of the following statements about trabecular bone is true?
   a. It accounts for about 80% of our skeleton.
   b. It forms the core of almost all of the bones of our skeleton.
   c. It is also called compact bone.
   d. It provides the scaffolding for cortical bone.

4. Which of the following individuals is most likely to require vitamin D supplements?
   a. a dark-skinned child living and playing outdoors in Hawaii
   b. a fair-skinned construction worker living in Florida
   c. a fair-skinned retired teacher living in a nursing home in Ohio
   d. None of the above individuals is likely to require vitamin D supplements.

5. Calcium is necessary for several body functions, including
   a. demineralization of bone, nerve transmission, and immune responses.
   b. cartilage structure, nerve transmission, and muscle contraction.
   c. structure of bone, nerve, and muscle tissue, immune responses, and muscle contraction.
   d. structure of bone, nerve transmission, and muscle contraction.

6. True or false? The process by which bone is formed through the action of osteoblasts and resorbed through the action of osteoclasts is called remodeling.

7. True or false? Moderate consumption of alcohol has been associated with increased bone density.

8. True or false? Although osteoporosis can lead to painful and debilitating fractures, it is not associated with an increased risk of premature death.

9. True or false? The amount of calcium we absorb depends upon our age, our calcium intake, the types of calcium-rich foods we eat, and our body's supply of vitamin D.

10. True or false? Our body absorbs vitamin D from sunlight.

11. Explain why people with diseases that cause a malabsorption of fat may suffer from deficiency of vitamins D and K.

12. Most people reach their peak height by the end of adolescence, maintain that height for several decades, and then start to lose height in their later years. Describe the two processes behind this phenomenon.

13. The morning after reading this chapter, you are eating your usual breakfast cereal when you notice that the Nutrition Facts Panel on the box states that one serving contains 100% of your DRI for calcium. In addition, you're eating the cereal with about ½ cup of skim milk. Does this meal ensure that your calcium needs for the day are met? Why or why not?

14. Your best friend has light skin and lives in Buffalo, New York. How much time does your friend need to spend out of doors with exposed skin on winter days to avoid the need for consuming vitamin D in the diet or from supplements?

15. Look back at the information you learned about Liz in the Nutri-Case introductions in Chapter 1, as well as in Chapters 5, 6, and 7. Identify aspects of Liz's nutrition and lifestyle that put her at increased risk for osteoporosis.

FIND THE QUACK

Wyn just got some bad news: her mom phoned to say that a routine bone scan ordered by her physician had shown that she has osteoporosis. Wyn was shocked, because her mom is only 51 years old, and she'd always thought of osteoporosis as a disease for "old ladies." Now Wyn decides to go online to see if she can learn more about osteoporosis. When she discovers the importance of calcium and vitamin D, she searches on "calcium supplements." That's when she finds a site promoting "a unique form of calcium from Pacific sea coral." She reads that this form of "coral calcium" is derived from remnants of coral that have broken off from coral reefs and are mined from ocean beds. The manufacturer makes the following claims for coral calcium:

- Coral calcium is absorbed into the body within 20 minutes, rather than within 6–8 hours like other calcium supplements.

- The calcium carbonate in coral calcium is 100% absorbable, whereas the calcium in milk is only 17% absorbable.

- The most important daily habits anyone can adopt to preserve their health are to consume coral calcium and get a minimum of 2 hours of sunlight on their face, without sunscreen.

- Calcium deficiency not only causes osteoporosis, but also makes the body acidic and leads to a host of other diseases, including heart disease, multiple sclerosis, and cancer. People who live on the Japanese island of Okinawa never experience cancer because there is coral calcium in their drinking water, which keeps their bodies alkaline and cancels out disease-causing acids.

- Coral calcium is only $19.95 for a 30-day supply.

1. Recall what you learned about digestion in Chapter 3. Do you think it is likely that coral calcium is absorbed into the body within 20 minutes? Why or why not?

2. Do you accept the claim that milk is 17% absorbable, but the calcium carbonate in coral calcium is 100% absorbable? Why or why not? If necessary, review both the Highlight box on page 374 and the Nutrition Label Activity on page 373.

3. Comment on the statement "The most important daily habits anyone can adopt to preserve their health are to consume coral calcium and get a minimum of 2 hours of sunlight on their face, without sunscreen."

4. Comment on the statement that calcium deficiency causes a host of diseases such as heart disease, multiple sclerosis, and cancer, and that Okinawans "never experience cancer because there is coral calcium in their drinking water, which keeps their bodies alkaline and cancels out disease-causing acids."

Answers can be found at www.aw-bc.com/thompson.

WEB LINKS

www.nlm.nih.gov/medlineplus
MEDLINE Plus Health Information

Search for rickets or osteomalacia to learn more about these vitamin D–deficiency diseases.

www.ada.org
American Dental Association

Look under "Your Oral Health" to learn more about the fluoridation of community water supplies and the use of fluoride-containing products.

www.nof.org
National Osteoporosis Foundation

Learn more about the causes, prevention, detection, and treatment of osteoporosis.

www.osteofound.org
International Osteoporosis Foundation

Find out more about this foundation and its mission to increase awareness and understanding of osteoporosis worldwide.

www.niams.nih.gov/bone
National Institutes of Health: Osteoporosis and Related Bone Diseases—National Resource Center

Access this site for additional resources and information on metabolic bone diseases including osteoporosis.

REFERENCES

1. Ball, J. W., and R. C. Bindler. 2003. *Pediatric Nursing: Caring for Children*. Upper Saddle River, NJ: Pearson Education.
2. Ho, A. Y. Y., and A. W. C. Kung. 2005. Determinants of peak bone mineral density and bone area in young women. *J. Bone Miner. Metab*. 23:470–475.
3. Chevalley, T., R. Rizzoli, D. Hans, S. Ferrari, and J. P. Bonjour. 2005. Interaction between calcium intake and menarcheal age on bone mass gain: an eight-year follow-up study from prepuberty to postmenarche. *J. Clin. Endocrinol. Metab*. 90:44–51.
4. Kindblom, J. M., M. Lorentzon, E. Norjavaara, A. Hellqvist, S. Nilsson, D. Mellström, and C. Ohlsson. 2006. Pubertal timing predicts previous fractures and BMD in young adult men: the GOOD study. *J. Bone Min. Res*. 21:790–795.
5. Zemel, M. B., W. Thompson, A. Milstead, K. Morris, and P. Campbell. 2004. Calcium and dairy acceleration of weight and fat loss during energy restriction in obese adults. *Obes. Res*. 12:582–590.
6. Bowen, J., M. Noakes, and P. M. Clifton. 2005. Effect of calcium and dairy foods in high protein, energy-restricted diets on weight loss and metabolic parameters in overweight adults. *Int. J. Obes*. 29:957–965.
7. Institute of Medicine, Food and Nutrition Board. 1997. *Dietary Reference Intakes for Calcium, Phosphorus, Magnesium, Vitamin D, and Fluoride*. Washington, DC: National Academies Press.
8. Nusser, S. M., A. L. Carriquiry, K. W. Dodd, and W. A. Fuller. 1996. A semiparametric transformation approach to estimating usual daily intake distributions. *J. Am. Stat. Assoc*. 91:1440–1449.
9. Massey, L. K., H. Roman-Smith, and R. A. Sutton. 1993. Effect of dietary oxalate and calcium on urinary oxalate and risk of formation of calcium oxalate kidney stones. *J. Am. Diet. Assoc*. 93:901–906.
10. Keller, J. L., A. J. Lanou, and N. D. Barnard. 2002. The consumer cost of calcium from food and supplements. *J. Am. Diet. Assoc*. 102:1669–1671.
11. Ross, E. A., N. J. Szabo, and I. R. Tebbett. 2000. Lead content of calcium supplements. *JAMA* 284:1425–1433.
12. Holick, M. F., L. Y. Matsuoka, and J. Wortsman. 1989. Age, vitamin D, and solar ultraviolet. *Lancet* 2:1104–1105.
13. Need, A. G., H. A. Morris, M. Horowitz, and C. Nordin. 1993. Effects of skin thickness, age, body fat, and sunlight on serum 25-hydroxyvitamin D. *Am. J. Clin. Nutr*. 58:882–885.
14. Florez, H., R. Martinez, W. Chacra, N. Strickman-Stein, and S. Levis. 2007. Outdoor exercise reduces the risk of hypovitaminosis D in the obese. *J. Steroid Biochem. Mol. Biol*. 103:679–681.
15. Holick, M. F. 2005. The vitamin D epidemic and its health consequences. *J. Nutr*. 135:2739S–2748S.
16. Holick, M. F. 1994. McCollum Award Lecture, 1994: Vitamin D: new horizons for the 21st century. *Am. J. Clin. Nutr*. 60:619–630.
17. Hollis, B. W. 2005. Circulating 25-hydroxyvitamin D levels indicative of vitamin D sufficiency: implications for establishing a new effective dietary intake recommendation for vitamin D. *J. Nutr*. 135:317–322.
18. Weaver, C. M., and J. C. Fleet. 2004. Vitamin D requirements: current and future. *Am. J. Clin. Nutr*. 80(suppl.):1735S–1739S.
19. Institute of Medicine, Food and Nutrition Board. 2002. *Dietary Reference Intakes for Vitamin A, Vitamin K, Arsenic, Boron, Chromium, Copper, Iodine, Iron, Manganese, Molybdenum, Nickel, Silicon, Vanadium, and Zinc*. Washington, DC: National Academies Press.
20. Feskanich, D., S. A. Korrick, S. L. Greenspan, H. N. Rosen, and G. A. Colditz. 1999. Moderate alcohol consumption and bone density among post-menopausal women. *J. Women's Health* 8:65–73.
21. Wyshak, G., R. E. Frisch, T. E. Albright, N. L. Albright, I. Schiff, and J. Witschi. 1989. Nonalcoholic carbonated beverage consumption and bone fractures among women former college athletes. *J. Orthop. Res*. 7:91–99.
22. Wyshak, G., and R. E. Frisch. 1994. Carbonated beverages, dietary calcium, the dietary calcium/phosphorus ratio, and bone fractures in girls and boys. *J. Adolesc. Health* 15:210–215.
23. Wyshak, G. 2000. Teenaged girls, carbonated beverage consumption, and bone fractures. *Arch. Pediatr. Adolesc. Med*. 154:610–613.
24. Heaney, R. P., and K. Rafferty. 2001. Carbonated beverages and urinary calcium excretion. *Am. J. Clin. Nutr*. 74:343–347.
25. Pak, C. Y., K. Sakhaee, B. Adams-Huet, V. Piziak, R. D. Peterson, and J. R. Poindexter. 1995. Treatment of postmenopausal osteoporosis with slow-release sodium fluoride. Final report of a randomized controlled trial. *Ann. Int. Med*. 123:401–408.
26. Reginster, J. Y., D. Felsenberg, I. Pavo, J. Stepan, J. Payer, H. Resch, C. C. Glüer, D. Mühlenbacher, D. Quail, H. Schmitt, and T. Nickelsen. 2003. Effect of raloxifene combined with monofluorophosphate as compared with monofluorophosphate alone in postmenopausal women with low bone mass: a randomized, controlled trial. *Osteoporosis Int*. 14:741–749.
27. Ringe, J. D., A. Dorst, H. Faber, C. Kipshoven, L. C. Rovati, and I. Setnikar. 2005. Efficacy of etidronate and sequential monofluorophosphate in severe postmenopausal osteoporosis: a pilot study. *Rheumatol. Int*. 25:296–300.
28. American Dietetic Association. 2005. Position of the American Dietetic Association: the impact of fluoride on health. *J. Am. Diet. Assoc*. 105:1620–1628.

29. U.S. Department of Health and Human Services. Public Health Service. 1991. *Review of Fluoride: Benefits and Risks.* Report of the Ad Hoc Subcommittee on Fluoride of the Committee to Coordinate Environmental Health and Related Programs. www.health.gov/environment/ReviewofFluoride/default.htm. (Accessed April 2007.)

30. International Osteoporosis Foundation. 2007. Facts and statistics about osteoporosis and its impact. www.iofbonehealth.org/facts-and-statistics.html. (Accessed April 2007.)

31. National Osteoporosis Foundation. 2004. Fast facts on osteoporosis. www.nof.org/osteoporosis/diseasefacts.htm. (Accessed April 2007.)

32. Laitinen, K., M. Valimaki, and P. Keto. 1991. Bone mineral density measured by dual-energy x-ray absorptiometry in healthy Finnish women. *Calcif. Tissue Int.* 48:224–231.

33. Holbrook, T. L., and E. Barrett-Connor. 1993. A prospective study of alcohol consumption and bone mineral density. *BMJ* 306:1506–1509.

34. Felson, D. T., Y. Zhang, M. T. Hannan, W. B. Kannel, and D. P. Kiel. 1995. Alcohol intake and bone mineral density in elderly men and women. The Framingham Study. *Am. J. Epidemiol.* 142:485–492.

35. Rapuri, P. B., J. C. Gallagher, K. E. Balhorn, and K. L. Ryschon. 2000. Alcohol intake and bone metabolism in elderly women. *Am. J. Clin. Nutr.* 72:1206–1213.

36. Massey, L. K. 2001. Is caffeine a risk factor for bone loss in the elderly? *Am. J. Clin. Nutr.* 74:569–570.

37. Rapuri, P. B., J. C. Gallagher, H. K. Kinyamu, and K. L. Ryschon. 2001. Caffeine intake increases the rate of bone loss in elderly women and interacts with vitamin D receptor genotypes. *Am. J. Clin. Nutr.* 74:694–700.

38. Devine A., R. A. Criddle, I. M. Dick, D. A. Kerr, and R. L. Prince. 1995. A longitudinal study of the effect of sodium and calcium intakes on regional bone density in post-menopausal women. *Am. J. Clin. Nutr.* 62:740–745.

39. Dawson-Hughes, B., and S. S. Harris. 2002. Calcium intake influences the association of protein intake with rates of bone loss in elderly men and women. *Am. J. Clin. Nutr.* 75:773–779.

40. Tucker, K. L., M. T. Hannan, H. Chen, L. A. Cupples, P. W. F. Wilson, and D. P. Kiel. 1999. Potassium, magnesium, and fruit and vegetable intakes are associated with greater bone mineral density in elderly men and women. *Am. J. Clin. Nutr.* 69:727–736.

41. Tucker, K. L., H. Chen, M. T. Hannan, L. A. Cupples, P. W. F. Wilson, D. Felson, and D. P. Kiel. 2002. Bone mineral density and dietary patterns in older adults: the Framingham Osteoporosis Study. *Am. J. Clin. Nutr.* 76:245–252.

42. South-Pal, J. E. 2001. Osteoporosis: Part II. Nonpharmacologic and pharmacologic treatment. *Am. Fam. Physician* 63:1121–1128.

43. Writing Group for the Women's Health Initiative Investigators. 2002. Risks and benefits of estrogen plus progestin in healthy postmenopausal women. Principal results from the Women's Health Initiative randomized control trial. *JAMA* 288:321–332.

NUTRITION DEBATE

Hormone Replacement Therapy—For Women at High Risk for Osteoporosis, Do the Benefits Outweigh the Potential Health Risks?

hormone replacement therapy (HRT) is a combination of estrogen and the hormone progestin. Research has consistently shown that HRT is effective in preventing and treating osteoporosis. It is also believed to reduce the less serious symptoms some menopausal women experience, including hot flashes, vaginal dryness, sleep disturbances, and memory loss. For many years, physicians viewed HRT as a safe and effective medication option, and prescriptions skyrocketed in the 1980s and 1990s. Indeed, it became standard medical practice to prescribe HRT to any menopausal woman who requested it. Then, in 2002, serious concerns arose over study results that indicated increased risks of breast cancer and other disease in women taking HRT. Those concerns raise a difficult question for women with low bone density and osteoporosis: are the benefits of HRT on bone density worth the increased risk of other diseases? We examine that question here.

Estrogen replacement medications come in a variety of forms for use by postmenopausal women.

The benefit of HRT is a reduced risk of osteoporosis and other symptoms of menopause.

Until the early 1990s, research had suggested that, in addition to its beneficial effect on bone density and menopausal symptoms, HRT lowered cholesterol levels and reduced a woman's risk for heart disease. However, much of the evidence supporting these benefits of HRT had been observational in nature, meaning that these studies were not actually designed to administer HRT and test its direct effect on health risks and benefits. In 1991, researchers involved in the Women's Health Initiative began designing clinical trials that would test the direct effects of HRT on risks for heart disease, various cancers, and bone fractures. The researchers hypothesized that women taking these hormones would have a lower risk of heart disease and hip fracture but higher rates of breast cancer. More than 160,000 women ranging in age from 50 to 79 years were recruited into this study, and researchers planned to follow these women during an average of 8.5 years.

Much to the surprise of many researchers and health professionals, the trials testing HRT had to be stopped early because the health risks to women on HRT exceeded the health benefits over an average follow-up of only 5 years.[43] Women taking HRT were found to have increased risk for breast cancer, heart disease, stroke, and pulmonary embolism, which is a clot that forms in the arteries of the lungs. These results became news headlines throughout the United States and around the world. Within weeks, hundreds of thousands of women had either stopped taking HRT or rushed to meet with their physicians to discuss their options.

Although these findings are certainly troubling, the risks of taking HRT may not be as high as many fear. The investigators report that during any 1 year, 10,000 women taking HRT may experience seven more heart disease–related events, eight more strokes, eight more cases of breast cancer, and eight more pulmonary emboli than women taking no hormone therapy. Moreover, the Women's Health Initiative trials found positive health effects of HRT, in that it decreased the number of hip, spine, and other osteoporosis-related fractures. For example, during any 1 year, 10,000 women on HRT will experience five fewer fractures of the hip than women not taking HRT. In addition, HRT decreased the risk for colorectal cancer. During 1 year, 10,000 women on HRT will experience six fewer cases of colorectal cancer.

Based on the data from the Women's Health Initiative trials, should a woman take HRT to combat osteoporosis and treat menopausal symptoms? This question can only be answered by the woman herself after consulting with her physician. HRT is still an effective treatment and prevention option for osteoporosis, and women at low risk for breast cancer and heart disease

Women should consider their personal risk factors as well as lifestyle traits, such as how much exercise they regularly participate in, before making a decision about HRT.

may decide to use this therapy. Women at high risk for breast cancer and heart disease may decide to avoid taking HRT and may select some other medication approved for the prevention or treatment of osteoporosis. In summary, working with their physician, women must weigh the benefits of reducing fracture risk with the increased risks of breast cancer and heart disease when considering HRT as a treatment option for osteoporosis and low bone density.

CHAPTER 10

CHAPTER OBJECTIVES

After reading this chapter you will be able to:

1. Describe how coenzymes enhance the activities of enzymes, pp. 402–403.

2. For each of the eight B-complex vitamins, describe their primary functions and their food sources, pp. 404–417.

3. Explain the importance of adequate folate intake for women of childbearing age, p. 413.

4. Describe the association between folate, vitamin B_{12}, and vascular disease, p. 413.

5. Identify at least two minerals that function as cofactors in energy metabolism, pp. 419 and 430–432.

6. Describe the four components of blood, p. 421.

7. Discuss the role that iron plays in oxygen transport, pp. 424–425.

8. Distinguish between iron-deficiency anemia, pernicious anemia, and macrocytic anemia, pp. 413–414 and 428–429.

TEST YOURSELF TRUE OR FALSE?

1. The B-complex vitamins are an important source of energy for our bodies. T or F

2. People consuming a vegan diet are at greater risk for micronutrient deficiencies than are people who eat foods of animal origin. T or F

3. Chromium supplements are consistently effective in reducing body fat and enhancing muscle mass. T or F

4. Iron deficiency is the most common nutrient deficiency in the world. T or F

5. Taking a daily multivitamin/mineral supplement is a waste of money. T or F

Test Yourself answers can be found after the Chapter Summary.

Nutrients Involved in Energy Metabolism and Blood Health

d r. Leslie Bernstein looked in astonishment at the 80-year-old man in his office. A leading gastroenterologist and professor of medicine at Albert Einstein College of Medicine in New York City, he had admired Pop Katz for years as one of his most healthy patients, a strict vegetarian and athlete who just weeks before had been going on 3-mile runs as if he were 40 years younger. Now he could barely stand. He was confused, cried easily, was wandering away from the house partially clothed, and had lost control of his bladder. Tests showed that he was not suffering from Alzheimer's disease, had not had a stroke, did not have a tumor or infection, and had no evidence of exposure to pesticides, metals, drugs, or other toxins. Blood tests were normal except that his red blood cells were slightly enlarged. Bernstein consulted with a neurologist, who diagnosed "rapidly progressive dementia of unknown origin."

Bernstein was unconvinced: "In a matter of weeks, a man who hadn't been sick for 80 years suddenly became demented. . . . 'Holy smoke!,' I thought, 'I'm an idiot! The man's been a vegetarian for 38 years. No meat. No fish. No eggs. No milk. He hasn't had any animal protein for decades. He has to be B_{12} deficient!'" Bernstein immediately tested Katz's blood, then gave him an injection of B_{12}. The blood test confirmed Bernstein's hunch: the level of B_{12} in Katz's blood was too low to measure. The morning after his injection, Katz could sit up without help. Within a week of continuing treatment, he could read, play card games, and hold his own in conversations. Unfortunately, the delay in diagnosis left some permanent neurological damage, including alterations in his personality and an inability to concentrate. Bernstein notes, "A diet free of animal protein can be healthful and safe, but it should be supplemented periodically with B_{12} by mouth or by injection."[1]

It was not until 1906, when the English biochemist F. G. Hopkins discovered what he called *accessory factors,* that scientists began to appreciate the many critical roles of micronutrients in maintaining human health. Vitamin B_{12}, for instance, was not isolated until 1948! In Chapters 7 through 9, we explored several key roles of vitamins and minerals, including regulation of fluids and nerve-impulse transmission, protection against the damage caused by oxidation, and maintenance of healthy bones. In this chapter, we conclude our exploration of the micronutrients with a discussion of two final roles: their contribution to the metabolism of carbohydrates, fats, and proteins and their role in the formation and maintenance of our blood.

How Do Our Bodies Regulate Energy Metabolism?

We explored the digestion and metabolism of carbohydrates, fats, and proteins in Chapters 3 through 6 of this text. In those chapters, you learned that the regulation of energy metabolism is a complex process involving numerous biological substances and chemical pathways. Here, we describe how the micronutrients we consume in our diet assist us in generating energy from the carbohydrates, fats, and proteins we eat along with them.

Our Bodies Require Vitamins and Minerals to Produce Energy

Although vitamins and minerals do not directly provide energy, we are unable to generate energy from the macronutrients without them. The B-complex vitamins are particularly important in assisting us with energy metabolism. Also referred to as the B vitamins, this group includes thiamin, riboflavin, vitamin B_6, niacin, folate, vitamin B_{12}, pantothenic acid, and biotin.

The primary role of the B-complex vitamins is to act as coenzymes. Recall from Chapter 6 that an *enzyme* is a protein that accelerates the rate of chemical reactions but is not used up or changed during the reaction. A **coenzyme** is a molecule that combines with an enzyme to activate it and help it do its job. FIGURE 10.1 illustrates

coenzyme A molecule that combines with an enzyme to activate it and help it do its job.

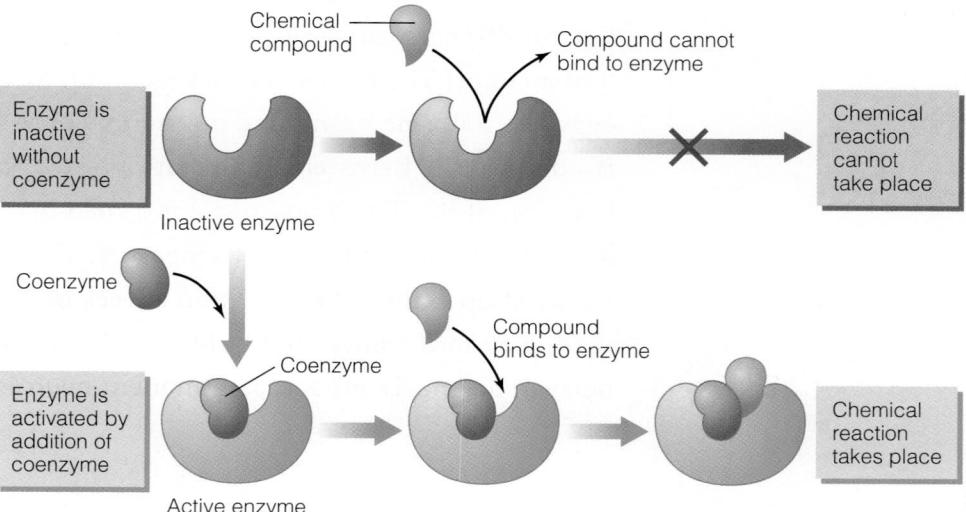

FIGURE 10.1 Coenzymes combine with enzymes to activate them, ensuring that the chemical reactions that depend upon these enzymes can occur.

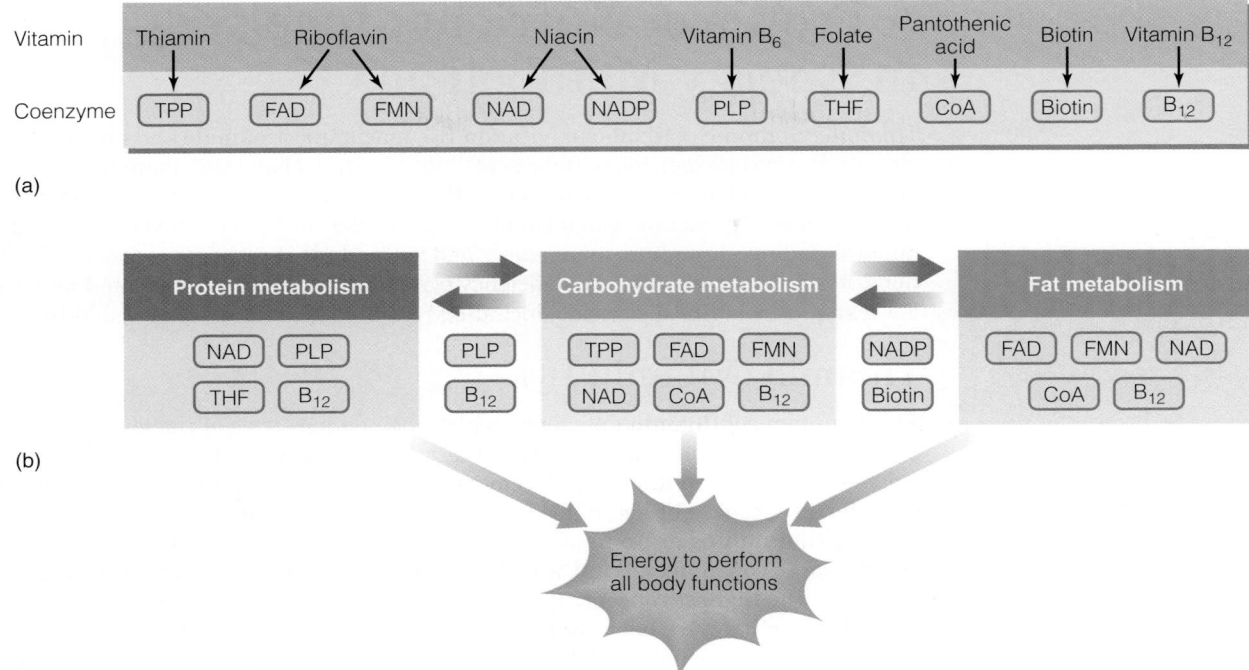

FIGURE 10.2 The B-complex vitamins play many important roles in the reactions involved in energy metabolism. **(a)** B-complex vitamins and the coenzymes they are a part of. **(b)** This chart illustrates many of the coenzymes essential for various metabolic functions; however, this is only a small sample of the thousands of roles that the B-complex vitamins serve in our bodies.

how coenzymes work. Without coenzymes, we would be unable to produce the energy necessary for sustaining life and supporting daily activities.

FIGURE 10.2 provides an overview of how some of the B-complex vitamins act as coenzymes to promote energy metabolism. For instance, thiamin is part of the coenzyme thiamin pyrophosphate, or TPP, which assists in the breakdown of glucose. Riboflavin is a part of two coenzymes, flavin mononucleotide (FMN) and flavin adenine dinucleotide (FAD), which help break down both glucose and fatty acids. The specific functions of each B-complex vitamin are described in detail shortly.

Some Micronutrients Assist with Nutrient Transport and Hormone Production

Some micronutrients promote energy metabolism by facilitating the transport of nutrients into the cells. For instance, the mineral chromium helps improve glucose uptake into cells. Other micronutrients assist in the production of hormones that regulate metabolic processes; the mineral iodine, for example, is necessary for synthesis of thyroid hormones, which regulate our metabolic rate and promote growth and development. The details of these processes and their related nutrients are discussed in the following section.

> **RECAP:** *Vitamins and minerals are not direct sources of energy, but they help generate energy from carbohydrates, fats, and proteins. Acting as coenzymes, nutrients such as the B-complex vitamins assist enzymes in metabolizing nutrients to produce energy. Minerals such as chromium and iodine assist with nutrient uptake into the cells and with regulating energy production and cell growth.*

A Profile of Nutrients Involved in Energy Metabolism

Thiamin (vitamin B_1), riboflavin (vitamin B_2), niacin (nicotinamide and nicotinic acid), vitamin B_6 (pyridoxine), folate (folic acid), vitamin B_{12} (cobalamin), pantothenic acid, and biotin are the nutrients identified as the B-complex vitamins. Other nutrients involved in energy metabolism include a vitamin-like substance called choline and the minerals iodine, chromium, manganese, and sulfur. In this section, we discuss the functions, food sources, toxicity, and deficiency symptoms for these vitamins and minerals. For a summary of this discussion, including recommended intakes, see Table 10.1.

Thiamin (Vitamin B_1)

The symptoms of thiamin deficiency, which include paralysis of the lower limbs, have been described throughout recorded history, but it was not until the 19th century, when steam-powered mills began removing the outer shell of grains, especially rice, that the disease was linked to food instead of a toxin or infection. At the time, it was thought that milling grain improved the quality of the grain and made it more acceptable to consumers. What wasn't known was that the outer layer of the grain contained the highest concentrations of B vitamins, especially thiamin.[2] Thus, most of the B vitamins were being removed and discarded as the grain was milled or the rice polished. It was not until 1885 that Dr. K. Takaki, a Japanese naval surgeon, discovered that he could prevent thiamin deficiency by improving the quality of the diets of seamen. Then in 1906, Dr. Eijkman, a Dutch medical doctor living in Java, and his colleague Dr. Grijns described how he could produce the symptoms of thiamin deficiency in chickens or pigeons by feeding them polished rice and could cure them by feeding back the rice bran that was removed during polishing.[2,3] Dr. Eijkman's successor and colleague was able to isolate the water-soluble substance in rice bran that was responsible for the cure. He called it thiamin. Because it was the first B-complex vitamin discovered, it is designated vitamin B_1.[2] Thiamin is part of the coenzyme thiamin pyrophosphate, or TPP. As a part of TPP, thiamin plays a critical role in the breakdown of glucose for energy and acts as a coenzyme in the metabolism of the branched-chain amino acids, which include leucine, isoleucine, and valine. TPP assists in producing DNA and RNA and plays a role in the synthesis of neurotransmitters, or chemicals important in the transmission of messages throughout the nervous system.

Good food sources of thiamin include enriched cereals and grains, whole-grain products, wheat germ and yeast extracts, ready-to-eat cereals, ham and other pork products, organ meats of most animals, and some green vegetables, including peas, asparagus, and okra (FIGURE 10.3 on page 407). Overall, whole grains are some of the best sources of thiamin, while more processed foods such as refined sugars and fats are the lowest sources. Unless milled grains are fortified (that is, the thiamin is added back), they are poor sources.

Because the B-complex vitamins are involved in most energy-generating processes, many of the symptoms of thiamin deficiency include a combination of fatigue, apathy, muscle weakness, and detriments in cognitive function (see Table 10.1). Thiamin-deficiency disease is called **beriberi.** In this disease, the body's inability to metabolize energy leads to muscle wasting and nerve damage; in later stages, patients may be unable to move at all. The heart muscle may also be affected, and the patient may die of heart failure. Beriberi is seen in countries in which unenriched, processed grains are a primary food source; for instance, beriberi was widespread in China when rice was processed and refined, and it still occurs in refugee camps and other settlements dependent on poor-quality food supplies. Beriberi is also seen in industrialized countries in people with heavy alcohol consumption and limited food intake. Chronic alcohol abuse is associated with a host of neurological symptoms, collectively called Wernicke-Korsakoff syndrome, in which thiamin intake is decreased and absorption and utilization impaired.[2] Although thiamin supplementation has been the treatment of choice for this

Ready-to-eat cereals are a good source of thiamin and other B-complex vitamins.

beriberi A disease caused by thiamin deficiency.

TABLE 10.1 Functions, Recommended Intakes, and Toxicity and Deficiency Symptoms of the Energy Nutrients

Nutrient	Primary Functions	Recommended Intake*	Toxicity Symptoms/ Side Effects	Deficiency Symptoms/ Side Effects
Thiamin (vitamin B_1)	Part of the coenzyme thiamin pyrophosphate (TPP) involved in carbohydrate metabolism Coenzyme involved in branched-chain amino acid metabolism	RDA for 19 years and older: Men = 1.2 mg/day Women = 1.1 mg/day	None known at this time	Beriberi, apathy, confusion and irritability, muscle weakness
Riboflavin (vitamin B_2)	Coenzymes including flavin mononucleotide (FMN) and flavin adenine dinucleotide (FAD), involved in oxidation–reduction reactions for metabolism of carbohydrates and fats	RDA for 19 years and older: Men = 1.3 mg/day Women = 1.1 mg/day	None known at this time	Ariboflavinosis, cheilosis (dry, cracked lips), angular stomatitis (inflammation of the mucous membranes of the mouth), seborrheic dermatitis (inflammation of oil glands in the skin)
Niacin (nicotinamide and nicotinic acid)	Coenzymes in carbohydrate and fatty acid metabolism, including nicotinamide adenine dinucleotide (NAD^+ and NADH) and nicotinamide adenine dinucleotide phosphate ($NADP^+$) Plays role in DNA replication and repair and cell differentiation	RDA for 19 years and older: Men = 16 mg/day Women = 14 mg/day UL: 35 mg/day for 19 years and older	Excessive supplementation causes: Flushing Liver dysfunction and damage Glucose intolerance Blurred vision and edema of eyes	Pellagra, pigmented rash, vomiting, constipation or diarrhea, bright red tongue, depression, fatigue
Vitamin B_6	Part of coenzyme (pyridoxal phosphate, or PLP) involved in amino acid metabolism, synthesis of blood cells, and carbohydrate metabolism	RDA for 19 to 50 years of age: Men and women = 1.3 mg/day RDA for 51 years and older: Men = 1.7 mg/day Women = 1.5 mg/day UL: 100 mg/day for 19 years and older	Excessive supplementation causes: Sensory neuropathy Lesions of the skin	Seborrheic dermatitis, microcytic anemia, convulsions, depression and confusion
Folate (folic acid)	Coenzyme tetrahydrofolate (THF) (or tetrahydrofolic acid, THFA) involved in DNA synthesis and amino acid metabolism Involved in the metabolism of homocysteine	RDA for 19 years and older: Men and women = 400 µg/day UL: 1,000 µg/day for 19 years and older	Excessive supplementation causes: A masking of symptoms of vitamin B_{12} deficiency Neurological damage	Macrocytic anemia, weakness and fatigue, elevated levels of homocysteine in the blood, neural tube defects in the developing fetus
Vitamin B_{12} (cobalamin)	Part of coenzymes that assist with formation of blood, nervous system function, and homocysteine metabolism	RDA for 19 years and older: Men and women = 2.4 µg/day	None known at this time	Pernicious anemia, diminished energy and low exercise tolerance, fatigue, tingling and numbness in extremities, abnormal gait, disorientation, dementia

*RDA, Recommended Dietary Allowance; AI, Adequate Intake; UL, Upper Limit. (*Continued*)

TABLE 10.1 Functions, Recommended Intakes, and Toxicity and Deficiency Symptoms of the Energy Nutrients (continued)

Nutrient	Primary Functions	Recommended Intake*	Toxicity Symptoms/Side Effects	Deficiency Symptoms/Side Effects
Pantothenic acid	Component of coenzymes (coenzyme A, or CoA) that assist with fatty acid metabolism	AI for 19 years and older: Men and women = 5 mg/day	None known at this time	Rare; only seen in people fed diets with virtually no pantothenic acid
Biotin	Component of coenzymes involved in carbohydrate, fat, and protein metabolism	AI for 19 years and older: Men and women = 30 µg/day	None known at this time	Red, scaly skin rash, depression, hallucinations, burning, tingling, tickling
Choline	Assists with homocysteine metabolism Accelerates the synthesis and release of the neurotransmitter acetylcholine Assists in synthesis of phospholipids and other components of cell membranes Assists in the transport and metabolism of fats and cholesterol	AI for 19 years and older: Men = 550 mg/day Women = 425 mg/day UL: 3.5 g/day for 19 years and older	Excessive supplementation causes: Fishy body odor Vomiting Excess salivation Sweating Diarrhea Low blood pressure	Increased fat accumulation in the liver, leading to liver damage
Iodine	Needed for the synthesis of thyroid hormones	RDA for 19 years and older = 150 µg/day UL: 1,100 µg/day for 19 years and older	Goiter	Goiter, hypothyroidism, cretinism in infant from iodine deficiency in pregnancy
Chromium	Enhances the ability of insulin to transport glucose into the cells	AI for 19 to 50 years: Men = 35 µg/day Women = 25 µg/day AI for 51 years and older: Men = 30 µg/day Women = 20 µg/day	None	Decreased glucose uptake and increased blood lipids
Manganese	Involved in energy metabolism, urea formation, bone and cartilage formation	AI for 19 years and older: Men = 2.3 mg/day Women = 1.8 mg/day	Neuromuscular problems such as muscle spasms and tremors	Poor growth and reproductive function Impaired bone growth

*RDA, Recommended Dietary Allowance; AI, Adequate Intake; UL, Upper Limit.

disease for over 50 years, there is still uncertainty about the appropriate dose and duration of supplementation.[4] There are no known adverse effects from consuming excess amounts of thiamin.

Riboflavin (Vitamin B$_2$)

The theory that there might be more than one vitamin in rice bran was first proposed in the early 1900s after researchers noticed that rats fed diets of polished rice had poor growth.[3] Finally, in 1917 researchers found that there were at least two vitamins in the extracts of rice polishing, one that cured beriberi and another that

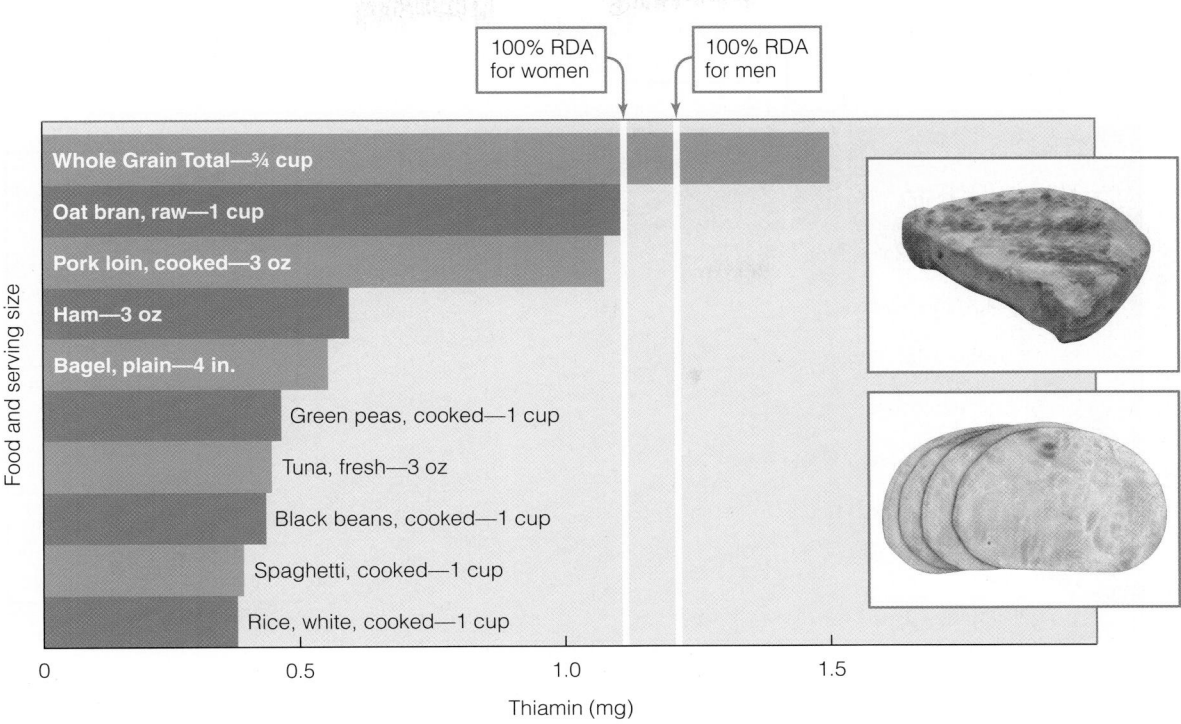

FIGURE 10.3   Common food sources of thiamin. The RDA for thiamin is 1.2 mg/day for men and 1.1 mg/day for women 19 years and older. (Data from U.S. Department of Agriculture, Agricultural Research Service, 2006, USDA Nutrient Database for Standard Reference, Release 19. Nutrient Data Laboratory Home Page, www.ars.usda.gov/ba/bhnrc/ndl.)

stimulated growth. The latter substance was first called vitamin B_2 and then named riboflavin for its ribose-like side chain and the yellow color it produced in water (*flavus* means yellow in Latin).[5]

Riboflavin is an important component of coenzymes that are involved in oxidation–reduction reactions occurring within the energy-producing metabolic pathways. These coenzymes, flavin mononucleotide (FMN) and flavin adenine dinucleotide (FAD), are involved in the metabolism of carbohydrates and fat. Riboflavin is also a part of the antioxidant enzyme glutathione peroxidase, thus assisting in the fight against oxidative damage.

Milk is a good source of riboflavin; however, riboflavin is destroyed when it is exposed to light. Thus, milk is generally stored in opaque containers to prevent the destruction of riboflavin. In the United States, meat and meat products, including poultry, fish, and milk and dairy products, are the most significant sources of dietary riboflavin.[6] However, green vegetables, such as broccoli, asparagus, and spinach, are also good sources. Finally, although whole grains are relatively low in riboflavin, fortification and enrichment of grains have increased the intake of riboflavin from these sources, especially ready-to-eat cereals and energy bars, which can provide 25–100% of the Daily Value (DV) for riboflavin in 1 serving (FIGURE 10.4).

There are no known adverse effects from consuming excess amounts of riboflavin. Because coenzymes derived from riboflavin are so widely distributed in metabolism, riboflavin deficiency, referred to as **ariboflavinosis,** lacks the specificity we see with other vitamins. However, riboflavin deficiency can have profound effects on energy production, which result in "nondescript" symptoms such as fatigue and muscle weakness. More advanced riboflavin deficiency can result in lips that are dry and scaly, inflammation and ulcers of the mucous membranes of the mouth and throat, irritated patches on the skin, changes in the cornea, anemia, and in some cases personality changes.[6] It is now known that cataract formation can be decreased by higher riboflavin intakes.[7] In addition, riboflavin is important in the metabolism

ariboflavinosis A condition caused by riboflavin deficiency.

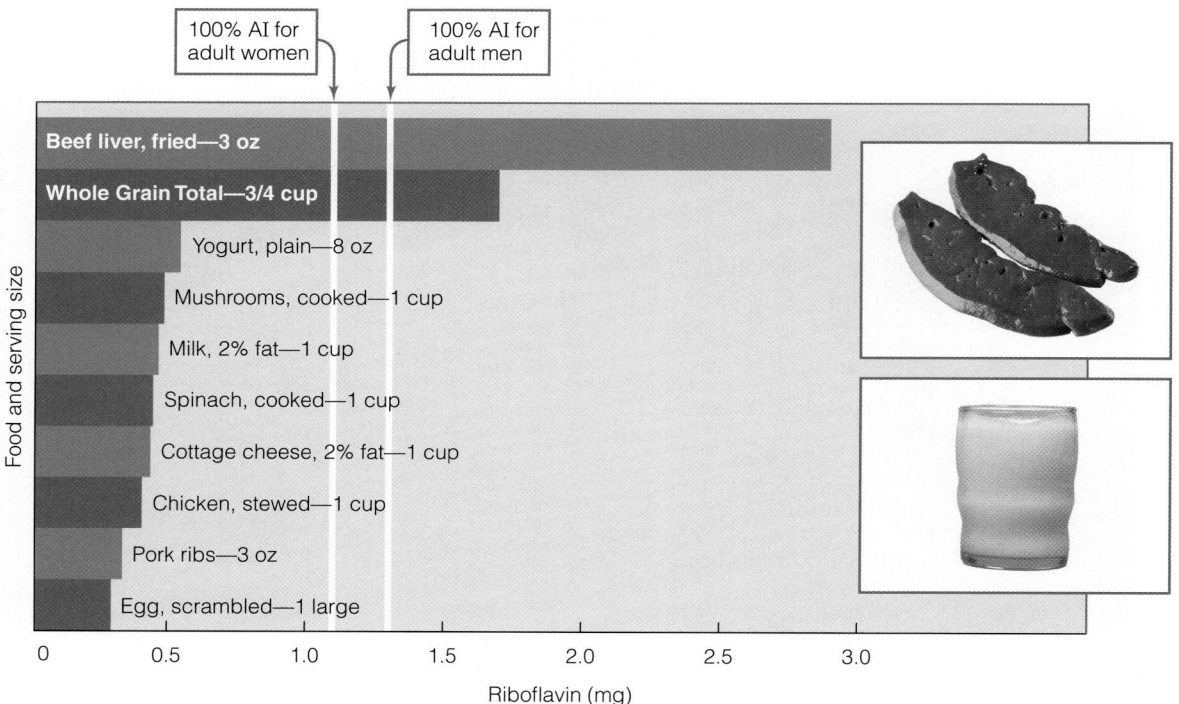

FIGURE 10.4 Common food sources of riboflavin. The RDA for riboflavin is 1.3 mg/day for men and 1.1 mg/day for women 19 years and older. (Data from U.S. Department of Agriculture, Agricultural Research Service, 2006, USDA Nutrient Database for Standard Reference, Release 19. Nutrient Data Laboratory Home Page, www.ars.usda.gov/ba/bhnrc/ndl.)

of four other vitamins: folic acid, vitamin B_6, vitamin K, and niacin.[6] Thus, a deficiency in riboflavin can affect a number of body systems.

Niacin

Pellagra, the deficiency of niacin, was first described in the 1700s in northern Spain but was also seen widely across the United States, Western and Eastern Europe, and the Middle East, where corn or maize was the dietary staple.[3] The term *pellagra* literally means raw skin.[8] The four characteristic symptoms—dermatitis, diarrhea, dementia, and death—are referred to as the *four Ds*. Individuals who develop the disease first complain of inflammation and soreness in the mouth, followed by red, raw skin (dermatitis) on areas exposed to sunlight. The disease then progresses to the digestive and nervous systems. The symptoms of this stage of the disease are diarrhea, vomiting, and dementia. At the present time, pellagra is rarely seen in industrialized countries, except in cases of chronic alcoholism. Pellagra is still found in impoverished areas of some developing nations. (For more information on pellagra, see the Highlight: Solving the Mystery of Pellagra, page 5.)

Corn-based diets are low in niacin and the amino acid tryptophan, which can be converted to niacin in the body. Niacin refers to the compounds nicotinamide and nicotinic acid, which are converted to active coenzymes that assist in the metabolism of carbohydrates and fatty acids for energy. Niacin also plays an important role in DNA replication and repair and in the process of cell differentiation. Thus, it is not surprising that a deficiency of niacin can disrupt so many systems in the body.

Niacin is widely distributed in foods, with good sources being yeast, meats, including fish and poultry, cereals, legumes, and seeds (FIGURE 10.5). Other foods such as milk, leafy vegetables, coffee, and tea can also add appreciable amounts of

pellagra A disease that results from severe niacin deficiency.

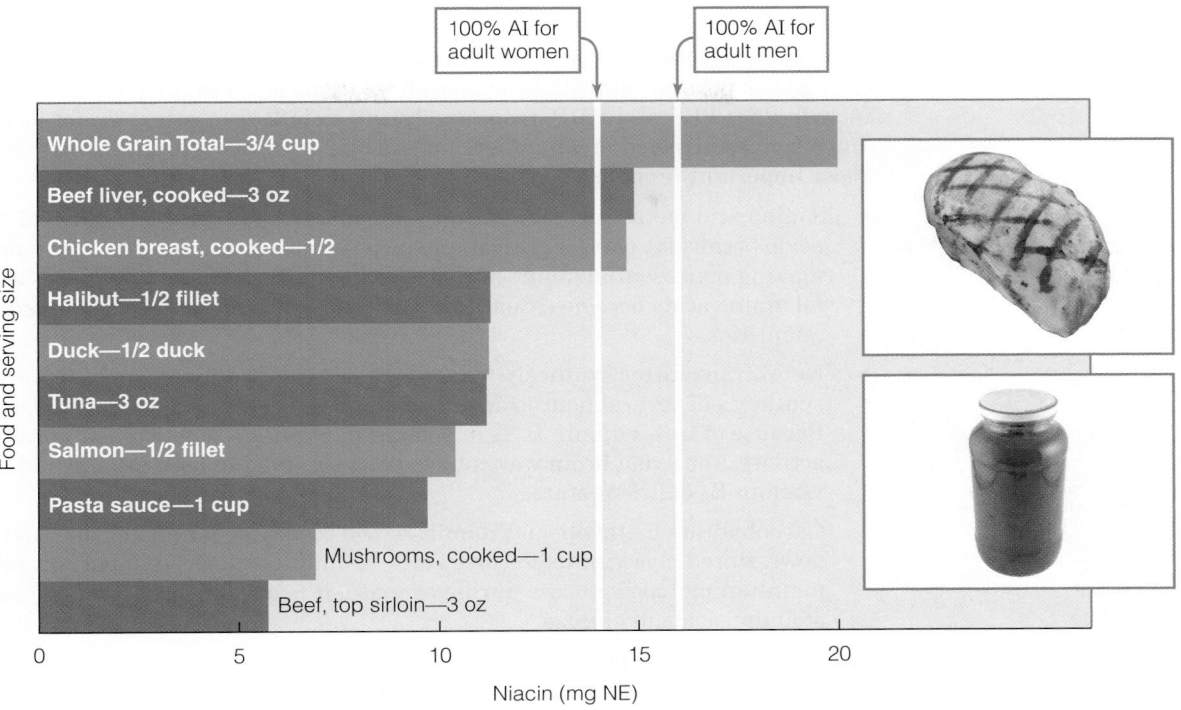

FIGURE 10.5   Common food sources of niacin. The RDA for niacin is 16 mg niacin equivalents (NE)/day for men and 14 mg NE/day for women 19 years and older. (Data from U.S. Department of Agriculture, Agricultural Research Service, 2006, USDA Nutrient Database for Standard Reference, Release 19. Nutrient Data Laboratory Home Page, www. ars.usda.gov/ba/bhnrc/ndl.)

riboflavin to the diet.[8] As with riboflavin, enriched or fortified breads, ready-to-eat cereals, and energy bars frequently provide 25–100% of the Daily Value for niacin.

Niacin can cause toxicity symptoms when taken in supplement form. These symptoms include *flushing,* which is defined as burning, tingling, and itching sensations accompanied by a reddened flush primarily on the face, arms, and chest. Liver damage, glucose intolerance, blurred vision, and edema of the eyes can be seen with very large doses of niacin taken over long periods of time.

> RECAP: *The B-complex vitamins include thiamin, riboflavin, niacin, vitamin B_6 (pyridoxine), folate, vitamin B_{12} (cobalamin), pantothenic acid, and biotin. Thiamin plays a critical role in the breakdown of glucose for energy and acts as a coenzyme in the metabolism of the branched-chain amino acids. Whole grains are good sources of thiamin. Thiamin-deficiency disease is called beriberi. Riboflavin is an important coenzyme involved in the metabolism of carbohydrates and fat. Milk, meats, and green vegetables are good sources of riboflavin. Riboflavin-deficiency disease is called ariboflavinosis. Niacin assists in the metabolism of carbohydrates and fatty acids for energy. It also plays an important role in DNA replication and repair and in cell differentiation. Corn-based diets can be low in niacin and can result in the deficiency disease pellagra.*

Vitamin B_6 (Pyridoxine)

Researchers discovered vitamin B_6 by ruling out deficiency of other B vitamins as the cause of a scaly dermatitis in rats.[3] They then discovered that B_6 deficiency was associated with convulsions in birds and later that infants fed formulas lacking B_6 also had convulsions and dermatitis.[9]

Functions of Vitamin B_6

Vitamin B_6 is actually a group of six related compounds: pyridoxine (PN), pyridoxal (PL), pyridoxamine (PM), and the phosphate forms of these compounds, which include PNP, PLP, and PMP (respectively). Vitamin B_6 is a coenzyme for more than 100 enzymes involved in a number of metabolic processes within the body. Some of these important functions are listed below.

- Amino acid metabolism. Vitamin B_6 is important for the metabolism of amino acids because it plays a critical role in transamination, which is a key process in making nonessential amino acids (see Chapter 6). Without adequate vitamin B_6, all amino acids become essential, as our bodies cannot make them in sufficient quantities.

- Neurotransmitter synthesis. Vitamin B_6 is a cofactor for enzymes involved in the synthesis of several neurotransmitters, which is also a transamination process. Because of this, vitamin B_6 is important in cognitive function and normal brain activity. Abnormal brain waves have been observed in both infants and adults in vitamin-B_6 deficient states.[10]

- Carbohydrate metabolism. Vitamin B_6 is a coenzyme for an enzyme that breaks down stored glycogen to glucose. Thus, vitamin B_6 plays an important role in maintaining blood glucose during exercise. It is also important for the conversion of amino acids to glucose.

- Heme synthesis. The synthesis of heme, required for the production of hemoglobin and thus the transport of oxygen, requires vitamin B_6. Chronic vitamin B_6 deficiency can lead to small red blood cells with inadequate amounts of hemoglobin, which is called *microcytic, hypochromic anemia*.[10] (This is discussed in more detail later in this chapter.)

- Immune function. Vitamin B_6 plays a role in maintaining the health and activity of lymphocytes and in producing adequate levels of antibodies in response to an immune challenge. The depression of immune function seen in vitamin B_6 deficiency may also be due to a reduction in vitamin B_6-dependent enzymes involved in DNA synthesis.

- Metabolism of other nutrients. Vitamin B_6 also plays a role in the metabolism of other nutrients, including niacin, folate, and carnitine.[10]

- Reduction of cardiovascular disease (CVD) risk. As discussed later in this chapter, high blood levels of homocysteine are considered an independent risk factor for CVD.[11] **Homocysteine** is a metabolic by-product of the metabolism of methionine, an essential amino acid. The enzymes involved in homocysteine metabolism require three key vitamins: folate, vitamin B_6, and vitamin B_{12}.[12] If they are not available to completely metabolize methoinine, blood levels of homocysteine increase. Adequate intakes of folate, vitamin B_6, and vitamin B_{12} can help keep blood levels of homocysteine low.

How Much Vitamin B_6 Should We Consume?

The recommended intakes for vitamin B_6 are listed in Table 10.1. Rich sources of vitamin B_6 are meats, including fish and poultry, eggs, dairy products, and peanut butter (FIGURE 10.6). Many vegetables, such as asparagus, potatoes, and carrots, fruits, especially bananas, and whole-grain cereals are also good sources of vitamin B_6. As with the other B vitamins discussed in this chapter, fortified or enriched grains, cereals, and energy bars can provide 25–100% of the daily value in 1 serving. Little vitamin B_6 is lost in storage or handling of foods, except the milling of grains; however, vitamin B_6 is sensitive to both heat and light so can easily be lost in cooking.

Vitamin B_6 supplements have been used to treat conditions such as premenstrual syndrome and carpal tunnel syndrome. You need to use caution, however, when using such supplements. Whereas consuming excess vitamin B_6 from food sources does not cause toxicity, excess B_6 from supplementing can result in nerve damage and lesions of the skin. A condition called *sensory neuropathy* (damage to the

Tuna is a good source of vitamin B_6.

homocysteine An amino acid that requires adequate levels of folate, vitamin B_6, and vitamin B_{12} for its metabolism. High levels of homocysteine in the blood are associated with an increased risk for vascular diseases such as cardiovascular disease.

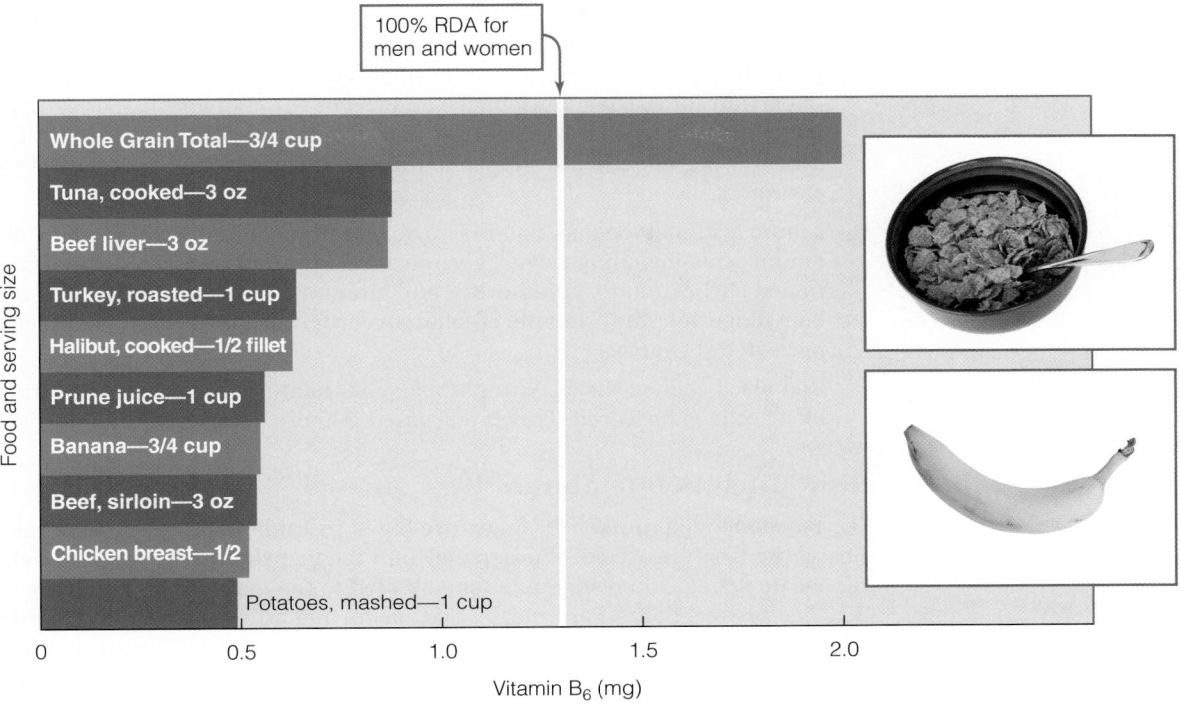

100% RDA for men and women

Whole Grain Total—3/4 cup

Tuna, cooked—3 oz

Beef liver—3 oz

Turkey, roasted—1 cup

Halibut, cooked—1/2 fillet

Prune juice—1 cup

Banana—3/4 cup

Beef, sirloin—3 oz

Chicken breast—1/2

Potatoes, mashed—1 cup

Food and serving size

0   0.5   1.0   1.5   2.0

Vitamin B$_6$ (mg)

FIGURE 10.6   Common food sources of vitamin B$_6$. The RDA for vitamin B$_6$ is 1.3 mg/day for men and women 19–50 years. (Data from U.S. Department of Agriculture, Agricultural Research Service, 2006, USDA Nutrient Database for Standard Reference, Release 19. Nutrient Data Laboratory Home Page, www.ars.usda.gov/ba/bhnrc/ndl.)

sensory nerves) has been documented in individuals taking high-dose B$_6$ supplements. The symptoms of sensory neuropathy include numbness and tingling involving the face, neck, hands, and feet, with difficulty manipulating objects and walking.

The symptoms of vitamin B$_6$ deficiency include anemia, convulsions, depression, confusion, and inflamed, irritated patches on the skin. Deficiency of vitamin B$_6$ has also been associated with a decreased ability to metabolize the amino acid methionine and a resultant increased risk for cardiovascular, cerebrovascular, and peripheral vascular disease. This condition also occurs with deficiency of folate and vitamin B$_{12}$, and is discussed in more detail in the next section.

Folate

Reports of symptoms we now recognize as folate deficiency go back two centuries.[13] By the late 1800s, a disorder associated with large red blood cells was characterized, but it wasn't until the 1930s that researchers understood that the condition was related to diet. It took another 40 years before researchers more fully understood the relationship between this blood abnormality and deficiency of folate, a substance found in many foods, especially leafy green vegetables. The name *folate* originated from the fact the vitamin is abundant in "foliage."[13]

Functions of Folate

Folate-requiring reactions in the body are collectively called *1-C metabolism*. This means folate is involved in adding "one-carbon units" to other organic compounds during the synthesis of new compounds or the modification of existing ones. Thus, the most basic cellular functions, such as the synthesis of DNA, require folate. Listed below are some of the functions that require folate.

- Nucleotide synthesis. Folate is required for the synthesis of thymidine and purines, which are needed for DNA synthesis. For this reason folate is important for cell division. Adequate intake is especially critical during the first few weeks of pregnancy, when the combined sperm–egg cell multiplies rapidly to form the primitive tissues and structures of the human body. Folate continues to be important for tissue maintenance and repair throughout life. For example, low folate may predispose normal tissues to increased risk of transformation into cancer cells, while folate supplementation appears to suppress the development of tumors.[14]

- Amino acid metabolism. Folate is involved in the metabolism of many of the amino acids including serine, glycine, histidine, and methionine. And as mentioned earlier, folate, vitamin B_{12}, and vitamin B_6 are required for the metabolism of methionine. The role of folate in cardiovascular disease is discussed in more detail shortly.

- Red blood cell synthesis. Without adequate folate, the synthesis of normal red blood cells is impaired. This is discussed in more detail shortly.

How Much Folate Should We Consume?

The recommended intakes for folate are listed in Table 10.1. The critical role of folate during the first few weeks of pregnancy and the fact that many women of childbearing age do not consume adequate amounts led to the mandatory fortification of enriched breads, flours, corn meals, rice, pasta, and other grain products with folic acid in 1998. Because of fortification, getting adequate folate in your diet is not difficult. The primary sources of folate in the American diet are ready-to-eat cereals, breads, and other grain products. Other good food sources include milk and eggs; oatmeal; meats, especially liver; fruits, such as bananas, grapefruit, oranges, pears, pineapple, and strawberries; juices of these fruits; and vegetables, including asparagus, green beans, peas, beets, broccoli, cauliflower, corn, tomatoes, lentils, spinach, and romaine lettuce (FIGURE 10.7).

Because folate is sensitive to heat, it can be lost when foods are cooked. It can also leach out into cooking water, which may then be discarded.

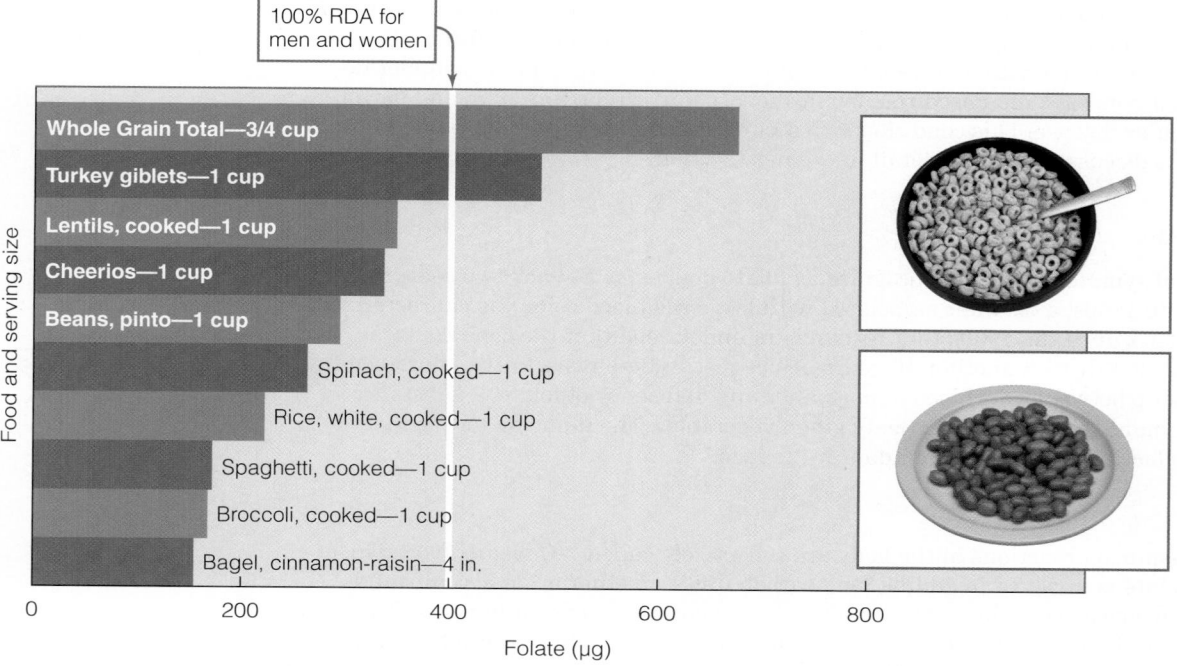

FIGURE 10.7 Common food sources of folate and folic acid. The RDA for folate is 400 µg/day for men and women. (Data from U.S. Department of Agriculture, Agricultural Research Service, 2006, USDA Nutrient Database for Standard Reference, Release 19. Nutrient Data Laboratory Home Page, www.ars.usda.gov/ba/bhnrc/ndl.)

What Happens If We Consume Too Much Folate?

Toxicity can occur when taking supplemental folate. One especially frustrating problem with folate toxicity is that it can mask a simultaneous vitamin B_{12} deficiency. This often results in failure to detect the B_{12} deficiency, and, as you saw in the chapter-opening case, a delay in diagnosis of B_{12} deficiency can contribute to severe damage to the nervous system. There do not appear to be any clear symptoms of folate toxicity independent from its interaction with vitamin B_{12} deficiency.

What Happens If We Don't Consume Enough Folate?

Folate deficiency can cause many adverse health effects, the three most significant of which are discussed here.

Neural Tube Defects.   A woman's requirement for folate substantially increases during pregnancy. This is because of the high rates of cell development needed for enlargement of the uterus, development of the placenta, expansion of the mother's red blood cells, and growth of the fetus. Inadequate folate intake during pregnancy is associated with major malformations in the fetus that are classified as neural tube defects.

Neural tube defects are the most common malformations of the central nervous system that occur during fetal development. The neural tube is formed by the fourth week of pregnancy, and it eventually develops into the brain and the spinal cord of the fetus. In a folate-deficient environment, the tube will fail to fold and close properly. The resultant defect in the newborn depends on the degree of failure and can range from protrusion of the spinal cord outside of the spinal column to a partial absence of brain tissue. Some forms of neural tube defects are minor and can be surgically repaired, while other forms are fatal. Neural tube defects are described in more detail in Chapter 19.

The challenging aspect of neural tube defects is that they occur very early in a woman's pregnancy, almost always before she knows she is pregnant. Thus, adequate folate intake is extremely important for all sexually active women of childbearing age, whether or not they intend to become pregnant. To prevent neural tube defects, it is recommended that all women capable of becoming pregnant consume 400 µg of folate daily from supplements, fortified foods, or both in addition to the folate they consume in their standard diet.[15]

Vascular Disease and Homocysteine.   As mentioned above, folate, vitamin B_6, and vitamin B_{12} are necessary for the complete metabolism of the essential amino acid methionine (**FIGURE 10.8**). When intakes of these nutrients are insufficient, the level of homocysteine, a by-product of methionine metabolism, increases in the blood. A thorough review of recent studies on this topic showed that elevated levels of homocysteine are associated with a 1.5 to 2 times greater risk for cardiovascular, cerebrovascular, and peripheral vascular diseases.[16] These diseases substantially increase a person's risk for a heart attack or stroke.

The exact mechanism by which elevated homocysteine levels increase the risk for vascular diseases is currently unknown. It has been speculated that homocysteine may damage the lining of blood vessels and stimulate the accumulation of plaque, which can lead to hardening of the arteries.[17] Homocysteine also increases blood clotting, which could lead to an increased risk of blocked arteries. Thus, by consuming adequate amounts of vitamin B_6, folate, and vitamin B_{12}, we may decrease our risk for a heart attack or stroke.

Macrocytic Anemia.   The term *anemia* literally means "without blood"; it is used to refer to any condition in which hemoglobin levels are low. Some anemias are caused by genetic problems. For instance, in Chapter 6 we discussed *sickle cell anemia,* a genetic disorder in which the red blood cells have a sickle shape. Another inherited anemia is *thalassemia,* a condition characterized by red blood cells that are small and short-lived. Other anemias are due to micronutrient deficiencies. These can be

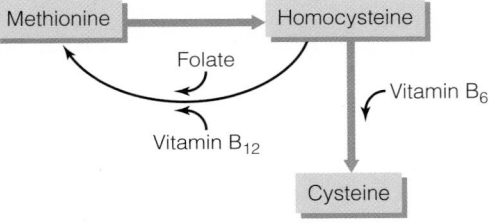

FIGURE 10.8   The metabolism of methionine, an essential amino acid, to homocysteine. Homocysteine can then be converted back to methionine through a vitamin B_{12}- and folate-dependent reaction or to cysteine through a vitamin B_6-dependent reaction. Cysteine is a nonessential amino acid important for making other biological compounds. Without these B vitamins, blood levels of homocysteine can increase. High levels of homocysteine are a risk factor for cardiovascular disease.

neural tube defects The most common malformations of the central nervous system that occur during fetal development. A folate deficiency can cause neural tube defects.

classified according to the general way they alter the size and shape of the red blood cells. Low iron, copper, and vitamin B_6 cause *microcytic anemia* (small red blood cells), while inadequate intakes of folate or vitamin B_{12} cause *macrocytic anemia* (large red blood cells). We discuss macrocytic anemia in more detail here.

Deficiency of either folate or vitamin B_{12} can impair DNA synthesis, which decreases the ability of blood cells to divide. If they cannot divide, differentiate, and mature, the cells remain large and immature precursors to red blood cells, known as *megaloblasts* (from *megalo,* meaning large, and *blast,* meaning a precursor cell). These immature cells contain inadequate hemoglobin; thus, their ability to transport oxygen is diminished. The resulting condition is sometimes referred to as *megaloblastic anemia*, but is more commonly called **macrocytic anemia** (from *macro,* meaning large, and *cyte,* meaning cell). Symptoms of macrocytic anemia are similar to those of other types of anemia, including weakness, fatigue, difficulty concentrating, irritability, headache, shortness of breath, and reduced exercise tolerance.

Vitamin B_{12} (Cobalamin)

In 1855, a clinician named Thomas Addison described a strange form of anemia in patients that left them feeling weak and exhausted.[18,19] To our knowledge, this is the first report describing the often fatal course of vitamin B_{12} deficiency, later called **pernicious anemia** (the word *pernicious* means causing great harm). Several decades passed before an "animal protein factor" was associated with the cobalt-containing vitamin B_{12}. The first clinical experiments in humans were done by Drs. Minot and Murphy in the 1920s. They fed patients with pernicious anemia large doses of liver and documented the improvement in their red blood cells.[19] For this work they were awarded the Nobel Prize in 1934. This work was extended by others who identified that some special "extrinsic factor" in the liver or meat was combined with an "intrinsic factor" in the stomach. When both of these factors were present, patients with pernicious anemia recovered. The final step in the identification of vitamin B_{12} as the extrinsic factor and in determining its structure was done by Dr. Dorothy Crowfoot Hodgkin, who was awarded the Nobel Prize for Chemistry in 1964.[19]

Functions of Vitamin B_{12}

Vitamin B_{12} is a coenzyme for two enzymes in the body that are part of two very important metabolic pathways.[18] First, vitamin B_{12} is important for the metabolism of methionine, an essential amino acid, and assists in the synthesis of biologic compounds such as creatine, phospholipids, neurotransmitters, DNA, and RNA. As with folate deficiency, a deficiency in vitamin B_{12} is most pronounced in rapidly dividing cells, such as the red blood cells, and results in a form of macrocytic anemia.

As noted earlier, adequate levels of folate, vitamin B_6, and vitamin B_{12} are necessary to prevent the buildup of homocysteine. A high level of homocysteine in the blood is related to an increased risk of heart disease.

The metabolic pathway involved in the metabolism of methionine also converts folate to its active form, which is a vitamin B_{12}-dependent process. Without vitamin B_{12}, folate becomes "trapped" in an inactive form and folate deficiency symptoms develop, even though adequate amounts of folate may be present in the diet.

Vitamin B_{12} is also important for the metabolism of certain abnormal fatty acids. When vitamin B_{12} is deficient in the diet, these abnormal fatty acids accumulate in the blood and are incorporated into cell membranes, including those in the nervous system, where they cause neurological problems. Also, as you saw in the chapter-opening scenario, B_{12} is essential for healthy functioning of the nervous system because it helps maintain the myelin sheath that coats nerve fibers. When this sheath is damaged or absent, the conduction of nervous signals is slowed, causing numerous neurological problems.

How Much Vitamin B_{12} Should We Consume?

The recommended intakes for vitamin B_{12} are listed in Table 10.1. Vitamin B_{12} is found primarily in animal products such as meats, fish, poultry, dairy products, and eggs and in fortified cereal products, such as ready-to-eat cereals (FIGURE 10.9). As dis-

macrocytic anemia A form of anemia manifested as the production of larger than normal red blood cells containing insufficient hemoglobin, which inhibits adequate transport of oxygen; also called megaloblastic anemia. Macrocytic anemia can be caused by a severe folate deficiency.

pernicious anemia A special form of anemia that is the primary cause of a vitamin B_{12} deficiency; occurs at the end stage of an autoimmune disorder that causes the loss of various cells in the stomach.

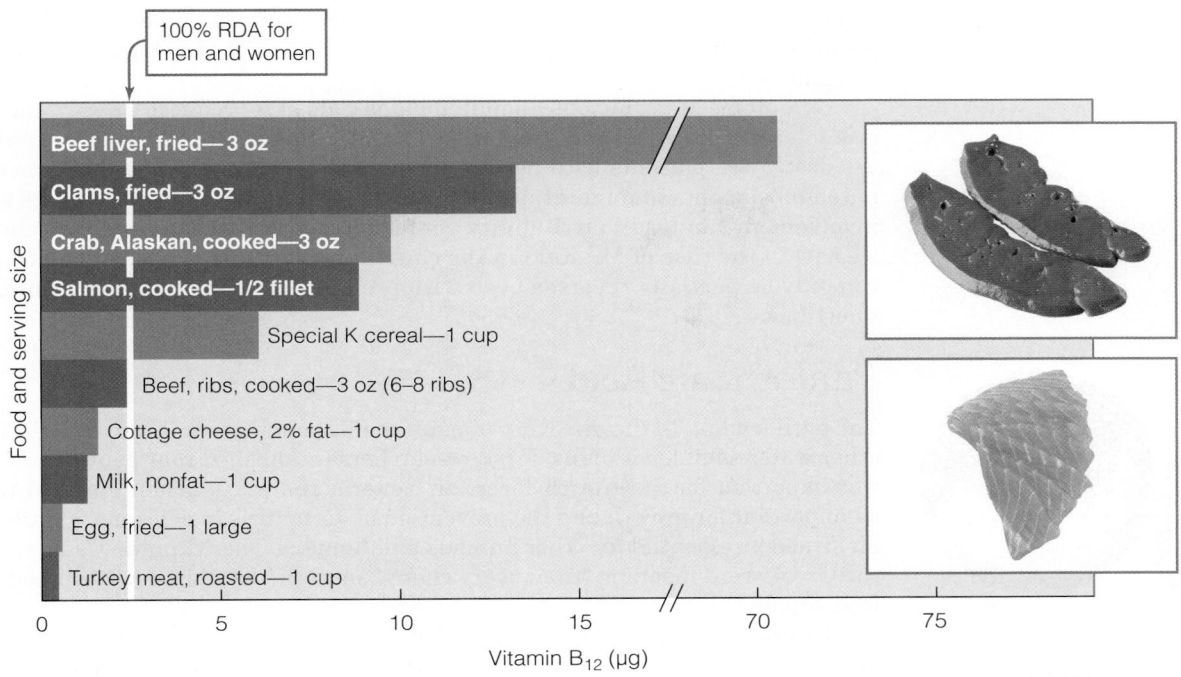

FIGURE 10.9   Common food sources of vitamin B$_{12}$. The RDA for vitamin B$_{12}$ is 2.4 μg/day for men and women. (Data from U.S. Department of Agriculture, Agricultural Research Service, 2006, USDA Nutrient Database for Standard Reference, Release 19. Nutrient Data Laboratory Home Page, www.ars.usda.gov/ba/bhnrc/ndl.)

cussed in Chapter 6, individuals consuming a vegan diet need to eat vegetable-based foods that are fortified with vitamin B$_{12}$ or take vitamin B$_{12}$ supplements or injections to ensure that they maintain adequate blood levels of this nutrient.

As we age, our sources of vitamin B$_{12}$ may need to change. Individuals younger than 51 years are generally able to meet the RDA for vitamin B$_{12}$ by consuming it in foods. However, it is estimated that about 10–30% of adults older than 50 years have a condition referred to as **atrophic gastritis** that results in low stomach acid secretion.[15] Since stomach acid separates food-bound vitamin B$_{12}$ from dietary proteins, if the acid content of the stomach is inadequate, then we cannot free up enough vitamin B$_{12}$ from food sources alone. Because atrophic gastritis can affect almost one-third of the older adult population, it is recommended that people older than 50 years of age consume foods fortified with vitamin B$_{12}$, take a vitamin B$_{12}$–containing supplement, or have periodic B$_{12}$ injections.

What Happens If We Consume Too Much Vitamin B$_{12}$?

There are no known adverse effects from consuming excess amounts of vitamin B$_{12}$ as either food or supplements.[15]

What Happens If We Don't Consume Enough Vitamin B$_{12}$?

The two primary causes of vitamin B$_{12}$ deficiency are insufficient intake and the inability to absorb the vitamin B$_{12}$ consumed. Either of these problems can result in the development of pernicious anemia, a special form of macrocytic anemia. The most common cause of the vitamin B$_{12}$ deficiency seen with pernicious anemia is lack of a protein called **intrinsic factor,** which is normally secreted by parietal cells in the stomach. Intrinsic factor binds to vitamin B$_{12}$ and aids its absorption in the small intestine. Without intrinsic factor, vitamin B$_{12}$ cannot cross the intestinal lining. Inadequate production of intrinsic factor occurs more commonly in older people, making them at higher risk for vitamin B$_{12}$ deficiency and pernicious anemia. It is also commonly seen in people with malabsorption disorders, as well as in people with tapeworm infestation of the gut, as the worms take up the vitamin B$_{12}$

Turkey contains vitamin B$_{12}$.

atrophic gastritis A condition that results in low stomach acid secretion; is estimated to occur in about 10–30% of adults older than 50 years.

intrinsic factor A protein secreted by cells of the stomach that binds to vitamin B$_{12}$ and aids its absorption in the small intestine.

before it can be absorbed by the intestines. Pernicious anemia can also occur in people who consume little or no vitamin B_{12} in their diets, such as people following a vegan diet.

Symptoms of pernicious anemia include pale skin, reduced energy and exercise tolerance, fatigue, and shortness of breath. In addition, because nerve cells are destroyed, patients with pernicious anemia lose the ability to perform coordinated movements and maintain their body's positioning. Central nervous system involvement can lead to irritability, confusion, depression, and even paranoia. As we saw in the case of Mr. Katz in the chapter opener, after onset, such symptoms can only be partially reversed even with prompt administration of vitamin B_{12} injections.

Pantothenic Acid

Shiitake mushrooms contain pantothenic acid.

The path leading to the discovery of pantothenic acid was similar to that for the other water-soluble vitamins. First, researchers established that pantothenic acid was important for the growth of certain bacteria and yeasts. Then they identified it as important for growth and the prevention of dermatitis in chickens. Finally, it was identified as essential for other animals and humans. The vitamin was named after the Greek word meaning "from everywhere," since the vitamin is widespread in the food supply.[20]

Pantothenic acid is a component of an important coenzyme that is required for all the energy-producing metabolic pathways. It is especially important for the breakdown and synthesis of fatty acids within the body. Thus, pantothenic acid assures that the foods we eat can be used for energy and that the excess energy we consume can be stored as fat.

The recommended intakes for pantothenic acid are listed in Table 10.1. Food sources include chicken, beef, egg yolks, potatoes, oat cereals, tomato products, whole grains, organ meats, and yeast. There are no known adverse effects from consuming excess amounts of pantothenic acid. Deficiencies of pantothenic acid are very rare.

Biotin

Early in the 1900s, it was observed that rats could maintain normal growth while being fed a diet containing cooked egg whites as the sole source of protein. About the same time, other researchers observed that if the egg whites were raw, rats developed diarrhea and skin problems.[3] The detrimental effects of feeding raw egg whites aroused great interest in the nutrition community. Could there be a toxic substance in raw egg whites that wasn't found in cooked egg whites? Experiments led to the discovery of biotin, which prevented the diarrhea and skin problems that occurred when raw egg whites were fed to rats. Raw egg whites contain a protein called avidin, which binds biotin in the gastrointestinal tract and prevents its absorption.

Biotin is a coenzyme for five important enzymes that are critical in the metabolism of carbohydrate, fat, and protein. It also plays an important role in gluconeogenesis.

The recommended intakes for biotin are listed in Table 10.1. The biotin content has been determined for very few foods, and these values are not reported in food composition tables or dietary analysis programs. Biotin appears to be widespread in foods, but is especially high in liver, egg yolks, and cooked cereals. Biotin is also produced by the intestinal flora in the gut, but its availability for absorption appears low.

There are no known adverse effects from consuming excess amounts of biotin. Biotin deficiencies are typically seen only in people who consume a large number of raw egg whites over long periods of time. Biotin deficiencies are also seen in people fed total parenteral nutrition (nutrients that are administered intravenously and bypass the gastrointestinal tract) that is not supplemented with biotin. Symptoms include thinning of hair; loss of hair color; development of red, scaly rash around the eyes, nose, and mouth; depression; lethargy; and hallucinations.

NUTRI-CASE LIZ

"Ever since my dance company folded after Christmas, I've been feeling exhausted. I know I should start auditioning for other companies, but it just seems too overwhelming right now. I'm cranky and spaced-out, and the least little thing makes me cry. Besides, I'm too fat to audition anywhere these days, because I'm so tired I've been skipping dance class. When I was still in bed at eleven o'clock this morning, my roommate told me I needed to start taking some B vitamins. She says that they give you energy. Maybe I'll ask her to drive me down to the health food store to buy some. It's only a mile away, but I don't think I have the energy to walk."

Is Liz's roommate correct when she asserts that B-complex vitamins "give you energy"? Considering what you've learned about Liz in previous Nutri-Case episodes, do you think it is likely that she'd benefit from taking B-complex vitamin supplements? Why or why not? What other concerns does her situation raise, and what additional advice might you give her?

RECAP: *Vitamin B$_6$ is a coenzyme for more than 100 enzymes involved in processes such as the metabolism of amino acids and carbohydrates and synthesis of neurotransmitters. It is widely found in meats, poultry, fish, dairy products, and certain fruits and vegetables. The most basic cellular functions, such as the synthesis of DNA as well as cell differentiation, require folate. Folate is widely found in green leafy vegetables and is added to breads, cereals, and other grain-based foods. Folate deficiency causes macrocytic anemia and can lead to neural tube defects in the developing fetus. Vitamin B$_{12}$ is essential for metabolism of methionine and certain abnormal fatty acids. Deficiency leads to pernicious anemia, a type of macrocytic anemia, and nervous system damage. Low intakes of vitamin B$_6$, folate, and vitamin B$_{12}$ are associated with elevated blood homocysteine levels, which increase the risk of cardiovascular, cerebrovascular, and peripheral vascular disease. Pantothenic acid is especially important for the breakdown and synthesis of fatty acids, whereas biotin is a coenzyme for enzymes that are critical in the metabolism of carbohydrate, fat, and protein.*

acetylcholine A neurotransmitter that is involved in many functions, including muscle movement and memory storage.

Choline

Choline is a vitamin-like substance found in many foods. It is typically grouped with the B-complex vitamins because of its role in assisting homocysteine metabolism (see Table 10.1). Choline also accelerates the synthesis and release of **acetylcholine,** a neurotransmitter that is involved in many functions, including muscle movement and memory storage. Choline is also necessary for the synthesis of phospholipids and other components of cell membranes; thus, choline plays a critical role in the structural integrity of cell membranes. Finally, choline plays an important role in the transport and metabolism of fats and cholesterol.

The recommended intakes for choline are listed in Table 10.1. The choline content of foods is not typically reported in nutrient databases. However, we do know that choline is widespread in foods, especially milk, liver, eggs, and peanuts. Inadequate intakes of choline can lead to increased fat accumulation in the liver, which eventually leads to liver damage. Excessive intake of supplemental choline results in various toxicity symptoms, including a fishy body odor, vomiting, excess salivation, sweating, diarrhea, and low blood pressure.

Choline is widespread in foods and can be found in eggs and milk.

FIGURE 10.10 Goiter, or enlargement of the thyroid gland, occurs with both iodine toxicity and deficiency.

Iodine

Iodine is a trace mineral needed to support energy regulation. Iodine is also unique in that it is the heaviest metal required for human nutrition, but it is responsible for just one function within the body, the synthesis of thyroid hormones.[21] Our bodies require thyroid hormones to regulate body temperature, maintain resting metabolic rate, and support reproduction and growth. Inorganic iodine, the form of iodine found in the earth's environment, occurs predominantly as iodide, while iodine, the oxidized from of iodide, is the form of the nutrient most common in food. The iodine content of crops depends on the level of iodide in the soil. Iodide-deficient soils are common in mountainous areas and areas that have experienced frequent flooding. In general, the level naturally found in most foods and beverages is low.

While our bodies need relatively little iodine, adequate amounts are necessary to maintain health. The recommended intakes are listed in Table 10.1. Very few foods naturally contain iodine. Saltwater foods tend to have higher amounts because marine animals concentrate iodine from seawater. Good food sources include saltwater fish, shrimp, iodized salt, white and whole-wheat breads made with iodized salt and bread conditioners, and milk and other dairy products. Interestingly, iodine is added to dairy cattle feed and used in sanitizing solutions in the dairy industry, making dairy foods an important source. In addition, a majority of households worldwide now use iodized salt. For many people, iodized salt is their only source of iodine, and approximately one-half a teaspoon meets the entire adult RDA for iodine.

Too much iodine blocks the synthesis of thyroid hormones. As the thyroid attempts to produce more hormones, it may enlarge, a condition known as **goiter** (FIGURE 10.10). (Goiter refers only to the enlarged thyroid gland, regardless of its cause.) Iodine toxicity generally occurs due to excessive supplementation.

Paradoxically, goiter is also the primary symptom of iodine deficiency. Iodine deficiency suppresses the production of thyroid hormones, leading to *hypothyroidism* (low levels of thyroid hormones) and goiter. Other symptoms of hypothyroidism are decreased body temperature, inability to tolerate cold environmental temperatures, weight gain, fatigue, and sluggishness. If a woman experiences iodine deficiency during pregnancy, her infant has a high risk of being born with a special form of mental retardation referred to as **cretinism.** In addition to mental retardation, these infants may suffer from stunted growth, deafness, and muteness.

Chromium

Chromium is a trace mineral that plays an important role in carbohydrate metabolism. You may be interested to learn that the chromium in our bodies is the same metal used in the chrome plating for cars.

Chromium enhances the ability of insulin to transport glucose from the bloodstream into cells. Chromium also plays important roles in the metabolism of RNA and DNA, in immune function, and in growth. Chromium supplements are marketed to reduce body fat and enhance muscle mass and have become popular with bodybuilders and other athletes interested in improving their body composition. The Nutrition Myth or Fact? box investigates whether taking supplemental chromium is effective in improving body composition.

We have only very small amounts of chromium in our bodies. Whether the U.S. diet provides adequate chromium is controversial; our bodies appear to store less chromium as we age.

The recommended intakes for chromium are listed in Table 10.1. Foods that have been identified as good sources of chromium include mushrooms, prunes, dark chocolate, nuts, whole grains, cereals, asparagus, brewer's yeast, some beers, and red wine. Dairy products are typically poor sources of chromium.

There appears to be no toxicity related to consuming chromium in the diet or in supplement form. Chromium deficiency appears to be uncommon in the United States. When induced in a research setting, chromium deficiency inhibits the uptake of glucose by the cells, causing a rise in blood glucose and insulin levels. Chromium deficiency can also result in elevated blood lipid levels and in damage to the brain and nervous system.

Our bodies contain very little chromium. Asparagus is a good dietary source of this trace mineral.

goiter Enlargement of the thyroid gland; can be caused by either iodine toxicity or deficiency.

cretinism A special form of mental retardation that occurs in infants when the mother experiences iodine deficiency during pregnancy.

NUTRITION MYTH OR FACT?

Can Chromium Supplements Enhance Body Composition?

Because athletes are always looking for a competitive edge, there are a multitude of supplements marketed and sold to enhance exercise performance and body composition. Chromium supplements, predominantly in the form of chromium picolinate, are popular with bodybuilders and weight lifters. This popularity stems from the claims that chromium increases muscle mass and muscle strength and decreases body fat.

An early study of chromium supplementation was promising, in that chromium use in both untrained men and football players was found to decrease body fat and increase muscle mass.[22] These findings caused a surge in popularity of chromium supplements and motivated many scientists across the United States to test the reproducibility of these early findings. The next study of chromium supplementation found no effects of chromium on muscle mass, body fat, or muscle strength.[23]

These contradictory reports led experts to closely examine the two studies and to design more sophisticated studies to assess the effect of chromium on body composition. There were a number of flaws in the methodology of these early studies. One major concern was that the chromium status of the research participants prior to the study was not measured or controlled. It was possible that the participants were

deficient in chromium; this deficiency could cause a more positive reaction to chromium than would be expected in people with normal chromium status.

A second major concern was that body composition was measured in these studies using the skinfold technique, in which calipers are used to measure the thickness of the skin and fat at various sites on the body. While this method gives a good general estimate of body fat in young, lean, healthy people, it is not sensitive to small changes in muscle mass. Thus, subsequent studies of chromium used more sophisticated methods of measuring body composition.

The results of research studies conducted over the past 10 years consistently show that chromium supplementation has no effect on muscle mass, body fat, or muscle strength in a variety of groups, including untrained college males and females, obese females, collegiate wrestlers, and older men and women.[24–30] Despite the overwhelming evidence to the contrary, many supplement companies still claim that chromium supplements enhance strength and muscle mass and reduce body fat. These claims result in millions of dollars of sales of supplements to consumers each year. Armed with this information, you can avoid being fooled by such an expensive nutrition myth.

Manganese

A trace mineral, manganese is a cofactor involved in energy metabolism and in the formation of urea, the primary component of urine. It also assists in the synthesis of the protein matrix found in bone tissue and in building cartilage, a tissue that supports joints. As reviewed in Chapter 8, manganese is also an integral component of superoxide dismutase, an antioxidant enzyme. Thus, manganese assists in the conversion of free radicals to less damaging substances, protecting our bodies from oxidative damage.

The recommended intakes for manganese are listed in Table 10.1. Manganese requirements are easily met, as this mineral is widespread in foods and is readily available in a varied diet. Whole-grain foods such as oat bran, wheat flour, whole-wheat spaghetti, and brown rice are good sources of manganese (FIGURE 10.11). Other foods that are good sources of manganese include pineapple, pine nuts, okra, spinach, and raspberries.

Okra is one of the many foods that contain manganese.

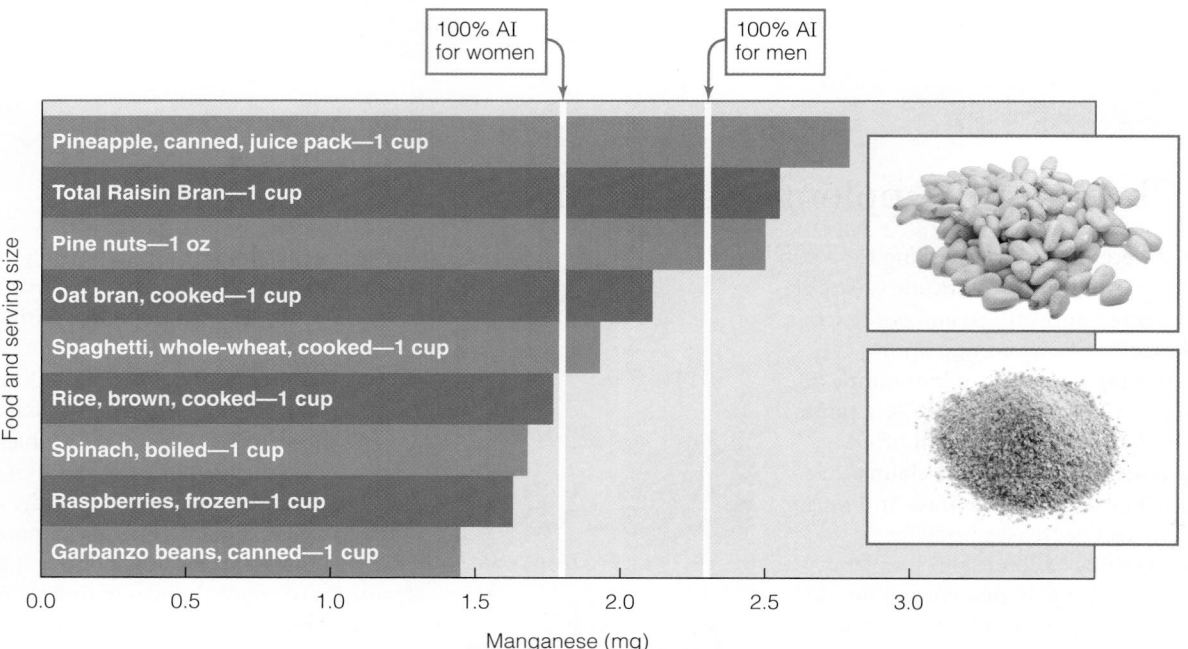

FIGURE 10.11 Common food sources of manganese. The AI for manganese is 2.3 mg/day for men and 1.8 mg/day for women. (Data from U.S. Department of Agriculture, Agricultural Research Service, 2006, USDA Nutrient Database for Standard Reference, Release 19. Nutrient Data Laboratory Home Page, www.ars.usda.gov/ba/bhnrc/ndl.)

Manganese toxicity can occur in occupational environments in which people inhale manganese dust and can also result from drinking water high in manganese. Toxicity results in impairment of the neuromuscular system, causing symptoms similar to those seen in Parkinson's disease, such as muscle spasms and tremors. Manganese deficiency is rare in humans. Symptoms of manganese deficiency include impaired growth and reproductive function, reduced bone density and impaired skeletal growth, impaired glucose and lipid metabolism, and skin rash.

Sulfur

Sulfur is a major mineral and a component of the B-complex vitamins thiamin and biotin. In addition, as part of the amino acids methionine and cysteine, sulfur helps stabilize the three-dimensional shapes of proteins. The liver requires sulfur to assist in the detoxification of alcohol and various drugs, and sulfur helps the body maintain acid–base balance.

We are able to synthesize ample sulfur from the protein-containing foods we eat; as a result, we do not need to consume sulfur in the diet, and there is no DRI for sulfur. There are no known toxicity or deficiency symptoms associated with sulfur.

RECAP: *Choline is a vitamin-like substance that assists in homocysteine metabolism and the production of acetylcholine. Iodine is necessary for the synthesis of thyroid hormones, which regulate metabolic rate and body temperature. Chromium enhances the transport of glucose into the cell, is important in the metabolism of RNA and DNA, and plays a role in immune function and growth. Manganese is involved in energy metabolism, the formation of urea, the synthesis of bone protein matrix and cartilage, and protection against free radicals. Sulfur is part of the B-complex vitamins thiamin and biotin and also part of the amino acids methionine and cysteine.*

Whole blood

Components separated by centrifuge

55% plasma (fluid portion of blood)

Less than 1% platelets and white blood cells (leukocytes)

45% red blood cells (erythrocytes)

FIGURE 10.12 Blood has four components, which are visible when the blood is drawn into a test tube and spun in a centrifuge. The bottom layer is the erythrocytes, or red blood cells. The milky layer above the erythrocytes contains the leukocytes and platelets. The yellow fluid on top is the plasma.

What Is the Role of Blood in Maintaining Health?

Blood is critical to maintaining life, as it transports virtually everything in our bodies. No matter how efficiently we metabolize carbohydrates, fats, and proteins, without healthy blood to transport those nutrients to our cells, we could not survive. In addition to transporting nutrients and oxygen to our cells to support life, blood removes the waste products generated from metabolism so that they can be properly excreted. Our health and our ability to perform daily activities are compromised if the quantity and quality of our blood are diminished.

Blood is actually a tissue, the only fluid tissue in our bodies. It has four components (**FIGURE 10.12**). **Erythrocytes,** or red blood cells, are the cells that transport oxygen. **Leukocytes,** or white blood cells, are the key to our immune function and protect us from infection and illness. **Platelets** are cell fragments that assist in the formation of blood clots and help stop bleeding. **Plasma** is the fluid portion of the blood, and it is needed to maintain adequate blood volume so that the blood can flow easily throughout our bodies.

Certain micronutrients play important roles in the maintenance of blood health through their actions as cofactors, coenzymes, and regulators of oxygen transport. These nutrients are discussed in detail in the following section.

A Profile of Nutrients That Maintain Healthy Blood

The nutrients recognized as playing a critical role in maintaining blood health include vitamin K, iron, zinc, and copper. A summary of the functions, requirements, and toxicity and deficiency symptoms of these nutrients is provided in Table 10.2.

Vitamin K

Vitamin K is a fat-soluble vitamin important for both bone and blood health. The role of vitamin K in the synthesis of proteins involved in maintaining bone density was

erythrocytes The red blood cells, which are the cells that transport oxygen in our blood.

leukocytes The white blood cells, which protect us from infection and illness.

platelets Cell fragments that assist in the formation of blood clots and help stop bleeding.

plasma The fluid portion of the blood; is needed to maintain adequate blood volume so that the blood can flow easily throughout our bodies.

TABLE 10.2 Functions, Recommended Intakes, and Toxicity and Deficiency Symptoms of Nutrients Involved in Maintaining Blood Health

Nutrient	Primary Functions	Recommended Intake*	Toxicity Symptoms/ Side Effects	Deficiency Symptoms/ Side Effects
Vitamin K	Coenzyme that assists in the synthesis of proteins involved in the coagulation of blood Coenzyme involved in the synthesis of proteins that assist in maintaining bone density	AI for 19 years and older: Men = 120 µg/day Women = 90 µg/day	None known at this time	Excessive bleeding or severe hemorrhaging due to inability to form blood clots Effect on bone health is controversial
Iron	As a component of hemoglobin, assists with oxygen transport in our blood As a component of myoglobin, assists in the transport of oxygen into muscle cells Cofactor for enzymes involved in energy metabolism Part of the antioxidant enzyme system that combats free radicals	RDA for 19 to 50 years: Men = 8 mg/day Women = 18 mg/day RDA for 51 years and older: Men = 8 mg/day Women = 8 mg/day RDA for pregnant females: 27 mg/day UL for 19 years and older: 45 mg/day	Nausea; vomiting, diarrhea; dizziness; confusion; rapid heartbeat; damage to heart, central nervous system, liver, kidneys; death	First stage of iron deficiency is marked by a decrease in iron stores with no physical symptoms Second stage of iron deficiency is marked by a decrease in iron transport, causing reduced work capacity Third stage of iron deficiency is marked by anemia, causing impaired work performance, general fatigue, pale skin, depressed immune function, impaired cognitive and nerve function, and impaired memory
Zinc	Cofactor that assists with hemoglobin production Part of superoxide dismutase antioxidant enzyme system that combats free radicals Assists enzymes in metabolizing carbohydrates, fats, and proteins and in activating vitamin A to facilitate vision Facilitates folding of proteins, which assists in gene regulation Plays role in cell replication and normal growth and sexual maturation Plays a role in proper development and function of immune system	RDA for 19 years and older: Men = 11 mg/day Women = 8 mg/day UL for 19 years and older: 40 mg/day	Intestinal pain and cramps, nausea, vomiting, loss of appetite, diarrhea, headaches, depressed immune function, decreased concentration of high-density lipoprotein, reduced absorption of copper	Growth retardation, diarrhea, delayed sexual maturation and impotence, eye and skin lesions, hair loss, impaired appetite, increased incidence of illness and infections

*RDA, Recommended Dietary Allowance; AI, Adequate Intake; UL, Upper Limit.

TABLE 10.2 Functions, Recommended Intakes, and Toxicity and Deficiency Symptoms of Nutrients Involved in Maintaining Blood Health (continued)

Nutrient	Primary Functions	Recommended Intake*	Toxicity Symptoms/ Side Effects	Deficiency Symptoms/ Side Effects
Copper	Cofactor in metabolic pathways that produce energy Coenzyme that assists in production of collagen and elastin Part of superoxide dismutase antioxidant enzyme system that combats free radicals Component of ceruloplasmin, which facilitates the proper transport of iron	RDA for 19 years of age and older: Men and Women = 900 µg/day UL for 19 years and older: 10 mg/day	Abdominal pain and cramps, nausea, diarrhea, vomiting, liver damage occurs in extreme cases that result from Wilson's disease and other rare disorders	Anemia, reduced levels of white blood cells, osteoporosis in infants and growing children

*RDA, Recommended Dietary Allowance; AI, Adequate Intake; UL, Upper Limit.

discussed in detail on page 381 in Chapter 9. In this section we focus primarily on its role in blood health.

Functions of Vitamin K

Vitamin K acts as a coenzyme that assists in the synthesis of a number of proteins that are involved in the coagulation of blood, including *prothrombin* and the *procoagulants, factors VII, IX,* and *X.* Without adequate vitamin K, blood does not clot properly: clotting time can be delayed, or clotting may even fail to occur. The failure of blood to clot can lead to increased bleeding from even minor wounds, as well as internal hemorrhaging.

How Much Vitamin K Should We Consume?

Our needs for vitamin K are relatively small, but intakes of this nutrient in the United States are highly variable because vitamin K is found in few foods.[31] Healthful intestinal bacteria produce vitamin K in our large intestine, providing us with an important non-dietary source of vitamin K.

The recommended intakes for vitamin K are listed in Table 10.2. There is no upper limit (UL) established for vitamin K at this time.[32]

Green, leafy vegetables are good sources of vitamin K. Examples include collard greens, spinach, broccoli, brussels sprouts, and cabbage. Soybean and canola oils are also good sources. Refer to FIGURE 9.13 (page 382) for a description of the vitamin K content of these foods.

What Happens If We Consume Too Much Vitamin K?

There are no known side effects associated with consuming large amounts of vitamin K from supplements or from food.[32] In the past, a synthetic form of vitamin K was used for therapeutic purposes and was shown to cause liver damage; this form is no longer used.

What Happens If We Don't Consume Enough Vitamin K?

Vitamin K deficiency inhibits our ability to form blood clots, resulting in excessive bleeding and even severe hemorrhaging in some cases. Vitamin K deficiency is rare in humans. People with diseases that cause malabsorption of fat, such as celiac disease, Crohn's disease, and cystic fibrosis, can suffer secondarily from a deficiency of

Blood clotting. Without enough vitamin K our blood will not clot properly.

Green, leafy vegetables are a good source of vitamin K.

hemoglobin The oxygen-carrying protein found in our red blood cells; almost two-thirds of all of the iron in our bodies is found in hemoglobin.

vitamin K. Newborns are typically given an injection of vitamin K at birth, as they lack the intestinal bacteria necessary to produce this nutrient.

As discussed in Chapter 9, the impact of vitamin K deficiency on bone health is controversial. Although a recent study found that low intakes of vitamin K were associated with a higher risk of bone fractures in women, there is not enough scientific evidence to strongly illustrate that vitamin K deficiency causes osteoporosis.[32,33]

> RECAP: *Blood is a fluid tissue composed of erythrocytes, leukocytes, plasma, and platelets. It transports nutrients and oxygen to our cells to support life and removes the waste products generated from metabolism. Vitamin K is a fat-soluble vitamin and coenzyme that is important for blood clotting and bone metabolism. Bacteria manufacture vitamin K in our large intestine.*

Iron

With few exceptions, iron is important for every known living organism. It is essential to cells, but can be toxic in high doses. Thus, the body needs to regulate iron levels carefully to be sure adequate iron is supplied to cover the essential functioning of biological processes, but prevent excess accumulation. Thus, iron is a trace mineral that is needed in very small amounts in our diets. Despite our relatively small need for iron, iron deficiency is the most common nutrient deficiency in the world.

Functions of Iron

Iron is a component of four primary iron-containing protein groups within the body, which carry out a number of important functions within the body. First, iron is a component of two oxygen-carrying proteins within the body: hemoglobin and myoglobin. **Hemoglobin** is the oxygen-carrying protein found in our red blood cells. In fact, almost two-thirds of all of the iron in our bodies is found in hemoglobin. As shown in FIGURE 10.13, the hemoglobin molecule consists of four polypeptide chains studded

FIGURE 10.13 Iron is contained in the heme portion of hemoglobin and myoglobin.

with four iron-containing **heme** groups. You know that we cannot survive for more than a few minutes without oxygen. Thus, hemoglobin's ability to transport oxygen throughout the body is absolutely critical to life. To carry oxygen, hemoglobin depends on the iron in its heme groups. Iron is able to bind with and release atoms such as oxygen, nitrogen, and sulfur very easily. It does this by transferring electrons to and from the other atoms as it moves between various oxidation states. In the bloodstream, iron acts as a shuttle, picking up oxygen from the environment, binding it during its transport in the bloodstream, and then dropping it off again in our tissues. Iron is also a component of **myoglobin,** a protein similar to hemoglobin but found in muscle cells. As a part of myoglobin, iron assists in the transport of oxygen into muscle cells.

Iron is found in a number of enzymes involved in energy production. Iron-requiring enzymes called *cytochromes* are electron carriers within the metabolic pathways that result in the production of energy from carbohydrates, fats, and protein. Iron is also part of a group of sulfur-containing enzymes that act as electron carriers. In addition, more than twelve different iron-containing proteins, including the cytochromes, are found in the mitochondria.[34] Iron is critical to the function of certain enzymes important to some immune cells and signaling pathways; thus, iron is required for humans to mount an effective immune response to pathogens.[34] Research over the last 30 years has also documented the importance of iron in central nervous system functions. Like vitamin B_{12}, iron is required for maintenance of the myelin sheath covering nerve fibers; as noted earlier, without adequate myelin, conduction of nerve impulses is slowed. Iron is also needed for the production of neurotransmitters including serotonin, norepinephrine, and dopamine. Moreover, iron is important for muscle function. Individuals who have poor iron status complain of lethargy, apathy, and listlessness, which may be independent of iron's role in oxygen delivery. Some of these complaints could be due to the impact of iron deficiency on the brain or on fuel metabolism. Finally, as you learned in Chapter 8, iron is a part of the antioxidant enzyme system that assists in fighting free radicals. Interestingly, excess iron can also act as a prooxidant and promote the production of free radicals.

How Is Iron Absorbed?

Our bodies contain relatively little iron; men have less than 4 g of iron in their bodies, while women have just over 2 g. Our bodies are capable of storing excess iron in two storage forms, **ferritin** and **hemosiderin.** The most common areas of iron storage in our bodies are the liver, bone marrow, intestinal mucosa, and spleen. Because iron is so important for life, our bodies recycle the iron lost when aging cells are broken down, especially cells high in iron like red blood cells. The liver and spleen are responsible for breaking down old red blood cells and recycling the components, including the iron. This iron-recycling program reduces the body's reliance on dietary iron. Each day, about 85% of the iron released from hemoglobin breakdown is reused by the body.

Our ability to absorb iron from the diet is influenced by a number of factors, including iron status, stomach acid content, the amount and type of iron in foods, and the presence of dietary factors that can either enhance or inhibit the absorption of iron. Absorption of iron is highest when our iron stores are low. Thus, people who have poor iron status, such as those with iron deficiency, pregnant women, or people who have recently experienced blood loss (including menstruation), have the highest iron absorption rates. In addition, adequate amounts of stomach acid are necessary for iron absorption. People with low levels of stomach acid, including many older adults, have a decreased ability to absorb iron.

The total amount of iron in your diet influences your absorption rate. People who consume low levels of dietary iron absorb more iron from their foods than those with higher dietary iron intakes. Our bodies can also detect when iron stores are high; when this occurs, less iron is absorbed from food.

The type of iron in the foods you eat is a major factor influencing your iron absorption. There are two types of iron found in foods: heme iron and non-heme iron. **Heme iron** is a part of hemoglobin and myoglobin and is found only in animal-based foods such as meat, fish, and poultry. **Non-heme iron** is the form of iron that is not

heme The iron-containing molecule found in hemoglobin.

myoglobin An iron-containing protein similar to hemoglobin except that it is found in muscle cells.

ferritin A storage form of iron in our bodies found primarily in the intestinal mucosa, spleen, bone marrow, and liver.

hemosiderin A storage form of iron in our bodies found primarily in the intestinal mucosa, spleen, bone marrow, and liver.

heme iron Iron that is a part of hemoglobin and myoglobin; found only in animal-based foods such as meat, fish, and poultry.

non-heme iron The form of iron that is not a part of hemoglobin or myoglobin; found in animal- and plant-based foods.

a part of hemoglobin or myoglobin. It is found in both plant-based and animal-based foods. Heme iron is much more absorbable than non-heme iron. Since the iron in animal-based foods is about 40% heme iron and 60% non-heme iron, animal-based foods are good sources of absorbable iron. In contrast, all of the iron found in plant-based foods is non-heme iron. Meat, fish, and poultry also contain a special **meat factor** that enhances the absorption of non-heme iron. Vitamin C (or ascorbic acid) also enhances the absorption of non-heme iron.

Dietary factors that impair iron absorption include phytates, polyphenols, vegetable proteins, and calcium. Phytates are found in legumes, rice, and whole grains. Polyphenols include tannins found in tea and coffee and are also present in oregano and red wine. Soybean protein and calcium inhibit iron absorption. Due to the variability of iron absorption as a result of these dietary factors, it is estimated that the bioavailability of iron from a vegan diet is approximately 10%, while it averages 18% for a mixed Western diet.[32]

How Much Iron Should We Consume?

The variability of iron availability from food sources was taken into consideration when estimating dietary recommendations for iron, which are listed in Table 10.2. Notice that the higher iron requirement for younger women is due to the excess iron and blood lost during menstruation.

A number of special circumstances can significantly affect iron requirements. These are identified in Table 10.3.

meat factor A special factor found in meat, fish, and poultry that enhances the absorption of non-heme iron.

TABLE 10.3 Special Circumstances Affecting Iron Status

Circumstances That Improve Iron Status	Circumstances That Diminish Iron Status
Use of oral contraceptives—use of oral contraceptives reduces menstrual blood loss in women.	Use of hormone replacement therapy—use of hormone replacement therapy in postmenopausal women can cause uterine bleeding, increasing iron requirements.
Breastfeeding—breastfeeding delays resumption of menstruation in new mothers so reduces menstrual blood loss. It is therefore an important health measure, especially in developing nations.	Eating a vegetarian diet—vegetarian diets, particularly vegan diets, contain no sources of heme iron or meat factor. Due to the low absorbability of non-heme iron, vegetarians have iron requirements that are 1.8 times higher than those of nonvegetarians.
Consumption of iron-containing foods and supplements.	Intestinal parasitic infection—approximately 1 billion people suffer from intestinal parasite infection. Many of these parasites cause intestinal bleeding and occur in countries in which iron intakes are inadequate. Iron-deficiency anemia is common in people with intestinal parasitic infection.
	Blood donation—blood donors have lower iron stores than nondonors; people who donate frequently, particularly premenopausal women, may require iron supplementation to counter the iron losses that occur with blood donation.
	Intense endurance exercise training—people engaging in intense endurance exercise appear to be at risk for poor iron status due to many factors, including suboptimal iron intake and increased iron loss in sweat and increased fecal losses.

Source: From "Dietary Reference Intakes for Vitamin A, Vitamin K, Arsenic, Boron, Chromium, Copper, Iodine, Manganese, Molybdenum, Nickel, Silicon, Vanadium, and Zinc," © 2002 by the National Academy of Sciences. Reprinted by permission.

SHOPPER'S GUIDE
Good Food Sources of Iron

Good food sources of heme iron include meats, poultry, and fish (FIGURE 10.14). Clams, oysters, and beef liver are particularly good sources of iron. Many breakfast cereals and breads are enriched with iron; although this iron is the non-heme type and less absorbable, it is still significant because these foods are a major part of the U.S. diet. Some vegetables and legumes are also good sources of iron, and the absorption of their non-heme iron can be enhanced by eating them with foods that contain the meat factor and heme iron, such as meat, fish and poultry, or with vitamin C–rich foods, such as citrus foods, red and green peppers, or broccoli.

FIGURE 10.14 Common food sources of iron. The RDA for iron is 8 mg/day for men and 18 mg/day for women aged 19 to 50 years. (Data from U.S. Department of Agriculture, Agricultural Research Service, 2006, USDA Nutrient Database for Standard Reference, Release 19. Nutrient Data Laboratory Home Page, www.ars.usda.gov/ba/bhnrc/ndl.)

Tips for Increasing Your Iron Intake

√ Shop for iron-fortified breads and breakfast cereals. Check the Nutrition Facts Panel!

√ When choosing nutrition bars, select brands that are fortified with iron.

√ Consume a food or beverage that is high in vitamin C along with plant or animal sources of iron. For instance, drink a glass of orange juice with your morning toast to increase the absorption of the non-heme iron in the bread. Or add chopped tomatoes to beans or lentils. Or sprinkle lemon juice on fish.

(Continued)

√ Add small amounts of meat, poultry, or fish to baked beans, vegetable soups, stir-fried vegetables, or salads to enhance the absorption of the non-heme iron in the plant-based foods.

√ Cook foods in cast-iron pans to significantly increase the iron content of foods: the iron in the pan will be absorbed into the food during the cooking process.

√ Avoid drinking red wine, coffee, or tea when eating iron-rich foods, as chemicals called polyphenols in these beverages will reduce iron absorption.

√ Avoid drinking cow's milk or soymilk with iron-rich foods, as both calcium and soybean protein inhibit iron absorption.

√ Avoid taking calcium supplements or zinc supplements with iron-rich foods, as these minerals decrease iron absorption.

What Happens If We Consume Too Much Iron?

Accidental iron overdose is the most common cause of poisoning deaths in children younger than 6 years of age in the United States.[35] It is important for parents to take the same precautions with dietary supplements as they would with other drugs, keeping them in a locked cabinet or well out of reach of children. Symptoms of iron toxicity include nausea, vomiting, diarrhea, dizziness, confusion, and rapid heartbeat. If iron toxicity is not treated quickly, significant damage to the heart, central nervous system, liver, and kidneys can result in death.

Adults who take iron supplements even at prescribed doses commonly experience constipation. Taking vitamin C with the iron supplement not only enhances absorption but also can help reduce constipation. Other gastrointestinal symptoms include nausea, vomiting, and diarrhea. As introduced in Chapter 8, some individuals suffer from a hereditary disorder called hemochromatosis. This disorder affects between 1 in 200 and 1 in 400 individuals of northern European descent.[36] Hemochromatosis is characterized by excessive absorption of dietary iron and altered iron storage. The accumulation of iron in these individuals over many years causes cirrhosis of the liver, liver cancer, heart attack and heart failure, diabetes, and arthritis. Men are more at risk for this disease than women due to the higher losses of iron in women through menstruation. Treatment includes reducing dietary intake of iron, avoiding high intakes of vitamin C, and withdrawing blood occasionally.

What Happens If We Don't Consume Enough Iron?

Iron deficiency is the most common nutrient deficiency in the world. People at particularly high risk for iron deficiency include infants and young children, adolescent girls, premenopausal women, and pregnant women. Refer to the Highlight box to learn more about the impact of iron deficiency on people around the world.

Iron deficiency progresses through three stages (FIGURE 10.15). The first stage of iron deficiency causes a decrease in iron *stores,* resulting in reduced levels of ferritin. During this first stage, there are generally no physical symptoms because hemoglobin levels are not yet affected. The second stage of iron deficiency causes a decrease in the *transport* of iron. This manifests as a reduction in the transport protein for iron, called **transferrin.** The production of heme also starts to decline during this stage, leading to symptoms of reduced work capacity. During the third and final stage of iron deficiency, **iron-deficiency anemia** results.

In iron-deficiency anemia, the production of normal, healthy red blood cells decreases. Red blood cells that are produced are smaller than normal and do not contain enough hemoglobin to transport adequate oxygen or to allow the proper transfer of electrons to produce energy. This type of anemia is often referred to as *microcytic*

transferrin The transport protein for iron.

iron-deficiency anemia A form of anemia that results from severe iron deficiency.

HIGHLIGHT

Iron Deficiency Around the World

Iron deficiency is the most common nutritional deficiency in the world. According to the World Health Organization, approximately 4 to 5 billion people, or 66–80% of the world's population, are iron deficient.[37] Because of its high prevalence worldwide, iron deficiency is considered an epidemic.

As you have learned in this chapter, severe iron deficiency results in anemia. Iron deficiency appears to be the main cause of anemia around the world. Other factors that can cause anemia include deficiencies of folate, vitamin B_{12}, and vitamin A and infections such as hookworm and malarial parasites. In fact, it is estimated that 2 billion people suffer from worm infections, while 300 to 500 million people suffer from malaria.

Those who are particularly susceptible to iron deficiency include people living in developing countries, pregnant women, and young children. But iron deficiency not only hurts individuals. Because it results in increased healthcare needs, premature death and resultant family breakdown, and lost work productivity, it also damages communities and entire nations.

Among children, the health consequences of iron-deficiency anemia are particularly devastating. They include:

- Premature birth
- Low birth weight
- Increased risk of infections
- Increased risk of premature death
- Impaired cognitive and physical development
- Behavioral problems and poor school performance

To date, it is still unclear whether iron supplementation in children already suffering from iron-deficiency anemia can effectively and consistently reverse the cognitive and behavioral damage that has occurred.[38]

The World Health Organization has developed a comprehensive plan to address all aspects of iron deficiency and anemia.[37] This plan is being implemented in developing countries that suffer high rates of iron deficiency and anemia. This plan involves:

1. increasing iron intake with iron supplements, iron-rich foods, and foods that enhance iron absorption,
2. controlling infections that cause anemia, including hookworm infections and malaria, and
3. improving overall nutritional status by controlling major nutrient deficiencies and improving the quality and diversity of people's diets.

By implementing this plan around the world, it is hoped that the devastating effects of iron deficiency can be reduced and potentially even eliminated.

Stage III, iron-deficiency anemia
- Decreased production of normal red blood cells
- Reduced production of heme
- Inadequate hemoglobin to transport oxygen
- Symptoms include pale skin, fatigue, reduced work performance, impaired immune and cognitive functions

Stage II, iron-deficiency erythropoiesis
- Decreased iron transport
- Reduced transferrin
- Reduced production of heme
- Physical symptoms include reduced work capacity

Stage I, iron depletion
- Decreased iron stores
- Reduced ferritin level
- No physical symptoms

FIGURE 10.15 Iron deficiency passes through three stages. The first stage is identified by decreased iron stores, or reduced ferritin levels. The second stage is identified by decreased iron transport, or a reduction in transferrin. The final stage of iron deficiency is iron-deficiency anemia, which is identified by decreased production of normal, healthy red blood cells and inadequate hemoglobin levels.

anemia (*micro,* meaning small, and *cyte,* meaning cell). As normal cellular death occurs over time, more and more healthy red blood cells are replaced by these deficient cells, and the classic symptoms of oxygen and energy deprivation develop. These symptoms include impaired work performance, general fatigue, pale skin, depressed immune function, impaired cognitive and nerve function, and impaired memory. Pregnant women with severe anemia are at higher risk for low-birth-weight infants, premature delivery, and increased infant mortality.

> RECAP: *Iron is a trace mineral that, as part of the hemoglobin protein, plays a major role in the transportation of oxygen in our blood. Iron is also a coenzyme in many metabolic pathways involved in energy production. Meat, fish, and poultry are good sources of heme iron, which is more absorbable than non-heme iron. Toxicity symptoms for iron range from nausea and vomiting to organ damage and potentially death. If left untreated, iron deficiency eventually leads to iron-deficiency anemia.*

Zinc

Zinc is a trace mineral that acts as a cofactor for approximately a hundred different enzymes. It thereby plays an important role in many physiologic processes in nearly every body system.

Functions of Zinc

As a cofactor, zinc assists in the production of hemoglobin, indirectly supporting the adequate transport of oxygen to our cells. Zinc is also part of the superoxide dismutase antioxidant enzyme system and thus helps fight the oxidative damage caused by free radicals. It assists enzymes in generating energy from carbohydrates, fats, and protein and in activating vitamin A in the retina of the eye.

Zinc also plays a role in facilitating the folding of proteins into biologically active molecules used in gene regulation. Thus, it is critical for cell replication and normal growth. In fact, zinc deficiency was discovered in the early 1960s when researchers were trying to determine the cause of severe growth retardation, anemia, and poorly developed testicles in a group of Middle Eastern men. These symptoms of zinc deficiency illustrate its critical role in normal growth and sexual maturation.

Zinc is vital for the proper development and functioning of the immune system. In fact, zinc has received so much attention for its contribution to immune system health that zinc lozenges have been formulated to fight the common cold. The Nutrition Debate at the end of this chapter explores the question of whether or not these lozenges are effective.

How Much Zinc Should We Consume?

As with iron, our need for zinc is relatively small, but our intakes are variable and absorption is influenced by a number of factors. Overall, zinc absorption is similar to that of iron, ranging from 10% to 35% of dietary zinc. People with poor zinc status absorb more zinc than individuals with optimal zinc status, and zinc absorption increases during times of growth, sexual development, and pregnancy.

Several dietary factors influence zinc absorption. High non-heme iron intakes can inhibit zinc absorption, which is a primary concern with iron supplements (which are non-heme), particularly during pregnancy and lactation. High intakes of heme iron appear to have no effect on zinc absorption. The phytates and fiber found in whole grains and beans strongly inhibit zinc absorption. In contrast, dietary protein, especially animal-based protein, enhances zinc absorption. It's not surprising, then, that the primary cause of the zinc deficiency in the Middle Eastern men just mentioned was their low consumption of meat and high consumption of beans and unleavened breads (also called *flat breads*). In leavening bread, the baker adds yeast to the dough. This not only makes the bread rise, but also helps reduce the phytate content of the bread.

The recommended intakes for zinc are listed in Table 10.2. Good food sources of zinc include red meats, some seafood, whole grains, and enriched grains and cereals. The dark meat of poultry has a higher content of zinc than white meat. As zinc is signif-

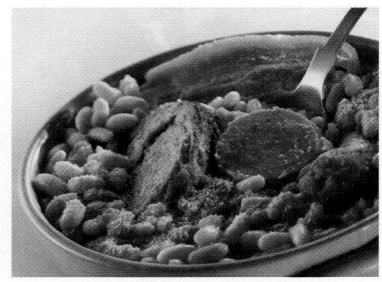

Zinc can be found in pork and beans.

FIGURE 10.16 Common food sources of zinc. The RDA for zinc is 11 mg/day for men and 8 mg/day for women. (Data from U.S. Department of Agriculture, Agricultural Research Service, 2006, USDA Nutrient Database for Standard Reference, Release 19. Nutrient Data Laboratory Home Page, www.ars.usda.gov/ba/bhnrc/ndl.)

icantly more absorbable from animal-based foods, zinc deficiency is a concern for people eating a vegan diet. FIGURE 10.16 shows various foods that are relatively high in zinc.

What Happens If We Consume Too Much Zinc?

Eating high amounts of dietary zinc does not appear to lead to toxicity. Zinc toxicity can occur from consuming zinc in supplement form and in fortified foods. Toxicity symptoms include intestinal pain and cramps, nausea, vomiting, loss of appetite, diarrhea, and headaches. Excessive zinc supplementation has also been shown to depress immune function and decrease high-density lipoprotein concentrations. High intakes of zinc can also reduce copper status, as zinc absorption interferes with the absorption of copper.

What Happens If We Don't Consume Enough Zinc?

Zinc deficiency is uncommon in the United States but occurs more often in countries in which people consume predominantly grain-based foods. Symptoms of zinc deficiency include growth retardation, diarrhea, delayed sexual maturation and impotence, eye and skin lesions, hair loss, and impaired appetite. As zinc is critical to a healthy immune system, zinc deficiency also results in increased incidence of infections and illnesses.

Copper

Copper is a trace mineral that functions as a cofactor in many physiologic reactions. Copper is widely distributed in foods, and copper deficiency is rare.

Copper functions as a cofactor in the metabolic pathways that produce energy, in the production of the connective tissues collagen and elastin, and as part of the superoxide dismutase enzyme system that fights the damage caused by free radicals. Copper is a component of *ceruloplasmin,* a protein that is critical for the proper transport of iron. If ceruloplasmin levels are inadequate, iron accumulation results, causing symptoms similar to those described with the genetic disorder hemochromatosis

Lobster is a food that contains copper.

(page 428). Copper is also necessary for the regulation of certain neurotransmitters important to brain function.

Copper needs are very small, and people who eat a varied diet can easily meet their requirements. As we saw with iron and zinc, people with low dietary copper intakes absorb more copper than people with high dietary intakes. Also recall that high zinc intakes can reduce copper absorption and, subsequently, copper status. In fact, zinc supplementation is used as a treatment for a rare disorder called Wilson's disease, in which copper toxicity occurs. High iron intakes can also interfere with copper absorption in infants.

The recommended intakes for copper are listed in Table 10.2. Good food sources of copper include organ meats, seafood, nuts, and seeds. Whole-grain foods are also relatively good sources. FIGURE 10.17 identifies some foods relatively high in copper.

The long-term effects of copper toxicity are not well studied in humans. Toxicity symptoms include abdominal pain and cramps, nausea, diarrhea, and vomiting. Liver damage occurs in the extreme cases of copper toxicity that occur with Wilson's disease and other health conditions associated with excessive copper levels.

Copper deficiency is rare but can occur in premature infants fed milk-based formulas and in adults fed prolonged formulated diets that are deficient in copper. Deficiency symptoms include anemia, reduced levels of white blood cells, and osteoporosis in infants and growing children.

> RECAP: *Zinc is a trace mineral that is a part of almost a hundred enzymes that impact virtually every body system. Zinc plays a critical role in hemoglobin synthesis, physical growth and sexual maturation, and immune function and assists in fighting the oxidative damage caused by free radicals. Copper is a trace mineral that functions as a cofactor in the metabolic pathways that produce energy, in the production of the connective tissues collagen and elastin, and as part of the superoxide dismutase enzyme system that fights the damage caused by free radicals. Copper is also a component of ceruloplasmin, a protein that is critical for the proper transport of iron.*

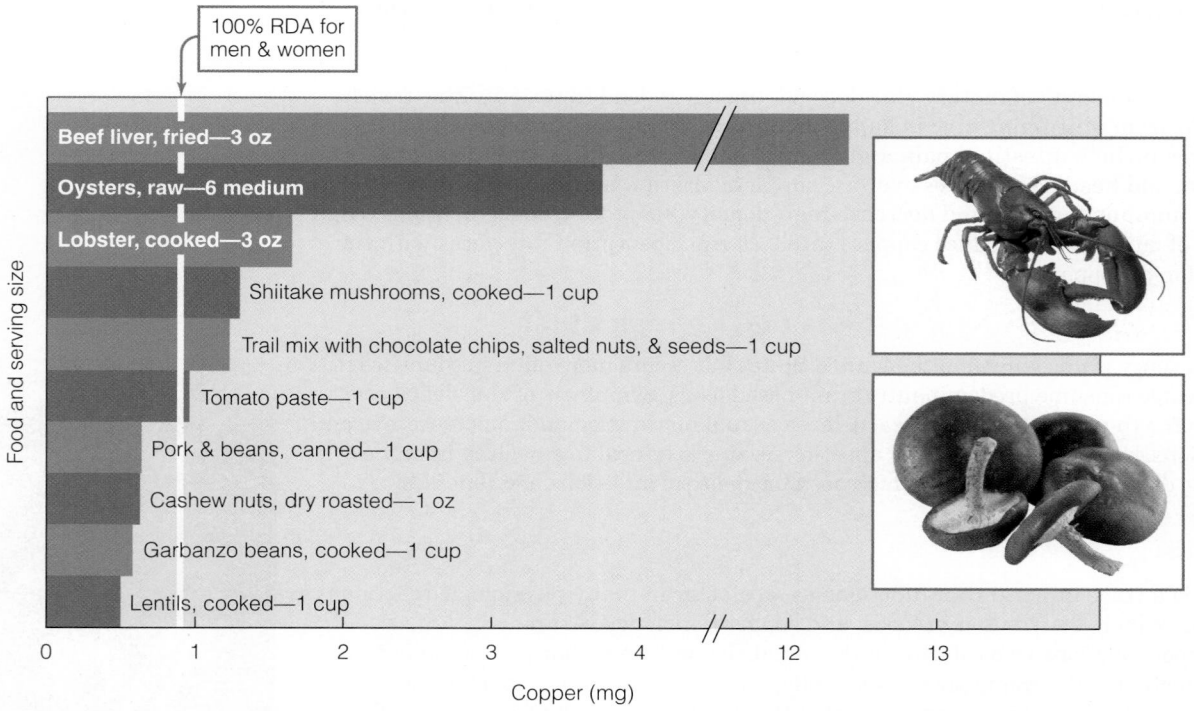

FIGURE 10.17 Common food sources of copper. The RDA for copper is 900 μg/day for men and women. (Data from U.S. Department of Agriculture, Agricultural Research Service, 2006, USDA Nutrient Database for Standard Reference, Release 19. Nutrient Data Laboratory Home Page, www.ars.usda.gov/ba/bhnrc/ndl.)

NUTRI-CASE THEO

" You know, I never thought I needed to take a multivitamin because I'm healthy and I eat lots of different kinds of foods. But now I've learned in my nutrition course about what all these vitamins and minerals do in the body, and I'm thinking, heck, maybe I should take one just for insurance. I mean, I use up a lot of fuel playing basketball and working out. Maybe if I popped a pill every day, I'd have an easier time keeping my weight up!"

Do you think Theo should take a multivitamin-mineral supplement "just for insurance"? Why or why not? Would taking one be likely to have any effect on Theo's weight?

CHAPTER SUMMARY

- The B-complex vitamins include thiamin, riboflavin, vitamin B_6, niacin, folate, vitamin B_{12}, pantothenic acid, and biotin.
- The primary role of the B-complex vitamins is to act as coenzymes. In this role, they activate enzymes and assist them in the metabolism of carbohydrates, fats, and amino acids; the repair and replication of DNA; cell differentiation; the formation and maintenance of the central nervous system; and the formation of blood.
- Thiamin is abundant in whole-grain foods; deficiency causes beriberi.
- Riboflavin is abundant in milk, meat, poultry, and fish, and some green vegetables; deficiency causes ariboflavinosis.
- Niacin is widely available, but may be inadequate in limited corn-based diets; deficiency of niacin causes pellagra.
- Vitamin B_6 is found in a variety of foods. Toxicity is possible with supplementation and causes sensory neuropathy.
- Folate is found in green vegetables and in fortified grain-based foods such as breads and cereals. Neural tube defects, which can result from inadequate folate intake during the first 4 weeks of pregnancy, are the most common malformations of the fetal central ner-

vous system. Some neural tube defects are minor and can be treated with surgery; other neural tube defects are fatal.

- Inadequate intakes of vitamin B_6, folate, and vitamin B_{12} are associated with elevated homocysteine levels and a greater risk of suffering from cardiovascular, cerebrovascular, and peripheral vascular diseases. These diseases significantly increase one's risk for a heart attack or stroke.
- Deficiency of folate causes macrocytic anemia, in which the red blood cells are large and immature. Symptoms include fatigue and weakness.
- Vitamin B_{12} is available only from animal-based foods, fortified foods, and supplements. Pernicious anemia can be caused by insufficient dietary intake of vitamin B_{12}, but is more commonly caused by insufficient levels of intrinsic factor secretion by the parietal cells of the stomach. Pernicious anemia causes reduced energy and exercise tolerance, as well as signs of nervous system damage, including impaired movement and cognitive and personality changes.
- Choline is a vitamin-like substance that assists with homocysteine metabolism. Choline also accelerates the synthesis and release of acetylcholine, a neurotransmitter that is involved in a variety of functions such as muscle function and memory storage.
- Iodine is a trace mineral needed for the synthesis of thyroid hormones. Thyroid hormones are integral to the

regulation of body temperature, maintenance of resting metabolic rate, and healthy reproduction and growth.

- Chromium is a trace mineral that enhances the ability of insulin to transport glucose from the bloodstream into the cell. Chromium is also necessary for the metabolism of RNA and DNA and supports normal growth and immune function.

- Manganese is a trace mineral that acts as a cofactor in energy metabolism and in the formation of urea. Manganese also assists in the synthesis of the protein matrix found in bone, assists in building cartilage, and is a component of the superoxide dismutase antioxidant enzyme system.

- Sulfur is a major mineral that is a component of the B-complex vitamins thiamin and biotin. It is also a part of the amino acids methionine and cysteine. Sulfur helps stabilize the three-dimensional shapes of proteins and helps the liver detoxify alcohol and various drugs.

- Blood is the only fluid tissue in our bodies. It has four components: erythrocytes, or red blood cells; leukocytes, or white blood cells; platelets; and plasma, or the fluid portion of our blood.

- Blood is critical for transporting oxygen and nutrients to our cells and for removing waste products from our cells so they can be properly excreted.

- Vitamin K is a fat-soluble vitamin that acts as a coenzyme assisting in the coagulation of blood. Vitamin K is also a coenzyme in the synthesis of proteins that assist in maintaining bone density.

- Iron is a trace mineral. Almost two-thirds of the iron in our bodies is found in hemoglobin, the oxygen-carrying protein in our blood. Iron is a cofactor for many of the enzymes involved in the metabolism of carbohydrates, fats, and protein. It is also a part of the superoxide dismutase antioxidant enzyme system that fights free radicals.

- Heme iron is found in animal-based foods and is more readily absorbed than non-heme iron found in plant-based foods.

- Zinc is a trace mineral that acts as a cofactor in the production of hemoglobin, in the superoxide dismutase antioxidant enzyme system, in the metabolism of carbohydrates, fats, and proteins, and in activating vitamin A in the retina. Zinc is also critical for cell reproduction and growth and for proper development and functioning of the immune system.

- Copper is a trace mineral that functions as a cofactor in the metabolic pathways that produce energy, in the production of collagen and elastin, and as part of the superoxide dismutase antioxidant enzyme system.

Copper is also a component of ceruloplasmin, a protein needed for the proper transport of iron.

- *Anemia* is a term that means "without blood." Severe iron deficiency results in iron-deficiency anemia, in which the production of normal, healthy red blood cells decreases and hemoglobin levels are inadequate. Symptoms include fatigue, weakness, and increased susceptibility to infection. A form of microcytic anemia, iron deficiency is the most common nutrient deficiency in the world.

TEST YOURSELF ANSWERS

1. **False.** B-complex vitamins do not directly provide energy for our bodies. However, they play critical roles in ensuring that our bodies are able to generate energy from carbohydrates, fats, and proteins.

2. **True.** People who consume a vegan diet need to pay particularly close attention to consuming enough vitamin B_{12}, iron, and zinc. In some cases, these individuals may need to take supplements to consume adequate amounts of these nutrients.

3. **False.** Research studies have failed to show any consistent effects of chromium supplements on reducing body fat or enhancing muscle mass.

4. **True.** This deficiency is particularly common in infants, children, and women of childbearing age.

5. **True and false!** For an individual who consumes a varied diet that provides adequate energy and nutrients, this statement is true. However, many people do not consume a varied diet that provides adequate levels of micronutrients, and others have health issues that increase their requirements or affect their ability to absorb micronutrients from food. For these individuals, a daily multivitamin/mineral supplement is not a waste of money and is important to optimize health.

REVIEW QUESTIONS

1. The B-complex vitamins include
   a. niacin, folate, and iodine.
   b. cobalamin, iodine, and chromium.
   c. manganese, riboflavin, and pyridoxine.
   d. thiamin, pantothenic acid, and biotin.

2. The micronutrient most closely associated with blood clotting is
   a. iron.
   b. vitamin K.
   c. zinc.
   d. vitamin B_{12}.

FIND THE QUACK

Like many menstruating women, Dionna has premenstrual syndrome, more commonly called PMS. For the 7 to 10 days preceding her monthly period, she experiences moodiness, fatigue, bloating, headaches, and strong cravings for sweet and salty foods. In fact, she blames PMS for her steady weight gain over the last several years. Surfing the Internet for a solution to her food cravings and other PMS-related symptoms, Dionna finds a supplements Web site promoting vitamin B_6 supplements for the treatment of PMS. Here is what it says:

- If you experience headache, fluid retention, breast tenderness, food cravings, depression, anxiety, or mood swings during the week to 2 weeks before your period, you probably have a vitamin B_6 deficiency.

- Used as recommended, our patented **PMS Formula** provides 152 mg per day of vitamin B_6 as pyridoxine.

- Our average customer rating for this product is five stars: A typical satisfied customer: "I used to feel so exhausted in the week before my period that I could barely drag myself through the days. Now I have energy to spare!" —Tasha from Santa Monica.

1. What is the RDA for vitamin B_6 for a woman Dionna's age (she is 19)? What is the UL? What percentage of each does the **PMS Formula** provide if used as recommended?

2. What, if any, health concerns might the level of vitamin B_6 recommended by this manufacturer raise?

3. Tasha from Santa Monica states that the **PMS Formula** has given her "energy to spare." Comment on the implication of her statement that B-complex vitamins give us energy.

4. The **PMS Formula** is patented; thus, it must have been tested for effectiveness and safety by U.S. government agencies. True or false?

Answers can be found at www.aw-bc.com/thompson.

3. Which of the following statements about iron is true?
   a. Iron is stored primarily in the liver, the blood vessel walls, and the heart muscle.
   b. Iron is a component of hemoglobin, myoglobin, and certain enzymes.
   c. Iron is a component of red blood cells, platelets, and plasma.
   d. Excess iron is stored primarily in the form of ferritin, cytochromes, and intrinsic factor.

4. Homocysteine is
   a. a by-product of glycolysis.
   b. a trace mineral.
   c. an amino acid.
   d. a B-complex vitamin.

5. Which of the following statements about choline is true?
   a. Choline is found exclusively in foods of animal origin.
   b. Choline is a B-complex vitamin that assists in homocysteine metabolism.
   c. Choline is a neurotransmitter that is involved in muscle movement and memory storage.
   d. Choline is necessary for the synthesis of phospholipids and other components of cell membranes.

6. True or false? Blood has four components: erythrocytes, leukocytes, platelets, and plasma.

7. True or false? There is no DRI for sulfur.

8. True or false? Iron is found only in foods of animal origin.

9. True or false? The best way for a pregnant woman to protect her fetus against neural tube defects is to begin taking a folate supplement as soon as she learns she is pregnant.

10. True or false? Wilson's disease occurs when copper deficiency allows accumulation of iron in the body.

11. In the chapter-opening story, Mr. Katz was given an injection of vitamin B_{12}. Why didn't his physician simply give him the vitamin in pill form?

12. Cassandra is 11 years old and has just begun menstruating. She and her family members are vegans (that is, they consume only plant-based foods). Explain why Cassandra's parents should be careful that their daughter consume not only adequate iron, but also adequate vitamin C.

13. Avery is a lacto-ovo-vegetarian. His typical daily diet includes milk, yogurt, cheese, eggs, nuts, seeds, legumes, whole grains, and a wide variety of fruits and

vegetables. He does not take any supplements. What, if any, micronutrients are likely to be inadequate in his diet?

14. Janine is 23 years old and engaged to be married. She is 40 pounds overweight and has hypertension, and her mother suffered a mild stroke recently, at age 45. For all these reasons, Janine is highly motivated to lose weight and has put herself on a strict low-carbohydrate diet recommended by a friend. She now scrupulously avoids breads, pastries, pasta, rice, and "starchy" fruits and vegetables. Identify two reasons why Janine should consider taking a folate supplement.

15. Create a simple flow chart showing how loss of intrinsic factor in an older adult can lead to symptoms of dementia.

WEB LINKS

www.ars.usda.gov/ba/bhnrc/ndl
Nutrient Data Laboratory Home Page

Click on Search to find reports listing food sources for selected nutrients.

www.anemia.com
Anemia Lifeline

Visit this site to learn about anemia and its various treatments.

www.unicef.org/nutrition/index_4050.html
UNICEF-Nutrition

This site provides information about micronutrient deficiencies in developing countries and the efforts to combat them.

www.thearc.org
The Arc

Search this site for "neural tube defects" and find a wealth of information on the development and prevention of these conditions.

REFERENCES

1. Bernstein, L. 2000. Dementia without a cause: Lack of vitamin B_{12} can cause dementia. *Discover* Magazine, February, 2000.
2. Bates, C. J. 2006. Thiamin. In: Bowman, B. A., and R. M. Russel, eds. *Present Knowledge in Nutrition,* 9th edn., pp. 242–249. Washington, DC: ILSI Press.
3. McCollum, E. V. 1957. *A History of Nutrition.* Boston, MA: Houghton Mifflin Co.
4. Day, E., P. Bentham, R. Callaghan, T. Kuruvilla, and S. George. 2004. Thiamine for Wernicke-Korsakoff Syndrome in people at risk from alcohol abuse (review). *Cochrane Database Syst. Rev.* 1:CD0040033.
5. McCormick, D. B. 2005. Riboflavin. In: Shils, M. E., M. Shike, A. C. Ross, B. Caballero, and R. Cousins, eds. *Modern Nutrition in Health and Disease,* 10th edn., pp. 434–441. Philadelphia, PA: Lippincott Williams & Wilkins.
6. Rivlin, R. S. 2006. Riboflavin. In: Bowman, B. A., and R. M. Russel, eds. *Present Knowledge in Nutrition,* 9th edn., pp. 250–259. Washington, DC: ILSI Press.

7. Jacques, P. F., A. Taylor, S. Moeller, et al. 2005. Long-term nutrient intake and 5-year change in nuclear lens opacities. *Arch. Ophthalmol.* 123:571–526.
8. Jacob, R. A. 2006. Niacin. In: Bowman, B. A., and R. M. Russel, eds. *Present Knowledge in Nutrition,* 9th edn., pp. 260–268. Washington, DC: ILSI Press.
9. Jukes, T. H. 1990. Nutrition science from vitamins to molecular biology. *Annual Reviews of Nutrition,* 10:1–10.
10. Mackey, A. D., S. R.Davis, and J. F. Gregory III. 2006. Vitamin B_6. In: Shils, M. E., M. Shike, A. C. Ross, B. Caballero, and R. Cousins, eds. *Modern Nutrition in Health and Disease,* 10th edn., pp. 452–461. Philadelphia, PA: Lippincott Williams & Wilkins.
11. Boushey, C. J., S. A. Beresford, G. S. Omenn, and A. G. Motulsky. 1995. A quantitative assessment of plasma homocysteine as a risk factor for vascular disease. Probable benefits of increasing folic acid intakes. *JAMA* 274:1049–1057.
12. Joubert, L. M., and M. M. Manore. 2006. Exercise, nutrition and homocysteine. *Int. J. Sport Nutr. Exer. Metab.* 16:341–361.
13. Carmel, R. 2006. Folic acid. In: Shils, M. E., M. Shike, A. C. Ross, B. Caballero, and R. Cousins, eds. *Modern Nutrition in Health and Disease,* 10th edn., pp. 470–481. Philadelphia, PA: Lippincott Williams & Wilkins.
14. Kim, Y. 2006. Does a high folate intake increase the risk of breast cancer? *Nutr. Rev.* 64(10):468–475.
15. Institute of Medicine, Food and Nutrition Board. 1998. *Dietary Reference Intakes for Thiamin, Riboflavin, Niacin, Vitamin B_6, Folate, Vitamin B_{12}, Pantothenic Acid, Biotin, and Choline.* Washington, DC: National Academies Press.
16. Beresford, S. A., and C. J. Boushey. 1997. Homocysteine, folic acid, and cardiovascular disease risk. In: Bendich, A., and R. J. Deckelbaum, eds. *Preventive Nutrition: The Comprehensive Guide for Health Professionals.* Totowa, NJ: Humana Press.
17. Mayer, E. L., D. W. Jacobsen, and K. Robinson. 1996. Homocysteine and coronary atherosclerosis. *J. Am. Coll. Cardiol.* 27:517–527.
18. Sabler, S. P. 2006. Vitamin B_{12}. In: Bowman, B. A., and R. M. Russel, eds. *Present Knowledge in Nutrition,* 9th edn., pp. 302–313. Washington, DC: ILSI Press.
19. Carmel, R. 2006. Cobalamin (vitamin B_{12}). In: Shils, M. E., M. Shike, A. C. Ross, B. Caballero, and R. Cousins, eds. *Modern Nutrition in Health and Disease,* 10th edn., pp. 482–497. Philadelphia, PA: Lippincott Williams & Wilkins.
20. Miller, W. J., L. M. Rogers, and R. B. Rubker, 2006. Pantothenic acid. In: Bowman, B. A., and R. M. Russel, eds. *Present Knowledge in Nutrition,* 9th edn., pp. 327–339.Washington, DC: ILSI Press.
21. Freake, H. C. 2000. Iodine. In: Stipanuk, M. H., ed. *Biochemical and Physiological Aspects of Human Nutrition,* pp. 761–781. Philadelphia, PA: W. B. Saunders Co.
22. Evans, G. W. 1989. The effect of chromium picolinate on insulin controlled parameters in humans. *Int. J. Biosoc. Med. Res.* 11:163–180.
23. Hasten, D. L., E. P. Rome, D. B. Franks, and M. Hegsted. 1992. Effects of chromium picolinate on beginning weight training students. *Int. J. Sports Nutr.* 2:343–350.
24. Lukaski, H. C., W. W. Bolonchuk, W. A. Siders, and D. B. Milne. 1996. Chromium supplementation and resistance training: effects on body composition, strength, and trace element status of men. *Am. J. Clin. Nutr.* 63:954–965.
25. Hallmark, M. A., T. H. Reynolds, C. A. DeSouza, C. O. Dotson, R. A. Anderson, and M. A. Rogers. 1996. Effects of chromium and resistive training on muscle strength and body composition. *Med. Sci. Sports Exerc.* 28:139–144.
26. Pasman, W. J., M. S. Westerterp-Plantenga, and W. H. Saris. 1997. The effectiveness of long-term supplementation of carbohydrate, chromium, fibre and caffeine on weight maintenance. *Int. J. Obes. Relat. Metab. Disord.* 21:1143–1151.

27. Walker, L. S., M. G. Bemben, D. A. Bemben, and A. W. Knehans. 1998. Chromium picolinate effects on body composition and muscular performance in wrestlers. *Med. Sci. Sports Exerc.* 30:1730–1737.

28. Campbell, W. W., L. J. Joseph, S. L. Davey, D. Cyr-Campbell, R. A. Anderson, and W. J. Evans. 1999. Effects of resistance training and chromium picolinate on body composition and skeletal muscle in older men. *J. Appl. Physiol.* 86:29–39.

29. Volpe, S. L., H. W. Huang, K. Larpadisorn, and I. I. Lesser. 2001. Effect of chromium supplementation and exercise on body composition, resting metabolic rate and selected biochemical parameters in moderately obese women following an exercise program. *J. Am. Coll. Nutr.* 20:293–306.

30. Campbell, W. W., L. J. O. Joseph, R. A. Anderson, S. L. Davey, J. Hinton, and W. J. Evans. 2002. Effects of resistive training and chromium picolinate on body composition and skeletal muscle size in older women. *Int. J. Sports Nutr. Exerc. Metab.* 12:125–135.

31. Booth, S. L., and J. W. Suttie. 1998. Dietary intake and adequacy of vitamin K. *J. Nutr.* 128:785–788.

32. Institute of Medicine, Food and Nutrition Board. 2001. *Dietary Reference Intakes for Vitamin A, Vitamin K, Arsenic, Boron, Chromium, Copper, Iodine, Iron, Manganese, Molybdenum, Nickel, Silicon, Vanadium, and Zinc.* Washington, DC: National Academies Press.

33. Feskanich, D., S. A. Korrick, S. L. Greenspan, H. N. Rosen, and G. A. Colditz. 1999. Moderate alcohol consumption and bone density among post-menopausal women. *J. Women's Health* 8:65–73.

34. Beard, J. 2006. Iron. In: Bowman, B. A., and R. M. Russel, eds. *Present Knowledge in Nutrition,* 9th edn., pp. 430–444. Washington, DC: ILSI Press.

35. U.S. Food and Drug Administration. 1997. *Preventing Iron Poisoning in Children.* FDA Backgrounder.www.cfsan. fda.gov/~dms/bgiron.html. (Accessed April 2007.)

36. Bacon, B. R., J. K. Olynyk, E. M. Brunt, R. S. Britton, and R. K. Wolff. 1999. HFE genotype in patients with hemochromatosis and other liver diseases. *Ann. Intern. Med.* 130:953–962.

37. Baltussen, R., C. Knai, and M. Sharan. 2004. Iron fortification and iron supplementation are cost-effective interventions to reduce iron deficiency in four subregions of the world. *J Nutr.* 134:2678–2684.

38. Grantham-McGregor, S., and C. Ani. 2001. A review of studies on the effect of iron deficiency on cognitive development in children. *J. Nutr.* 131:649S–668S.

39. National Institute of Allergy and Infectious Diseases, National Institutes of Health. 2001. *The Common Cold.* www.niaid.nih. gov/factsheets/cold.htm. (Accessed April 2007.)

40. Prasad, A. 1996. Zinc: the biology and therapeutics of an ion. *Ann. Intern. Med.* 125:142–143.

41. Jackson, J. L., E. Lesho, and C. Peterson. 2000. Zinc and the common cold: A meta-analysis revisited. *J. Nutr.* 130:1512S–1515S.

NUTRITION DEBATE

Do Zinc Lozenges Help Fight the Common Cold?

the common cold has plagued human beings since the beginning of time. It is estimated that approximately 1 billion colds occur in the United States each year.[39] Children suffer from six to ten colds each year, and adults average two to four per year. Although colds are typically benign, they result in significant absenteeism from work and cause discomfort and stress. Finding a cure for the common cold has been at the forefront of modern medicine for many years.

The most frequent causes of the adult colds are viruses called coronaviruses; rhinovirus is another virus that causes about one-third of all adult colds. It is estimated that there are more than 200 viruses that can cause a cold. Because a cold can be caused by so many different viruses, finding treatments or potential cures for a cold is extremely challenging.

The role of zinc in the health of our immune system is well known. Zinc has been shown to inhibit the replication of rhinovirus and other viruses that cause the common cold, thus leading to speculation that taking zinc supplements may reduce the length and severity of colds.[40] Consequently, zinc lozenges were formulated as a means of providing potential relief from cold symptoms. These lozenges are readily found in most drugstores.

Does taking zinc in lozenge form actually reduce the length and severity of a cold? Over the past 20 years, numerous research studies have been conducted to try to answer this question. Unfortunately, the results of these studies are inconclusive because about half have found that zinc lozenges do reduce the length and severity of a cold, while about half find that zinc lozenges have no effect on cold symptoms or duration.[41] Some reasons that various studies report different effects of zinc on a cold include:

- Inability to truly "blind" participants to the treatment—Because zinc lozenges have a unique taste, it may be difficult to keep the research participants uninformed as to whether they are getting zinc lozenges or a

Zinc lozenges come in different formulations and dosages.

placebo. Knowing which lozenge they are taking could lead participants to report biased results.

- Self-reported symptoms are subject to inaccuracy— Many studies had the research participants self-report changes in symptoms, which may be inaccurate and influenced by mood and other emotional factors.

- Wide variety of viruses that cause a cold—Because more than 200 viruses can cause a cold, it is highly unlikely that zinc can combat all of these viruses. It is possible that people who do not respond favorably to zinc lozenges are suffering from a cold virus that cannot be treated with zinc.

- Differences in zinc formulations and dosages—The type of zinc formulation and the dosages of zinc consumed by study participants differed across studies. These differences most likely contributed to various responses across studies. It is estimated that for zinc to be effective, at least 80 mg of zinc should be consumed each day, and that people should begin using zinc lozenges within 48 hours of onset of cold symptoms. This level of zinc is nearly ten times the RDA and can decrease the absorption of copper and iron if continued for long periods of time. Also, sweeteners and flavorings found in many zinc lozenges, such as citric acid, sorbitol, and mannitol, may bind the zinc and inhibit its ability to be absorbed into the body, limiting its effectiveness.

- Another consideration is that supplements may provide excessive zinc and impair immune function. One experimental study showed that 300 mg/day of supplemental zinc reduced lymphocyte response and decreased destruction of bacteria by immune cells called neutrophils. This amount is about six tablets of a zinc gluconate pill that has 50 mg of elemental zinc.

Based on what you have learned here, do you think taking zinc lozenges can be effective in fighting the common cold? Have you ever tried zinc lozenges, and did you find them effective? Even if you only have about a 50% chance of reducing the length and severity of your cold by taking zinc lozenges, would you do it? Because there is no conclusive evidence supporting or refuting the effectiveness of zinc lozenges on the common cold, the debate on whether people should take them to treat their colds will most likely continue for many years.

One word of caution: If you decide to use zinc lozenges, more is not better. Excessive or prolonged zinc supplementation can cause other mineral imbalances. Check the label of the product you are using, and do not exceed its recommended dosage or duration of use.

The congestion, fatigue, and other symptoms of the common cold cause absenteeism from work or school as well as personal discomfort.

CHAPTER 11

CHAPTER OBJECTIVES

After reading this chapter you will be able to:

1. Define what is meant by a healthful weight, p. 442.

2. Define the terms *underweight*, *overweight*, *obesity*, and *morbid obesity* and discuss the health risks of each of these conditions, pp. 442, 468, 470–471.

3. List at least three methods that can be used to assess your body composition or risk for overweight, pp. 442–447.

4. Identify and discuss the three components of energy expenditure, pp. 448–452.

5. List and describe at least two theories that link genetic influences to control of body weight, pp. 452–454.

6. Discuss at least two societal factors that influence our body weight, pp. 457–458.

7. Develop an action plan for healthful weight loss, pp. 463–466.

8. List and describe three treatment options for obesity, pp. 466–467, 473–474.

TEST YOURSELF TRUE OR FALSE?

1. Being underweight can be just as detrimental to our health as being obese. T or F

2. Obesity is a condition that is simply caused by people eating too much food and not getting enough exercise. T or F

3. Getting my body composition measured at the local fitness club will give me an accurate assessment of my body fat level. T or F

4. Although a majority of Americans are overweight, only about 10% of Americans are obese. T or F

5. People who are moderately overweight and physically active should be considered healthy. T or F

Test Yourself answers can be found after the Chapter Summary.

Achieving and Maintaining a Healthful Body Weight

a s a teenager, she won a full athletic scholarship to Syracuse University, where she was honored for her "significant contribution to women's athletics and to the sport of rowing." After graduating, she became a television reporter and anchor for an NBC station in Flagstaff, Arizona. Then she went into modeling, and soon her face smiled out from the covers of fashion magazines, cosmetics ads, even a billboard in Times Square. Now considered a "supermodel," she hosts her own television show and has her own Web site, her own clothing line, and even a collection of dolls. *People* magazine has twice selected her as one of the "50 Most Beautiful People" and *Glamour* magazine named her "Woman of the Year." So who is she? Her name is Emme Aronson . . . and, by the way, her average weight is 190 pounds.

Emme describes herself as "very well-proportioned." She focuses not on maintaining a certain weight, but instead on keeping healthy and fit. So she eats when she's hungry and works out regularly. Observing that "We live in a society that is based on the attainment of unrealistic beauty," Emme works hard to get out the message that self-esteem should not be contingent on size. She frequently speaks to young people about body image concerns, and recently published her first children's book, *What Are You Hungry For?*, to encourage children to celebrate their individuality. Characteristically, she says of herself, "I don't know if I'll ever be perfect, but I'm happy with who I am."[1,2]

Are you happy with your weight, shape, body composition, and fitness? If not, what needs to change—your attitude, your diet, your level of physical activity? What role do diet and physical activity play in maintaining a healthful body weight? How much of your body size and shape is due to genetics?

What influence does society—including food advertising—have on your weight? And if you decide that you do need to lose weight, what's the best way to do it? In this chapter, we will explore these questions and provide some answers.

What Is a Healthful Body Weight?

As you begin to think about achieving and maintaining a healthful weight, it's important to make sure you understand what a healthful body weight actually means. We can define a healthful weight as all of the following:[3]

- A weight that is appropriate for your age and physical development
- A weight that you can achieve and sustain without severely curtailing your food intake or constantly dieting
- A weight that is compatible with normal blood pressure, lipid levels, and glucose tolerance
- A weight that is based upon your genetic background and family history of body shape and weight
- A weight that promotes good eating habits and allows you to participate in regular physical activity
- A weight that is acceptable to you

As you can see, a healthful weight is not one at which a person must be extremely thin or overly muscular. In addition, there is no one particular body type that can be defined as healthful. Thus, achieving a healthful body weight should not be dictated by the latest fad or current societal expectations of what is acceptable.

Now that we know what a healthful body weight is, let's look at some terms applying to underweight and overweight. Physicians, nutritionists, and other scientists define **underweight** as having too little body fat to maintain health, causing a person to have a weight that is below an acceptably defined standard for a given height. **Overweight** is defined as having a moderate amount of excess body fat, resulting in a person having a weight that is greater than some accepted standard for a given height but is not considered obese. **Obesity** is defined as having an excess body fat that adversely affects health, resulting in a person having a weight that is substantially greater than some accepted standard for a given height. People can also suffer from **morbid obesity**; in this case, their body weights exceed 100% of normal, putting them at very high risk for serious health consequences. In the next section we discuss how these terms are defined using certain indicators of body weight and body fat.

How Can You Evaluate Your Body Weight?

Various methods are available to help you determine whether or not you are currently maintaining a healthful body weight. Let's review a few of these methods.

Determine Your Body Mass Index (BMI)

Body mass index (BMI, or *Quetelet's index*) is a commonly used index representing the ratio of a person's body weight to the square of his or her height. You can calculate your BMI using the following equation:

$$\text{BMI (kg/m}^2) = \text{weight (kg)} / \text{height (m)}^2$$

For those less familiar with the metric system, there is an equation to calculate BMI using weight in pounds and height in inches:

$$\text{BMI (kg/m}^2) = [\text{weight (lb)} / \text{height (in.)}^2] \times 703$$

A healthful body weight varies from person to person.

underweight Having too little body fat to maintain health, causing a person to have a weight that is below an acceptably defined standard for a given height.

overweight Having a moderate amount of excess body fat, resulting in a person having a weight that is greater than some accepted standard but is not considered obese.

obesity Having an excess body fat that adversely affects health, resulting in a person having a weight that is substantially greater than some accepted standard for a given height.

morbid obesity A condition in which a person's body weight exceeds 100% of normal, putting him or her at very high risk for serious health consequences.

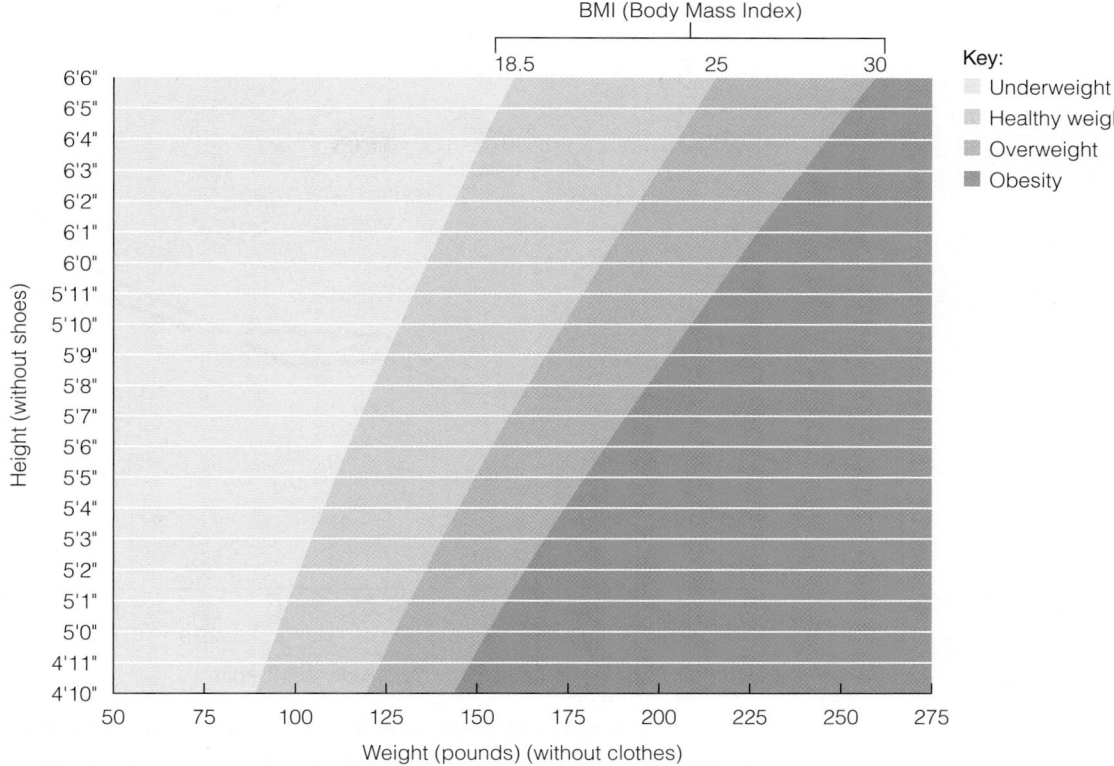

FIGURE 11.1 Measure your body mass index (BMI) using this graph. To determine your BMI, find the value for your height on the left and follow this line to the right until it intersects with the value for your weight on the bottom axis. The area on the graph where these two points intersect is your BMI.

A less exact but often useful method is to use the graph in FIGURE 11.1, which shows approximate BMIs for your height and weight and whether your BMI is in a healthful range. You can also calculate your BMI on the Internet using the BMI calculator found at *www.nhlbisupport.com/bmi*.

Why Is BMI Important?

Your body mass index provides an important clue to your overall health. Research studies show that a person's risk for type 2 diabetes, high blood pressure, heart disease, and other diseases largely increases when BMI is above a value of 30. On the other hand, having a very low BMI, defined as a value below 18.5, is also associated with increased risk of health problems and death.

FIGURE 11.2 shows how the *mortality rate,* or death rate, from all diseases increases significantly above a value of 30. Having a BMI value within the healthful range means that your risk of dying prematurely is within the expected average. If your BMI value falls outside of this range, either higher or lower, your risk of dying prematurely becomes greater than the average risk. For example, men with a BMI equal to or greater than 35 kg/m^2 have a risk of dying prematurely that is more than twice that of men with a BMI value in the range of 22 to 25 kg/m^2.

Theo always worries about being too thin, and he wonders if he is underweight. Theo calculates his BMI (see the calculations in the You Do the Math box on page 445) and is surprised to find that it is 22 kg/m^2 and falls within the healthy range.

Limitations of BMI

While calculating your BMI can be very helpful in estimating your health risk, this method has a number of limitations that should be taken into consideration. BMI

body mass index (BMI) A measurement representing the ratio of a person's body weight to his or her height.

FIGURE 11.2 Increased body mass index is associated with an increased risk for premature mortality. These results pertain only to U.S. adults who have never smoked and have no history of disease. (Adapted from Calle, E. E., M. J. Thun, J. M. Petrelli, C. Rodriguez, and C. W. Heath, Jr. 1999. Body-mass index and mortality in a prospective cohort of U.S. adults. *N. Engl. J. Med.* 341:1097–1105.)

BMI is not an accurate indicator of overweight for certain populations, including heavily muscled people.

cannot tell us how much of a person's body mass is composed of fat, nor can it give us an indication of where on the body excess fat is stored. As we'll discuss shortly, upper body fat stores increase the risk of chronic disease more than fat stores in the lower body. A person's age affects his or her BMI; BMI does not give a fair indication of overweight or obesity in people over the age of 65 years, as the BMI standards are based on data from younger people, and BMI does not accurately reflect the differential rates of bone and muscle loss in older people. BMI also cannot reflect differences in bone and muscle growth in children. Recent research indicates that BMI is more strongly associated with height in young people; thus, taller children are more likely to be identified as overweight or obese, even though they may not have higher levels of body fat.[4]

BMI also does not take into account physical and metabolic differences between people of different ethnic backgrounds. At the same BMI, people from different ethnic backgrounds will have different levels of body fat. For instance, African American and Polynesian people have less body fat than whites at the same BMI value, while Indonesians, Thais, and Ethiopians have more body fat than whites at the same BMI value.[5] There is also evidence that, even at the same BMI level, Asian, Hispanic, and African American women have a higher risk for diabetes than white women.[6] The same study also found that when Asian and Hispanic women gained weight, their risk of developing diabetes over a 20-year period was approximately twice as high as it was for white and African American women who gained the same amount of weight.

Finally, BMI is limited when used with people who have a disproportionately higher muscle mass for a given height. People who fall into this category include some athletes and pregnant and lactating women. For example, one of Theo's friends, Randy, is a 23-year-old weight lifter who is 5'7" and weighs 210 pounds. According to

YOU DO THE MATH

Calculating Your Body Mass Index

Calculate your personal BMI value based on your height and weight. Let's use Theo's values as an example:

BMI = weight (kg)/height(m)^2

1. Theo's weight is 200 pounds. To convert his weight to kilograms, divide his weight in pounds by 2.2 pounds per kilogram:

200 lb/2.2 lb/kg = 90.91 kg

2. Theo's height is 6 feet 8 inches, or 80 inches. To convert his height to meters, multiply his height in inches by 0.0254 meters per inch:

80 in. × 0.0254 m/in. = 2.03 m

3. Find the square of his height in meters:

2.03 m × 2.03 m = 4.13 m^2

4. Then, divide his weight in kilograms by his height in meters squared to get his BMI value:

90.91 kg / 4.13 m^2 = 22.01 kg/m^2

Is Theo underweight according to this BMI value? As you can see in Figure 11.1, this value shows that he is maintaining a normal, healthful weight!

our BMI calculations, Randy's BMI is 32.9, placing him in the obese and high-risk category for many diseases. Is Randy really obese? In cases such as his, an assessment of body composition is necessary.

Measure Your Body Composition

There are many methods available to assess your **body composition,** or the amount of body fat (or *adipose tissue*) and lean body mass (or *lean tissue*) you have. FIGURE 11.3 lists and describes some of the more common methods used to assess body composition. It is important to remember that measuring body composition provides only an estimate of your body fat and lean body mass, meaning that we cannot measure your exact level of these tissues. Because the range of error of these methods can be from 3% to more than 20%, body composition results should not be used as the only indicator of health status.

Let's return to Randy, whose BMI of 32.9 kg/m^2 places him in the obese category. Is he overweight? Randy trains with weights 4 days per week, rides the exercise bike for about 30 minutes per session three times per week, and does not take drugs, smoke cigarettes, or drink alcohol. Through his local gym, Randy contacted a trained technician who assesses body composition. The results of his skinfold measurements show that his body fat is 9%. This value is within the healthful range for men. Randy is an example of a person whose BMI appears very high but who is not actually obese.

Assess Your Fat Distribution Patterns

To evaluate the health of your current body weight, it is also helpful to consider the way fat is distributed throughout your body. This is because your fat distribution pattern is known to affect your risk for various diseases. FIGURE 11.4 on page 447 shows two types of fat patterning. *Apple-shaped fat patterning*, or upper-body obesity, is known to significantly increase a person's risk for many chronic diseases such as type 2 diabetes, heart disease, and high blood pressure. It is thought that the apple-shaped patterning causes problems with the metabolism of fat and carbohydrate, leading to unhealthful changes in blood cholesterol, insulin, glucose, and blood pressure. In contrast, *pear-shaped fat patterning*, or lower-body obesity, does not seem to significantly

body composition The ratio of a person's body fat to lean body mass.

Method		Limitations

Underwater weighing:
Considered the most accurate method. Estimates body fat within a 2–3% margin of error. This means that if your underwater weighing test shows you have 20% body fat, this value could be no lower than 17% and no higher than 23%. Used primarily for research purposes.

- Must be comfortable in water.
- Requires trained technician and specialized equipment.
- Does not work well with obese people.
- Must abstain from food for at least 8 hours and from exercise for at least 12 hours prior to testing.

Skinfolds:
Involves "pinching" a person's fold of skin (with its underlying layer of fat) at various locations of the body. The fold is measured using a specially designed caliper. When performed by a skilled technician, it can estimate body fat with an error of 3–4%. This means that if your skinfold test shows you have 20% body fat, your actual value could be as low as 16% or as high as 24%.

- Less accurate unless technician is well trained.
- Proper prediction equation must be used to improve accuracy.
- Person being measured may not want to be touched or may not want to expose their skin.
- Cannot be used to measure obese people, as their skinfolds are too large for the caliper.

Bioelectrical impedance analysis (BIA):
Inolves sending a very low level of electrical current through a person's body. As water is a good conductor of electricity and lean body mass is made up of mostly water, the rate at which the electricity is conducted gives an indication of a person's lean body mass and body fat. This method can be done while lying down, with electrodes attached to the feet, hands, and the BIA machine. Hand-held and standing models (that look like bathroom scales) are now available. Under the best of circumstances, BIA can estimate body fat with an error of 3–4%.

- Less accurate.
- Body fluid levels must be normal.
- Proper prediction equation must be used to improve accuracy.
- Should not eat for 4 hours and should not exercise for 12 hours prior to the test.
- No alcohol should be consumed within 48 hours of the test.
- Females should not be measured if they are retaining water because of menstrual cycle changes.

Dual-energy X-ray absorptiometry (DXA):
The technology is based on using very low level x-ray to differentiate between bone tissue, soft (or lean) tissue, and fat (or adipose) tissue. It involves lying for about 30 minutes on a specialized bed fully clothed, with all metal objects removed. The margin of error for predicting body fat ranges from 2% to 4%.

- Expensive; requires trained technician with specialized equipment.
- Cannot be used to measure extremely tall, short, or obese people as they do not fit properly within the scanning area.

Bod Pod:
A machine that uses air displacement to measure body compostition. This machine is a large, egg-shaped chamber made from fiberglass. The person being measured sits in the machine wearing a swimsuit. The door is closed and the machine measures how much air is displaced. This value is used to calculate body composition. It appears promising as an easier and equally accurate alternative to underwater weighing in many populations, but it may overestimate body fat in some African American men.

- Expensive.
- Less accurate in some populations.

FIGURE 11.3 Overview of various body composition assessment methods.

increase your risk for chronic diseases. Women tend to store fat in their lower body, and men in their abdominal region. In 2004, a study involving more than 10,000 people found that 64% of women are pear-shaped and 38% of men are apple-shaped.[7]

You can use the following three-step method to determine your type of fat patterning:

1. Ask a friend to measure the circumference of your natural waist, that is, the narrowest part of your torso as observed from the front (FIGURE 11.5a).

2. Now have that friend measure your hip circumference at the maximal width of the buttocks as observed from the side (FIGURE 11.5b).

3. Now divide the waist value by the hip value. This measurement is called your *waist-to-hip ratio*. For example, if your natural waist is 30 inches and your hips are 40 inches, then your waist-to-hip ratio is 30 divided by 40, which equals 0.75.

Once you figure out your ratio, how do you interpret it? An increased risk for chronic disease is associated with the following waist-to-hip ratios:

• In men, a ratio higher than 0.90.

• In women, a ratio higher than 0.80.

These ratios suggest an apple-shaped fat distribution pattern. In addition, waist circumference alone can indicate your risk for chronic disease. For males, your risk of chronic disease is increased if your waist circumference is above 40 inches (or 102 cm). For females, your risk is increased at measurements above 35 inches (or 88 cm).

> RECAP: *Body mass index, body composition, and the waist-to-hip ratio and waist circumference are tools that can help you evaluate the health of your current body weight. None of these methods is completely accurate, but most may be used appropriately as general health indicators.*

What Makes Us Gain and Lose Weight?

Have you ever wondered why some people are thin and others are overweight, even though they seem to eat about the same diet? If so, you're not alone. For hundreds of years, researchers have puzzled over what makes us gain and lose weight. In this section, we explore some information and current theories that may shed some light on this question.

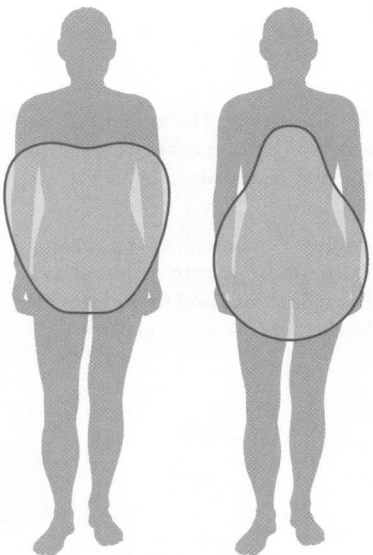

(a) Apple-shaped fat patterning (b) Pear-shaped fat patterning

FIGURE 11.4 Fat distribution patterns. **(a)** An apple-shaped fat distribution pattern increases an individual's risk for many chronic diseases. **(b)** A pear-shaped distribution pattern does not seem to be associated with an increased risk for chronic disease.

FIGURE 11.5 Determining your type of fat patterning. **(a)** Measure the circumference of your natural waist. **(b)** Measure the circumference of your hips at the maximal width of the buttocks as observed from the side. Dividing the waist value by the hip value gives you your waist-to-hip ratio.

We Gain or Lose Weight When Our Energy Intake and Expenditure Are Out of Balance

energy intake The amount of food a person eats; in other words, it is the number of kilocalories consumed.

energy expenditure The energy the body expends to maintain its basic functions and to perform all levels of movement and activity.

Fluctuations in body weight are a result of changes in our **energy intake** (the food we eat) and our **energy expenditure** (the amount of energy we expend at rest and during physical activity). This relationship between what we eat and what we do is defined by the energy balance equation:

Energy balance occurs when energy intake = energy expenditure

This means that our energy is balanced when we consume the same amount of energy that we burn each day. FIGURE 11.6 shows how our weight changes when we

FIGURE 11.6 Energy balance describes the relationship between the food we eat and the energy we burn each day. **(a)** Weight loss occurs when food intake is less than energy output. **(b)** Weight gain occurs when food intake is greater than energy output. **(c)** We maintain our body weight when food intake equals energy output.

change either side of this equation. From this figure, you can see that in order to lose body weight, we must expend more energy than we consume. In contrast, to gain weight, we must consume more energy than we expend. Finding the proper balance between energy intake and expenditure allows us to maintain a healthful body weight.

Energy Intake Is the Food We Eat Each Day

Energy intake is equal to the amount of energy in the food we eat each day. This value includes all foods and beverages. Daily energy intake is expressed as *kilocalories per day* (*kcal/day,* or *kcal/d*). Energy intake can be estimated manually by using food composition tables or computerized dietary analysis programs. The energy content of each food is a function of the amount of carbohydrate, fat, protein, and alcohol that each food contains; vitamins and minerals have no energy value, so they contribute zero kilocalories to our energy intake.

Remember that the energy value of carbohydrate and protein is 4 kcal/g and the energy value of fat is 9 kcal/g. The energy value of alcohol is 7 kcal/g. By multiplying the energy value (in kcal/g) by the amount of the nutrient (in grams), you can calculate how much energy is in a particular food. For instance, 1 cup of quick oatmeal has an energy value of 142 kcal. How is this energy value derived? One cup of oatmeal contains 6 g of protein, 25 g of carbohydrate, and 2 g of fat. Using the energy values for each nutrient, you can calculate the total energy content of oatmeal:

6 g protein × 4 kcal/g = 24 kcal from protein
25 g carbohydrate × 4 kcal/g = 100 kcal from carbohydrate
2 g fat × 9 kcal/g = 18 kcal from fat
Total kcal for 1 cup oatmeal = 24 kcal + 100 kcal + 18 kcal = 142 kcal

When someone's total daily energy intake exceeds the amount of energy that person expends, then weight gain results. An excess intake of approximately 3,500 kcal will result in a gain of 1 pound. Without exercise, this gain will likely be fat.

Energy Expenditure Includes More Than Just Physical Activity

Energy expenditure (also known as energy output) is the energy our body expends to maintain its basic functions and to perform all levels of movement and activity. Total 24-hour energy expenditure is calculated by estimating the energy used during rest and as a result of physical activity. There are three components of energy expenditure: basal metabolic rate (BMR), thermic effect of food (TEF), and energy cost of physical activity (FIGURE 11.7).

Our Basal Metabolic Rate Is Our Energy Expenditure at Rest. **Basal metabolic rate,** or **BMR,** is the energy we expend just to maintain our body's *basal,* or *resting,* functions. These functions include respiration, circulation, maintaining body temperature, synthesis of new cells and tissues, secretion of hormones, and nervous system activity. The majority of our energy output each day (about 60–75%) is a result of our BMR. This means that 60–75% of our energy output goes to fuel the basic activities of staying alive, aside from any physical activity.

BMR varies widely among people. The primary determinant of our BMR is the amount of lean body mass that we have. People with a higher lean body mass have a higher BMR, as lean body mass is more metabolically active than body fat. Thus, it takes more energy to support this active tissue. One common assumption is that obese people have a depressed BMR. This is usually not the case. Most studies of obese people show that the amount of energy they expend for every kilogram of lean body mass is similar to that of a non-obese person. In general, people who weigh more also have more lean body mass and consequently have a *higher* BMR. See FIGURE 11.8 for an example of how lean body mass can vary for people with different body weights and body fat levels.

BMR decreases with age, approximately 3–5% per decade after age 30. This age-related decrease results partly from hormonal changes, but much of this change is due to the loss of lean body mass resulting from physical inactivity. Thus, a large proportion

The energy provided by a bowl of oatmeal is derived from its protein, carbohydrate, and fat content.

Components of energy expenditure

FIGURE 11.7 The components of energy expenditure include basal metabolic rate (BMR), the thermic effect of food (TEF), and the energy cost of physical activity. BMR accounts for 60–75% of our total energy output, whereas TEF and physical activity together account for 25–40%.

basal metabolic rate (BMR) The energy the body expends to maintain its fundamental physiologic functions.

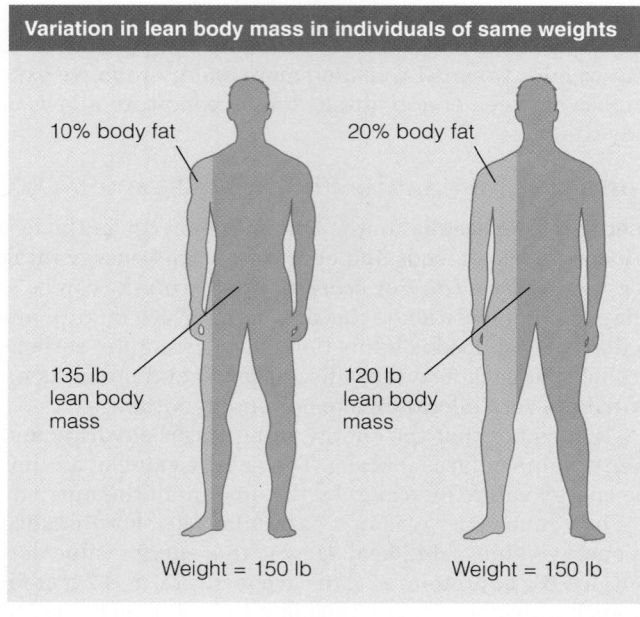

(a)

(b)

FIGURE 11.8 Lean body mass varies in people with different body weights and body fat levels. **(a)** The person on the left has a higher body weight, body fat, and lean body mass than the person on the right. **(b)** The two people are the same weight, but the person on the right has more body fat and less lean body mass than the person on the left.

TABLE 11.1   Factors Affecting Basal Metabolic Rate (BMR)

Factors That Increase BMR	Factors That Decrease BMR
Higher lean body mass	Lower lean body mass
Greater height (more surface area)	Lower height
Younger age	Older age
Elevated levels of thyroid hormone	Depressed levels of thyroid hormone
Stress	Starvation or fasting
Male gender	Female gender
Pregnancy and lactation	
Certain drugs such as stimulants, caffeine, and tobacco	

of this decrease may be prevented with regular physical activity. There are other factors that can affect a person's BMR, and some of these are listed in Table 11.1.

How can you estimate the amount of energy you expend for your BMR? Of the many equations that can be used, one of the simplest ways to estimate your BMR is to multiply your body weight in kilograms by 1.0 kcal per kilogram of body weight per hour for men or by 0.9 kcal per kilogram of body weight per hour for women. A little later in this chapter you will have an opportunity to calculate your BMR and determine your total daily energy needs.

The Thermic Effect of Food Is the Energy Expended to Process Food.   The **thermic effect of food (TEF)** is the energy we expend as a result of processing the food we eat. A certain amount of energy is needed to digest, absorb, transport, metabolize, and store the nutrients we eat. The TEF is equal to about 5–10% of the energy content of a meal, a relatively small amount. Thus, if a meal contains 500 kcal, the thermic effect of processing that meal is about 25 to 50 kcal. These values apply to

thermic effect of food (TEF) The energy expended as a result of processing food consumed.

eating what is referred to as a mixed diet, or a diet containing a mixture of carbohydrate, fat, and protein. Most of us eat some combination of these nutrients throughout the day. Individually, the processing of each nutrient takes a different amount of energy. While fat requires very little energy to digest, transport, and store in our cells, protein and carbohydrate require relatively more energy to process.

At one time, it was thought that obese people had a blunted (or reduced) TEF, which was thought to contribute to their obesity. We now know that errors associated with measuring the TEF make our previous assumptions about its link to obesity questionable. One of the most important contributors to obesity in industrialized countries is having an inactive lifestyle, which significantly reduces the energy output due to physical activity, our next topic.

The Energy Cost of Physical Activity Is Highly Variable. The **energy cost of physical activity** represents about 15–35% of our total energy output each day. This is the energy that we expend due to any movement or work above basal levels. This includes lower-intensity activities such as sitting, standing, and walking and higher-intensity activities such as running, skiing, and bicycling. One of the most obvious ways to increase how much energy we expend as a result of physical activity is to do more activities for a longer period of time.

Table 11.2 lists the energy costs for certain activities. As you can see, activities such as running, swimming, and cross-country skiing that involve moving our larger

Brisk walking expends energy.

energy cost of physical activity
The energy that is expended on body movement and muscular work above basal levels.

TABLE 11.2 Energy Costs of Various Physical Activities

Activity	Intensity	Energy Cost (kcal/kg body weight/min)
Sitting, knitting/sewing	Light	0.026
Cooking or food preparation (standing or sitting)	Light	0.035
Walking, shopping	Light	0.04
Walking, 2 mph (slow pace)	Light	0.044
Cleaning (dusting, straightening up, vacuuming, changing linen, carrying out trash)	Moderate	0.044
Stretching—Hatha yoga	Moderate	0.044
Weight lifting (free weights, Nautilus, or universal type)	Light or moderate	0.052
Bicycling < 10 mph	Leisure (work or pleasure)	0.07
Walking, 4 mph (brisk pace)	Moderate	0.088
Aerobics	Low impact	0.088
Weight lifting (free weights, Nautilus, or universal type)	Vigorous	0.105
Bicycling, 12 to 13.9 mph	Moderate	0.14
Running, 5 mph (12 minutes per mile)	Moderate	0.14
Running, 6 mph (10 minutes per mile)	Moderate	0.175
Running, 8.6 mph (7 minutes per mile)	Vigorous	0.245

Source: Ainsworth, B. E., W. L. Haskell, M. C. Whitt, M. L. Irwin, A. M. Swartz, S. J. Strath, W. L. O'Brien, D. R. Bassett, Jr., K. H. Schmitz, P. O. Emplaincourt, D. R. Jacobs, Jr., and A. S. Leon. 2000. Compendium of physical activities: an update of activity codes and MET intensities. *Med. Sci. Sports Exerc.* 32:S498–S516. Reprinted by permission of Lippencott, Williams & Wilkins.

muscle groups (or more parts of the body) require more energy. The amount of energy we expend during activities is also affected by our body size, the intensity of the activity, and how long we perform the activity. This is why the values in Table 11.2 are expressed as kilocalories of energy per kilogram of body weight per minute.

Using the energy value for running at 6 miles per hour (or a 10-minute-per-mile running pace) for 30 minutes, let's calculate how much energy Theo would expend doing this activity:

- Theo's body weight (in kg) = 200 lb/2.2 lb/kg = 90.91 kg

- Energy cost of running at 6 mph = 0.175 kcal/kg body weight/min

- At Theo's weight, the energy cost of running per minute = 0.175 kcal/kg body weight/min × 90.91 kg = 15.91 kcal/min

- If Theo runs at this pace for 30 minutes, his total energy output = 15.91 kcal/min × 30 min = 477 kcal

Given everything we've discussed so far, you're probably asking yourself, "How many kilocalories do I need each day to maintain my current weight?" This question is not always easy to answer, as our energy needs fluctuate from day to day according to our activity level, environmental conditions, and other factors such as the amount and type of food we eat and our intake of caffeine, which temporarily increases our BMR. However, you can get a general estimate of how much energy your body needs to maintain your present weight. The You Do the Math box describes how you can estimate your total daily energy needs.

> RECAP: *The energy balance equation relates food intake to energy expenditure. Eating more energy than you expend causes weight gain, while eating less energy than you expend causes weight loss. The three components of energy expenditure are basal metabolic rate, the thermic effect of food, and the energy cost of physical activity.*

Genetic Factors Affect Body Weight

Our genetic background influences our height, weight, body shape, and metabolic rate. A classic study shows that the body weights of adults who were adopted as children are similar to the weights of their biological parents, not their adoptive parents.[8] FIGURE 11.9 shows that about 25% of our body fat is accounted for by genetic influences. Two theories linking genetics with our body weight are the thrifty gene theory and the set-point theory.

The Thrifty Gene Theory

The **thrifty gene theory** suggests that some people possess a gene (or genes) that causes them to be energetically thrifty. This means that at rest and even during active times these individuals expend less energy than people who do not possess this gene. The proposed purpose of this gene is to protect a person from starving to death during times of extreme food shortages. This theory has been applied to some Native American tribes, as these societies were exposed to centuries of feast or famine. Those with a thrifty metabolism survived when little food was available, and this trait was passed on to future generations. Although an actual thrifty gene (or genes) has not yet been identified, researchers continue to study this explanation as a potential cause of obesity.

If this theory were true, think about how people who possess this thrifty gene might respond to today's environment. Low levels of physical activity, inexpensive food sources that are high in fat and energy, and excessively large serving sizes are the norm in our society. People with a thrifty metabolism would experience a great amount of weight gain, and their bodies would be more resistant to weight loss. Theoretically, having thrifty genetics would be advantageous during times of minimal food resources; however, this state could lead to very high levels of obesity in times of plenty.

Percent (%) contribution to body fat

FIGURE 11.9 Research indicates that about 25% of our body fat is accounted for by our genetic heritage. However, nongenetic factors such as diet and exercise play a much larger role.

thrifty gene theory A theory that suggests that some people possess a gene (or genes) that causes them to be energetically thrifty, resulting in them expending less energy at rest and during physical activity.

YOU DO THE MATH

Calculating BMR and Total Daily Energy Needs

One potential way to estimate how much energy you need each day is to record your total food and beverage intake for a defined period of time, such as 3 or 7 days. You can then use a food composition table or computer dietary assessment program to estimate the amount of energy you eat each day. Assuming that your body weight is stable over this period of time, your average daily energy intake should represent how much energy you need to maintain your present weight.

Unfortunately, many studies of energy intake in humans have shown that dietary records estimating energy needs are not very accurate. Most studies show that humans underestimate the amount of energy they eat by 10–30%. Overweight people tend to underestimate by an even higher margin, at the same time overestimating the amount of activity they do. This means that someone who really eats about 2,000 kcal/day may record eating only 1,400 to 1,800 kcal/day. So one reason many people are confused about their ability to lose weight is that they are eating more than they realize.

A simpler and more accurate way to estimate your total daily energy needs is to calculate your BMR, and then add the amount of energy you expend as a result of your activity level. Refer to the example below to learn how to do this. As the energy cost for the thermic effect of food is very small, you don't need to include it in your calculations.

1. *Calculate your BMR:* If you are a man, you will need to multiply your body weight in kilograms by 1 kcal per kilogram body weight per hour. Assuming you weigh 175 pounds, your body weight in kilograms would be 175 lb/2.2 lb/kg = 79.5 kg. Next, multiply your weight in kilograms by 1 kcal per kilogram body weight per hour:

$$1 \text{ kcal/kg body weight/hour} \times 79.5 \text{ kg}$$
$$= 79.5 \text{ kcal/hour}$$

Calculate your BMR for the total day (or 24 hours):

$$79.5 \text{ kcal/hour} \times 24 \text{ hours/day}$$
$$= 1,909 \text{ kcal/day}$$

(If you are a woman, multiply your body weight in kg by 0.9 kcal/kg body weight/hour.)

2. *Estimate your activity level by selecting the description that most closely fits your general lifestyle.* The energy cost of activities is expressed as a percentage of your BMR. Refer to the values in the following table when estimating your own energy output.

	Men	Women
Sedentary/Inactive Involves mostly sitting, driving, or very low levels of activity.	25–40%	25–35%
Lightly Active Involves a lot of sitting; may also involve some walking, moving around, and light lifting.	50–70%	40–60%
Moderately Active Involves work plus intentional exercise such as an hour of walking or cycling 4 to 5 days per week; may have a job requiring some physical labor.	65–80%	50–70%
Heavily Active Involves a great deal of physical labor, such as roofing, carpentry work, and/or regular heavy lifting and digging.	90–120%	80–100%
Exceptionally Active Involves a lot of physical activities for work and intentional exercise. Also applies to athletes who train for many hours each day, such as triathletes and marathon runners or other competitive athletes performing heavy, regular training.	130–145%	110–130%

3. *Multiply your BMR by the decimal equivalent of the lower and higher percentage values for your activity level.* Let's use the man referred to in step 1. He is a college student who lives on campus. He walks to classes located throughout campus, carries his book bag, and spends most of his time reading and writing. He does not exercise on a regular basis. His lifestyle would be defined as lightly active, meaning he expends 50–70% of his BMR each day in activities. You want to calculate how much energy he expends at both ends of this activity level. How many kcal does this equal?

$$1,909 \text{ kcal/day} \times 0.50 \text{ (or 50\%)} = 955 \text{ kcal/day}$$
$$1,909 \text{ kcal/day} \times 0.70 \text{ (or 70\%)} = 1,336 \text{ kcal/day}$$

These calculations show that this man expends about 955 to 1,336 kcal/day doing daily activities.

4. *Calculate total daily energy output by adding together BMR and the energy needed to perform daily activities.* In this man's case, his total daily energy output is:

$$1,909 \text{ kcal/day} + 955 \text{ kcal/day} = 2,864 \text{ kcal/day}$$
or
$$1,909 \text{ kcal/day} + 1,336 \text{ kcal/day} = 3,245 \text{ kcal/day}$$

Assuming this man is maintaining his present weight, he requires between 2,864 and 3,245 kcal/day to stay in energy balance!

The Set-Point Theory

The **set-point theory** suggests that our bodies are designed to maintain our weight within a narrow range, or at a "set point." In many cases, our bodies appear to respond in such a way as to maintain our present weight. When we dramatically reduce energy intake (such as with fasting or strict diets), our body responds with physiologic changes that cause our BMR to drop. This causes a significant slowing of our energy output. In addition, being physically active while fasting or starving is difficult because we just don't have the energy for it. These two mechanisms of energy conservation may contribute to some of the rebound weight gain many dieters experience after they quit dieting.

Conversely, overeating in some people may cause an increase in BMR and is thought to be associated with an increased thermic effect of food as well as an increase in spontaneous movements, or fidgeting. This in turn increases energy output and prevents weight gain. These changes may explain how some people fail to gain all of the weight expected from eating excess food. We don't eat the exact same amount of food each day; some days we overeat, other days we eat less. When you think about how much our daily energy intake fluctuates (about 20% above and below our average monthly intake), our ability to maintain a certain weight over long periods of time suggests that there is some evidence to support the set-point theory.

Can we change our weight set point? It appears that, when we maintain changes in our diet and activity level over a long period of time, weight change does occur. This is obvious in the case of obesity, since many people become obese during middle adulthood, and they are not able to maintain the lower body weight they had as a younger adult. Also, many people do successfully lose weight and maintain that weight loss over long periods of time. Thus, the set-point theory cannot entirely account for our body's resistance to weight loss. An interesting study on weight gain in twins demonstrates how genetics may affect our tendency to maintain a set point; this study is reviewed in the accompanying Highlight box.

set-point theory A theory that suggests that the body raises or lowers energy expenditure in response to increased and decreased food intake and physical activity. This action serves to maintain an individual's body weight within a narrow range.

> RECAP: *Many factors affect our ability to gain and lose weight. Our genetic background influences our height, weight, body shape, and metabolic rate. The thrifty gene theory suggests that some people possess a thrifty gene, or set of genes, that causes them to expend less energy at rest and during physical activity than people who do not have this gene. The set-point theory suggests that our bodies are designed to maintain weight within a narrow range, also called a set point.*

Behaviors learned as a child can affect adult weight and physical activity patterns.

Lifestyle Choices Adopted in Childhood Influence Adult Weight

In addition to genetic factors, the environmental factors present in our childhood can influence our food choices, activity level, and other behaviors as adults and cause us to weigh more or less than others of similar body type. For example, children who are very physically active and eat healthful diets that do not contain a lot of excess fat and sugar are less likely to be overweight or obese as children. In contrast, children who spend most of their time on the computer or watching television and who eat a lot of foods that contain excess fat and sugar are more likely to be overweight or obese as children. When these patterns are carried into adulthood, they can result in adult overweight and obesity. We know that being overweight or obese as a child can be detrimental to our health as we age, as childhood overweight has been shown to significantly increase a person's risk of heart disease and premature death in adulthood.[10]

HIGHLIGHT

Overfeeding Responses of Identical Twins

A classic study done by researchers at Laval University in Quebec, Canada, shows how genetics plays a role in our responses to overeating.[9] Twelve pairs of male identical twins volunteered to stay in a dormitory where they were supervised 24 hours a day for 120 consecutive days. Researchers measured how much energy each man needed to maintain his body weight at the beginning of the study. For 100 days, the subjects were fed 1,000 kcal more per day than they needed to maintain body weight. Daily physical activity was limited, but each person was allowed to walk outdoors for 30 minutes each day, read, watch television and videos, and play cards and video games. The research staff stayed with these men to ensure that they did not stray from the study protocol.

The average weight gain experienced by this group of men was almost 18 pounds. Although they were all overfed enough energy to gain about 26 pounds, the average weight gain was 8 pounds less than expected. These men gained mostly fat but also gained about 6 pounds of lean body mass. Interestingly, there was a very wide range of weight gained. One man gained only about 9.5 pounds, while another man gained more than 29 pounds! Keep in mind that the food these men ate and the activities they performed were tightly controlled.

This study shows that when people overeat by the same amount of food, they can gain very different amounts of weight and body fat. While each twin gained a similar amount of weight to his twin pair, there was a lot of difference in how each set of twins responded. It is suggested that those more resistant to weight gain when they overeat have the ability to increase BMR, store more excess energy as lean body mass instead of fat, and increase spontaneous movements such as fidgeting. Thus, genetic differences may explain why some people have a better ability to maintain a certain weight set point than others.

Composition of the Diet Affects Fat Storage

As previously discussed, when we eat more energy than we expend, we gain weight. Most people eat what is referred to as a "mixed" diet, meaning it contains a mix of carbohydrate, fat, and protein. Scientists used to think that people would gain the same amount of weight if they ate too much food of any type, but now there is evidence to support the theory that when we overeat dietary fat, we store it much more easily as adipose tissue than we do either carbohydrate or protein.[11] This may be due to the fact that eating fat doesn't cause much of an increase in metabolic rate, and the body stores fat in the form of adipose tissue quite easily. In contrast, when we overeat protein or carbohydrate, our body's initial response is to use this extra food for energy, storage, or the building of tissues, with a smaller amount of the excess stored as fat. This does not mean, however, that you can eat as many low-fat foods as you want and not gain weight! Consistently overeating protein or carbohydrate will also lead to weight gain. Instead, maintain a balanced diet combining fat, carbohydrate, and protein and reduce your dietary fat to less than 35% of total energy. This strategy may help reduce your storage of fat energy as adipose tissue.

A balanced diet contains protein, carbohydrate, and fat.

Physiologic Factors Influence Body Weight

Numerous physiologic factors affect body weight, including hunger, specific proteins, hormones, and blood glucose levels. These various factors contribute to the complexities of weight regulation. We discuss some of these factors in the following paragraphs.

Hunger

As introduced in Chapter 3, *hunger* is the innate, physiologic drive or need to eat. Physical signals such as a growling stomach and lightheadedness indicate when one is hungry. This drive for food is triggered by physiologic changes such as low blood glucose that affect chemicals in the brain. The hypothalamus plays an important role in hunger regulation. Special hypothalamic cells referred to as *feeding cells* respond to conditions of low blood glucose, causing hunger and driving a person to eat. Once one has eaten and the body has responded accordingly, other centers in the hypothalamus are triggered, and the desire to eat is reduced. The state reached in which there is no longer a desire to eat is referred to as *satiety*. It may be that some people have an insufficient satiety mechanism, which prevents them from feeling full after a meal, allowing them to overeat.

Proteins

Leptin is a protein that is produced by adipose cells and functions as a hormone. First discovered in mice, leptin acts to reduce food intake and cause a decrease in body weight and body fat. A gene called the *ob* gene (obesity gene) codes for the production of leptin. Obese mice were found to have a genetic mutation in the *ob* gene. This mutation reduces the ability of adipose cells to synthesize leptin in sufficient amounts; therefore, food intake increases dramatically, energy output is reduced, and weight gain occurs.

When these findings were first published, a great deal of excitement was generated about how leptin might decrease obesity in humans. Unfortunately, studies have shown that although obese mice respond positively to leptin injections, obese humans do not. Instead, they tend to have very high amounts of leptin in their bodies and are insensitive to leptin's effects. In truth, we have just begun to learn about leptin and its role in the human body. Researchers are currently studying its role in starvation and overeating, and it appears it might play a role in cardiovascular and kidney complications that result from obesity and related diseases.

In addition to leptin, numerous proteins affect the regulation of appetite and storage of body fat. Primary among these is **ghrelin,** a protein synthesized in the stomach. It acts as a hormone and plays an important role in appetite regulation through its actions in the hypothalamus. Ghrelin stimulates appetite and increases the amount of food one eats. Ghrelin levels increase before a meal and fall within about 1 hour after a meal. This action indicates that ghrelin may be a primary contributor to both hunger and satiety. Ghrelin levels appear to increase after weight loss, and researchers speculate that this factor could help to explain why people who have lost weight have difficulty keeping it off.[12] We noted earlier that obese people seem to lose their sensitivity to leptin, but this is not true for ghrelin: obese people are just as sensitive to the effects of ghrelin as non-obese people.[13] For this reason, potential mechanisms that can block the actions of ghrelin are currently a prime target of research into the treatment of obesity.

Peptide YY, or **PYY,** is a protein produced in the gastrointestinal tract. It is released after a meal, in amounts proportional to the energy content of the meal. In contrast with ghrelin, PYY decreases appetite and inhibits food intake in animals and humans.[14] Interestingly, obese individuals have lower levels of PYY when they are fasting and also show less of an increase in PYY after a meal than non-obese individuals, which suggests that PYY may be important in the manifestation and maintenance of obesity.[15]

Recall from Chapter 3 that mitochondria are organelles within cells that generate ATP. Uncoupling proteins found in the inner mitochondrial membrane of a variety of human cells (including skeletal muscle cells and adipose cells) may influence body weight. These proteins uncouple the oxidation of fat from ATP formation; when this occurs, the oxidation of fat produces heat instead of ATP. This production of heat increases energy expenditure and results in less storage of excess energy. Thus, a person with more uncoupling proteins or a higher activity of these proteins would be more resistant to weight gain and obesity. The role of uncoupling proteins in human obesity is currently under research.

leptin A hormone that is produced by body fat that acts to reduce food intake and to decrease body weight and body fat.

ghrelin A protein synthesized in the stomach that acts as a hormone and plays an important role in appetite regulation by stimulating appetite.

peptide YY (PYY) A protein produced in the gastrointestinal tract that is released after a meal in amounts proportional to the energy content of the meal; it decreases appetite and inhibits food intake.

Other Physiologic Factors

Various other physiologic factors known to increase satiety (or decrease food intake) include:

- Hormones such as serotonin and cholecystokinin (CCK). Serotonin is made from the amino acid tryptophan, and CCK is produced by the intestinal cells and stimulates the gallbladder to secrete bile.

- An increase in blood glucose levels, such as that normally seen after the consumption of a meal.

- Stomach expansion.

- Nutrient absorption from the small intestine.

Other physiologic factors that can decrease satiety (or increase food intake) include:

- Hormones such as beta-endorphins. Beta-endorphins increase a sense of pleasure while eating, which can increase food intake.

- Neuropeptide Y, an amino acid–containing compound produced in the hypothalamus. Neuropeptide Y stimulates appetite.

- Decreased blood glucose levels, such as the decrease that occurs after an overnight fast.

Psychological and Social Factors Influence Behavior and Body Weight

We explored in Chapter 3 the concept that *appetite* can be experienced in the absence of hunger. Appetite may therefore be considered a psychological drive to eat, being stimulated by learned preferences for food and particular situations that promote eating. For instance, some people learn as children to love or hate certain foods. This may explain why foods such as frogs' legs, cactus, and cultured yeast extract (Marmite) appeal to people in certain cultures who were raised on them but are almost never adopted into the diet as new foods by an adult. Others may follow learned behaviors related to timing and size of meals. In addition, the sight and fragrance of certain foods stimulate the pleasure centers of the brain, whether or not we happen to be hungry at the time. Mood can also affect appetite, as some people will eat more or less if they feel depressed or happy. As you can imagine, appetite leads many people to overeat.

Food preferences often depend on culture. Some cultures enjoy foods such as frogs' legs, while others do not.

Social factors can encourage people to overeat or choose high-energy foods. For example, pressure from family and friends to eat the way they do and easy access to large servings of inexpensive and high-fat foods contribute to overeating. Think about how you might eat differently when you attend a birthday celebration with family or friends. Perhaps you are offered hot dogs, pizza, birthday cake, ice cream, or other foods that are relatively high in fat and energy. The pressure to overeat on holidays is also high, as family members or friends offer extra servings of favorite holiday foods and follow a very large meal with a rich dessert.

Americans also have numerous opportunities to overeat because of easy access throughout the day to foods high in fat and energy. Vending machines selling junk foods are everywhere: at some schools, in business offices, and even at fitness centers. Shopping malls are filled with fast-food restaurants, where inexpensive, large serving sizes are the norm. Food manufacturers are producing products in ever-larger serving sizes: For instance, in 2005, the Mars candy company introduced a supersize version of M&M's candy, with each piece about 55% larger than the standard-size M&M's. Other supersize examples include the Monster Thickburger from Hardee's restaurant, the Full House XL pizza from Pizza Hut, and the Enormous Omelet Sandwich from Burger King.[16] Serving sizes have become so large that many Americans are suffering

Easy access or fast foods may be inexpensive and filling, but are often high in fat and sugar.

from "portion distortion." To test your understanding of a serving size, take the "Portion Distortion" interactive quiz from the National Institutes of Health at **http://hp2010.nhlbihin.net/portion**. Even foods traditionally considered healthful, such as some brands of peanut butter, yogurt, chicken soup, and milk, are often filled with added sugars and other ingredients that are high in energy. This easy access to large servings of high-energy meals and snacks leads many people to consume excess energy.

Social factors can also cause people to be less physically active. For instance, we don't even have to spend time or energy preparing food anymore, as everything either is ready to serve or requires just a few minutes to cook in a microwave oven. Other social factors restricting physical activity include living in an unsafe community, watching a lot of television, coping with family, community, and work responsibilities that do not involve physical activity, and living in an area with harsh weather conditions. Many overweight people identify such factors as major barriers to maintaining a healthful body weight, and research seems to confirm their influence. There is growing evidence that sedentary behaviors such as television watching are associated with obesity in both children and adults. A study of 11- to 13-year-old schoolchildren found that children who watched more than 2 hours of television per night were more likely to be overweight or obese than children who watched less than 2 hours of television per night. Interestingly, adults who reported an increase in television watching of 20 hours per week (approximately 3 hours per day) over a 9-year period had a significant increase in waist circumference, indicating significant weight gain.[17]

On the other hand, social pressures to maintain a lean body are great enough to encourage many people to undereat or to avoid foods that are perceived as "bad," especially fats. Our society ridicules and often ostracizes overweight people, many of whom face discrimination in many areas of their lives, including employment. Media images of waiflike fashion models and men in tight jeans with muscular chests and abdomens encourage many people—especially adolescents and young adults—to skip meals, resort to crash diets, and exercise obsessively. Even some people of normal body weight push themselves to achieve an unrealistic and unattainable weight goal, in the process threatening their health and even their lives.

It should be clear that how a person gains, loses, and maintains body weight is a complex matter. Most people who are overweight have tried several weight-loss programs but have been unsuccessful in maintaining long-term weight loss. A significant number of these people have consequently given up all weight-loss attempts. Some even suffer from severe depression related to their body weight. Should we condemn these people as failures and continue to pressure them to lose weight? Should people who are overweight but otherwise healthy (for example, having low blood pressure, cholesterol, triglycerides, and glucose levels) be advised to lose weight? The Nutrition Debate at the end of this chapter addresses these issues and provides an opportunity to discuss how we should deal with the growing concerns and prejudices related to obesity in our society.

> RECAP: *A person's diet and activity patterns as a child influence his or her body weight as an adult. The macronutrient composition of the diet influences the storage of body fat, and physiologic factors such as hunger, leptin, ghrelin, peptide YY, uncoupling proteins, and various hormones impact body weight by their effects on satiety, appetite, and energy expenditure. Psychological and social factors influencing weight include the ready availability of large portions of high-energy foods, lack of physical activity, and too much television watching. Prejudices and social pressures against those who are overweight and obese can drive people to use unhealthful and even dangerous methods to achieve an unrealistic body weight.*

NUTRI-CASE HANNAH

" My mom says the YMCA is having a swim camp at the lake during spring break and I can go if I want, but I told her "no thanks." When she asked why not, I said "cause it's for little kids," but that's not the real reason. The real reason is that, when I went last year, the other kids picked on me so bad the whole time. I had a real pretty swimsuit, but one of the boys said it was bigger than his grandma's. The girls were even meaner, especially when I was changing in the locker room, calling me "fatty" and "elephant" and even worse stuff I won't repeat. I'd just as soon stay home and watch television during spring break."

Think back to your own childhood. Were you ever teased for some aspect of yourself that you felt unable to change? Can Hannah change her weight? Given what you have learned about her and her mother, Judy, thus far in this book, can you identify obstacles to weight loss that she might face? If you were Judy, would you encourage her to attend the swim camp despite her feelings? Why or why not? How might organizations that work with children, such as schools, YMCAs, scout troops, and church-based groups, increase their leaders' awareness of social stigmatization of overweight children and reduce incidents of teasing and other insensitivity?

How Can You Achieve and Maintain a Healthful Body Weight?

Achieving and maintaining a healthful body weight involve three primary strategies (Table 11.3):

- Gradual changes in energy intake
- Incorporation of regular and appropriate physical activity
- Application of behavior modification techniques

In this section, we first discuss popular diet plans, which may or may not incorporate these strategies. We then explain how to design a personalized weight-loss plan that includes all three of them. Finally, we review the use of prescribed medications and dietary supplements in losing weight.

If You Decide to Follow a Popular Diet Plan, Choose One Based on the Three Strategies

With the assistance of MyPyramid and the information in this book, you are ready to design your own personalized diet plan. If you'd feel more comfortable following an established plan, however, an unlimited number are available. How can you know whether or not it is based on sound dietary principles, and whether its promise of long-term weight loss will prove true for *you*? Look to the three strategies just identified: Does the plan promote gradual reductions in energy intake? Does it advocate increased physical activity? Does it include strategies for modifying your eating and activity-related behaviors? Reputable diet plans incorporate all of these strategies. Unfortunately, many dieters are drawn to fad diets, which do not.

TABLE 11.3   Recommendations for a Sound Weight-Loss Plan

Dietary Recommendations	Physical Activity Recommendations	Behavior Modification Recommendations
Reasonable weight loss is defined as 0.5 to 2 pounds per week. To achieve this, energy intake should be reduced from 250 to no more than 1,000 kcal/day of present intake. A weight-loss plan should never provide less than a total of 1,200 kcal/day.	A long-term goal for physical activity should be a minimum of 30 minutes of moderate physical activity most, or preferably all, days of the week. Doing 45 minutes or more of an activity such as walking at least 5 days per week is ideal.	Shop only when you are not hungry, eat only at set times in one location, refuse to buy problem foods, and avoid vending machines, convenience stores, and fast-food restaurants.
Total fat intake should be 15–25% of total energy intake.		Suppress inappropriate behaviors by taking small food portions, eating foods on smaller serving dishes so they appear larger, and avoiding feelings of deprivation by eating regular meals throughout the day.
Saturated fat intake should be 5–10% of total energy intake.		
Monounsaturated fat intake should be 10–15% of total energy intake.		Strengthen appropriate behaviors by sharing food with others, learning appropriate serving sizes, planning healthful snacks, scheduling walks and other physical activities with friends, and keeping clothes and equipment for physical activity in convenient places.
Polyunsaturated fat intake should be no more than 10% of total energy intake.		
Cholesterol intake should be less than 300 mg/day.		
Protein intake should be approximately 15–20% of total energy intake.		Repeat desired behaviors by slowing down eating, always using utensils, leaving food on your plate, moving more throughout the day, and joining groups that are physically active.
Carbohydrate intake should be around 55% of total energy intake, with less than 10% of energy intake coming from simple sugars.		
Fiber intake should be 25 to 35 g/day.		Reward yourself for positive behaviors by getting a massage, buying new clothes or tickets to nonfood amusements, taking a walk, or reading a book (for fun).
Calcium intake should be 1,000 to 1,500 mg/day.		
		Use the "buddy" system by exercising with a friend or relative and/or calling this support person when you need an extra boost to stay motivated.
		Don't punish yourself if you deviate from your plan (and you will—everyone does). Ask others to avoid responding to any slips you make.

Source: Adapted from National Heart, Lung, and Blood Institute Expert Panel, National Institutes of Health. 1998. *Clinical Guidelines on the Identification, Evaluation, and Treatment of Overweight and Obesity in Adults.* Washington, DC: Government Printing Office.

Avoid Fad Diets

Beware of fad diets! They are simply what their name implies—fads that do not result in long-term, healthful weight changes. To be precise, fad diets are programs that enjoy short-term popularity and are sold based on a marketing gimmick that appeals to the public's desires and fears. Of the hundreds of such diets on the market today, most will "die" within a year, only to be born again as a "new and improved" fad diet. The goal of the person or company designing and marketing a fad diet is to make money. How can you tell if the program you are interested in qualifies as a fad diet? Here are some pointers to help you:

- The promoters of the diet claim that the program is new, improved, or based on some new discovery; however, no scientific data are available to support these claims.

- The program is touted for its ability to promote rapid weight loss or body fat loss, usually more than 2 pounds per week, and may include the claim that weight loss can be achieved with little or no physical exercise.

- The diet includes special foods and supplements, many of which are expensive and/or difficult to find or can be purchased only from the diet promoter. Common recommendations for these diets include avoiding certain foods, eating only a special combination of certain foods, or including magic foods in the diet that "burn" fat and speed up metabolism.

- The diet may include a rigid menu that must be followed daily or may limit participants to eating a few select foods each day. Variety and balance are discouraged, and restriction of certain foods (such as fruits and vegetables) is encouraged.

- Many programs promote supplemental foods and/or nutritional supplements that are described as critical to the success of the diet. They usually include claims that these supplements can cure or prevent a variety of health ailments or that the diet can stop the aging process.

The success of fad diets lies in their ability to appeal to the concerns of many people: being overweight or not being muscular enough; reducing the effects of aging such as wrinkles, loose skin, and tissue damage; and eating anything you want and still losing weight. In a world where many of us feel we have to meet a certain physical standard to be attractive and "good enough," these types of diets flourish: it is estimated that we currently spend more than $33 billion on fad diets each year.[18] Unfortunately, the only people who usually benefit from them are their marketers, who can become very wealthy promoting programs that are highly ineffectual.

Diets Focusing on Macronutrient Composition May or May Not Work for You

A comprehensive review of the currently available evidence shows that achieving a negative energy balance is the major factor in successful weight loss.[19] The macronutrient composition of a diet does not appear to affect the amount of weight lost. However, the three main types of weight-loss diets that have been most seriously and comprehensively researched all encourage increased consumption of certain macronutrients and restrict the consumption of others. Provided here is a brief review of these three main types and their general effects on weight loss and health parameters.[19]

Moderate-Fat, High-Carbohydrate, Moderate-Protein Diets. Moderate-fat, high-carbohydrate, moderate-protein diets that are balanced in nutrients typically contain 20–30% of total energy intake as fat, 55–60% of total energy intake as carbohydrate, and 15–20% of energy intake as protein. These diets include Weight Watchers, Jenny Craig, and others that follow the general guidelines of the DASH diet and the USDA MyPyramid. All of these diet plans emphasize that weight loss occurs when energy intake is lower than energy expenditure. The goal is gradual weight loss, or about 1 to 2 lb of body weight per week. Typical energy deficits are between 500 and 1,000 kcal/day. It is recommended that women eat no less than 1,000 to 1,200 kcal/day and that men consume no less than 1,200 to 1,400 kcal/day. Regular physical activity is encouraged.

To date, these types of low-energy diets have been researched more than any others. There is a substantial amount of high-quality scientific evidence (from randomized controlled trials) that they are effective in decreasing body weight. In addition,

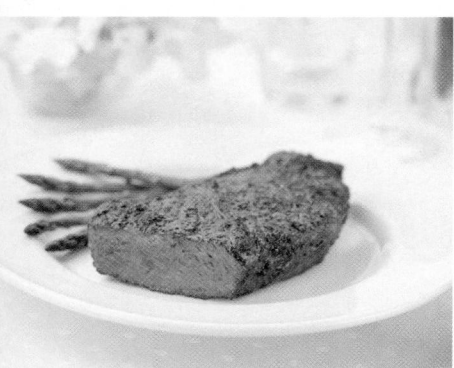

"Low-carb" diets may lead to weight loss but are nutritionally inadequate and can cause negative side effects.

the people who lose weight on these diets also decrease their LDL-cholesterol, reduce their blood triglyceride levels, and decrease their blood pressure. The diets are nutritionally adequate if the individual's food choices follow the guidelines of MyPyramid. If the individual's food choices are not varied and balanced, the diets may be low in nutrients such as fiber, zinc, calcium, iron, and vitamin B$_{12}$. Under these circumstances, supplementation is needed.

High-Fat, Low-Carbohydrate, High-Protein Diets. High-fat, low-carbohydrate, high-protein diets cycle in and out of popularity on a regular basis. By definition, these types of diets generally contain about 55–65% of total energy intake as fat and less than 100 g of carbohydrate per day, with the balance of daily energy intake as protein. Examples of these types of diets include Dr. Atkins' Diet Revolution, the Carbohydrate Addict's Diet, Life Without Bread, Sugar Busters, and Protein Power. These diets minimize the role of restricting total energy intake on weight loss. They instead advise participants to restrict carbohydrate intake, proposing that carbohydrates are addictive and that they cause significant overeating, insulin surges leading to excessive fat storage, and an overall metabolic imbalance that leads to obesity. The goal is to reduce carbohydrates enough to cause ketosis, which will decrease blood glucose and insulin levels and reduce appetite.

Countless people claim to have lost substantial weight on these types of diets; however, quality scientific studies of these diets are just beginning to be conducted. Based on the current limited evidence, it appears that individuals in both free-living conditions and experimental studies do lose weight with high-fat, low-carbohydrate, high-protein diets. In addition, it appears that those people who lose weight may also experience positive metabolic changes such as decreased blood lipid levels, decreased blood pressure, and decreased blood glucose and insulin. However, this evidence is based on the results of relatively few nonrandomized or observational studies. In addition, the amount of weight loss and improvements in metabolic health measured with these diets are no greater than those seen with higher-carbohydrate diets. Long-term compliance on these diets also appears to be similar to that of other types of diets and may be more affected by psychological factors than by the macronutrient composition of the diet. In addition, high-fat, low-carbohydrate, high-protein diets are nutritionally inadequate and require supplementation. Finally, reported side effects of these diets include constipation, diarrhea, ketone breath, headaches, insomnia, nausea, fatigue, and thirst. Thus, these diets must be approached cautiously, especially if you have any health concerns.

Low-Fat and Very-Low-Fat Diets. Low-fat diets contain 11–19% of total energy as fat, whereas very-low-fat diets contain less than 10% of total energy as fat. Both of these types of diets are high in carbohydrate and moderate in protein. Examples of these types of diets include Dr. Dean Ornish's Program for Reversing Heart Disease and the New Pritikin Program. These diets do not focus on total energy intake but emphasize eating foods higher in complex carbohydrates and fiber. The Ornish diet is vegetarian, whereas the Pritikin diet allows 3.5 oz of lean meat per day. Consumption of sugar and white flour is very limited. Regular physical activity is a key component of these diets.

These programs were not originally designed for weight loss but rather were developed to decrease or reverse heart disease. Also, these diets are not popular with consumers, as people view them as too restrictive and difficult to follow. Thus, there are limited data on their effects. However, high-quality evidence suggests that people following these diets do lose weight, and some data suggest that these diets may also decrease LDL-cholesterol, blood triglyceride levels, glucose, insulin levels, and blood pressure. Few side effects have been reported on these diets; the most common is flatus that typically decreases over time. Low-fat diets are low in vitamin B$_{12}$, and very-low-fat diets are low in essential fatty acids, vitamins B$_{12}$ and E, and zinc. Thus, supplementation is needed. These types of diets are not considered safe for people with diabetes who are insulin dependent (either type 1 or type 2) or for people with carbohydrate-malabsorption illnesses.

Low-fat and very-low-fat diets emphasize eating foods higher in complex carbohydrates and fiber.

If You Decide to Design Your Own Diet Plan, Include the Three Strategies

As we noted earlier, a healthful and effective weight-loss plan involves a modest reduction in energy intake, incorporating physical activity into each day, and practicing changes in behavior that can assist you in reducing your energy intake and increasing your energy expenditure. Below are some guidelines for designing your own personalized diet plan that incorporates these strategies.

Set Realistic Goals

The first key to safe and effective weight loss is setting realistic goals related to how much weight to lose and how quickly (or slowly) to lose it. Although making gradual changes in body weight is frustrating for most people, this slower change is much more effective in maintaining weight loss over the long term. Ask yourself the question, "How long did it take me to gain this extra weight?" If you are like most people, your answer is that it took 1 or more years, not just a few months. A fair expectation for weight loss is similarly gradual: experts recommend a pace of about 0.5 to 2 pounds per week. Your weight-loss goals should also take into consideration any health-related concerns you may have. After checking with your physician, you may decide initially to set a goal of simply maintaining your current weight and preventing additional weight gain. After your weight has remained stable for several weeks, you might then write down realistic goals for weight loss.

Goals that are more likely to be realistic and achievable share the following characteristics:

- They are specific. Telling yourself "I will eat less this week" is not helpful because the goal is not specific. An example of a specific goal is "I will eat only half of my restaurant entrée tonight and take the rest home and eat it tomorrow for lunch."

- They are reasonable. If you are not presently physically active, it would be unreasonable to set of a goal of exercising for 30 minutes every day. A more reasonable goal would be to exercise for 15 minutes per day, 3 days per week. Once you've achieved that goal, you can increase the frequency, intensity, and time of exercise according to the improvements in fitness that you have experienced.

- They are measurable. Effective goals are ones you can measure. An example is "I will lose at least half a pound this week," or "I will substitute drinking water for my regular soft drink at lunch each day this week." Thus, recording your specific, reasonable goals and measuring them will help you to better determine whether you are achieving them.

By monitoring your progress regularly you can determine whether you are meeting your goals or whether you need to revise them based on accomplishments or challenges that arise.

Eat Smaller Portions of Lower-Fat Foods

One of the most challenging issues related to food is understanding what a healthful portion size is and how to reduce the portion sizes of foods that we eat. As discussed in Chapter 2, the portion sizes of foods have expanded considerably over the past 40 years, and people trying to lose weight find it very challenging because of the large portion sizes offered and sold in restaurants and grocery stores.

Recent studies indicate that when children and adults are presented with large portion sizes of foods and beverages, they eat more energy overall and do not respond to cues of fullness.[20,21] Thus, it has been suggested that effective weight-loss strategies include reducing both the portion size and energy density of foods consumed, and replacing energy-dense beverages with low-calorie or non-calorie beverages.[21]

What specific changes can you make to reduce your energy intake and stay healthy? Here are some helpful suggestions:

1. Follow the serving sizes recommended in MyPyramid (pages 54–56). Making this change involves understanding what constitutes a serving size and measuring foods to determine whether they meet or exceed the recommended serving size.

2. Reduce the amount of foods that are high in fat and energy from your daily diet. People trying to lose weight should aim for a total fat intake of 15–25% of total energy intake. This goal can be achieved by eliminating extra fats such as butter, margarine, and mayonnaise and snack foods such as ice cream, doughnuts, and cakes. Save these foods as occasional special treats. Select lower-fat versions of the foods listed in MyPyramid. This means selecting leaner cuts of meat (such as the white meat of poultry and extra-lean ground beef) and reduced-fat or skim dairy products, and selecting lower-fat preparation methods (such as baking and broiling instead of frying). It also means switching from a sugar-filled beverage to a low-calorie or non-calorie beverage during and between meals.

3. Consume foods that are relatively low in energy density. This includes foods such as salads (with low- or non-calorie dressings), fruits, vegetables, and soups (broth-based). These foods are low in energy and high in fiber, water, and nutrients. Because they contain relatively more water and fiber than more energy-dense foods, they allow a person to feel satiated without having to consume large amounts of energy.

FIGURE 11.10 illustrates two sets of meals, one higher in energy and one lower in energy. You can see from this figure that simple changes to a meal, such as choosing lower-fat dairy products, smaller portion sizes, and foods that are relatively less dense in energy, can reduce energy intake without sacrificing taste, pleasure, or nutritional quality!

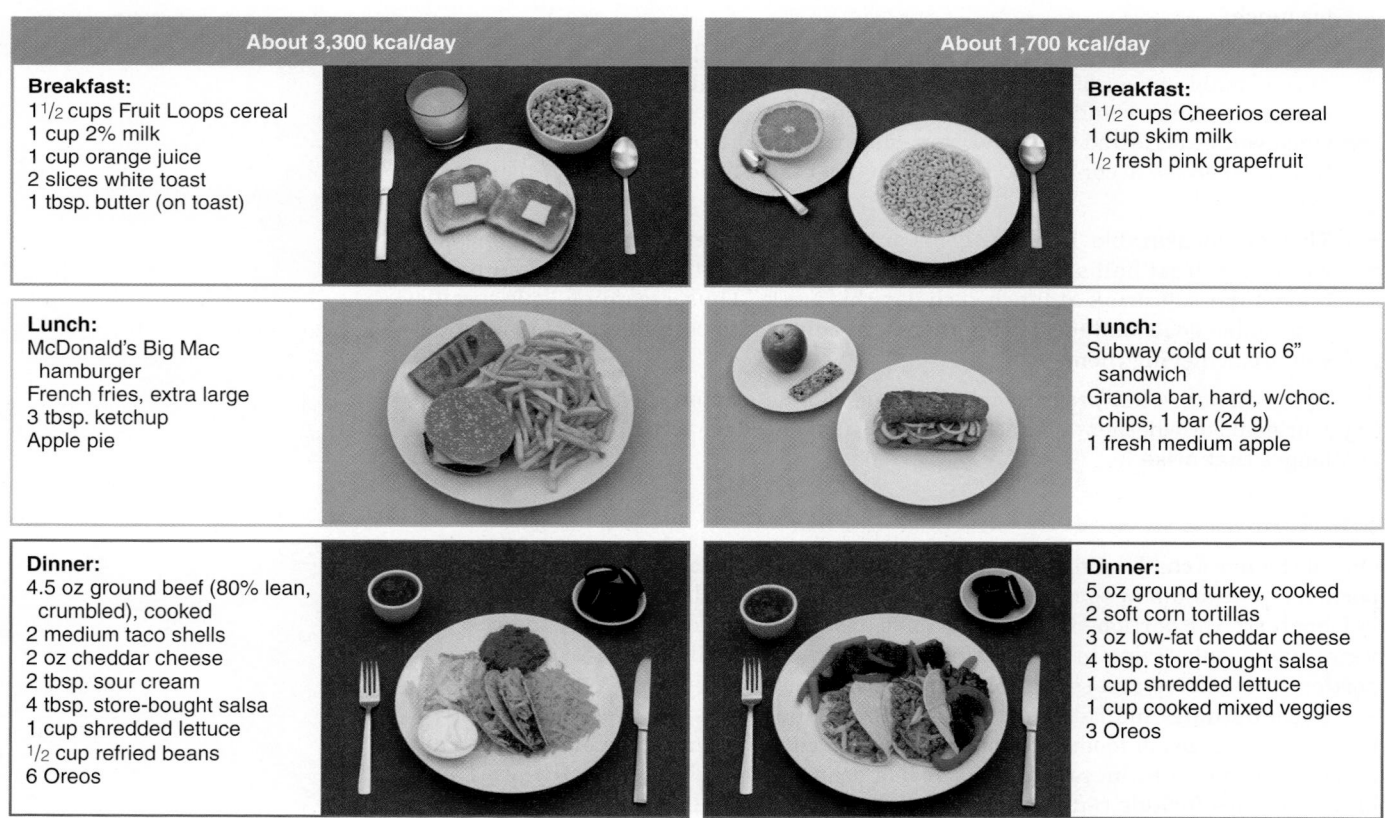

About 3,300 kcal/day	About 1,700 kcal/day
Breakfast: 1 1/2 cups Fruit Loops cereal 1 cup 2% milk 1 cup orange juice 2 slices white toast 1 tbsp. butter (on toast)	**Breakfast:** 1 1/2 cups Cheerios cereal 1 cup skim milk 1/2 fresh pink grapefruit
Lunch: McDonald's Big Mac hamburger French fries, extra large 3 tbsp. ketchup Apple pie	**Lunch:** Subway cold cut trio 6" sandwich Granola bar, hard, w/choc. chips, 1 bar (24 g) 1 fresh medium apple
Dinner: 4.5 oz ground beef (80% lean, crumbled), cooked 2 medium taco shells 2 oz cheddar cheese 2 tbsp. sour cream 4 tbsp. store-bought salsa 1 cup shredded lettuce 1/2 cup refried beans 6 Oreos	**Dinner:** 5 oz ground turkey, cooked 2 soft corn tortillas 3 oz low-fat cheddar cheese 4 tbsp. store-bought salsa 1 cup shredded lettuce 1 cup cooked mixed veggies 3 Oreos

FIGURE 11.10 The energy density of two sets of meals. The set on the left is higher in energy density, while the set on the right is lower in energy density and the preferred choice for a person trying to lose weight.

Participate in Regular Physical Activity

As compared to the previous version of the USDA Food Guide Pyramid, MyPyramid places far greater emphasis on the role of physical activity in maintaining a healthful weight. Why is being physically active so important for achieving changes in body weight and for maintaining a healthful body weight? Of course, we expend extra energy during physical activity, but there's more to it than that because exercise alone (without a reduction of energy intake) does not result in dramatic decreases in body weight. Instead, one of the most important reasons for being regularly active is that it helps us maintain or increase our lean body mass and our BMR. In contrast, energy restriction alone causes us to lose lean body mass. As you've learned, the more lean body mass we have, the more energy we expend over the long term.

The National Weight Control Registry is an ongoing project documenting the habits of people who have lost at least 30 pounds and kept their weight off for at least 1 year. Of the 784 people studied thus far, the average weight loss was 66 pounds, and the group maintained the minimum weight-loss criteria of 30 pounds for more than 5 years.[22] Almost all of the people (89%) reported changing both physical activity and dietary intake to lose weight and maintain weight loss. No one form of exercise seems to be most effective, but many people report doing some form of aerobic exercise (such as bicycling, walking, running, aerobic dance, step aerobics, or hiking) and weight lifting at least 45 minutes most days of the week. In fact, on average, this group expended more than 2,800 kcal each week through physical activity! While very few weight-loss studies have documented long-term maintenance of weight loss, those that have find that only people who are regularly active are able to maintain most of their weight loss.

In addition to expending energy and maintaining lean body mass and BMR, regular physical activity improves our mood, results in a higher quality of sleep, increases self-esteem, and gives us a sense of accomplishment (see Chapter 13 for more benefits of regular physical activity). All of these changes enhance our ability to engage in long-term healthful lifestyle behaviors.

Incorporate Appropriate Behavior Modifications into Daily Life

Successful weight loss and long-term maintenance of a healthful weight requires people to modify their behaviors. Some of the behavior modifications related to food and physical activity have been discussed in the previous sections. Here are a few more tips on modifying behavior that will assist you in losing weight and maintaining a healthful weight:

- Eat only at set times in one location. Do not eat while studying, working, driving, watching television, and so forth.

- Keep a log of what you eat, when, and why. Try to identify social or emotional cues that cause you to overeat, such as getting a poor grade on an exam or feeling lonely. Then strategize about non-food-related ways to cope, such as phoning a sympathetic friend.

- Save high-fat, high-kilocalorie snack foods such as ice cream, donuts, and cakes for occasional special treats.

- Avoid buying problem foods, that is, foods that you may have difficulty eating in moderate amounts.

- Avoid purchasing high-fat, high-sugar food from vending machines and convenience stores.

- Serve your food portions on smaller dishes so they appear larger.

- Avoid feelings of deprivation by eating small, regular meals throughout the day.

- Whether at home or dining out, share food with others.

- Prepare healthful snacks to take along with you so that you won't be tempted by foods from vending machines, fast-food restaurants, and so forth.

- Chew food slowly, taking at least 20 minutes to eat a full meal, and stopping at once if you begin to feel full.

- Always use appropriate utensils.
- Leave food on your plate or store it for the next meal.

Weight Loss Can Be Enhanced with Prescribed Medications

The biggest complaint about the recommendations for healthful weight loss is that they are difficult to maintain. Many people are looking for a "magic bullet" that will allow them to lose weight quickly and easily, requiring little sustained effort on their part to achieve their weight goals. Other people have tried to follow healthful weight-loss suggestions for years and have not been successful. In response to these challenges, prescription drugs have been developed to assist people with weight loss. These drugs typically act as appetite suppressants and may also increase satiety.

Weight-loss medications should be used only with proper supervision from a physician. One reason physician involvement is so critical is that many drugs developed for weight loss have side effects. Some have even proven deadly. Fenfluramine (brand name Pondimin), dexfenfluramine (brand name Redux), and a combination of phentermine and fenfluramine (called "phen-fen") are appetite-suppressing drugs that were banned from the market in 1996. These drugs, while resulting in more weight loss than diet alone, were found to cause two life-threatening conditions: primary pulmonary hypertension and valvular heart disease. Although these drugs were banned many years ago, they still serve as examples illustrating that the treatment of obesity through pharmacological means is neither simple nor risk-free.

Two Prescribed Medications Are Available.   Two prescription weight-loss drugs are currently available, and their long-term safety and efficacy are still being explored. Sibutramine (brand name Meridia) is an appetite suppressant that can cause increased heart rate and blood pressure in some people. Because many people who are overweight or obese have high blood pressure and are at increased risk for heart disease, these side effects could limit the widespread use of this drug. However, in one study, combining sibutramine therapy with medically supervised aerobic exercise and a low-fat diet resulted in significant weight loss and a significant decrease in heart rate and blood pressure.[23] In addition to increased blood pressure, side effects of sibutramine include dry mouth, anorexia, constipation, insomnia, dizziness, and nausea. Orlistat (brand name Xenical) is a drug that acts to inhibit the absorption of dietary fat from the intestinal tract, which can result in weight loss in some people. Recent research shows that orlistat results in significant weight loss in obese adolescents, and adults experience significant weight loss and improved blood lipid profiles when orlistat is combined with an energy-restricted diet.[24,25] The side effects of orlistat include abdominal pain, fatty and loose stools, leaky stools, flatulence, and decreased absorption of fat-soluble nutrients such as vitamins E and D.

For Whom Are Prescription Weight-Loss Medications Prescribed?   Because the use of prescribed weight-loss medications is associated with side effects and a certain level of risk, for whom are such medications justified? The answer is, for people who are severely obese. That's because the health risks of severe obesity override the risks of the medications. Specifically, prescription weight-loss medications are advised for people who have:

- a BMI greater than or equal to 30 kg/m^2
- a BMI greater than or equal to 27 kg/m^2 who also have other significant health risk factors such as heart disease, high blood pressure, and type 2 diabetes.

These medications should be used only while under a physician's supervision so that progress and health risks can be closely monitored. They are most effective when combined with a program that supports energy restriction, regular exercise, and increasing physical activity throughout the day.

Using Dietary Supplements to Lose Weight Is Controversial

Over-the-counter medications and dietary supplements are also marketed for weight loss. It is important to remember that the Food and Drug Administration

(FDA) requires prescription drugs and over-the-counter medications to undergo rigorous testing for safety and effectiveness before they can be released onto the market, but the FDA does not have a similar level of control over the development of dietary supplements. Thus, dangerous or ineffective supplements can be marketed and sold without meeting the FDA's strict safety and quality standards. Moreover, the FDA can pull a dietary supplement from the shelves only if it can prove that the supplement is dangerous. They cannot force the makers of an ineffective but harmless supplement to stop selling it. Recently, two reviews of various supplements and alternative treatments for weight loss were published.[26,27] Both concluded that there is insufficient evidence to support the use of the following products widely marketed to enhance weight loss: chromium, spirulina (or blue-green algae), ginseng, chitosan (derived from the exoskeleton of crustaceans), green tea, and psyllium (a source of fiber). Yet these products continue their brisk sales to people desperate to lose weight.

Many products marketed for weight loss do indeed increase metabolic rate and decrease appetite; however, they prompt these effects because they contain *stimulants*, substances that speed up physiologic processes. Stimulants commonly found in weight-loss supplements include caffeine, phenylpropanolamine (PPA), and ephedrine. Use of these substances is controversial and may be dangerous, as abnormal increases in heart rate and blood pressure can occur.

In addition to being a stimulant, caffeine is addictive; nevertheless, it is legal and unregulated in most countries and is considered safe when consumed in moderate amounts (up to the equivalent of 3 to 4 cups of coffee). The extent to which it affects people is influenced by their tolerance for caffeine, the amount consumed, and their body weight. In most adults, a moderate amount of caffeine causes positive mood changes and increased alertness. Its effects on the body include increased heart rate, blood pressure, and urine output. Adverse effects of high doses of caffeine include nervousness, irritability, anxiety, muscle twitching and tremors, headaches, elevated blood pressure, and irregular or rapid heartbeat. Long-term overuse of high doses of caffeine can lead to sleep and anxiety disorders that require clinical attention. Caffeine overdose can be fatal; however, the lethal dose of caffeine is estimated to be about 150 to 200 mg/kg body weight, which is about equivalent to the amount of caffeine contained in 80 to 100 cups of coffee. As this volume of coffee is very difficult to consume, deaths due to caffeine have occurred primarily as a result of taking caffeine tablets.

Phenylpropanolamine (PPA) is another stimulant found in supplements marketed for weight loss. In the year 2000, the FDA banned over-the-counter medications containing PPA in response to the deaths of several women who experienced brain hemorrhage after taking the prescribed dose. Consumers were instructed to throw away any medications in their homes that contained PPA. However, PPA may still be present in dietary supplements marketed for weight loss, as these are beyond FDA control.

Ephedrine use has also been associated with dangerous elevations in heart rate, blood pressure, and death. Ephedra has been banned by the International Olympic Committee for many years, and the FDA banned the manufacture and sale of ephedra in the United States in 2004 because of its potentially fatal side effects. In April 2005, a federal judge in Utah struck down this FDA ban. The judge's ruling stated that the FDA had failed to prove that low doses of ephedra were dangerous. The FDA appealed this ruling, and the U.S. Court of Appeals eventually ruled in favor of the FDA's original ban of ephedra. As a result of this ruling it is illegal to sell ephedra-containing supplements in the United States, and ephedra continues to be banned by international, national, and collegiate sports governing bodies. Some herbal supplement producers still include *ma huang*, the so-called herbal ephedra, in their weight-loss products; however, *ma huang* is simply the Chinese name for ephedra. Some herbal weight-loss supplements contain a combination of *ma huang*, caffeine, and aspirin. As you can see, using weight-loss dietary supplements entails serious health risks.

> RECAP: *Achieving and maintaining a healthful body weight involves gradual reductions in energy intake, such as by eating smaller portion sizes and limiting dietary fat; incorporating regular physical activity; and applying appropriate behavioral modification techniques. Fad diets do not incorporate these strategies and do not result in long-term, healthful weight change. Diets based on macronutrient composition may promote long-term weight loss, but some have unhealthful side effects. When necessary, drugs can be used to reduce obesity with a doctor's prescription and supervision. Using dietary supplements to lose weight is controversial and can be dangerous in some instances.*

What Disorders Are Related to Energy Intake?

At the beginning of this chapter, we provided some definitions of underweight, overweight, obesity, and morbid obesity. Let's take a closer look at these disorders.

Underweight

As defined earlier in this chapter, underweight occurs when a person has too little body fat to maintain health. People with a BMI of less than 18.5 kg/m² are typically considered underweight. Being underweight can be just as unhealthful as being obese, because it increases the risk for infections and illness and impairs the body's ability to recover. Some people are healthy but underweight because of their genetics and/or because they are very physically active and consume adequate energy to maintain their underweight status, but not enough to gain weight. In others, underweight is due to heavy smoking, an underlying disease such as cancer or HIV infection, or an eating disorder such as anorexia nervosa (see Chapter 15).

Safe and Effective Weight Gain

With so much emphasis in the United States on obesity and weight loss, some find it surprising that many people are trying to gain weight. People looking to gain weight include those who are underweight to the extent that it is compromising their health and many athletes who are attempting to increase strength and power for competition.

To gain weight, people must eat more energy than they expend. While overeating large amounts of foods high in saturated fats (such as bacon, sausage, and cheese) can cause weight gain, doing this without exercising is not considered healthful because most of the weight gained is fat, and high-fat diets increase our risks for cardiovascular and other diseases. Unless there are medical reasons to eat a high-fat diet, it is recommended that people trying to gain weight eat a diet that is relatively low in dietary fat (less than 30% of total calories) and relatively high in complex carbohydrates (55% of total calories). Recommendations for weight gain include:

- Eat a diet that includes about 500 to 1,000 kcal/day more than is needed to maintain present body weight. Although we don't know exactly how much extra energy is needed to gain 1 pound, estimates range from 3,000 to 3,500 kcal. Thus, eating 500 to 1,000 kcal/day in excess should result in a gain of 1 to 2 pounds of weight each week.

- Eat frequently, including meals and numerous snacks throughout the day. Many underweight people do not take the time to eat often enough.

- Avoid the use of tobacco products, as they depress appetite and increase metabolic rate, and both of these effects oppose weight gain. Tobacco use also causes lung, mouth, and esophageal cancers.

- Exercise regularly and incorporate weight lifting or some other form of resistance training into your exercise routine. This form of exercise is most effective in increasing muscle mass. Performing aerobic exercise (such as walking, running, bicycling, or swimming) at least 30 minutes for 3 days per week will help maintain a healthy cardiovascular system.

Eating frequent nutrient- and energy-dense snacks can help promote weight gain.

The key to gaining weight is to eat frequent meals throughout the day and to select energy-dense foods. When selecting foods that are higher in fat, make sure you select foods higher in polyunsaturated and monounsaturated fats (such as peanut butter, olive and canola oils, and avocados). For instance, smoothies and milkshakes made with low-fat milk or yogurt are a great way to take in a lot of energy. Eating peanut butter with fruit or celery and including salad dressings on your salad are other ways to increase the energy density of foods. The biggest challenge to weight gain is setting aside time to eat; by packing a lot of foods to take with you throughout the day, you can enhance your opportunities to eat more.

NUTRI-CASE THEO

" I'm sick and tired of everybody everywhere complaining about how they can't lose weight even though they're starving themselves and feel hungry all the time. Nobody talks about people like me, who have exactly the opposite problem. I keep super-busy, I'm almost never hungry, and I can't keep weight on! It's especially bad right now because it's basketball season: no matter what I do, the pounds peel off! For breakfast this morning, I had bacon and eggs. For lunch, I'll probably eat a couple of ham sandwiches. Then a protein bar after practice, and for dinner, I'll probably go out for burgers with my friends. What more can I do? Don't tell me to eat between meals because, like I said, I'm just not that hungry."

Given what you've learned about energy balance and weight management, what if any problems do you perceive with Theo's food intake today? What might you advise him to change about his food choices that might help stimulate his appetite? What else might he do to gain weight?

Protein Supplements Do Not Increase Muscle Growth or Strength

As with weight loss, there are many products marketed for weight gain. One of the most common claims is that these products are *anabolic,* that is, that they increase muscle mass. These products include amino acid and protein supplements, anabolic steroids, and *androstenedione,* a substance that became very popular after baseball player Mark McGwire claimed he used this product during the time he was breaking home run records. Do these substances really work?

A growing body of evidence exists to show that amino acid and protein supplements do not enhance muscle gain or result in improvements in strength.[28] Anabolic steroids can increase body weight and muscle mass, but are known to cause major health problems. Although the case of Mark McGwire may seem to suggest that androstenedione is an extremely effective product for building muscle mass, gaining strength, and improving performance, several studies report that this product did not have any benefits.[29–31] Protein supplements and androstenedione are legal to sell in the United States, but these and other potentially anabolic substances are banned by the National Football League, the National Collegiate Athletic Association, and the International Olympic Committee.

The health consequences of using protein supplements are unknown. As just noted, the health consequences of using anabolic steroids are severe. They include unhealthful changes in blood cholesterol, mood disturbances (such as anger leading to violence), testicular shrinkage and breast enlargement in men, and irreversible clitoral enlargement in women (see Chapter 13 for a more detailed discussion of

Protein powders or amino acid supplements will not enhance muscle growth or make you stronger.

anabolic steroid use). Androstenedione causes unhealthful changes in high-density and low-density lipoprotein (HDL and LDL) levels in middle-aged men, potentially increasing their risk for heart disease.[30] We also know that buying these substances can have a substantial slenderizing effect—on your wallet!

> RECAP: *Weight gain can be achieved by eating more and performing weight lifting and aerobic exercise. Protein and amino acid supplements and androstenedione do not increase muscle growth or strength, and their potential side effects are unknown. Anabolic steroid use can increase body weight and muscle mass but is known to cause major health problems.*

Overweight

Overweight is defined as having a moderate amount of excess body fat, resulting in a person having a weight for a given height that is greater than some accepted standard but is not considered obese. People with a BMI between 25 and 29.9 kg/m² are considered to be overweight. Being overweight does not appear to be as detrimental to our health as being obese, but some of the health risks of overweight include an increased risk for high blood pressure, heart disease, type 2 diabetes, sleep disorders, osteoarthritis, gallstones, and gynecological abnormalities.[32] It is also more likely that overweight people will become obese, which can lead to an even higher risk for these diseases and for premature death. Because of these concerns, health professionals recommend that overweight individuals adopt a lifestyle that incorporates healthful eating and regular physical activity in an attempt to prevent additional weight gain, to reduce body weight to the normal level, and/or to support long-term health even if body weight is not significantly reduced.

Obesity and Morbid Obesity

Obesity is defined as having an excess body fat that adversely affects health, resulting in a person having a weight for a given height that is substantially greater than some accepted standard. People with a BMI between 30 and 39.9 kg/m² are considered obese. Morbid obesity occurs when a person's body weight exceeds 100% of normal; people who are morbidly obese have a BMI greater than or equal to 40 kg/m².

Both overweight and obesity are now considered an epidemic in the United States. It is estimated that about 34% of adults 20 years and older are overweight, and another 32% are obese.[33] Obesity rates have increased more than 50% over the past 20 years. This alarming rise in obesity is a major health concern because it is linked to many chronic diseases and adverse health conditions. These include:

- Hypertension
- Dyslipidemia, including elevated total cholesterol, triglycerides, and LDL-cholesterol, and decreased HDL-cholesterol
- Type 2 diabetes
- Heart disease
- Stroke
- Gallbladder disease
- Osteoarthritis
- Sleep apnea
- Certain cancers such as colon, breast, endometrial, and gallbladder
- Menstrual irregularities and infertility
- Gestational diabetes, premature fetal deaths, neural tube defects, and complications during labor and delivery
- Depression

Obesity is also associated with an increased risk of premature death: mortality rates for people with a BMI of 30 kg/m² or higher are 50–100% above the rates for those with a BMI between 20 and 25 kg/m². As we discussed in Chapter 1, several of the leading causes of death in the United States are associated with obesity (see page 6).

It has been estimated that the financial costs associated with obesity total more than $99 billion. These costs affect not just the person with obesity, but all of society, as they increase the costs of health care and medications, reduce productivity because of days of lost work, and reduce future earnings because of premature death.

Ironically, up to 40% of women and 25% of men are dieting at any given time. How can obesity rates be so high when there are so many people dieting? Certainly some people dieting are actually at a normal or even below-normal weight, and these people account for a small percentage of this total. However, a telephone survey of American adults with a history of obesity found that only about 20% had been successful in achieving and maintaining at least a 10% weight loss for a minimum of 1 year.[34] These results suggest that while some obese individuals are able to lose weight and maintain weight loss, about 80% of obese people who are dieting are somehow failing to lose weight or to maintain long-term weight loss. Why?

Obesity Is a Multifactorial Disease

Obesity is known as a **multifactorial disease,** meaning that there are many things that cause it. This makes obesity extremely difficult to treat. Although it is certainly true that obesity, like overweight, is caused by eating more energy than is expended, it is also true that some people are more susceptible to becoming obese than others. In addition, as we saw with the twin study, some people are more resistant to weight loss and maintaining weight loss than others. Research on the causes and best treatments of obesity is ongoing, but let's explore some current theories.

Genetic and Physiologic Factors.   Because a person's genetic background influences his or her height, weight, body shape, and metabolic rate, it can also affect a person's risk for obesity. Some obesity experts point out that, if proved, the existence of a thrifty gene or genes (discussed earlier) would show that obese people have a genetic tendency to expend less energy both at rest and during physical activity. Other researchers are working to determine whether the set-point theory can partially explain why many obese people are very resistant to weight loss. As we learn more about genetics, we will gain a greater understanding of the role it plays in the development and treatment of obesity.

We also discussed earlier several physiologic factors that may influence an individual's experience of hunger and satiation. These include the proteins leptin, ghrelin, PYY, and uncoupling proteins. Other physiologic factors such as beta-endorphins, neuropeptide Y, and decreased blood glucose can reduce satiety or increase hunger, theoretically promoting overeating and weight gain.

Childhood Overweight and Obesity Are Linked to Adult Obesity.   The prevalence of overweight in children and adolescents is increasing at an alarming rate in the United States (FIGURE 11.11). There was a time when having extra "baby fat" was considered good for the child. We assumed that childhood overweight and obesity were temporary and that the child would grow out of it. While it is important for children to have a certain minimum level of body fat to maintain health and to grow properly, researchers are now concerned that overweight and obesity are harming children's health and increasing their risk of overweight and obesity in adulthood.

Health data demonstrate that obese children are already showing signs of disease while they are young, including elevated blood pressure, high cholesterol levels, and changes in insulin and glucose metabolism that may increase the risk for type 2 diabetes (formerly known as *adult onset diabetes*). In some communities, children as young as 5 years of age have been diagnosed with type 2 diabetes. Unfortunately, many of these children are maintaining these disease risk factors into adulthood.

Does being an obese child guarantee that obesity will be maintained during adulthood? Although some children who are obese grow up to have a normal body weight, it has been estimated that about 70% of children who are obese maintain

multifactorial disease Any disease that may be attributable to one or more of a variety of causes.

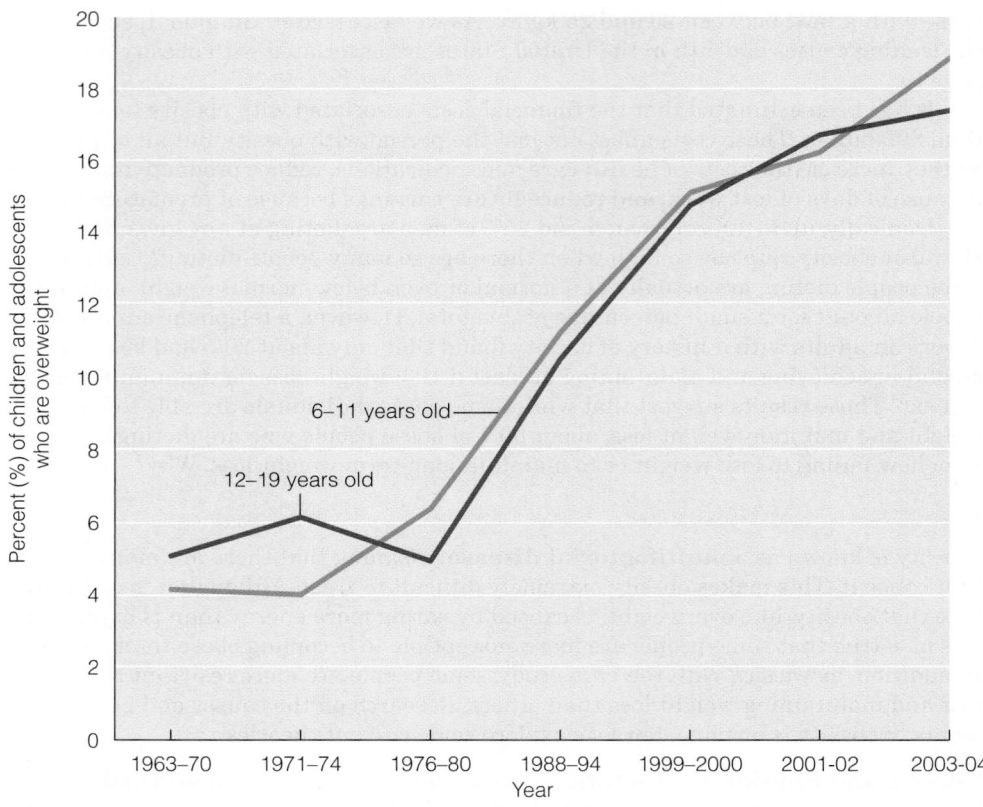

FIGURE 11.11   Increases in childhood and adolescent overweight from 1963 to 2004. (Adapted from Centers for Disease Control and Prevention. National Center for Health Statistics. 2007. Prevalence of overweight among children and adolescents: United States, 2003–2004. www.cdc.gov/nchs/products/pubs/pubd/hestats/overweight/overwght_child_03.htm.)

Adequate physical activity is instrumental in preventing childhood obesity.

their higher weight as adults.[35] Obviously, this has important consequences for their health.

It has been suggested that there are three critical periods in childhood during which substantial weight gain can increase the risk of obesity and related diseases in adulthood:

- Gestation and early infancy
- The period of weight gain (called *adiposity rebound*) that occurs between 5 and 7 years of age
- Adolescence (or puberty)

Having either one or two overweight parents increases the risk of obesity by two to four times.[36] This may be explained in part by genetics and in part by unhealthful eating patterns or lack of physical activity within the family.

Certainly, low physical activity levels are an important contributor to childhood obesity. There was a time when children played outdoors regularly and when physical education was offered daily in school. In today's society, many children cannot play outdoors due to safety concerns and lack of recreational facilities, and few schools have the resources to regularly offer physical education to children. In addition, many popular activities for children today are sedentary in nature, including playing video games, watching television, using the computer, and playing with hand-held electronic games. Childhood and adolescence are critical times for forming activity habits, but many young people today are not getting an opportunity to be physically active. This will likely have a significant impact on their physical activity levels and potential for obesity as adults.

Obesity Treatment Is Challenging

The first line of defense in treating obesity is a low-calorie diet and regular physical activity. Overweight and obese individuals should work with their healthcare practitioner to design and maintain a low-fat diet (less than 30% of total energy from fat) that has a deficit of 500 to 1,000 kcal/day.[32] Physical activity should be increased gradually so that the person can build to a program in which he or she is exercising at least 30 minutes per day, five times per week. The Institute of Medicine concurs that 30 minutes a day, five times a week is the minimum amount of physical activity needed, but up to 60 minutes per day may be necessary for many people to lose weight and to sustain a body weight in the healthy range over the long term.[37]

As discussed earlier in this chapter, changing entrenched dietary and activity patterns is challenging, and prescription medications are sometimes used to treat resistant cases of obesity in adults and children. Again, these medications should be used only while under a physician's supervision, and they appear to be most effective when combined with energy restriction and regular physical activity.

For people who are morbidly obese, surgery may be recommended. Generally, surgery is advised in people with a BMI greater than or equal to 40 kg/m^2 or in people with a BMI greater than or equal to 35 kg/m^2 who have other life-threatening conditions such as diabetes, hypertension, or elevated cholesterol levels.[38] The three most common types of weight-loss surgery performed are gastroplasty, gastric bypass, and gastric banding (FIGURE 11.12).

- *Vertical banded gastroplasty* involves partitioning or "stapling" a small section of the stomach to reduce total food intake.

- *Gastric bypass surgery* involves attaching the lower part of the small intestine to the stomach, so that food bypasses most of the stomach and the duodenum of the small intestine. This results in both a smaller stomach pouch, which restricts food intake, and significantly less absorption of food in the intestine.

- *Gastric banding* is a relatively new procedure is which stomach size is reduced using a constricting band, thus restricting food intake.

Surgery is considered a last resort for morbidly obese people who have not been able to lose weight with energy restriction and exercise. This is because risks of surgery in people with morbid obesity are extremely high. They include increased

   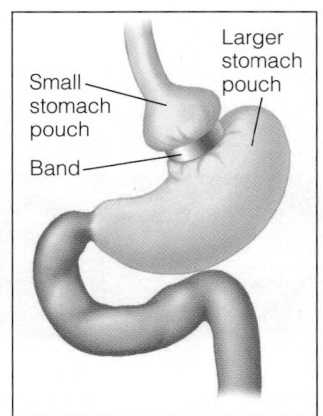

(a) Normal anatomy   (b) Vertical banded gastroplasty   (c) Gastric bypass   (d) Gastric banding

FIGURE 11.12 Various forms of surgery alter the normal anatomy of the gastrointestinal tract **(a)** to result in weight loss. Vertical banded gastroplasty **(b)**, gastric bypass **(c)**, and gastric banding **(d)** are three surgical procedures used to reduce morbid obesity.

infections, higher formation of blood clots, and more adverse reactions to anesthesia. After the surgery, these people may face a lifetime of problems with chronic diarrhea, vomiting, intolerance to dairy products and other foods, dehydration, and nutritional deficiencies resulting from alterations in nutrient digestion and absorption. Thus, the potential benefits of the procedure must outweigh the risks. It is critical that each surgery candidate is carefully screened by a trained physician. If the immediate threat of serious disease and death is more dangerous than the risks associated with surgery, then the procedure is justified.

Are these surgical procedures successful in reducing obesity? About one-third to one-half of people who received obesity surgery lose significant amounts of weight and keep this weight off for at least 5 years. The reasons that one-half to two-thirds do not experience long-term success include:

- inability to eat less over time, even with a smaller stomach
- loosening of staples and gastric bands and enlargement of stomach pouch
- failure to survive the surgery or the postoperative recovery period

Liposuction removes fat cells from specific areas of the body.

Although these surgical procedures may seem extremely risky, those who survive the surgery, lose weight, and maintain much of this weight loss over time reduce their risk for type 2 diabetes and cardiovascular disease, and may even improve their ability to stay physically active over a prolonged period of time.[39]

Liposuction is a cosmetic surgical procedure that removes fat cells from localized areas in the body. It is not recommended or typically used to treat obesity or morbid obesity. Instead, it is often used by normal or mildly overweight people to "spot reduce" fat from various areas of the body. This procedure is not without risks; blood clots, skin and nerve damage, adverse drug reactions, and perforation injuries can and do occur as a result of liposuction. It can also result in deformations in the area where the fat is removed. This procedure is not the solution to long-term weight loss, as the millions of fat cells that remain in the body after liposuction enlarge if the person continues to overeat. In addition, although liposuction may reduce the fat content of a localized area, it does not reduce a person's risk for the diseases that are more common among overweight or obese people. Only traditional weight loss with diet and exercise can reduce body fat and the risks for chronic diseases.

> RECAP: *Obesity is defined as a BMI of 30 or greater. Morbid obesity is a BMI greater than or equal to 40 kg/m². Obesity has many causes, including genetics and physiologic factors. In addition, childhood obesity is strongly associated with adult obesity. Treatments for overweight, obesity, and morbid obesity include low-calorie, low-fat diets in combination with regular physical activity, weight-loss prescription medications, and/or weight-loss surgery.*

CHAPTER SUMMARY

- Definitions of a healthful body weight include one that is appropriate for someone's age and level of development, promotes healthful blood lipids and glucose, can be achieved and sustained without constant dieting, promotes good eating habits, and allows for regular physical activity.

- Body mass index (BMI) is an index of weight per height squared. It is useful to indicate health risks associated with overweight and obesity in groups of people.

- Underweight is defined as having too little body fat to maintain health, causing a person to have a weight for a given height that is below an acceptably defined standard. A BMI below 18.5 is considered underweight.

- Overweight is defined as having a moderate amount of excess body fat, resulting in a person having a weight for a given height that is greater than some accepted standard but is not considered obese. A BMI of 25 to 29.9 is considered overweight.

- Obesity is defined as having excess body fat that adversely affects health, resulting in a person having a weight for a given height that is substantially greater than some accepted standard. A BMI of 30 to 39.9 is considered obese. Morbid obesity occurs when a person's body weight exceeds 100% of normal, which puts him or her at very high risk for serious health consequences. A BMI of 40 or above is considered morbidly obese.

- Body composition assessment involves estimating the proportions of a person's body fat (or adipose tissue) and lean body mass. Methods include underwater weighing, skinfold measures, bioelectrical impedance analysis, near infrared reactance, and the Bod Pod.

- The waist-to-hip ratio and waist circumference are used to determine patterns of fat storage. People with large waists (as compared to the hips) have an apple-shaped fat pattern. People with large hips (as compared to the waist) have a pear-shaped fat pattern. Having an apple-shaped pattern increases your risk for heart disease, type 2 diabetes, and other chronic diseases.

- We lose or gain weight based on changes in our energy intake, the food we eat, and our energy expenditure (both at rest and when physically active).

- Basal metabolic rate (BMR) is the energy needed to maintain the body's resting functions. BMR accounts for 60–75% of our total daily energy needs.

- The thermic effect of food is the energy we expend to process the food we eat. It accounts for 5–10% of the energy content of a meal and is higher for processing proteins and carbohydrates than for fats.

- The energy cost of physical activity represents energy that we expend for physical movement or work we do above basal levels. It accounts for 15–35% of our total daily energy output.

- Our genetic heritage influences the risk for obesity, and factors such as possessing a thrifty gene (or genes) or maintaining a weight set point may affect a person's risk for obesity.

- Being overweight or obese as a child can lead to adult obesity, and childhood obesity is linked with the risk for heart disease, type 2 diabetes, and premature death later in adulthood.

- Eating a diet proportionally higher in fat may increase the risk for obesity, as dietary fat is stored more easily as adipose tissue than is dietary carbohydrate or protein.

- Physiologic factors that contribute to obesity include alterations in various proteins and hormones that influence hunger and satiety, including leptin, ghrelin, peptide YY, uncoupling proteins, beta-endorphins, serotonin, and cholecystokinin.

- Social factors that may contribute to obesity include pressure to eat from family and peers, easy access to inexpensive and high-fat foods, watching too much television, and not taking time to exercise. Mood and emotional state also affect appetite.

- Fad diets are weight-loss programs that enjoy short-term popularity and are sold based on a marketing gimmick that appeals to the public's desires and fears. They typically promise rapid weight loss, often without increased physical activity or long-term behavioral modification, and rarely result in long-term maintenance of weight loss.

- Diet plans that restrict intake of certain macronutrients can help many people lose weight, but some have unhealthful side effects.

- A sound weight-loss plan involves gradual reduction in energy intake, incorporating physical activity into each day, and practicing changes in behavior that can assist in meeting realistic weight change goals.

- Prescription drugs can be used to assist with weight loss when the risks of obesity override the risks associated with the medications.

- Various dietary supplements are marketed as weight-loss products. Many of these products cause dangerous changes in heart rate and blood pressure. Unlike prescription drugs, these products are not strictly regulated by the FDA.

- Being underweight can be dangerous to one's health, and wasting (or starvation) among children is still a health crisis in many developing countries.

- Most of the products marketed for weight gain have been shown to be ineffective. The risks associated with these products are not well documented; many of these may have no effect on a person's weight and are simply a waste of money. Healthful weight gain involves consuming more energy than expended by selecting ample servings of nutritious, high-energy foods and exercising regularly by including resistance training and aerobic exercise.

- Approximately 34% of American adults are overweight and 32% are obese. Overweight is not as detrimental to health as obesity, but it is associated with an increased risk for high blood pressure, heart disease, type 2 diabetes, sleep disorders, osteoarthritis, gallstones, and gynecological abnormalities.

- Obesity and morbid obesity are associated with significantly increased risks for many diseases and for premature death. Obesity can be treated with low-energy diets and regular physical activity, prescription medications, and surgery when necessary.

TEST YOURSELF ANSWERS

1. **True.** Being underweight increases our risk for illness and premature death and in many cases can be just as unhealthful as being obese.

2. **False.** Obesity is a multifactorial disease with many contributing factors. Although eating too much food and not getting enough exercise can lead to being overweight and obese, the disease of obesity is complex and is not simply caused by overeating.

3. **False.** Body composition assessments can help give us a general idea of our body fat levels, but most methods are not extremely accurate.

4. **False.** According to the Centers for Disease Control and Prevention, in 2003–2004 approximately 33% of all adults in the United States were considered obese.

5. **True.** Health can be defined in many ways. An individual who is overweight, but who exercises regularly and has no additional risk factors for various diseases such as heart disease and type 2 diabetes, is considered a healthy person.

REVIEW QUESTIONS

1. The ratio of a person's body weight to height is represented as his or her
   a. body composition.
   b. basal metabolic rate.
   c. bioelectrical impedance.
   d. body mass index.

2. The body's total daily energy expenditure includes
   a. basal metabolic rate, thermal effect of food, and effect of physical activity.
   b. basal metabolic rate, movement, standing, and sleeping.
   c. effect of physical activity, standing, and sleeping.
   d. body mass index, thermal effect of food, and effect of physical activity.

3. All people gain weight when they
   a. eat a high-fat diet (>30% fat).
   b. take in more energy than they expend.
   c. fail to exercise.
   d. take in less energy than they expend.

4. The set-point theory proposes that
   a. obese people have a gene not found in slender people that regulates their weight so that it always hovers near a given set point.
   b. obese people have a gene that causes them to be energetically thrifty.
   c. all people have a genetic set point for their body weight.
   d. all people have a hormone that regulates their weight so that it always hovers near a given set point.

5. Our innate, physiologic drive to eat is called
   a. hunger.
   b. appetite.
   c. satiety.
   d. our basal metabolic rate.

6. True or false? Pear-shaped fat patterning is known to increase a person's risk for many chronic diseases, including diabetes and heart disease.

7. True or false? One pound of fat is equal to about 3,500 kcal.

8. True or false? Weight-loss medications are typically prescribed for people who have a body mass index greater than or equal to 18.5 kg/m^2.

9. True or false? Recommendations for weight gain include avoiding both aerobic and resistance exercise for the duration of the weight-gain program.

10. True or false? More than half of the people in the United States are currently either overweight or obese.

11. Identify at least four characteristics of a healthful weight.

12. Describe a sound weight-loss program, including recommendations for diet, physical activity, and behavioral modifications.

13. Can you increase your basal metabolic rate? Is it wise to try? Defend your answer.

14. Research at least three societal factors that may have influenced the rise in childhood and adolescent overweight in the United States since 1963 (see Figure 11.11). Consider the effect of advances in technology as well as changes in food production, distribution, and marketing that have occurred.

15. Your friend Misty joins you for lunch and confesses that she is discouraged about her weight. She says that she has been trying "really hard" for 3 months to lose weight, but that no matter what she does, she cannot drop below 148 pounds. Based on her height, you know Misty is not overweight, and she exercises regularly. What questions would you suggest she think about? How would you advise her?

FIND THE QUACK

Jeff is an account executive for a telecommunications business. His long hours leave him little time to exercise, and his frequent travel means too many fattening restaurant meals. Thus, his weight has been creeping steadily upward and as a result he has high blood pressure. He's shopping for groceries one evening when he notices a colorful display at the end of an aisle. Bright signs surrounding stacks of slender, elegant bottles are promoting a new soft drink called GingerSlim that promises to increase body metabolism and burn calories. Intrigued, Jeff accepts the sample a saleswoman hands him, along with a pamphlet. While sipping the beverage, which tastes like a strong ginger ale, Jeff reads the following in the product brochure:

- GingerSlim is a calorie-burning soft drink that works by increasing the body's basal metabolic rate (BMR). An increased BMR burns more calories.

- On average, BMR increases 10% for 1 to 3 hours after consuming GingerSlim.

- GingerSlim is itself almost completely calorie-free (4 calories per 8-oz bottle). It is a patented blend of pure water, ginger, caffeine, a sugar substitute, and a private blend of herbs and spices that rev up your metabolism.

- GingerSlim can be safely consumed up to three times a day to maintain your increased BMR.

When Jeff reads the fine print on the back of the brochure, he discovers that each 8-oz bottle of GingerSlim contains 210 mg of caffeine. He also notices a small area of boxed text at the bottom. It reads: "These statements have not been evaluated by the Food and Drug Administration. This product is not intended to diagnose, treat, cure, or prevent any disease." Jeff notes the price of GingerSlim on the display: it's "On Special" for $4.99 for a four-pack.

1. An 8-oz cup of brewed coffee contains an average of 85 mg of caffeine. Approximately how many cups of coffee does the amount of caffeine in an 8-oz bottle of GingerSlim represent?

2. If Jeff were to drink the recommended three bottles of GingerSlim per day, how much caffeine would he consume?

3. Jeff normally starts his day with one cup of brewed coffee. He then switches to bottled water, juices, and caffeine-free sodas. Predict how Jeff might feel if he starts consuming three bottles of GingerSlim per day. Predict the effects, if any, that the beverage might have on his long-term health and his weight.

4. Jeff's morning coffee, for which he uses canned coffee, costs him approximately 20¢ per 8-oz cup. How much would Jeff pay to brew coffee containing the same amount of caffeine as in a bottle of GingerSlim? (Reminder: One bottle of GingerSlim costs approximately $1.25 and contains 210 mg caffeine.) Do you think GingerSlim offers anything that is worth the increased price? Why or why not?

Answers can be found at www.aw-bc.com/thompson.

WEB LINKS

http://hp2010.nhlbihin.net/portion
National Institutes of Health Portion Distortion Site

Take the "Portion Distortion" quiz and find out how changing portion sizes influences body weight.

www.nhlbisupport.com/bmi
National Heart, Lung, and Blood Institute BMI Calculator

Calculate your body mass index (BMI) on the Internet.

www.ftc.gov/bcp/index.shtml
Federal Trade Commission Consumer Protection

Click on Consumer Information and then Diet, Health, and Fitness to find how to avoid false weight-loss claims.

www.consumer.gov/weightloss
Partnership for Healthy Weight Management

Visit this site to learn about successful strategies for achieving and maintaining a healthy weight.

www.eatright.org
American Dietetic Association

Go to this site to learn more about fad diets.

www2.niddk.nih.gov/HealthEducation/HealthNutrition
National Institute of Diabetes and Digestive and Kidney Diseases

Visit this site to find out more about healthy weight loss and its positive effects on diabetes risk.

www.sne.org

Society for Nutrition Education

Click on Resources and Relationships and then Weight Realities Resources for additional resources related to positive attitudes about body image and healthful alternatives to dieting.

www.oa.org

Overeaters Anonymous

Visit this site to learn about ways to reduce compulsive overeating.

REFERENCES

1. Emme. 2007. Bio profile; books. http://emmestyle.com. (Accessed July 2007.)
2. PBS. 2004. Beyond the scale. *Healthweek*. www.pbs.org/healthweek/featurep3_428.htm. (Accessed February 2004.)
3. Manore, M. M., and J. Thompson. 2000. *Sport Nutrition for Health and Performance*. Champaign, IL: Human Kinetics.
4. Wang, Y. 2004. Epidemiology of childhood obesity—methodological aspects and guidelines: what is new? *Int. J. Obes.* 23:S21–S28.
5. Deurenberg, P., M. Yap, and W. A. van Staveren. 1998. Body mass index and percent body fat: a meta analysis among different ethnic groups. *Int. J. Obes.* 22:1164–1171.
6. Shai, I., R. Jiang, J. E. Manson, M. J. Stampfer, W. C. Willett, G. A. Colditz, and F. B. Hu. 2006. Ethnicity, obesity, and risk of type 2 diabetes in women. *Diabet. Care* 29:1585–1590.
7. Zernike, K. 2004. U.S. body survey, head to toe, finds signs of expansion. *The New York Times,* March 1, section 1, page 12.
8. Stunkard, A. J., T. I. A. Sorensen, C. Hanis, T. W. Teasdale, R. Chakraborty, W. J. Schull, and F. Schulsinger. 1986. An adoption study of human obesity. *N. Engl. J. Med.* 314:193–198.
9. Bouchard, C., A. Tremblay, J. P. Després, A. Nadeau, P. J. Lupien, G. Thériault, J. Dussault, S. Moorjani, S. Pinault, and G. Fournier. 1990. The response to long-term overfeeding in identical twins. *N. Engl. J. Med.* 322:1477–1482.
10. Gunnell, D. J., S. J. Frankel, K. Nanchahal, T. J. Peters, and G. Davey Smith. 1998. Childhood obesity and adult cardiovascular mortality: a 57-y follow-up study based on the Boyd Orr cohort. *Am. J. Clin. Nutr.* 67:1111–1118.
11. Hellerstein, M. 2001. No common energy currency: de novo lipogenesis as the road less traveled. *Am. J. Clin. Nutr.* 74:707–708.
12. Cummings, D. E., D. S. Weigle, R. S. Frayo, P. A. Breen, M. K. Ma, E. P. Dellinger, and J. Q. Purnell. 2002. Plasma ghrelin levels after diet-induced weight loss or gastric bypass surgery. *N. Engl. J. Med.* 346:1623–1630.
13. Druce, M. R., A. M. Wren, A. J. Park, J. E. Milton, M. Patterson, G. Frost, M. A. Ghatei, C. Small, and S. R. Bloom. 2005. Ghrelin increases food intake in obese as well as lean subjects. *Int. J. Obes.* 29:1130–1136.
14. Batterham, R. L., M. A. Cowley, C. J. Small, H. Herzog, M. A. Cohen, C. L. Dakin, A. M. Wren, A. E. Brynes, M. J. Low, M. A. Ghatel, R. D. Cone, and S. R. Bloom. 2002. Gut hormone PYY3-36 physiologically inhibits food intake. *Nature* 418:650–664.
15. Batterham, R. L., M. A. Cohen, S. M. Ellis, C. W. Le Roux, D. J. Withers, G. S. Frost, M. A. Ghatei, and S. R. Bloom. 2003. Inhibition of food intake in obese subjects by peptide YY3-36. *N. Engl. J. Med.* 349:941–948.
16. Elliott, S. 2005. Calories? Hah! Munch some mega M&M's. *The New York Times,* August 5, section C5.
17. Koh-Banerjee, P., N. F. Chu, D. Spiegelman, B. Rosner, G. Colditz, W. Willett, and E. Rimm. 2003. Prospective study of the association of changes in dietary intake, physical activity, alcohol consumption, and smoking with 9-y gain in waist circumference among 16,587 U.S. men. *Am. J. Clin. Nutr.* 78:719–727.
18. American Dietetic Association. 2002. Position of the American Dietetic Association: food and nutrition misinformation. *J. Am. Diet. Assoc.* 102(2):260–266.
19. Freedman, M. R., J. King, and E. Kennedy. 2001. Popular diets: a scientific review. *Obes. Res.* 9(suppl. 1):1S–40S.
20. Ello-Martin, J. A., J. H. Ledikwe, and B. J. Rolls. 2005. The influence of food portion size and energy density on energy intake: implications for weight management. *Am. J. Clin. Nutr.* 82(suppl.):236S–241S.
21. Flood, J. E., L. S. Roe, and B. J. Rolls. 2006. The effect of increased beverage portion size on energy intake at a meal. *J. Am. Diet. Assoc.* 106:1984–1990.
22. Klem, M. L., R. R. Wing, M. T. McGuire, H. M. Seagle, and J. O. Hill. 1997. A descriptive study of individuals successful at long-term maintenance of substantial weight loss. *Am. J. Clin. Nutr.* 66:239–246.
23. Bérubé-Parent, S., D. Prud'homme, S. St-Pierre, E. Doucet, and A. Tremblay. 2001. Obesity treatment with a progressive clinical tri-therapy combining sibutramine and a supervised diet-exercise intervention. *Int. J. Obes.* 25:1144–1153.
24. Chanoine, J.-P., S. Hampl, C. Jensen, M. Boldrin, and J. Hauptman. 2005. Effect of orlistat on weight and body composition in obese adolescents. A randomized controlled trial. *JAMA* 293(23):2873–2883.
25. Hutton, B., and D. Fergusson. 2004. Changes in body weight and serum lipid profile in obese patients treated with orlistat in addition to a hypocaloric diet: a systemic review of randomized clinical trials. *Am. J. Clin. Nutr.* 80:1461–1468.
26. Saper, R. B., D. M. Eisenberg, and R. S. Phillips. 2004. Common dietary supplements for weight loss. *Am. Fam. Phys.* 70(9):1731–1738.
27. Allison, D. B., K. R. Fontaine, S. Heshka, J. L. Mentore, and S. B. Heymsfield. 2001. Alternative treatments for weight loss: a critical review. *Crit. Rev. Food Sci. Nutr.* 41(1):1–28.
28. Kreider, R. B., V. Miriel, and E. Bertun. 1993. Amino acid supplementation and exercise performance. *Sports Med.* 16:190–209.
29. Joyner, M. J. 2000. Over-the-counter supplements and strength training. *Exerc. Sport Sci. Rev.* 28:2–3.
30. Broeder, C. E., J. Quindry, K. Brittingham, L. Panton, J. Thomson, S. Appakondu, K. Breuel, R. Byrd, J. Douglas, C. Earnest, C. Mitchell, M. Olson, T. Roy, and C. Yarlagadda. 2000. The Andro Project: physiological and hormonal influences of androstenedione supplementation in men 35 to 65 years old participating in a high-intensity resistance training program. *Arch. Int. Med.* 160:3093–3104.
31. Brown, G. A., M. D. Vukovich, T. A. Reifenrath, N. L. Uhl, K. A. Parsons, R. L. Sharp, and D. S. King. 2000. Effects of anabolic precursors on serum testosterone concentrations and adaptations to resistance training in young men. *Intl. J. Sport Nutr. Ex. Metab.* 10:340–359.
32. U.S. Department of Health and Human Services. National Institutes of Health. 2007. National Heart Lung and Blood Institute Diseases and Conditions Index. Overweight and Obesity. www.nhlbi.nih.gov/health/dci/Diseases/obe/obe_risks.html.
33. Centers for Disease Control and Prevention (CDC). National Center for Health Statistics. 2007. Prevalence of overweight and obesity among adults: United States, 2003–2004. www.cdc.gov/nchs/products/pubs/pubd/hestats/overweight/overwght_adult_03.htm. (Accessed July 2007.)

34. McGuire, M. T., R. R. Wing, and J. O. Hill. 1999. The prevalence of weight loss maintenance among American adults. *Int. J. Obes.* 23:1314–1319.

35. Torgan, C. 2002. Childhood obesity on the rise. The NIH Word on Health. www.nih.gov/news/WordonHealth/jun2002/childhoodobesity.htm. (Accessed July 2007.)

36. Dietz, W. H. 1994. Critical periods in childhood for the development of obesity. *Am. J. Clin. Nutr.* 59:955–959.

37. Institute of Medicine. Food and Nutrition Board. 2002. *Dietary Reference Intakes for Energy, Carbohydrate, Fiber, Fat, Fatty Acids, Cholesterol, Protein, and Amino Acids (Macronutrients).* Washington, DC: National Academies Press.

38. National Institutes of Health. National Heart, Lung, and Blood Institute. 1998. Clinical Guidelines on the Identification, Evaluation, and Treatment of Overweight and Obesity in Adults. Executive Summary. www.nhlbi.nih.gov/guidelines/obesity/ob_exsum.pdf. (Accessed July 2007.)

39. Sjöström, L., A.-K. Lindroos, M. Peltonen, J. Torgerson, C. Bouchard, B. Carlsson, S. Dahlgren, B. Larsson, K. Narbro, C. D. Sjöström, M. Sullivan, and H. Wedel. 2004. Lifestyle, diabetes, and cardiovascular risk factors 10 years after bariatric surgery. *N. Engl. J. Med.* 351(26):2683–2693.

40. Dillon, S. 2007. Sorority evictions raise issue of looks and bias. *The New York Times,* February 25, section 1, page 17.

41. American Obesity Association. 2002. Discrimination. http://obesity1.tempdomainname.com/discrimination/employment.shtml.

42. Drewnowski, A., and N. Darmon. 2005. The economics of obesity: dietary energy and energy cost. *Am. J. Clin. Nutr.* 82:265S–273S.

43. Blair, S. N., and S. Brodney. 1999. Effects of physical inactivity and obesity on morbidity and mortality: current evidence and research issues. *Med. Sci. Sports Exerc.* 31(11; suppl. 1): S646–S662.

44. Bacon, L., N. L. Keim, M. D. Van Loan, M. Derricote, B. Gale, A. Kazaks, and J. S. Stern. 2002. Evaluating a 'non-diet' wellness intervention for improvement of metabolic fitness, psychological well-being and eating and activity behaviors. *Int. J. Obes. Relat. Metab. Disord.* 26(6):854–865.

NUTRITION DEBATE

The Obesity Epidemic: Who Is to Blame?

Although prejudice of all kinds still exists, our society espouses values of tolerance and compassion toward all people, despite their disease state, religious beliefs, sexual orientation, or racial and ethnic background. However, there seems to be one group of people against whom prejudice is still acceptable: obese people. They remain the punch line of many jokes, are socially ostracized, and experience widespread harassment and embarrassment at work, at school, and in other avenues of life. The recent efforts of airlines to deny flights to individuals who are too large to fit in standard airline seats, or to require them to buy two seats per person, are only two examples of how our society deals with obesity. To many people, these efforts by the airlines make perfect business sense, but others perceive such measures as demeaning, punitive, and overtly prejudicial. Recently, a group of overweight university women were evicted from their sorority house. Although the sorority claims these women lacked commitment to recruitment goals, the students and many others claim that they were discriminated against because they are overweight and have a physical appearance that was not considered acceptable by the sorority.[40] The American Obesity Association also reports that overweight and obese individuals are paid less than their normal weight colleagues and are discriminated against during both the hiring and promotion processes.[41]

Students who claim a sorority discriminated against members because of their weights.

As you have learned in this chapter, obesity is a complex, multifactorial disease, just as heart disease and diabetes are diseases. Although factors within an individual's control, such as overeating and doing too little exercise, are certainly part of the picture, genetics, physiology, and psychological and social factors also contribute. For instance, is it an individual's "fault" if he works long hours at a sedentary job and spends early mornings and evenings caring for elderly parents? Or if she is too poor to find housing in a safe neighborhood where she could go for walks outside, or to afford membership in a fitness club? Should we blame obese children whose schools provide no physical education and whose school lunches are high in fat and energy? Are inner-city residents to blame when their neighborhood grocery store closes and is replaced by a fast-food restaurant? Who is to blame for the increasing portion sizes in many restaurants, or for the sugar added to many seemingly wholesome foods from peanut butter to bottled water? Whose fault is it that the price of fresh fruits and vegetables increased 120% in the United States between 1985 and 2000, whereas the price of cooking oils and soft drinks increased less than 40%?[42] Finally, does eating healthfully and exercising regularly guarantee that a person will be thin? Most people do not understand the complex social, economic, and physiologic issues surrounding obesity and instead view it simply as a condition that results from being lazy and lacking the willpower to turn down fattening foods. Thus, some people feel justified in discriminating against people who struggle with obesity.

As we continue to learn about the causes of obesity, and to search for prevention and treatment measures that work, our society must take measures to reduce the social stigma of living with this disease. Such measures might begin with education: through public service announcements, teacher training, and other public efforts, we need to teach both children and adults what they can do to prevent obesity personally, as well as what efforts they can make as consumers to reduce portion sizes and lobby for more nutritious food choices. We also need to publicly acknowledge the fact that certain factors in obesity lie beyond an individual's control. Other measures to increase public acceptance include recent marketing campaigns using more overweight men and women in print and television advertisements and increasing public awareness of regulations prohibiting job and housing discrimination based on weight.

Recently, some compelling arguments have been put forth stating that we should stop our obsession with weight and switch our focus to health. There is strong evidence that having a higher cardiorespiratory fitness level reduces premature mortality rates and obesity-associated disease risk factors independent of a person's level of overweight or obesity.[43] What this means is that physically fit overweight or obese people have a lower risk of premature death and a lower risk for obesity-related

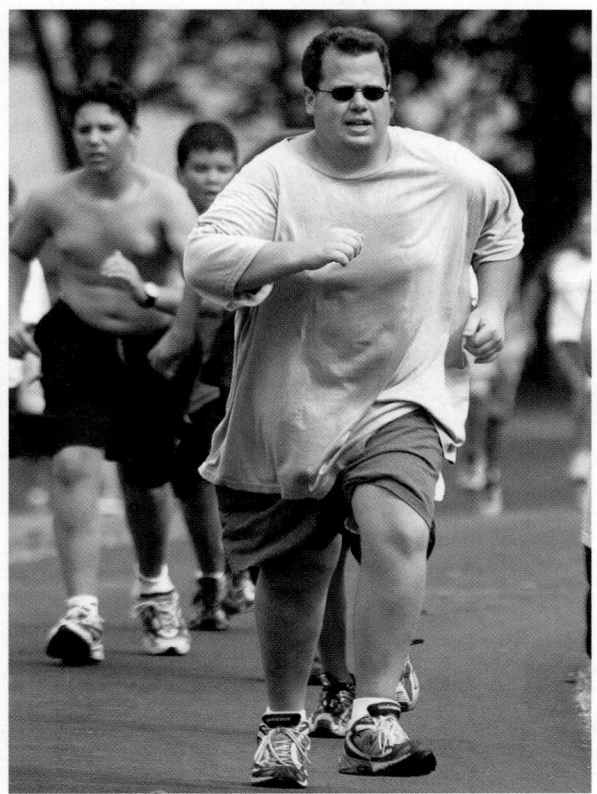

Overweight people can be physically fit and receive the health benefits of fitness.

chronic diseases than unfit overweight or obese people and also a lower risk than unfit people whose body weight is considered normal. So contrary to popular belief, people can be "fit and fat." Thus, there appears to be no clear-cut evidence to define the "best" body weight to improve health and prolong life, and experts question whether it makes sense to spend limited healthcare resources encouraging individuals who are moderately overweight, particularly those with no significant disease risk factors, to meet a predefined "ideal" weight. As a result, many nutrition and exercise professionals are proposing that we encourage a healthful lifestyle defined by eating a balanced diet and staying physically active on a regular basis and stop defining health by body weight.

Another compelling reason to focus on health rather than weight is the inability of most dieters to maintain long-term weight loss. Although more than $30 billion is spent every year on weight-loss efforts, the average weight loss is only about 10% of body weight, and most of the weight lost is regained within 5 years. In response to such discouraging statistics, a group of researchers at the

University of California, Davis, developed a non-diet approach to obesity. The UC Davis program, called "Health at Every Size," taught participants how to eat in response to internal hunger cues, distinguish between healthful and non-healthful foods, increase their body acceptance, and enjoy physical activity. By the end of the study, the group showed a significant decrease in total cholesterol, LDL-cholesterol, and systolic blood pressure. Also by the end of the study, the group had nearly quadrupled their level of physical activity and demonstrated significant improvements in self-esteem.[44] In contrast, a control group of dieters sustained no significant reduction in total or LDL-cholesterol or blood pressure and no increase in physical activity. Their initial loss of an average of 5% of body weight also was not sustained, and their self-esteem had worsened by the end of the study. Thus, despite the fact that the "Health at Every Size" program participants did not lose weight, their sustained improvements in health, physical activity, and self-esteem support the claim that healthcare resources should focus on helping people increase fitness rather than reduce fatness.

In recent years, some professional organizations have begun to embrace a new way of thinking about the definition of ideal body weight and the negative effects of dieting. For instance, "About Face" is a media literacy organization focused on the impact that mass media has on the mental, emotional, and physical well-being of girls. "Bullying" is a Web site written by students on the topic of bullying and weight prejudice among youth. The U.S. Department of Health and Human Services sponsors a Web site called "Girl Power!" which is a national education campaign aimed to encourage and motivate 9- to 14-year-old girls to make the most of their lives using targeted health messages. The Society for Nutrition Education has formed a division called "Weight Realities" to assist dietitians, nutrition educators, and the general public about coping with unrealistic body image expectations and an unhealthful pursuit of thinness. Refer to the Web site at **www.sne.org/weightrealitiesdivision.htm** to gain access to these Web links and other resources related to positive attitudes about body image and healthful alternatives to dieting.

Earlier, we identified a few measures for reducing the social stigma of obesity. What other measures can you think of? How can we deal with practical concerns such as small airline and movie theater seats, narrow department store aisles, and discrimination in employment, health insurance, education, and housing? Can you think of ways we can be more compassionate toward obese family members, friends, and acquaintances and support them in their quest for health? As the obesity epidemic continues to grow, our need to answer these questions becomes more critical.

CHAPTER 12

CHAPTER OBJECTIVES

After reading this chapter you will be able to:

1. Distinguish among physical activity for health, for fitness, and for performance.

2. Describe the benefits of regular physical activity, including improvements in physical health, mental health, stress management, and life span.

3. Explain the components of an aerobic exercise program, a strength-training program, and a stretching program.

4. Summarize ways to prevent and treat common fitness injuries.

5. Summarize the key components of a personal fitness program, and design a program that works for you.

TEST YOURSELF

1. Can exercise really reduce stress?

2. What types of exercises can I do to strengthen my muscles?

3. How can I motivate myself to exercise more?

4. Is it better to eat before or after exercising?

5. How do I choose a good running shoe?

Personal Fitness: Improving Health Through Exercise

a century ago in the United States, most people had to perform heavy physical labor on a daily basis just to survive. However, science and technology have transformed our lives since then. Today most adults in our country lead sedentary lifestyles and perform little physical labor or exercise. Students are no different; a recent survey indicated that 30 percent of college women and 24 percent of college men participate in no moderate or vigorous physical activities.[1] The growing percentage of Americans who live sedentary lives has been linked to dramatic increases in the incidence of obesity, diabetes, and other chronic diseases.[2] More than 134 million Americans are overweight or obese, 65 million have high blood pressure, 16 million have coronary artery disease, 21 million have diabetes, and approximately 54 million have "pre-diabetes."[3]

Decades of research show that physical activity has tremendous health-promoting and disease-preventing benefits. Now is an excellent time to develop exercise habits that will improve the quality and duration of your life.

Exercise does not have to involve going to the gym; activities such as playing with your dog do count toward your daily physical activity.

Physical Activity for Health, Fitness, and Performance

Generally speaking, **physical activity** is defined as any bodily movement that is produced by the contraction of skeletal muscles and that substantially increases energy expenditure.[4] Walking, swimming, heavy lifting, and housework are all examples of physical activity. Physical activities also may vary by intensity. For example, walking to class may require little effort, but walking to class up a hill while carrying a heavy backpack makes the activity more intense. There are three general categories of physical activity defined by the purpose for which they are done: physical activity for health, physical activity for fitness, and physical activity for performance.

Physical Activity for Health

Just about everyone can improve general health by increasing overall physical activity. Simply adding more physical movement to your day can benefit your health. A physically active lifestyle might include choices such as parking farther away from your destination, taking walking breaks while studying, or taking the stairs instead of the elevator. In addition to these incidental ways to increase activity, there are lots of ways you can enjoy being physically active in recreation. Going dancing, playing Frisbee, or walking your dog are all good examples.

The good thing about lifestyle physical activity is that you don't necessarily have to sustain your activity for an extended period of time to get a health benefit. Research shows that accumulating activity throughout the day can contribute to overall health and well-being. In their 2007 updated recommendations for adults, the ACSM and AHA stated that to promote and maintain good health, adults under age 65 should perform 30 minutes of moderate-intensity activity 5 days a week. This activity is in addition to the light-intensity activities of daily life and can be accumulated in bouts of at least 10 minutes. In their 2008 physical activity guidelines, the U.S. Department of Health and Human Services made a similar recommendation of 150 minutes of moderate physical activity per week, preferably spread throughout the week and performed in episodes of at least 10 minutes.[5]

Physical Activity for Fitness

The term **exercise** is a bit more specific than *physical activity*. Although all exercise is physical activity, not all physical activity may be exercise. For example, walking from your car to class is physical activity, but going for a brisk 30-minute walk is considered exercise. *Exercise* is defined as planned, structured, and repetitive bodily movement done to improve or maintain one or more components of physical fitness, such as endurance, flexibility, and strength.[6] **Physical fitness** is the ability to perform moderate to vigorous levels of physical activity on a regular basis without excessive fatigue. Table 12.1 identifies the major health-related components of physical fitness.

To become physically fit, you must increase the frequency, intensity, and duration of your exercise. Both the Centers for Disease Control and Prevention (CDC) and the American College of Sports Medicine (ACSM) recommend that adults

physical activity Any bodily movement that is produced by the contraction of skeletal muscles and that substantially increases energy expenditure

exercise Planned, structured, and repetitive bodily movement done to improve or maintain one or more components of physical fitness

physical fitness The ability to perform regular moderate to vigorous levels of physical activity without excessive fatigue

TABLE 12.1   Components of Physical Fitness

Cardiorespiratory fitness	Ability to sustain aerobic whole-body activity for a prolonged period of time
Muscular strength	Maximum force able to be exerted by single contraction of a muscle or muscle group
Muscular endurance	Ability to perform high-intensity muscle contractions repeatedly without fatiguing
Flexibility	Ability to move joints freely through their full range of motion
Body composition	The amount and relative proportions and distribution of fat mass and fat-free mass in the body

engage in moderate-intensity physical activities for at least 30 minutes on most days of the week or vigorous-intensity exercise for at least 20 minutes three times a week (or some combination of the two).[7] This amount of physical activity can improve your overall health and can result in some cardiovascular improvements. If you want to improve your cardiorespiratory fitness even more, the ACSM and CDC recommend you perform vigorous physical activities (e.g., jogging or running, circuit weight training, singles tennis) at least 3 days per week for at least 20 minutes at a time; if losing weight is your goal, you need to add 60 to 90 minutes of moderate to vigorous exercise to your daily routine.

Everyone can attain cardiovascular fitness and muscular endurance.

Some people have physical limitations that make achieving these recommendations difficult, but they can still be physically active and reap the benefits of a regular exercise program. For example, a woman with arthritis in the knee and hip joints might not be able to jog without extreme pain, but she can engage in water exercise in a swimming pool. The water will help relieve much of the stress on her joints, and she can improve her range of motion. Similarly, a man who uses a wheelchair may be unable to walk or run, but he can stay physically fit by playing wheelchair basketball.

Physical Activity for Performance

People who want to take their fitness level one step further can add exercise to improve performance. Programs can be designed to increase speed, strength, endurance, or specific muscle strength. Examples include plyometrics to improve control and speed in changing directions, and interval training to improve power and cardiovascular fitness.

Performance training is meant for those who already have a high physical fitness level and are training to enhance some aspect of their ability. Those who engage in this level of activity will achieve a high level of fitness but are also more prone to injury and overtraining.

[*WHAT DO YOU THINK? Which of the three categories of physical activity best describes your motivation for being physically active: health, fitness, or performance? What physical activities could you do to improve your health, fitness, or performance?*

Benefits of Regular Physical Activity

Regular physical activity has been shown to improve more than 50 different physiological, metabolic, and psychological aspects of human life. FIGURE 12.1 summarizes some of the major health-related benefits of regular physical activity and exercise.

Improved Cardiorespiratory Fitness

Exercise is good for the heart and lungs. It can reduce the risk for heart-related diseases, and it can improve blood flow and make performing everyday tasks much easier. Something as mundane as carrying a bag of groceries up a flight of stairs can leave someone with poor cardiorespiratory fitness winded and fatigued, while someone who's in better shape could make several trips without breaking a sweat.

Cardiorespiratory fitness is the ability to perform exercise using large-muscle groups at moderate to high intensity for prolonged periods.[8] Because it requires the cardiovascular and respiratory systems to supply oxygen to the body during sustained physical activity, it is a good indicator of overall health. Low levels of cardiorespiratory fitness are associated with increased risk of premature death and disease.[9]

Regular exercise makes the cardiovascular and respiratory systems more efficient by enlarging the heart muscle, enabling more blood to be pumped with each stroke, and increasing the number of *capillaries* (small blood vessels that allow gas exchange between blood and surrounding tissues) in trained skeletal muscles, which

cardiorespiratory fitness The ability of the heart, lungs, and blood vessels to supply oxygen to skeletal muscles during sustained physical activity

Brain
• Reduces stress and improves mood
• Decreases risk of depression
• Decreases anxiety
• Improves concentration
• Increases oxygen and nutrients to the brain

Breasts
• Decreases risk of breast cancer in women

Lungs
• Improves respiratory capacity
• Improves ability to extract oxygen from the air

Colon
• Decreases risk of colon cancer

Muscles
• Increases muscle strength and tone
• Improves energy production and extraction of oxygen by muscle cells
• Improves muscle endurance and coordination

Bones
• Increases bone density
• Strengthens bones
• Decreases risk of osteoporosis

Thyroid
• Increases rate of metabolism

Heart
• Decreases risk of heart disease
• Strengthens the heart
• Increases volume of blood pumped to the body
• Lowers resting heart rate

Pancreas
• Reduces risk of type 2 diabetes

Subcutaneous fat tissues
• Decreases body fat stores

Joints
• Increases range of motion
• Reduces the pain and swelling of arthritis

Arteries
• Increases levels of good cholesterol (HDL)
• Decreases resting blood pressure
• Decreases risk of atherosclerosis
• Improves circulation

FIGURE 12.1 Some health benefits of regular exercise.

supply more blood to working muscles. Exercise also improves the respiratory system by increasing the amount of oxygen that is inhaled and distributed to body tissues.[10]

Reduced Risk of Heart Disease

Exercise significantly lowers the risk of coronary heart disease.[11] Your heart is a muscular organ made up of highly specialized tissue. Because muscles become stronger and more efficient with use, regular exercise strengthens the heart, enabling it to pump more blood with each beat. This increased efficiency means that the heart requires fewer beats per minute to circulate blood throughout the body. A stronger, more efficient heart is better able to meet the ordinary demands of life.

Prevention of Hypertension

Blood pressure refers to the force exerted by blood against blood vessel walls, generated by the heart's pumping action. *Hypertension,* the medical term for abnormally high blood pressure, is a significant risk factor for cardiovascular disease and stroke. It is particularly prevalent in adult African Americans. People with consistently elevated blood pressure are more susceptible to heart disease and die at a younger age than people with normal blood pressure. Studies report that moderate exercise can reduce both diastolic and systolic blood pressure by 7 mm Hg.[12]

Improved Blood Lipid and Lipoprotein Profile

Regular exercise is known to increase the number of high-density lipoproteins (HDLs, or "good" cholesterol) and decrease the number of low-density lipoproteins (LDLs, or "bad" cholesterol) in the blood.[13] Higher HDL levels are associated with lower risk for artery disease, because they remove some of the "bad" cholesterol from artery walls and hence reduce clogging. Similarly, high levels of LDLs are associated with higher risk for artery disease, because they carry cholesterol in the blood and deposit it along blood vessel walls. The bottom line: Regular exercise lowers the risk of cardiovascular disease.

Reduced Cancer Risk

Regular physical activity appears to lower the risk for some types of cancer, particularly breast cancer. Research on exercise and breast cancer risk has found that the earlier in life a woman starts to exercise, the lower the breast cancer risk.[14]

Regular exercise is also associated with lower risk for colon cancer. One theory is that exercise decreases intestinal transit time. Experts say that because physical activity makes food move more quickly through your digestive system, there is less time for the body to absorb potential carcinogens and for potential carcinogens to be in contact with the digestive tract. Physical activity also decreases the levels of prosta-glandins, substances found in cells of the large intestine that are implicated in cancer.[15] Exercise's effect on prostate and ovarian cancer is unclear. Some studies point to protective effects, but more research is needed.[16]

Improved Bone Mass

A common affliction among older adults is **osteoporosis,** a disease characterized by low bone mass and deterioration of bone tissue, which increase fracture risk. Bone, like other human tissues, responds to the demands placed upon it. Women (and men) have much to gain by remaining physically active as they age—bone mass levels are significantly higher among active than among sedentary women.[17] Regular weight-bearing exercise, when combined with a balanced diet containing adequate calcium, helps keep bones healthy.

Improved Weight Control

Many people start exercising because they want to lose weight. Level of physical activity has a direct effect upon metabolic rate and can raise it for several hours following a vigorous workout. This increase in metabolic rate can reduce body fat and

osteoporosis A disease characterized by low bone mass and deterioration of bone tissue, which increases risk of fracture increase lean muscle mass. Having a healthy fat to lean muscle ratio is associated with a better cardiovascular risk profile.[18] An effective method for losing weight combines regular endurance-type exercises with a moderate decrease in food intake. In addition to helping you lose weight, increased physical activity also improves your chances of keeping the weight off.[19]

The ACSM recommends 30 minutes of moderate physical activity daily with an intake of between 1,500 and 2,000 calories per day.[20] Although exercise and dietary changes work best for weight loss, research shows that exercise alone can reduce obesity. For example, in a study of obese men, those who exercised at a moderate intensity for 60 minutes five times a week with no dietary changes significantly decreased their body fat and increased muscle mass.[21] However, remember that if you want to lose weight only through physical activity, you must spend more time exercising than if you also reduce your caloric intake.

Prevention of Diabetes

Noninsulin-dependent diabetes (type 2 diabetes) is a complex disorder that affects millions of Americans, many of whom have no idea they have the disease. Risk factors include obesity, high blood pressure, and high cholesterol, as well as a family history of the disease.[22] Physicians suggest exercise combined with weight loss and a healthy diet to help prevent diabetes. In a major national clinical trial, researchers found that exercising 150 minutes per week while eating fewer calories and less fat could prevent or delay the onset of type 2 diabetes.[23] Some researchers say that increasing physical activity is one of the most effective strategies both for preventing and managing type 2 diabetes.[24]

Improved Immunity

Regular, consistent exercise promotes a healthy immune system. Research shows that moderate exercise gives the immune system a temporary boost in the production of cells that attack bacteria.[25] But whereas moderate amounts of exercise can be beneficial, extreme exercise may actually be detrimental. For example, athletes engaging in marathon-type events or very intense physical training have an increased risk of colds and flu.[26]

Just how exercise alters immunity is not well understood. We do know that brisk exercise temporarily increases the number of white blood cells (WBCs), which are responsible for fighting infection.[27] The largest changes in immunity are seen in people who are sedentary and begin a moderately energetic program. Because their fitness level is low when they embark on an exercise program, they gain a large number of WBCs. Interestingly, those who participate in regular, long-term heavy exercise, such as marathon runners, experience a decrease in their immune function. If you are feeling worn down, your body could be telling you to take a break and prevent overtraining.

Can exercise really reduce stress? **?**

Improved Mental Health and Stress Management

People who engage in regular physical activity also notice psychological benefits. Regular vigorous exercise has been shown to "burn off" the chemical by-products of the stress response and increase endorphins, giving your mood a natural boost. Regular exercise improves a person's physical appearance by toning and developing muscles and reducing body fat. Feeling good about personal appearance boosts self-esteem. At the same time, as exercisers come to appreciate the improved strength, skills, and flexibility that accompany fitness, they often become less obsessed with physical appearance.[28]

Longer Life Span

Several large studies that followed groups of people over time found that those who exercised or who were more fit lived longer. In a study of over 5,000 middle-aged and older Americans, researchers found that those who had moderate to high levels of activity lived 1.3 to 3.7 years longer than those who got little exercise. Study subjects who exercised at a more intense level outlived sedentary subjects by 3.5 to 3.7 years.[29]

Cardiorespiratory Fitness

There are many options for improving cardiorespiratory fitness. Swimming, cycling, jogging, and in-line skating are just a few options for **aerobic exercise.** The term *aerobic* means "with oxygen" and describes any type of exercise—typically performed at moderate levels of intensity for extended periods of time—that increases your heart rate. A person in good shape has an above-average **aerobic capacity**—a term used to describe the functional status of the cardiorespiratory system (heart, lungs, blood vessels). Aerobic capacity (commonly written as VO_{2max}) is defined as the maximum volume of oxygen the muscles consume during exercise.

To measure your maximal aerobic capacity, an exercise physiologist or physician will typically perform a **graded exercise test** (sometimes called a *stress test*). This diagnostic exam evaluates your level of fitness, heart rate, and blood pressure response to activity and the adequacy of blood supply to your heart. The test is performed on a treadmill or a stationary bicycle. Participants start out slowly and gradually increase the speed, resistance, or elevation. Generally, the higher your cardiorespiratory endurance level, the more oxygen you can transport to exercising muscles and the longer you can exercise without becoming exhausted. In other words, the higher the VO_{2max} value, the higher your level of aerobic fitness.

You can test your own cardiorespiratory fitness by using either the 1.5-mile walk or run endurance test described in the Assess Yourself box on page 343. However, do not take this test if you are just starting to exercise. Progress slowly through a walking/jogging program at low intensities before measuring your fitness with one of these tests. If you have any medical conditions such as asthma, diabetes, heart disease, or obesity, consult your physician before beginning any exercise program.

Aerobic Fitness Programs

The most beneficial aerobic exercises are activities involving all the large muscle groups of your body—for example, swimming, cross-country skiing, and rowing. If you have been sedentary for quite a while, simply initiating a physical activity program may be the hardest task you'll face. The key is to begin at a very low intensity, progress slowly, and stay with it!

There are three main components to an aerobic exercise program: frequency, intensity, and duration. The characteristics of these components vary by individual exercise goals and beginning fitness level. These same dimensions also apply to the other components of fitness: muscular strength, muscular endurance, and flexibility; you can remember them with the acronym FITT, which stands for *frequency, intensity, time (duration),* and *type* of activity. FIGURE 12.2 shows how the FITT principle can be applied to the different fitness components.

Determining Exercise Frequency

To best improve your cardiovascular endurance, you must vigorously exercise at least three times a week. If you are a newcomer to exercise, you can still make improvements by doing less intense exercise but doing it more days a week, following the recommendations from the CDC and the ACSM for moderate physical activity 5 days a week.

Determining Exercise Intensity

There are several ways to measure exercise intensity. One of the main ways is using your **target heart rate** zone. To calculate your target heart rate zone, start by subtracting your age from 220 to find your maximum heart rate. Your target heart rate zone is a certain range of this maximum heart rate. For moderate-intensity physical activity, you should work out at 50 to 70 percent of your maximum heart rate. Thus, if you are 20 years old, your 50 percent target heart rate would be:

$$(220 - 20) \times 0.50, \text{ or } 100 \text{ beats per minute (bpm)}.$$

aerobic exercise Any type of exercise that increases heart rate

aerobic capacity The current functional status of a person's cardiovascular system; measured as VO_{2max}

graded exercise test A test of aerobic capacity administered by a physician, exercise physiologist, or other trained person; two common forms are the treadmill running test and the stationary bike test

target heart rate Percentage of maximum heart rate (220 minus age); heart rate is taken during aerobic exercise to check whether exercise intensity is at the desired level

	Cardiorespiratory endurance	Strength	Flexibility
Frequency	3–5 days a week	2–3 nonconsecutive days a week	Minimum of 2–3 days a week
Intensity	55/65–90% of maximum heart rate	70–85% of maximal resistance. Sufficient resistance to enhance strength and endurance	Sufficient to develop and maintain full range of motion
Time	20–60 minutes continuous aerobic activity	1 or more sets (8–12 repetitions) of 8–10 exercises conditioning all the major muscle groups	2–4 repetitions of each stretch held for 15–30 seconds
Type	Continuous aerobic activity that uses large-muscle groups	Resistance exercises in a full range of motion for all major muscle groups	Stretching for all major joints and muscle groups

FIGURE 12.2 The FITT principle applied to health-related components of fitness.
Source: Adapted from "Position Stand on the Recommended Quantity and Quality of Exercise for Developing and Maintaining Cardiorespiratory and Muscular Fitness and Flexibility in Adults," *Medicine and Science in Sports and Exercise* 30, no. 6 (1998): 975–91. Copyright © 1998 American College of Sports Medicine.

To determine 70 percent of a 20-year-old's maximum heart rate, you would use the following calculations:

$$(220 - 20) \times 0.70, \text{ or } 140 \text{ beats per minute.}$$

Thus, for a moderately intense cardiovascular workout, a 20-year-old would try to maintain aerobic exercise at an intensity of 100 to 140 bpm, or 50 to 70 percent of his or her maximum heart rate.

For more vigorous activities (e.g., running), aim for 70 to 85 percent of your maximum heart rate. People in poor physical condition should set a target heart rate between 40 and 50 percent of maximum and gradually increase the target rate in 5 percent increments.

Once you know your target heart zone, you can take your pulse during your workout to determine how close you are to this value. As you exercise, lightly place your index and middle fingers (don't use your thumb) on your radial artery (inside your wrist, on the thumb side). Using a watch or a clock, take your pulse for 6 seconds and multiply this number by 10 (just add a zero to your count) to get the number of beats per minute. Your pulse should be within a range of 5 beats per minute above or below your target heart rate. If necessary, adjust the pace or intensity of your workout to achieve your target heart rate.

SKILLS FOR BEHAVIOR CHANGE

Tips for Fitting Fitness in Your Life

Busy schedules, schoolwork, part-time jobs, family obligations, and social plans can make it difficult to find time and motivation to be physically active. If you're having trouble fitting exercise in, try some of these tips from the ACSM and AHA:

√ *Do a little at a time. Exercising for 10 minutes three times over the course of a day can be just as effective as exercising for 30 minutes straight.*

√ *Mix it up. You don't need to do the same amount of activity at the same intensity every day. If you take a brisk 30-minute walk 2 days a week and jog for 20 minutes 2 other days, you'll still meet the recommended guidelines.*

√ *Mark it on your schedule. Look for breaks of at least 10 minutes long in your daily schedule and block them off for a little exercise. Set aside specific days and times to exercise and make it part of your routine.*

√ *Make it a social affair. Ask friends, family members, or coworkers to join you during your exercise. Having company will add fun to your routine and will help keep you motivated.*

Another way of determining intensity is to use Borg's rating of perceived exertion (RPE) scale, as shown in FIGURE 12.3. Perceived exertion is how hard you feel you are working, based on your heart rate, increased breathing rate, sweating, and muscle fatigue. This scale uses a rating from 6 (no exertion at all) to 20 (maximal exertion). This method corresponds to heart rate for most people. Experts agree that RPE ratings of 12 to 14 correspond to moderate-intensity activity and 15 to 17 for vigorous activity.

The easiest, but least scientific, method of measuring exercise intensity is the "talk test." If you are exercising moderately, you should be able to carry on a conversation comfortably. If you are too out of breath to talk, you are exercising vigorously.

Determining Exercise Duration

Duration refers to the number of minutes of activity performed during any one session. To achieve health benefits, the ACSM recommends that vigorous activities be performed for at least 20 minutes at a time, and moderate activities for at least 30 minutes at a time.[30]

The lower your activity's intensity, the longer duration you'll need to get the same caloric expenditure. The number of calories burned is higher for a person who weighs more and lower for someone who weighs less.[31] Aim to expend 300 to 500 calories per exercise session, with an eventual weekly goal of 1,500 to 2,000 calories. As you progress, add to your exercise load by increasing duration or intensity, but not both at the same time. From week to week, don't increase duration or intensity by more than 10 percent.

Many of the health benefits associated with cardiorespiratory fitness (such as lower blood pressure) may take several months to achieve; don't expect improvements overnight. However, any physical activity of low to moderate intensity will benefit your overall health almost from the start (FIGURE 12.4). See the Skills for Behavior Change box for ways to fit more physical activity into your life.

6	No exertion at all
7	Extremely light
8	
9	Very light
10	
11	Light
12	
13	Somewhat hard
14	
15	Hard (heavy)
16	
17	Very hard
18	
19	Extremely hard
20	Maximal exertion

Target Heart Rate for Most People — 12–16

FIGURE 12.3 Rating of Perceived Exertion (RPE) scale.

Source: Borg-RPE-scale ® from G. Borg, *Borg's Perceived Exertion and Pain Scales* (Champaign, IL: Human Kinetics, 1998). © Gunnar Borg, 1970, 1985, 1994, 1998. Used with permission of Dr. G. Borg. See further credit information on page 517.

WOMEN'S HEALTH

Gender Differences in Exercise

Exercise is good for everyone's health, but research shows that there are differences in the way men and women choose, participate in, and react to exercise. Overall, men have higher rates of physical activity than women in all age groups. A national survey found that 73 percent of high school-age boys report regular physical activity, compared with 60 percent of girls. Also, almost 50 percent of girls reported *not* playing on a sports team, compared with 38 percent of boys. Gender differences in participation are also reported in college-age men and women. According to the American College Health Association (ACHA), national college health assessment, fewer women than men report participating in regular exercise 3 or more days per week. The difference is even more pronounced in the adult population. Only 24 percent of American women report getting recommended amounts of vigorous physical activity, compared with 33 percent of American men.

Why such differences? There are several reasons, including socialization, physiology, and access. In the past, women were not encouraged to exercise because it was thought that physical exertion would cause damage to their bodies, especially their reproductive organs. Women were also thought to be physiologically incapable of feats such as weight lifting or endurance running. This is not ancient history, considering that the marathon for women was only added to the Olympics in 1984!

Even though it is now known that exercise is beneficial—not detrimental—to the health of women, there are several physiological differences between men and women that account for performance differences, if not participation ones. First, aerobic capacity differs. While there are many women with a significantly higher VO_{2max} level than many men, on average, there is a 43 percent difference between the VO_{2max} level in a young, untrained man and a young, untrained woman. Part of this difference is explained by the fact that in general, men have larger hearts which relates to more capacity. Also, men may have higher levels of blood hemoglobin, which affects oxygen-carrying ability of the blood. Exercise performance can also be affected by percentage of body fat. Overall, women have an average body fat percentage of 25 percent, with men averaging 15 percent.

Muscle strength also can differ between men and women. While studies show that there is no difference in "muscle quality"—a muscle cell in a man is the same as a

muscle cell in a woman—there are strength and power differences, which are a function of muscle *quantity*. Flexibility is another area in which men and women differ, with women having greater hip and elbow flexibility. Relaxin is a hormone to increase flexibility and, unlike men, women have receptor sites for this hormone in their anterior cruciate ligament in the knee and their pubic ligaments.

The results of resistance training in men and women are quite different. Women do not develop muscle to the extent that men do because of differences in testosterone levels in their blood. Before puberty, testosterone levels are similar for both boys and girls. During adolescence, testosterone levels in boys increase dramatically (about tenfold), while testosterone levels in girls remain unchanged. Muscles will become larger (hypertrophy) as a result of resistance-training exercise, but typically this change is less dramatic in women because of their lower testosterone levels.

Women and men exhibit general differences in exercise preferences. From adolescence through adulthood, males are attracted to more competitive activities while females are motivated by the social opportunities that the activities provide. Adult women are more likely to participate in activities such as walking or gardening for exercise than men. Additionally, women appear to be motivated by potential appearance improvements. Another difference is that environmental perceptions seem to affect women more than men. For example, perceptions of safety and crime may be a barrier to jogging around campus for women, but not for men. Differences aside, exercise has health-promoting and disease-preventing benefits for both men and women.

Sources: Centers for Disease Control and Prevention, "Behavioral Risk Factor Surveillance System Prevalence Data." Physical Activity, 2007. http://apps.nccd.cdc.gov/BRFSS; National Center for Health Statistics, *Health, United States, 2007, with Chartbook on Trends in the Health of Americans* (Hyattsville, MD: 2007); S. Seiler, J. J. De Koning, and C. Foster, "The Fall and Rise of the Gender Difference In Elite Anaerobic Performance 1952–2006," *Medicine and Science in Sports and Exercise* 39, no. 3 (2007): 534–40; E. Blaak, "Gender Differences in Fat Metabolism," *Current Opinion in Clinical Nutrition and Metabolic Care* 4, no. 6 (2001): 499–502; J. Reed and B. Ainsworth, "Perceptions of Safety and Crime Affects Women," *Journal of American College Health* 56, no. 2 (2007): 199–204; E. Sohn, "No Bending or Twisting," *U.S. News and World Report,* June 3, 2004; J. R. Sirard, K. A. Pfeiffer, and R. R. Pate, "Motivational Factors Associated with Sports Program Participation in Middle School Students," *Journal of Adolescent Health* 38, no. 6 (2006): 696–703; T. Kurz, *Scientifically Stretching: A Guide to Flexibility Training.* 4th ed. (Island Pond, VT: Stadion Publishing Company, Inc., 2003).

Overload

The overload principle is the foundation of strength training. *Overload* doesn't mean forcing a muscle or muscle group to do too much, which could result in injuries; rather, it's requiring muscles to do more than they are used to doing. Everyone begins a resistance-training program with an initial level of strength. To become stronger, you must regularly create a degree of tension in your muscles that is greater than you are accustomed to. Tension is created by resistance provided by weights such as barbells or dumb-bells, elastic bands, specially designed machines, or the body's weight. Progressively overloading your muscles will cause them to adapt to a new level, thus becoming stronger.

Resistance-training exercises cause microscopic damage (tears) to muscle fibers, and the rebuilding process that increases the muscle's size and capacity takes about 24 to 48 hours. Thus, resistance-training exercise programs should include at least 1 day of rest and recovery between workouts before you overload the same muscles again.

Specificity of Training

According to the specificity principle, the effects of resistance-exercise training are specific to the muscles being exercised; only that muscle or muscle group responds to the demands placed upon it. For example, if you regularly do curls, the muscles involved—your biceps—will become larger and stronger, but the other muscles in your body won't change. Also note that if you only exercise certain muscle groups, you may put opposing muscle groups at increased risk for injury. For example, overworking your quadriceps but neglecting your hamstrings can put you at risk for a hamstring muscle pull.

Variation

Variation is a fundamental principle in strength training. This principle supports the need for changes in one or more parts of your workout routine over time to allow for the training effects to remain at an optimal level. It has been shown that varying duration and intensity is most effective for long-term results.

Reversibility

Another important principle is reversibility. Reversibility means that if you stop putting demands on your body, the body responds by deconditioning. Even after 4 days without training, muscles begin to revert back to their untrained state. The saying "use it or lose it" is applicable when it comes to strength (or cardiorespiratory) training.

Strength Training Elements

There are several elements you should consider when developing a strength-training routine, including the following:

What types of exercises can I do to strengthen my muscles?

- *Exercise selection.* Exercises that work a single joint (e.g., chest presses) are effective for building muscle strength, but multiple-joint exercises (e.g., a squat coupled with an overhead press) are some of the most effective for increasing overall muscle strength. The ACSM recommends that both exercise types be included in a strength-training program, with an emphasis on multiple-joint exercises for maximizing muscle strength.[34]

- *Exercise order.* The sequence of exercises can affect your results. When training all major muscle groups in a workout, complete large-muscle exercises before small-muscle-group exercises, multiple-joint exercises before single-joint exercises, and high-intensity exercises before lower-intensity exercises.

- *Sets and repetitions.* One element that is very important in strength training is how much weight to lift and how many times to lift it to achieve your fitness goals. The SAID principle refers to "specific adaptation to imposed demand." More simply put, the types of demands that you put on your body will result in the kind of adaptation that will follow. For example, if your strength training goal is to become stronger and increase muscle size, a program with three to six sets of four to eight repetitions at approximately 85 percent of your 1 RM would be effective. If your goal is to tone your muscles without a major increase in muscle size, a program that includes 8 to 12 repetitions would be sufficient. When you can comfortably and correctly complete 12 repetitions, increase the weight load by 10 percent.[35]

- *Rest periods.* The amount of rest between exercises is key to an effective strength-training workout. Resting in between exercises can reduce fatigue and help maintain performance and safety in subsequent sets. A rest period of 2 to 3 minutes is recommended for multiple-joint exercises that use large-muscle groups (squats with overhead presses) and a rest period of 1 to 2 minutes for single-joint exercises or for strength exercises using machines.

Methods of Providing Resistance

There are four commonly used resistance-exercise methods: body-weight resistance and fixed, variable, and accommodating resistance devices.

Body-Weight Resistance (Calisthenics)

Strength and endurance training doesn't have to involve equipment. You can use your own body weight to develop skeletal muscle fitness. Calisthenics (such as push-ups and chin-ups) use part or all of your body weight to offer resistance during exercise. Although they are less effective than other resistance methods in developing large muscle mass and strength, calisthenics improve general muscular fitness and muscle tone and maintain a level of muscular strength.

Fixed Resistance

Fixed-resistance exercises provide a constant amount of resistance throughout the full range of movement. Free weights, such as barbells and dumbbells, and some machines provide fixed resistance because their weight, or the amount of resistance, does not change during an exercise. Fixed-resistance equipment has the potential to strengthen all the major muscle groups in the body.

There are several advantages of using free weights. First, they require more balance and coordination. Also, free weights tend to recruit more muscle groups for action and promote more activity of the joint and stabilizer muscles. From a financial perspective, free weights are relatively inexpensive and can provide a great muscle workout.

Variable Resistance

Variable-resistance equipment alters the resistance a muscle encounters during a movement, so the muscle's effort is more consistent throughout the full range of motion. Variable-resistance equipment provides a more controlled motion and specifically isolates certain muscle groups and is often used for rehabilitation of muscle injuries. Some of these machines are expensive and too big to move easily, but others are affordable and more portable.

Accommodating-Resistance

Accommodating resistance devices, sometimes called *isokinetic machines,* maintain a constant speed through the range of motion. The exerciser performs at a maximal level of effort, while the device controls the exercise's speed. The machine is set to a particular speed, and muscles being exercised must move at a rate faster than or equal to that speed in order to encounter resistance.[36] These machines are often used in rehabilitation settings, but many health clubs have them as well.

Core Strength Training

The body's core muscles are the foundation for movement. These muscles are the deep back and abdominal muscles that attach to the spine and pelvis. The contraction of these muscles provides the basis of support for movements of the upper and lower body and powerful movements of the extremities. A weak core increases your

A stability ball is one type of equipment that is excellent for increasing core body strength.

chances for poor posture, lower back pain, and muscle injuries. A strong core gives you a more stable center of gravity and a more stable platform for movements, thus reducing the chance of injury.

You can develop core strength by simple calisthenics, using fitness equipment such as a stability ball, or taking an exercise class like yoga or Pilates. Holding yourself in a plank or "up" push-up position and doing abdominal curl-ups are two examples of calisthenic exercises to increase core strength. Experts recommend doing core-strengthening activities at least three times per week.[37]

Strength Training Benefits

Does strength training offer any benefits beyond simply getting stronger? Indeed, regular strength training can reduce the occurrence of lower back pain and joint and muscle injuries. It can also postpone loss of muscle tissue due to aging and a sedentary lifestyle and help prevent osteoporosis.

Strength training enhances muscle definition and tone and improves personal appearance. This, in turn, enhances self-esteem. Strength training even has a hidden benefit: muscle tissue burns calories faster than most other tissues, even when it is resting. So, increasing your muscle mass can help boost your metabolism and maintain a healthy weight.

Increased awareness of these and other benefits of strength training and muscle development have led to a proliferation of "performance-enhancing" drugs and supplements. In recent years, the use of such drugs has become a major problem on college campuses and among athletes (see the Health Headlines box on page 498).

> WHAT DO YOU THINK? *What types of resistance equipment are currently available to you?* • *Based on what you've read, what actions can you take to increase your muscular strength? Your muscular endurance?* • *How would you measure your improvement?*

Flexibility

Improved **flexibility**—a measure of the range of motion, or the amount of movement possible, at a particular joint—can give you a sense of well-being, help you deal with stress better, and stop your joints from hurting as much as they used to. Stretching exercises are the main way to improve flexibility. Improving the range of motion enhances efficiency, extent of movement, and posture. Today, stretching exercises are extremely popular, both because they are effective and because people can begin them at virtually any age and enjoy them for a lifetime. Flexibility exercises are effective in reducing the incidence and severity of lower back problems and muscle or tendon injuries that can occur during sports and everyday physical activities.[38] Improved flexibility also means less tension and pressure on joints, resulting in less joint pain and joint deterioration.[39] See the Assess Yourself box on page 511 for one way to measure your flexibility.

Flexibility is enhanced by the controlled stretching of muscles and muscle attachments that act on a particular joint. Each muscle involved in a stretching exercise is attached to the skeleton by tendons. The goal of stretching is to decrease the resistance of a muscle and its tendons to tension—that is, to reduce resistance to being stretched. Stretching exercises gradually result in greater flexibility. They involve stretching a muscle or muscle group to a point of slight discomfort and holding that position for 30 seconds or more. When a muscle is stretched, a part of the muscle records the change in length and sends a signal to the spine. This triggers the stretch reflex, which

flexibility The measure of the range of motion, or the amount of movement possible, at a particular joint attempts to resist the change in muscle length by causing the stretched muscle to contract. One reason for holding a stretch for a prolonged period is that the muscle becomes accustomed to the new length and reduces signaling. Gradually, you can train your muscles to allow greater lengthening. For many people, a regular program of stretching exercises enhances psychological and physical well-being.

Types of Stretching

Static stretching techniques involve the slow, gradual stretching of muscles and their tendons, then holding them at a point. During this holding period—the stretch—participants may feel mild discomfort and a warm sensation in the stretched muscles. Static stretching exercises involve specialized tension receptors in our muscles. When done properly, these exercises slightly lessen the sensitivity of tension receptors, which allows the muscle to relax and be stretched to greater length.[40] The stretch is followed by a slow return to the starting position.

Three major styles of stretching exercise have become widely practiced in the United States and other Western countries: yoga, tai chi, and Pilates. All three emphasize a joining of mind and body as a result of intense concentration on breathing and body position. As mentioned earlier in the section on strength training, these styles of exercise are also an excellent way to improve core body strength.

Yoga

One of the most popular fitness and static stretching activities, **yoga** originated in India about 5,000 years ago. Yoga blends the mental and physical aspects of exercise, a union of mind and body that participants find relaxing and satisfying. Done regularly, its combination of mental focus and physical effort improves flexibility, vitality, posture, agility, and coordination.

Yoga focuses attention on controlled breathing and purely physical exercise. In addition to its mental dimensions, yoga incorporates a complex array of static stretching exercises expressed as postures (*asanas*). Over 200 postures exist, but only about 50 are commonly practiced. During a session, participants move to different asanas and hold them for 30 seconds or more. Yoga enhances flexibility and has the great advantage of being flexible itself—asanas and combinations of asanas can be changed and adjusted for young and old and to accommodate people with physical limitations or disabilities. Asanas can also be combined to provide even conditioned athletes with challenging sessions.

A typical yoga session will move the spine and joints through their full range of motion. Yoga postures lengthen, strengthen, and balance musculature, leading to increased flexibility, stamina, and strength—and many people report a psychological sense of general well-being, too. Some popular styles of yoga include Hatha, Iyengar, Ashtanga, and Bikram.

Tai chi

Tai chi is an ancient Chinese form of exercise that, like yoga, combines stretching, balance, coordination, and meditation. It is designed to increase range of motion and flexibility while reducing muscular tension. Based on Chi Kung, a Taoist philosophy dedicated to spiritual growth and good health, tai chi was developed about AD 1000 by monks who wanted to defend themselves against bandits and warlords. It involves a series of positions called *forms* that are performed continuously. Both yoga and tai chi are excellent for improving flexibility and muscular coordination.

Pilates

Compared with yoga and tai chi, **Pilates** is the new kid on the exercise block. It was developed by Joseph Pilates, who came from Germany to New York City in 1926. Shortly after his arrival, he introduced his exercise methodology, which emphasizes flexibility, coordination, core strength, and muscle tone. Pilates combines stretching with movement against resistance, which is frequently aided by devices such as tension springs or heavy rubber bands.

static stretching Techniques that gradually lengthen a muscle to an elongated position (to the point of discomfort) and holding that position for 10 to 30 seconds

yoga A variety of Indian traditions geared toward self-discipline and the realization of unity; includes forms of exercise that promote balance, coordination, flexibility, and meditation through postures and breathing exercises

tai chi An ancient Chinese form of exercise, originally developed as a martial art, that promotes balance, coordination, flexibility, and stress reduction through a series of flowing postures and movements

Pilates Exercise program developed by Joseph Pilates that combines stretching with movement against resistance

HEALTH HEADLINES

Performance-Enhancing Drugs: The Magic Bullet?

It seems as if every year, newspaper headlines declare that certain elite athletes are being reprimanded for using performance-enhancing drugs. But it is not just professional athletes who turn to performance enhancing drugs to "step up their game." For some athletes, both amateur and professional alike, gaining the competitive edge by taking performance-enhancing drugs seems like just another training strategy. What these athletes don't realize is that these drugs affect more than performance. Becoming faster or stronger may be a short-term benefit but there are side effects and health risks to taking these drugs. Legal risks also stem from the fact that many of these drugs are illegal without medical prescriptions. Listed below are some of the major types of drugs used for performance enhancement.

ANABOLIC STEROIDS

Athletes take anabolic steroids to increase their muscle mass and strength. The presence of the hormone testosterone—the main anabolic steroid—in the body has two main effects: anabolic effects that promote muscle building, and androgenic effects that promote male traits such as facial hair and a deep voice. Synthetic versions of this hormone do have some medicinal purposes in treating AIDS and rare types of anemia, but athletes often use doses much higher than are medically prescribed. Men who use this steroid can develop prominent breasts, baldness, shrunken testicles, a higher voice, and infertility. Side effects for women include a deeper voice, increased body hair, baldness, and increased appetite. Both sexes can suffer from severe acne, liver abnormalities and tumors, high LDL cholesterol and low HDL cholesterol, aggressive behavior, and drug dependence.

ANDROSTENEDIONE

Androstenedione is a hormone produced by the adrenal glands, ovaries, and testes and converted by the body into testosterone in men and estradiol in women. The synthetic version is marketed to increase the body's production of testosterone, thus enhancing training levels of athletes. The claims have been refuted by scientific studies, and androstenedione is now listed as a controlled substance whose use is banned by most sports associations. Side effects from this drug are similar to those of anabolic steroids.

CREATINE

Creatine monohydrate is a compound produced by the body that helps release energy in muscles. It is marketed as a nutritional supplement and readily available at many retail stores. Some research shows that creatine can produce small gains in short-term bursts of power. Research does not support any benefits to aerobic or endurance activities. Some side effects of creatine include stomach cramps, muscle cramps, nausea, vomiting, diarrhea, and risk of dehydration. High doses may increase risk of damage to the kidneys, liver, and heart.

STIMULANTS

Stimulants are drugs that affect the central nervous system by increasing heart rate, blood pressure, and metabolism. These drugs can reduce fatigue, suppress appetite, and increase alertness. The illegal drugs cocaine and methamphetamine are both stimulants, as are some drugs sold in pharmacies, such as pseudoephedrine which is found in many cold and allergy remedies. Caffeine, the active ingredient in coffee, tea, and many soft drinks, is also a stimulant. Athletes have been known to use caffeine to decrease fatigue and increase aggressiveness. Side effects of such use of caffeine and over-the-counter stimulants include nervousness and irritability, insomnia, and psychological dependence.

DIURETICS

Diuretics are drugs that change the balance of fluids in the body, temporarily decreasing body weight. Athletes often use diuretics when they want to compete in a lighter weight class. High doses of this drug may result in electrolyte imbalance leading to muscle cramps, exhaustion, potassium deficiency, and heart problems.

Sources: Mayo Clinic Staff, "Taking Performance-Enhancing Drugs: Are You Risking Your Health?," Mayo Clinic, December 26, 2006, http://mayoclinic.com/health/performance-drugs-enhancing/hq01105; A. A. Walter et al., "Effects of Creatine Loading on Electromyographic Fatigue Threshold in Cycle Ergometry in College-Age Men," *International Journal of Sport Nutrition and Exercise Metabolism* 18, no. 2 (2008): 142–51.

Pilates differs from yoga and tai chi, because it includes a component designed to increase strength. The method consists of a sequence of carefully performed movements. Some are carried out on specially designed equipment, while others can be performed on mats. Each exercise stretches and strengthens the muscles involved and has a specific breathing pattern associated with it.

Stretching Methods Not Recommended

There are several ways to stretch that are no longer recommended due to the high risk of improper positioning and potential for injury. *Ballistic stretching* involves stretching the limb into an extended position with repeated bouncing movements. Because your muscles do not get a chance to recover and prepare for the stretch, injuries such as ruptured tendons or torn ligaments may occur, especially in novice exercisers. *Dynamic stretching* uses more controlled momentum to stretch a muscle than ballistic stretching. It usually combines a static stretch with movement. While this type of stretch is often used in sports training and therapy sessions, it is not recommended for use without a trainer due to the difficulty in knowing the correct body positioning and the speed at which the movement should occur.

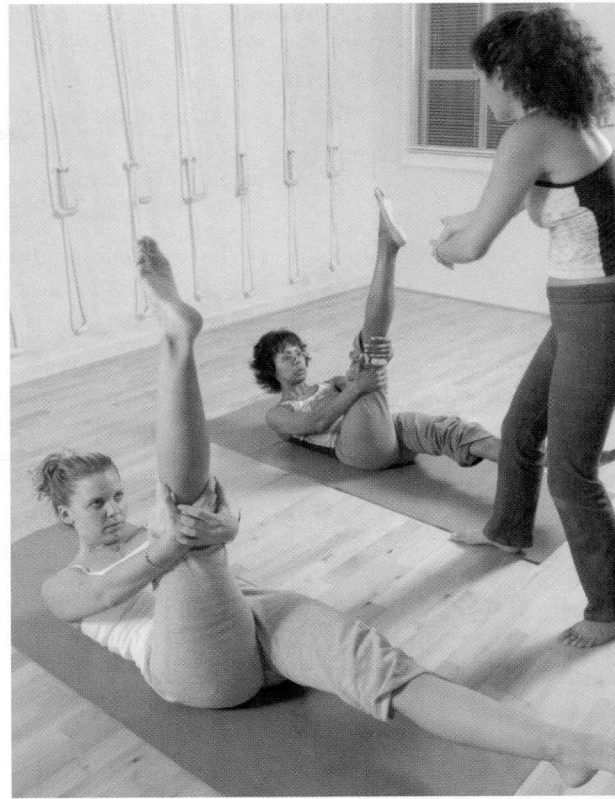

Pilates and other styles of exercise that strengthen core body muscles can also enhance flexibility and help lower stress levels.

Body Composition

Body composition is the fifth and final component of a comprehensive fitness program. It describes the relative proportions of lean tissue (muscle, bone, water, organs) and fat tissue in the body. Body composition parameters that can be influenced by regular physical activity include total body mass, fat mass, fat-free mass, and regional fat distribution. Aerobic activities that improve cardiovascular endurance also help improve body composition, because they expend calories and contribute to and help maintain weight loss. There are many ways to assess body composition. These range from simple (e.g., height–weight charts) to complex (e.g., underwater weighing).

Creating Your Own Fitness Program

Now that you know the benefits of improved physical fitness and the components that make up a physical fitness program, you can begin devising your own plan to become more physically fit.

Overcoming Common Obstacles to Exercise

The first step in forming a fitness program is identifying any hurdles that may keep you from getting started. There are many reasons why people do not exercise, ranging from personal ("I don't have time") to environmental ("I don't have a safe place to exercise"). You also may be reluctant to start exercising if you are overweight or out of shape.

What keeps you from being more active? Is it time? Do you lack a support group? Is the gym inconvenient, or do you lack money for a membership or equipment? Perhaps you're ready to begin but just can't get started. Once you've evaluated why you don't move more, look at Table 12.2 to determine how you can overcome your hurdles.

How can I motivate myself to exercise more? **?**

body composition The relative proportions of lean tissue (muscle, bone, water, organs) and fat tissue in the body

TABLE 12.2 Overcoming Obstacles to Physical Activity

Obstacles	Possible Solutions
Lack of time	• Take a good look at your schedule. Can you find three 30-minute time slots in your week? • Multitask. Read while riding an exercise bike or listen to lecture tapes while walking. • Exercise during your lunch breaks or between classes. • Select activities that require minimal time, such as brisk walking or jogging.
Social influence	• Invite family and friends to exercise with you. • Join a class to meet new people who share your exercise interests. • Explain the importance of exercise to people who may not support your efforts.
Lack of motivation, willpower, or energy	• Write your planned workout time in your schedule book. • Enlist the help of an exercise partner to make you accountable for working out. • Give yourself an incentive. • Schedule your workouts when you feel most energetic. • Remind yourself that exercise can give you more energy.
Lack of resources	• Select an activity that requires minimal equipment, such as walking, jogging, jumping rope, or calisthenics. • Identify inexpensive resources on campus or in the community.

Source: National Center for Chronic Disease Prevention and Health Promotion, "How Can I Overcome Barriers to Physical Activity?" 2003, www.cdc.gov/nccdphp/dnpa/physical/life/overcome.htm.

Identifying Your Fitness Goals

The next step in creating your fitness program is identifying your fitness goals. Do you want to improve your quality of life? Lose weight? Train for an upcoming 5K race? Think about a timeline for your goals. Do you want to be able to jog 3 miles before spring break? Hike across campus next semester with a heavy backpack and not be out of breath? Once you develop a specific goal, you can create a plan to help you achieve that goal.

Perhaps your most vital goal will be to become committed to fitness for the long haul—to establish a realistic schedule of diverse exercise activities that you can maintain and enjoy throughout your life.

Designing Your Program

DIDyouKNOW?

Fifty percent of people who start an exercise program drop out within the first six months.

There are several factors to consider that will boost your chances of successfully achieving your fitness goal. First, choose an activity that is appropriate for you. For example, don't plan on swimming if the pool is difficult to access. Choose activities that you like to do. If you hate to run, don't choose running as your exercise. Be creative in your activity choice; try something new! There are many different classes (e.g., salsa aerobics, boot camp classes) that can keep you motivated. If you don't like one activity, you can always try another.

Your plan should include very specific ways to incorporate physical activity into your lifestyle. When will you exercise? For how long? At what intensity? How often? As you make specific goals, keep in mind the FITT principle and the recommendations in FIGURE 12.2 on page 490.

You may also find that writing out these goals and putting them in your daily planner, as you would any other activity, will help you keep to your schedule. Lack of time is the number one reason given for not exercising. By looking at your weekly schedule, you can identify segments of time that work for you.

SKILLS FOR BEHAVIOR CHANGE

Establishing and Maintaining an Exercise Routine

The most successful exercise program is one that is realistic and appropriate for your skill level and needs.

√ *Start slow. For the sedentary, first-time exerciser, any type and amount of physical activity will be a step in the right direction. If you are extremely overweight or are out of condition, you might be able to walk for only 5 minutes at a time. Don't be discouraged; you're on your way!*

√ *Make only one life change at a time. Success with one major behavioral change will encourage you to make other positive changes.*

√ *Set reasonable expectations for yourself and your fitness program. Many people become exercise dropouts because their expectations were too high to begin with.*

√ *Choose a specific time to exercise and stick with it. Learning to establish priorities and keeping to a schedule are vital steps toward improved fitness. Try exercising at different times of the day to learn what schedule works best for you.*

√ *Keep a record of your progress. Include various facts about your physical activities (duration, intensity) and chronicle your emotions and personal achievements as you progress.*

√ *Take lapses in stride. Physical deconditioning—a decline in fitness level—occurs at about the same rate as physical conditioning. Renew your commitment to fitness, and restart your exercise program.*

Reevaluate your fitness goal and action plan after 30 days. This time period should give you a good idea of whether the program is working for you. Make changes if necessary, and then make a plan to reevaluate after another 30-day period. See the Skills for Behavior Change box for more tips on starting and maintaining an exercise plan.

Fitness Program Components

Good fitness programs are designed to improve or maintain cardiorespiratory fitness, flexibility, muscular strength and endurance, and body composition. A comprehensive program could include a warm-up period of easy walking, followed by stretching activities to improve flexibility, then selected strength-development exercises, followed by an aerobic activity for 20 minutes or more, and concluding with a cool-down period of gentle flexibility exercises.

Warming Up and Stretching

Warming up and stretching prepares your body for exercise and provides a transition from rest to physical activity. A 5 minute warm-up may consist of a 5-minute brisk walk to ease your cardiovascular system into more vigorous activity and to increase blood flow to the exercising muscles. This 5-minute warm-up can increase the temperature and elasticity of muscles and connective tissue, making stretching more effective. Add 5 to 10 minutes of stretching to your fitness routine and you'll be ready to go! FIGURE 12.5 shows a selection of exercises that will stretch the major muscle groups and can be used as a warm-up for other physical activities and exercise programs.

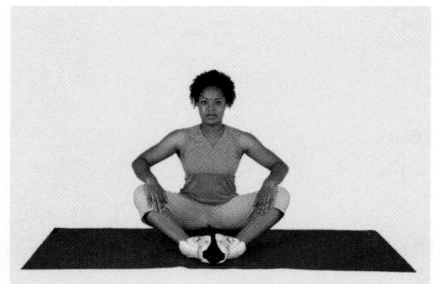
(a) Stretching the inside of the thighs

(b) Stretching the upper arm and the side of the trunk

(c) Stretching the triceps

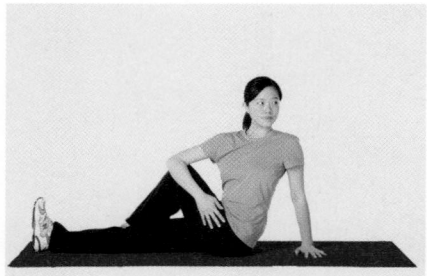
(d) Stretching the trunk and the hip

(e) Stretching the hip, back of the thigh, and the calf

(f) Stretching the front of the thigh and the hip flexor

FIGURE 12.5 Stretching exercises to improve flexibility.
Use these stretches as part of your warm-up and cool-down. Hold each one for 10 to 30 seconds, and repeat four times on each side. After only a few weeks of regular stretching, you'll begin to have more flexibility.

Resistance Training

When beginning a resistance exercise program, always consider your age, fitness level, and personal goals. Strength-training exercises are done in a set, or a single series of multiple repetitions using the same resistance. For both men and women under the age of 50, the ACSM recommends working major muscle groups with at least one set of eight to ten different exercises 2 to 3 days per week.[41] Weight loads should be at a level to allow up to 8 to 12 repetitions. Beginners should use lighter weights and complete 10 to 15 repetitions. Remember, experts suggest allowing at least 1 day of rest and recovery between workouts of any specific muscle group. Additional ACMS guidelines for creating a **resistance-training program** include the following:

- Exercises in the program should be of sufficient intensity to enhance strength and muscular endurance and to maintain fat-free mass.

- The program should be progressive and individualized, and provide a stimulus (overload) to all major muscle groups in the body.

- The exercise sequence should include large- before-small-muscle-group exercise, multiple-joint exercise before single-joint exercises, and higher-intensity before lower-intensity exercises.

- Performing eight to ten exercises that train the major muscle groups 2 to 3 days per week is recommended.

- The amount of weight used and number of repetitions vary by the individual's target goal, physical capacity, and training status.

Cardiorespiratory Training

You should spend the greatest proportion of exercise time developing cardiorespiratory fitness. Choose an aerobic activity you will like. Many people find cross training—alternate-day participation in two or more aerobic activities (such as jogging and

resistance-training program
A regular program of exercises designed to improve muscular strength and endurance in the major muscle groups

swimming)—more enjoyable than long-term participation in only one activity. Cross training is also beneficial, because it strengthens a variety of muscles, thus helping you avoid overuse injuries to muscles and joints.

Jogging, walking, cycling, rowing, step aerobics, and cross-country skiing are all excellent activities for developing cardiorespiratory fitness. Most colleges have recreation centers where students can use stair-climbing machines, stationary bicycles, treadmills, rowing machines, and ski-simulators.

Cooling Down and Stretching

Just as you ease into a workout with a warm-up, you should slowly transition from activity to rest. Devote at least 5 minutes of your workout to a gradual slowdown, decreasing the intensity of your activity. Be sure to stretch the major muscle groups to help reduce the amount of soreness from exercise.

Choosing Exercise Equipment and Facilities

If you have a treadmill that you use as a clothes rack or belong to a gym you haven't visited in months, you are not alone. Many people buy great equipment and don't get motivated to use it, but others buy services and equipment that don't have a ghost's chance of being useful. As with so many other products, consumers need to carefully evaluate advertising claims for fitness products. See the Green Guide on page 506 for ideas on how to be green when selecting fitness products.

SKILLS FOR BEHAVIOR CHANGE

Evaluating Fitness Products

Fitness products are a multimillion-dollar industry, but some may make fantastic claims that sound too good to be true. To get the most out of your investment, choose wisely and follow these guidelines from the Federal Trade Commission:

√ Ignore claims that an exercise machine or device can provide lasting, "no sweat" results in a short time.

√ Question claims that can "target" or burn fat off a particular part of the body.

√ Read the fine print. Advertised results may be based on more than just using a machine; they may also be based on caloric restriction.

√ Be skeptical of testimonials and before-and-after pictures of "satisfied" customers.

√ Calculate the cost and find out details about any shipping and handling fees, sales tax, delivery and set-up charges, or long-term commitments.

√ Get details on warranties, guarantees, and return policies.

√ Check out the company's customer support and service sections. Call the number to see how helpful the person on the other end really is.

√ Ask around. Get tips from friends or store personnel.

√ Try before you buy. You may be able to try out items at a gym or borrow one from someone before you invest in it.

√ Do your research. Check out consumer reports or online resources for the best product ratings and reviews.

Fitness Centers

There are a lot of benefits to joining a fitness or health club. Many fitness centers offer personal training, state-of-the-art equipment, and a variety of group exercise programs. Most campuses include recreational facilities, so start your search for a workout center there. Visit the facilities, find out when they are open, and consider whether they are convenient for you and offer classes and equipment that interest you.

If you want to join a private health club, shop around at several facilities before making a decision. You should carefully consider the convenience of the clubs and how using them will fit into your schedule. Visit the clubs during the hours you'd be most likely to use it so you can see how crowded it is. Tour the club and observe classes. A good club should offer a complete workout; they should have a variety of aerobic exercising machines (such as treadmills, stationary bikes, and elliptical machines) and a complete set of strength-training machines, free weights, mats for stretching, and aerobics classes. The club should also have plenty of well-trained and qualified staff. Take note of the staff during your visit to see if they seem friendly and helpful. Ask about the training of the personnel—including training in first aid and CPR—and inquire about the options for working with a personal trainer.

Finally, before you decide on a club, carefully weigh the financial implications. Find out what membership benefits are and whether there are student rates or other discounts available to you. Steer clear of clubs that pressure you to make a long-term commitment or don't offer a trial membership or a grace period during which you can get a refund.

Popular and Practical Exercise Equipment

There are many useful exercise products that can take your exercise program to the next level—they can provide variety, allowing you to work out at home, or encourage you to monitor your progress. Remember, however, that no equipment is ever a quick fix—in order to see changes in your fitness and health, you must do the work yourself. See the Skills for Behavior Change box for general tips on evaluating fitness equipment.

Heart Rate Monitors

Fitness enthusiasts use heart rate monitors to become aware of their heart rate and training intensity and to push performance higher. These monitors usually have a strap with a sensor that is placed around the chest and a watchlike readout on the wrist. Monitors cost between $50 and $200 and can provide instant feedback about the intensity of your workouts. Heart rate monitors provide a more technical way to measure heart rate than the fingers-to-the-wrist method.

Stability Balls

Stabilizing yourself on a ball strengthens core muscles. If you sit on the ball and do arm or shoulder exercises, you work your abdominals as well as your arms and shoulders. High-quality balls are made of burst-resistant vinyl and are independently tested to withstand as much as 600 pounds while still retaining their shape and usefulness.

Choose a ball that is suited to both your weight and height. To determine if the ball is right for you, sit on it. Your feet should be flat on the floor, your weight distributed evenly, and your knees should be at a 90-degree or slightly greater angle. Be sure to inflate the ball to the right height and use it properly, both for safety reasons and to ensure maximum workout results. Read the package carefully to be certain that if the ball is punctured, it will not drop you to the ground (high-quality balls are designed to deflate slowly if punctured, to minimize the risk of injury). Prices range from $25 to $50.

Pedometers

Pedometers offer features such as monitoring calories burned, counting number of steps, and keeping track of distance and speed. They are usually small and easy to use, and they can help you figure out how far you've gone on your daily walk/run or

NUTRITION AND EXERCISE **505**

measure how many steps you take on an average day. They can be an excellent motivator. Before you buy a pedometer, make sure it's simple to use and has an easy-to-read display. The unit should be accurate in its count when you wear it correctly—you may have to experiment with where to wear it. Distance accuracy depends on setting your stride length correctly. Some pedometers even come with a computer program to upload your step and distance records. Prices range from $20 to $100.

Balance Boards

When doing strengthening moves on a balance board, your core muscles contract, thus working your abs and other muscle groups. Athletes who regularly train with balance boards improve agility and reaction skills and ankle strength. This greatly decreases the risk of ankle injury during play, while improving coordination and overall athletic ability. For less-athletic types, working out on the balance board can reduce your chances of tripping and falling in everyday life. The cost is $40 to $80.

Resistance Bands

These bands are usually rubber or elastic material with handles that can be used to work the muscles without weights. The bands can provide various ways to improve muscular endurance and strength, flexibility, and range of motion. They are lightweight, portable, and can add variety to gym workouts. They are also compact and easy to pack when traveling. You can buy bands in varying degrees of resistance, depending on your fitness level or exercise goal, for $5 to $15.

Nutrition and Exercise

Getting the right "fuel" for your workouts is important for good health and effective exercise.[42] To make the most of your workouts, make sure you eat enough carbohydrates, which are the body's chief source of fuel. Your body stores carbohydrates as glycogen primarily in the muscles and liver. Your muscles use stored glycogen when needed for energy. Protein plays a role in muscle repair and growth. Most people can get enough protein from meat, dairy products, and nuts and don't need additional supplements. Fats are also important, as they are an additional fuel source for muscles.

When you eat is almost as important as what you eat. Eating a large meal before exercising can slow you down. Upset stomach, cramping, and diarrhea can result from your muscles having to compete with your digestive system for energy. Leave at least 3 to 4 hours between eating a large meal and exercising. On the other hand, not eating at all before a workout can also have negative repercussions. Low blood sugar levels that result from not eating can cause weakness and slow reaction time. A light snack may be beneficial before your workout. After your workout, help your muscles recover by eating a meal that contains both protein and carbohydrates.

In addition to eating well, staying hydrated is also crucial for active individuals to maintain a healthy, fully functional body. How much fluid do you need to stay well hydrated? The ACSM, along with the National Athletic Trainers Association, recommend consuming 14 to 22 ounces of fluid 2 hours prior to exercise. Drinking fluids during exercise is also important. For intense exercise, you should drink about 6 to 12 ounces per 15 to 20 minutes.[43]

What are the best fluids to drink? For exercise sessions lasting less than 1 hour, plain water is sufficient for rehydration. If your exercise session exceeds 1 hour, consider a sports drink containing electrolytes. Athletes such as marathon runners use these drinks to maintain their electrolyte balance.[44] The electrolytes in these products are minerals and ions such as sodium and potassium that are needed for proper functioning of your nervous and muscular systems. For athletes in endurance events lasting over 4 hours, the overconsumption of plain water can dilute the sodium concentration in the blood with potentially fatal results, an effect called **hyponatremia.**

Is it better to eat before or after exercising?

hyponatremia The overconsumption of plain water, which leads to a dilution of sodium concentration in the blood and can have fatal results

GREEN GUIDE

GUIDE   GREEN   GRE
GUIDE

Exercise and planned physical

activity are important in reducing and preventing risks for debilitating conditions such as obesity, heart disease, osteoporosis, and diabetes. However, there has been concern that the booming fitness industry is no friend of the environment. Be part of the solution by going green at the gym and in your workouts:

- Fitness facilities are getting on the ecofriendly bandwagon. Call around and ask questions about facilities' environmental commitments and ecofriendly strategies. Some questions to ask are: Is the building green? What is the LEED score? Do they use eco-responsible light fixtures and light bulbs? What is the recycling plan? Do they launder towels and other fabrics with ecofriendly detergents and water-conserving washers?

- Get outside! By exercising outdoors and avoiding electrically driven exercise equipment like treadmills and elliptical machines, you are reducing your carbon footprint and reducing health risks. Consider taking public transportation to a hiking trail, ride a bicycle to get groceries, ride a paddleboat on a lake (don't forget the life vest), or walk the dog to get your morning coffee (just remember to bring your own mug!).

- If joining a gym or going outdoors is not an option, consider using exercise equipment at home that is powered by you. Purchase preowned dumbbells, barbells, tubing, jump ropes, self-powered exercise machines, and other self-powered exercise equipment. For preowned equipment, consider contacting a local preowned fitness equipment retailer or explore

resources online such as www.playitagainsports.com or www.usedgymequipment.com. You will be reducing waste caused by discarded exercise equipment and minimizing your carbon footprint, and you will be preventing disease and illness in the future!

- When purchasing exercise clothing, investigate organic cottons, hemp, and other environmentally responsible fabrics. Purchase goods manufactured by companies that avoid toxic dye and process industrial wastes responsibly.

- Recycle! When you wear out your clothing or shoes, give it a second life by finding an organization that will recycle it. A brief search on the Internet reveals a wide variety of organizations and equipment suppliers that recycle shoes for needy runners and for athletic surfaces. For example, Patagonia recycles exercise clothing and turns it into new athletic wear, and Nike has an athletic shoe recycling program that uses your old shoes to create basketball courts, running tracks, and safe playgrounds.

- Use a PVC-free yoga mat or a yoga mat made from natural products. Production of PVC (polyvinyl chloride), commonly found in many plastics, releases cancer-causing dioxins into the environment. Also avoid yoga mats with phlalates used to increase the pliability of the mat, as these chemicals are thought to disrupt hormones and harm one's health. Carry your mat in a hemp or organic cotton bag to further minimize your impact on the environment.

Fitness-Related Injuries

Enthusiastic but out-of-shape beginners often injure themselves by doing too much too soon. Experienced athletes develop *overtraining syndrome* by engaging in systematic and progressive increases in training without getting enough rest and recovery time. Eventually, performance begins to decline and training sessions become increasingly difficult. Adequate rest, good nutrition, and rehydration are important to sustain or improve fitness levels.

There are two basic types of injuries stemming from fitness-related activities: overuse and traumatic injuries. **Overuse injuries** are due to cumulative, day-after-day stresses placed on tendons, bones, and ligaments during exercise. These injuries occur most often in repetitive activities such as swimming, running, bicycling, and step aerobics. The forces that occur normally during physical activity are not enough to cause a ligament sprain or muscle strain, but when these forces are applied daily for weeks or months, they can result in an injury. Common sites of overuse injuries are the leg, knee, shoulder, and elbow joints.

overuse injuries Injuries that result from the cumulative effects of day-after-day stresses placed on tendons, muscles, and joints

Traumatic injuries occur suddenly and violently, typically by accident. Typical traumatic injuries are broken bones, torn ligaments and muscles, contusions, and lacerations. Some traumatic injuries occur quickly and are difficult to avoid—for example, spraining your ankle by landing on another person's foot after jumping up for a rebound in basketball. If your traumatic injury causes a noticeable loss of function and immediate pain or pain that does not go away after 30 minutes, consult a physician.

Preventing Injuries

There are steps you can take to reduce your risk of over-use or traumatic injuries. Beyond the common sense mentioned earlier, identifying and using only the proper gear and equipment, and making sure they're always in fully functional condition, can help you avoid an injury.

Appropriate Footwear

Shoes are made to protect the foot from sport-specific movements. Proper footwear can decrease the likelihood of foot, knee, or back injuries.

When you purchase athletic shoes, the two most important factors to consider are (1) how well they fit and (2) the activity for which you'll need them. Feet come in all shapes and sizes. A good fit is essential for comfort and performance. To get the best fit, shop at a sports or fitness specialty store where there is a large selection and salespeople who are trained in properly fitting athletic shoes. Try on shoes later in the day when your feet are largest, and check to make sure there is a little extra room in the toe and that the width is appropriate. Because different activities place different stresses on your feet and joints, you should choose shoes specifically designed for your sport or activity. Shoes of any type should be replaced once they lose their cushioning. Continuing to use a shoe that is worn out will increase your risk of injury.

For individuals looking for quality running shoes, the shoes' ability to absorb shock is critical. Biomechanics research has revealed that running is a collision sport—with each stride, the runner's foot collides with the ground with a force three to five times the runner's body weight.[45] The force not absorbed by the running shoe is transmitted upward into the foot, leg, thigh, and back. Our bodies can absorb forces such as these but may be injured by the cumulative effect of repetitive impacts (such as running 40 miles per week). There are several other key components as well (see **FIGURE 12.6**).

Appropriate Protective Equipment

Some activities require special protective equipment to reduce chances of injury. Eye injuries can occur in virtually all fitness-related activities, although some are more risky than others. As many as 90 percent of the eye injuries resulting from racquetball and squash could be prevented by wearing appropriate eye protection—for example, goggles with polycarbonate lenses.[46]

Nearly 100 million people in the United States ride bikes for pleasure, fitness, or competition. Wearing a helmet while bicycle riding is an important safety precaution. An estimated 45 to 88 percent of head injuries among cyclists can be prevented by wearing a helmet. The direct medical costs from cyclists' failure to wear helmets is $8.1 million a year.[47] Cyclists aren't the only ones who should be wearing helmets. People who skateboard, use kick-scooters, or snowboard should also wear helmets. Look for helmets that meet the standards established by the American National Standards Institute and the Snell Memorial Foundation.

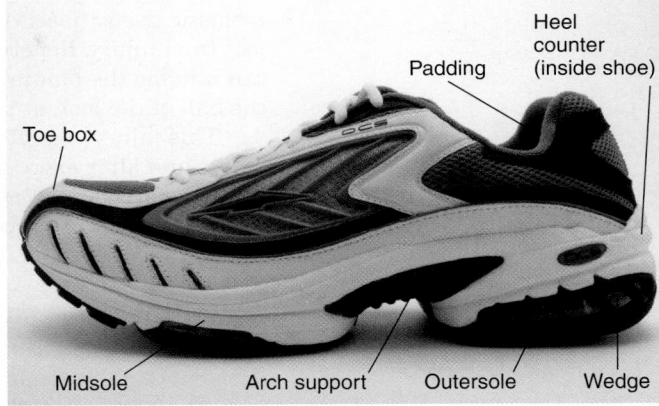

FIGURE 12.6 Anatomy of a running shoe. The midsole of your shoe is one of the most important factors in comfort. To evaluate the midsole's flexibility, hold the shoe lengthwise between the index fingers of your right and left hand. When you push on both ends of the shoe, it should bend easily at the midsole. If the force exerted by your index fingers cannot bend the shoe, its midsole is probably too rigid and will be painful.

How do I choose a good running shoe?

traumatic injuries Injuries that are accidental and occur suddenly and violently (such as fractured bones, ruptured tendons, and sprained ligaments)

Common Overuse Injuries

Three of the most common overuse injuries are plantar fasciitis, shin splints, and runner's knee.

Plantar Fasciitis

Plantar fasciitis is an inflammation of the plantar fascia, a broad band of dense, inelastic tissue (fascia) that protects the nerves, blood vessels, and muscles of the foot from injury. Repetitive weight-bearing movements such as walking and running can inflame the plantar fascia. Common symptoms are pain and tenderness under the ball of the foot, at the heel, or at both locations.[48]

This injury can often be prevented by regularly stretching the plantar fascia before and after exercise and by wearing athletic shoes with good arch support and shock absorbency. Stretch the plantar fascia by slowly pulling all five toes upward, holding for 10 to 15 seconds, and repeating this three to five times on each foot.

Shin Splints

A general term for any pain that occurs below the knee and above the ankle is *shin splints*. This broad description includes more than 20 different medical conditions. Problems can be due to muscles, bones, or attachments from muscle to bone. Typically, there is pain and swelling along the middle of the shin in the soft tissues, not the bone.

Sedentary people who start a new weight-bearing exercise program are at the greatest risk for shin splints, though even well-conditioned aerobic exercisers who rapidly increase their distance or pace may also develop them.[49] Running is the most frequent cause of shin splints, but those who do a great deal of walking (such as mail carriers and restaurant workers) may also develop this injury.

To help prevent shin splints, wear athletic shoes with good arch support and shock absorbency. Also, gradually increase training intensity and vary your routine. If the pain continues, see your physician. You may need to substitute a nonweight-bearing activity such as swimming during your recovery period.

Runner's Knee

Runner's knee describes a series of problems involving the muscles, tendons, and ligaments around the knee. The main symptom of this kind of injury is the pain experienced when downward pressure is applied to the kneecap after the knee is straightened fully. Symptoms include pain, swelling, redness, and tenderness around the kneecap.[50] If you have these symptoms, your physician will probably recommend that you stop running for a few weeks and reduce activities that compress the kneecap (for example, exercise on a stair-climbing machine or doing squats with heavy resistance) until you no longer feel any pain.

Treatment of Fitness-Related Injuries

RICE Acronym for rest, ice, compression, and elevation; the standard first-aid treatment for traumatic and overuse injuries

First-aid treatment for virtually all personal fitness injuries involves **RICE: r**est, **i**ce, **c**ompression, and **e**levation. *Rest,* the first component of this treatment, is required to avoid further irritation of the injured body part. *Ice* is applied to relieve pain and constrict the blood vessels to stop any internal or external bleeding. Never apply ice cubes, reusable gel ice packs, chemical cold packs, or other forms of cold directly to your skin. Instead, place a layer of wet toweling or elastic bandage between the ice and your skin. Ice should be applied to a new injury for approximately 20 minutes every hour for the first 24 to 72 hours. *Compression* of the injured body part can be accomplished with a 4- or 6-inch-wide elastic bandage; this applies indirect pressure to damaged blood vessels to help stop bleeding. Be careful, though, that the compression wrap does not interfere with normal blood flow. Throbbing or pain in the hand or foot indicates that the compression wrap should be loosened. *Elevation* of an injured extremity above the level of your heart also helps to control internal or external bleeding by making the blood flow upward to reach the injured area.

Exercising in the Heat

Heat stress, which includes several potentially fatal illnesses resulting from excessive core body temperature, should be a concern whenever you are exercising in warm, humid weather. In these conditions, your body's rate of heat production can exceed its ability to cool itself.

You can help prevent heat stress by following certain precautions. First, proper acclimatization to hot and/or humid climates is essential. The process of heat acclimatization, which increases your body's cooling efficiency, requires about 10 to 14 days of gradually increasing activity in the hot environment. Second, avoid dehydration by replacing the fluids you lose during and after exercise. Third, wear clothing appropriate for your activity and the environment. And finally, use common sense—for example, on a day when the temperature is 85°F and the humidity is 80 percent, postpone your usual lunchtime run until the cool of evening.

The three different heat stress illnesses—heat cramps, heat exhaustion, and heatstroke—are progressive in severity. **Heat cramps** (heat-related muscle cramps), the least serious problem, can usually be prevented by warm-ups, adequate fluid replacement, and a diet that includes the electrolytes lost during sweating (sodium and potassium). **Heat exhaustion** is caused by excessive water loss resulting from prolonged exercise or work. Symptoms of heat exhaustion include nausea, headache, fatigue, dizziness and faintness, and, paradoxically, goose bumps and chills. If you are suffering from heat exhaustion, your skin will be cool and moist, because the body's cooling system has faltered and circulation has slowed. **Heatstroke,** often called *sunstroke,* is responsible for at least 240 deaths in the United States each year. The condition triggers a series of metabolic events that may result in irreversible injury or death.[51] Heat stroke occurs during vigorous exercise when the body's heat production significantly exceeds its cooling capacities. Body core temperature can rise from normal (98.6°F) to 105°F to 110°F within minutes after the body's cooling mechanism shuts down. Rapidly increasing core temperature can cause brain damage, permanent disability, and death. Common signs of heatstroke are dry, hot, and usually red skin; very high body temperature; and rapid heart rate.

If you experience any of the symptoms mentioned here, stop exercising immediately, move to the shade or a cool spot to rest, and drink large amounts of cool fluids. Be aware that heat stress can also result from prolonged sauna, hot tub, or steam bath exposure, or performing activity in lots of heavy clothing and equipment, such as a football uniform.[52]

Exercising in the Cold

When you exercise in cool weather, especially in windy conditions, your body's rate of heat loss is frequently greater than its rate of heat production. These conditions may lead to **hypothermia**—a potentially fatal condition resulting from abnormally low body core temperature, which occurs when body heat is lost faster than it is produced. Temperatures need not be frigid for hypothermia to occur; it can also result from prolonged, vigorous exercise in 40°F to 50°F temperatures, particularly if there is rain, snow, or a strong wind.

In mild cases of hypothermia, as body core temperature drops from the normal 98.6°F to about 93.2°F, you will begin to shiver. Shivering—the involuntary contraction of nearly every muscle in the body—increases body temperature by using the heat given off by muscle activity. You may also experience cold hands and feet, poor judgment, apathy, and amnesia. Shivering ceases in most hypothermia victims as body core temperatures drop to between 87°F and 90°F, a sign that the body has lost its ability to generate heat. Death usually occurs at body core temperatures between 75°F and 80°F.[53]

To prevent hypothermia, analyze weather conditions and your risk of hypothermia before you undertake an outdoor physical activity. Remember that wind and humidity are as significant as temperature. Have a friend join you for cold weather outdoor activities and wear layers of appropriate clothing to prevent excessive heat loss (polypropylene or woolen undergarments, a windproof outer garment, and a wool

---

heat cramps Muscle cramps that occur during or following exercise in warm or hot weather

heat exhaustion A heat stress illness caused by significant dehydration resulting from exercise in warm or hot conditions

heatstroke A deadly heat stress illness resulting from dehydration and overexertion in warm or hot conditions

hypothermia Potentially fatal condition caused by abnormally low body core temperature

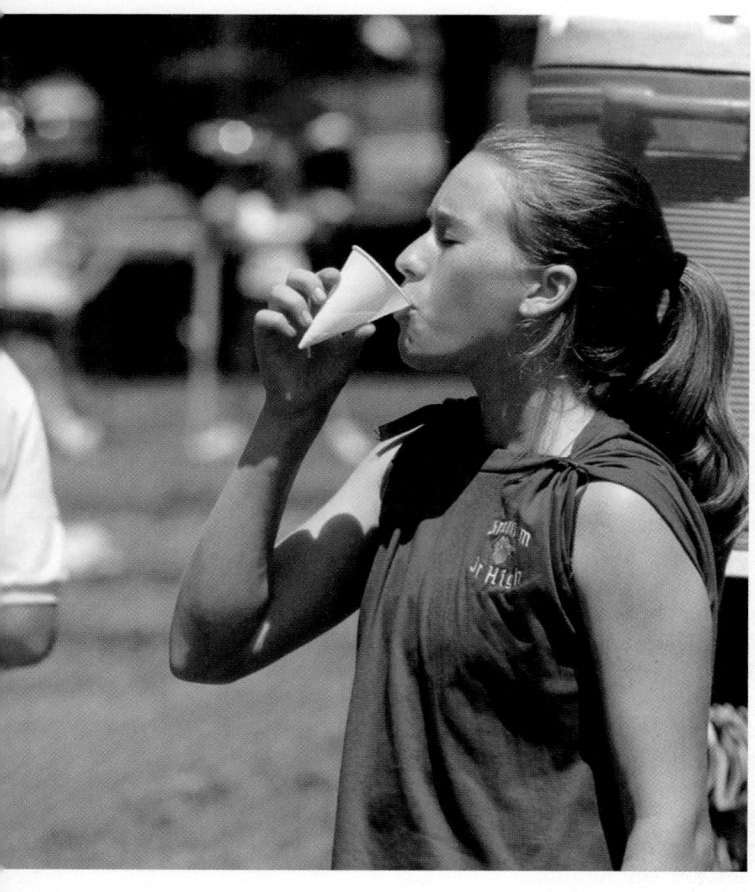

Staying hydrated is especially important when exercising in hot or cold weather, whether to avoid heat exhaustion, heatstroke, or hypothermia.

hat and gloves). Keep your head, hands, and feet warm. Don't allow yourself to become dehydrated. Thirst is suppressed in cold environments, so drink plenty of fluids even if you're not thirsty.[54]

Preventing Cramps

Although most of us have experienced the quick, intense pain of muscle cramps, they are poorly understood. A cramp is an involuntary and forcibly contracted muscle that does not relax. Cramps in legs, feet, arms, abdomen, and along the rib cage are common. A cramp can last a few seconds to 15 minutes or longer. There are several theories about cramping. According to the overexertion theory, when a muscle gets tired, the numerous muscle fibers that comprise it fail to contract in a synchronized rhythm, probably because of overstimulation from the nerves that trigger the muscles to contract.[55] Other theories relate cramping to dehydration. Dehydration may occur simply if someone doesn't consume sufficient liquids to compensate for loss in urine and sweat. Even if dehydration is not the only cause, it is clearly a problem for those who exercise and perspire heavily. Drinking enough fluids before, during, and after such activity is important.

If you get cramps, massaging, stretching, putting pressure on the muscle that is cramping, and deep breathing are generally useful remedies.

ASSESS YOURSELF

Fill out this assessment online at
www.pearsonhighered.com/myhealthlab
or www.pearsonhighered.com/donatelle.

How Physically Fit Are You?

PART ONE: Evaluating Your Muscular Endurance (the 1-minute Sit-Up Test)

Abdominal muscle strength and endurance are important for core stability and back support. This sit-up test measures the strength and endurance of your abdominals and hip flexor muscles.

Description/Procedure

Lie on a carpeted or cushioned floor with your knees bent at approximately right angles and your feet flat on the ground. Rest your hands on your thighs. Squeeze your stomach, push your back flat, and raise yourself high enough for your hands to slide along your thighs to touch the tops of your knees. Don't pull with your neck or head, and keep your lower back on the floor. Then return to the starting position. Have a partner time you and count how many sit-ups you can do in 1 minute.

Fitness Category	Men Age 18–25	Age 26–35	Age 36–45	Age 46–55	Age 56–65	Age 65+	Women Age 18–25	Age 26–35	Age 36–45	Age 46–55	Age 56–65	Age 65+
Excellent	>49	>45	>41	>35	>31	>28	>43	>39	>33	>27	>24	>23
Good	44–49	40–45	35–41	29–35	25–31	22–28	37–43	33–39	27–33	22–27	18–24	17–23
Above average	39–43	35–39	30–34	25–28	21–24	19–21	33–36	29–32	23–26	18–21	13–17	14–16
Average	35–38	31–34	27–29	22–24	17–20	15–18	29–32	25–28	19–22	14–17	10–12	11–13
Below average	31–34	29–30	23–26	18–21	13–16	11–14	25–28	21–24	15–18	10–13	7–9	5–10
Poor	25–30	22–28	17–22	13–17	9–12	7–10	18–24	13–20	7–14	5–9	3–6	2–4
Very poor	<25	<22	<17	<9	<9	<7	<18	<20	<7	<5	<3	<2

Source: Golding et al., *The Y's Way to Physical Fitness,* 1991.

PART TWO: Evaluating Your Flexibility (the Sit-and-Reach Test)

This test measures the flexibility of the lower back and hamstring muscles.

Description/Procedure

Sit on the floor with your legs straight out in front of you, toes pointed up. Place a yardstick between your feet on the floor so that the 23 centimeter mark is at your heels. Hold your knees flat against the floor. With hands on top of each other and palms facing down, reach forward along the measure of the yardstick, as far as possible. Take three practice stretches. On the fourth stretch, hold for 2 seconds, and record the distance you reach. Make sure that you make no jerky movements and that your finger-tips remain level and your legs flat. Record the score to the nearest centimeter as the distance before (negative) or beyond (positive) the toes. Because your toes are the 23 centimeter mark, you need to subtract 23 from your measurement to calculate your score. The table below gives you a guide for expected scores (in centimeters).

Flexibility Level	Men	Women
Super	>27	>30
Excellent	+17 to +27	+21 to +30
Good	+6 to +16	+11 to +20
Average	0 to +5	+1 to +10
Fair	−8 to −1	−7 to 0
Poor	−19 to −9	−14 to −8
Very poor	< −20	< −15

Continued

PART THREE: Evaluating Your Cardiorespiratory Endurance

This test assesses your cardiorespiratory endurance level.

Description/Procedure

Find a local track, typically one-quarter mile per lap, to perform your test. You may either run or walk for 1.5 miles; use a stopwatch to measure how long it takes to reach that distance. If you become extremely fatigued during the test, slow your pace or walk—do not overstress yourself! If you feel faint or nauseated or experience any unusual pains in your upper body, stop and notify your instructor. Use the chart below to estimate your cardiorespiratory fitness level based on your age and sex. Note that women have lower standards for each fitness category, because they have higher levels of essential fat than men do.

Fitness Category	Men Age 18–29	Age 30–39	Age 40–49	Age 50+	Women Age 18–29	Age 30–39	Age 40–49	Age 50+
Good	<11:27	<12:06	<12:32	<13:50	<13.24	<14.03	<14:29	<15:21
Adequate	11:28–12:58	12:07–13:37	12:33–14:03	13:25–15:21	13:25–14:55	14:04–15:21	14:30–15:47	15:22–16:39
Borderline	12:59–13:25	13:38–14:04	14:04–14:30	14:56–15:48	14:56–15:22	15.22–15:48	15:48–16:14	16:40–17:06
Poor	>13:25	>14:04	>14:30	>15:22	>15:22	>15:48	>16:14	>17:06

Source: From E. T. Howley and B. D. Franks, *Health Fitness Instructor's Handbook.* 4th ed., p. 75, Table 5.2. Copyright © 2003 by Edward T. Howley and B. Don Franks. Reprinted with permission from Human Kinetics (Champaign, IL).

Make It Happen!

The Assess Yourself activity helped you determine your current fitness levels. Your results may indicate that you should take steps to improve one or more components of your physical fitness.

Today, you can:

- Go for a brisk walk after dinner, or take your dog on an extra long evening walk.

- Visit your campus fitness facility and familiarize yourself with the equipment and resources. Find out what classes they offer, and take home a copy of the schedule so you can fit in a class or two when possible.

- Take a stretch break. Spend 5 minutes in between homework projects or just before bed doing some whole-body stretches to release tension.

Within the next 2 weeks, you can:

- Shop for comfortable workout clothes or running shoes.

- Investigate team sport leagues in your area. Is there an intramural basketball, volleyball, or ultimate Frisbee program on your campus? Think about which activities you might enjoy, and try them out.

- Ask a friend to join you in your workout once a week. Agree upon a date and time in advance so you'll both be committed to following through.

By the end of the semester, you can:

- Establish a regular routine of exercising at least three times a week. Mark your exercise times on your calendar and keep a log to track your progress. After you've been exercising regularly for a month or so, try taking the fitness assessments again.

- Take your workouts to the next level. If you have been working out at home, try making a regular habit of going to a gym or participating in an exercise class. If you are walking, perhaps try intermittent jogging or sign up for a fitness event like a charity 5K.

- Get involved with a regularly scheduled group activity, such as a dance class, a hiking club, a martial arts school, or an intramural soccer team. Combining social activity with physical activity will help keep you motivated and will enrich your life with new friends and skills.

TAKING CHARGE

CHAPTER SUMMARY

- The physiological benefits of regular physical activity include reduced risk of heart attack, some cancers, hypertension, and diabetes; and improved blood profile, skeletal mass, weight control, immunity to disease, mental health and stress management, and physical fitness. Regular physical activity can also increase life span.

- For general health benefits, every adult should participate in moderate-intensity activities for 30 minutes at least 5 days a week. For improvements in cardiorespiratory fitness, you should work out aerobically for at least 20 minutes, a minimum of 3 days per week. Exercise intensity involves working out a target heart rate. The longer the exercise period, the more calories burned and the greater the improvement in cardiorespiratory fitness.

- Three key principles for developing muscular strength and endurance are overload, specificity of training, and variation. The different types of muscle actions include isometric, concentric, and eccentric. Resistance-training programs include body weight resistance (calisthenics), fixed resistance, variable resistance, and accommodating-resistance devices.

- Flexibility exercises should involve static stretching performed in sets of two to four repetitions held for 15 to 30 seconds, at least 2 to 3 days a week. Popular forms of stretching exercise include yoga, tai chi, and Pilates.

- Planning a fitness program involves setting goals and designing a program to achieve these goals. A comprehensive program would include a warm-up period, stretching activities, strength-development exercises, an aerobic activity, and a cool-down period.

- Fitness injuries are generally caused by overuse or trauma; the most common are plantar fasciitis, shin splints, and runner's knee. Proper footwear and equipment can help prevent injuries. Exercise in the heat or cold requires special precautions.

REVIEW QUESTIONS

1. The maximum volume of oxygen consumed by the muscles during exercise defines
   a. target heart rate.
   b. muscular strength.
   c. aerobic capacity.
   d. muscular endurance.

2. What is physical fitness?
   a. The ability to respond to routine physical demands
   b. Having enough reserves after working out to cope with a sudden challenge
   c. Both aerobic and muscular strength
   d. All of the above

3. Which type of cancer may be prevented by being physically active?
   a. Skin
   b. Lung
   c. Colon
   d. Liver

4. Flexibility is the range of motion around
   a. specific bones.
   b. specific joints.
   c. the hips and pelvis.
   d. the muscles.

5. The "talk test" measures
   a. exercise intensity.
   b. exercise duration.
   c. exercise frequency.
   d. metabolism.

6. An example of aerobic exercise is
   a. brisk walking.
   b. bench pressing weights.
   c. stretching exercises.
   d. yoga breathing.

7. Theresa wants to lower her ratio of fat weight to her total body weight. She wants to work on her
   a. flexibility.
   b. muscular endurance.
   c. muscular strength.
   d. body composition.

8. Miguel is a cross-country runner and is therefore able to sustain moderate-intensity, whole-body activity for extended periods of time. This ability relates to what component of physical fitness?
   a. Flexibility
   b. Body composition
   c. Cardiorespiratory fitness
   d. Muscular strength and endurance

9. Janice has been lifting 95 pounds while doing three sets of ten leg curls. To become stronger, she began lifting 105 pounds while doing leg curls. What principle of strength development does this represent?
   a. Reversibility
   b. Overload
   c. Flexibility
   d. Specificity of training

10. Joel enjoys various types of fitness exercises. He alternates his training days with jogging, cycling, and step aerobics. This type of training is called
    a. cardiac fitness training.
    b. static training.
    c. cross training.
    d. multisport training.

QUESTIONS FOR DISCUSSION AND REFLECTION

1. How do you define *physical fitness*? What are the key components of a physical fitness program? What might you need to consider when beginning a fitness program?

2. How would you determine the proper intensity and duration of an exercise program? How often should exercise sessions be scheduled?

3. Why is stretching vital to improving physical flexibility? Why is flexibility important in everyday activities?

4. Identify at least four physiological and psychological benefits of physical fitness. How would you promote these benefits to nonexercisers?

5. Describe the different types of resistance employed in an exercise program. What are the benefits of each type?

6. Your roommate has decided to start running first thing in the morning in an effort to lose weight, tone muscles, and improve cardiorespiratory fitness. What advice would you give to make sure your roommate gets off to a good start and doesn't get injured?

7. What key components would you include in a fitness program for yourself?

ACCESSING YOUR HEALTH ON THE INTERNET

The following websites explore further topics and issues related to personal health. You'll also find links to each organization's website on the Companion Website for *Access to Health,* Green Edition, at www.pearsonhighered.com/donatelle.

1. *ACSM Online.* A link with the American College of Sports Medicine and all its resources. www.acsm.org

2. *American Council on Exercise.* Information on exercise and disease prevention. www.acefitness.org

3. *Centers for Disease Control and Prevention, National Center for Chronic Disease Prevention and Health Promotion, Division of Nutrition and Physical Activity.* A resource for current information on exercise and health. www.cdc.gov/nccdphp/dnpa

4. *National Strength and Conditioning Association.* A resource for personal trainers and others interested in conditioning and fitness. www.nsca-lift.org

5. *The President's Council on Physical Fitness and Sports.* Provides information on fitness programs. www.fitness.gov

FURTHER READING

S. K. Powers and S. L. Dodd, *Total Fitness and Wellness.* 5th ed. (San Francisco: Benjamin Cummings, 2009).

A complete guide to improving all areas of fitness, including being a smart health consumer, specific exercises for improving fitness and the links between nutrition and fitness.

S. Schlosberg, *The Ultimate Workout Log: An Exercise Diary for Everyone.* 3d ed. (Boston: Houghton Mifflin, 2005).

A 6-month log that also provides fitness definitions, training tips, and motivational quotes.

T. D. Fahey, *Super Fitness for Sports, Conditioning, and Health* (Boston: Allyn & Bacon, 2000).

A brief guide to developing fitness that emphasizes training techniques for improving sports performance.

REFERENCES

1. American College Health Association, *American College Health Association—National College Health Assessment (ACHA-NCHA) Reference Group Data Report Fall 2007* (Baltimore: American College Health Association, 2008).

2. Ibid.; National Center for Chronic Disease Prevention and Health Promotion, "Physical Activity for Everyone," Centers for Disease Control and Prevention, updated March 2008, www.cdc.gov/nccdphp/dnpa/physical/everyone/health/index.htm.

3. American Diabetes Association, "Total Prevalence of Diabetes and Pre-diabetes," American Diabetes Association, www.diabetes.org/diabetes-statistics/prevalence.jsp; American Heart Association, *Heart Disease and Stroke Statistics—2008 Update* (Dallas: American Heart Association, 2008).

4. U.S. Department of Health and Human Services, *Physical Activity and Health: A Report of the Surgeon General* (Atlanta: Centers for Disease Control, National Center for Chronic Disease Prevention and Health Promotion, 1996).

5. W. L. Haskell et al., "Physical Activity and Public Health: Updated Recommendation for Adults from the American College of Sports Medicine and the American Heart Association," *Medicine and Science in Sports and Exercise* 39, no. 8 (2007): 1423–34; U.S. Department of Health and Human Services, *2008 Physical Activity Guidelines for Americans* (Washington, DC: U.S. Department of Health and Human Services, 2008) ODPHP Publication no. U0036.

6. W. L. Haskell et al., "Physical Activity and Public Health," 2007.

7. National Center for Chronic Disease Prevention and Health Promotion, "Physical Activity for Everyone;" W. L. Haskell et al., "Physical Activity and Public Health," 2007.

8. V. H. Heyward, *Advanced Fitness Assessment and Prescription.* 5th ed. (Champaign, IL: Human Kinetics, 2006).

9. X. Sui, M. J. Lamonte, and S. N. Blair, "Cardiorespiratory Fitness and Risk of Nonfatal Cardiovascular Disease in Women and Men with Hypertension," *American Journal of Hypertension* 20, no. 6 (2007): 608–15.

10. A. Colin et al., "Cardiorespiratory Fitness, Physical Activity, and Arterial Stiffness: The Northern Ireland Young Hearts Project," *Hypertension* 44 (2004): 721–26.

11. G. A. Kelley and K. S. Kelley, "Efficacy of Aerobic Exercise on Coronary Heart Disease Risk Factors," *Preventive Cardiology* 11, no. 2 (2008): 71–75.

12. American Heart Association, "The Number of Adults in the U.S. with High Blood Pressure Rose in the Last Decade," 2004, www.americanheart.org/presenter.jhtml?identifier=3024254; W. Wang et al., "A Longitudinal Study of Hypertension Risk Factors and Their Relation to Cardiovascular Disease," *Hypertension* 47 (2006): 403; American College of Sports Medicine, *ACSM's Certification Review.* 2nd ed. (Lippincott Williams & Wilkins, 2006).

13. American Stroke Association, "American Heart Association: Cholesterol," 2006, www.strokeassociation.org.

14. G. A. Colditz et al., "Physical Activity and Risk of Breast Cancer in Premenopausal Women," *British Journal of Cancer* 89, no. 5 (2003): 847–51; A. K. Samad et al., "A Meta-Analysis of the Association of Physical Activity with Risk of Colorectal Cancer," *Colorectal Disease* 7, no. 3 (2005): 204–13; L. Bernstein et al., "Lifetime Recreational Exercise Activity and Breast Cancer Risk Among Black and White Women," *Journal of the National Cancer Institute* 77, no. 22 (2005): 1671–79.

15. T. J. Key et al., "Diet, Nutrition, and the Prevention of Cancer," *Public Health Nutrition,* no. 1A (February 7, 2004): 187–200.

16. Harvard Medical School, "Supplements vs. Exercise for Heart Disease and Cancer: The 'Vitamins' in Your Legs," *Harvard Men's Health Watch* 12, no. 4 (2007): 1–4.

17. K. J. Stewart et al., "Exercise Effects on Bone Mineral Density Relationships to Changes in Fitness and Fatness," *American Journal of Preventive Medicine* 28, no. 5 (2005): 453–60; W. McArdle, F. Katch, and V. Katch, *Exercise Physiology.* 6th ed. (Philadelphia: Lippincott Williams and Wilkins, 2006), 60–65.

18. Division of Nutrition, Physical Activity and Obesity, "About BMI for Adults," National Center for Chronic Disease Prevention and Health Promotion, updated May 2007, www.cdc.gov/nccdphp/dnpa/bmi/adult_BMI/about_adult_BMI.htm.

19. University of Colorado Health Sciences Center, "National Weight Control Registry," www.uchsc.edu/nutrition/WyattJortberg/nwcr.htm.

20. W. L. Haskell et al., "Physical Activity and Public Health," 2007.

21. S. Lee et al., "Exercise without Weight Loss Is an Effective Strategy for Obesity Reduction in Obese Individuals With or Without Type 2 Diabetes," *Journal of Applied Physiology* 99, no. 3 (2005): 1220–25.

22. American Diabetes Association, "Diabetes Risk Test," 2004, www.diabetes.org/risk-test.jsp.

23. National Diabetes Information Clearinghouse, "Diabetes Prevention Program," NIH Publication no. 06-5099, August 2006.

24. J. O. Hill et al., "Physical Activity and Managing Obesity and Type 2 Diabetes," *Nestle Nutrition Workshop Series: Clinical & Performance Program* 11 (2006): 183–91.

25. T. Kizaki et al., "Adaptations of Macrophages to Exercise Training Improves Innate Immunity," *Biochemical and Biophysical Research Communications* 372, no. 1 (2008): 152–56.

26. E. Tiollier et al., "Intense Training: Mucosal Immunity and Incidence of Respiratory Infections," *European Journal of Applied Physiology* 93, no. 4 (2006): 421–28.

27. B. F. Burke, "Exercise and Immunity," *MedLine Plus,* National Institutes of Health, updated May 2008, www.nlm.nih.gov/medlineplus/ency/article/007165.htm.

28. L. M. Hays, T. M. Damush, and D. O. Clark, "Relationships Between Exercise Self-Definitions and Exercise Participation among Urban Women in Primary Care," *Journal of Cardiovascular Nursing* 20, no. 1 (2005): 9–17.

29. U.S. Department of Health and Human Services, *Physical Activity and Health: A Report of the Surgeon General,* 1996; O. H. Franco et al., "Effects of Physical Activity on Life Expectancy with Cardiovascular Disease," *Archives of Internal Medicine* 165, no. 20 (2005): 2355–60.

30. W. L. Haskell et al., "Physical Activity and Public Health," 2007.

31. Centers for Disease Control and Prevention, "Calories/Hour Expended in Common Physical Activities," 2006, www.cdc.gov/nccdphp/dnpa/spotlights/calories_per_hour_table.htm.

32. American College Health Association, *American College Health Association—National College Health Assessment,* 2008.

33. W. J. Kraemer et al., "Progression Models in Resistance Training for Healthy Adults, American College of Sports Medicine Position Stand," *Medicine and Science in Sports and Exercise* 34, no. 2 (2002): 364–80.

34. Ibid.

35. Ibid.

36. American Council on Exercise, *Personal Trainer Manual: Resource for Fitness Professionals.* 3rd ed. (Indianapolis: American College of Sports Medicine, 2003).

37. Mayo Clinic Staff, "Core Exercises: Beyond Your Average Abs Routine," Mayo Clinic, October 5, 2007, www.mayoclinic.com/health/core-exercises/SM00071.

38. P. A. Adler and B. L. Roberts, "The Use of Tai Chi to Improve Health in Older Adults," *Orthopedic Nursing* 25, no. 2 (2006): 122–26.

39. Arthritis Foundation, "Exercise and Arthritis," 2007, www.arthritis.org/conditions/exercise.

40. J. W. Smith, "Flexibility Basics: Physiology, Research, and Current Guidelines," *ACSM Certified News* 14, no. 3 (2004): 7–9.

41. American College of Sports Medicine, *ACSM Certification Review, 2006* (Philadelphia: Lippincott Williams and Wilkins, 2005).

42. Mayo Clinic Staff, "Eating and Exercise: Time It Right to Maximize Your Workout," Mayo Clinic, December 26, 2006, www.mayoclinic.com/health/exercise/HQ00594_D.

43. Dieticians in Sports and Exercise Nutrition, "Fluid and Hydration in Sport," 2004, www.disen.org/nutrition/pages-to-edit/fluids.htm.

44. S. M. Shirreffs et al., "Fluid and Electrolyte Needs for Preparation and Recovery from Training and Competition," *Journal of Sports Science* 22, no. 1 (2004): 57–63.

45. U. G. Kersting and G. P. Bruggemann, "Midsole Material-Related Force Control During Heel-Toe Running," *Research in Sports Medicine* 14, no. 1 (2006): 1–17.

46. American Academy of Ophthalmology, "Play Sports Safely—Use Eye Protection," American Academy of Ophthalmology, 2003.

47. Bicycle Helmet Safety Institute, "Helmet-Related Statistics," revised 2007, www.helmets.org/stats.htm.

48. D. Ritchie, "Plantar Fasciitis: Treatment Pearls," American Academy of Podiatric Sports Medicine, Accessed June 2008, www.aapsm.org/plantar_fasciitis.html.

49. J. Story and T. C. Cymet, "Shin Splints: Painful to Have and to Treat," *Comprehensive Therapy* 32, no. 3 (2006): 192–95.

50. American Academy of Orthopaedic Surgeons, "Runner's Knee," reviewed August 2007, http://orthoinfo.aaos.org/topic.cfm?topic=A00382&return_link=0.

51. J. L. Glazer, "Management of Heat Stroke and Heat Exhaustion," *American Family Physician* 71, no. 11 (2005): 2141.

52. International Fitness Association, *Aerobics and Fitness Institute Certification Coursebook* (Orlando: International Fitness Association, 2004).

53. R. Curtis, *Outdoor Action Guide to Hypothermia and Cold Weather Injuries* (Atlanta: Centers for Disease Control and Prevention, 2006).

54. American Council on Exercise, *Exercising in the Cold, 2006* (Indianapolis: American Council on Exercise, 2006).

55. N. Clark, "Muscle Cramps: Do They Cramp Your Style?" *Newsletter of the American College of Sports Medicine,* no. 7 (Summer 2001).

56. Borg-RPE-scale ® from G. Borg, (1998), Borg's Perceived Exertion and Pain Scales. Champaign, IL: Human Kinetics. © Gunnar Borg, 1970, 1985, 1994, 1998. Used with permission of Dr. G. Borg. For correct usage of the scale the exact design and instructions given in Borg's folders must be followed: The BORG-RPE SCALE ®, a method for measuring perceived exertion. © G. Borg, 1994, 2003. Order folders and scales from: Borg Products, Inc., "BPU," Joseph V. Myers III, 1579F, Monroe Drive, #416, Atlanta, GA 30324.

CHAPTER 13

CHAPTER OBJECTIVES

After reading this chapter you will be able to:

1. Explain the differences between physical activity and exercise, p. 520.

2. List at least four health benefits of being physically active on a regular basis, pp. 520–521.

3. Define the four components of fitness, pp. 520–521.

4. Describe the FIT principle and calculate your maximal and training heart rate range, pp. 524–527.

5. List and describe at least three processes we use to break down fuels to support physical activity, pp. 529–535.

6. Discuss at least three changes in nutrient needs that can occur in response to an increase in physical activity or vigorous exercise training, pp. 535–547.

7. Define the heat illnesses, including heat syncope, heat cramps, heat exhaustion, and heatstroke, pp. 544–545.

8. Define the term *ergogenic aids* and discuss the potential benefits and risks of at least four ergogenic aids that are currently on the market, pp. 548–552.

TEST YOURSELF TRUE OR FALSE

1. *Physical activity* and *exercise* mean basically the same thing and are terms that can be used interchangeably. **T or F**

2. Despite the multitude of health benefits of participating in regular physical activity, more than half of all Americans are insufficiently active. **T or F**

3. To achieve fitness, a person needs to exercise at least 1 hour each day. **T or F**

4. Eating extra protein helps us to build muscle. **T or F**

5. Most ergogenic aids are not effective, and many can be dangerous or cause serious health consequences. **T or F**

Test Yourself answers can be found after the Chapter Summary.

Nutrition and Physical Activity: Keys to Good Health

1

I n the summer of 2005, Frank Levine of Pennsylvania and Mary Haines of Connecticut each won two gold medals in their class in track and field at the National Senior Games. Levine clocked 5:24.90 in the 800-meter run and 11:27.54 in the 1500 meter. Haines won the 200-meter dash in 2:00.35 and the 1500 meter in 21:15.06. If their performance times don't amaze you, perhaps they will when you consider these athletes' ages: at the time they gave these winning performances, both were 91 years old!

There's no doubt about it: regular physical activity dramatically improves our strength, stamina, health, and quality of life. But what qualifies as "regular physical activity"? In other words, how much do we need to do to reap the benefits? And if we do become more active, does our diet have to change, too?

Healthy eating practices and regular physical activity are like two sides of the same coin, interacting in a variety of ways to improve our strength and stamina and to increase our resistance to many chronic diseases and acute illnesses. In fact, the nutrition and physical activity recommendations for reducing your risk of heart disease also reduce your risk of high blood pressure, type 2 diabetes, obesity, and some forms of cancer! In this chapter, we define physical activity, identify its many benefits, and discuss the nutrients needed to maintain an active life.

Taken from: *Nutrition: An Applied Approach,* Second Edition, by Janice Thompson and Melinda Manore

Why Engage in Physical Activity?

A lot of people are looking for a "magic pill" that will help them maintain weight loss, reduce their risk of diseases, make them feel better, and improve their quality of sleep. Although many people are not aware of it, regular physical activity is this magic pill. **Physical activity** describes any movement produced by muscles that increases energy expenditure. Different categories of physical activity include occupational, household, leisure-time, and transportation.[1] **Leisure-time physical activity** is any activity not related to a person's occupation and includes competitive sports, planned exercise training, and recreational activities such as hiking, walking, and bicycling. **Exercise** is therefore considered a subcategory of leisure-time physical activity and refers to activity that is purposeful, planned, and structured.[2]

One of the most important benefits of regular physical activity is that it increases our physical fitness. **Physical fitness** is a state of being that arises largely from the interaction between nutrition and physical activity. It is defined as the ability to carry out daily tasks with vigor and alertness, without undue fatigue, and with ample energy to enjoy leisure-time pursuits and meet unforeseen emergencies.[1] Physical fitness has many components (Table 13.1).[3] These include **cardiorespiratory fitness,** which is defined as the ability of the heart, lungs, and circulatory system to efficiently supply oxygen and nutrients to working muscles. **Musculoskeletal fitness** involves fitness of both the muscles and bones and includes muscular strength and muscular endurance. **Muscular strength** is the maximal force or tension level that can be produced by a muscle group, and **muscular endurance** is the ability of a muscle to maintain submaximal force levels for extended periods of time. **Flexibility** is the ability to move a joint fluidly through the complete range of motion, and **body composition** is the amount of bone, muscle, and fat tissue in the body. Although many people are interested in improving their physical fitness, some are more interested in maintaining general fitness, while others are interested in achieving higher levels of fitness to optimize their athletic performance.

Other benefits of regular physical activity include the following:

- *Reduces our risks for, and complications of, heart disease, stroke, and high blood pressure:* Regular physical activity increases high-density lipoprotein cholesterol (HDL, the "good" cholesterol) and lowers triglycerides in the blood, improves the strength of the heart, helps maintain healthy blood pressure, and limits the progression of atherosclerosis (or hardening of the arteries).

- *Reduces our risk for obesity:* Regular physical activity maintains lean body mass and promotes more healthful levels of body fat, may help in appetite control, and increases energy expenditure and the use of fat as an energy source.

physical activity Any movement produced by muscles that increases energy expenditure; includes occupational, household, leisure-time, and transportation activities.

leisure-time physical activity Any activity not related to a person's occupation; includes competitive sports, recreational activities, and planned exercise training.

exercise A subcategory of leisure-time physical activity; any activity that is purposeful, planned, and structured.

physical fitness The ability to carry out daily tasks with vigor and alertness, without undue fatigue, and with ample energy to enjoy leisure-time pursuits and meet unforeseen emergencies.

cardiorespiratory fitness Fitness of the heart and lungs; achieved through regular participation in aerobic-type activities.

musculoskeletal fitness Fitness of the muscles and bones.

muscular strength A subcomponent of musculoskeletal fitness defined as the maximal force or tension level that can be produced by a muscle group.

muscular endurance A subcomponent of musculoskeletal fitness defined as the ability of a muscle to maintain submaximal force levels for extended periods of time.

flexibility The ability to move a joint through its full range of motion.

body composition The amount of bone, muscle, and fat tissue in the body.

Hiking is a leisure-time physical activity that can contribute to your physical fitness.

TABLE 13.1 The Components of Fitness

Fitness Component	Examples of Activities One Can Do to Achieve Fitness in Each Component
Cardiorespiratory	Aerobic-type activities such as walking, running, swimming, cross-country skiing
Musculoskeletal fitness:	Resistance training, weight lifting, calisthenics, sit-ups, push-ups
Muscular strength	Weightlifting or related activities using heavier weights with few repetitions
Muscular endurance	Weight lifting or related activities using lighter weights with greater number of repetitions
Flexibility	Stretching exercises, yoga
Body composition	Aerobic exercise and resistance training

- *Reduces our risk for type 2 diabetes:* Regular physical activity enhances the action of insulin, which improves the cells' uptake of glucose from the blood, and can improve blood glucose control in people with diabetes, which in turn reduces the risk for, or delays the onset of, diabetes-related complications.

- *Potential reduction in our risk for colon cancer:* Although the exact role that physical activity may play in reducing colon cancer risk is still unknown, we do know that regular physical activity enhances gastric motility, which reduces transit time of potential cancer-causing agents through the gut.

- *Reduces our risk for osteoporosis:* Regular physical activity strengthens bones and enhances muscular strength and flexibility, thereby reducing the likelihood of falls and the incidence of fractures and other injuries when falls occur.

Regular physical activity is also known to improve our sleep patterns, reduce our risk for upper respiratory infections by improving immune function, and reduce anxiety and mental stress. It also can be effective in treating mild and moderate depression. In women receiving chemotherapy treatment for breast cancer, regular physical activity may reduce fatigue.[4] During pregnancy, regular physical activity helps maintain the mother's fitness and muscle tone and helps control weight gain. It is also associated with lower fetal distress during labor, shorter labor, lower risk of cesarean birth, and improved recovery for the mother after the birth.[5]

Despite the plethora of benefits derived from regular physical activity, most people find that this magic pill is not easy to swallow. In fact, most people in the United States are physically inactive. The Centers for Disease Control and Prevention report that over half of all U.S. adults do not do enough physical activity to meet national health recommendations, and almost 16% of adults in the United States admit to doing no leisure-time physical activity at all (FIGURE 13.1).[6] These statistics mirror the reported increases in obesity, heart disease, and type 2 diabetes in industrialized countries.

This trend toward inadequate physical activity levels is also occurring in young people. Only 17% of middle and junior high schools and only 2% of senior high schools require daily physical activity for all students.[7] Low rates of voluntary participation in physical education (PE) compound this problem, as less than 30% of high school students participate in daily PE. Since our habits related to eating and physical activity are formed early in life, it is imperative that we provide opportunities for children and adolescents to engage in regular, enjoyable physical activity. An active lifestyle during childhood increases the likelihood of a healthier life as an adult.

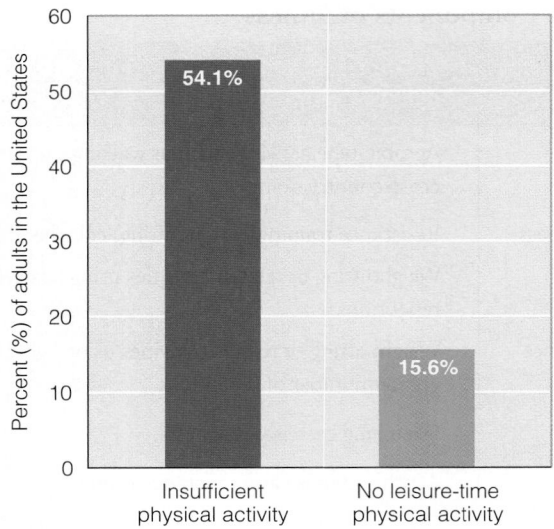

FIGURE 13.1 Rates of physical inactivity in the United States. Over 50% of the U.S. population do not do enough physical activity to meet national health recommendations, and almost 16% report doing no leisure-time physical activity. (From Centers for Disease Control and Prevention (CDC). 2005. Adult participation in recommended levels of physical activity—United States, 2001 and 2003. *Morbid. Mortal. Wkly. Rep.* 54(47):1208–1212.)

> RECAP: *Physical activity is any movement produced by muscles that increases energy expenditure. Physical fitness is the ability to carry out daily tasks with vigor and alertness, without undue fatigue, and with ample energy to enjoy leisure-time pursuits and meet unforeseen emergencies. Physical activity provides a multitude of health benefits, including reducing our risks for obesity and many chronic diseases and relieving anxiety and stress. Despite the many health benefits of physical activity, most people in the United States, including many children, are inactive.*

What Is a Sound Fitness Program?

There are several widely recognized qualities of a sound fitness program, as well as guidelines to help you design one that is right for you. These are explored here.

A Sound Fitness Program Meets Your Personal Goals

A fitness program may be ideal for someone else, but that doesn't necessarily mean it is right for you. Before you design or evaluate any program, you need to know what you intend to get from it; in other words, you need to define your personal fitness goals. Do you want to prevent osteoporosis, diabetes, or another chronic disease that runs in your family? Do you simply want to increase your energy and stamina? Or do you intend to compete in athletic events? Each of these scenarios would require a very different fitness program.

For example, if you want to train for athletic competition, a traditional approach that includes planned, purposive exercise sessions under the guidance of a trainer or coach would probably be most beneficial. Or, if you want to achieve cardiorespiratory fitness, you would likely be advised to participate in an aerobics class at least three times per week, or jog for at least 20 minutes three times per week.

In contrast, if your goal were to maintain your overall health, you might do better to follow the 1996 report of the Surgeon General on achieving health through regular physical activity.[1] This report emphasizes that significant health benefits, including reducing your risk for chronic diseases (such as heart disease, osteoporosis, and type 2 diabetes), can be achieved by participating in a moderate amount of physical activity (such as 30 minutes of gardening, 15 minutes of jogging, or 45 minutes of basketball) on most, if not all, days of the week. These health benefits occur even when the time spent performing the physical activities is cumulative (for example, brisk walking for 10 minutes three times per day). While these guidelines are appropriate for achieving health benefits, they are not necessarily of sufficient intensity and duration to improve physical fitness.

Recently, the Institute of Medicine published guidelines that state that the minimum amount of physical activity that should be done each day to maintain health and fitness is 60 minutes, not 30 minutes as published in the Surgeon General's report.[1,8] This discrepancy in fitness guidelines has caused some confusion among consumers. Refer to the Nutrition Debate at the end of this chapter to learn more about this controversy.

Moderate physical activity, such as gardening, helps maintain overall health.

A Sound Fitness Program Is Fun and Includes Variety and Consistency

One of the most important goals for everyone is fun; unless you enjoy being active, you will find it very difficult to maintain your physical fitness. What activities do you consider fun? If you enjoy the outdoors, hiking, camping, fishing, and rock climbing are potential activities for you. If you would rather exercise with friends on your lunch break, walking, climbing stairs, and bicycle riding may be more appropriate. Or you may find it more enjoyable to stay indoors and use the programs and equipment at your local fitness club . . . or purchase your own treadmill and free weights.

Variety is critical to maintaining your fitness. While some people enjoy doing similar activities day after day, most of us get bored with the same fitness routine. Incorporating a variety of activities into your fitness program will help maintain your interest and increase your enjoyment while you are active. Variety can be achieved by combining indoor and outdoor activities throughout the week, taking a different route when you walk each day, watching a movie or reading a book while you ride a stationary bicycle or walk on a treadmill, or participating in different activities each week such as walking, bicycling, swimming, taking the stairs, hiking, and gardening. This smorgasbord of activities can increase your activity level without leading to monotony and boredom.

Fortunately, a fun and useful tool has been developed to help you increase the variety of your physical activity choices (**FIGURE 13.2**). Similar in shape to the previous USDA Food Guide Pyramid, the **Physical Activity Pyramid** makes recommendations for the type and amount of activity that should be done weekly to increase your physical activity level. The bottom of the pyramid describes activities that should be done every day, including walking more, taking the stairs instead of the elevator, and working in your garden. Aerobic types of exercises (such as bicycling and brisk walking) and recreational activities (such as soccer, tennis, and basketball) should be done three to five times each week, for at least 20 or 30 minutes. Flexibility, strength, and leisure activities should be done two to three times each week. The top of the pyramid emphasizes things we should do less of, including watching TV, playing computer games, or sitting for more than 30 minutes at one time.

Watching television or reading can provide variety while running on a treadmill.

It is important to understand that you cannot do just one activity to achieve overall fitness. Refer back to Table 13.1, and notice that different activities are listed as examples to achieve the various components of fitness. There is simply not one activity that we can do to achieve overall fitness because physical fitness is specific to each component. For instance, participating in aerobic-type activities will improve our cardiorespiratory fitness but will do little to improve muscular strength. To

Physical Activity Pyramid A pyramid similar to the previous USDA Food Guide Pyramid that makes recommendations for the type and amount of activity that should be done weekly to increase physical activity levels.

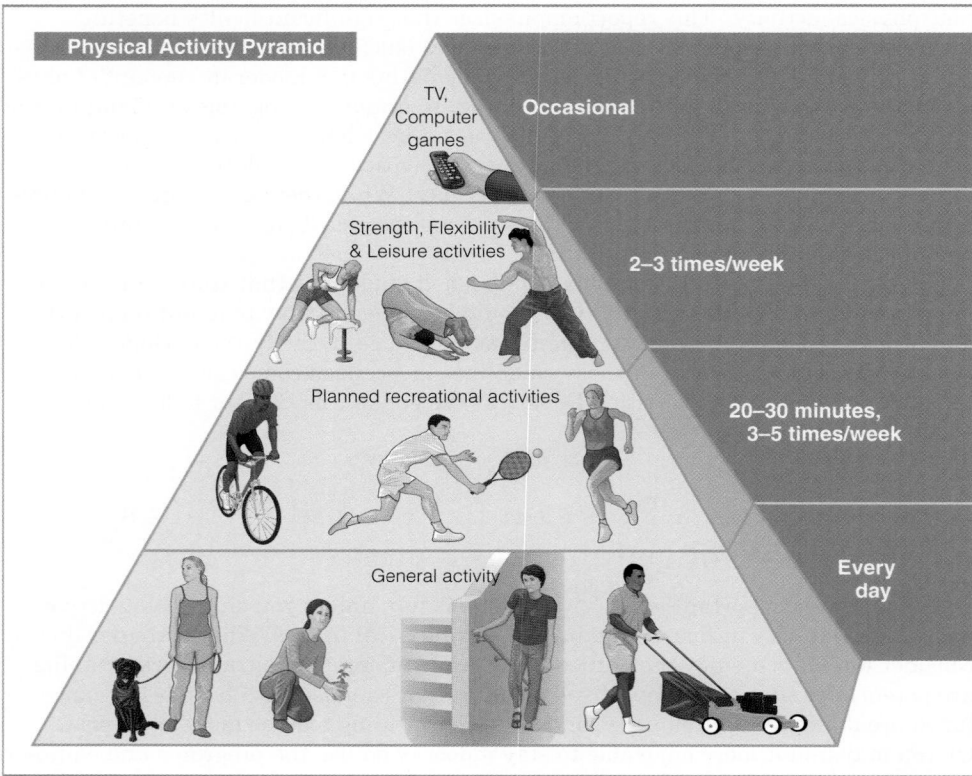

FIGURE 13.2 You can use this Physical Activity Pyramid as a guide to increase your level of physical activity. (From Corbin, C. B., and R. D. Pangrazi. 1998. Physical Activity Pyramid rebuffs peak experience. *ACSM's Health Fitness J.* 2(1). Copyright © 1998. Used with permission.)

achieve that goal, we must participate in some form of **resistance training,** or exercises in which our muscles work against resistance. Flexibility is achieved by participating in stretching activities. By following the recommendations put forth in the Physical Activity Pyramid, you can achieve physical fitness in all components.

A Sound Fitness Program Appropriately Overloads the Body

In order to improve your fitness level, you must place an extra physical demand on your body. This is referred to as the **overload principle.** A word of caution is in order here: *the overload principle does not advocate subjecting your body to inappropriately high stress* because this can lead to exhaustion and injuries. In contrast, an appropriate overload on various body systems will result in healthy improvements in fitness.

To achieve an appropriate overload, you should consider three factors, collectively known as the **FIT principle:** *f*requency, *i*ntensity, and *t*ime of activity. You can use the FIT principle to design either a general physical fitness program or a performance-based exercise program. FIGURE 13.3 shows how the FIT principle applies to a cardiorespiratory, musculoskeletal, and flexibility fitness program.

Let's consider each of the FIT principle's three factors in more detail.

Frequency

Frequency refers to the number of activity sessions per week. Depending upon your goals for fitness, the frequency of your activities will vary. To achieve cardiorespiratory fitness, you should train more than 2 days per week. On the other hand, training more than 5 days per week does not cause significant gains in fitness but can

resistance training Exercises in which our muscles act against resistance.

overload principle Placing an extra physical demand on your body in order to improve your fitness level.

FIT principle The principle used to achieve an appropriate overload for physical training. Stands for frequency, intensity, and time of activity.

frequency Refers to the number of activity sessions per week you perform.

	Frequency	Intensity	Time
Cardiorespiratory fitness	3–5 days per week	64–90% maximal heart rate	At least 20 consecutive minutes
Muscular fitness	2–3 days per week	70–85% maximal weight you can lift	1–3 sets of 8–12 lifts* for each set *A minimum of 8–10 exercises involving the major muscle groups such as arms, shoulders, chest, abdomen, back, hips, and legs is recommended.
Flexibility	2–4 days per week	Stretching through full range of motion	2–4 repetitions per stretch* *Hold each stretch for 15–30 seconds.

FIGURE 13.3 Using the FIT principle to achieve cardiorespiratory and musculoskeletal fitness and flexibility.

substantially increase your risk for injury. Training 3 to 5 days per week appears optimal to achieve and maintain cardiorespiratory fitness. In contrast, only 2 to 3 days are needed to achieve musculoskeletal fitness.

Think about Theo's goals for fitness during the off-season and the frequency needed to achieve these goals. He is interested in maintaining his general physical fitness so he can continue to play basketball, and he also wants to significantly improve muscular strength and size. Using the Physical Activity Pyramid as a guide, Theo should do the activities suggested for every day and those prescribed three to five times a week. To further improve muscular strength and size, Theo should weight lift at least 2 to 3 days each week. With this type of program, Theo will be able to reach his goals. Theo should also regularly participate in flexibility activities to enhance his quality of training and to prevent potential injuries.

Intensity

Intensity refers to the amount of effort expended or, to put it another way, how difficult the activity is to perform. In general, **low-intensity activities** are those that cause very mild increases in breathing, sweating, and heart rate, while **moderate-intensity activities** cause moderate increases in these responses. **Vigorous-intensity activities** produce significant increases in breathing, sweating, and heart rate so that talking is difficult when exercising at a vigorous intensity.

Traditionally, heart rate has been used to indicate level of intensity during aerobic activities. **FIGURE 13.4** shows an example of a heart rate training chart. You can calculate the range of exercise intensity that is appropriate for you by estimating your **maximal heart rate,** which is the rate at which your heart beats during maximal intensity exercise (see the You Do the Math box on page 527). Maximal heart rate is estimated by subtracting your age from 220 and is described in more

intensity Refers to the amount of effort expended during the activity, or how difficult the activity is to perform.

low-intensity activities Activities that cause very mild increases in breathing, sweating, and heart rate.

moderate-intensity activities Activities that cause moderate increases in breathing, sweating, and heart rate.

vigorous-intensity activities Activities that produce significant increases in breathing, sweating, and heart rate; talking is difficult when exercising at a vigorous intensity.

maximal heart rate The rate at which your heart beats during maximal-intensity exercise.

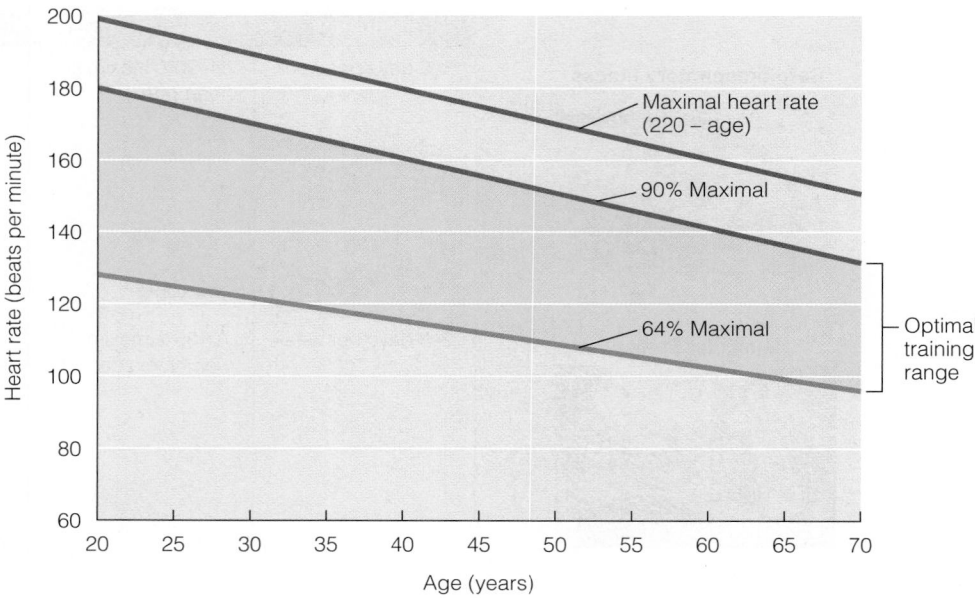

FIGURE 13.4 This heart rate training chart can be used to estimate your aerobic exercise intensity. The top line indicates the predicted maximal heart rate value for a person's age (220 – age). The shaded area represents the heart rate values that fall between 64% and 90% of maximal heart rate, which is the range generally recommended to achieve aerobic fitness.

Testing in a fitness lab is the most accurate way to determine maximal heart rate.

time of activity How long each exercise session lasts.

detail below. For achieving and maintaining physical fitness, the intensity range typically recommended is 64–90% of your estimated maximal heart rate. People who are older or who have been inactive for a long time may want to exercise at the lower end of the range. Those who are more physically fit or are striving for a more rapid improvement in fitness may want to exercise at the higher end of the range. Competitive athletes generally train at a higher intensity, around 80–95% of their maximal heart rate.

Although the calculation *220 – age* has been used extensively for years to predict maximal heart rate, it was never intended to accurately represent everyone's true maximal heart rate or to be used as the standard of aerobic training intensity. The most accurate way to determine your own maximal heart rate is to complete a maximal exercise test in a fitness laboratory; however, this test is not commonly conducted with the general public and can be very expensive. Although not completely accurate, the estimated maximal heart rate method can still be used to give you a general idea of your aerobic training range.

Time of Activity

Time of activity refers to how long each session lasts. To achieve general health, you can do multiple short bouts of activity that add up to 30 minutes each day. However, to achieve higher levels of fitness, it is important that the activities be done for at least 20 to 30 consecutive minutes.

For example, let's say you want to compete in triathlons. To be successful during the running segment of the triathlon, you will need to be able to run quickly for at least 3 miles. Thus, it is appropriate for you to train so that you can complete 3 miles during one session and still have enough energy to swim and bicycle during the race. Running for two or three 10-minute sessions each day would not be a sufficient overload to prepare you for this competition. You will need to consistently train at a

YOU DO THE MATH %

Calculating Your Maximal and Training Heart Rate Range

Judy was recently diagnosed with type 2 diabetes, and her healthcare provider has recommended she begin an exercise program. She is considered obese according to her body mass index, and she has not been regularly active since she was a teenager. Judy's goals are to improve her cardiorespiratory fitness and achieve and maintain a more healthful weight. Fortunately, Valley Hospital, where she works as a nurse's aide, recently opened a small fitness center for the use of its employees. Judy plans to begin by either walking on the treadmill or riding the stationary bicycle at the fitness center during her lunch break.

Judy needs to exercise at an intensity that will help her improve her cardiorespiratory fitness and lose weight. She is 38 years of age, is obese, has type 2 diabetes, and has been approved to do moderate-intensity activity by her healthcare provider. Even though she does a lot of walking and lifting in her work as a nurse's aide, her doctor has recommended that she set her exercise intensity range to begin at a heart rate that is slightly lower than the currently recommended minimal intensity of 64%. Based on this information, Judy should set her training heart rate range between 50% and 75% of her maximal heart rate.

Let's calculate Judy's maximal heart rate values:

- Maximal heart rate: 220 – age = 220 – 38 = 182 beats per minute (bpm)
- Lower end of intensity range: 50% of 182 bpm = 0.50 × 182 bpm = 91 bpm

- Higher end of intensity range: 75% of 182 bpm = 0.75 × 182 bpm = 137 bpm

Because Judy is a trained nurse's aide, she is skilled at measuring a heart rate, or pulse. To measure your own pulse:

- Place your second (index) and third (middle) finger on the inside of your wrist, just below the wrist crease and near the thumb. Press lightly to feel your pulse. Don't press too hard, or you will occlude the artery and be unable to feel its pulsation.
- If you can't feel your pulse at your wrist, try the carotid artery at the neck. This is located below your ear, on the side of your neck directly below your jaw. Press lightly against your neck under the jaw bone to find your pulse.
- Begin counting your pulse with the count of "zero," then count each beat for 15 seconds.
- Multiply that value by 4 to estimate heart rate over 1 minute.
- Do not take your pulse with your thumb, as it has its own pulse, which would prevent you from getting an accurate estimate of your heart rate.

As you can see from the calculations above, when Judy walks on the treadmill or rides the bicycle, her heart rate should be between 91 and 137 bpm; this will put her in her aerobic training zone and allow her to achieve cardiorespiratory fitness. It will also assist in weight loss.

distance of 3 miles; you will also benefit from running longer distances. In contrast, bicycling for 10 minutes two or three times each day would be appropriate for someone like Judy to achieve her health-related cardiorespiratory fitness goal.

Table 13.2 compares the guidelines for achieving health to those for achieving physical fitness. The guidelines you follow will depend on your personal goals. These recommendations apply to people of all ages, and following either set will allow you to improve and maintain your health. For people with established disease, these guidelines may help postpone complications and reduce their reliance on medications. People with heart disease, high blood pressure, diabetes, osteoporosis, or arthritis should get approval to exercise from their healthcare practitioner prior to starting a fitness program. In addition, a medical evaluation should be conducted before starting an exercise program for an apparently healthy but currently inactive man 40 years or older or woman 50 years or older.

TABLE 13.2 Physical Activity Guidelines for Achieving Health versus Physical Fitness

	Health	Physical Fitness
Frequency	Daily	2–5 days per week (3–5 days for cardiorespiratory fitness, 2–3 days for muscular fitness and flexibility)
Intensity	Any level	64–90% of maximal heart rate
Time	Accumulation of a minimum of 30 minutes each day	20–60 minutes of continuous or intermittent activity
Type	Any activity	Aerobic-type activities, resistance exercises to enhance muscular strength and endurance, and flexibility exercises

Source: Adapted from American College of Sports Medicine (ACSM). 2006. *ACSM's Guidelines for Exercise Testing and Prescription,* 7th edn. Philadelphia: Lippincott Williams and Wilkins; and U.S. Department of Health and Human Services. 1996. *Physical Activity and Health: A Report of the Surgeon General.* Atlanta, GA: U.S. Department of Health and Human Services, Centers for Disease Control and Prevention, National Center for Chronic Disease Prevention and Health Promotion.

A Sound Fitness Plan Includes a Warm-Up and a Cool-Down Period

Stretching should be included in the warm-up before and the cool-down after exercise.

warm-up Also called preliminary exercise; includes activities that prepare you for an exercise bout, including stretching, calisthenics, and movements specific to the exercise bout.

cool-down Activities done after an exercise session is completed; should be gradual and allow your body to slowly recover from exercise.

To properly prepare for and recover from an exercise session, warm-up and cool-down activities should be performed. **Warm-up,** also called preliminary exercise, includes general activities (such as stretching and calisthenics) and specific activities that prepare you for the actual activity (such as jogging or swinging a golf club). Your warm-up should be brief (5 to 10 minutes), gradual, and sufficient to increase muscle and body temperature but should not cause fatigue or deplete energy stores.

Warming up prior to exercise is important, as it properly prepares the muscles for exertion by increasing blood flow and temperature. It may also help to prepare a person psychologically for the exercise session or athletic event.

Cool-down activities are done after the exercise session is completed. Similar to the warm-up, the cool-down should be gradual and allow your body to slowly recover. Your cool-down should include some of the same activities you performed during the exercise session but done at a low intensity, and you should allow ample time for stretching. Cooling down after exercise assists in the prevention of injury and may help reduce muscle soreness.

RECAP: *A sound fitness program must meet your personal fitness goals, such as reducing your risks for disease or preparing for athletic competition. It should be fun and include variety and consistency to help you maintain interest and achieve fitness in all components. It must also place an extra physical demand, or an overload, on your body. To achieve appropriate overload, follow the FIT principle: Frequency refers to the number of activity sessions per week. Intensity refers to how difficult the activity is to perform. Time refers to how long each activity session lasts. Warm-up exercises prepare the muscles for exertion by increasing blood flow and temperature. Cool-down activities assist in the prevention of injury and may help reduce muscle soreness.*

NUTRI-CASE: JUDY

" I can't remember a time in my life when I wasn't trying to lose weight. But nothing ever works, and when I go off a diet, I always end up fatter than I started out! Last week I had my annual check-up and my doctor confirmed what I already knew—I'm obese! She also said my weight is contributing to my diabetes symptoms, and that my blood pressure is high, too. Being a nurse's aide, I see every day the health problems caused by obesity. Still, like I told my doctor, knowing how bad it is doesn't help me to lose the weight and keep it off. So we talked about some "slow and steady" strategies for losing weight: I promised I'd do a better job of watching my diet, take the medications she prescribed, and start working out at the new fitness center here at the hospital. I checked it out on my lunch break today, and I guess it's okay. They have a couple of treadmills and stationary bikes right in front of a big TV so you can watch the soaps while you work out. Still, I'm not really sure what I'm supposed to do or how many times a week or how long. I mean, if I only had to lose 5 pounds, that would be easy. But I've got to lose 50! And I only get half an hour for lunch!"

Imagine that you were a trainer at the Valley Hospital employee fitness center, and Judy told you about her weight loss and fitness goals. Applying the FIT principle, recommend a physical activity program that includes an appropriate:

- number of times per 5-day work week
- intensity
- duration of activity
- variety of activity.

If you get stuck, don't forget the You Do the Math box and Table 13.2!

What Fuels Our Activities?

In order to perform exercise, or muscular work, we must be able to generate energy. The common currency of energy for virtually all cells in the body is **ATP**, or **adenosine triphosphate.** As you might guess from its name, a molecule of ATP includes an organic compound called adenosine and three phosphate groups **(FIGURE 13.5).** When one of the phosphates is cleaved, or broken away, from ATP, energy is released. The products remaining after this reaction are adenosine diphosphate (ADP) and an independent inorganic phosphate group (P_i). In a mirror image of this reaction, the body regenerates ATP by adding a phosphate group back to ADP. In this way, we continually provide energy to our cells.

The amount of ATP stored in a muscle cell is very limited; it can keep the muscle active for only about 1 to 3 seconds. Thus, we need to generate ATP from other sources to fuel activities for longer periods of time. Fortunately, we are able to generate ATP from the breakdown of carbohydrate, fat, and protein, providing our cells with a variety of sources from which to receive energy. The primary energy systems we rely upon to provide energy for physical activities are the adenosine triphosphate–creatine phosphate (ATP-CP) energy system and the anaerobic and aerobic breakdown of carbohydrates. Our bodies also generate energy from the breakdown of

adenosine triphosphate (ATP)
The common currency of energy for virtually all cells of the body.

FIGURE 13.5 Structure of adenosine triphosphate (ATP). Energy is produced when ATP is split into adenosine diphosphate (ADP) and inorganic phosphate (P_i).

FIGURE 13.6 When the compound creatine phosphate (CP) is broken down into a molecule of creatine and an independent phosphate molecule, energy is released. This energy, along with the independent phosphate molecule, can then be used to regenerate ATP.

fats. As you will see, the type, intensity, and duration of the activities we perform determine the amount of ATP we need and therefore the energy system we use.

The ATP-CP Energy System Uses Creatine Phosphate to Regenerate ATP

As we said, muscle cells store only enough ATP to maintain activity for 1 to 3 seconds. When more energy is needed, a high-energy compound called **creatine phosphate (CP)** (also called **phosphocreatine, or PCr**) can be broken down to support the regeneration of ATP (FIGURE 13.6). Because this reaction can occur in the absence of oxygen, it is referred to as an **anaerobic** reaction (meaning "without oxygen").

Muscle tissue contains about four to six times as much CP as ATP, but there is still not enough CP available to fuel activities longer than 2 minutes. We tend to use CP the most during very intense, short bouts of activity such as lifting, jumping, and sprinting (FIGURE 13.7). Together, our stores of ATP and CP can support a *maximal* physical effort for only about 3 to 15 seconds. We must rely on other energy sources, such as carbohydrate and fat, to support activities of longer duration.

creatine phosphate (CP) A high-energy compound that can be broken down for energy and used to regenerate ATP.

anaerobic Means "without oxygen." Term used to refer to metabolic reactions that occur in the absence of oxygen.

Activity	Percent (%) contribution to energy to perform activity
Sprint start (0–3 sec)	100% ATP/CP
100-m dash (10–12 sec)	50% ATP/CP / 50% Carbohydrate
1500-m race (4–6 min)	6% ATP/CP / 94% Carbohydrate
10-km race (32–40 min)	100% Carbohydrate
Marathon (2.5–3 hr)	5% Other / 20% Fat / 75% Carbohydrate
Day-long hike (5.5–7 hr)	65% Fat / 35% Carbohydrate

FIGURE 13.7 The relative contributions of ATP-CP, carbohydrate, and fat to activities of various durations and intensities.

> RECAP: *Adenosine triphosphate, or ATP, is the common energy source for all cells of the body. When one of the phosphate groups is cleaved from the ATP molecule, energy is released. The amount of ATP stored in a muscle cell can keep a muscle active for only about 1 to 3 seconds. For activities of maximal physical effort lasting about 3 to 15 seconds, creatine phosphate can be broken down to provide energy and support the regeneration of ATP. To support activities that last longer than 2 minutes, we must derive energy from the breakdown of carbohydrates, fats, and protein.*

The Breakdown of Carbohydrates Provides Energy for Brief and Long-Term Exercise

When our bodies cannot generate enough ATP from the breakdown of CP to fully support our efforts, we need an energy source that we can use quickly to produce

FIGURE 13.8 The breakdown of one molecule of glucose, or the process of glycolysis, yields two molecules of pyruvic acid and two ATP molecules. The further metabolism of pyruvic acid in the presence of insufficient oxygen (anaerobic process) results in the production of lactic acid. The metabolism of pyruvic acid in the presence of adequate oxygen (aerobic process) yields 36 to 38 molecules of ATP.

ATP. The breakdown of carbohydrates, specifically glucose, provides this quick energy in a process called **glycolysis.** The most common source of glucose during exercise comes from glycogen stored in the muscles and glucose found in the blood. As shown in **FIGURE 13.8**, for every glucose molecule that goes through glycolysis, two ATP molecules are produced. The primary end product of glycolysis is **pyruvic acid.**

When oxygen availability is limited in the cell, pyruvic acid is converted to **lactic acid.** For years it was assumed that lactic acid was a useless, even potentially toxic, by-product of high-intensity exercise. We now know that lactic acid is an important intermediate of glucose breakdown and that it plays a critical role in supplying fuel for working muscles, the heart, and resting tissues (see the Nutrition Myth or Fact? box: Does Lactic Acid Cause Muscle Fatigue and Soreness?).

The major advantage of glycolysis is that it is the fastest way that we can regenerate ATP for exercise, other than the ATP-CP system. However, this high rate of ATP production can be sustained only for a brief period of time, generally less than 3 minutes. To perform exercise that lasts longer than 3 minutes, we must rely on the aerobic energy system to provide adequate ATP.

To generate even more ATP molecules, pyruvic acid can go through additional metabolic pathways in the presence of oxygen (see **FIGURE 13.8**). Although this process is slower than glycolysis occurring under anaerobic conditions, the breakdown of 1 glucose molecule going through aerobic metabolism yields 36 to 38 ATP molecules for energy, while the anaerobic process yields only 2 ATP molecules. Thus, this aerobic process supplies 18 times more energy! Another advantage of the aerobic process is that it does not result in the significant production of acids and other compounds that contribute to muscle fatigue, which means that a low-intensity activity can be performed for hours. Aerobic metabolism of glucose is the primary source of fuel for our muscles during activities lasting from 3 minutes to 4 hours (see **FIGURE 13.7**).

glycolysis The breakdown of glucose; yields two ATP molecules and two pyruvic acid molecules for each molecule of glucose.

pyruvic acid The primary end product of glycolysis.

lactic acid A compound that results when pyruvic acid is metabolized in the presence of insufficient oxygen.

NUTRITION MYTH OR FACT?

Does Lactic Acid Cause Muscle Fatigue and Soreness?

Theo and his teammates won their basketball game last night, but just barely. With two of the players sick, Theo got more court time than usual, and when he got back to the dorm, he could hardly get his legs to carry him up the stairs. This morning, Theo's muscles ache all over, and he wonders if a build-up of lactic acid is to blame.

Lactic acid is a by-product of glycolysis. For many years, both scientists and athletes believed that lactic acid causes muscle fatigue and soreness. Does recent scientific evidence support this belief?

The exact causes of muscle fatigue are not known, and there appear to be many contributing factors. Recent evidence suggests that fatigue may be due not only to the accumulation of many acids and other metabolic by-products but also to the depletion of creatine phosphate and changes in calcium in the cells that affect muscle contraction. Depletion of muscle glycogen, liver glycogen, and blood glucose, as well as psychological factors, can all contribute to fatigue.[9] Thus, it appears that lactic acid only contributes to fatigue and does not cause fatigue independently.

So what factors cause muscle soreness? As with fatigue, there are probably many factors. It is hypothesized that soreness usually results from microscopic tears in the muscle fibers as a result of strenuous exercise. This damage triggers an inflammatory reaction that causes an influx of fluid and various chemicals to the damaged area. These substances work to remove damaged tissue and initiate tissue repair, but they may also stimulate pain.[9] However, it appears highly unlikely that lactic acid is an independent cause of muscle soreness.

Recent studies indicate that lactic acid is produced even under aerobic conditions! This means it is produced at rest as well as during exercise of any intensity. The reasons for this constant production of lactic acid are still being studied. What we do know is that lactic acid is an important fuel for resting tissues and for working cardiac and skeletal muscles. That's right—skeletal muscles not only *produce* lactic acid, but also *use* it for energy, both directly and after it is converted into glucose and glycogen in the liver.[9,10] We also know that endurance training improves the muscles' ability to use lactic acid for energy. Thus, contrary to being a waste product of glucose metabolism, lactic acid is actually an important energy source for muscle cells during rest and exercise.

As you learned in Chapter 4, we can store only a limited amount of glycogen in our bodies. An average, well-nourished man who weighs about 154 pounds (70 kg) can store about 200 to 500 g of muscle glycogen, which is equal to 800 to 2000 kcal of energy. Although trained athletes can store more muscle glycogen than the average person, there is still not enough glycogen stored in our bodies to provide an unlimited energy supply for long-term activities. Thus, we also need a fuel source that is very abundant and can be broken down under aerobic conditions so that it can support activities of lower intensity and longer duration. This fuel source is fat.

> RECAP: *To support activities that last from 30 seconds to less than 3 minutes, energy is produced from the breakdown of glucose, called glycolysis. Two ATP molecules are produced for every glucose molecule broken down, and pyruvic acid is the primary end product of this reaction. Lactic acid is formed when pyruvic acid is metabolized under anaerobic conditions. To support activities that last from 3 minutes to 4 hours, energy is produced from the aerobic metabolism of pyruvic acid. During this process, pyruvic acid is broken down in the presence of oxygen, and each molecule can yield 36 to 38 ATP molecules.*

Aerobic Breakdown of Fats Supports Exercise of Low Intensity and Long Duration

When we refer to fat as a fuel source, we mean the triglyceride molecule, which is the primary storage form of fat in our cells. As you learned in Chapter 5, a triglyceride molecule is composed of a glycerol backbone attached to three fatty acid molecules (see **FIGURE 5.1**, page 172). It is these fatty acid molecules that provide much of the energy we need to support long-term activity. Fatty acids are classified by their length, that is, by the number of carbons they contain. The longer the fatty acid, the more ATP that can be generated from its breakdown. For instance, palmitic acid is a fatty acid with 16 carbons. If palmitic acid is broken down completely, it yields 129 ATP molecules! Obviously, far more energy is produced from this one fatty acid molecule than from the aerobic breakdown of a glucose molecule.

There are two major advantages of using fat as a fuel. First, fat is a very abundant energy source, even in lean people. For example, a man who weighs 154 pounds (70 kg) who has a body fat level of 10% has approximately 15 pounds of body fat, which is equivalent to more than 50,000 kcal of energy! This is significantly more energy than can be provided by his stored muscle glycogen (800 to 2,000 kcal). Second, fat provides 9 kcal of energy per gram, while carbohydrate provides only 4 kcal of energy per gram, which means that fat supplies more than twice as much energy per gram as carbohydrate. The primary disadvantage of using fat as a fuel is that the breakdown process is relatively slow; thus, fat is used predominantly as a fuel source during activities of lower intensity and longer duration. Fat is also our primary energy source during rest, sitting, and standing in place.

What specific activities are primarily fueled by fat? Walking long distances uses fat stores, as do other low- to moderate-intensity forms of exercise. Fat is also an important fuel source during endurance events such as marathons (26.2 miles) and ultra-marathon races (49.9 miles). Endurance exercise training improves our ability to use fat for energy, which may be one reason that people who exercise regularly tend to have lower body fat levels than people who do not exercise.

It is important to remember that we are almost always using some combination of carbohydrate and fat for energy. At rest, we use very little carbohydrate, relying mostly on fat. During maximal exercise (at 100% effort), we are using mostly carbohydrate and very little fat. However, most activities we do each day involve some use of both fuels (**FIGURE 13.9**).

When it comes to eating properly to support regular physical activity or exercise training, the nutrient to focus on is carbohydrate. This is because most people store

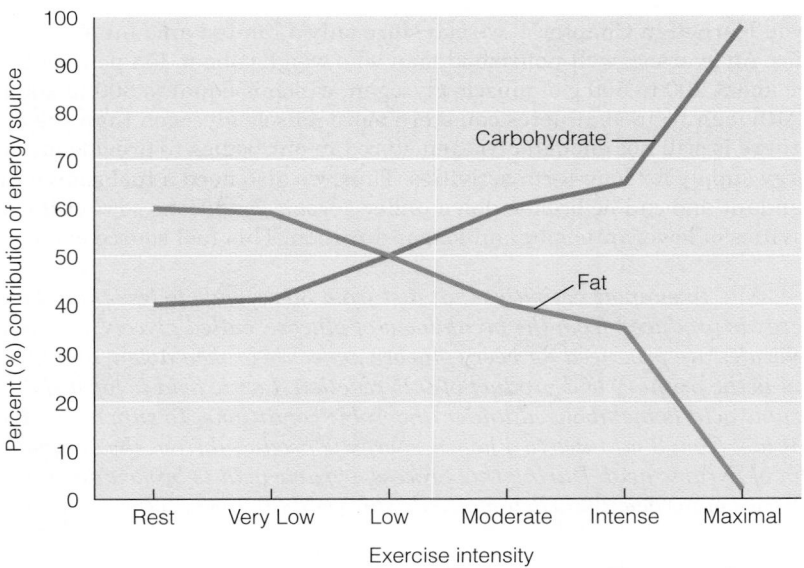

FIGURE 13.9 For most daily activities, including exercise, we use a mixture of carbohydrate and fat for energy. At lower exercise intensities, we rely more on fat as a fuel source. As exercise intensity increases, we rely more on carbohydrate for energy. (Based on Brooks, G. A., and J. Mercier. 1994. Balance of carbohydrate and lipid utilization during exercise: the "crossover" concept. *J. Appl. Physiol.* 76(6):2253–2261.)

more than enough fat to support exercise, whereas our storage of carbohydrate is limited. It is especially important that we maintain adequate stores of glycogen for moderate to intense exercise. Dietary recommendations for fat, carbohydrate, and protein are reviewed later in this chapter (pages 536–543).

> RECAP: *Fat can be broken down aerobically to support activities of low intensity and long duration. When a triglyceride molecule is broken down, the amount of energy derived depends upon the length of the fatty acid chain. The two major advantages of using fat as a fuel is that it is an abundant energy source and it provides more than twice the energy per gram as compared to carbohydrate. The primary disadvantage of using fat as a fuel is that the breakdown process is relatively slow so it cannot support quick, high-intensity activities.*

Amino Acids Are Not Major Sources of Fuel During Exercise

Proteins, or more specifically amino acids, are not major energy sources during exercise. As discussed in Chapter 6, amino acids can be used directly for energy if necessary, but they are more often used to make glucose to maintain our blood glucose levels during exercise. Amino acids also help build and repair tissues after exercise. Depending upon the intensity and duration of the activity, amino acids may contribute about 3–6% of the energy needed.[11]

Given this, why is it that so many people are concerned about their protein intakes? As you learned in Chapter 6, our muscles are not stimulated to grow when we eat extra dietary protein. Only appropriate physical training can stimulate our muscles to grow and strengthen. Thus, while we need enough dietary protein to support activity and recovery, consuming very high amounts does not provide an added benefit. The protein needs of athletes are only slightly higher than the needs of non-athletes, and most of us eat more than enough protein to support even the highest requirements for competitive athletes! Thus, there is generally no need for recreationally active people or even competitive athletes to consume protein or amino acid supplements.

> RECAP: *Amino acids may contribute from 3% to 6% of the energy needed during exercise, depending upon the intensity and duration of the activity. Amino acids help build and repair tissues after exercise. We generally consume more than enough protein in our diets to support regular exercise, and there is typically no need for protein or amino acid supplementation even for competitive athletes.*

What Kind of Diet Supports Physical Activity?

Lots of people wonder, "Do my nutrient needs change if I become more physically active?" The answer to this question depends upon the type, intensity, and duration of the activity in which you participate. It is not necessarily true that our requirement for every nutrient is greater if we are physically active.

People who are performing moderate-intensity daily activities for health can follow the dietary guidelines put forth in the Dietary Guidelines for Americans. For smaller or less-active people, the lower end of the range of recommendations for each food group may be appropriate. For larger or more-active people, the higher end of the range is suggested. Modifications may need to be made for people who exercise vigorously every day, particularly for athletes training for competition. Table 13.3 provides an overview of the nutrients that can be affected by regular, vigorous exercise training. Each of these nutrients is described in more detail in the following section.[12]

TABLE 13.3   Suggested Intakes of Nutrients to Support Vigorous Exercise

Nutrient	Functions	Suggested Intake
Energy	Supports exercise, activities of daily living, and basic body functions	Depends upon body size and the type, intensity, and duration of activity. For many female athletes: 1,800 to 3,500 kcal/day For many male athletes: 2,500 to 7,500 kcal/day
Carbohydrate	Provides energy, maintains adequate muscle glycogen and blood glucose; high complex carbohydrate foods provide vitamins and minerals	At least 55% of total energy intake Depending upon sport and gender, 6-10 g of carbohydrate per kg body weight per day
Fat	Provides energy, fat-soluble vitamins, and essential fatty acids; supports production of hormones and transport of nutrients	15-25% of total energy intake
Protein	Helps build and maintain muscle; provides building material for glucose; energy source during endurance exercise; aids recovery from exercise	12-20% of total energy intake Endurance athletes: 1.4-1.6 g per kg body weight Strength athletes: 1.0-1.7 g per kg body weight
Water	Maintains temperature regulation (adequate cooling); maintains blood volume and blood pressure; supports all cell functions	Consume fluid before, during, and after exercise Consume enough to maintain body weight Consume at least 8 cups (or 64 fl. oz) of water daily to maintain regular health and activity Athletes may need up to 10 liters (or 170 fl. oz) every day; more is required if exercising in a hot environment
B vitamins	Critical for energy production from carbohydrate, fat, and protein	May need slightly more (one to two times the RDA) for thiamin, riboflavin, and vitamin B_6
Calcium	Builds and maintains bone mass; assists with nervous system function, muscle contraction, hormone function, and transport of nutrients across cell membrane	Meet the current AI: 14-18 years: 1,300 mg/day 19-50 years: 1,000 mg/day 51 and older: 1,200 mg/day
Iron	Primarily responsible for the transport of oxygen in blood to cells; assists with energy production	Consume at least the RDA: Males: 14-18 years: 11 mg/day 19 and older: 8 mg/day Females: 14-18 years: 15 mg/day 19-50 years: 18 mg/day 51 and older: 8 mg/day

Vigorous Exercise Increases Energy Needs

Athletes generally have higher energy needs than moderately physically active or sedentary people. The amount of extra energy needed to support regular training is determined by the type, intensity, and duration of the activity. In addition, the energy needs of male athletes are higher than those of female athletes because male athletes weigh more, have more muscle mass, and expend more energy during activity than women. This is relative, of course: a large woman who trains 3 to 5 hours each day will probably need more energy than a small man who trains 1 hour each day. The energy needs of athletes can range from only 1,500 to 1,800 kcal/day for a small female gymnast to more than 7,500 kcal/day for a male cyclist competing in the Tour de France cross-country cycling race!

FIGURE 13.10 shows a sample of meals that total 1,800 kcal per day and 4,000 kcal per day, with the carbohydrate content of these meals meeting more than 60% of total energy intake. As you can see, athletes who need more than 4,000 kcal per day need to consume very large quantities of food. However, the heavy demands of daily physical training, work, school, and family responsibilities often leave these athletes with little time to eat adequately. Thus,

Small snacks can be helpful to meet daily energy demands.

1,800 kcal/day	4,000 kcal/day
1½ cup Cheerios 4 oz skim milk 1 medium banana 8 fl. oz orange juice	3 cups Cheerios 8 fl. oz skim milk 1 medium banana 2 slices whole-wheat toast 1 tbsp. butter 16 fl. oz orange juice

Turkey sandwich with:
  2 slices whole-wheat bread
  3 oz turkey lunch meat
  1 oz Swiss cheese slice
  1 leaf iceberg lettuce
  2 slices tomato
1 cup tomato soup
  (made with water)
	Two turkey sandwiches with:
	  2 slices whole wheat bread
	  3 oz turkey lunch meat
	  1 oz Swiss cheese slice
	  1 leaf iceberg lettuce
	  2 slices tomato
	2 cups tomato soup
	  (made with water)
	Two 8-oz containers of
	  low-fat fruit yogurt
	24 fl. oz of Gatorade

4 oz grilled skinless
  chicken breast
1½ cup mixed salad greens
1 tbsp. French salad dressing
1 cup steamed broccoli
1 cup cooked brown rice
8 fl. oz skim milk
	6 oz grilled skinless
	  chicken breast
	3 cups mixed salad greens
	3 tbsp. French salad dressing
	2 cups cooked
	  spaghetti noodles
	1 cup spaghetti sauce
	  with meat
	16 fl. oz skim milk

FIGURE 13.10 High-carbohydrate (approximately 60% of total energy) meals that contain approximately 1,800 kcal/day (on left) and 4,000 kcal/day (on right). Athletes must plan their meals carefully to meet energy demands, particularly those with very high energy needs.

many athletes meet their energy demands by planning regular meals and snacks and **grazing** (eating small meals throughout the day) consistently. They may also take advantage of the energy-dense snack foods and meal replacements specifically designed for athletes participating in vigorous training. These steps help athletes to maintain their blood glucose and energy stores.

If an athlete is losing body weight, then his or her energy intake is inadequate. Conversely, weight gain may indicate that energy intake is too high. Weight maintenance is generally recommended to maximize performance. If weight loss is warranted, food intake should be lowered no more than 200 to 500 kcal/day, and athletes should try to lose weight prior to the competitive season if at all possible. Weight gain may be necessary for some athletes and can usually be accomplished by consuming 500 to 700 kcal/day more than needed for weight maintenance. The extra energy should come from a healthy balance of carbohydrate (55–60% of total energy intake), fat (25–30% of total energy intake), and protein (10–20% of total energy intake).

Many athletes are concerned about their weight for reasons of performance or physical appearance. Jockeys, boxers, wrestlers, judo athletes, and others are required to "make weight," or meet a predefined weight category. Others, such as distance runners, gymnasts, figure skaters, and dancers, are required to maintain a very lean figure for performance and aesthetic reasons. These athletes tend to eat less energy than they need to support vigorous training, which puts them at risk for inadequate intakes of all nutrients. These athletes are at a higher risk of suffering from health consequences resulting from poor energy and nutrient intake, including eating disorders, osteoporosis, menstrual disturbances, dehydration, heat and physical injuries, and even death.

RECAP: *The type, intensity, and duration of activities you participate in will determine your nutrient needs. Vigorous-intensity exercise requires extra energy, and male athletes typically need more energy than female athletes because of their higher muscle mass and larger body weight. Weight maintenance is recommended to maximize athletic performance. Some athletes who are concerned with making a competitive weight or with the aesthetic demands of their sport may be at risk for poor energy and nutrient intakes.*

grazing Consistently eating small meals throughout the day; done by many athletes to meet their high energy demands.

Carbohydrate Needs Increase for Many Active People

As you know, carbohydrate (in the form of glucose) is one of the primary sources of energy needed to support exercise. Both endurance athletes and strength athletes require adequate carbohydrate to maintain their glycogen stores and provide quick energy.

How Much of an Athlete's Diet Should Be Carbohydrates?

You may recall from Chapter 4 that the AMDR for carbohydrates is 45–65% of total energy intake. Athletes should consume at least 55% of their total energy intake as carbohydrates, which falls within this recommended range. Athletes who are participating in strength-type activities, sprinting, or other explosive-type events, or are not training for more than 1 hour each day, may find that consuming 50% of their total energy intake as carbohydrate is sufficient.

To illustrate how inadequate carbohydrate affects glycogen stores, let's see what happens to Theo when he participates in a study designed to determine how carbohydrate intake affects glycogen stores during a period of heavy training. Theo was asked to come to the exercise laboratory at the university and ride a stationary bicycle for 2 hours a day for three consecutive days at 75% of his maximal heart rate. Before and after

Fruit and vegetable juices can be a good source of carbohydrates.

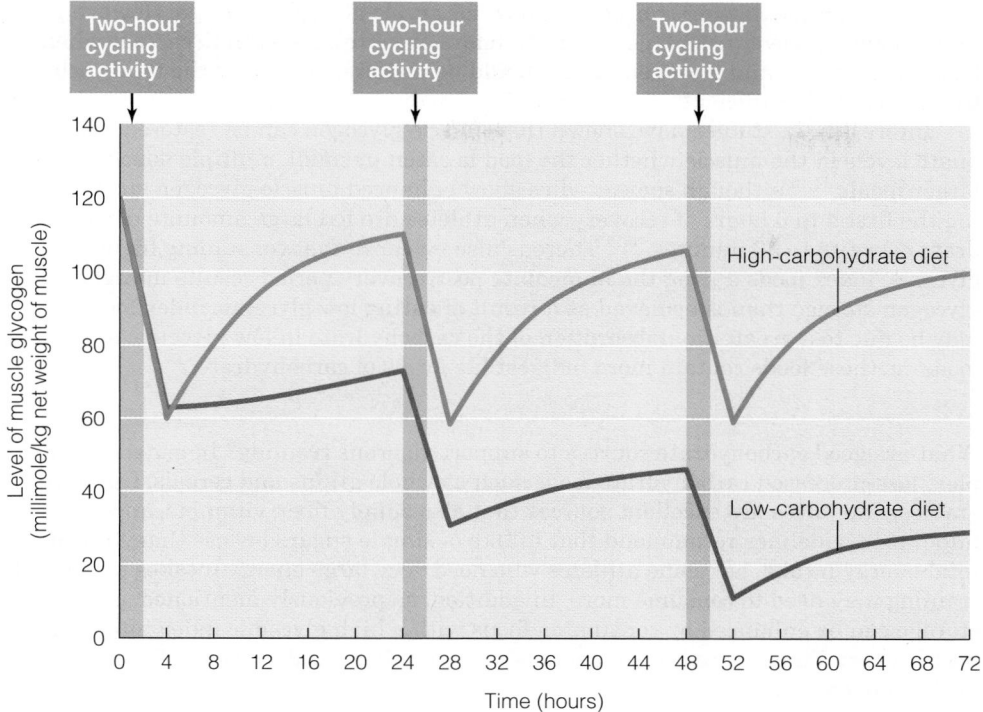

FIGURE 13.11 The effects of a low-carbohydrate diet on muscle glycogen stores. When a low-carbohydrate diet is consumed, glycogen stores cannot be restored during a period of regular vigorous training. (Adapted from Costill, D. L., and J. M. Miller. 1980. Nutrition for endurance sport: CHO and fluid balance. *Int. J. Sports Med.* 1:2–14. Copyright © 1980 Georg Thieme Verlag. Used with permission.)

each ride, samples of muscle tissue were taken from his thighs to determine the amount of glycogen stored in the working muscles. Theo performed these rides on two different occasions—once when he had eaten a high-carbohydrate diet (80% of total energy intake) and again when he had eaten a moderate-carbohydrate diet (40% of total energy intake). As you can see in FIGURE 13.11, Theo's muscle glycogen levels decreased dramatically after each training session. More importantly, his muscle glycogen levels did not recover to baseline levels over the 3 days when Theo ate the lower-carbohydrate diet. He was able to maintain his muscle glycogen levels only when he was eating the higher-carbohydrate diet. Theo also told the researchers that completing the 2-hour rides was much more difficult when he had eaten the moderate-carbohydrate diet as compared to when he ate the diet that was higher in carbohydrate.

When Should Carbohydrates Be Consumed?

It is important for athletes not only to consume enough carbohydrate to maintain glycogen stores, but also to time their intake optimally. Our bodies store glycogen very rapidly during the first 24 hours of recovery from exercise, with the highest storage rates occurring during the first few hours.[13] Higher carbohydrate intakes during the first 24 hours of recovery from exercise are associated with higher amounts of glucose being stored as muscle glycogen. It is recommended that a daily carbohydrate intake of approximately 7 to 10 g of carbohydrate per kg body weight will optimize muscle glycogen stores in many athletes. However, this need could be much greater in athletes who are training heavily daily, as they have less time to recover and require more carbohydrate to support both training and storage needs.

If an athlete has to perform or participate in training bouts that are scheduled less than 8 hours apart, then he or she should try to consume enough carbohydrate in the few hours following training to allow for ample glycogen storage. However, with a longer recovery time (generally 12 hours or more), the athlete can eat when he or she chooses, and glycogen levels should be restored as long as the total carbohydrate eaten is sufficient.

Interestingly, studies have shown that muscle glycogen can be restored to adequate levels in the muscle whether the food is eaten in small, multiple snacks or in larger meals,[14,15] although some studies show enhanced muscle glycogen storage during the first 4 to 6 hours of recovery when athletes are fed large amounts of carbohydrate every 15 to 30 minutes.[16,17] There is also evidence that consuming high glycemic index foods during the immediate postrecovery period results in higher glycogen storage than is achieved as a result of eating low glycemic index foods. This may be due to a greater malabsorption of the carbohydrate in low glycemic index foods, as these foods contain more indigestible forms of carbohydrate.[13]

What Food Sources of Carbohydrates Are Good for Athletes?

What are good carbohydrate sources to support vigorous training? In general, complex, less-processed carbohydrate foods such as whole grains and cereals, fruits, vegetables, and juices are excellent sources that also supply fiber, vitamins, and minerals. Guidelines recommend that intake of simple sugars be less than 10% of total energy intake, but some athletes who need very large energy intakes to support training may need to consume more. In addition, as previously mentioned, glycogen storage can be enhanced by consuming foods with a high glycemic index immediately postrecovery. Thus, there are advantages to consuming a wide variety of carbohydrate sources.

As a result of time constraints, many athletes have difficulties consuming enough food to meet carbohydrate demands. Many beverages and snack bars have therefore been designed to assist athletes with increasing carbohydrate intake. Some of these are listed in Table 13.4, along with other simple, inexpensive foods that contain 50 to 100 g of carbohydrate.

When Does Carbohydrate Loading Make Sense?

As you know, carbohydrate is a critical energy source to support exercise, particularly endurance-type activities. Because of the importance of carbohydrates as an exercise fuel and our limited capacity to store them, discovering ways to maximize our storage of carbohydrates has been at the forefront of sports nutrition research for many years. The practice of **carbohydrate loading,** also called *glycogen loading,* involves altering both exercise duration and carbohydrate intake such that the amount of muscle glycogen is maximized. Table 13.5 reviews a schedule for carbohydrate loading for an endurance athlete. Athletes who may benefit from maximizing muscle glycogen stores include those competing in marathons, ultra-marathons, long-distance swimming, cross-country skiing, and triathlons. Athletes who compete in baseball, American football, 10-kilometer runs, walking, hiking, weightlifting, and most swimming events will not gain any performance benefits from this practice, nor will people who regularly participate in moderately intense physical activities to maintain fitness.

It is important to emphasize that carbohydrate loading does not always improve performance. There are many adverse side effects of this practice, including extreme gastrointestinal distress, particularly diarrhea. We store water along with the extra glycogen in our muscles, which leaves many athletes feeling heavy and sluggish. Athletes who want to try carbohydrate loading should experiment prior to competition to determine whether it is an acceptable and beneficial approach for them.[18]

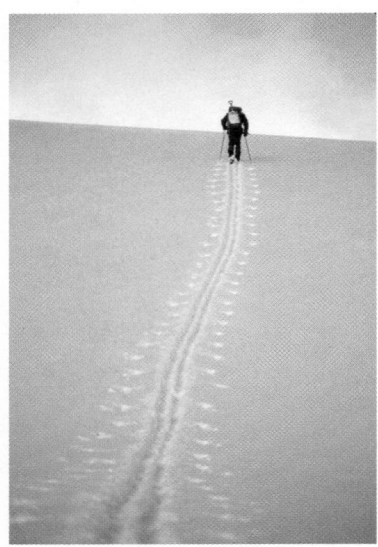

Carbohydrate loading may benefit endurance athletes, such as cross-country skiers.

carbohydrate loading Also known as glycogen loading. A process that involves altering training and carbohydrate intake so that muscle glycogen storage is maximized.

> RECAP: *Carbohydrate needs increase for active people. In general, athletes should consume 55–60% of their total energy as carbohydrate. Consuming carbohydrate sources within the first few hours of recovery can maximize carbohydrate storage rates. Good food sources of carbohydrates for active people include whole grains and cereals, fruits, vegetables, and juices. Carbohydrate loading involves altering physical training and the diet such that the storage of muscle glycogen is maximized in an attempt to enhance endurance performance.*

TABLE 13.4   Carbohydrate and Total Energy in Various Foods and Sports Bars

Food	Amount	Carbohydrate (g)	Energy from Carbohydrate (%)	Total Energy (kcal)
Sweetened applesauce	1 cup	50	97	207
Large apple	1 each	50	82	248
Saltine crackers	8 each			
Whole-wheat bread	1 oz slice	50	71	282
Jelly	4 tsp.			
Skim milk	12 fl. oz			
Spaghetti (cooked)	1 cup	50	75	268
Tomato sauce	¼ cup			
Brown rice (cooked)	1 cup	100	88	450
Mixed vegetables	½ cup			
Apple juice	12 fl. oz			
Grape-Nuts cereal	½ cup	100	84	473
Raisins	⅜ cup			
Skim milk	8 fl. oz			
Clif Bar (chocolate chip)	2.4 oz	45	72	250
Meta-Rx (fudge brownie)	3.53 oz	48	60	320
Power Bar (chocolate)	2.25 oz	42	75	225
PR Bar Ironman	2 oz	24	42	230

Source: Adapted from Manore, M., and J. Thompson. 2000. *Sport Nutrition for Health and Performance,* page 118, Table 4.5. © 2000 by Melinda Manore and Janice Thompson. Reprinted with permission from Human Kinetics (Champaign, IL).

TABLE 13.5   Recommended Carbohydrate Loading Procedure for Endurance Athletes

Days Prior to Event	Exercise Duration (minutes)	Carbohydrate Content of Diet (grams per kilogram of body weight)
6	90	5
5	40	5
4	40	5
3	20	10
2	20	10
1	None (rest day)	10
Day of Race	Competition	Precompetition food and fluid

Source: Adapted from Coleman, E. 2006. Carbohydrate and exercise. In: Dunford, M., ed. *Sports Nutrition,* 4th edn. Chicago, IL: The American Dietetic Association. Used with permission.

Moderate Fat Consumption Is Enough to Support Most Activities

As you have learned, fat is an important energy source for both moderate physical activity and vigorous endurance training. When athletes reach a physically trained state, they are able to use more fat for energy; in other words, they become better "fat burners." This can also occur in people who are not athletes but who regularly participate in aerobic-type fitness activities. This training effect occurs for a number of reasons, including an increase in the number and activity of various enzymes involved in fat metabolism, improved ability of the muscle to store fat, and improved ability to extract fat from the blood for use during exercise. By using fat as a fuel, athletes can spare carbohydrate so they can use it during prolonged, intense training or competition.

Many athletes concerned with body weight and physical appearance believe they should eat less than 15% of their total energy intake as fat, but this is inadequate for vigorous activity. Instead, a fat intake of 15–25% of total energy intake is generally recommended for most athletes, with less than 10% of total energy intake as saturated fat. These same recommendations can also be followed by people who are not competitive athletes. Recall from Chapter 5 that fat provides not only energy, but also fat-soluble vitamins and essential fatty acids that are critical to maintaining general health. If fat consumption is too low, inadequate levels of these can eventually prove detrimental to training and performance. Athletes who have chronic disease risk factors such as high blood lipids, high blood pressure, or unhealthful blood glucose levels should work with their physician to adjust their intake of fat and carbohydrate according to their health risks.

> RECAP: *Athletes and physically active people use more fat than carbohydrates for energy because they experience an increase in the number and activity of the enzymes involved in fat metabolism, and they have an improved ability to store fat and extract it from the blood for use during exercise. A dietary fat intake of 15–25% is generally recommended for athletes, with less than 10% of total energy intake as saturated fat.*

Active People Need More Protein Than Do Inactive People, but Many Already Eat Enough

The protein intakes suggested for competitive athletes and moderately active people are given in Table 13.6. Competitive male and female endurance athletes are those individuals who train 5 to 7 days per week for more than an hour each day; many of

TABLE 13.6 **Estimated Protein Requirements for Athletes**

Group	Protein Requirements (grams per kilogram body weight)
Competitive male and female athletes	1.4–1.6
Moderate-intensity endurance athletes	1.2
Recreational endurance athletes	0.8–1.0
Football, power sports players	1.4–1.7
Resistance athletes, weight lifters (early training)	1.5–1.7
Resistance athletes, weight lifters (steady-state training)	1.0–1.2

Source: Tarnopolsky, M. 2006. Protein and amino acid needs for training and bulking up. In: Burke, L. and Deakin, V., eds. *Clinical Sports Nutrition*, 3rd edn. Sydney, Australia: McGraw-Hill, p. 109.

these individuals may train for 3 to 6 hours per day. These athletes need protein in amounts similar to strength athletes, while the needs of moderate-intensity endurance athletes are slightly higher than the current RDA of 0.8 g of protein per kg body weight. Moderate-intensity endurance athletes are people exercising four to five times per week for 45 to 60 minutes each time; these individuals may compete in community races and other activities. Recreational endurance athletes are people who exercise four to five times per week for 30 minutes at less than 60% of their maximal effort. These individuals have a protein need that is equal to, or slightly higher than, the needs of sedentary people. Strength athletes who are already trained need less protein than those who are initiating training. Studies do not support the contention that consuming more than 2 g of protein per kg body weight improves protein synthesis, muscle strength, or performance.[11]

As we mentioned earlier, most inactive people and many athletes in the United States consume more than enough protein to support their needs.[18] However, some athletes do not consume enough protein; these typically include individuals with very low energy intakes, vegetarians or vegans who do not consume high-protein food sources, and young athletes who are growing and are not aware of their higher protein needs.

In 1995, Dr. Barry Sears published *The Zone: A Dietary Road Map,* a book that claims numerous benefits of a high-protein, low-carbohydrate diet for athletes.[19] Although this book was published a number of years ago, many of the principles it espoused are still being recommended to both athletes and non-athletes today. As you learned in Chapter 6, low-carbohydrate, high-protein diets are quite popular, especially among people who want to lose weight (see Nutrition Debate in Chapter 6, page 249). Unlike many of the current high-protein diets, the Zone Diet was developed and marketed specifically for competitive athletes. It recommends that athletes eat a 40–30–30 diet, or one composed of 40% carbohydrate, 30% fat, and 30% protein. Dr. Sears claims that high-carbohydrate diets impair athletic performance because of unhealthy effects of insulin. These claims have never been supported by research—in fact, many of Dr. Sears' claims are not consistent with human physiology. The primary problem with the Zone Diet for athletes is that it is too low in both energy and carbohydrate to support training and performance.

As described in Chapter 6, high-quality protein sources include lean meats, poultry, fish, eggs and egg whites, low-fat dairy products, legumes, and soy products. By following the Dietary Guidelines for Americans and meeting energy needs, people of all fitness levels can consume more than enough protein without the use of supplements or specially formulated foods.

RECAP: *Protein needs can be higher for athletes and active people. However, most people in the United States already consume more than twice their daily needs for protein. Athletes at risk for low protein intakes include those with low-energy intakes, vegetarians or vegans who do not consume high-protein food sources, and young athletes who are growing and not aware of their higher protein needs. Although low-carbohydrate, high-protein diets have been marketed to athletes, these diets are generally too low in carbohydrate and energy to support regular training and competition.*

Regular Exercise Increases Our Need for Fluids

A detailed discussion of fluid and electrolyte balance is provided in Chapter 7. In this chapter, we will briefly review some of the basic functions of water and its role during exercise.

Functions of Water

Water serves many important functions in the body. It is:

- A lubricant that bathes the tissues and cells
- A transport medium for nutrients, hormones, and waste products

Water is essential for maintaining fluid balance and preventing dehydration.

evaporative cooling Another term for sweating, which is the primary way in which we dissipate heat.

heat syncope Dizziness that occurs when people stand for too long in the heat or when they stop suddenly after a race or stand suddenly from a lying position; results from blood pooling in the lower extremities.

heat cramps Muscle spasms that occur several hours after strenuous exercise; most often occur when sweat losses and fluid intakes are high, urine volume is low, and sodium intake is inadequate.

heat exhaustion A heat illness that is characterized by excessive sweating, weakness, nausea, dizziness, headache, and difficulty concentrating. Unchecked heat exhaustion can lead to heatstroke.

heatstroke A potentially fatal heat illness that is characterized by hot, dry skin, rapid heart rate, vomiting, diarrhea, body temperature greater than or equal to 104°F, hallucinations, and coma.

- An important component of many chemical reactions, particularly those related to energy production

- A structural part of body tissues such as proteins and glycogen

- A vital component in temperature regulation; without adequate water, we cannot cool our bodies properly through sweating and thereby can experience severe heat illness and even death.

Cooling Mechanisms

When you exercise, your body generates heat. In fact, heat production can increase 15 to 20 times during heavy exercise! The primary way in which we dissipate this heat is through sweating, which is also called **evaporative cooling.** When body temperature rises, more blood (which contains water) flows to the surface of the skin. Heat is carried in this way from the core of our bodies to the surface of our skin. By sweating, the water (and body heat) leaves our bodies and the air around us picks up the evaporating water from our skin, cooling our bodies.

Dehydration and Heat-Related Illnesses

Exercising in extreme heat and humidity is very dangerous for two reasons: the extreme heat dramatically raises body temperature, and the high humidity prohibits evaporative cooling. During periods of high humidity, the environmental air is so saturated with water that it is unable to pull the water from the surface of our skin. Under these conditions, we are unable to cool ourselves adequately, and heat illnesses are likely to occur. It is important to remember that dehydration significantly increases our risk for heat illnesses. General signs of dehydration for adults and children were introduced in Chapter 3 and are listed in Table 3.1 (see page 107). In Table 13.7, specific signs of dehydration during heavy exercise are listed.

Heat illnesses include heat syncope, heat cramps, heat exhaustion, and heatstroke. **Heat syncope** is dizziness that occurs when people stand for too long in the heat, and the blood pools in their lower extremities rather than fully supplying their brains. It can also occur when people stop suddenly after a race or stand suddenly from a lying position. **Heat cramps** are muscle spasms that occur several hours after strenuous exercise. They occur during times when sweat losses and fluid intakes are high, sodium intake is inadequate to replace these losses, and urine volume is low. These cramps generally are felt in the legs, arms, or abdomen after a person cools down from exercise.

Heat exhaustion and **heatstroke** occur on a continuum, with unchecked heat exhaustion leading to heatstroke. Early signs of heat exhaustion include excessive sweating, weakness, nausea, dizziness, headache, and difficulty concentrating. As this condition progresses, consciousness becomes impaired. Signs that a person is progressing to heatstroke are hot, dry skin, rapid heart rate, vomiting, diarrhea, body temperature greater than or equal to 104°F, hallucinations, and coma. It is critical that a person gets proper medical care, or death can result. These illnesses occur because during exercise in the heat, our muscles and skin are constantly competing for blood flow. When there is no longer enough blood flow to simultaneously provide adequate blood to our muscles and to our skin, muscle blood flow takes priority over

TABLE 13.7 Signs of Dehydration During Heavy Exercise

Decreases In:	Increases In:
Exercise performance	Heart rate at a given exercise intensity
Urine output (and urine is dark yellow or brown in color)	Level of perceived exertion during exercise
Appetite	Fatigue and weakness
Ability to mentally concentrate	Headache and dizziness

the skin, which prevents us from cooling ourselves. Body temperature during these conditions becomes dangerously high, and the dehydration that occurs during this situation worsens this overheating condition. Heat cramps and heat exhaustion are highly likely to occur, and heatstroke is possible with prolonged exposure or exercise in environmental temperatures between 90 and 130°F; heatstroke is highly likely in temperatures of at least 130°F.[20]

Guidelines for Proper Fluid Replacement

How can we prevent dehydration and heat illnesses? Obviously, adequate fluid intake is critical before, during, and after exercise. Unfortunately, our thirst mechanism cannot be relied upon to signal when we need to drink. If we rely only on our feelings of thirst, we will not consume enough fluid to support exercise.

General fluid replacement recommendations are based on maintaining body weight. As discussed in Chapter 7, athletes who are training and competing in hot environments should weigh themselves before and after the training session or event and should regain the weight lost over the subsequent 24-hour period. They should avoid losing more than 2–3% of body weight during exercise, as performance can be impaired with fluid losses as small as 1% of body weight.

Table 13.8 reviews guidelines for proper fluid replacement. For activities lasting less than 1 hour, plain water is generally adequate to replace fluid losses. However, for training and competition lasting longer than 1 hour in any weather, sport beverages containing carbohydrates and electrolytes are recommended. These beverages are also recommended for people who will not drink enough water because they don't like the taste. If drinking these beverages will guarantee adequate hydration, they are appropriate to use. For more specific information about sport beverages, refer to pages 299–301.

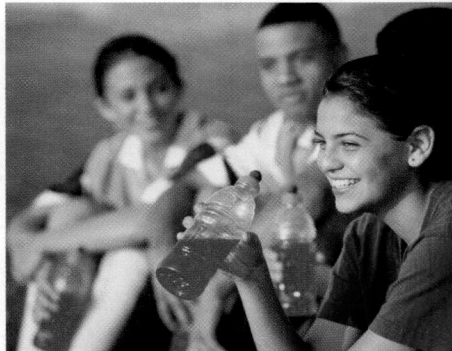

Drinking sports beverages during training and competition lasting more than 1 hour replaces fluid, carbohydrates, and electrolytes.

> RECAP: *Regular exercise increases our fluid needs. Fluid is critical to cool our internal body temperature and prevent heat illnesses. Dehydration is a serious threat during exercise in extreme heat and high humidity. Heat illnesses include heat syncope, heat cramps, heat exhaustion, and heatstroke. Adequate fluid intake before, during, and after exercise is critical to prevent heat illnesses.*

Inadequate Intakes of Some Vitamins and Minerals Can Diminish Health and Performance

When individuals train vigorously for athletic events, their requirements for certain vitamins and minerals may be altered. Many highly active people do not eat enough food or a variety of foods that allows them to consume enough of these nutrients, yet it is imperative that active people do their very best to eat an adequate, varied, and balanced diet to try and meet the increased needs associated with vigorous training.

B Vitamins

The B-complex vitamins are directly involved in energy metabolism (see pages 404–416). There is reliable evidence that the requirements of active people for thiamin, riboflavin, and vitamin B_6 may be slightly higher than the current RDA.[18] However, these increased needs are easily met by consuming adequate energy and a lot of complex carbohydrates, fruits, and vegetables. Athletes and physically active people at risk for poor B-complex vitamin status are those who consume inadequate energy or who consume mostly refined carbohydrate foods such as soda pop and sugary snacks. Vegan athletes and active individuals may be at risk for inadequate intake of vitamin B_{12}; food sources enriched with this nutrient include soy and cereal products.

Calcium and the Female Athlete Triad

Calcium supports proper muscle contraction and ensures bone health (see pages 366–372). Calcium intakes are inadequate for most women in the United States, including both sedentary and active women. This is most likely due to the failure to consume foods that are high in calcium, particularly dairy products. While vigorous training does not appear to increase our need for calcium, we need to consume

TABLE 13.8 Guidelines for Fluid Replacement

Activity Level	Environment	Fluid Requirements (liters per day)
Sedentary	Cool	2–3
Active	Cool	3–6
Sedentary	Warm	3–5
Active	Warm	5–10

Before Exercise or Competition:

- Drink adequate fluids during the 24 hours before event; should be able to maintain body weight
- Slowly drink about 0.17 to 0.24 fl. oz per kg body weight of water or a sports drink at least 4 hours prior to exercise or event to allow time for excretion of excess fluid prior to event
- Slowly drink another 0.10 to 0.17 fl. oz per kg body weight about 2 hours before the event
- Consuming beverages with sodium and/or small amounts of salted snacks at a meal will help stimulate thirst and retain fluids consumed

During Exercise or Competition:

- Drink early and regularly throughout event to sufficiently replace all water lost through sweating
- Amount and rate of fluid replacement depend on individual sweating rate, exercise duration, weather conditions, and opportunities to drink
- Fluids should be cooler than the environmental temperature and flavored to enhance taste and promote fluid replacement

During Exercise or Competition That Lasts More Than 1 Hour:

- Fluid replacement beverage should contain 5–10% carbohydrate to maintain blood glucose levels; sodium and other electrolytes should be included in the beverage in amounts of 0.5–0.7 g of sodium per liter of water to replace the sodium lost by sweating

Following Exercise or Competition:

- Consume about 3 cups of fluid for each pound of body weight lost
- Fluids after exercise should contain water to restore hydration status, carbohydrates to replenish glycogen stores, and electrolytes (for example, sodium and potassium) to speed rehydration
- Consume enough fluid to permit regular urination and to ensure the urine color is very light or light yellow in color; drinking about 125–150% of fluid loss is usually sufficient to ensure complete rehydration

In General:

- Products that contain fructose should be limited, as these may cause gastrointestinal distress
- Caffeine and alcohol should be avoided, as these products increase urine output and reduce fluid retention
- Carbonated beverages should be avoided, as they reduce the desire for fluid intake due to stomach fullness

Source: Adapted from Murray, R. 1997. Drink more! Advice from a world class expert. *ACSM's Health and Fitness Journal* 1:19–23; American College of Sports Medicine Position Stand. 2007. Exercise and fluid replacement. *Med. Sci. Sports Exerc.* 39(2):377–390; Casa, D. J., L. E. Armstrong, S. K. Hillman, S. J. Montain, R. V. Reiff, B. S. E. Rich, W. O. Roberts, and J. A. Stone. 2000. National Athletic Trainers' Association position statement: fluid replacement for athletes. *J. Athlet. Train.* 35:212–224.

amenorrhea Lack of menstruation for at least 3 consecutive months in the absence of pregnancy.

enough calcium to support bone health. If we do not, stress fractures and severe loss of bone can result.

Some female athletes suffer from what is referred to as the female athlete triad (see Chapter 15 for more details). The triad includes three syndromes: disordered eating, menstrual dysfunction, especially **amenorrhea** (lack of menstruation for at least 3 consecutive months in the absence of pregnancy), and osteoporosis. In this triad, nutritional inadequacies from disordered eating behaviors cause irregularities in the menstrual cycle; these in turn cause hormonal disturbances that lead to a significant loss of bone mass. Reduction in bone mass may cause *osteoporosis,* a disease in which the bones become porous and break easily (see page 388). Thus, the athlete is at high risk for fractures. Consuming the recommended amounts of calcium can help prevent osteoporosis. For female athletes who are physically small and consume lower energy intakes, supplementation may be needed to meet current recommendations.

Iron

Iron is a part of the hemoglobin molecule and is critical for the transport of oxygen in our blood to our cells and working muscles. Iron also is involved in energy production. Research has shown that active individuals lose more iron in the sweat, feces, and urine than do inactive individuals and that endurance runners lose iron when their red blood cells break down in their feet due to the high impact of running.[21] Female athletes and non-athletes lose more iron than male athletes because of menstrual blood losses, and females in general tend to eat less iron in their diet. Vegetarian athletes and active people may also consume less iron. Thus, many athletes and active people are at higher risk of iron deficiency. Depending upon its severity, poor iron status can impair athletic performance and our ability to maintain regular physical activity.

Not all athletes suffer from iron deficiency. A phenomenon known as *sports anemia* was identified in the 1960s. Sports anemia is not true anemia, but a transient decrease in iron stores that occurs at the start of an exercise program for some people, and it is also seen in athletes who increase their training intensity. Exercise training increases the amount of water in our blood (called *plasma volume*); however, the amount of hemoglobin does not increase until later into the training period. Thus, the iron content in the blood appears to be low but instead is falsely depressed due to increases in plasma volume. Sports anemia, since it is not true anemia, does not affect performance.

The stages of iron deficiency are described on pages 428–430. In general, it appears that physically active females are at relatively high risk of suffering from the first stage of iron depletion, in which iron stores are low.[22,23] Because of this it is suggested that blood tests of iron stores and monitoring dietary iron intakes be routinely done for active females.[18] In some cases, iron needs cannot be met through the diet, and supplementation is necessary. Iron supplementation should be done with a physician's approval and proper medical supervision.

> RECAP: *Some athletes may have a greater need for certain vitamins and minerals. Active people may need more thiamin, riboflavin, and vitamin B_6 than inactive people. Exercise itself does not increase our calcium needs, but most women, including active women, do not consume enough calcium. Some female athletes suffer from the female athlete triad, a condition that involves the interaction of disordered eating, menstrual dysfunction, and osteoporosis. Many active individuals require more iron, particularly female athletes and vegetarian athletes.*

NUTRI-CASE THEO

" Ever since I did that cycling test in the fitness lab, I've been watching my carbohydrates. Lately, I've been topping 500 g of carbs a day. But now I'm beginning to wonder, am I getting enough protein? I'm starting to feel really wiped out, especially after games. We've won four out of the last five games, and I'm giving it everything I've got, but today I was really dragging myself through practice. I'm eating about 150 g of protein a day, but I think I'm going to try one of those protein powders they sell at my gym. I guess I just feel like, when I'm competing, I need some added insurance."

Theo's weight averages about 190 pounds during basketball season. Given what you've learned about the role of the energy nutrients in vigorous physical activity, what do you think might be causing Theo to feel "wiped out"? Would you recommend that Theo try the protein supplement? What other strategies might be helpful for him to consider?

Are Ergogenic Aids Necessary for Active People?

Many competitive athletes and even some recreationally active people continually search for that something extra that will enhance their performance. **Ergogenic aids** are substances used to improve exercise and athletic performance. For example, nutrition supplements can be classified as ergogenic aids, as can anabolic steroids and other pharmaceuticals. Interestingly, people report using ergogenic aids not only to enhance athletic performance, but also to improve their physical appearance, prevent or treat injuries, treat diseases, and help them cope with stress. Some people even report using them because of peer pressure!

As you have learned in this chapter, adequate nutrition is critical to athletic performance and to regular physical activity, and products such as sports bars and beverages can assist athletes with maintaining their competitive edge. However, as we will explore shortly, many of these products are not effective, some are dangerous, and most are very expensive. For the average consumer, it is virtually impossible to track the latest research findings for these products. In addition, many have not been adequately studied, and unsubstantiated false claims surrounding them are rampant. How can you become a more educated consumer about ergogenic aids?

Lightsey and Attaway describe the most common deceptive practices used to sell ergogenic aids.[24] Although this article was published more than 15 years ago, the practices reviewed are still commonly used, and the article is as timely today as it was when it was published. These practices are identified and discussed in the accompanying Highlight box: Nine Deceptive Practices Used to Market Ergogenic Aids. You should know that, in many cases, research done on a product is misrepresented or is conducted by an inexperienced investigator. It is important that independent laboratories conduct some of the research, as they are more likely to be unbiased. Many companies claim that research is being conducted but state that the findings cannot be shared with the public. This is a warning sign, as there is no need to hide research findings. The use of a celebrity spokesperson is also very common, as celebrity testimonials help to sell products. However, many times this spokesperson is simply being paid to endorse the product and does not actually use it. Finally, it is critical that consumers realize that a patent on a product does not guarantee the effectiveness or safety of that product. Patents are granted solely to distinguish differences among products; indeed, they can be granted for a product that has never been scientifically tested for effectiveness or safety.

New ergogenic aids are available virtually every month, and keeping track of these substances is a daunting task. It is therefore not possible to discuss every available product in this chapter. However, a brief review of a number of currently popular ergogenic aids is provided.

Anabolic substances are often marketed to people wishing to increase muscle size, but many cause harmful side effects.

Anabolic Products Are Touted as Muscle and Strength Enhancers

Many ergogenic aids are said to be **anabolic,** meaning that they build muscle and increase strength. Most anabolic substances promise to increase testosterone, which is the hormone that is associated with male sex characteristics and that increases muscle size and strength. Although some anabolic substances are effective, they are generally associated with harmful side effects.

Anabolic Steroids

Anabolic steroids are testosterone-based drugs that have been used extensively by strength and power athletes. Anabolic steroids are known to be effective in increasing muscle size, strength, power, and speed. These products are illegal in the United States, and their use is banned by all major collegiate and professional sports organizations, in addition to both the U.S. and the International Olympic Committees. Proven long-term and irreversible effects of steroid use include infertility; early clo-

ergogenic aids Substances used to improve exercise and athletic performance.

anabolic Refers to a substance that builds muscle and increases strength.

HIGHLIGHT

Nine Deceptive Practices Used to Market Ergogenic Aids

1. **General misrepresentation of research:**
   - Published research is taken out of context or findings are applied in an unproven manner.
   - Claims that the product is university tested may be true, but the investigator may be inexperienced or the manufacturer may control all aspects of the study.
   - Research may not have been done, but the company falsely claims it has been conducted.

2. **Company claims that research is currently being done:** Although many companies claim they are doing properly controlled research, most are unable to provide specific information about this research.

3. **Company claims that research is not available for public review:** Consumers have a right to obtain proof about performance claims, and there is no rationale to support hiding research findings.

4. **Testimonials:** Celebrities who endorse a product may be doing so only for the money. Testimonials can be faked, bought, and exaggerated. If the product does work for that person, it may be due to the placebo effect, discussed on page 22 (in Chapter 1). The **placebo effect** means that even though a product has been proven to have no physiologic benefits, a person believes so strongly in the product that his or her performance improves. It is estimated that there is a 40% chance that any substance will enhance mental or physical performance through the placebo effect.

5. **Patents:** These are granted to indicate distinguishable differences among products. Patents do not indicate effectiveness or safety of a product and can be given without any research being done on a product.

6. **Inappropriately referenced research:**
   - References may include poorly designed and inadequately controlled studies.
   - The company may refer to research that was published in another country and is not accessible in the United States or may base claims on unsubstantiated rumors or unconfirmed reports.
   - The company may cite outdated research that has been proven wrong or fail to quote studies that do not support their claims.

7. **Media approaches:** Advertising modes include infomercials and mass-media marketing videos. While the Federal Trade Commission (FTC) regulates false claims in advertising, products are generally investigated only if they pose significant danger to the public.

8. **Mail-order fitness evaluations:** Used to attract consumers to the company's products. Most of these evaluations are not specific enough to be useful to the consumer, and their accuracy is highly questionable.

9. **Anabolic measurements:** Some companies perform in-house tests of hair and blood to give consumers information on protein balance. Many times these tests are used inappropriately and only to sell their ergogenic products. The test results may be inaccurate or may indicate nutritional deficiencies that can be remedied with proper nutrition.

Source: All information adapted from Lightsey, D. M., and J. R. Attaway. Deceptive tactics used in marketing purported erogenic aids. *National Strength Conditioning Association Journal.* 14(2), © 1992. National Strength and Conditioining Association. Reprinted by permission of Alliance Communications Group, a division of Allen Press, Inc.

---

sure of the plates of the long bones, resulting in permanent shortened stature; shriveled testicles, enlarged breast tissue (that can be removed only surgically), and other signs of "feminization" in men; enlarged clitoris, facial hair growth, and other signs of "masculinization" in women; increased risk of certain forms of cancer; liver damage; unhealthful changes in blood lipids; hypertension; severe acne; hair thinning or baldness; and depression, delusions, sleep disturbances, and extreme anger (so-called *roid rage*).

Androstenedione and Dehydroepiandrosterone

Androstenedione ("andro") and dehydroepiandrosterone (DHEA) are precursors of testosterone. Manufacturers of these products claim that taking them will increase testosterone levels and muscle strength. As we noted in Chapter 11, androstenedione became very popular after baseball player Mark McGwire claimed he used it during

placebo effect An experience of symptom relief, improved athletic perfromance, or other benefit following the administration of a therapy proven to have no scientific value, and thought to be due to a belief that the therapy is effective.

the time he was breaking home run records. A national survey found that, in 2002, about one of every forty high-school seniors had used it in the past year.[25] Contrary to popular claims, recent studies have found that neither androstenedione nor DHEA increases testosterone levels, and androstenedione has been shown to increase the risk of heart disease in men aged 35 to 65 years.[26] There are no studies that support claims that these products improve strength or increase muscle mass.

Gamma-Hydroxybutyric Acid

Gamma-hydroxybutyric acid, or GHB, has been promoted as an alternative to anabolic steroids for building muscle. The production and sale of GHB have never been approved in the United States; however, it was illegally produced and sold on the black market. For many users, GHB caused only dizziness, tremors, or vomiting, but others experienced severe side effects, including seizures. Many people were hospitalized and some died.

After GHB was banned, a similar product (gamma-butyrolactone, or GBL) was marketed in its place. This product was also found to be dangerous and was removed from the market. Recently, another replacement product called BD, or 1,4-butanediol, was banned because it has caused at least seventy-one deaths, with forty more under investigation. BD is an industrial solvent and is listed on ingredient labels as tetramethylene glycol, butylene glycol, or sucol-B. Side effects include wild, aggressive behavior, nausea, incontinence, and sudden loss of consciousness.

Creatine

Creatine is a supplement that has become wildly popular with strength and power athletes. Creatine, or creatine phosphate, is found in meat and fish and stored in our muscles. As described earlier in this chapter, we use creatine phosphate (or CP) to regenerate ATP. By taking creatine supplements, it is hypothesized that more CP is available to replenish ATP, which will prolong a person's ability to train and perform in short-term, explosive activities such as weight lifting and sprinting. Between 1994 and 2007, more than 700 research articles related to creatine and exercise in humans were published. These studies indicate that creatine does not enhance performance in aerobic-type events, but does enhance sprint performance in swimming, running, and cycling.[26–30] Other studies have shown that creatine increases the work performed and the amount of strength gained during resistance exercise.[29,31,32] Currently, creatine is not banned by any sports governing bodies, and many collegiate sports programs readily provide creatine supplements for their athletes.

In January 2001, the *New York Times* reported that the French government claimed that creatine use could lead to cancer.[33] The news spread quickly across national and international news organizations and over the Internet. These claims were found to be false, as there are absolutely no studies in humans that suggest an increased risk of cancer with creatine use. In fact, there are numerous studies that show an anticancer effect of creatine.[34,35] Although side effects such as dehydration, muscle cramps, and gastrointestinal disturbances have been reported with creatine use, we have very little information on how long-term use of creatine impacts health. A recent study by Schilling and colleagues found that the incidence of muscle cramps, injuries, or other side effects for athletes who had never used creatine was similar to that in those using creatine up to 4 years.[36] Further research is needed to determine the effectiveness and safety of creatine use over prolonged periods of time.

> RECAP: *Ergogenic aids are substances used to improve exercise and athletic performance. Anabolic steroids are effective in increasing muscle size, power, and strength, but they are illegal and can cause serious health consequences. Androstenedione and dehydroepiandrosterone are precursors of testosterone; neither of these products has been shown to effectively increase testosterone levels or to increase strength or muscle mass. Gamma-hydroxybutyric acid and its replacement products have been banned because of severe and sometimes fatal side effects. Creatine supplements are popular and can enhance sprint performance in swimming, running, and cycling. Little is known about their long-term use.*

Some Products Are Said to Optimize Fuel Use During Exercise

Certain ergogenic aids are touted as increasing energy levels and improving athletic performance by optimizing our use of fat, carbohydrate, and protein. The products reviewed here include caffeine, ephedrine, carnitine, chromium, and ribose.

Caffeine

As discussed in Chapter 11, caffeine is a stimulant that makes us feel more alert and energetic, decreasing feelings of fatigue during exercise. Caffeine has been shown to increase the use of fat as a fuel during endurance exercise, which spares muscle glycogen and improves performance.[37,38] It should be recognized that caffeine is a controlled or restricted drug in the athletic world, and athletes can be banned from Olympic competition if urine caffeine levels are too high. However, the amount of caffeine that is banned is quite high, and athletes would need to consume caffeine in pill form to reach this level. Side effects of caffeine use include increased blood pressure, increased heart rate, dizziness, insomnia, headache, and gastrointestinal distress.

Ephedrine

Ephedrine, also known as ephedra, Chinese ephedra, or *ma huang*, is a strong stimulant marketed as a weight-loss supplement and energy enhancer. In reality, many products sold as Chinese ephedra (or herbal ephedra) contain ephedrine from the laboratory and other stimulants such as caffeine. The use of ephedra supplements does not appear to enhance performance, but supplements containing both caffeine and ephedra have been shown to prolong the amount of exercise that can be done until exhaustion is reached.[39] Ephedra is known to reduce body weight and body fat in sedentary women, but its impact on weight loss and body fat levels in athletes is unknown. Side effects of ephedra use include headaches, nausea, nervousness, anxiety, irregular heart rate, and high blood pressure, and at least seventeen deaths have been attributed to its use.[40] As discussed in Chapter 11, it is currently illegal to sell ephedra-containing supplements in the United States.

Ephedrine is made from the herb *Ephedra sinica* (Chinese ephedra).

Carnitine

Carnitine is a compound made from amino acids that is found in the mitochondrial membrane of our cells. Carnitine helps shuttle fatty acids into the mitochondria so they can be used for energy. In theory, it has been proposed that exercise training depletes our cells of carnitine and that supplementation should increase the amount of carnitine in our cell membranes. By increasing cellular levels of carnitine, we should be able to improve the use of fat as a fuel source. Thus, carnitine is marketed not only as a performance-enhancing substance, but also as a "fat burner." Research studies of carnitine supplementation do not support these claims, as neither the transport of fatty acids nor their oxidation appears to be enhanced with supplementation.[41,42] Use of carnitine supplements has not been associated with significant side effects.

Chromium

Chromium is a trace mineral that enhances insulin's action of increasing the transport of amino acids into the cell (see Chapter 10). It is found in whole-grain foods, cheese, nuts, mushrooms, and asparagus. It is theorized that many people are chromium deficient and that supplementation will enhance the uptake of amino acids into muscle cells, which will increase muscle growth and strength. Like carnitine, chromium is marketed as a fat burner, as it is speculated that its effect on insulin stimulates the brain to decrease food intake.[40] Chromium supplements are available as chromium picolinate and chromium nicotinate. Early studies of chromium supplementation showed promise, but more recent, better-designed studies do not support any benefit of chromium supplementation on muscle mass, muscle strength, body fat, or exercise performance.[43]

Ribose

Ribose is a five-carbon sugar that is critical to the production of ATP. Ribose supplementation is claimed to improve athletic performance by increasing work output and by promoting a faster recovery time from vigorous training. While ribose has been shown to improve exercise tolerance in patients with heart disease,[44] several studies have reported that ribose supplementation has no impact on athletic performance.[45–47]

From this review of ergogenic aids, you can see that most of these products are not effective in enhancing athletic performance or in optimizing muscle strength or body composition. It is important to be a savvy consumer when examining these products to make sure you are not wasting your money or putting your health at risk by using them.

> RECAP: *Caffeine is a stimulant that increases the use of fat during exercise; caffeine is a banned substance in the athletic world due to its potential impact on performance. Ephedrine is a stimulant that has been banned from the United States due to its potentially fatal side effects. Carnitine helps shuttle fatty acids into our mitochondria so they can be used for energy. Carnitine supplements do not enhance fat utilization during exercise or improve athletic performance. Chromium is a trace mineral that is marketed as a fat burner, but chromium supplements do not appear to enhance body composition or athletic performance. Ribose supplementation is claimed to increase work output and promote faster recovery time from training, but no studies have yet been done in athletes to support these claims.*

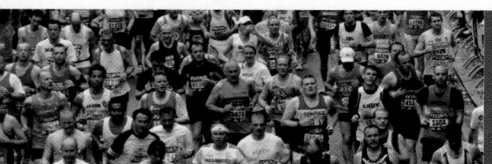

CHAPTER SUMMARY

- Physical activity is any movement produced by muscles that increases energy expenditure. It includes occupational, household, leisure-time, and transportation activities.

- Leisure-time physical activity is any activity not related to a person's occupation and includes competitive sports and recreational activities. Exercise is a subcategory of leisure-time physical activity and is purposeful, planned, and structured.

- Physical fitness has many components and is defined as the ability to carry out daily tasks with vigor and alertness, without undue fatigue, and with ample energy to enjoy leisure-time pursuits and meet unforeseen emergencies.

- Physical activity provides a multitude of health benefits, including reducing our risks for heart disease, stroke, high blood pressure, obesity, type 2 diabetes, and osteoporosis. Despite these benefits, most Americans are inactive.

- The components of fitness include cardiorespiratory fitness, musculoskeletal fitness (which includes muscular strength and endurance), flexibility, and body composition. Physical fitness is specific to each one of these components.

- To achieve the appropriate overload for fitness, the FIT principle should be followed (frequency, intensity, and time of activity). Frequency refers to the number of activity sessions per week. Intensity refers to how difficult the activity is to perform. Time refers to how long each activity session lasts.

- Warm-up, or preliminary exercise, is important to get prepared for exercise. Warm-up exercises prepare the muscles for exertion by increasing blood flow and temperature.

- Cool-down activities are done after an exercise session is complete. Cool-down activities assist in the prevention of injury and may help reduce muscle soreness.

- Adenosine triphosphate, or ATP, is the common energy source for all cells of the body. The amount of ATP stored in a muscle cell is limited and can keep a muscle active for only about 1 to 3 seconds.

- For maximal-effort activities lasting about 3 to 15 seconds, creatine phosphate can be broken down in an anaerobic reaction to provide energy and support the regeneration of ATP.

- To support activities that last from 30 seconds to less than 3 minutes, energy is produced from glycolysis. Glycolysis produces two ATP molecules for every glucose molecule broken down. Pyruvic acid is the final end product of glycolysis.

- The further metabolism of pyruvic acid in the presence of adequate oxygen provides energy for activities that last from 3 minutes to 4 hours. During this aerobic process, each molecule of glucose can yield 36 to 38 ATP molecules.

- Fat can be broken down aerobically to support activities of low intensity and long duration. Fat is an abundant energy source and it provides more than twice the energy per gram as compared to carbohydrate, but its breakdown process is relatively slow, and it cannot support quick, high-intensity activities.

- Amino acids can be used to make glucose to maintain our blood glucose levels during exercise and can contribute from 3–6% of the energy needed during exercise. Amino acids also help build and repair tissues after exercise.

- Vigorous intensity exercise requires extra energy, and male athletes typically need more energy than female athletes because of their higher muscle mass and larger body weight. Athletes who are concerned with making a competitive weight or with the aesthetic demands of their sport may be at risk for poor energy and nutrient intakes.

- It is generally recommended that athletes consume 55–60% of their total energy as carbohydrate.

- Carbohydrate loading involves altering physical training and the diet such that the storage of muscle glycogen is maximized in an attempt to enhance endurance performance.

- A dietary fat intake of 15–25% is generally recommended for athletes, with less than 10% of total energy intake as saturated fat.

- Protein needs can be higher for athletes and regularly active people, but most people in the United States already consume more than twice their daily needs for protein.

- Athletes at risk for low protein intakes include those with low energy intakes, vegetarians or vegans who do not consume high-protein food sources, and young athletes who are growing and not aware of their higher protein needs.

- Regular exercise increases our fluid needs to help cool our internal body temperature and prevent heat illnesses. Heat illnesses include heat syncope, heat cramps, heat exhaustion, and heatstroke. Adequate fluid intake before, during, and after exercise will help prevent heat illnesses.

- Active people may need more thiamin, riboflavin, and vitamin B_6 than inactive people. Most women, including active women, do not consume enough calcium. Many active individuals also require more iron, particularly female athletes and vegetarian athletes.

- Ergogenic aids are substances used to improve exercise and athletic performance, improve physical appearance, prevent or treat injuries, treat diseases, or cope with stress. Many ergogenic aids are not effective, some are dangerous, and most are expensive.

TEST YOURSELF ANSWERS

1. **False.** *Physical activity* refers to any movement produced by muscles that increases energy expenditure, while *exercise* is a subcategory of leisure-time physical activity and refers to activity that is planned, purposeful, and structured.

2. **True.** About 54% of Americans are insufficiently active, and almost 16% report doing no leisure activity at all.

3. **False.** Each person has to design a fitness program based on his or her own interests and needs. Depending upon his or her fitness goals, being active 20 to 30 minutes each day could be enough for a given individual.

4. **False**. Our muscles are not stimulated to grow when we eat extra protein, whether as food or supplements. Weight-bearing exercise appropriately stresses the body and produces increased muscle mass and strength.

5. **True**. Most ergogenic aids are ineffective or do not produce the results that are advertised. Many ergogenic aids, such as anabolic steroids and ephedrine, can actually cause serious health consequences and can even cause death in some instances.

REVIEW QUESTIONS

1. For achieving and maintaining cardiorespiratory fitness, the intensity range typically recommended is
   a. 25–50% of your estimated maximal heart rate.
   b. 35–75% of your estimated maximal heart rate.
   c. 64–90% of your estimated maximal heart rate.
   d. 75–95% of your estimated maximal heart rate.

2. The amount of ATP stored in a muscle cell can keep a muscle active for about
   a. 1 to 3 seconds.
   b. 10 to 30 seconds.
   c. 1 to 3 minutes.
   d. 1 to 3 hours.

3. To support a long afternoon of gardening, the body predominantly uses which nutrient for energy?
   a. carbohydrate
   b. fat
   c. amino acids
   d. lactic acid

4. Creatine
   a. seems to enhance performance in aerobic-type events.
   b. appears to increase an individual's risk for bladder cancer.
   c. seems to increase strength gained in resistance exercise.
   d. is stored in our liver.

5. Athletes participating in an intense athletic competition lasting more than 1 hour should
   a. drink caffeinated beverages to improve their performance while maintaining their hydration.
   b. drink plain warm water copiously both before and during the event in response to fluid losses from sweating and desire to drink.
   c. drink plain ice water both before and during the event in response to thirst.
   d. drink a beverage containing carbohydrate and electrolytes both before and during the event in amounts that balance hydration with energy, carbohydrate, and electrolyte needs.

6. True or false? A sound fitness program overloads the body.

FIND THE QUACK

When Brian joined the track team his first year in high school, he found his passion. Now in his third year of college, he's built a reputation as a winning distance runner, and he has several medals to prove it. One day his friend Jim, who is the track team's top sprinter, tells him about creatine supplements. Jim says that since he started using them several weeks ago, his performance times have improved. With an intercollegiate marathon event approaching, Brian is looking to improve his performance, so he goes online to check out the creatine supplements Web site Jim recommends. Here's what he learns:

- Creatine is an amino acid synthesized by the body that plays a vital role in anaerobic energy production by regenerating ATP in skeletal muscle.

- Creatine supplementation has been shown in several controlled studies to increase muscle stores of creatine and to improve performance in athletes whose sports rely heavily on the creatine phosphate anaerobic energy pathway. (The article cites six recent studies published in academic journals.)

- Creatine supplementation is most effective for performance of intense bursts of activity.

- The manufacturer has on file more than 1,000 testimonials from satisfied customers whose athletic performance improved after taking creatine supplements.

- The recommended dosage for an athlete's "loading phase" varies according to gender, weight, and other factors, but a general recommendation is to consume four to five doses of 5 g each per day, for 5 to 7 days. This will fill the muscles' creatine phosphate stores to capacity. After this, a reduced maintenance dose of approximately 2–5 g/day is recommended. Taken as recommended, the supplements cost as little as $1 a day!

1. Explain what the Web site article means by "the creatine phosphate anaerobic energy pathway."

2. Brian is a distance runner. Would you recommend he purchase creatine supplements? Why or why not?

3. Brian's track teammate Jim is a sprinter. Do you think it's possible that he has experienced physiologic benefits from creatine supplementation, or do you think his increased performance times are due to the placebo effect? Explain.

4. Of the nine deceptive practices used to market ergogenic aids, how many were employed by the creatine supplements Web site? Is this Web site an example of quackery? Why or why not?

Answers can be found at www.aw-bc.com/thompson.

7. True or false? A dietary fat intake of 15–25% is generally recommended for athletes.

8. True or false? Carbohydrate loading involves altering the duration and intensity of exercise and intake of carbohydrate such that the storage of fat is minimized.

9. True or false? Sports anemia is a chronic decrease in iron stores that occurs in some athletes who have been training intensely for several months to years.

10. True or false? FIT stands for frequency, intensity, and time.

11. Write a plan for a weekly activity/exercise routine that does the following:
    a. meets your personal fitness goals
    b. is fun for you to do
    c. includes variety and consistency
    d. uses all components of the FIT principle
    e. includes a warm-up and cool-down period

12. Determine how many grams of carbohydrate, protein, and fat you need to consume daily to support the activity/exercise routine you described in the previous question.

13. You decide to start training for your school's annual marathon. After studying this chapter, which of the following preparation strategies would you pursue, and why?
    a. use of B vitamin supplements
    b. use of creatine supplements
    c. use of sports beverages
    d. carbohydrate loading

14. Given what you have learned about Gustavo in the Nutri-Cases in previous chapters, would you advise him to begin a planned exercise program of low to moderate intensity? Why or why not? If so, what steps should he take before starting an exercise program?

15. Marisa and Conrad are students at the same city college. Marisa walks to and from school each morning from her home seven blocks away. Conrad lives in a suburb 12 miles away and drives to school. Marisa, an early childhood education major, covers the lunch shift, 2 hours a day, at the college's day care center, cleaning up the lunchroom and supervising the children in the playground. Conrad, an accounting major, works in his department office 2 hours a day, entering data into computer spreadsheets. On weekends, Marisa and her sister walk downtown and go shopping. Conrad goes to the movies with his friends. Neither Marisa nor Conrad participates in sports or scheduled exercise sessions. Marisa has maintained a normal, healthful weight throughout the school year, but in the same period of time, Conrad has gained several pounds. Identify at least two factors that might play a role in Marisa's and Conrad's current weight.

WEB LINKS

www.americanheart.org
American Heart Association

The Healthy Lifestyle section of this site has sections on health tools, exercise and fitness, healthy diet, managing your lifestyle, and more.

www.acsm.org
American College of Sports Medicine

Click on "General Public" for guidelines on healthful aerobic activity and calculating your exercise heart rate range. You can also click on the "Fit Society Page" section to access ACSM's Fit Society Page newsletter.

www.mypyramid.gov/pyramid/physical_activity.html
USDA MyPyramid Inside the Pyramid

Visit this site to learn more about physical activity and how to find ways to incorporate more physical activity into your daily life.

www.webmd.com
WebMD Health

Visit this site to learn about a variety of lifestyle topics, including fitness and exercise.

www.hhs.gov
U.S. Department of Health and Human Services

Review this site for multiple statistics on health, exercise, and weight as well as information on supplements, wellness, and more.

http://win.niddk.nih.gov/publications/physical.htm
Weight-control Information Network

Find out more about healthy fitness programs from this Web site produced by the National Institute of Diabetes and Digestive and Kidney Diseases.

http://dietary-supplements.info.nih.gov
NIH Office of Dietary Supplements

Look on this National Institutes of Health site to learn more about the health effects of specific nutritional supplements.

www.nal.usda.gov/fnic/etext/ds_ergogenic.html
Food and Nutrition Information Center

Visit this site for links to detailed information about ergogenic aids and sports nutrition.

http://nutrition.arizona.edu/new
Nutrition Exercise Wellness

Check this University of Arizona site for information for athletes on nutrition, fluid intake, and ergogenic aids.

REFERENCES

1. U.S. Department of Health and Human Services. 1996. *Physical Activity and Health: A Report of the Surgeon General.* Atlanta, GA: U.S. Department of Health and Human Services, Centers for Disease Control and Prevention, National Centers for Chronic Disease Prevention and Health Promotion.

2. Caspersen, C. J., K. E. Powell, and G. M. Christensen. 1985. Physical activity, exercise, and physical fitness: definitions and distinctions for health-related research. *Publ. Health Rep.* 100:126–131.

3. Heyward, V. H. 2002. *Advanced Fitness Assessment and Exercise Prescription,* 4th edn. Champaign, IL: Human Kinetics.

4. Schwartz, A. L., M. Mori, R. Gao, L. M. Nail, and M. E. King. 2001. Exercise reduces daily fatigue in women with breast cancer receiving chemotherapy. *Med. Sci. Sports Exerc.* 33:718–723.

5. Olds, S. B., M. L. London, P. W. Ladewig, and M. R. Davidson. 2003. *Maternal-Newborn Nursing and Women's Health Care,* 7th edn. Upper Saddle River, NJ: Prentice Hall Health.

6. Centers for Disease Control and Prevention (CDC). 2005. Adult participation in recommended levels of physical activity—United States, 2001 and 2003. *Morbid. Mortal. Wkly. Rep.* 54(47):1208–1212.

7. U.S. Department of Health and Human Services. 2000, January. *Healthy People 2010* (conference edn., 2 vols.). Washington, DC: U.S. Department of Health and Human Services.

8. Institute of Medicine, Food and Nutrition Board. 2002. *Dietary Reference Intakes for Energy, Carbohydrates, Fiber, Fat, Protein and Amino Acids (Macronutrients).* Washington, DC: National Academies Press.

9. Brooks, G. A. 2000. Intra- and extra-cellular lactate shuttles. *Med. Sci. Sports Exerc.* 32:790–799.

10. Gladden, L. B. 2000. Muscle as a consumer of lactate. *Med. Sci. Sports Exerc.* 32:764–771.

11. Tarnopolsky, M. 2006. Protein and amino acid needs for training and bulking up. In: Burke, L., and Deakin, V., eds. *Clinical Sports Nutrition,* 3rd edn. Sydney, Australia: McGraw-Hill, pp. 73–98.

12. American College of Sports Medicine, American Dietetic Association, and Dietitians of Canada. 2000. Nutrition and athletic performance. Joint position statement. *Med. Sci. Sports Exerc.* 32:2130–2145.

13. Burke, L. 2006. Nutrition for recovery after competition and training. In: Burke, L., and Deakin, V., eds. *Clinical Sports Nutrition,* 3rd ed. Sydney, Australia: McGraw-Hill, pp. 415–440.

14. Burke, L. M. 1996. Nutrition for post-exercise recovery. *Aust. J. Sci. Med. Sports* 29(1):3–10.

15. Costill, D. L., W. M. Sherman, W. J. Fink, C. Maresh, M. Witten, and J. M. Miller. 1981. The role of dietary carbohydrates in muscle glycogen resynthesis after strenuous running. *Am. J. Clin. Nutr.* 34:1831–1836.

16. van Hall, G., S. M. Shirreffs, and J. A. L. Calbert. 2000. Muscle glycogen resynthesis during recovery from cycle exercise: no effect of additional protein ingestion. *J. Appl. Physiol.* 88:1631–1636.

17. Jentjens, R. L., L. J. C. van Loon, C. H. Mann, A. J. M. Wagenmakers, and A. E. Jeukendrup. 2001. Addition of protein and amino acids to carbohydrates does not enhance postexercise muscle glycogen synthesis. *J. Appl. Physiol.* 91:839–846.

18. Manore, M., and J. Thompson. 2000. *Sports Nutrition for Health and Performance.* Champaign, IL: Human Kinetics.

19. Sears, B. 1995. *The Zone: A Dietary Road Map.* New York: HarperCollins Publishers.

20. National Weather Service Forecast Office. 2006. Heat Index. www.crh.noaa.gov/pub/heat.php.

21. Weaver, C. M., and S. Rajaram. 1992. Exercise and iron status. *J. Nutr.* 122:782–787.

22. Haymes, E. M. 1998. Trace minerals and exercise. In: Wolinsky, I., ed. *Nutrition and Exercise and Sport.* Boca Raton, FL: CRC Press, pp. 1997–2218.

23. Haymes, E. M., and P. M. Clarkson. 1998. Minerals and trace minerals. In: Berming, J. R., and Steen, S. N., eds. *Nutrition and Sport and Exercise.* Gaithersburg, MD: Aspen Publishers, pp. 77–107.

24. Lightsey, D. M., and J. R. Attaway. 1992. Deceptive tactics used in marketing purported ergogenic aids. *Natl. Strength Cond. Assoc. J.* 14:26–31.

25. Food and Drug Administration (FDA). 2004. HHS Launches Crackdown on Products Containing Andro. www.fda.gov/bbs/topics/news/2004/hhs_031104.html. (Accessed July 2007.)

26. Broeder, C. E., J. Quindry, K. Brittingham, L. Panton, J. Thomson, S. Appakondu, K. Breuel, R. Byrd, J. Douglas, C. Earnest, C. Mitchell, M. Olson, T. Roy, and C. Yarlagadda. 2000. The Andro Project: physiological and hormonal influences of androstenedione supplementation in men 35 to 65 years old participating in a high-intensity resistance training program. *Arch. Intern. Med.* 160:3093–3104.

27. Balsom, P. D., K. Söderlund, B. Sjödin, and B. Ekblom. 1995. Skeletal muscle metabolism during short duration high-intensity exercise: influence of creatine supplementation. *Acta Physiol. Scand.* 1154:303–310.

28. Grindstaff, P. D., R. Kreider, R. Bishop, M. Wilson, L. Wood, C. Alexander, and A. Almada. 1997. Effects of creatine supplementation on repetitive sprint performance and body composition in competitive swimmers. *Int. J. Sport Nutr.* 7:330–346.

29. Kreider, R. B., M. Ferreira, M. Wilson, P. Grindstaff, S. Plisk, J. Reinardy, E. Cantler, and A. L. Almada. 1998. Effects of creatine supplementation on body composition, strength, and sprint performance. *Med. Sci. Sports Exerc.* 30:73–82.

30. Tarnopolsky, M. A., and D. P. MacLennan. 2000. Creatine monohydrate supplementation enhances high-intensity exercise performance in males and females. *Int. J. Sport Nutr. Exerc. Metab.* 10:452–463.

31. Kreider, R., M. Ferreira, M. Wilson, and A. L. Almada. 1999. Effects of calcium beta-hydroxy-beta-methylbutyrate (HMB) supplementation during resistance-training on markers of catabolism, body composition and strength. *Int. J. Sports Med.* 20(8):503–509.

32. Volek, J. S., N. D. Duncan, S. A. Mazzetti, R. S. Staron, M. Putukian, A. L. Gomez, D. R. Pearson, W. J. Fink, and W. J. Kraemer. 1999. Performance and muscle fiber adaptations to creatine supplementation and heavy resistance training. *Med. Sci. Sports Exerc.* 31:1147–1156.

33. Reuters. 2001. Creatine use could lead to cancer, French government reports. *New York Times,* January 25.

34. Jeong, K. S., S. J. Park, C. S. Lee, T. W. Kim, S. H. Kim, S. Y. Ryu, B. H. Williams, R. L. Veech, and Y. S. Lee. 2000. Effects of cyclocreatine in rat hepatocarcinogenesis model. *Anticancer Res.* 20(3A):1627–1633.

35. Ara, G., L. M. Gravelin, R. Kaddurah-Daouk, and B. A. Teicher. 1998. Antitumor activity of creatine analogs produced by alterations in pancreatic hormones and glucose metabolism. *In Vivo* 12:223–231.

36. Schilling, B. K., M. H. Stone, A. Utter, J. T. Kearney, M. Johnson, R. Coglianese, L. Smith, H. S. O'Bryant, A. C. Fry, M. Starks, R. Keith, and M. E. Stone. 2001. Creatine supplementation and health variables: a retrospective study. *Med. Sci. Sports Exerc.* 33:183–188.

37. Anderson, M. E., C. R. Bruce, S. F. Fraser, N. K. Stepto, R. Klein, W. G. Hopkins, and J. A. Hawley. 2000. Improved 2000-meter rowing performance in competitive oarswomen after caffeine ingestion. *Int. J. Sport Nutr. Exerc. Metab.* 10:464–475.

38. Spriet, L. L., and R. A. Howlett. 2000. Caffeine. In: Maughan, R. J., ed. *Nutrition in Sport.* Oxford: Blackwell Science, pp. 379–392.

39. Bucci, L. 2000. Selected herbals and human exercise performance. *Am. J. Clin. Nutr.* 72:624S–636S.

40. Williams, M. H. 1998. *The Ergogenics Edge.* Champaign, IL: Human Kinetics.

41. Hawley, J. A. 2002. Effect of increased fat availability on metabolism and exercise capacity. *Med. Sci. Sports Exerc.* 34(9):1485–1491.

42. Heinonen, O. J. 1996. Carnitine and physical exercise. *Sports Med.* 22:109–132.

43. Vincent, J. B. 2003. The potential value and toxicity of chromium picolinate as a nutritional supplement, weight loss agent and muscle development agent. *Sports Med.* 33(3):213–230.

44. Pliml, W., T. von Arnim, A. Stablein, H. Hofmann, H. G. Zimmer, and E. Erdmann. 1992. Effects of ribose on exercise-induced ischaemia in stable coronary artery disease. *Lancet* 340(8818):507–510.

45. Earnest, C. P., G. M. Morss, F. Wyatt, A. N. Jordan, S. Colson, T. S. Church, Y. Fitzgerald, L. Autrey, R. Jurca, and A. Lucia. 2004. Effects of a commercial herbal-based formula on exercise performance in cyclists. *Med. Sci. Sports Exerc.* 36(3):504–509.

46. Hellsten, Y., L. Skadhauge, and J. Bangsbo. 2004. Effect of ribose supplementation on resynthesis of adenine nucleotides after intense intermittent training in humans. *Am. J. Physiol. Regul. Integr. Comp. Physiol.* 286:R182–R188.

47. Kreider, R. B., C. Melton, M. Greenwood, C. Rasmussen, J. Lundberg, C. Earnest, and A. Almada. 2003. Effects of oral D-ribose supplementation on anaerobic capacity and selected metabolic markers in healthy males. *Int. J. Sport Nutr. Exerc. Metab.* 13(1):76–86.

48. King, A. C., W. L. Haskell, C. B. Taylor, H. C. Kraemer, and R. F. DeBusk. 1991. Group- vs. home-based exercise training in healthy older men and women: a community-based clinical trial. *JAMA* 266:1535–1542.

49. Kohrt, W. M., M. T. Malley, A. R. Coggan, R. J. Spina, T. Ogawa, A. A. Ehsani, R. E. Bourey, W. H. Martin, 3rd, and J. O. Holloszy. 1991. Effects of gender, age, and fitness level on response of Vo_{2max} to training in 60–71 yr olds. *J. Appl. Physiol.* 71:2004–2011.

50. LaCroix, A. Z., S. G. Leveille, J. A. Hecht, L. C. Grothaus, and E. H. Wagner. 1996. Does walking decrease the risk of cardiovascular disease hospitalizations and death in older adults? *J. Am. Geriatr. Soc.* 44:113–120.

51. Blair, S. N., H. W. Kohl III, C. E. Barlow, R. S. Paffenbarger Jr., L. W. Gibbons, and C. A. Macera. 1995. Changes in physical fitness and all-cause mortality: a prospective study of healthy and unhealthy men. *JAMA* 273:1093–1098.

52. Paffenbarger, R. S., Jr., R. T. Hyde, A. L. Wing, and C.-C. Hsieh. 1986. Physical activity, all-cause mortality, and longevity of college alumni. *N. Engl. J. Med.* 314:605–613.

53. Leon, A. S., J. Connett, D. R. Jacobs Jr., and R. Rauramaa. 1987. Leisure-time physical activity levels and risk of coronary heart disease and death: the Multiple Risk Factor Intervention Trial. *JAMA* 258:2388–2395.

54. Slattery, M. L., D. R. Jacobs Jr., and M. Z. Nichaman. 1989. Leisure-time physical activity and coronary heart disease death: the U.S. Railroad Study. *Circulation* 79:304–311.

55. Helmrich, S. P., D. R. Ragland, R. W. Leung, and R. S. Paffenbarger Jr. 1991. Physical activity and reduced occurrence of non-insulin-dependent diabetes mellitus. *N. Engl. J. Med.* 325:147–152.

How Much Physical Activity Is Enough?

Y our aerobics instructor tells you to work out at your target heart rate for 20 minutes a day, whereas your doctor tells you to walk for half an hour three or four times a week. A magazine article exhorts you to work out to the point of exhaustion, while a new weight-loss book claims that you can be perfectly healthy without ever breaking a sweat. And as if these mixed messages about what constitutes "regular physical activity" weren't enough, a recent report from the Institute of Medicine, which contributed to the 2005 revision of the Dietary Guidelines for Americans, has inadvertently added to the confusion. In this report, it is recommended that Americans should be active 60 minutes per day to optimize health.[8] This message appears contradictory to the Surgeon General's report published in 1996, in which it was recommended that Americans need to accumulate 30 minutes of physical activity on most, if not all, days of the week to optimize health.[1]

The publication of the report by the Institute of Medicine resulted in an immediate firestorm of responses from various health organizations condemning the recommendations. A similar response greeted the publication in 2005 of the revised Dietary Guidelines for Americans, which included some of the Institute of Medicine recommendations. The primary concern of these organizations was that consumers would be confused about how much physical activity was enough and that this confusion would result in frustration and lead to people giving up on participating in any physical activity. Another concern was that 60 minutes of physical activity each day is too much to ask a population in which over half are already insufficiently active.

So how much activity is really enough? To try to answer this question, let's take a closer look at how the reports of the Surgeon General and Institute of Medicine differ. The Surgeon General's report considers a combination of what we have learned from exercise training studies and from population-based epidemiological studies. *Exercise training studies* involve taking individuals, putting them through a clearly defined training program, and assessing fitness and health outcomes. These studies consistently show that less fit and older individuals can significantly improve their cardiorespiratory fitness and reduce their risk for chronic diseases by participating in moderate levels of physical activity.[48,49] In contrast, *population-based epidemiological studies* compare self-reports of physical activity and/or fitness to rates of illness and mortality.[50,51] In other words, the direct effect of exercise training is not being assessed in these studies; instead, they assess only the relationship between level of physical activity/fitness and rates of disease and premature death. These studies show that unfit, sedentary people suffer from the highest rates of disease and premature mortality and that increased physical activity significantly correlates to decreased risks for chronic diseases and premature mortality.

One challenge highlighted in the Surgeon General's report was how to determine the exact dose of exercise needed to improve physical fitness and health. The authors of this report clearly state that using epidemiological studies to determine this dose is problematic. However, some studies indicate that expending an average of 150 kcal/day, which is equivalent to about 30 minutes of moderate physical activity per day, is associated with significant reductions in disease risk and premature mortality.[52–55] This information was used to shape the recommendations put forth in the Surgeon General's report. It is important to emphasize that these recommendations are intended for individuals who are currently inactive. They are not intended to apply to individuals who are already physically active and doing more activity that results in moderate to high fitness levels. In fact, the Surgeon General's report emphasizes that additional health and fitness benefits will result by doing more moderate-intensity physical activity or by substituting vigorous physical activities for those that are moderate in intensity.

In contrast, the Institute of Medicine based their physical activity recommendations on the assumption of a healthful energy balance, in which energy intake should

Older and less fit individuals can improve their health and physical fitness with moderate daily activity.

be equal to the energy expenditure associated with maintaining a healthful body weight. Thus, this group of experts examined studies that measured the amount of energy people expend to maintain a BMI of 18.5 to 25 kg/m^2. After reviewing a large number of studies that assessed energy expenditure and BMI, the Institute of Medicine concluded that participating in about 60 minutes of moderately intense physical activity per day will move people from a very sedentary to an active lifestyle and will allow them to maintain a healthful body weight.

Although this recommendation appears to be very different from that from the Surgeon General's report, and may seem unrealistic, the Institute of Medicine emphasizes that this recommendation includes all activities a person does above resting levels, including gardening, dog walking, housekeeping, and shopping.

So are these two recommendations really that different? Probably not. The Surgeon General's recommendation is based on associations among self-reported physical activity levels, physical fitness levels, and disease and mortality rates. Its report clearly states that 30 minutes per day, most days of the week, is the minimum amount of physical activity recommended to improve physical fitness and optimize health. The Institute of Medicine's recommendation is based on studies that precisely determined an energy expenditure associated with a healthful body weight. Its report more clearly defines how much physical activity is needed to maintain a healthful weight and does not focus specifically on disease risk or premature

mortality. It is commonly recognized by nutrition and exercise experts and other health professionals that weight loss and healthful weight maintenance is easier to achieve in people who do more physical activity each day, not less.

So how much physical activity is enough for you? To answer this question, you must determine what your fitness goals are and how you can best achieve them. For weight loss and maintenance of weight loss and to train for athletic competition, you will need to be active for at least 60 minutes each day to achieve your goals. To move from a sedentary to a relatively fit person and to improve your health status, doing at least 30 minutes of moderate physical activity each day will be sufficient. Thus, there is no one right answer to this question for everyone. By considering your health status, current fitness level, personal interests, the time you have available, and your fitness goals, you can determine the right amount of physical activity to meet your goals.

The amount of daily physical activity you should participate in is determined by your personal fitness goals.

CHAPTER 14

TEST YOURSELF TRUE OR FALSE?

1. All stress is bad for your health and should be eliminated. T or F

2. Chronic stress increases your risk for heart disease. T or F

3. Many everyday situations can cause you to feel stressed. T or F

4. Good time management can help you manage stress. T or F

5. Your personality has no effect on your level of stress. T or F

Test Yourself answers can be found after the Chapter Summary.

Stress Management

do you tend to get sick during finals, or do you have difficulty sleeping when a big term paper is due? Does a fight with your boyfriend or girlfriend leave you unfocused? Do you feel muscle tension while sitting frustrated in rush-hour traffic? These familiar, everyday situations often lead to stress and the negative physical symptoms associated with stress. On the other hand, you may have noticed that if you do not feel some stress before a test, competition or performance, you do not do your best. A certain amount of stress is good. The goal is not to eliminate all stress, but to manage it well so it does not have a negative impact on your health and performance.

Have you thought about the specific physical responses your body undergoes during a period of stress? Are you aware of the potential long-term effects stress can have on your health? We will discuss these topics and more in this chapter as we analyze the complex topics of stress and stress management.

Taken from: *Total Fitness Update, Media Update,* Fifth Edition, by Scott K. Powers, Stephen L. Dodd, Erica M. Jackson

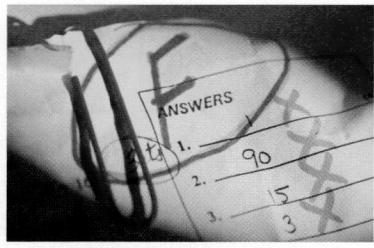

CONSIDER THIS!
In one survey, 33% of students experienced stress to the point that their academic performance was negatively affected.

stress A state of physical and mental tension in response to a situation that is perceived as a threat or challenge.

stressor A factor that produces stress.

stress response The physiological and behavioral changes that take place when a person is presented with a stressor.

eustress A stress level that results in improved performance; also called *positive stress.*

distress Negative stress that is harmful to performance.

What Are Stress and the Stress Response?

Most people are familiar with the term *stress*, but few are aware of its precise definition. Let's find out how scientists define the term.

Defining Stress

During **stress,** the body is in a state of mental and physical tension, and the balance (homeostasis) of the body's systems is disrupted. Stress is caused by one or more **stressors,** which can be physical (such as an injury) or mental (such as emotional distress resulting from a personal relationship). Regardless of the nature of the stressor, the body's physiological and mental responses usually include feelings of strain, tension, and anxiety. Our bodies' reactions to stress, called the **stress response,** prepare us to deal with stressors so balance can be restored. People are stressed by numerous stressors during daily life, and different people are stressed by different things. For example, you might find a long commute to work stressful, but someone else might enjoy the alone time.

There are different classifications of stressors, and each can affect our behaviors, health, and life. Stressors can be acute (such as the death of a loved one), cumulative (such as a series of events that lead to a breakup with a boyfriend or girlfriend), or chronic (such as daily job- or school-related pressures). Although it is clear that chronic or extreme stress is unhealthy, some degree of stress is required to maximize performance. For any type of "performance" activity there is an optimal level of stress that pushes us to perform and excel. This level is specific to the individual, and it is motivating and energizing. Stress that is positive and that is associated with improved performance is called **eustress.**

Although some level of stress is desirable and beneficial, too much stress or poorly managed stress can have a negative impact on health and lead to poor performance and decisions. This idea is illustrated in FIGURE 14.1. When we are out of the range that leads to optimal performance, stress can have a negative impact. This negative stress is called **distress.** For example, regular exercise can be described as a positive stressor. However, regular exercise at very high frequency or intensity increases the risk for injury and emotional tension, and it can be considered a negative stressor because performance often suffers.

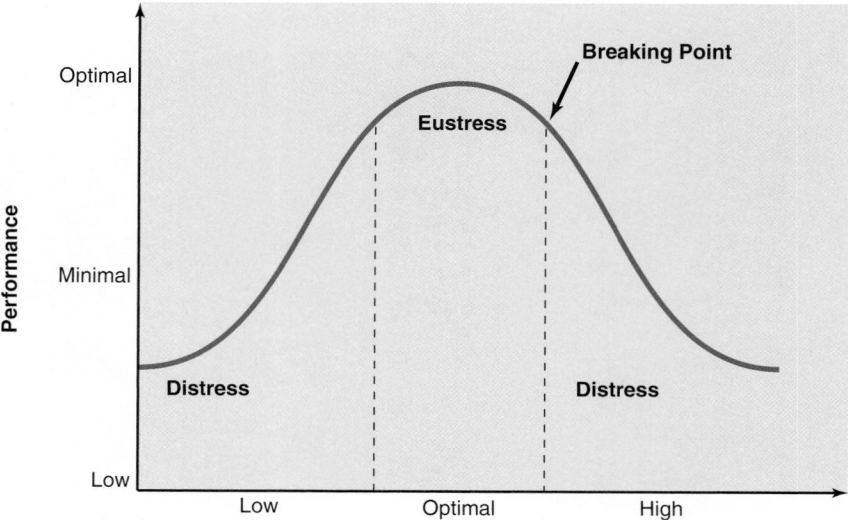

FIGURE 14.1 Eustress is positive stress that helps you achieve optimal performance. Distress (negative stress) hurts performance. Too much or too little stress also hurts performance.

Physiological Changes of the Stress Response

You are driving home, and another driver runs a stop sign and just barely misses hitting your car. Your body will have a set of predictable reactions to this acute stressor: Your heart rate increases, your senses heighten, and **endorphins** are released, to name a few of the changes that take place. These reactions are part of the stress response. The body's responses to stress are mediated by an area in the brain called the *hypothalamus* and are initiated when the hormones **epinephrine, norepinephrine**, and **cortisol** are released into the bloodstream. The hormones cause a number of physiological changes, some of which are illustrated in FIGURE 14.2. Hence the two body systems primarily responsible for the changes that occur during the stress response are the *nervous system* and the **endocrine system.**

Your nervous system controls both your voluntary movements (such as your raising your hand in class) and your involuntary bodily processes (such as your heartbeat and digestion). The involuntary actions are controlled by the **autonomic nervous system.** There are two branches of the autonomic nervous system, the **parasympathetic** branch and the **sympathetic** branch. The parasympathetic branch is in control of body processes and functions when you are relaxed or resting. Maintaining your resting heart rate and blood pressure, growth, digestion, and storing energy are examples of processes under control of the parasympathetic nervous system. The sympathetic branch is the excitatory division of the autonomic nervous system. This branch is activated when you need to react and produce energy. The increase in heart rate, faster breathing, perspiration, and initial release of epinephrine are some of the changes produced by the activation of the sympathetic division.

As part of the stress response, the sympathetic nervous system activates the endocrine system, which in turn releases hormones. The main stress hormone

endorphins A group of hormones (endogenous opioids, or "painkillers") released during the stress response.

epinephrine A hormone secreted by the inner core (medulla) of the adrenal gland; also called *adrenaline*.

norepinephrine A hormone secreted by the inner core (medulla) of the adrenal gland.

cortisol A hormone secreted by the outer layer (cortex) of the adrenal gland.

endocrine system Series of glands and tissues in the body that secrete hormones to regulate bodily processes.

autonomic nervous system The branch of the nervous system that controls basic bodily functions that do not require conscious thought; includes the parasympathetic and sympathetic branches.

parasympathetic branch The division of the autonomic nervous system that is dominant at rest and controls the energy conservation and restoration processes.

sympathetic branch The division of the autonomic nervous system that is in control when we need to react or respond to challenges; the excitatory branch.

Eyes
Pupils dilate so vision is better

Lungs
Lungs dilate for increased air movement

Liver
Sugar is released to provide energy

Stored Fat
Stored fat is broken down for energy

Skin
Perspiration increases for better cooling

Brain
Endorphins released to block pain

Ears
Hearing becomes more acute

Heart
Increased heart rate for improved circulation and breathing

Digestive System
Sphincters relax and digestion stops

Spleen
Spleen releases more red blood cells

Blood
Blood vessels constrict and blood pressure increases

FIGURE 14.2 The body's physiological responses to stress.

released by the system is cortisol. This hormone is more predominant during distress and prolonged stress situations. Cortisol helps make glucose and break down fat for energy, increase the production of epinephrine and norepinephrine, and suppress an immune response.

The Fight-or-Flight Response

Together the responses of the autonomic nervous system and the endocrine system make up the **fight-or-flight response.** This initial response to stress was first discovered by Harvard physiologist Walter Canon (1) and later elaborated on by the biologist Hans Selye (2). Canon described the stress response as an inborn, automatic, and primitive response designed to prepare individuals to face (fight) or run away (flight) from any type of perceived threat or challenge to survival. According to Canon, once a person perceives a threat, the brain initiates a sequence of physiological and physical changes that ready the body for action. However, the challenge does not have to be a matter of life or death. The stressors we are presented with in everyday life can also evoke the fight-or-flight response.

Imagine you are at home asleep and the telephone rings. You answer the phone and hear your professor's voice asking why you did not take the final exam. You look at your clock and realize you overslept and missed class! Suddenly your heart is racing, you are sweating profusely, your blood pressure rises, and your hands become cold and clammy. These responses prepare you to deal with the threatening or stressful situation. Do you try to explain the situation to your professor (fight) or quickly hang up and never return to school again (flight)?

Your body has "activation" responses to enable you to fight or flee (Figure 14.2). In addition to the changes already mentioned, blood is directed away from the digestive tract and redirected into the muscles to provide extra energy for fighting or fleeing. You will have an increased awareness of your surroundings, quickened impulses, and diminished pain perception. Your body physically and mentally prepares to "battle" the stressor. After you successfully cope with your stressor or no longer perceive it as threatening, the body returns to homeostasis. However, if the situation is not resolved, you will stay in this aroused state.

During the fight-or-flight response, people are in an "attack mode" and are focused on short-term "survival." Primitive people were required to exert physical activity while fighting or fleeing from wild animals, and physical exertion related to the act of fighting or fleeing would rid the body of excess levels of stress hormones, allowing it to return to homeostasis. However, today's modern stressors, such as congested roads, too few parking spaces, missing an exam, bouncing a check, or having an argument with your significant other, do not typically require physical exertion. People living highly stressful lives can experience chronic stress in which they have some level of arousal from stress almost constantly. There is often no release from these stressors in the form of physical exertion, and over time the stress hormones accumulate in the body, causing illness and chronic disease. We'll discuss the relationship between chronic stress and disease later in the chapter.

Make sure you know . . .

- Stress is a mental and physical response to situations we perceive as pressures or challenges.

- Stressors can come from many sources, and they can be positive (eustress) or negative (distress). Some degree of stress is required to maximize performance.

- The autonomic nervous system and the endocrine system are responsible for the changes that occur during the stress response. The parasympathetic branch of the autonomic nervous system is in control at rest, and the sympathetic branch is activated when you need to react. Cortisol is the main stress hormone produced by the endocrine system.

- The changes in the body that occur during the stress response prepare our bodies to fight or flee the stressful situation. These responses are collectively referred to as the fight-or-flight response.

fight-or-flight response A series of physiological reactions by the body to prepare to combat a real or perceived threat.

What Factors Affect Your Stress Level?

Although everyone feels stress, life events and situations do not affect everyone the same way. Our personalities, past experiences, and gender are three influences on the way we perceive situations and cope with stress. For example, your grandmother who recently recovered from a hip fracture might experience stress when she enters a setting with a lot of stairs and uneven terrain. However, as a young healthy adult, you do not find that environment threatening. You might have the tendency to freak out during finals, whereas your roommate remains calm. We will discuss some of the factors that impact your ability to handle stressful situations next.

Personality Behavior Patterns

People's different reactions to the same stressful situation can be due to personality differences and how they have learned to respond.

There are many different ways to describe personalities and behavior patterns. Note that although there is no one specific (or completely reliable) way of identifying stress-prone personality patterns, one of the most common, and easily interpreted, classification groupings describes individuals as having characteristics that fit into one of four behavior pattern categories: Type A, Type B, Type C, and Type D (Table 14.1). This classification system describes the four most common behavior patterns.

People who exhibit Type A behavior pattern (TABP) are highly motivated, time-conscious, hard-driving, impatient, and sometimes hostile, cynical, and angry. They have a heightened response to stress, and their hostility and anger, especially if repressed, place them at a greater risk for heart disease (3, 4). Individuals with Type B behavior pattern are easygoing, nonaggressive, and patient, and they are not prone to hostile episodes like their TABP counterparts. People with Type B behavior pattern are less likely to perceive everyday annoyances as significant stressors and are at low risk for heart disease from stress.

Most people have heard of TABP and Type B behavior pattern, but you might not be familiar with the other behavior patterns. People with Type C behavior pattern have many of the positive qualities of TABP. They are confident, highly motivated, and competitive. However, individuals with Type C behavior pattern typically do not express the hostility and anger seen with TABP, and they use their personality characteristics to maintain a constant level of emotional control and to channel their ambition into creative directions. People with Type C behavior pattern have the positive characteristics of TABP but do not express their negative emotions and feelings in the same manner. As a result, individuals with Type C behavior pattern experience the same low risk for stress-related heart disease as do those with Type B behavior pattern. However, a person with Type C behavior pattern who keeps emotions in and does not express them can face a higher risk for heart disease.

TABLE 14.1 Personality Behavior Patterns and Their Risks for Heart Disease

Personality Behavior Pattern	Qualities	Risk for Heart Disease
A	Impatient, competitive, aggressive, highly motivated, and sometimes hostile	High
B	Patient, with low aggression, and easygoing	Low
C	Competitive, highly motivated, high level of confidence, and constant level of emotional control	Low
D	Negative, anxious, worried, and socially inhibited	High

CONSIDER THIS!
About 15% of college students say their academic performance has been impaired because of Internet use or computer games.

Individuals with Type D behavior pattern also are considered to be at greater risk for stress-related disease. These individuals are prone to worry and anxiety and also tend to be socially inhibited and uneasy when interacting with others. Their social clumsiness results in a chronic state of anxiety, which places them at greater risk for heart disease (5, 6). You can see a summary of the different personality behavior patterns, and their corresponding risks for heart disease, in Table 14.1.

Past Experiences

Discovering aspects of one's personality can be interesting and entertaining, but we must keep in mind that ultimately it is our perception of a stressor and the way we react to it that will determine any resulting health effects. We learn from our experiences, and what we learn can help us respond more positively in future situations. For example, finals time is a common stressor. You would expect a person with TABP to be extremely stressed during the time leading up to finals. However, a person with TABP who has learned that too much stress leads to unfocused study time and poor grades might plan to manage and structure study time weeks in advance to avoid the last-minute stress. Likewise, a student with type B behavior who performed poorly in the past because she was too relaxed during finals and did not prepare well might learn to prepare more diligently for future finals to improve her performance.

Gender

Gender is another factor that impacts the way we react to stressors. There are no sex differences in the physiological responses to stress, but gender might affect the way we perceive situations and how we react to stressors. For example, our society has traditionally deemed it more acceptable for women to express their emotions openly. Therefore, a woman might feel more comfortable discussing stressors and be better able to cope with them than a man who has been socialized to "keep his feelings in." Conversely, a woman might have been taught that certain responses, such as explosive anger, are not "ladylike" and therefore refrain from expressing her anger, leading to greater stress. Participating in activities outside traditional gender roles also might produce stress. A man who decides to be a stay-at-home dad or work from home so his wife can pursue her career, for example, might experience higher levels of stress because his choice does not fit with societal norms. Gender-related reactions to stress also might vary in different cultures.

Regardless of your personality characteristics, past experiences, and gender, you can learn ways to deal with the stress in your life, and the first step is to examine your stress level. A convenient way to do this is to complete a questionnaire designed to evaluate your stress level, such as Laboratory 14.1. If the results suggest that you are under unhealthy levels of stress, you should implement stress management and stress reduction techniques.

Common Causes of Stress

Recognizing the everyday life situations that contribute to your stress level is important in managing stress. The pressure of performing well in your classes, along with competing deadlines for papers, projects, and tests, can be a source of stress, especially if you do not have strong time management skills. Choosing a major and planning for your future after graduation are also stressful processes. Making use of career services and talking with your professors and faculty advisors can help you find the best options for your strengths and interests.

Interpersonal relationships often change when you enter college. If you move to go to college, getting connected within the college community and developing new relationships can be a source of stress. Leaving family and friends also can be a challenge. If you did not have to move, your existing relationships still might be affected as you balance your time with schoolwork, new friends, and other responsibilities of college life.

Financial responsibilities can be a source of stress in many stages of life. Costs associated with college tuition, fees, and books are high, and you may have to rely on student loans to assist with college expenses. Work-study and other college programs can relieve some of the financial burden but place additional demands on your already limited time. Maybe you are among the many students who have to work during the school year and summers to make money for school. These work demands can be a significant source of stress, because they affect relationships, time, and schoolwork. Also, when selecting your major, you have to consider job opportunities and earning potential of the career paths that interest you. The need to attend graduate school or take low-paying or nonpaying internships can further add to financial strain and stress. Budgeting and planning for expenses are important skills to develop. Avoiding credit card debt also reduces stress of the financial burden of college.

Other common college stressors include traffic, parking on campus, and adjusting to college life. (See the Closer Look box on page 568 for a discussion of road rage, one common source of traffic stress). Students who are married with families have the combined stresses of managing home and family responsibilities with the demands of school. Nontraditional students—for example, people who have returned to school after several years—may feel out of place and experience additional stress related to those feelings. In addition to balancing the demands of school, work, and relationships, some students engage in leisure activities, such as spending time on the Internet, which affect productivity and, in turn, may lead to stress. Students with disabilities are likely to face stressors in learning to navigate a college campus that might not adequately accommodate their specific disabilities.

College life comes with stressors from many sources.

Make sure you know . . .

- Personality can impact the way we perceive situations and respond to stress. Type A and Type D behavior patterns are associated with higher risk for heart disease.

- Past experiences and gender also influence our reactions to situations we perceive as stressful.

- College life can present many stressors. Some of the most common include academic responsibilities, poor time management, the demands of relationships, and finances.

Stress and Health

Chronic (persistent) stress is related to some of the most significant health problems in the United States. Heart disease, depression, and migraines are all associated with stress and have significant direct and indirect health care costs. Stress is a risk factor for depression and anxiety, and up to 25% of the U.S. adult population suffers from these and other mental health problems every year (7). Approximately 75–90% of all physician visits are for stress-related complaints, and millions of people take medication for stress-related illnesses (8). From a medical standpoint, stress can affect both emotional and physical health. Chronic stress has been linked to elevated blood pressure, heart disease, hormonal imbalances, reduced resistance to disease, and emotional disorders (9–11) (FIGURE 14.3).

Stress-related problems cost both businesses and government billions of dollars every year in the form of employee absenteeism and health care costs. Stress can suppress the immune system, making a person more susceptible to illness. Acute stress also can impact productivity. Headaches and tension might cause a person to miss work or class or be less focused. Therefore, stress is a major health problem that affects individual lives and the economy as a whole.

FIGURE 14.3 Chronic stress can have negative effects on both physical and mental health.

general adaptation syndrome A pattern of responses to stress that consists of an alarm stage, a resistance stage, and an exhaustion stage.

Hans Selye developed one of the earliest scientific theories to explain the relationship between stress and disease. Selye proposed that humans adapt to stress in a response he termed the **general adaptation syndrome,** which involves three stages: an alarm stage, a resistance stage, and an exhaustion stage (2).

During the alarm stage, the fight-or-flight response, discussed earlier, occurs. There is a release of the stress hormones, and their effects on the body can cause anxiety, headaches, and disrupted patterns of sleeping and eating (2). During this phase, the body is more susceptible to disease and more prone to injury.

With continued exposure to stress, the individual reaches the resistance stage. During this stage, the body's resistance to stress is higher than normal, and mechanisms are activated that allow the body to resist disease effectively. In short, the resistance stage represents an improved ability to cope with stress (2).

However, if the stress persists, the individual reaches the exhaustion stage. Note that "exhaustion" in this sense refers to the depletion of the physical and psychological resources to cope with stress that occurs with chronic exposure to stress. Selye suggests that the body is vulnerable to disease during this stage because the resources for responding to stress are depleted. During this phase, physical symptoms that appeared in the alarm stage can reappear, but they now are more serious and can sometimes compromise health.

A CLOSER LOOK

Road Rage

WHAT IS ROAD RAGE?

Road rage refers to extreme acts of aggression resulting from disagreements between drivers. Typical road rage behaviors include tailgating, headlight flashing, obscene gestures, deliberately blocking other vehicles, verbal abuse, and its most extreme form—physical assault. According to estimates, aggressive driving injures or kills at least 1500 people each year. Road rage is a serious problem and a criminal offense.

WHAT CAUSES ROAD RAGE?

For many of us, driving is our most stressful daily activity. Roadways are crowded, and we must deal with all levels of drivers—good and bad. Everyone makes traffic mistakes at times, whether intentionally or unintentionally. Often, road rage starts as a simple misunderstanding between drivers and then escalates into a more serious situation. Usually, the driving incident is not the immediate cause of anger. For some, mounting professional or personal troubles, plus

frustration over another driver's "stupid" mistakes, is enough to cause them to erupt in anger. Drivers in a "bad mood" before they get behind the wheel are more likely to have strong reactions to the actions of other drivers. Researchers believe that some personality characteristics are more prone to aggressive driving.

If you drive aggressively, the following tips can help you reduce your traffic stress:

- Avoid driving during times of heaviest congestion.
- Allow yourself plenty of time so you do not have to speed, run traffic lights, or roll through stop signs.
- Drive in comfort. Use your air conditioner, get a comfortable seat cover, and listen to classical music during your drive. Do not listen to emotionally stimulating radio talk shows. Enjoy audio books.
- Do not drive when you are angry or upset.
- When in traffic, concentrate on being relaxed. Practice breathing for relaxation.

Although Selye's model of adaptation to stress is still viewed as an important contribution to our understanding of the stress response, newer research findings have improved our understanding of the relationship between stress and disease. We now know that the underlying cause of many stress-related diseases is the body's inability to respond to stress the normal way, not because of depletion of resources. The repeated and/or prolonged response to stress results in the continual activation of the nervous, endocrine, and immune systems. This long-term activation includes the continual release of stress hormones, including cortisol.

The ideas of **allostasis** and **allostatic load** are better explanations of the relationship between stress and disease. Allostasis refers to the body's ability to change and adapt in stressful situations. With long-term stress, we do not adapt as well. The allostatic load is the point at which there is too much stress, which taxes the system's stress response (12). The constant level of activation or the repeated activation causes stress response to become inefficient.

allostasis The ability to maintain homeostasis through change.

allostatic load The inability to respond appropriately to stress; leads to compromised health.

STEPS FOR BEHAVIOR CHANGE

How Well Do You Manage Your Time?

Take the quiz below to find out whether you are a good time manager.

Y   N

☐   ☐   Do you procrastinate?

☐   ☐   Do you take on more responsibilities than you can handle?

☐   ☐   Are you consistently late for class, appointments, or work?

☐   ☐   Do you need more hours in the day to accomplish all of your daily tasks?

☐   ☐   Do you have little time for fun with friends or family?

If you answered yes to most or all of these questions, you can probably use some tips for better time management.

Tips to Improve Your Time Management Skills, Reduce Stress, and Increase Productivity

☑ Plan ahead. Plan your day by using a PDA or daily planner to organize tasks. Make a schedule you are able to implement, and allow time for unscheduled events and delays.

☑ Delegate responsibility. If you are involved with clubs or group projects, share and delegate responsibility to lower stress. Also, learn to say no to activities that prevent you from achieving your goals. Before accepting a new responsibility, complete your current task or eliminate an unnecessary project.

☑ Establish goals. Establish a list of goals you plan to accomplish. Include short- and long-term goals.

☑ Prioritize. List your tasks in order of their importance (high priority to low priority), and then follow that list. Establish a daily goal of accomplishing the three most important tasks on your priority list.

☑ Schedule time for you. Find time each day to relax and do something you enjoy. Regularly evaluate your ratio of work time to home and leisure time, and make sure you maintain balance.

STEPS FOR BEHAVIOR CHANGE

Are You Getting Enough Sleep?

Making sure that you get enough sleep will help you effectively deal with your daily stressors and may also help improve your grades. Answer these questions to find out whether you are getting enough sleep.

Y N

☐ ☐ Do you fall asleep as soon as your head hits the pillow?

☐ ☐ Do you find yourself dozing in class or at other inappropriate times of the day?

☐ ☐ Do you frequently take naps during the day?

☐ ☐ Do you have an irregular bedtime?

☐ ☐ Do you "binge" sleep on the weekend?

☐ ☐ Do you have difficulty waking in the morning?

If you answered yes to more than two of the above questions, you may not be getting enough sleep at night.

Tips to Help You Get Consistent, Restful Sleep

☑ Avoid drinking caffeinated beverages after 4:00 PM.

☑ Avoid stimulating reading or television/movies in the evening. Instead, try meditating or listening to soothing music to help you unwind and relax.

☑ Keep a regular bedtime.

☑ Avoid disrupting your regular sleep pattern. Long naps during the day and using the weekend to play "catch up" on sleep missed during the week can disrupt sleep patterns.

☑ Use bright light in the morning to help you wake up.

☑ Sleep in a comfortable environment. A cool, dark room with little noise is recommended for a good night of sleep.

One's risk of developing a stress-related illness increases because high levels of cortisol in the blood impair the immune system's ability to fight infections over time (12–15). As you have realized by now, prolonged stress places an individual at greater risk for illness and other associated problems. As a result, understanding and implementing stress management skills are important for maintaining a high level of wellness.

Make sure you know . . .

- Depression and anxiety have a significant impact on the U.S. adult population, and stress is a risk factor for both conditions.

- General adaptation syndrome, which includes alarm, resistance, and exhaustion stages, was one of the first theories proposed about the relationship between stress and disease.

- The concept of the allostatic load is that long-term and repeated exposure to stress and the continual activation of the stress response compromise health.

How Can You Manage Stress?

Once you know your stress level, you can cope with stress by using stress management techniques. There are two general steps to managing stress: Reduce the amount of stress in your life, and cope with stress by improving your ability to relax (16). Let's discuss each of these steps individually.

Manage Stressors

The first significant way to lower the impact of stress on your life is to reduce the number of stressors you encounter (see the Closer Look box, page 573). Although you will not be able to avoid all sources of stress, you can eliminate many "unnecessary" forms of stress. The first step is to recognize those factors that produce daily stress. Use Laboratory 14.1 to assess your stressors and to help determine which ones you can most readily work to eliminate, avoid, or better manage. Getting adequate amounts of rest and sleep and exercising regularly, are also important factors in managing your stress levels.

One example of a stressor that you can eliminate is overcommitment, a frequent cause of stress in college students. If you plan your time carefully and prioritize your activities, you can avoid feeling overwhelmed by having too much to do and not enough time to do it. You can plan a daily schedule that allows you to accomplish the things you need to without being distracted by less important activities. The Steps for Behavior Change box on page 569 can help you determine how well you manage your time.

Another common stressor that you may be able to better manage is financial pressure. You cannot eliminate the high costs associated with paying tuition, rent (or room and board), or buying textbooks and materials, but you can strive to minimize the amount of debt you accrue as a student, particularly credit card debt. Avoiding overuse of credit cards and developing a budget are two very important strategies for preventing excessive debt. Look for ways to reduce your everyday costs, and do not buy the expensive clothes or gadgets if you do not have the money to pay for them, no matter how popular they may be.

Rest and Sleep

One of the most effective means of reducing stress and tension is to get an adequate amount of rest and sleep. How much sleep do you need? Although individual needs vary greatly, adults typically need 7 to 9 hours of restful sleep per night. Because of the body's natural hormonal rhythms, you should also try to go to bed at approximately the same time every night. See the Steps for Behavior Change box on page 570 to help determine whether you're getting enough sleep.

In addition to a good night's sleep, 15 to 30 minutes of rest during the day can help reduce stress. You can do this by simply putting your feet up on a desk or table and closing your eyes. A well-rested body is the best protection against stress and fatigue.

Exercise

Light to moderate exercise can reduce many types of stress and anxiety. Even if you are not an experienced exerciser, you can benefit from the calm feeling that comes after an exercise session. The recommended types of exercise for optimal stress reduction are low-to-moderate-intensity aerobic exercises, such as brisk walking, swimming, and cycling. The guidelines for this type of exercise prescription are presented in Chapter 3. Yoga, tai-chi, and Pilates are other popular types of exercise that help you reduce stress and relax. Many gyms and health clubs offer classes in these forms of exercise.

FIGURE 14.4 Rest, exercise, and meditation are all techniques you can use to reduce your stress level.

Studies have shown that exercise is a very effective for stress reduction (17–19). FIGURE 14.4 compares the effects of a 30-minute session of exercise (running) to other common forms of stress reduction: rest, reading, and meditation. In this study, meditation provided the greatest stress reduction, with exercise finishing a close second (17). Other studies have shown that exercise reduces stress about as much as other types of relaxation techniques (20). Also, the relaxing effects of exercise can last for hours after an exercise session (21).

Although we consistently see that people feel more relaxed after exercise, we do not know exactly how exercise reduces stress. Several ideas have been proposed. One theory is that exercise causes the brain to release several natural tranquilizers (endorphins), which can produce a calming effect (22). Another theory is that exercise may be a diversion or break from your stressors and worries of life. The improved physical fitness and self-image that you enjoy as a result of regular exercise also increases your resistance to stress. A final possibility is that all of these factors may contribute to the beneficial effects of exercise on stress management. The next time you feel stressed, try exercising; you will feel and look better as a result.

Use Relaxation Techniques to Cope with Stress

Stress management techniques can help reduce the potentially harmful effects of stress. Most of these techniques are designed to relax you and thereby reduce your stress level. When trying to relax, ask yourself two questions: (a) What prevents me from relaxing? And (b) What am I not doing that could help me relax? (9). Your answers can help you determine how and where to focus your efforts to manage your stress. Lowering your levels of stress and practicing effective stress management techniques will increase your overall level of wellness (14). The following are some of the more common approaches used in stress management.

Progressive Relaxation

Progressive relaxation is a stress reduction technique that uses exercises to reduce muscle tension. (Muscle tension is a common symptom of stress.) You practice the technique while sitting quietly or lying down. First you contract muscle groups, and then you relax them one at a time, beginning with your feet and then moving up your body to your hands and neck, until you achieve a complete state of muscle relaxation. You can find specific directions for one progressive relaxation exercise in the Closer Look box on page 574.

The proponents of progressive relaxation techniques argue that relaxing the muscles in this manner will also relax the mind and therefore relieve stress. The theory behind this concept is that an anxious (stressed) mind cannot exist in a relaxed body.

A CLOSER LOOK

How Much Stress Is Too Much?

The number of stressors that each of us can deal with, as well as our reaction to the stressors, is very individual. Even so, there are some common signs of being overstressed. People who experience chronic stress or very high levels of stress and its associated feelings of anxiety can experience **burnout** (21). If you recognize any of the following warning signals of burnout in your own life, begin practicing the stress management techniques offered in this chapter.

1. *Changes in sleeping patterns.* You might sleep too much or too little. Also, you might have trouble falling asleep and/or staying asleep. Waking up during the night with difficulty returning to sleep is especially a concern. During these periods of waking, you typically find yourself thinking about events or activities that are causing you stress.

2. *Changes in eating habits.* You either overeat or undereat. During stressful times some people gain weight, especially in the abdominal area. However, others lose weight. Once again, this response is highly individual.

3. *Greater susceptibility to illness.* You begin to notice more frequent headaches (migraines), stomachaches, muscle tension, and other aches or pains. Over time you may be more susceptible to colds or other viral and bacterial infections. In addition, you do not recover as quickly as you once did.

4. *Intense cravings.* Specific cravings depend on your preferences and habits. Common cravings include coffee (caffeine), cigarettes, alcohol, and special "comfort" foods, such as chocolate, ice cream, and other high-fat, high-calorie foods. You might find that to relieve your anxiety, it takes larger quantities of these substances than you would normally use or consume. Sometimes the behavior or food does not relieve the negative feelings caused by stress.

5. *Increased feelings of hopelessness and exhaustion.* Over time, the lack of sleep, coupled with the ever-increasing unhealthy lifestyle and its negative consequences, can make you to want to "give up." If you get to this point, you may find yourself thinking about dropping a class, quitting your job or school, leaving your mate, moving, or doing anything that may relieve some of the stress in your life.

Breathing Exercises

Breathing exercises can also help you relax. The following is a sample step-by-step breathing exercise for reducing stress:

1. Assume a comfortable position, sitting or lying down, with your eyes closed.

2. Begin to slowly inhale and exhale. Count from 1 to 3 during each inhalation and each exhalation to maintain a slow and regular breathing pattern.

3. Next, combine stretching and breathing to provide greater relaxation and stress reduction. For example, stretch your arms toward the ceiling as you inhale, then lower your arms as you exhale.

   Try this exercise for 5 to 15 minutes in a quiet room.

Meditation

Meditation has been practiced for ages to help people relax and achieve inner peace. There are many types of meditation, and there is no scientific evidence that one form is superior to another. Most types of meditation have the same common elements: sitting quietly for 15 to 20 minutes twice a day, concentrating on a single word or image, and breathing slowly and regularly. The goal is to achieve a complete state of physical and mental relaxation.

burnout The loss of physical, emotional, and mental energy, which, if ignored, can lead to emotional exhaustion and withdrawal.

meditation A method of relaxation that involves sitting quietly, focusing on a word or image, and breathing slowly.

A CLOSER LOOK

A CLOSER LOOK A CLOSER LOOK A CLOSER LOOK

Progressive Relaxation Training

There are many types of progressive relaxation training methods, and over 200 different exercises have been described. The basic technique involves contracting and relaxing muscle groups, starting in your lower body and moving toward your upper body. The following technique is one of the many forms that you can use.

1. Find a quiet, comfortable, and private place. Remove your shoes. Wear loose, comfortable clothing, or loosen any tight clothing. The first few times you can expect emerging thoughts and emotions to distract your attempts to relax. After some practice, you will be able block distractions. Listening to soothing music during your relaxation sessions is one way to help you relax and filter distractions; there are many commercial relaxation music CDs available. You may also read the instructions into a tape recorder and use them to guide you through your relaxation session. Using this strategy you will avoid having to remember the steps involved.

2. Assume a relaxed position (either sitting or lying down). Close your eyes, and begin by focusing on your breathing. Become aware of how it feels to breathe in and breathe out. Breathe deeply and slowly through your nose, and imagine that you are breathing in good, healing air and breathing out stress and muscle tension. While developing your breathing you may find it useful to inhale to a count of 7, 1-2-3-4-5-6-7, and exhale to the same count. Breathe this way several minutes before starting your progressive relaxation exercise.

3. Without speaking, focus on relaxing each part of your body. You are consciously "telling" each part of your body to relax. Contracting the muscles in each body part first and then relaxing them can help you to feel the difference, because sometimes we are not aware of tension we carry in our muscles. Do not move on to the next area until you have relaxed the part you are focusing on.

Proceed by relaxing your body in the following order:

a. Toes of left foot
b. Toes of right foot
c. Left foot
d. Right foot
e. Left ankle
f. Right ankle
g. Lower left leg
h. Lower right leg
i. Left thigh
j. Right thigh
k. Buttocks
l. Abdomen
m. Chest
n. Left shoulder
o. Right shoulder
p. Left arm
q. Left hand
r. Left fingers
s. Right arm
t. Right hand
u. Right fingers
v. Neck
w. Face

4. Now you should be completely relaxed. Continue breathing for the next few minutes. Try not to let your mind wander—remain in this relaxed state.

5. At the end of your session, take a deep breath. Slowly bring yourself out of your relaxed state. Stand up and stretch. You should feel renewed and refreshed.

Although beginning a successful program may require the help of an experienced instructor, the following is a brief overview of how to practice meditation:

1. First, choose a word or sound, called a *mantra*, to repeat during the meditation. The idea of using a mantra is that this word or sound should become your symbol of complete relaxation. Choose a mantra that has little emotional significance for you, such as the word *red*.

2. Next, find a quiet area and sit comfortably with your eyes closed. Take several deep breaths, and concentrate on relaxing; let your body go limp.

3. Concentrate on your mantra. This means that you should not hear or think about anything else. Repeat your mantra over and over again in your mind, and relax. Avoid distracting thoughts, and focus only on the mantra.

4. After 15 to 20 minutes of concentration on the mantra, open your eyes, and begin to move your thoughts away from the mantra. End the session by making a fist with both hands and saying to yourself that you are alert and refreshed.

Visualization

Visualization (sometimes called *imagery*) uses mental pictures to reduce stress. The idea is to create an appealing mental image (such as a quiet mountain setting) that promotes relaxation and reduces stress. To practice visualization, follow the instructions presented for meditation, but substitute a relaxing mental scene for the mantra. If you fail to reach a complete state of relaxation after your first several sessions, do not be discouraged. Achieving complete relaxation with this technique may require numerous practice sessions.

Develop Spiritual Wellness

Spiritual wellness is associated with better recovery from illness and improved mental health. Spiritual wellness can provide a sense of peace. People who report high levels of spiritual wellness often practice behaviors such as prayer, meditation, or enjoying the beauty of nature to reduce stress and anxiety.

Develop a Support Network

Having a network of friends and family to help you cope with stressors can help to reduce or eliminate stress. Sometimes just talking through your stressful situation can help you think more clearly about the situation and develop an effective plan to address your stressors. Others who have your best interest as a concern will likely help you with a plan for stress management. When you are dealing with stressors that cannot be eliminated, your network will be there for support while you work through your period of stress.

Avoid Counterproductive Behaviors

Some people choose poor health behaviors, such as smoking cigarettes or drinking alcohol, in an attempt to manage stress. However, these behaviors are counterproductive and can lead to more cumulative stress in the long term.

Using Tobacco

Many people say that they smoke cigarettes "to relax," but the nicotine in cigarettes and other tobacco products is actually a stimulant that produces responses similar to the fight-or-flight response. Additionally, nicotine is an addictive substance that has serious long-term effects. As discussed earlier, smoking is the leading cause of preventable death, increasing the risk for lung and other types of cancer and the risk for heart disease. Smoking and tobacco also are very costly habits.

Using Alcohol or Other Drugs

Using alcohol or other substances might make you briefly forget about problems or stressors, but these behaviors do not eliminate or reduce the stressor. In some cases they might add to your level of stress. Alcohol (especially binge drinking) or drug use can affect your sleep patterns and productivity. Using alcohol or other substances to solve or cope with your problems can lead to abuse. Even legal substances, such as caffeine, also can cause problems instead of solving them.

Assuming a relaxed position in a quiet setting is central to several relaxation techniques.

visualization A relaxation technique that uses appealing mental images to promote relaxation and reduce stress; also called *imagery*.

CONSUMER CORNER

Can Nutritional Supplements Reduce Emotional Stress?

Currently, there is no scientific evidence that any specific nutritional supplement, including megadoses of vitamins, will reduce emotional stress. According to researchers at the University of Texas Southwestern Medical Center at Dallas, most "stress formulas" contain B vitamins, such as niacin and riboflavin, which are meant to aid in recovery from physical stress (e.g., injuries), not emotional stress. The B vitamins are sometimes used to supplement the diets of people recovering from surgery. However, emotional stress does not increase the body's energy or nutrient needs, so taking vitamins will not calm us down.

Getting plenty of rest and exercising regularly, combined with a healthy diet, are the best ways to deal with emotional stress. Combining healthy lifestyle practices with stress management techniques such as those offered in this chapter can help you deal with life's stressors.

Although numerous nutritional products are marketed as stress relievers, none have been proven effective for stress reduction.

Disordered Eating Patterns

Disordered eating patterns are eating patterns that are not healthy, but that do not meet the clinical definitions for eating disorders. These patterns can lead to the development of an eating disorder. Undereating or overeating can be disordered eating. Skipping meals will result in lack of nutrients and energy, which can affect how well you can focus and cope with stressors. Overeating, binge eating, or using "comfort foods" to cope with stress can lead to weight gain and health problems. Also, blood glucose levels can be affected, resulting in fluctuations in your energy levels and decreased ability to focus on managing your stress.

Make sure you know . . .

- The two general steps involved in stress management are reducing the sources of stress and using relaxation techniques to help you cope with stress.

- The ideal way to lessen the effects of stress on your life is to reduce the sources of stress.

- Getting more rest and sleep; engaging in exercise; and practicing progressive muscle relaxation, breathing exercises, meditation, and visualization are some of the many relaxation techniques that can help you cope with stress.

- Developing your spiritual and social wellness can be very important in managing stress.

- Adopting unhealthy behaviors, such as smoking or drinking alcohol, to relax will lead to higher levels of stress in the long term.

CHAPTER SUMMARY

1. Stress is defined as a physiological and mental response to things in our environment that we perceive as threatening. Any factor that produces stress is called a stressor.
2. Excessive stress or poorly managed stress can lead to headaches, digestive problems, heart disease, and mental health problems.
3. The autonomic nervous system consists of the parasympathetic and sympathetic branches and works with the endocrine system to produce the stress response. The combined physiological responses of these systems result in the fight-or-flight response, which prepares the body to fight or flee.
4. Common stressors include academic and financial responsibilities, managing interpersonal relationships, and everyday life hassles.
5. Personality factors, past experiences, and gender can affect the way we perceive situations and behave in response to stressors.
6. Two steps in managing stress are to reduce stressors in your life and to learn to cope with stress by improving your ability to relax.
7. Common relaxation techniques to reduce stress include rest and sleep, exercise, progressive relaxation, breathing exercises, meditation, visualization. Developing spiritual wellness and a social network can also help you better manage stress. Avoiding unhealthy habits for reducing stress is key to maintaining manageable stress levels.

TEST YOURSELF ANSWERS

1. **False.** Everyone experiences some stress and a certain amount is necessary for optimal performance.
2. **True.** A person with chronic stress experiences some level of stress response on a consistent basis with little relief. This consistent activation of the systems involved in the stress response can increase the risk for heart disease.
3. **True.** You probably know that certain significant events, such as a death, finals, or the end of a relationship, cause stress. However, a number of everyday annoyances, such as rush-hour traffic, waiting in line, or being late, can also be a significant source of stress for some people.
4. **True.** Good time management skills can help you use time more effectively and reduce the stress of deadlines, being late, and procrastination.
5. **False.** Personality characteristics influence the way we perceive situations and the way we respond to stressful situations. Our past experiences and gender also impact our level of stress.

STUDY QUESTIONS

1. Which of the following is a physical symptom of stress?
   a. muscle tension
   b. headaches
   c. anxiety
   d. all of the above

2. Positive stress that is associated with optimal performance is called _____.
   a. distress
   b. visualization
   c. eustress
   d. productive stress

3. Which of the following is not a hormone that is part of the stress response?
   a. dopamine
   b. cortisol
   c. epinephrine
   d. norepinephrine

4. Common stressors include _____.
   a. financial responsibilities
   b. interpersonal relationship problems
   c. academic pressures
   d. all of the above

5. Which of the following is not a healthy way to cope with stress?
   a. exercise
   b. alcohol
   c. meditation
   d. progressive muscle relaxation

6. Define *stress.* Define *stressor,* and name common stressors.

7. Why is stress management important to health?

8. List the steps in stress management. Identify some common stress management (relaxation) techniques.

9. Discuss the concept of eustress.

10. Explain potential ways exercise is useful in reducing stress.

11. List the key guidelines for the development of a time management program.

SUGGESTED READING

Atkinson, D. *Live Right! Beating Stress in College and Beyond*. San Francisco: Benjamin Cummings, 2008.

Barrett, S., W. Jarvis, M. Kroeger, and W. London. *Consumer Health: A Guide to Intelligent Decisions*, 7th ed. New York: McGraw-Hill, 2002.

Benson, H. *The Relaxation Response*. New York: Avon, Wholecare, 2000.

Daniel, E. (Ed.). *Annual Editions: Health*, 25th ed. Guilford, CT: McGraw-Hill, 2004.

Donatelle, R. *Health: The Basics*, 8th ed. San Francisco: Benjamin Cummings, 2009.

Greenberg, J. *Comprehensive Stress Management*, 10th ed. Dubuque, IA: McGraw-Hill, 2006.

REFERENCES

1. Canon, W. *The Wisdom of the Body*. New York: Norton Publishing, 1932.

2. Selye, H. *The Stress of Life*, revised edition. New York: McGraw-Hill, 1978.

3. Friedman, M., and R. H. Rosenman. Type A behavior pattern: Its association with coronary heart disease. *Annals of Clinical Research* 3(6):300–312, 1971.

4. Knox, S. S., G. Wiedner, A. Adelman, S. M. Stoney, and R. C. Ellison. Hostility and physiological risk in the National Heart, Lung, and Blood Institute Family Heart Study. *Archives of Internal Medicine* 164(22): 2442–2448, 2004.

5. DeFruyt, F., and J. Denollet. Type D personality: A five factor model perspective. *Psychology and Health* 17(5): 671–683, 2002.

6. Albus, C., J. Jordan, and C. Herrmann-Lingen. Screening for psychosocial risk factors in patients with coronary heart disease—Recommendations for clinical practice. *European Journal of Cardiovascular Rehabilitation* 11(1):75–79, 2004.

7. Kessler, R. C., W. T Chui, O. Demler, K. R. Merikangas, and E. E. Walters. Prevalence, severity, and comorbidity of 12-month DSM-IV disorders in the National Comorbidity Survey Replication Study. *Archives of General Psychiatry* 62:590–592, 2005.

8. American Psychological Association HelpCenter. How does stress affect us? www.apahelpcenter.org, accessed May 2007.

9. Weil, A. Stress and relaxation: An introduction. www.drweil.com/drw/u/id/ART00534, accessed June 2007.

10. Margen, S., et al. (Eds.). *The Wellness Encyclopedia*. Boston: Houghton Mifflin, 1992.

11. Lovallo, W. R. *Stress and Health: Biological and Psychological Interactions*. Thousand Oaks, CA: Sage Publications, 1997.

12. McEwen, B. S. Allostasis and allostatic load: Implications for neuropsychopharmacology. *Neuropsychopharmacology* 22:108–124, 2000.

13. Abercrombie, H., et al. Flattened cortisol rhythms in metastatic breast cancer patients. *Psychoneuroendocrinology* 29(8):1082–1092, 2004.

14. Holroyd, K. A., et al. Management of chronic tension-type headache with tricyclic antidepressant medication, stress management therapy, and their combination: A randomized trial. *Journal of the American Medical Association* 285(17):2208–2215, 2001.

15. Sewitch, M., et al. Psychological distress, social support, and disease activity in patients with inflammatory bowel disease. *American Journal of Gastroenterology* 96(5): 1470–1479, 2001.

16. Howley, E., and B. D. Franks. *The Fitness Professional's Handbook*, 5th ed. Champaign, IL: Human Kinetics, 2007.

17. Tsai, J. C., et al. The beneficial effects of tai chi chuan on blood pressure and lipid profile and anxiety status in a randomized controlled trial. *Journal of Alternative Complementary Medicine* 9(5):747–754, 2003.

18. Berger, B., and D. Owen. Stress reduction and mood enhancement in four exercise modes: Swimming, body conditioning, hatha yoga, and fencing. *Research Quarterly for Exercise and Sport* 59:148–159, 1988.

19. Oliver, S., and D. Alfermann. Effects of physical exercise on resources evaluation, body self-concept and well-being among older adults. *Anxiety, Stress, and Coping* 15(3):311–320, 2002.

20. Breus, M. J., and P. J. O'Connor. Exercise-induced anxiolysis: A test of the "time out" hypothesis in high anxious females. *Medicine and Science in Sports and Exercise* 30(7):1107–1112, 1998.

21. Petruzzello, S. J., D. M. Landers, B. D. Hatfield, K. A. Kubitz, and W. Salazar. Meta-analysis on the anxiety-reducing effects of acute and chronic exercise: Outcomes and mechanisms. *Sports Medicine* 11:143–182, 1991.

22. Farrell, P. Enkephalins, catecholamines, and psychological mood alterations: Effects of prolonged exercise. *Medicine and Science in Sports and Exercise* 19:347–353, 1987.

WEB LINKS

For links to the organizations and websites listed below, visit The Total Fitness and Wellness Website at www.pearsonhighered.com/powers.

American College Counseling Association
Offers information related to counseling and college students.

American College Health Association (ACHA)
Offers health-related information for college students.

National Institute of Mental Health
Working to improve mental health through biomedical research on mind, brain, and behavior.

Weil Lifestyle
Provides a wide range of wellness information.

Mayo Clinic Health
Contains wide-ranging information about stress, diet, fitness, and mental health.

American Medical Association
Includes many sources of information about a wide variety of medical problems, including stress-related disorders.

WebMD
Contains information about a wide variety of diseases and medical problems, including stress-related disorders.

American Psychological Association
Provides information on stress management and psychological disorders.

VIDEOS

Log on to **www.pearsonhighered.com/powers** to view these chapter-related videos.

Stress Management
The Multi-tasking Myth
Stress at Work and Home

CHAPTER OBJECTIVES

After reading this chapter you will be able to:

1. Explain what is meant by the statement that eating behaviors occur along a continuum, pp. 582–583.

2. Compare and contrast disordered eating behaviors and true clinical eating disorders, pp. 582–584.

3. Identify at least four factors that may contribute to the development of an eating disorder, pp. 584–587.

4. Create a table listing the symptoms and health risks of anorexia nervosa, bulimia nervosa, binge-eating disorder, night-eating syndrome, and chronic dieting, pp. 588–599.

5. Discuss the steps you can use when discussing an eating disorder with a friend or family member, p. 591.

6. List the three components of the female athlete triad and explain how they are interconnected, pp. 601–604.

7. Describe the various treatment options available for people with anorexia nervosa or bulimia nervosa, pp. 604–607.

8. Discuss ways of preventing the development of eating disorders and disordered eating, p. 607.

TEST YOURSELF TRUE OR FALSE?

1. Only females get eating disorders. T or F

2. No one ever recovers from an eating disorder. T or F

3. In most cases, eating disorders develop in response to overcontrolling parents. T or F

4. Disordered eating behaviors may lead to the development of a true eating disorder. T or F

5. Obesity can be associated with an eating disorder. T or F

Test Yourself answers can be found after the Chapter Summary.

Disordered Eating

On August 2, 2006, Uruguayan fashion model Luisel Ramos collapsed during a fashion show while returning to her dressing room from the runway. Just 22 years old, she was pronounced dead of heart failure brought on by anorexia nervosa, a condition of self-imposed starvation. Family members say that, in the months prior to her death, she had adopted a diet of lettuce leaves and Diet Coke, and at 5'9" tall, her weight had dropped to just 98 pounds. The following month, Madrid's "Fashion Week" responded to Ramos' death by banning from its runway fashion models who could not meet a minimum weight-height standard, a body mass index (BMI) of at least 18.0 kg/m^2. At the time of her death, Ramos' BMI was 14.5 kg/m^2. Although the Madrid restriction was praised by many in the fashion industry and adopted by other shows, it did not prevent further tragedies: Two months later, a 21-year-old Brazilian model, Ana Carolina Reston, died from anorexia nervosa, and in February 2007, 18-year-old Eliana Ramos followed her sister Luisel to the grave. Also a fashion model, she too suffered a heart attack suspected to have been brought on by "malnutrition."

Ana Carolina Reston, one of a string of models who have recently died due to eating disorders.

Do only fashion models develop eating disorders, or do they occur in people like you? When does normal dieting cross the line into disordered eating? Are there any early warning signs that would tip you off that a friend was crossing that line? If you noticed the signs in a friend or family member, would you confront him or her? If so, what would you say?

This chapter will discuss the continuum of eating behaviors and the negative consequences of moving from more normal to disordered to abnormal eating behaviors. First, we describe eating behaviors and body image as a continuum. We then discuss specific eating disorders and disordered eating behaviors that commonly occur in adolescents and adults. We also discuss the female athlete triad. Finally, we review the various treatment options available to those with an eating disorder.

Eating Behaviors Occur on a Continuum

Over the last 20 years, food availability and lifestyle choices have changed so dramatically that it is difficult to describe "normal eating behaviors." The days of a nuclear family sitting down to a home-cooked meal together every evening at 6:00 PM seem part of our culture's distant past. Nowadays, our schedules are crammed with classes, jobs, and activities, and our meals are often packaged or eaten out. Skipping meals, eating at odd times, and trying a variety of fad diets are all behaviors commonly accepted as normal. So when does normal eating in a disorderly life cross over into disordered eating or a medically diagnosed eating disorder?

This question is tricky to answer because eating behaviors occur on a *continuum*, a spectrum that can't be divided neatly into parts. An example is a rainbow—where exactly does the red end and the orange begin? Thinking about eating behaviors as a continuum makes it easier to understand how a person could progress from relatively normal eating behaviors to a pattern that is disordered. For instance, let's say that for several years you've skipped breakfast in favor of a mid-morning snack, but now you find yourself avoiding the cafeteria until early afternoon. Is this normal? To answer that question, you'd need to consider your feelings about food and your **body image**—the way you perceive your body.

Feelings About Food and Body Image Influence Eating Behaviors

Take a moment to study the Eating Issues and Body Image Continuum in FIGURE 15.1. Which of the five columns best describes your feelings about food and your body? If you find yourself identifying with the statements on the left side of the continuum, you probably have few issues with food or body image. Most likely you accept your body size and view food as a normal part of maintaining your health and fueling your daily physical activity. As you progress to the right side of the continuum, food and body image become bigger issues, with food restriction becoming the norm. If you identify with the statements on the far right, you are probably afraid of eating and dislike your body. If so, what can you do to begin to move toward the left side of the continuum? How can you begin to develop a more healthful approach to food selection and to view your body in a more positive light? Before you can begin to find solutions, you need to understand the many complex factors that contribute to eating disorders and disordered eating and the differences between these terms.

Eating Disorders and Disordered Eating Patterns Are Not the Same Thing

The media, consumers, and health professionals frequently use the terms *eating disorder* and *disordered eating* interchangeably. Do they mean the same thing? The answer is no! An **eating disorder** is a psychiatric condition that must be diagnosed by a physician and involves extreme body dissatisfaction and long-term eating patterns that negatively affect body functioning. The behaviors of someone with an eating disorder typically include severe food restriction, obsessive exercising, self-induced vomiting, and/or laxative abuse. Before a physician can diagnose an eating disorder, the patient's condition and behavior must meet specific diagnostic crite-

Hectic schedules often force us to grab a quick meal "on the go."

body image A person's perception of his or her body's appearance and functioning.

eating disorder A psychiatric disorder characterized by severe disturbances in body image and eating behaviors. Anorexia nervosa and bulimia nervosa are two examples of eating disorders for which specific diagnostic criteria must be present for diagnosis.

• I am not concerned about what others think regarding what and how much I eat. • When I am upset or depressed I eat whatever I am hungry for without any guilt or shame. • I feel no guilt or shame no matter how much I eat or what I eat. • Food is an important part of my life but only occupies a small part of my time. • I trust my body to tell me what and how much to eat.	• I pay attention to what I eat in order to maintain a healthy body. • I may weigh more than what I like, but I enjoy eating and balance my pleasure with eating with my concern for a healthy body. • I am moderate and flexible in goals for eating well. • I try to follow Dietary Guidelines for healthy eating.	• I think about food a lot. • I feel I don't eat well most of the time. • It's hard for me to enjoy eating with others. • I feel ashamed when I eat more than others or more than what I feel I should be eating. • I am afraid of getting fat. • I wish I could change how much I want to eat and what I am hungry for.	• I have tried diet pills, laxatives, vomiting or extra time exercising in order to lose or maintain my weight. • I have fasted or avoided eating for long periods of time in order to lose or maintain my weight. • I feel strong when I can restrict how much I eat. • Eating more than I wanted to makes me feel out of control.	• I regularly stuff myself and then exercise, vomit, use diet pills or laxatives to get rid of the food or calories. • My friends/family tell me I am too thin. • I am terrified of eating fat. • When I let myself eat, I have a hard time controlling the amount of food I eat. • I am afraid to eat in front of others.
FOOD IS NOT AN ISSUE	**CONCERNED WELL**	**FOOD PREOCCUPIED/ OBSESSED**	**DISRUPTIVE EATING PATTERNS**	**EATING DISORDERED**
BODY OWNERSHIP	**BODY ACCEPTANCE**	**BODY PREOCCUPIED/ OBSESSED**	**DISTORTED BODY IMAGE**	**BODY HATE/ DISASSOCIATION**
• Body image is not an issue for me. • My body is beautiful to me. • My feelings about my body are not influenced by society's concept of an ideal body shape. • I know that the significant others in my life will always find me attractive. • I trust my body to find the weight it needs to be at so I can move and feel confident of my physical body.	• I base my body image equally on social norms and my own self-concept. • I pay attention to my body and my appearance because it is important to me, but it only occupies a small part of my day. • I nourish my body so it has the strength and energy to achieve my physical goals. • I am able to assert myself and maintain a healthy body without losing my self-esteem.	• I spend a significant time viewing my body in the mirror. • I spend a significant time comparing my body to others. • I have days when I feel fat. • I am preoccupied with my body. • I accept society's ideal body shape and size as the best body shape and size. • I'd be more attractive if I was thinner, more muscular, etc...	• I spend a significant amount of time exercising and dieting to change my body. • My body shape and size keeps me from dating or finding someone who will treat me the way I want to be treated. • I have considered changing or have changed my body shape and size through surgical means so I can accept myself. • I wish I could change the way I look in the mirror.	• I often feel separated and distant from my body—as if it belongs to someone else. • I hate my body and I often isolate myself from others. • I don't see anything positive or even neutral about my body shape and size. • I don't believe others when they tell me I look OK. • I hate the way I look in the mirror.

FIGURE 15.1 The Eating Issues and Body Image Continuum. The progression from normal eating to eating disorders occurs on a continuum. People whose responses fall to the far left of the continuum have normal eating patterns and do not suffer from an eating disorder. People whose responses fall to the far right of the continuum most likely suffer from an eating disorder such as anorexia nervosa or bulimia nervosa. (From Smiley/King/Avery: Campus Health Service. Original Continuum, C. Shisslak: Preventive Medicine and Public Health. Copyright © 1997 Arizona Board of Regents. Used with permission.)

ria outlined by the American Psychiatric Association's (APA's) *Diagnostic and Statistical Manual of Mental Disorders (DSM-IV)*.[1]

The two most commonly diagnosed eating disorders are anorexia nervosa and bulimia nervosa. *Anorexia nervosa* is a potentially life-threatening eating disorder that is characterized by self-starvation, which eventually leads to severe nutrient deficiencies. In contrast, *bulimia nervosa* is characterized by recurrent episodes of extreme overeating and compensatory behaviors to prevent weight gain, such as self-induced vomiting, misuse of laxatives, fasting, or excessive exercise. Both disorders will be discussed in detail later in the chapter.

In contrast, **disordered eating** is a general term used to describe a variety of abnormal or atypical eating behaviors that people use to achieve or maintain a lower

disordered eating General term used to describe a variety of abnormal or atypical eating behaviors that are used to keep or maintain a lower body weight but are not severe enough to make the person seriously ill.

body weight. These behaviors may be as simple as going on and off diets or as extreme as refusing to eat any fat. Such behaviors don't usually continue for long enough to make the person seriously ill, nor do they significantly disrupt the person's normal routine. In fact, most people who engage in disordered eating behaviors from time to time don't consider what they're doing unusual or particularly unhealthful. However, sometimes such behaviors disturb individuals or their loved ones enough to cause them to seek medical care. The American Psychiatric Association's *DSM–IV* diagnosis that would apply to these individuals is "Eating Disorders Not Otherwise Specified" (EDNOS).[1,2] It is estimated that one-third of all people treated for eating disorders receive a diagnosis of EDNOS.[3] As we have said, not all atypical eating behaviors qualify as EDNOS; thus, we use the more inclusive term *disordered eating* throughout the remainder of this chapter.

> RECAP: *Eating behaviors occur along a continuum from normal to somewhat abnormal to disordered. Our feelings about food and our body images influence our eating behaviors. True eating disorders are psychiatric conditions characterized by long-term behavior patterns that negatively affect body functioning, whereas disordered eating is a more general term applicable to any of a variety of abnormal or atypical eating behaviors that may not seriously impair health or functioning.*

What Factors Contribute to the Development of Eating Disorders?

The factors that result in the development of an eating disorder are very complex, but research indicates that a number of psychological, interpersonal, social, genetic, and biological factors may contribute in any particular individual (Table 15.1).

Family Environment Influences Eating Behavior

Most of us recognize that family conditioning influences our eating behaviors. During childhood, our parents and other family members provided most of the food we ate, limiting our choices and influencing our developing concept of how much food to eat, when, how often, and so forth. As we grew, our families developed unique mealtime rituals. For example, perhaps your family never sat down together at a meal, and you

TABLE 15.1   Risk Factors That May Contribute to the Development of an Eating Disorder

Psychological Factors	Interpersonal Factors	Social Factors	Genetic and Biological Factors*
Low self-esteem	Troubled family and personal relationships	Cultural pressures to be "thin" and the high value placed on a "perfect body"	Chemical imbalances that control hunger, appetite, and digestion
Feelings of inadequacy or lack of control over life	Difficulty expressing emotions and feelings	Narrow definitions of beauty that include women and men of only a certain body size	Possible gene or set of genes that predisposes an individual
Depression, anxiety, anger, or loneliness	History of being teased or ridiculed based on size or weight	Cultural norms that value people on the basis of physical appearances and not inner qualities and strengths	
	History of physical or sexual abuse		

*These factors are still under investigation.
Source: Adapted from National Eating Disorders Association (NEDA), © 2002. Causes of Eating Disorders. www.nationaleatingdisorders.org/p.asp?WebPage_ID5286&Profile_ID541144.

were responsible for getting your own meals. Or perhaps your family insisted on a shared mealtime, and one family member was responsible for preparing the meal for the whole family. We also had experiences that caused us to associate food with particular family members or shared activities. Maybe you really like hot oatmeal with brown sugar and raisins on winter days because your grandmother prepared this for you when you visited for the holidays. Because of such family patterns, rituals, and associations, our response to food and our eating behaviors are to some extent conditioned. Thus, it is not difficult to believe that the family eating environment might contribute to the development of an eating disorder.

Researchers have examined a number of family-related factors to determine whether or not they contribute to the development of eating disorders. Currently, there are no data to suggest that family size or birth order is influential. Research on siblings, however, does show a greater likelihood of developing an eating disorder if a sibling also has an eating disorder. The precise reason for this is unclear. Family structure and patterns of interaction have also been implicated. Based on observational studies, compared to "normal" families, families with an anorexic member show more rigidity in their family structure, less clear interpersonal boundaries, and a tendency to avoid open discussions on topics of disagreement. Conversely, families with a member diagnosed with bulimia nervosa have a less stable family organization, are less nurturing, and are more angry and disruptive than "normal" families.[4b] In addition, childhood physical or sexual abuse can increase the risk of an eating disorder developing in a child.[3] In short, family conditioning, structure, and patterns of interaction, including abuse, can influence the development of an eating disorder.

Family environment influences when, what, and how much we eat.

Sociocultural Values Shape Identity and Self-Esteem

Although many people believe that eating disorders did not exist prior to the 20th century, written records in Europe have documented instances of eating disorders for hundreds of years. The problem began to capture medical and media attention in the United States in 1893, when James Hendrie Lloyd published the first clinical description of a "fasting girl." Still, it was not until the 1960s that anorexia nervosa was associated with the specific diagnostic criteria we use today, and bulimia nervosa was only recognized by the APA as distinct from anorexia nervosa and from obesity in 1970.[4a] The APA developed these specific definitions and diagnostic criteria in response to a need, as the number of patients consulting physicians for treatment of an eating disorder increased dramatically in the decades following World War II.

Evidence suggesting that Western sociocultural values have contributed to this surge in eating disorders is hard to deny. For instance, consider the fact that eating disorders are significantly more common in white females in Western societies than in other women worldwide. This may be due in part to our culture's valuing of slenderness, not only for aesthetic reasons, but also because Westerners tend to consider it as an indication that the person is self-disciplined, a generally valued characteristic. Westerners also associate slenderness with health and often with wealth. In contrast, until quite recently, the prevailing view in developing societies has been that excess body fat is desirable as a sign of material abundance.

Only limited research has examined the prevalence of eating disorders in nonwhite populations and in non-Western cultures; thus, we have a lot to learn about how culture affects the development of eating disorders. However, as cross-cultural interactions increase, some researchers hypothesize that non-Western cultures will adapt Western norms for beauty, and this may increase the development of eating disorders in those cultures.

The members of society with whom we most often interact—our family members, friends, teachers, and coworkers—also influence the way we see ourselves. Their comments related to our body weight or shape can be particularly hurtful—enough so to cause some people to start down the path of disordered eating. This is what happened to gymnast Christy Henrich: After failing to make the 1988 Olympic team, Christy was told by a U.S. judge that, at 4'11" tall and 98 pounds, she was too fat. She began dieting and exercising obsessively, and despite medical intervention, her weight plummeted to a low of 47 pounds. She died of complications from anorexia

Former gymnast Christy Henrich and her fiancé, a year before she died.

nervosa in 1994. Individuals with bulimia nervosa also report that they perceive greater pressure from their peers to be thin than do controls, while research shows that peer teasing about weight increases body dissatisfaction and eating disturbances.[5] Thus, our comments to others regarding their weight do count.

Unrealistic Media Images Affect Body Image

As media saturation has increased over the last century, so has the incidence of eating disorders among white women.[6] Every day, we are confronted with advertisements in which computer-enhanced images of lean, beautiful women promote everything from beer to cars (FIGURE 15.2). Most adult men and women understand that these images are unrealistic, but adolescents, who are still developing a sense of their identity and body image, lack the same ability to distance themselves from what they see.[7] Adolescent girls are likely to compare themselves unfavorably to these "perfect" female bodies and to develop a negative body image as a result. Also, as we explored at the beginning of this chapter, the "hot look" in fashion modeling until recently has been that of an emaciated waif (FIGURE 15.3). Adolescents lack the cognitive maturity to recognize that such extreme underweight is incompatible with good health. Since body image influences eating behaviors, it is not unlikely that the barrage of rail-thin models may be contributing to an increase in eating disorders. Unfortunately, scientific evidence demonstrating whether the media is *causing* increased eating disorders is difficult to obtain.

Certain Personality Traits Are Associated with Eating Disorders

Researchers have long been interested in the question of whether certain personalities predispose individuals to the development of an eating disorder. The reverse question has also been asked: Does an eating disorder modify personality traits, making changes in personality a consequence of the disorder instead of a cause?

A number of studies suggest that people with anorexia nervosa exhibit increased rates of obsessive-compulsive disorder (OCD), which is an inherited illness characterized by intrusive thoughts and/or compulsions to repeat certain behaviors in a certain way.[8] The increased incidence of OCD occurs not only in individuals with eating

FIGURE 15.2 Photos of celebrities or models are often airbrushed or altered to "enhance" physical appearance. Unfortunately, many people believe that these are accurate images and strive to reach this unrealistic level of physical beauty.

disorders but also in their families. For example, one child may have anorexia nervosa while another child has OCD.

Other personality traits associated with anorexia nervosa are perfectionism, a tendency to be socially inhibited, compliance, and emotional restraint.[9] Unfortunately, these traits are frequently observed only in individuals who are very ill and in a state of starvation, which may affect personality. Thus, it is difficult to determine whether personality is the cause or the effect of the disorder. For example, research shows that perfectionism is high in malnourished individuals and takes a long time to change after recovery.[9]

In contrast to individuals with anorexia nervosa, individuals with bulimia nervosa tend to be more impulsive, have low self-esteem, and demonstrate an extroverted erratic personality style that seeks attention and admiration. For example, a comparison of diaries kept by individuals with bulimia nervosa and healthy controls indicated that those with bulimia nervosa showed greater self-criticism and deterioration in mood following a stressful interpersonal interaction.[10] In individuals with bulimia nervosa, negative moods are more likely to cause overeating than food restriction.[9] Finally, individuals with bulimia nervosa are more likely to practice substance abuse and suffer from anxiety disorders.

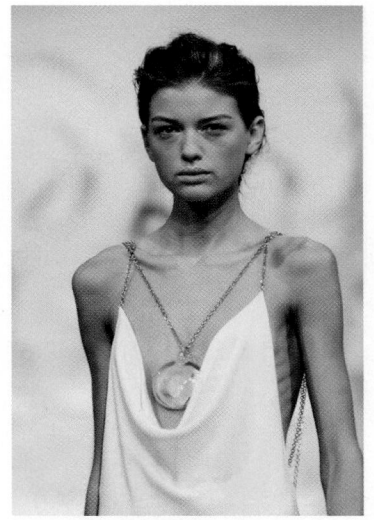

FIGURE 15.3 Until recently, the "in" look among runway models required extreme emaciation, often achieved by self-starvation and/or drug abuse.

Genetic and Biological Factors May Contribute to Eating Disorders

Overall, the diagnosis of anorexia nervosa and bulimia nervosa is several times more common in biological relatives who also have the diagnosis than in the general population.[11] This observation would imply that existence of some mechanism of transmission of the disease occurs within families; however, it is difficult to separate the impact of genetic and environmental components in many studies.

One way to address this issue is to look at the incidence of eating disorders in twins. The heritability of bulimia nervosa was examined in this way in a series of studies from the Virginia Twin Registry.[12] The studies found that heritability and specific environmental influences each accounted for approximately 50% of the variability in who was diagnosed with bulimia nervosa. Similarly, research on twins with anorexia nervosa has determined that if one twin develops anorexia nervosa, there is a 50–75% chance that the other twin will also develop an eating disorder, even if the twins are raised in different households.[13] Although researchers now have strong evidence suggesting that a specific gene or sets of genes may influence the development of eating disorders, no candidate genes have been identified at this time.

Biological factors may also play a role in the development of eating disorders, although this hypothesis is under investigation. Currently, researchers are looking at imbalances in the chemicals that control hunger, appetite, and digestion. Among these are hormones produced in the central nervous system, such as serotonin, dopamine, and cholecystokinin, and a protein called ghrelin, which is released from the stomach and small intestine.[14,15] These are discussed in more detail in Chapter 11.

RECAP: *A number of factors are thought to influence the development of eating disorders. These factors include family environment, society, culture, the media, personality, genetic makeup, and biological factors. However, the combination of factors triggering the development of an eating disorder in any individual is probably unique.*

What Does an Eating Disorder Look Like?

An eating disorder can be defined as a "persistent disturbance of eating behavior which significantly impairs physical health or psychosocial functioning."[16] As we will discuss below, anorexia nervosa and bulimia nervosa fit this description.

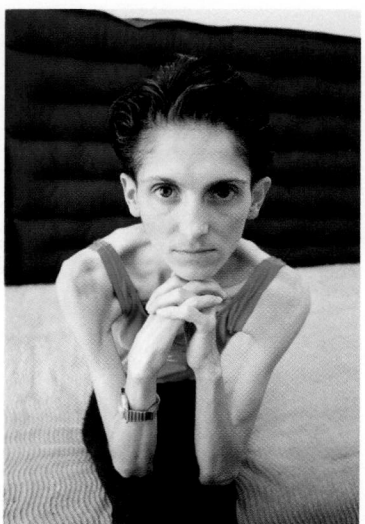

FIGURE 15.4 People with anorexia nervosa experience an extreme drive for thinness, resulting in potentially fatal weight loss.

anorexia nervosa A serious, potentially life-threatening eating disorder that is characterized by self-starvation, which eventually leads to a deficiency in energy and essential nutrients that are required by the body to function normally. For an individual to be considered to have anorexia nervosa, he or she must be medically diagnosed by a physician and meet specific diagnostic criteria.

amenorrhea The absence of a menstrual period. Primary amenorrhea is the absence of menstruation by the age of 16 years in a girl who has secondary sex characteristics, while secondary amenorrhea is the absence of the menstrual period for 3 or more months after menarche. The presence of amenorrhea is a criterion for the diagnosis of anorexia nervosa.

Anorexia Nervosa Is a Potentially Deadly Eating Disorder

Anorexia nervosa is a medical disorder in which an individual uses a number of unhealthful practices to maintain a body weight less than 85% of expected, as based on height and weight. According to the APA, 90–95% of individuals with anorexia nervosa are young girls or women.[1] Approximately 0.5–1% of U.S. females develop anorexia, and between 5% and 20% of these will die from complications of the disorder within 10 years of initial diagnosis.[3] These statistics make anorexia nervosa the most common and deadly psychiatric disorder diagnosed in women and the leading cause of death in females between the ages of 15 and 24 years.[3] Anorexia nervosa also occurs in males, but the prevalence is much lower than in females.[17]

Symptoms of Anorexia Nervosa

For people who develop anorexia nervosa, the trigger factors that initiated the disorder may differ widely, but the results are the same: extremely restrictive eating practices that lead to self-starvation (FIGURE 15.4). These individuals have such an intense drive for thinness and need for weight loss that they may fast completely, restrict energy intake to only a few calories per day, or eliminate all but one or two food groups from their diet. They also have an intense fear of weight gain or becoming fat, even though they are underweight. In anorexic individuals, small amounts of weight gain (for example, 1 or 2 pounds) trigger high stress and anxiety.

Amenorrhea (no menstrual periods for at least 3 months) is a feature of anorexia nervosa in females. *Primary amenorrhea* occurs when a girl has not yet begun to menstruate by age 16, even though she has secondary sex characteristics; *secondary amenorrhea* is the absence of a menstrual period for 3 or more months after menarche. It occurs when a young woman consumes insufficient energy to maintain normal body functions.

The *DSM-IV* identifies the following conditions of anorexia nervosa (reprinted with permission from the *Diagnostic and Statistical Manual of Mental Disorders, Text Revision*, © 2000 American Psychiatric Association):

- Refusal to maintain body weight at or above a minimally normal weight for age and height

- Intense fear of gaining weight or becoming fat, even though considered underweight by all medical criteria

- Disturbance in the way in which one's body weight or shape is experienced, undue influence of body weight or shape on self-evaluation, or denial of the seriousness of the current low body weight

- Amenorrhea in females who are past puberty. Amenorrhea is defined as the absence of at least three consecutive menstrual cycles. A woman is considered to have amenorrhea if her periods occur only when given hormones, such as estrogen or oral contraceptives.

Do you know anyone who might have anorexia nervosa? How can you tell? Table 15.2 lists behavioral, emotional, mental, and physical signs of anorexia nervosa that you might look for in someone you suspect may have this disorder. Remember, one person may not display all of these characteristics, but you may observe one or two characteristics in each category.

Health Risks of Anorexia Nervosa

Left untreated, anorexia nervosa eventually leads to a deficiency in energy and other nutrients that are required by the body to function normally. During this period of self-imposed starvation, the body will use stored fat and lean tissue (for example, organ and muscle tissue) as energy sources to maintain brain tissue and vital body functions. The body will also shut down or reduce nonvital body functions to conserve energy. For example, the menstrual cycle will stop, thus conserving the energy

TABLE 15.2 Behavioral, Emotional, Mental, and Physical Signs of Anorexia Nervosa

Behavioral Signs	Emotional and Mental Signs	Physical Signs
Avoids eating situations	Depression, social isolation, low self-esteem and self-worth	Low body weight
Weighs self frequently		Lack of energy and fatigue
Monitors food intake carefully, develops rigid food rituals, avoids certain foods	Controlling, perfectionistic, rigid, and inflexible	Unsteady gait
	Low sex drive	Complains of being cold or having tingling in hands and feet
Unhappy with body size	Inability to concentrate; insomnia	Thinning of hair or hair loss
Denial of hunger		Excessive exercise

required for normal periods and eliminating the chance of pregnancy during a period when there are inadequate nutrients to support a growing fetus. In children and adolescents, growth slows or stops because the body does not have enough energy to support the formation of new tissue.

In addition, people with anorexia nervosa may have many of the following health problems (FIGURE 15.5). The severity of these problems will depend on the length of time they have had the disorder and the degree of weight loss that has occurred.

- Electrolyte imbalances—These imbalances can lead to irregular heartbeats, heart failure, and death. The role of electrolytes in our health is discussed in detail in Chapter 7.

- Cardiovascular problems—Rapid heart rate, low blood pressure, dizziness, and fainting can all occur as a result of starvation.

- Gastrointestinal problems—The gastrointestinal tract can become weak and lose its ability to function. These changes result in irritable bowel syndrome, constipation, loss of peristalsis, and delayed emptying of food from the intestines. People with anorexia nervosa frequently complain of stomach pain.

- Bone problems—The malnutrition that accompanies starvation can deprive the body of bone-building nutrients such as calcium. The amenorrhea that occurs is associated with a decrease in estrogen production, which causes poor bone health and can lead to osteoporosis (see Chapter 9).

- Muscle and organ wasting—Chronic undernutrition reduces the body's ability to build, repair, and maintain its protein tissues. Eventually, the body begins to use these tissues as an energy source.

- Reproduction—Undernutrition also causes the body to suppress reproductive hormones so that pregnancy does not occur.

- Skin, hair, and nails—In response to undernutrition, the skin becomes increasingly dry and fragile, hair thins, and nails become brittle.

Because the best chances for recovery occur when an individual receives intensive treatment early, it is important to recognize the early warning signs of anorexia nervosa. Use these warning signs as a guide to help identify those at risk for anorexia nervosa and to encourage them to seek help. Discussing a friend's eating disorder can be difficult. It is important to choose an appropriate time and place to raise your concerns, and that you listen closely and with great sensitivity to the person's feelings. The Highlight box: Discussing an Eating Disorder with a Friend or Family Member: What Do You Say? on page 591 outlines an approach you might use in confronting a friend or family member who might have an eating disorder.

Skin/hair/nails:
- Hair becomes thin, dry, and brittle; hair loss occurs
- Skin is dry, easily bruised, and discolored
- Nails turn brittle

Blood and immune system:
- Anemia
- Compromised immune system increases risk of infection

Kidneys:
- Dehydration
- Electrolyte abnormalities that can be life-threatening
- Chronic renal failure

Reproductive function:
- Disruption of sex hormone production, resulting in menstrual dysfunction and amenorrhea in females
- Infertility

Muscle:
- Loss of muscle tissue as the body uses the muscles as an energy source

Brain:
- Altered levels of serotonin and other neurotransmitters
- Alteration in glucose metabolism
- Mood changes

Thyroid gland:
- Abnormal thyroid levels due to starvation

Heart:
- Low blood pressure and abnormal heart rate contribute to dizziness and fainting
- Abnormal electrocardiogram (ECG)
- Sudden death due to ventricular arrhythmias

Gastrointestinal system:
- Abdominal pain and bloating caused by slowed gastric emptying and intestinal motility
- Acute pancreatitis
- Constipation

Bone:
- Decreased bone mineral density (osteopenia)
- Decreased ability to absorb calcium due to low estrogen levels
- Decreased intake of bone-building nutrients due to starvation
- Increased loss of bone due to elevated cortisol levels

FIGURE 15.5 Impact of anorexia nervosa on the body.

bulimia nervosa A serious eating disorder characterized by recurrent episodes of binge eating and recurrent inappropriate compensatory behaviors (such as self-induced vomiting; misuse of laxatives, diuretics, enemas, or other medications; fasting; or excessive exercise) in order to prevent weight gain.

binge eating Consumption of a large amount of food in a short period of time, usually accompanied by a feeling of loss of self-control.

purging An attempt to rid the body of unwanted food by vomiting or other compensatory means, such as excessive exercise, fasting, or laxative abuse.

> RECAP: *Anorexia nervosa is a severe, life-threatening disorder in which the person refuses to maintain a minimally normal body weight, is intensely afraid of gaining weight, and exhibits a significant distortion in the perception of body size and shape. Knowing the early warning signs of anorexia nervosa can help you identify friends and family members at risk for this disorder.*

Bulimia Nervosa Is Characterized by Binging and Purging

Bulimia nervosa is an eating disorder characterized by repeated episodes of **binge eating,** followed by some form of **purging.** While binge eating, the person feels a loss of self-control, including an inability to end the binge once it has started.[18] At the same time, the person feels a sense of euphoria not unlike a drug-induced high. For practical purposes, a binge is usually determined on an individual basis, but generally it is a quantity of food that would be large for the individual, compared to what other people eat, and for the time period and social occasion.[18] For example, a person may eat a dozen brownies with 2 quarts of ice cream in 30 minutes. Binge episodes occur an average of twice a week or more.[1] An individual with bulimia ner-

HIGHLIGHT

HIGHLIGHT HIGHLIGHT HIGHLIGHT HIGHLIGHT HIGHLIGHT

Discussing an Eating Disorder with a Friend or Family Member: What Do You Say?

Background: Before approaching a friend or family member you suspect to have an eating disorder, learn as much as possible as you can about the eating disorder. Make sure you know the difference between the facts and myths about eating disorders. Locate a health professional specializing in eating disorders to whom you can refer your friend, and be ready to go with your friend if he or she does not want to go alone. If you are at a university or college, check with your local health center to see if they have an eating disorder team or can recommend someone to you. Set the stage for your discussion by finding a relaxed and private setting.

Steps to use in your discussion:

- Schedule a time to talk. Set aside a time and place for a private discussion where you can share your concerns openly and honestly in a caring and supportive way. Make sure the setting is quiet and away from other distractions.
- Communicate your concerns. Share your memories and knowledge of specific times when you felt concerned about your friend's eating or exercise behaviors. Explain that you think these things may indicate that there could be a problem that needs professional attention.

- Ask your friend to explore these concerns with a counselor, doctor, nutritionist, or other health professional who is knowledgeable about eating issues.
- Avoid conflicts or a "battle of the wills" with your friend. If your friend refuses to acknowledge that there is a problem, restate your feelings and the reasons for them and leave yourself open and available as a supportive listener.
- Avoid placing shame, blame, or guilt on your friend regarding his or her actions or attitudes. Do not use accusatory "you" statements such as, "You just need to eat" or "You are acting irresponsibly." Instead use "I" statements such as "I am concerned about you because you refuse to eat breakfast and lunch" or "It makes me afraid when I hear you vomit."
- Avoid giving simple solutions. For example, "If you would just stop, everything would be fine."
- Express your continued support. Remind your friend that you care and want your friend to be healthy and happy.

Source: Adapted from National Eating Disorders Association. 2002. Communication: What Should I Say? Used with permission.

---

vosa typically purges after most episodes, but not necessarily on every occasion, and weight gain as a result of binge eating can be significant.

The prevalence of bulimia nervosa is higher than anorexia nervosa; it is estimated to affect 1–4% of women. Like anorexia nervosa, bulimia nervosa is found predominantly in women, with the male–female prevalence ratio ranging from 1:6 to 1:10.[19] This means that for every one male diagnosed with bulimia nervosa, six to ten females are diagnosed. The mortality rate is much lower than for anorexia nervosa, with 1% of patients dying within 10 years of diagnosis.[3] Statistics on bulimia nervosa are somewhat misleading, because about half of anorexic individuals will also be diagnosed with bulimia at some point. Thus, many of the women who die of anorexia nervosa may also have bulimia.

Although the prevalence of bulimia nervosa is much higher in women than in men, rates for men are higher in some predominantly thin-build male sports in which participants are encouraged to maintain a low body weight (for example, horse racing, wrestling, crew, and gymnastics).[17] Individuals in these sports typically do not have all the characteristics of bulimia nervosa, however, and the purging behaviors they practice typically stop once the sport is discontinued.

The binge–purge pattern of disordered eating may begin as an infrequent occurrence in which a person attempts to deal with unwanted food in a social situation. For example, friends are having a pizza party and the person wants to join in but

Men who participate in "thin-build" sports, such as jockeys, have a higher risk for bulimia nervosa than men who do not.

feels guilty about eating so much food. So upon returning home, the person induces vomiting, takes laxatives, or stays up late exercising to burn off the extra calories. What may begin as an isolated incident can develop into a daily event, with purging occurring even after the person has eaten only a small amount of food. Binging and purging behaviors can also be triggered by periods of dieting: depriving oneself of adequate food and energy for a long period of time requires tremendous self-control, and when the control fails, such as if the person "cheats" even once, he or she can quickly lose any ability to deal with food rationally.

Many people with bulimia engage in vomiting as a way of purging unwanted foods. Others abuse laxatives, diuretics, or enemas. These methods do not, of course, rid the body of all of the energy consumed, because some absorption occurs before they take effect. Some people purge with excessive exercise; for example, after a binge a runner may increase her daily mileage to equal the "calculated" energy content of the binge. Some people with bulimia fast for a day or two until they feel they have compensated for the extra calories from the binge.[18]

Symptoms of Bulimia Nervosa

As with anorexia nervosa, the *DMV-IV* has identified conditions of bulimia nervosa (reprinted with permission from the *Diagnostic and Statistical Manual of Mental Disorders, Text Revision*, © 2000 American Psychiatric Association):

* Recurrent episodes of binge eating (for example, eating a large amount of food in a short period of time, such as within 2 hours) (FIGURE 15.6)

* Recurrent inappropriate compensatory behavior in order to prevent weight gain, such as self-induced vomiting; misuse of laxatives, diuretics, enemas, or other medications; fasting; or excessive exercise

* Binge eating occurs on average at least twice a week for 3 months

* Body shape and weight unduly influence self-evaluation

* The disturbance does not occur exclusively during episodes of anorexia nervosa. Some individuals will have periods of binge eating and then periods of starvation, which makes classification of their disorder difficult.

How can you tell if a family member or friend has bulimia nervosa? The National Eating Disorders Association identifies the following early warning signs (Table 15.3):

* Disappearance of large amounts of food in a short period of time, or the existence of wrappers or containers indicating the consumption of large amounts of food

* Frequent trips to the bathroom after a meal, signs or smells of vomiting, presence of wrappers or packages of laxatives or diuretics

* Excessive exercising

* Visual signs such as unusual swelling of the cheeks or jaw area, which is due to the swelling of the salivary glands as they increase saliva production to coat the mouth and esophagus and protect them from stomach acid; calluses on the back of the hands and knuckles from trauma during self-induced vomiting; and/or discoloration of the teeth from contact with stomach acids

* Withdrawal from usual friends and family

* Statements and behaviors indicating that weight loss, dieting, and control of food are becoming primary concerns

To learn more about the realities of having bulimia nervosa, refer to the Highlight box: A Day in the Life of a Bulimic on page 594.

Health Risks of Bulimia Nervosa

The destructive behaviors of bulimia nervosa can lead to illness and even death. The most common health consequences associated with bulimia nervosa are the following:

* Electrolyte imbalance—This can lead to irregular heartbeat and even heart failure and death. The electrolyte imbalance seen in bulimia nervosa is caused by

FIGURE 15.6 People who suffer from bulimia nervosa can consume relatively large amounts of food in brief periods of time.

TABLE 15.3 Behavioral, Emotional, Mental, and Physical Signs of Bulimia Nervosa

Behavioral Signs	Emotional and Mental Signs	Physical Signs
Binge eating at least twice a week for 3 months	Body weight and shape influence self-esteem	Disappearance of large amounts of food
Vomiting, misuse of medications such as laxatives, fasting, or excessive exercise in response to binge eating	Withdrawal from family and friends	Frequent trips to the bathroom
	Statements that weight loss or dieting are of primary concern	Excessive exercise
	Low self-esteem and/or depression	Swelling of cheeks or jaw area
		Tooth decay and tooth staining
		Calluses on hands
		Complaints of gastrointestinal discomfort or pain

dehydration and the loss of potassium and sodium from the body with frequent vomiting.

- Gastrointestinal problems—Inflammation, ulceration, and possible rupture of the esophagus and stomach from frequent binging and vomiting. Chronic irregular bowel movements and constipation may result in people with bulimia who regularly abuse laxatives.

- Dental problems—Tooth decay and staining and mouth sores from stomach acids released during frequent vomiting.

- Calluses on the back of the hands and knuckles from self-induced vomiting.

- Swelling of the cheeks or jaw area from recurrent vomiting.

As with anorexia nervosa, the chance of recovery from bulimia nervosa increases, and the negative effects on health decrease, if the disorder is detected at an early stage. Familiarity with the warning signs of bulimia nervosa can help you identify friends and family members who might be at risk.

> **RECAP:** *Bulimia nervosa is a severe, life-threatening disorder characterized by recurrent episodes of binge eating followed by self-induced vomiting or another method of purging (for example, laxatives, diuretics, excessive exercise, fasting) in an attempt to avoid weight gain. Knowing the early warning signs of bulimia nervosa can help you identify friends and family members who may be at risk.*

What Does Disordered Eating Look Like?

As we discussed earlier, a variety of unhealthful behaviors constitute disordered eating. Chronic overeating and chronic dieting are the milder and more common forms and fall in the middle of the eating issues continuum (see Figure 15.1, page 583). As one progresses to the right of the continuum, a more severe pattern of disordered eating can occur. If it becomes habitual and rigid, these behavior patterns may constitute what is called **Eating Disorders Not Otherwise Specified (EDNOS)**. It is estimated that 3–6% of middle school–aged females and 2–24% of high school–aged

Eating Disorders Not Otherwise Specified (EDNOS) A group of atypical eating disorders that meet the definition of an eating disorder but not the strict criteria for anorexia nervosa or bulimia nervosa

HIGHLIGHT

A Day in the Life of a Bulimic

Hi, my name is Katie.* Through high school and my first 2 years of college, I suffered from bulimia nervosa and used exercise as a method of purging. Initially, I was able to keep it a secret because people saw me eat meals, and I looked normal because I had learned to purge my calories through exercise. After a few years, I knew I had a problem and so did people around me. My excessive exercise is what clued in my friends and family. Below, I give you an example of what a typical day was like for me during my first 2 years of college.

5:30 AM

Alarm goes off. I ate too much yesterday. I was the only one to finish my plate of food at dinner. I must get up and go running. If I can run this morning and eat only a small bowl of cereal at breakfast then everything that happened last night won't matter.

6:10 AM

Two miles in 15:45 minutes. That's horrible. What is my problem? OK, if I won't run fast enough, I'll just have to increase my miles. Instead of running 3 miles, I'm going to run 5. Why are my legs so heavy? I've got to run faster than this.

8:30 AM

The run was pathetic. It wasn't even worth going out. If I just skip going to the cafeteria, then I won't eat breakfast. That's what I should do. No breakfast today. Just get to class and then you'll be OK until lunch.

9:00 AM

Oh no, there's Julie. I know she's going to ask me to go into the cafeteria with her. I can't. Katie, do not let yourself go in to the cafeteria, no matter what Julie says or does. Just wait 3 more hours until lunch. Don't go.

9:25 AM

I can't believe I went to the cafeteria with Julie. Of course, they were serving my favorite scones and I ate two! They are huge—there must be 400 calories in each of them. I'm so utterly disgusting. Julie does not even understand how hard that is for me. I'm so mad at myself. After class, I'll go to the gym. Katie, do not worry about the scones. You can get rid of them by taking the kickboxing class after your workout.

1:00 PM

If I can walk straight past the cafeteria and not eat lunch, I can get home faster, and get to the gym sooner.

1:15 PM

I did it—I walked past the cafeteria. Not eating lunch is going to make my workout feel so much better. I'll drink a diet Coke first and then I'll go.

2:30 PM

Three hundred calories burned on the treadmill and 400 burned on the elliptical machine. That's 700 calories! If I go to the kickboxing class, then I can stop thinking about the scones I ate for breakfast and I'll be able to eat a normal dinner with my roommates.

4:00 PM

I'm exhausted. I've got to lie down.

4:15 PM

I can't lie down. You don't burn calories while you're sleeping. Get up!

5:00 PM

I'm so dizzy. I hate that feeling, but I love it at the same time. It's good to know that I was strong enough to deny myself food long enough to feel dizzy. I get such a sense of strength from feeling so weak, it's strange. I'm safe to go to dinner now as long as I don't eat any dessert afterwards.

7:00 PM

It's amazing how normal I can act when I eat dinner. Even my roommates don't have any idea how hard it is for me to just enjoy a meal with them. I ate my complete dinner and took seconds—I couldn't believe I kept eating. I will add a couple of miles to my run in the morning to make up for the extra 300 calories. I'm too tired to think about it now.

8:30 PM

I've got to go to bed. I can't move my body. I can't concentrate on my homework. I don't know when I'm ever going to get caught up in my classes. I'll have to read some after I run in the morning. I have to do better tomorrow—more exercise and less food.

*Not her real name. This true story was submitted by a student of one of the authors.

females have some type of disordered eating behavior, with the incidence in college-aged athletes and active women being much higher.[3] A number of specific eating disorders fall under the larger category of EDNOS, such as binge-eating disorder and night-eating syndrome, both of which are discussed below. Finally, at the end of this section we discuss chronic dieting, which can lead to EDNOS or more severe eating disorders if left unchecked.

Binge-Eating Disorder Can Cause Significant Weight Gain

When was the last time a friend or relative confessed to you about "going on an eating binge"? Most likely, they explained that the behavior followed some sort of stressful event, such as a problem at work, the break-up of a relationship, or a poor grade on an exam. As we noted earlier, binge eating is defined as the consumption of a large amount of food *in a short period of time*. This time factor distinguishes binge eating from "continual snacking" or "grazing." Many people have one or two binge episodes every year or so, in response to stress. But when the behavior occurs an average of twice a week or more, the person is categorized in the *DSM-IV* as having a **binge-eating disorder**.[1]

The prevalence of binge-eating disorder is estimated to be 2–3% of the adult population and 8% of the obese population; however, some obesity treatment programs report that 20–40% of their patients suffer from this disorder.[20] In contrast to anorexia nervosa and bulimia nervosa, binge-eating disorder is also common in men (in an approximate ratio of 1.5 female to 1 male) and minority groups.

Symptoms of Binge-Eating Disorder

Not surprisingly, people with binge-eating disorder are often overweight. This is not only because of the amount of food they eat, but also because they do not end the binge by purging themselves of the food. In the absence of purging, the increased energy intake that occurs with each binge can significantly increase the person's overall energy intake and contribute to weight gain. Some evidence suggests that a large proportion of people who suffer from binge-eating disorder (35–55%) experienced their first binge-eating episode prior to beginning a diet.[20] As in bulimia nervosa, individuals suffering from binge-eating disorder have a sense of lack of control during the binge episode and cannot will themselves to stop eating. The *DSM-IV* diagnostic criteria for binge-eating disorder are listed below (reprinted with permission from the *Diagnostics and Statistical Manual of Mental Disorders, Text Revision,* © 2000 American Psychiatric Association):[1]

- There are recurrent episodes of binge eating.

- The binge-eating episodes are associated with three (or more) of the following:

    1. eating much more rapidly than normal

    2. eating until feeling uncomfortably full

    3. eating large amounts of food when not feeling physically hungry

    4. eating alone because of being embarrassed by how much one is eating

    5. feeling disgusted with oneself, depressed, or guilty after overeating

- Marked distress regarding binge eating is present.

- The binge eating occurs, on average, at least 2 days a week for 6 weeks.

- The binge eating is not associated with the regular use of inappropriate compensatory behaviors (for example, purging, excessive exercise, fasting) and does not occur exclusively during the course of anorexia nervosa or bulimia nervosa.

In addition, individuals who suffer from binge-eating disorder generally have chaotic eating behaviors, have low levels of dietary restraint (for example, when food is available they cannot resist), and may suffer from chronic overeating behaviors (for example, regularly overeating but without losing control). As you would expect, our

binge-eating disorder A disorder characterized by binge eating an average of twice a week or more.

current food environment, which offers an abundance of good-tasting, cheap food any time of the day, makes it difficult for people with binge-eating disorder to avoid food triggers.

People with binge-eating disorder frequently suffer from negative self-esteem, are distressed over their eating behaviors and body size, and have dysfunctional attitudes about their weight and shape.[20] Depression is reported in 50–60% of people with binge-eating disorder. Substance abuse and anxiety disorders are also common.

Health Risks of Binge-Eating Disorder

Not surprisingly, the destructive overeating behaviors of people suffering from binge-eating disorder can have long-term health consequences. First, the increased energy intake associated with each binge significantly increases a person's risk of being overweight or obese. As discussed in detail in Chapter 11, obesity in turn increases the risk of other health problems such as heart disease, high blood pressure, stroke, diabetes, and arthritis. Second, the types of foods individuals typically consume during a binge episode are high in fat and sugar, which can increase blood lipids. Third, the stress associated with binge eating can have psychological consequences, such as low self-esteem, avoidance of social contact, depression, and negative thoughts related to body size. Constantly battling the negative thought processes that occur following each binge can be overwhelming and increase stress levels. In general, there is a high level of psychological distress associated with this disorder.

> RECAP: *Binge-eating disorder, a form of EDNOS, is characterized by recurrent episodes of compulsive overeating or binge eating. The binge occurs on average two times a week but is not associated with the regular use of inappropriate compensatory behaviors (including vomiting, fasting, excessive exercise) seen in bulimia nervosa. Many people suffering from binge-eating disorder are overweight and experience psychological distress, including depression.*

Night-Eating Syndrome Can Lead to Obesity

Night-eating syndrome was first described in 1955, by Dr. Albert Stunkard, one of the world's leading experts in eating disorders.[21] He identified a group of patients who were not hungry in the morning, but spent the evening and night eating and also reported insomnia. Like binge-eating disorder, night-eating syndrome is associated with obesity: approximately 10% of obese individuals enrolled in weight-loss clinics and 25% of patients undergoing surgical treatment of obesity have the disorder.[21] Night-eating disorder occurs in approximately 5% of individuals who are being treated for insomnia.

Symptoms of Night-Eating Syndrome

The distinguishing characteristic of night-eating syndrome is the time during which most of the day's energy intake occurs. Night eaters eat relatively little during the day, consuming the majority of their energy between 8:00 PM and 6:00 AM. They even get up in the night to eat. In a 1999 study, researchers found that whereas controls consumed 74% of their energy intake by 6:00 PM, night eaters had consumed only 37% by 6:00 PM.[22]

Night eating is also characterized by a depressed mood, which appears to get worse as the day progresses, and by insomnia.[23] These symptoms can be explained in part by the differences in brain neurotransmitters and hormones in the night eater compared to controls. For example, individuals with night-eating syndrome have lower levels of melatonin, a hormone associated with maintaining sleep patterns, and higher levels of cortisol, a hormone associated with stress.[22] In short, night eaters appear to have a unique combination of three disorders: an eating disorder, a sleep disorder, and a mood disorder.[22]

Unlike individuals with bulimia nervosa, night eaters exhibit no compensatory behaviors. Although they don't binge, their intake from snacking throughout the evening and night can represent more calories than those consumed during a single binge-eating episode.[23]

Someone with night-eating syndrome consumes most of his or her daily energy between 8 PM and 6 AM.

night-eating syndrome A disorder characterized by intake of the majority of the day's energy between 8:00 PM and 6:00 AM. Individuals with this eating disorder also experience mood and sleep disorders.

Health Risks of Night-Eating Syndrome

Night-eating syndrome is important clinically because of its association with obesity, which increases the risk for several chronic diseases, including heart disease, high blood pressure, stroke, type 2 diabetes, and arthritis. Obesity also increases the risk for sleep apnea, which can further disrupt the night eater's already abnormal sleeping pattern. However, night eating is still a newly described eating disorder: the APA does not yet list it in the *DSM*, so no uniform definition exists. Once researchers can agree on a definition and diagnostic criteria, the research necessary to determine the prevalence of the disorder, mechanisms of treatment, and long-term health effects can be done.

> RECAP: *Night-eating syndrome is a newly described eating disorder characterized by morning anorexia, evening eating lasting most of the night, insomnia, and depression. As with binge-eating disorder and bulimia nervosa, many people suffering from night-eating disorder are overweight.*

Chronic Dieting Is a Common Pattern of Disordered Eating

Do you find yourself dieting every January to make up for holiday eating or dieting every spring in preparation for beach season? If so, you're not alone. Many people diet occasionally to lose those 3 or 4 extra pounds, and their behavior certainly doesn't qualify as disordered eating. But at some point for some people, those occasional weight-loss diets become habitual, and a cycle of chronic dieting begins. **Chronic dieting** is usually defined as consistently and successfully restricting energy intake to maintain an average or below average body weight.[24] The chronic

chronic dieting Consistently and successfully restricting energy intake to maintain an average or below average body weight.

After several rounds of dieting and then regaining the weight, Oprah Winfrey has stated that she is now comfortable with her weight. Here are two extreme examples of her weight cycling. At left, Oprah in 1988, after losing 67 pounds. At right, in 1992, having regained the weight.

dieter is often referred to as a "restrained eater" in the research literature and may be at risk for poor health and nutrition.

Conversely, **weight cycling** or "yo-yo" dieting occurs when a person who is normal weight or overweight successfully diets to lose weight, then regains the lost weight, and then repeats the cycle all over again.[24] One reason why weight cyclers are thought to be unsuccessful at maintaining long-term weight loss is their failure to make permanent lifestyle changes in their eating and exercise behaviors.

Although energy restriction during the dieting phase can be severe, weight cycling is unlikely to cause serious illness unless the diet is long and unmonitored by a physician. This is because the person overeats during the non-dieting phase, restoring the body's nutritional status. The long-term health consequences associated with this type of dieting, such as increased risk of heart disease, remain controversial. However, everyone agrees that there is a great deal of physiological stress associated with losing and then regaining weight.

Symptoms of Chronic Dieting

How can you tell if someone is a chronic dieter? What characteristics would you look for? Remember the eating continuum (see FIGURE 15.1, page 583)? Notice that as you move from column 3 to column 4, the comments related to dieting and body image become more extreme. That means that people who chronically diet are very aware of what they are eating and may constantly have negative thoughts related to food. If they allow themselves to eat foods they feel are "bad," they become upset with themselves for having so little self-control. Understandably, chronic dieters experience a lot of stress related to eating, and research has shown that their production of the stress hormone cortisol is higher. Some of the symptoms you may observe in a friend or family member who is chronically dieting are related to this increased stress. Below are listed some of the signs of chronic dieting behavior:

Dietary Patterns/Eating Behaviors

- Preoccupation with food, calories, and/or weight
- Strict dieting
- Classifies foods as "good" or "bad"

Exercise/Training Patterns

- Relentless, excessive exercise to help expend energy
- Chronically fatigued and finds it hard to exercise

Psychological Functioning

- Loss of concentration
- Mood swings
- Overly concerned with comparing themselves with others (body shape, training regime)
- Increased criticism of body size or shape

Health Risks of Chronic Dieting

Serious health problems may arise for individuals who chronically restrict their energy intake, especially if they are expending high amounts of energy in exercise. In fact, the female athlete triad (discussed on pages 601–604) is one example of a serious health consequence that can arise from chronic energy restriction in active females. Some other health risks associated with chronic dieting include the following:[25,26]

- Poor nutrient and energy intakes—If you restrict energy intake to less than 1,600 to 1,800 kcal/day, it is almost impossible to get adequate nutrients (pro-

weight cycling The condition of successfully dieting to lose weight, regaining the weight, and repeating the cycle again.

tein, carbohydrates, vitamins, and minerals), even if you are inactive. In general, inactive women need at least 1,600 kcal/day to maintain weight. Recreationally active females (females who exercise 6 to 10 hours a week) typically need 2,200 to 2,500 kcal/day for weight maintenance, while active males may need 2,800 to 3,500 kcal/day. For the competitive athlete who exercises more than 10 hours per week, energy requirements are at least 2,500 to 2,800 kcal/day for females and 3,500 to 4,000 kcal/day for males to maintain body weight. Both inactive and active individuals who restrict energy intake in order to lose weight will frequently have poor vitamin and mineral intakes, especially calcium, magnesium, iron, zinc, B-complex vitamins, and antioxidants. Individuals who diet need to carefully select the foods they eat to make sure their micronutrient needs are met. They may also need to consider taking a multivitamin-mineral supplement.

- Decreased total daily energy expenditure—It is well documented that as you severely restrict energy intake, your basal metabolic rate (BMR) decreases faster than your weight. As you know, your BMR represents the amount of energy required to keep your body functioning at rest—up to 75% of the energy you expend each day. Thus, as dieting reduces your BMR, you need an even greater energy restriction to bring about the weight loss you want. A more reasonable approach to weight loss is to increase energy expenditure (by about 300 to 500 kcal/day on 4 to 5 days per week) using both endurance and strength training, while only moderately decreasing energy intake (no more than 300 to 500 kcal/day). This decrease can usually be achieved by altering food choices and serving size, without counting calories. When this more moderate approach to weight loss is used, more fat tissue is lost, while decreases in lean tissue and BMR are minimized. See the Highlight box: How Does Severe Dieting Alter Basal Metabolic Rate (BMR)?

- Decreased ability to exercise—Remember that in order to maintain body weight, you must consume enough energy to fuel basic metabolism, the building and repair of muscle tissue, activities of daily living, and exercise. Females of reproductive age must also cover the energy costs of menstruation, while children and adolescents need extra energy to fuel their growth. If, in addition, you are trying to maintain an exercise or training program or are competing regularly in sports or dance, you need even more energy. Chronic dieting reduces the level of nutrients available to cover these energy costs. At the same time, it dramatically increases an individual's risk of injury and the time it takes to recover from injury, and reduces both the ability to concentrate and exercise performance.[28] In athletes, a number of psychological stresses are reported with severe dieting, such as increased depression, obsession with food and body weight, increased incidence of binge–purge eating behaviors, increased stress of constantly trying to "make weight" or maintain an unrealistic body weight, and increased risk of developing an eating disorder.[28,29]

- Increased risk of developing a psychiatric eating disorder—One fact that eating disorder specialists agree on is that chronic dieting can lead to more severe forms of disordered eating, including anorexia nervosa. As individuals become more and more restrictive in their dieting behaviors, they move further to the right on the eating continuum and their perception of what constitutes normal eating behaviors becomes more distorted.

RECAP: *An individual who consistently and successfully restricts energy intake to maintain an average or below average body weight is considered a chronic dieter. Because this type of behavior can last for years, the long-term health consequences may be poor nutrient status, loss of lean tissue, poor bone health, fatigue, and decreased ability to exercise. Chronic dieters are also at risk for developing a more severe eating disorder such as anorexia nervosa or bulimia nervosa.*

HIGHLIGHT

How Does Severe Dieting Alter Basal Metabolic Rate (BMR)?

Researchers at the University of Nebraska-Kearney looked at the effect of severe dieting (520 kcal/day) and exercise on changes in BMR and lean tissue in obese females.[27] This classic study is especially interesting because researchers studied both aerobic and weight-training types of exercise. The researchers recruited 115 sedentary female subjects, who were then randomly assigned to one of six exercise groups for a 12-week period. Each of the six exercise groups was fed the same low-energy diet (520 kcal/day), and the researchers monitored all exercise. The exercise consisted of no exercise, aerobic exercise, strength-training exercise, or a combination of aerobic and strength-training exercise administered in different ways.

The researchers found that all groups lost weight, as you would expect on such a low-calorie diet, but total weight loss did not differ between the groups and ranged from 16.7% to 22.3% of the individual's initial body weight. All individuals also lost similar amounts of body fat, ranging from 6.9% to 9.3%. As expected, BMR decreased as a result of the diet and exercise. Interestingly, the greatest decrease in BMR (240 kcal/day decrease; 13.5% decrease) was seen in the dieters who did both aerobic and strength-training exercise (FIGURE 15.7). However, the amount of lean tissue lost in this group was similar to that lost in the other five groups (approximately 4 kg, or 9 pounds).

This study shows that severe energy restriction reduces BMR and that exercise does not slow the decrease of lean tissue or BMR compared to dieting without exercise. The exercise group had the highest energy expenditure and the greatest decrease in BMR during the 12-week dieting period because they had the greatest energy deficit. Thus, the body decreases BMR to conserve energy when our energy intake is low and our energy expenditure is high.

If you're trying to lose weight, the lesson here is to decrease your energy intake modestly, say by 300–500 kcal/day, while increasing energy expenditure by a similarly moderate amount. In this way, you'll achieve a total energy deficit of about 600–1,000 kcal/day. The exact degree of energy deficit you aim for should reflect your body size, current level of daily physical activity, and other health issues. As an example, let's say you begin increasing your energy expenditure by about 300 kcal/day and reducing your energy intake by about the same amount. This is equivalent to adding about 3 miles of walking throughout your day, while skipping the bowl of ice cream each night. By maintaining these modest changes, you should be able to lose about 1 pound a week. This modest deficit should not prompt a dramatic reduction in your BMR, and you should be able to maintain your lower weight as long as you continue your healthful behaviors. Thus, one of the benefits of gradual weight loss is that you lose little lean body mass, which helps you maintain your BMR, while most of the weight loss is fat mass. In addition, you gain all the health benefits of physical activity, such as improved cardiac function, strength, and fitness.

FIGURE 15.7 Obese women who combined severe dieting with exercise experienced a significant decrease in basal metabolic rate. This decrease in basal metabolic rate can inhibit weight loss over the long term. (From J. E. Donnelly, D. J. Jacobsen, J. M. Jakicic, and J. E. Whatley. 1994. Very low calorie diet with concurrent versus delayed and sequential exercise. *Int. J. Obesity* 18: 469–475. Used with permission.)

NUTRI-CASE HANNAH

" This morning, my mom and I each had half a grapefruit for breakfast. I asked her for my Cocoa Puffs, but she said we need to lose some weight, so she was trying this new grapefruit diet. "Oh great," I think, "here we go again!" She's always trying some stupid diet, and they never work. Then she gets all depressed and eats chips and cookies and stuff. The worst thing is, when she goes on a diet, she makes me do it, too. And now here it is not even close to lunch time, and I'm starving!"

If you could counsel Hannah's mother, Judy, about her eating behaviors, what would you say? Specifically, what information might persuade her to change her pattern of disordered eating? What weight-loss strategies might be more effective than her current behaviors? Which of these strategies would be appropriate for Judy and Hannah to pursue together?

What Is the Female Athlete Triad?

The **female athlete triad** is a term used to describe a serious syndrome that consists of three medical disorders frequently seen in female athletes: disordered eating, menstrual dysfunction such as amenorrhea, and osteoporosis (FIGURE 15.8). The American College of Sports Medicine issued a position stand on the female athlete triad in 1997, which emphasized the seriousness of this syndrome in active women and girls and delineated its three components.[30] These are discussed in more detail shortly.

Sports That Emphasize Leanness Increase the Risk for the Female Athlete Triad

Sports that emphasize leanness or a thin body build may place a young girl or woman at risk for the female athlete triad. The American College of Sports Medicine has identified these sports and activities as follows:[30]

- Sports that have subjective performance scoring, such as dance, skating, diving, and gymnastics
- Endurance sports that emphasize a lean build and/or a low body weight, such as long-distance running, cycling, and cross-country skiing
- Sports that require the athlete to wear body-contouring or body-revealing clothing, such as gymnastics, swimming, volleyball, aerobics, track, and dance
- Sports that require athletes to weigh in or that use weight-specific categories for participation, such as horse racing, martial arts, and rowing
- Sports that emphasize a preadolescent body build for success, such as gymnastics, figure skating, and diving

Three Disorders Characterize the Female Athlete Triad

Like women throughout our society, many female athletes feel pressure to conform to a certain ideal body shape and size; however, their source of pressure is twofold. These women experience the general social and cultural demands placed on women

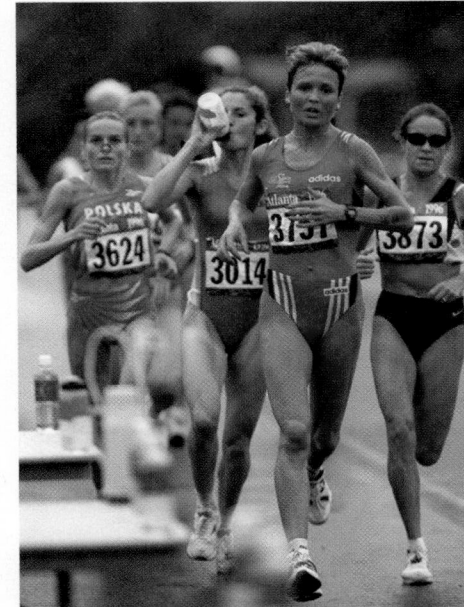

Sports that emphasize leanness or require the athlete to wear body-contouring clothing increase the risk for the female athlete triad.

female athlete triad A serious syndrome that consists of three medical disorders frequently seen in female athletes: disordered eating, menstrual dysfunction, especially amenorrhea, and osteoporosis.

FIGURE 15.8 The female athlete triad is a syndrome composed of three coexisting disorders: disordered eating, menstrual dysfunction such as amenorrhea, and osteoporosis.

to be thin, but also experience pressure from their coach, teammates, judges, and/or spectators to meet weight standards or body size expectations for their sport. Failure to meet these standards can result in severe consequences such as being cut from the team, losing an athletic scholarship, or being eliminated from competition.

As the pressure to be thin mounts, some female athletes begin to engage in disordered eating behaviors. The resulting energy deficit may disrupt the menstrual cycle and result in amenorrhea. Without a normal menstrual cycle and adequate reproductive hormones, which play an important role in bone health, osteoporosis can result. Thus, for many female athletes, disordered eating is the event that leads to amenorrhea and osteoporosis. In the following sections we describe each of the components of the female athlete triad.

Disordered Eating

The first component of the female athlete triad is disordered eating. The way that intense pressure to be thin can increase the incidence of disordered eating was illustrated in a study of military personnel in a military weight-management program who were required to achieve and maintain low body weight in order to keep their jobs.[31] These individuals engaged in bulimic weight-loss behaviors two to five times more often than volunteers in a civilian weight-management program. Thus, under pressures to lose weight or face possible discharge, these soldiers resorted to excessive and unhealthful weight-loss measures. This study can easily be applied to the female athlete who is required to lose weight to make the team or to please a coach or parent. When the stakes are high, female athletes frequently turn to harmful dieting practices to achieve their weight-loss goal.

A number of risk factors may predispose active women to disordered eating, including a history of chronic dieting, an increase in exercise due to training or competition, a stressful event, or the pressure to maintain a low body weight.[31,32] In addition, active women frequently avoid consumption of animal-based foods and strictly limit their fat intake, and these factors can increase their risk even further.[28]

Table 15.2 (see page 589) lists some of the signs and symptoms that an active individual, either male or female, may not be eating enough.

Menstrual Dysfunction

The second component of the female athlete triad is menstrual dysfunction, such as irregular periods, amenorrhea, or failure to ovulate. As we discussed earlier, energy restriction combined with high levels of physical activity can disrupt the menstrual cycle. Research suggests that the menstrual dysfunction may be attributable in part to periods of negative energy balance, when high energy expenditure due to exercise and psychological or physical stress is combined with inadequate energy intake.[26,33] The prevalence of exercise-induced menstrual dysfunction may be as high as 50% in female athletes.[28,33]

Osteoporosis

The final component of the female athlete triad is osteoporosis, which was defined in Chapter 9 as loss of bone mineral density. Female athletes with menstrual dysfunction typically display reduced levels of the reproductive hormones estrogen and progesterone. When estrogen levels in the body are low, it is difficult for bone to retain calcium, and gradual loss of bone mass occurs. Research shows that in the lumbar region of the spine, bone mineral density is reduced by about 14% in amenorrheic athletes compared to athletes with regular menstrual cycles, and by as much as 27% compared to normally menstruating sedentary women.[33] Loss of bone mineral density also increases the risk of muscle and bone injuries, such as stress fractures. Thus, despite the positive stimulus of exercise on bone, the hormonal changes associated with menstrual dysfunction compromise bone mineral density and increase the risk for fracture.

NUTRI-CASE LIZ

" I used to dance with a really cool modern company, where everybody looked sort of healthy and "real." No waifs! When they folded after Christmas, I was really bummed, but this spring, I'm planning to audition for the City Ballet. My best friend dances with them, and she told me that they won't even look at anybody over 100 pounds. That means I have 3 months to lose 8 pounds. With morning and afternoon dance classes, teaching, and school performances, I've got the exercise part down, but I've had to put myself on a pretty strict diet, too. Most days, I come in under 1,200 calories, though some days I cheat and then I feel so out of control. Last week, my dance teacher stopped me after class and asked me whether or not I was menstruating. I thought that was a pretty weird question, so I just said sure, but then when I thought about it, I realized that I haven't had my period for a couple of months now. And I do feel tired a lot. But the audition is only a week away, and after that I can relax a little. I still have 1 pound to go, but I'm going to try a juice fast this weekend. I've just got to make it into the City Ballet!"

What factors increase Liz's risk for the female athlete triad? If you were to explain to her about osteoporosis, stress fractures, and increased injuries, do you think that this might change her disordered eating behaviors? Why or why not? What, if anything, do you think Liz's dance teacher should do? Why is intervention even necessary, since the audition is only a week away?

Recognizing and Treating the Female Athlete Triad Can Be Challenging

Recognition of an athlete with one or more of the components of the female athlete triad can be difficult, especially if the athlete is reluctant to be honest when questioned about the symptoms. For this reason, familiarity with the early warning signs is critical. These include excessive dieting and/or weight loss, excessive exercise, stress fractures, and self-esteem that appears to be dictated by body weight and shape. You may not know whether a female friend or teammate is experiencing irregular periods, but you might overhear her commenting negatively on her body or see her head off to the gym after eating only a lettuce salad for lunch.

Treating an athlete requires a multidisciplinary approach. This means that the sports medicine team, nutritionist, exercise physiologist, psychologist, coach, trainer, parents, friends of the athlete, and the athlete all must work together. As with any health problem, prevention is the best treatment. Thus, recognition of the risk factors by the sports medicine team and education of athletes, coaches, and parents are imperative. If the athlete is having trouble with weight and body shape issues, care should be taken to deal with these issues before they develop into something more serious.

RECAP: *The female athlete triad is a syndrome consisting of three distinct disorders: disordered eating, menstrual dysfunction, and osteoporosis. It is initiated when energy intake is reduced to the point of disrupting the menstrual cycle. When menstrual cycles become irregular or cease, there is a significant decrease in estrogen, a reproductive hormone that improves calcium absorption and the maintenance of healthy bones. Eventually, osteoporosis develops.*

What Therapies Work for People with an Eating Disorder?

Recognition and treatment of someone with an eating disorder can be difficult, especially if the person is reluctant to answer questions about the symptoms and does not want treatment. Since eating disorders can be triggered by any number of factors (discussed earlier), multiple issues may need to be addressed in treatment.

Most Treatment Programs Use a Team Approach

Most treatment programs use a multidisciplinary team-management approach that incorporates medical and nutritional management, psychological treatment, and a number of other therapies, depending on the individual problems and issues that need to be addressed.

Team treatment begins with a physical examination, diagnosis, and identification of underlying causes or trigger factors. The team then meets to decide on the approach each member will use in working with the patient.[34] At this time the team may choose to develop a contract for treatment that is then signed by the patient. Team members meet individually with the patient and as a team to determine the progress being made and the next steps in the treatment process. Team members may also meet with family and friends of the patient and involve them in the treatment plan; this is especially true if the patient is still living at home. Discussed below are the various steps and options that are available.

Treatment Options Vary According to Several Factors

The services available to treat eating disorders range from intensive hospitalization to varied levels of outpatient care (FIGURE 15.9). Many factors influence the type of program selected, including the patient's medical condition, options available, personal preference of the individual and family members involved, and affordability. Of these factors, the patient's medical condition is the most important: an individual who is severely underweight, displays signs of malnutrition, is medically unstable

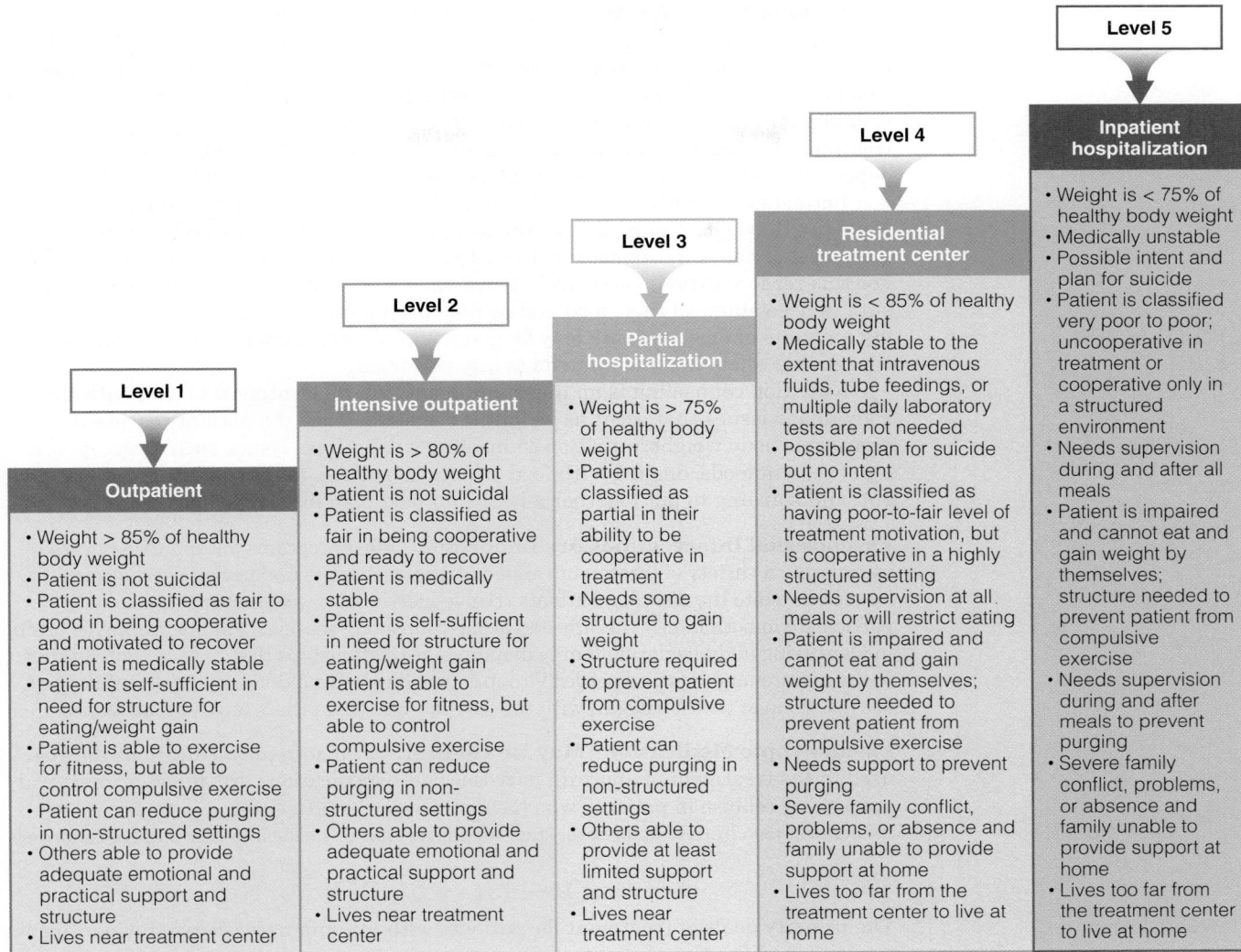

FIGURE 15.9 Five levels of care for eating disorders. An appropriate level is chosen for each patient based on the severity and type of eating disorder as well as social factors. (Adapted from the American Psychiatric Association. 2005. *Practice Guidelines for the Treatment of Patients with Eating Disorders, 2nd edn.* Washington, DC: American Psychiatric Publishing. Used with permission.)

(for example, has elevated pulse rate, low blood pressure, inability to maintain core body temperature, abnormal blood electrolytes), or is suicidal may require immediate hospitalization to stabilize his or her condition and initiate refeeding. Patients may be hospitalized for several days until stabilized, and then transferred to a residential care facility specifically dedicated to treating people with eating disorders.

Conversely, patients who are underweight but are still medically stable may enter an outpatient program designed to meet their specific needs. Some outpatient programs are extremely intensive, requiring patients to come in each day for treatment, while others are less rigorous, requiring only weekly visits for meetings with a psychiatrist or eating disorder specialist.

Treatment Options for Patients with Anorexia Nervosa

The goals of treatment for patients with anorexia nervosa are to restore the patient to a healthy weight, treat any physical complications that may be present, motivate the patient to restore healthful eating habits and lifestyle patterns, correct any dysfunctional feelings related to the patient's eating disorder, treat associated psychiatric conditions, enlist the aid of family and friends to support the patient's healing, and prevent relapse. Nutritional rehabilitation, psychosocial interventions, and medications are the therapies most commonly used to reach these goals.

Nutritional Therapies Are Critical in Anorexia Nervosa Treatment. The goals of nutritional therapies are to restore the individual to a healthy body weight and resolve the nutrition-related eating issues. For hospitalized patients, the expected weight gain per week ranges from 1 to 3 pounds. For outpatient settings, the expected weight gain is much lower (0.5 to 1 pound/week). During the weight gain phase of a treatment program, energy intake goals may be set at 1,000 to 1,600 kcal/day, depending on body size, severity of the disease, and achievable levels of intake.

Patients frequently try a variety of methods to avoid consuming the food presented to them. They may discard the food, vomit, exercise excessively, or engage in a high level of nonexercise motor activity to eliminate the energy they just consumed. For this reason, patients are carefully watched by hospital staff or parents to make sure they swallow all their food and do not spit it out or vomit. In addition to increasing amounts of food, patients may be given vitamin and mineral supplements to ensure that adequate micronutrients are consumed.

Nutrition counseling is an important aspect of the treatment to deal with the body image issues that occur as weight is regained. Once the patient reaches an acceptable body weight, nutrition counseling will address issues such as acceptability of certain foods, dealing with food situations such as family gatherings and eating out, and learning to put together a healthful food plan for weight maintenance.

Psychosocial Interventions Are Important. Most programs for anorexia nervosa incorporate a variety of treatments aimed at addressing the underlying psychological issues related to the disorder. Patients receive individual psychotherapy and usually participate in both family therapy and group counseling sessions. Family therapy is useful in identifying and alleviating family dynamics or relationships that may be contributing to the maintenance of the disorder. Group counseling helps individuals realize that they are not alone in their struggles with the disorder and that others have similar issues.

Psychotropic Medications May Be Helpful. Psychotropic medications may be used in the treatment of anorexia nervosa. These medications are aimed primarily at preventing relapse in patients who have undergone treatment and in treating associated psychiatric disorders, such as depression or obsessive-compulsive disorder.

Treatment Options for Patients with Bulimia Nervosa

The primary goals of treatment for patients with bulimia nervosa are the identification and modification of events, behaviors, or environments that trigger binging and purging behaviors. As with anorexia nervosa, a variety of approaches are used to reach these goals. The most common include nutritional rehabilitation, psychosocial interventions, and medications.

Nutrition Counseling Is Critical in Bulimia Nervosa Treatment. Most individuals with bulimia nervosa are of normal weight or overweight, so restoring body weight is generally not the focus of treatment as it is with anorexia nervosa. Instead, nutrition counseling generally focuses on identifying and dealing with events and feelings that trigger binging, reducing purging, and establishing eating behaviors that can maintain a healthful body weight. In addition, nutrition counseling will address negative feelings about foods and the fear associated with uncontrolled binge eating of foods.

Psychosocial Interventions Are Important. Cognitive therapy that helps patients monitor and alter their thought patterns related to eating issues and body image has been shown to be the most effective form of treatment for bulimia nervosa. Behavior modification can help patients stop a binge episode from occurring or interrupt one in progress. As with anorexia nervosa, both group therapy and family therapy are important. These approaches help identify food issues, body image concerns, interpersonal conflicts, difficulties with anger and aggression management, family dysfunctions, and coping styles that contribute to the disorder.

Antidepressant Medications May Be Helpful. The treatment of bulimia nervosa frequently includes the use of antidepressant medications. These are prescribed to alleviate the symptoms of depression, anxiety, obsessions, and overriding impulses that trigger a binge-and-purge event.

> RECAP: *Treatments for patients with an eating disorder may combine a variety of therapies, including feeding patients, nutritional counseling, individual psychotherapy, family therapy, support groups, and medications. Individuals may progress through various levels of treatment (for example, hospitalization to weekly outpatient counseling) over a period of months or years. Some individuals need ongoing counseling and medications to help prevent a recurrence of their eating disorder.*

How Can We Prevent Eating Disorders and Disordered Eating?

We have suggested throughout this book that, rather than trying to achieve an unrealistic body weight, you try to achieve a weight that is healthful for you and one that you can maintain for life. This process requires you to think about your genetics, current body size and shape, environment, social life, exercise habits, health concerns, and psychological factors. A healthful weight is one that can be realistically maintained, allows for involvement in physical activity, and reduces risk factors for chronic disease. It is dangerous to strive for a body weight that you cannot maintain except by constant dieting or by resorting to disordered eating behaviors. See Chapter 11 for practical advice on identifying and maintaining a healthful body weight. In addition, at the end of this chapter is a list of Web links to additional resources related to dieting and eating disorders.

As we noted earlier, it is difficult to delineate precisely what factors precipitate the development of eating disorders. Nevertheless, research does suggest that the following techniques may be useful in prevention:[35]

- Reducing peer and family weight-related criticism and teasing; educating parents and teachers about the destructiveness of such behavior

- Teaching children and adolescents that changes of body shape and size are a natural part of human development

- Improving media literacy skills and helping children and adolescents identify unrealistic body images and subliminal messages

- Establishing public policies related to media messages about body weight and size aimed at children and adolescents

- Identifying body weight and image concerns among children and adolescents early in the developmental years

- Encouraging participation in physical activity and sports early in life to help prevent excessive weight gain

- Establishing healthy eating behaviors within the home, school, and social environments, both for adults and for children; making positive changes in the food environment to reduce unlimited access to high-fat, high-sugar foods in large portions; finding alternative rewards for successful behaviors to replace the use of food (for example, snacks, candy, sweets, fast food) and sedentary behavior (for example, more time at the computer or in front of the television) as rewards

- Establishing opportunities for activity throughout the day, at work, at school, and during periods of leisure time; encouraging the development of walking programs that allow children and adolescents to walk safely to school and within their neighborhoods

- Modeling of healthful diet and exercise habits by parents

- Commenting positively on attributes of children's and adolescents' bodies that are not related to appearance, such as strength, flexibility, endurance, and gross and fine motor skills

It is most healthful to maintain a body weight that is appropriate for your body type, that allows you to be involved in physical activity, and that reduces risk factors for chronic disease.

Encouraging an active lifestyle early on helps to prevent excessive weight gain and eating disorders.

[
RECAP: *The prevention of eating disorders and disordered eating is a relatively new topic of research; thus, researchers are still developing models for prevention. The current goals of eating disorder prevention programs are to identify precipitating factors in the home, school, and social environment and to implement strategies to reduce or eliminate these factors.*

CHAPTER SUMMARY

- Eating behaviors occur along a continuum from normal to somewhat abnormal to disordered. Our feelings about food and our body image influence our eating behaviors.

- An eating disorder is a psychiatric disorder characterized by extreme body dissatisfaction and long-term eating patterns that negatively affect body functioning.

- Disordered eating is a general term used to describe a variety of abnormal or atypical eating behaviors that are used to achieve or maintain a lower body weight.

- The most common clinically diagnosed eating disorders in the United States are anorexia nervosa, bulimia nervosa, and EDNOS.

- A number of factors are thought to contribute to the development of eating disorders, including family environment, social and cultural factors, the media, personality traits, and genetics and biological factors.

- Anorexia nervosa is a medical disorder in which an individual uses severe food restriction and other practices to maintain a body weight that is less than 85% of the expected weight.

- Health risks associated with anorexia nervosa include electrolyte imbalance, cardiovascular and gastrointestinal problems, malnutrition, and poor bone health. Between 5% and 20% of people with anorexia will die from complications of the disorder within 10 years of initial diagnosis.

- Bulimia nervosa is an eating disorder characterized by recurrent episodes of binge eating, followed by some form of purging.

- The health consequences associated with bulimia nervosa include electrolyte imbalance, dental decay and mouth sores, gastrointestinal ulcerations from binging and vomiting, and constipation. Bulimia nervosa results in death in 1% of patients within 10 years of diagnosis.

- Eating Disorders Not Otherwise Specified (EDNOS) is defined as those conditions that meet the definition of an eating disorder but not the criteria for anorexia nervosa or bulimia nervosa.

- Binge-eating disorder is a type of EDNOS characterized by the consumption of a large amount of food in a short period of time (such as within 2 hours) without compensatory behaviors.

- Increased rates of obesity, cardiovascular disease, diabetes, hypertension, cancer, and depression are associated with binge-eating disorder.

- Night-eating syndrome is a type of eating disorder in which individuals consume the majority of their energy between 8:00 PM and 6:00 AM. Individuals with this eating disorder also experience mood and sleep disorders.

- Chronic dieting is defined as consistently and successfully restricting energy intake to maintain an average or below average body weight.

- Some of the health consequences of chronic dieting may include the following: poor energy and nutrient intakes, poor nutritional status, decreased metabolic rate and total daily energy expenditure, increased psychological stress, increased risk of developing a clinical eating disorder, and increased risk of exercise-induced menstrual dysfunction.

- The female athlete triad is a syndrome characterized by the presence of three coexisting disorders: disordered eating, menstrual dysfunction, especially amenorrhea, and osteoporosis.

- Treatment of a clinical eating disorder typically involves a team approach that includes nutritional management, psychological treatment, medications, and other treatment options as necessary.

- Patients with life-threatening symptoms are hospitalized until their vital signs become stable. They are then typically transferred to an inpatient facility specializing in the treatment of patients with eating disorders. Patients with less severe symptoms typically receive outpatient care that may range from intensive daily appointments to weekly sessions.

• Strategies for preventing eating disorders include interventions to promote children's and adolescents' self-esteem and to help them develop and maintain healthful eating behaviors and exercise habits throughout life.

TEST YOURSELF ANSWERS

1. **False.** Males also are diagnosed with eating disorders, but the incidence for males is much lower than for females.

2. **False.** People can and do recover from medically diagnosed eating disorders, with the best outcomes occurring in those who seek and get treatment early in their illness.

3. **False.** A number of factors may play a role in the development of an eating disorder in any one individual, and researchers no longer believe that the family or home environment is the primary contributor.

4. **True.** As eating behaviors become more and more atypical, there is an increased risk of a clinical eating disorder developing.

5. **True.** Individuals who suffer from bulimia nervosa and binge-eating disorder may be obese. This is especially true of individuals who suffer from binge-eating disorder because they do not purge the extra energy consumed during the binge-eating episode. Overall, 8% of obese people have a problem with binge eating, and some clinics report the incidence to be as high as 20–40% of their obese clients.

REVIEW QUESTIONS

1. Damage to the esophagus, dental decay, and electrolyte imbalances are health risks of what disorder?
   a. binge-eating disorder
   b. bulimia nervosa
   c. chronic dieting
   d. night-eating syndrome

2. Chronic dieting
   a. increases your risk of developing a psychiatric eating disorder.
   b. increases your basal metabolic rate.
   c. is a psychiatric eating disorder.
   d. is a characteristic of bulimia nervosa.

3. The components of the female athlete triad are
   a. disordered eating, amenorrhea, and osteoarthritis.
   b. anorexia nervosa, bulimia nervosa, and increased injuries.
   c. anorexia nervosa, premenstrual syndrome, and osteoporosis.
   d. disordered eating, menstrual dysfunction, and osteoporosis.

4. One recommended strategy for maintaining a healthful body image is to
   a. exercise regularly.
   b. read sports magazines.
   c. reduce your fat intake to no more than 10% of your daily energy consumption.
   d. reduce your intake of sweets to no more than one "treat" a day.

5. Which of the following statements reflects a distorted body image?
   a. I am afraid that if I eat whenever I am hungry I will get fat.
   b. I wish I could change the way I look in the mirror.
   c. My friends tell me I am too thin.
   d. I think about food a lot.

6. True or false? People with binge-eating disorder typically purge to compensate for the binge.

7. True or false? Media images of idealized female bodies are known to cause eating disorders in some adolescent girls.

8. True or false? Insomnia is associated with night-eating syndrome.

9. True or false? People with anorexia typically claim to be ravenously hungry, but then fail to eat.

10. True or false? Chronic overeating is the common name for binge-eating disorder.

11. Explain why there is some truth to the saying that the more you diet, the harder it is to lose weight.

12. Create a flow chart showing how restricted energy intake in female athletes can eventually lead to a fracture.

13. Compare and contrast anorexia nervosa and bulimia nervosa. In what ways are they similar? In what ways are they different?

14. You start a new aerobics class and make friends with another student named Kashi. Although Kashi wears oversized clothes in class, you notice right away that she is extremely thin. After class, you go out for coffee and are surprised when Kashi eats two large pastries with her skim-milk latte. Propose at least two theories as to what might be going on with Kashi.

15. You've noticed that your friend Carlo, who is on your crew team, has been losing a lot of weight over the last few months. Today you sit next to him in class and notice that his cheeks look swollen and the knuckles on the back of his right hand are scabbed. After class, you ask him if he is feeling okay and he frowns. "Never felt better!" he says—and abruptly walks away. What might you do next?

FIND THE QUACK

When Petra left her home in the Czech Republic a year ago to enroll in an acting school in Los Angeles, she viewed her figure as curvaceous. Now when she looks in the mirror, she sees herself as fat. Convinced that she has been turned down at auditions because of her weight, she has tried diet pills, a soup fast, a juice fast, and exercising for 2 or more hours each day, but the weight hasn't been coming off fast enough. A classmate suggested vomiting to rid herself of unwanted calories, but she couldn't make herself do it. At a step aerobics class, she sees a flyer recommending colon cleansing. It lists a Web site address where Petra can learn more about the process and order a "Colon Cleansing Tonic." The flyer states that this is not an enema, but a "pleasant-tasting laxative tonic," and that regular use of this "tonic" will take weight off and keep it off. When Petra gets home, she goes online to the site. Here is what she reads:

- Your colon can contain up to 25 pounds of undigested food and trapped fecal matter. Over time, these ferment and release toxins throughout your body.

- If you don't naturally have a bowel movement after every meal, then your intestines are very likely blocked. If you have difficulty losing weight, low energy, headaches, insomnia, bloating, or constipation, you almost certainly need to cleanse your colon.

- Our patented "Colon Cleansing Tonic" will flush up to 25 pounds from your body. Taken daily, it will help you maintain your new figure and trimmer waistline. It will also increase your energy level, relieve headaches, help you sleep better, and prevent diseases of the digestive system.

- "Colon Cleansing Tonic" was developed by a chemist and a nutritionist. It is a pleasant-tasting syrup containing a proprietary blend of organically grown herbs, roots, and other medicinals chosen for their colon-cleansing power.

- "Colon Cleansing Tonic" is easy to use. Simply mix 2 tablespoons with a cup of pure water and drink each morning upon rising. Never before has it been so easy to eliminate up to 25 pounds of trapped wastes and toxins from your body! A 30-day supply is available for a limited time at the special price of just $29.99! That's less than a dollar a day to a slimmer, healthier you!

1. Petra is 5′7″ tall. When she entered acting school, she weighed 133 pounds. She now weighs 119 pounds. Currently, what is Petra's BMI (see Chapter 11)? Is she overweight? What if any inconsistencies do you notice between her feelings about herself and her actual weight, both 1 year ago and now?

2. Comment on the Web site's statements that "Colon Cleansing Tonic was developed by a chemist and a nutritionist" and that it is a "patented" formula containing a "proprietary" blend of ingredients.

3. You learned in Chapter 3 about the normal functions of digestion and elimination. Comment on the Web site's assertion that "If you don't naturally have a bowel movement after every meal, then your intestines are very likely blocked."

4. Do you think it is possible that Petra's intestines are holding "up to 25 pounds of undigested food and trapped fecal matter"? Why or why not? If the "Colon Cleansing Tonic" is actually a very strong laxative, and Petra were to ingest the recommended dose daily, what do you think she might experience? Hint: Laxative abuse can cause diarrhea, the complications of which are discussed in Chapter 3.

Answers can be found at www.aw-bc.com/thompson.

WEB LINKS

www.massgeneral.org/harriscenter
Massachusetts General Hospital, Harris Center

This site provides information about current eating disorder research, as well as sections on understanding eating disorders and resources for those with eating disorders.

www.nimh.nih.gov
National Institute of Mental Health (NIMH)

Search this site for "disordered eating" or "eating disorders" to find numerous articles on the subject.

www.anad.org

National Association of Anorexia Nervosa and Associated Disorders

Visit this site for information and resources about eating disorders for the public and professional eating disorder specialists.

www.nationaleatingdisorders.org

National Eating Disorders Association

This site is dedicated to expanding public understanding of eating disorders and promoting access to treatment for those affected and support for their families.

www.menstuff.org/issues/byissue/eatingdisorders.html

Menstuff Eating Disorders

A resource for men about eating disorders. Contains information about male anorexia and eating disorders in general, self-assessments, disordered eating statistics, and prevention information.

www.somethingfishy.org

Something Fishy Website on Eating Disorders

A comprehensive Web site about the dangers of eating disorders, eating disorder treatment, and signs and symptoms of disorders. This site includes first-hand survivors' stories and online chats.

www.eatright.org

American Dietetic Association

Visit this site to learn about healthy eating habits.

www.aedweb.org

Academy for Eating Disorders

An organization of professionals dedicated to the best-practice, evidence-based care of individuals suffering from eating disorders.

www.iaedp.com

International Association of Eating Disorders Professionals

Offers education and training in the field of eating disorders, promotes public awareness of eating disorders, and assists in prevention efforts.

www.naafa.org

National Association to Advance Fat Acceptance (NAAFA)

The NAAFA is an organization dedicated to improving the quality of life of overweight people. This site provides public education about the issues of overweight and obesity, news and newsletters, and member support.

www.about-face.org

About Face

A Web site that promotes positive self-esteem among females of all ages, sizes, races, and backgrounds. This site encourages education, activism, and outreach.

REFERENCES

1. American Psychiatric Association (APA). 1994. *Diagnostic and Statistical Manual of Mental Disorders (DSM-IV)*, 4th edn. Washington, DC: American Psychiatric Association.
2. Walsh, B. T., and D. M. Garner. 1997. *Diagnostic Issues. Handbook of Treatment for Eating Disorders*, 2nd edn. New York: Guilford Press.
3. Patrick, L. 2002. Eating disorders: a review of the literature with emphasis on medical complication and clinical nutrition. *Altern. Med. Rev.* 7(3):184–202.
4a. Vandereycken, W. 2002. History of anorexia nervosa and bulimia nervosa. In: D. G. Fairburn and K. D. Brownell, eds. *Eating Disorders and Obesity: A Comprehensive Handbook*, 2nd edn., pp. 151–154. New York: Guilford Press.
4b. Vandereycken, W. 2002. Families of patients with eating disorders. In: D. G. Fairburn and K. D. Brownell, eds. *Eating Disorders and Obesity: A Comprehensive Handbook*, 2nd edn., pp. 215–220. New York: Guilford Press.
5. Stice, E. 2002. Sociocultural influences on body image and eating disturbances. In: D. G. Fairburn and K. D. Brownell, eds. *Eating Disorders and Obesity: A Comprehensive Handbook*, 2nd edn., pp. 103–107. New York: Guilford Press.
6. Striegel-Moore, R. H., and L. Smolak. 2002. Gender, ethnicity, and eating disorders. In: D. G. Fairburn and K. D. Brownell, eds. *Eating Disorders and Obesity: A Comprehensive Handbook*, 2nd edn., pp. 251–255. New York: Guilford Press.
7. Steinberg, L. 2002. *Adolescence*, 6th edn. New York: McGraw-Hill.
8. Lilenfeld, L. R. R., S. Wonderlich, L. P. Riso, R. Crosby, and J. Mitchell. 2005. Eating disorders and personality: a methodological and empirical review. *Clin. Psychol. Rev.* 26(3): 299–320.
9. Wonderlich, S. A. 2002. Personality and eating disorders. In: D. G. Fairburn and K. D. Brownell, eds. *Eating Disorders and Obesity: A Comprehensive Handbook*, 2nd edn., pp. 204–209. New York: Guilford Press.
10. Steiger, H., P. M. Lehoux, and L. Gauvin. 1999. Impulsivity, dietary control and the urge to binge in bulimic syndromes. *Inter. J. Eating Disord.* 26:261–274.
11. Strober, M., and C. M. Bulik. 2002. Genetic epidemiology of eating disorders. In: D. G. Fairburn and K. D. Brownell, eds. *Eating Disorders and Obesity: A Comprehensive Handbook*, 2nd edn., pp. 238–242. New York: Guilford Press.
12. Kendler, K. S., C. MacLean, M. Neal, R. Kessler, A. Heath, and L. Eaves. 1991. The genetic epidemiology of bulimia nervosa. *Am. J. Psychiatry* 148:1627–1637.
13. Klump, K. L., S. Wonderlich, P. Lehoux, L. R. R. Lilenfeld, and C. M. Bulik. 2002. Does environment matter? A review of non-shared environment and eating disorders. *Int. J. Eating Disord.* 31:118–135.
14. Bailor, U. F., and W. H. Kaye. 2003. A review of neuropeptide and neuroendocrine dysregulation in anorexia and bulimia nervosa. *Curr. Drug Target CNS Neurol. Disord.* 2:53–59.
15. Tanaka, M., T. Naruo, N. Nagai, N. Kuroki, T. Shiiya, M. Nakazato, S. Matsukura, and S. Nozoe. 2003. Habitual binge/purge behavior influences circulating ghrelin levels in eating disorders. *J. Psychiat. Res.* 37:17–22.
16. Fairburn, C. G., and T. B. Walsh. 2002. Atypcial eating disorders. In: D. G. Fairburn and K. D. Brownell, eds. *Eating Disorders and Obesity: A Comprehensive Handbook*, 2nd edn., pp. 171–177. New York: Guilford Press.
17. Robb, A. S., and M. J. Dadson. 2002. Eating disorders in males. *Child Adolesc. Psychiatr. Clin. N. Am.* 11:399–418.

18. Garfinkel, P. E. 2002. Classification and diagnosis of eating disorders. In: D. G. Fairburn and K. D. Brownell, eds. *Eating Disorders and Obesity: A Comprehensive Handbook*, 2nd edn., pp. 155–161. New York: Guilford Press.

19. Yager, J., M. J. Devlin, K. A. Halmi, D. B. Herzog, J. E. Mitchell, P. S. Powers, and K. J. Zerbe. 2005. Guideline Watch: *Practice Guidelines for the Treatment of Patients with Eating Disorders*, 2nd edn. Arlington, VA: American Psychiatric Association.

20. Grilo, C. M. 2002. Binge eating disorder. In: D. G. Fairburn and K. D. Brownell, eds. *Eating Disorders and Obesity: A Comprehensive Handbook*, 2nd edn., pp. 178–182. New York: Guilford Press.

21. Stunkard, A. J. 2002. Night eating syndrome. In: D. G. Fairburn and K. D. Brownell, eds. *Eating Disorders and Obesity: A Comprehensive Handbook*, 2nd edn., pp. 183–187. New York: Guilford Press.

22. Birketvedt, G., J. Florholmen, J. Sundsfjord, B. Osterud, D. Binges, W. Bilker, and A. J. Stunkard. 1999. Behavioral and neuroendocrine characteristics of the night-eating syndrome. *J. Am. Med. Assoc.* 282:657–663.

23. O'Reardon, J. P., A. Peshek, K. C. Allison. 2005. Night eating syndrome: diagnosis, epidemiology and management. *CNS Drugs* 19(12):997–1008.

24. Manore, M. M. 1996. Chronic dieting in active women: what are the health consequences? *Women's Health Issues* 6(6):332–341.

25. Manore, M. M. 1998. Running on empty: health consequences of chronic dieting in active women. *ACMS Health Fitness J.* 2(2):24–31.

26. Manore, M. M. 2002. Dietary recommendations and athletic menstrual dysfunction. *Sports Med.* 32(14):887–901.

27. Donnelly, J. E., D. J. Jacobsen, J. M. Jakicic, and J. E. Whatley. 1994. Very low calorie diet with concurrent versus delayed and sequential exercise. *Int. J. Obesity* 18:469–475.

28. Beals, K. A., and M. M. Manore. 1998. Nutritional status of female athletes with subclinical eating disorders. *J. Am. Diet. Assoc.* 98:419–425.

29. Beals, K. A., and M. M. Manore. 2002. Disordered eating and menstrual dysfunction in female collegiate athletes. *Int. J. Sport Nutr. Exerc. Metab.* 12:281–293.

30. Otis, C. L., B. Drinkwater, M. Johnson, A. Loucks, and J. Wilmore. 1997. American College of Sports Medicine Position Stand: the female athlete triad. *Med. Sci. Sports Exerc.* 29:i–ix.

31. Peterson, A. L., W. Talcott, W. J. Kelleher, and S. D. Smith. 1995. Bulimic weight-loss behaviors in military versus civilian weight-management programs. *Military Med.* 160:616–620.

32. Sundgot-Borgen, J. 1994. Risk and trigger factors for the development of eating disorders in female elite athletes. *Med. Sci. Sport Exerc.* 26:414–419.

33. Dueck, C. A., M. M. Manore, and K. S. Matt. 1996. Role of energy balance in athletic menstrual dysfunction. *Int. J. Sport Nutr.* 6:90–116.

34. Joy, E., N. Clark, M. L. Ireland, J. Martie, A. Nattiv, and S. Varechok. 1997. Team management of the female athlete triad. Part 2: Optimal treatment and prevention tactics. *Physician Sports Med.* 25(4):55–69.

35. Piran, N. 2002. Prevention of eating disorders. In: D. G. Fairburn and K. D. Brownell, eds. *Eating Disorders and Obesity: A Comprehensive Handbook*, 2nd edn., pp. 367–371. New York: Guilford Press.

36. Beals, K. A. 2003. Mirror, mirror on the wall, who is the most muscular one of all? Disordered eating and body image disturbances in male athletes. *ACSM Health and Fitness J.* 7(2):6–11.

37. Beals, K. A. 2004. *Disordered Eating in Athletes: A Comprehensive Guide for Health Professionals*. Champaign, IL: Human Kinetics.

38. Woodside, D. B., P. E. Garfinkel, E. Lin, P. Goering, A. S. Kaplan, D. S. Goldbloom, and S. H. Kennedy. 2001. Comparisons of men with full or partial eating disorders, men without eating disorders, and women with eating disorders in the community. *Am. J. Psychiatry* 158(4):570–574.

39. Anorexia Nervosa and Related Eating Disorders, Inc. (ANRED). 2002. Males with eating disorders. www.anred.com/males.html. (Accessed August 2007.)

40. Andersen, A. E. 1992. Eating disorders in male athletes: A special case? In: Brownell, K. D., J. Rodin, and J. H. Wilmore, eds. *Eating, Body Weight and Performance in Athletes: Disorders of Modern Society*, pp. 172–188. Philadelphia, PA: Lea and Febiger.

41. Carlat, D. J., C. A. Camargo, and D. B. Herzog. 1997. Eating disorders in males: a report on 135 patients. *Am. J. Psychiatry* 154(8):1127–1132.

42. Andersen, R. E., S. J. Bartlett, G. D. Morgan, and K. D. Brownell. 1995. Weight loss, psychological and nutritional patterns in competitive male body builders. *Int. J. Eating Disord.* 18:49–57.

43. Nemeroff, C. J., R. I. Stein, N. S. Diehl, and K. M. Smilack. 1994. From the Cleavers to the Clintons: role choices and body orientation as reflected in magazine article content. *Int. J. Eating Disord.* 16:167–176.

44. Mangweth, B., H. G. Pope, G. Kemmler, C. Ebenbichler, A. Hausmann, C. DeCol, B. Kreutner, J. Kinzl, and W. Biebl. 2001. Body image and psychopathology in male bodybuilders. *Psychother. Psychosom.* 70:38–43.

45. Andersen, A. E. 2001, Spring. Eating disorders in males: gender divergence management. *Currents* 2(2). University of Iowa Health Care. www.uihealthcare.com/news/currents/vol2issue2/eatingdisordersinmen.html. (Accessed August 2007.)

46. Pope, H. G., K. A. Phillips, and R. Olivardia. 2000. *The Adonis Complex: The Secret Crisis of Male Body Obsession*. New York: The Free Press.

47. Pope, H. G., and D. L. Katz. 1994. Psychiatric and medical effects of anabolic-androgenic steroid use: a controlled study of 160 athletes. *Arch. Gen. Psychiatry* 51:375–382.

NUTRITION DEBATE

Eating Disorders in Men: Are They Different?

david was tired of being called "fat boy." But the real motivation behind his weight loss was his coach's end-of-season threat: if he didn't lose at least 20 pounds, he wouldn't make the soccer team again next year. David couldn't imagine his life without soccer, so he started cutting back on his snacks and running a couple of mornings a week at the gym. He lost 2 pounds, but it took him 4 weeks. Discouraged by the slow pace, he eliminated all snacking, put less on his plate at mealtimes, and ran every day, first 2 miles, then 3, then 5. The weight started dropping more dramatically, and he loved the high he got from "running on empty." Four months into his program, he'd lost all 20 pounds, and added weight training to his program. By the time the soccer season started, he'd lost 32 pounds, and his coach rewarded him with more time on the field. He knew he should cut back on the dieting

and exercise now that he was in practice every day, but something made him keep at it. Every time he went to the gym, he saw guys more trim, more buff than he was. And he was determined to become like them. No one was ever going to call him "fat boy" again.

Like many people, you might find it hard to believe that "real men" like David develop eating disorders . . . or if they do, their disorders must be somehow different, right? To explore this question, let's take a look at what research has revealed about similarities and differences between men and women with eating disorders.

Comparing Men and Women with Eating Disorders

Until about a decade ago, little research was conducted on eating disorders in males.[36,38] Recently, however, eating disorder experts have begun to examine the gender differences debate in detail and have discovered that "men with eating disorders are very similar to women with eating disorders on most variables."[38] Or, to put it more simply, no current evidence suggests that eating disorders in males are atypical or somehow different from the eating disorders experienced by females.[39] Following is a list of what *is* currently known regarding the similarities and differences between males and females with eating disorders.

Predisposing Factors, Personality Traits, and Dieting History Are Similar

Many of the factors that appear to predispose an individual to an eating disorder are similar for males and females. For example, both have a high probability of coming from families with mental illness and/or have a personal history of mental illness.[36,37,40,41] Both males and females are also frequently connected with some type of social group, such as a family, peer group, or sports team, in which leanness is encouraged.[42] In addition, media studies suggest that males are increasingly becoming the target of articles and ads promoting dieting and an ideal of lean muscularity that is difficult to achieve.[43]

Unlike women, males with eating disorders are likely to have a history of being overweight.

Both males and females with eating disorders, especially anorexia nervosa, tend to be perfectionists, goal oriented, and introverted.[9,37] However, as with women, the extent to which these personality traits are effects of the illness rather than risk factors is not clear.[38]

Finally, dieting is one of the most powerful eating disorder triggers for both males and females.[39] Eating disorders in both males and females typically develop after a period of dieting that becomes increasingly stringent (in anorexia nervosa) or increasingly erratic (in bulimia nervosa).

History of Overweight, Triggers for Dieting, and Methods of Weight Loss Are Different

We discussed in this chapter the fact that females with eating disorders say they *feel* fat even though they typically are normal weight or even underweight before they develop the disorder. In contrast, males who develop eating disorders are more likely to have actually *been* overweight or even obese.[17,37] Thus, the male's fear of "getting fat again" is based on reality. In addition, males with disordered eating are less concerned with actual body weight (scale weight) than females but are more concerned with body composition (percentage of muscle mass compared to fat mass). For example, Mangweth and colleagues found that male bodybuilders obsessed with eating and exercising focused on gaining muscle mass, as opposed to losing fat or weight, and were preoccupied with body image.[44]

Whereas dieting itself is a common trigger for eating disorders in both males and females, research suggests that the factors *initiating* the dieting behavior are different.[40] There appear to be four reasons why males diet: to improve athletic performance, to avoid being teased for being fat, to avoid obesity-related illnesses observed in male family members, and to improve a homosexual relationship.[45] Similar factors are rarely reported by women.

The methods that men and women use to achieve weight loss also appear to differ. Males are more likely to use excessive exercise as a means of weight control, while females use more passive methods such as severe energy restriction, vomiting, and laxative abuse. These weight control differences may stem from the societal biases surrounding dieting and male behavior; that is, dieting is considered to be more acceptable for women, whereas the overwhelming sociocultural belief is that "real men don't diet."[37]

Reverse Anorexia Nervosa: The New Male Eating Disorder?

Is there an eating disorder unique to men? Recently, some eating disorder experts who work with men have suggested that there is. Observing men who are distressed by the idea that they are not sufficiently lean and muscular, who spend long hours lifting weights, and who follow an extremely restrictive diet, they have defined a disorder called *reverse anorexia nervosa*. (The disorder is also

Men are more likely than women to exercise excessively in an effort to control their weight.

called *muscle dysphoria* or *muscle dysmorphia*.) Men with reverse anorexia nervosa perceive themselves as small and frail even though they are actually quite large and muscular. Thus, like men with true anorexia nervosa, they suffer from a body image distortion, but it is reversed. No matter how "buff" or "chiseled" they become, their biology cannot match their idealized body size and shape.[45]

There are other "reversals" in these men compared to men with anorexia and other eating disorders. For instance, men with reverse anorexia nervosa frequently abuse performance-enhancing drugs: in one study, approximately half of the participants reported using anabolic steroids.[46]Additionally, whereas people with anorexia eat little of anything, men with reverse anorexia tend to consume excessive high-protein foods and dietary supplements, especially products like protein powders that promise increased muscle mass and weight gain.[47]

On the other hand, men with reverse anorexia share some characteristics with men and women with other eating disorders. For instance, they too report "feeling fat" and engage in the same behaviors that indicate an obsession with appearance (such as looking in the mirror). They also express significant discomfort with the idea of having to expose their body to others (for example, taking off their clothes in the locker room) and have increased rates of mental illness.[46]

There are some outward indications that someone may be struggling with reverse anorexia nervosa. Not all of them apply to all men with the disorder. If you notice any of the following behaviors in a friend or relative, talk about it with him and let him know that help is available.

- Rigid and excessive schedule of weight training
- Strict adherence to a high-protein, muscle-enhancing diet
- Use of anabolic steroids, protein powders, or other muscle-enhancing drugs or supplements
- Poor attendance at work, school, or sports activities because of interference with rigid weight-training schedule
- Avoidance of social engagements where the person will not be able to follow his strict diet
- Avoidance of situations in which the person would have to expose his body to others
- Frequent and critical self-evaluation of body composition

Do you know anyone who might have reverse anorexia nervosa? If you do, maybe you're wondering how you can tell whether your friend's concern about his body size is extreme or a simple enthusiasm for weight lifting. The warning signs listed above may help. If you think they apply to your friend, talk to him about it. Whereas reverse anorexia nervosa isn't typically life threatening, it can certainly cause distress and despair, as well as all of the health problems associated with use of anabolic steroids and other harmful "bodybuilding" supplements (see Chapter 13). Therapy—especially participation in an all-male support group—can help.

CHAPTER 16

WHAT DO YOU THINK?

Evan is a college sophomore who likes to bet on football with his friends. Most of the time his bets have been small—$5 here, $10 there. Lately, he's been spending more time and money on betting. He and his roommate have running bets on all aspects of the weekly football contests, leading to increased gambling expenditures that reached $100 over the past weekend. For the first time, Evan dipped into his savings to cover his bets. He's also been skipping his evening class since it's on a Monday night and pro football is on TV. He received D's on two recent tests. His roommate has been less willing to bet with him because of Evan's increasing irritability when he loses.

Is Evan addicted to gambling? What signs of possible addiction is he exhibiting? Should his roommate confront him more directly about his gambling? If so, how would you suggest approaching the issue?

Kelly is at home for the summer after her first year of college. She notices that alcohol is a constant presence in her family. Kelly's father has used alcohol for as long as she can remember. He has never been arrested or been violent, but he spends most evenings at the local bar. When Kelly came home this year during school vacations, she felt hurt that her father spent time at the bar rather than with her, but she never said anything. Kelly's mother doesn't directly discuss his drinking, but she gives him the "cold shoulder" the day after a particularly long visit to the bar.

Is Kelly's father dependent on alcohol? How has his drinking affected Kelly? What communication patterns are present in the family that either help or hinder dealing with the issue? How might Kelly's family history affect her own decisions about alcohol?

Addictions and Addictive Behavior: Threats to Wellness

t isn't difficult these days to find numerous high-profile cases of compulsive and destructive behavior. Stories of celebrities and politicians struggling with addictions to alcohol, drugs, and sex are splashed in the headlines and profiled on television news programs. But millions of "everyday" people throughout the world are staging their own battles with addiction as well. (See the Health in a Diverse World box.) Addictions can be perplexing, since many potentially addictive activities may actually enhance the lives of the people who engage in them moderately. The most commonly recognized objects of addiction besides alcohol and drugs are food, sex, relationships, spending money, work, exercise, gambling, and using the Internet.

Taken from: *Decisions for Healthy Living*, by B.E. Pruitt and Jane J. Stein

Obsession with a substance or a behavior, even a generally positive activity such as exercise, can eventually develop into an addiction.

Defining Addiction

Addiction is continued involvement with a substance or activity despite ongoing negative consequences. Addictive behaviors initially provide a sense of pleasure or stability that is beyond the addict's power to achieve in other ways. Eventually, the addicted person needs to be involved in the behavior in order to feel normal.

Physiological dependence is only one indicator of addiction. Psychological dynamics play an important role, which explains why behaviors not related to the use of chemicals—gambling, for example—may also be addictive. In fact, psychological and physiological dependence are so intertwined that it is not really possible to separate the two. For every psychological state, there is a corresponding physiological state. In other words, everything you feel is tied to a chemical process occurring in your body.[1] Thus, addictions once thought to be entirely psychological in nature are now understood to have physiological components.

To be addictive, a behavior must have the potential to produce a positive mood change. Chemicals are responsible for the most profound addictions, not only because they produce dramatic mood changes, but also because they cause cellular changes to which the body adapts so well that it eventually requires the chemical in order to function normally. Yet other behaviors, such as gambling, spending money, working, and sex, also create changes at the cellular level along with positive mood changes. Although the mechanism is not well understood, all forms of addiction probably reflect dysfunction of certain biochemical systems in the brain.[2]

Traditionally, diagnosis of an addiction was limited to drug addiction and was based on three criteria: (1) the presence of an abstinence syndrome, or **withdrawal**—a series of temporary physical and psychological symptoms that occurs when the addicted person abruptly stops using the drug; (2) an associated pattern of pathological behavior (deterioration in work performance, relationships, and social interaction); and (3) **relapse,** the tendency to return to the addictive behavior after a period of abstinence.

Furthermore, until recently, health professionals were unwilling to diagnose an addiction until medical symptoms appeared in the patient. Now we know that although withdrawal, pathological behavior, relapse, and medical symptoms are valid indicators of addiction, they do not characterize all addictive behavior.

Habit versus Addiction

How do we distinguish between a harmless habit and an addiction? The stereotypical image of the addict is of someone desperately seeking a fix 24 hours a day. People have the notion that if you aren't doing the behavior every day, then you're not addicted. The reality is somewhere between these two extremes.

Addiction certainly involves elements of **habit,** a repeated behavior in which the repetition may be unconscious. A habit can be annoying, but it can be broken without too much discomfort by simply becoming aware of its presence and choosing not to do it. Addiction also involves repetition of a behavior, but the repetition occurs by **compulsion,** and considerable discomfort is experienced if the behavior is not performed. An addiction is a habit that has gotten out of control and has negative health effects.

To understand addiction, we need to look beyond the amount and frequency of the behavior, for what happens when a person is involved in the behavior is far more meaningful. For example, someone who drinks only rarely, and then in moderation, may experience personality changes, blackouts (drug-induced amnesia), and other negative consequences (e.g., failing a test, missing an important appointment, getting into a fight) that would never have occurred had the person not taken a few

addiction Continued involvement with a substance or activity despite ongoing negative consequences.

withdrawal A series of temporary physical and biopsychosocial symptoms that occur when the addict abruptly abstains from an addictive chemical or behavior.

relapse The tendency to return to the addictive behavior after a period of abstinence.

habit A repeated behavior in which the repetition may be unconscious.

compulsion Obsessive preoccupation with a behavior and an overwhelming need to perform it.

HEALTH IN A DIVERSE WORLD

HEALTH IN A DIVERSE WORLD

Addiction across Cultures

Although alcohol is considered the typical drug of addiction in the United States, many countries are struggling with epidemic rates of dependence on other drugs. In fact, demand for addiction treatment services is increasing in many nations. Here's a look at some current drug addiction treatment data from around the world:

- In India, more people are seeking treatment for heroin addiction, based on estimates that up to 1 million Indians became addicted to the substance during the 1980s.
- Political upheaval and the resulting disintegration of the family appear to be strongly related to rising drug abuse. A study in Ireland found that as many as 10 percent of young people (ages 15–20) in Dublin were addicted to heroin.
- In the Americas as a whole, cocaine and cocaine derivatives account for almost 60 percent of the demand for drug treatment.

- In contrast, in European nations, opiates, primarily heroin, are the drug of choice for nearly three-quarters of individuals seeking treatment.
- Opiates are also the drug of choice for about two-thirds of addicted individuals in Asian nations.
- Amphetamine use is higher in Nordic nations such as Sweden and Finland, where it accounts for 20 percent and 40 percent of treatment needs, respectively.
- Treatment for cannabis (marijuana, hashish) dependence is much higher in the Caribbean, including Jamaica, where it accounts for over 50 percent of treatment demand.

Sources: From "The Social Impact of Drug Abuse," 1995, United Nations Office for Drug Control and Crime Prevention, New York; and "Global Illicit Drug Trends," 1999, United Nations Office for Drug Control and Crime Prevention, New York.

---

drinks. On the other hand, someone who has a few martinis every evening may never do anything out of character while under the influence of alcohol but may become irritable, manipulative, and aggressive without those regular drinks. For both of these people, alcohol appears to perform a function (mood control) that people should be able to perform without the aid of chemicals, which is a possible sign of addiction. Habits are behaviors that occur through choice and typically do not cause negative health consequences. In contrast, no one decides to become addicted, even though people make choices that contribute to the development of an addiction.

Signs of Addiction

If you asked 10 people to define addiction, you would quite possibly get 10 different responses. Studies show that all animals share the same basic pleasure and reward circuits in the brain that turn on when they come into contact with addictive substances or engage in something pleasurable, such as eating or orgasm. We all engage in potentially addictive behaviors to some extent because some are essential to our survival and are highly reinforcing, such as eating, drinking, and sex. At some point along the continuum, however, some individuals are not able to engage in these or other behaviors moderately and become addicted.

Although different opinions exist as to the cause of addiction, most experts agree on some universal signs of addiction. All addictions are characterized by four common symptoms: (1) compulsion, which is characterized by **obsession,** or excessive preoccupation with the behavior and an overwhelming need to perform it; (2) **loss of control,** or the inability to predict reliably whether any isolated occurrence of the behavior will be healthy or damaging; (3) **negative consequences,** such as physical damage, legal trouble, financial problems, academic failure, and family dissolution, which do not occur with healthy involvement in any behavior; and (4) **denial,** or the inability to perceive that the behavior is self-destructive.

obsession Excessive preoccupation with an addictive object or behavior.

loss of control Inability to predict reliably whether a particular instance of involvement with the addictive object or behavior will be healthy or damaging.

negative consequences Physical damage, legal trouble, financial ruin, academic failure, family dissolution, and other severe problems associated with addiction.

denial Inability to perceive or accurately interpret the effects of the addictive behavior.

These four components are present in all addictions, whether chemical or behavioral.

> WHAT DO YOU THINK? *Have you ever seen signs of addiction in a friend or family member? What types of negative consequences have you witnessed? Can you think of any habits you have that could potentially become addictive?*

The Addictive Process

Addiction is a process that evolves over time. It begins when a person repeatedly seeks the illusion of relief to avoid unpleasant feelings or situations. This pattern is known as **nurturing through avoidance** and is a maladaptive way of taking care of emotional needs. As a person becomes increasingly dependent on the addictive behavior, there is a corresponding deterioration in relationships with family, friends, and coworkers; in performance at work or school; and in personal life. Eventually, addicts do not find the addictive behavior pleasurable but consider it preferable to the unhappy realities they are seeking to escape. FIGURE 16.1 illustrates the cycle of psychological addiction.

The Physiology of Addiction

nurturing through avoidance Repeatedly seeking the illusion of relief to avoid unpleasant feelings or situations, a maladaptive way of taking care of emotional needs.

neurotransmitters Biochemical messengers that exert influence at specific receptor sites on nerve cells.

Virtually all intellectual, emotional, and behavioral functions occur as a result of biochemical interactions between nerve cells in the body. Biochemical messengers, called **neurotransmitters,** exert their influence at specific receptor sites on nerve cells. Drug use and chronic stress can alter these receptor sites and cause the production and breakdown of neurotransmitters.

Mood-altering chemicals, for example, fill up the receptor sites for the body's natural "feel-good" neurotransmitters (endorphins) so that nerve cells are fooled into believing they have enough neurotransmitters and shut down production of these

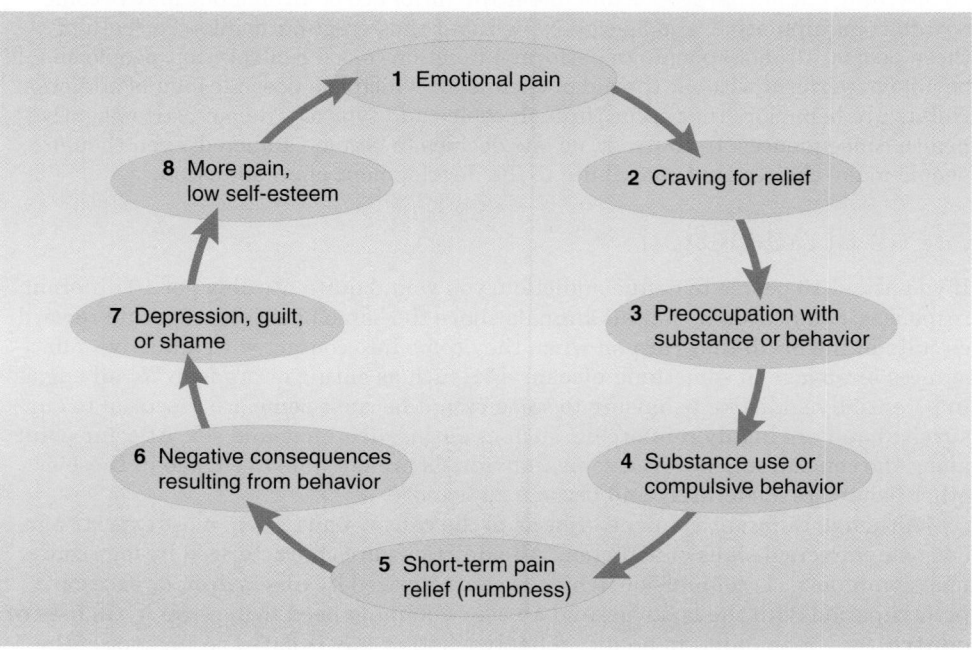

FIGURE 16.1 Cycle of psychological addiction.
Source: Adapted from R. Goldberg, *Drugs Across the Spectrum,* 3rd ed., 2000. Reprinted with permission of Wadsworth, a division of Thomson Learning.

substances temporarily. When the drug use stops, those receptor sites become emptied, resulting in uncomfortable feelings that remain until the body resumes neurotransmitter production or the person consumes more of the drug. Some people's bodies always produce insufficient quantities of these neurotransmitters, so they naturally seek out chemicals such as alcohol as substitutes, or they pursue behaviors such as exercise that increase natural production. Thus, we may be "wired" to seek out substances or experiences that increase pleasure or reduce discomfort.

Mood-altering substances and experiences produce **tolerance,** a phenomenon in which progressively larger doses of a drug or more intense involvement in an experience are needed to obtain the desired effects. All of us develop some degree of tolerance to any mood-altering experience. But because addicts tend to seek intense mood-altering experiences, they eventually increase the amount and intensity to the point of causing negative side effects.

Withdrawal is another phenomenon associated with mood-altering experiences. The drug or activity replaces or causes an effect that the body should normally provide on its own. If the experience is repeated often enough, the body adjusts: It starts to require the drug or experience to obtain the effect it used to be able to produce itself, but no longer can. Stopping the behavior will therefore cause a withdrawal syndrome.

Withdrawal symptoms of chemical dependencies are generally the opposite of the effects of the drug being withdrawn. For example, a cocaine addict experiences a characteristic "crash" (depression and lethargy), while a barbiturate addict experiences trembling, irritability, and convulsions upon withdrawal. Withdrawal symptoms for addictive behaviors are usually less dramatic. They usually involve psychological discomforts such as anxiety, depression, irritability, guilt, anger, and frustration, with an underlying preoccupation with or craving for another exposure to the behavior.

Withdrawal syndromes range from mild to severe. The most severe form of withdrawal syndrome is delirium tremens (DTs), which occurs in approximately 5 percent of dependent individuals withdrawing from alcohol.

A Model of Addiction

Theories abound concerning the cause of addictions, and most of them focus on a single causative factor. Biological or disease models have been proposed since ancient times. However, it has become clear through time that psychological and environmental factors may also be involved in the development of addiction. The most effective treatment today is being provided by those who rely on the **biopsychosocial model of addiction,** which proposes that addiction is caused by a variety of factors operating together, thereby lending credibility to all the other theories. The biopsychosocial model is not a compromise solution to a theoretical controversy. Rather, it represents a reasonable comprehension of all that we have learned about addiction.

Biological or Disease Influences

Studies show that people addicted to mood-altering substances metabolize these substances differently than nonaddicted people do. For example, studies of adult children of alcoholics have found that these people have abnormal concentrations or activity of various neurotransmitters related to mood—specifically norepinephrine, serotonin, endorphin, and enkephalin.[3] Abnormal levels of any of these neurotransmitters may create a biochemically based mood disorder. To obtain relief from the disorder, people may turn to mood-altering chemicals or behaviors.

Genetic studies support a genetic influence for addiction. It has been known for centuries that alcoholism runs in families. Research on family members and twins has repeatedly confirmed the existence of a genetic factor in alcoholism. In the past decade, other studies have shown that the children of drug-addicted parents are more likely to engage in addictive behaviors than are the children of nonaddicted parents. These findings hold true whether or not the children lived with their addicted parents.[4]

tolerance Phenomenon in which progressively larger doses of a drug or more intense involvement in a behavior is needed to produce the desired effects.

biopsychosocial model of addiction Theory of the relationship between an addict's biological (genetic) nature and psychological and environmental influences.

Environmental Influences

Cultural expectations and mores help determine whether people engage in certain behaviors. For example, although many native Italians use alcohol abundantly, there is a low incidence of alcoholism in this culture. Low rates of alcoholism typically exist in cultures such as the Italian one, where children are gradually introduced to alcohol in diluted amounts, on special occasions, and within a strong family group. There is deep disapproval of intoxication, which is not viewed as socially acceptable, stylish, or funny.[5] Such cultural traditions and values are not widespread in the United States, where the incidence of alcohol addiction and alcohol-related problems is very high.

Societal attitudes and messages also influence addictive behavior. The media's emphasis on appearance and the "ideal body" plays a significant role in exercise addiction. Media messages associating alcohol use with holidays, celebrations, romance, sports, and special achievements make it difficult for some people to believe it is possible to have fun without using substances. Societal glorification of money and materialism can lead to work addiction, which is often admired. Societal changes, in turn, influence individual norms. People living in cities characterized by rapid social change or social disorganization often feel less connected to social, religious, and civic institutions. The resulting disenfranchisement leads to increased destructive behaviors, including addiction.[6]

Social learning theory proposes that people learn behaviors by watching role models—parents, caregivers, and significant others. The effects of modeling, imitation, and identification with behavior from early childhood on are well documented. Modeling is especially influential when it involves behavior that is mood-altering. Many studies show that modeling by parents and by idolized celebrities exerts a profound influence on young people.[7]

On an individual level, major stressful life events, such as marriage, divorce, change in work status, and death of a loved one, may trigger addictive behaviors. The death of a spouse is the most common trigger event for excessive drinking among the elderly. Traumatic events in general often instigate addictive behaviors, as traumatized people seek to medicate their pain—pain they may not even be aware of because they've repressed it. One thing that makes addictive behaviors so powerfully attractive is that they reliably alleviate personal pain. However, the relief of pain from addictive behaviors is only temporary; addictive behaviors cause more pain than they relieve. Family members whose needs for love, security, and affirmation are not consistently met; who are refused permission to express their feelings, desires, or needs; and who frequently submerge their personalities to "keep the peace" are prone to addiction. Children whose parents are not consistently available to them (physically or emotionally); who are subjected to sexual abuse, physical abuse, neglect, or abandonment; or who receive inconsistent or disparaging messages about their self-worth may experience psychosocial or physical illness and addiction in adulthood.

Psychological Factors

A person's individual psychological makeup also factors into the potential for addiction. People with low self-esteem, a tendency toward risk-taking behavior, or poor coping skills are more likely to develop addictive patterns of behavior. Individuals who consistently look outside themselves (who have an external locus of control) for solutions and explanations for life events are more likely to experience addiction.[8]

The complexity of addiction and consistent evidence of multiple contributing factors lead us to conclude that addiction is not the result of a single influence but rather of a variety of influences working together. Biological, psychological, and environmental factors all contribute to its development. Although one factor may play a larger role than another in a specific individual, a single factor is rarely sufficient to explain an addiction. FIGURE 16.2 lists risk factors for addiction.

social learning theory Theory that people learn behaviors by watching role models—parents, caregivers, and significant others.

WHAT DO YOU THINK? *Which factors discussed in this section do you think play the biggest role in addiction? Do you think some addictions have a biological basis? Why?*

Biological Factors	Psychological Factors	Environmental Factors
• Unusual early response to the substance or experience (e.g., easy development of tolerance to alcohol)	• Low self-esteem	• Ready access to the substance or experience
• Attention deficit/hyperactivity disorder and other learning disabilities	• External locus of control (looking outside oneself for solutions)	• Abusive or neglectful home environment
• Biologically based mood disorders (depression and bipolar disorders)	• Passivity	• Peer norms
• Addiction among biological family members	• Posttraumatic stress disorders (victims of abuse or other trauma)	• Misperception of peer norms
		• Membership in an alienated, oppressed, or marginalized group
		• Life events, including chronic or acute stressors

FIGURE 16.2   Risk factors for addiction.

Types of Addiction

It is difficult to document the incidence of addictions of any kind because involvement with a chemical or a behavior does not, by itself, indicate addiction. Nevertheless, many studies on morbidity and mortality associated with a substance or behavior provide reasonable estimates. Another indication of the possible prevalence of addictions is that an estimated 10 million people are actively involved in self-help groups in the United States,[9] although, of course, not all of these groups address addiction.

Clearly, tobacco, alcohol, and other drugs are addictive, and addictions to these drugs create multiple problems for addicted individuals as well as their families and society. In this chapter we examine the fundamental concepts and process of addiction, as well as its associated problems. Later chapters in this book will discuss specific addictions. Our discussion of specific forms of addiction focuses on what are commonly called **process addictions**—behaviors known to be addictive because they are mood-altering, such as money, work, exercise, Internet, and sexual addictions.

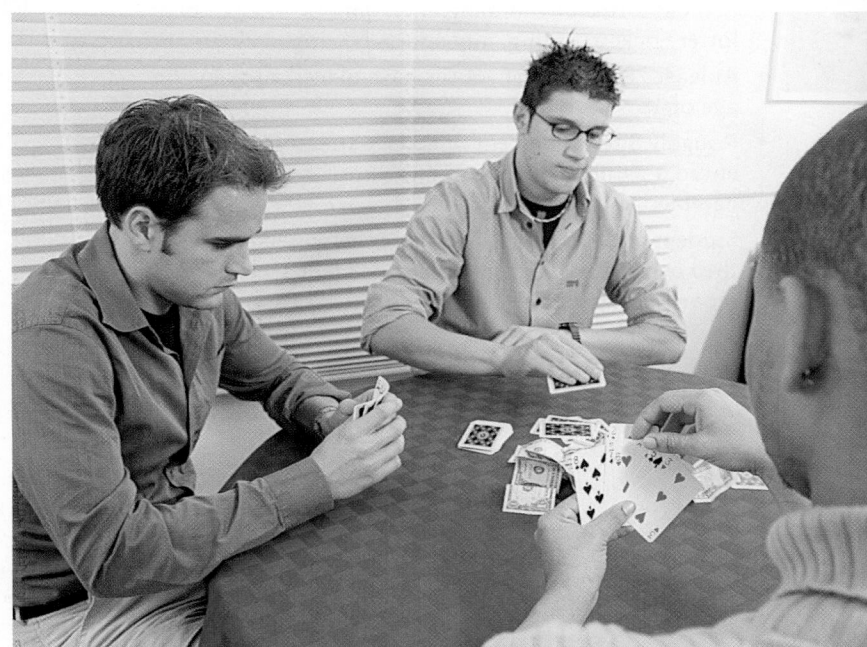

Though many people gamble occasionally as a form of recreation, others become addicted and may face grave financial and personal consequences.

Money Addictions

Money addictions include compulsive gambling, spending, and borrowing. Research has shown that, among susceptible individuals, the various money addictions produce profound mood elevations resulting from synthesis of the neurotransmitters that regulate stimulation, excitement, and pleasure.[10] Money addicts develop tolerance and also experience the phenomenon of withdrawal. Withdrawal symptoms include extreme restlessness, agitation, insomnia, depression, anxiety, and anger.[11] Money addictions are common to both genders and across all ages, races, religions, and socioeconomic groups.

process addictions Behaviors such as money addictions, work addiction, exercise addiction, and sex addictions that are known to be addictive because they are mood-altering.

REALITY CHECK

Gambling and College Students

The Final Four, the Super Bowl, Saturday college football games—there are numerous opportunities for gambling, and recent trends tell us that many college students are taking part. The National Collegiate Athletic Association (NCAA) estimated that during March Madness (the men's college basketball tournament) each year, there are over 1.2 million active gambling pools, with over $2.5 billion gambled. More and more of these dollars are coming from the pockets of college students. There is growing evidence, in fact, that betting on college campuses is interfering with some students' financial and academic futures. Consider the following:

- Almost 80 percent of college students have participated in most forms of gambling, including casino gambling, lottery tickets, racing, and sports betting.
- At least 78 percent of youths have placed a bet by the age of 18.
- Roughly 8 to 20 percent of college students have experienced a gambling problem and about 4.8 percent have gambled compulsively.
- Student athletes have come under increased scrutiny for their association with gambling. Student athletes who report having gambled also report risk-taking behaviors.

- The three most common reasons college students give for gambling are risk, the chance to make money, and the excitement.

Although most college students who gamble are able to do so without developing a problem, warning signs of problem gambling include:

- Missing class or work to participate in gambling.
- Spending more money than intended on bets.
- Lying to roommates, friends, and family about betting, amounts spent, and losses.
- Using tuition money, savings, or money set aside for living expenses to bet.
- Taking cash advances on credit cards or dipping into savings for betting money.

Source: "Sports Betting by College Students: Who Bets and How Often?" by T. J. Knapp, 1998, *College Student Journal* 32 (2); "Survey on College Gambling," by Penn State University, November 1999; "I Can Make That Shot!" *The Wager,* March 6, 2002, 7 (2) (see http://www.thewager.org).

Compulsive Gambling

Gambling is a healthy form of recreation and entertainment for millions of Americans. Most people who gamble do so casually and moderately to experience the excitement of anticipating a win.

But over 5 million Americans are **compulsive gamblers** (addicted to gambling), and 15 million more are considered to be at risk for developing a gambling addiction.[12]

Men are more likely to have gambling problems than women are. Gambling prevalence is also higher among lower-income individuals, those who are divorced, African Americans, and individuals residing within 50 miles of a casino. Residents of southern states, where opportunities to gamble have increased significantly in the past 20 years, also have higher problem gambling rates.[13] For these people, gambling is a compulsion that rules, and often ruins, their lives (see the Reality Check box). While casual gamblers can stop anytime they wish and are capable of seeing the necessity to do so, compulsive gamblers are unable to control the urge to gamble even in the face of devastating consequences: high debt, legal problems, and the loss of everything meaningful, including homes, families, jobs, health—and even their lives. Cardiovascular problems affect 38 percent of compulsive gamblers, and their suicide rate is 20 times higher than that of the general population.[14]

Compulsive Shopping and Borrowing

Although compulsive spending has been a pervasive problem in the United States for some time, a more insidious form of the addiction lurks in the new "plastic generation." Credit card companies entice you with fantasies of having it all, right now—whether or not you can afford it.

compulsive gambler A person addicted to gambling.

The credit card companies seem to be succeeding. There are 400 million Master-Cards and Visas out there. Add to that cable shopping stations, catalog shopping, and now e-commerce, or shopping over the Internet, and the opportunity to overspend is greater than ever before. The resulting debt from all this spending is phenomenal. Bankruptcies, formerly a last resort, have become almost run of the mill—almost 1.3 million were recorded for 2000. On average, compulsive spenders are $23,000 in debt, usually in the form of credit card debt or mortgages against their homes.[15]

Although most people can manage debt with careful planning, some use spending to meet emotional needs they can't fulfill elsewhere. Anxiety, self-doubt, and anger all lead to spending as a way of coping with daily stressors. College students may be particularly vulnerable to spending problems because advertisers and credit card companies heavily target them.

Compulsive gambling and shopping can frequently lead to compulsive borrowing to help support the addiction. Irresponsible investments and purchases lead to debts that the addict tries to repay by borrowing more. Compulsive debtors borrow money repeatedly from family, friends, or institutions in spite of the problems this causes. While most people incur overwhelming debt through a combination of hardship and ignorance about financial management, compulsive debtors incur debt primarily as a result of buying or gambling behaviors in which they have engaged to relieve painful feelings.

Work Addiction

In order to understand work addiction, we need to understand the concept of healthy work. Healthy work provides a sense of identity, helps develop our strengths, and is a means of satisfaction, accomplishment, and mastery of problems. Healthy workers may work passionately for long hours. Although they have occasional projects that keep them away from family, friends, and personal interests for short periods of time, they generally maintain balance in their lives and full control of their schedules. Healthy work does not "consume" the worker.

Conversely, **work addiction** is the compulsive use of work and the work persona to fulfill needs of intimacy, power, and success. It is characterized by obsession, perfectionism, rigidity, fear, anxiety, feelings of inadequacy, low self-esteem, and alienation. Work addiction is more than being unable to relax when not doing something considered "productive." It is the pursuit of the "work persona"—the image that work addicts wish to project onto others.

work addiction The compulsive use of work and the work persona to fulfill needs for intimacy, power, and success.

Work addiction is found among all age, racial, and socioeconomic groups, but it typically develops in people in their 40s and 50s. Male work addicts outnumber female work addicts, but women are catching up fast as they gain more equality in the workforce.

Although work addicts tend to be admired in our society, the effects on individuals and those around them are far reaching. Work addiction is a major source of marital discord and family breakup. In fact, most work addicts come from homes that were alcoholic, rigid, violent, or otherwise dysfunctional. A survey of grandchildren of alcoholics revealed that 64 percent identified work addiction as the most common compulsion in one or both of their parents.[16]

Whether or not they lose their families, work addicts do compromise their emotional and physical health. They may become emotionally crippled, losing the communication and human interaction skills critical to living and working with other people. They are often riddled with guilt and chronic fear—of failure, boredom, laziness, persecution, or being found out. Because they are unable to relax and play, they commonly suffer from chronic fatigue. The excessive pumping of adrenaline that is part of the addiction causes fatigue, hypertension and other cardiovascular diseases, nervousness, trembling, and increased sweating. Work addicts commonly suffer from disorders of the gastrointestinal tract, and they often report a feeling of pressure in the chest, constricted breathing, dizziness, and lightheadedness. FIGURE 16.3 identifies other typical signs of work addiction.

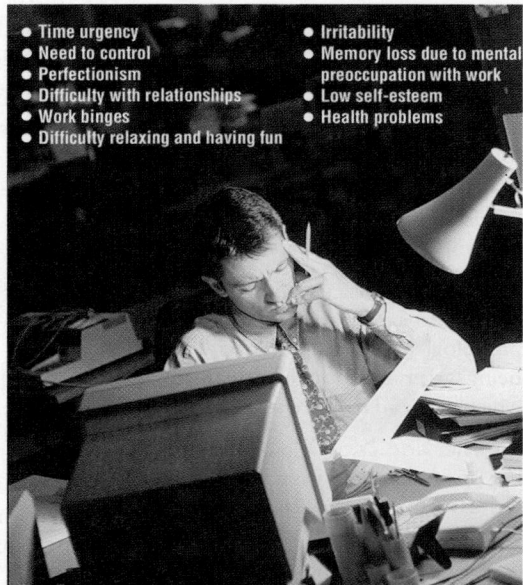

- Time urgency
- Need to control
- Perfectionism
- Difficulty with relationships
- Work binges
- Difficulty relaxing and having fun
- Irritability
- Memory loss due to mental preoccupation with work
- Low self-esteem
- Health problems

FIGURE 16.3 Signs of work addiction.

Exercise Addiction

It may seem odd that a personal health text that advocates exercise would also identify it as a potential addiction. Yet, as a powerful mood enhancer, exercise can be addictive. Statistics on the incidence of this addiction are not available, but it is clear that a large portion of America's 2 million people with anorexia and/or bulimia use exercise as a purge instead of or in addition to self-induced vomiting.

Addictive exercisers abuse exercise in the same way that alcoholics abuse alcohol or addictive spenders abuse money. They use it compulsively to try to meet needs that cannot truly be met by an object or activity: nurturance, intimacy, self-esteem, and self-competency. As a result, addictive exercise results in negative consequences similar to those found in other addictions: alienation of family and friends, injuries from overdoing it, and a craving for more.

Traditionally, women have been perceived as more at risk for exercise addiction. However, evidence is growing that more men are developing unhealthy exercise patterns. Media images promoting "six-pack abs" and lean, muscular male bodies have influenced society's view of the masculine ideal. However, that body type is as unrealistic for most men as the stick-thin fashion model figure is for most women. Meanwhile, more men are abusing steroids and overexercising to attain the desired frame. **Muscle dysmorphia,** sometimes referred to as "bigarexia," is a pathological preoccupation with being larger and more muscular.[17] Sufferers view themselves as small and weak even though they may be quite the opposite.[18] Consequences of muscle dysmorphia include excessive weight lifting and exercising as well as steroid or supplement abuse.

Internet Addiction

There are enormous numbers of Internet users in the United States, with virtually unlimited access to all types of information.[19] It is no wonder that Internet use is becoming a serious problem for some people. **Internet addiction** is a blanket term that encompasses various compulsive behaviors related to computer use. They include viewing sexually explicit materials, playing fantasy games or other computer games, online stock trading, and spending hours in chatrooms or on discussion boards.

Current research indicates that the Internet can be addictive for several reasons:

- *It is accessible.* A person doesn't have to travel or leave the house to chat with people, shop, trade, or play games.

- *It provides control.* A person can trade stocks without a broker, and online auction sites allow users to bid on items without an auctioneer. The Internet also provides the illusion of privacy, meaning that people feel more comfortable having open or explicit conversations that they might not have face to face.

- *It is exciting.* Placing the winning bet, watching stocks rise, winning a fantasy game, and making the highest bid all provide a rush of excitement that reinforces the behavior.[20]

Psychologists and other treatment professionals report an increase in the number of clients who exhibit symptoms of Internet addiction and experience subsequent problems in their relationships, work, and other areas of their lives.[21] See the Assess Yourself box to analyze your Internet use.

Sexual Addiction

Everyone needs love and intimacy, but the sexual practices of people addicted to sex involve neither. In **sexual addiction,** people confuse the intensity of physical arousal with intimacy.[22] They do not feel nurtured by the person with whom they have sex but by the activity itself. Likewise, they are incapable of nurturing another because sex, not the person, is the object of their affection. In fact, people with sexual addictions do not necessarily seek partners to obtain sexual arousal; they may be satisfied by masturbation, whether alone or during phone sex or while reading or

addictive exercisers People who exercise compulsively to try to meet needs of nurturance, intimacy, self-esteem, and self-competency.

muscle dysmorphia Sometimes referred to as "bigarexia," a pathological preoccupation with being larger and more muscular, which can lead to exercise addiction.

internet addiction Compulsive use of computer activities such as fantasy games, online shopping, and chatrooms.

sexual addiction Compulsive involvement in sexual activity.

Are You Addicted to the Internet?

How do you know if you're already addicted or rapidly tumbling toward trouble? Everyone's situation is different, and it's not simply a matter of time spent online. Some people indicate they are addicted with only 20 hours of Internet use, while others who spend much more time online insist it is not a problem for them. It's more important to measure the damage your Internet use causes in your life. What conflicts have emerged in family, relationships, work, or school?

Let's find out. This simple exercise will help you in two ways: (1) If you already know or strongly believe you are addicted to the Internet, this guide will assist you in identifying the areas in your life most impacted by your excessive Net use; and (2) If you're not sure whether you are addicted or not, this will help determine the answer and begin to assess the damage done. Remember, when answering, consider only the time you spend online for nonacademic or non-job-related purposes.

Circle the answer that most closely describes your behavior:

1. How often do you find that you stay online longer than you intended?
   1 = Rarely
   2 = Occasionally
   3 = Frequently
   4 = Often
   5 = Always

2. How often do you neglect household chores to spend more time online?
   1 = Rarely
   2 = Occasionally
   3 = Frequently
   4 = Often
   5 = Always

3. How often do you prefer the excitement of the Internet to intimacy with your partner?
   1 = Rarely
   2 = Occasionally
   3 = Frequently
   4 = Often
   5 = Always

4. How often do you form new relationships with fellow online users?
   1 = Rarely
   2 = Occasionally
   3 = Frequently
   4 = Often
   5 = Always

5. How often do others in your life complain to you about the amount of time you spend online?
   1 = Rarely
   2 = Occasionally
   3 = Frequently
   4 = Often
   5 = Always

6. How often do your grades or school work suffer because of the amount of time you spend online?
   1 = Rarely
   2 = Occasionally
   3 = Frequently
   4 = Often
   5 = Always

7. How often do you check your e-mail before something else that you need to do?
   1 = Rarely
   2 = Occasionally
   3 = Frequently
   4 = Often
   5 = Always

8. How often does your job performance or productivity suffer because of the Internet?
   1 = Rarely
   2 = Occasionally
   3 = Frequently
   4 = Often
   5 = Always

9. How often do you become defensive or secretive when anyone else asks you what you do online?
   1 = Rarely
   2 = Occasionally
   3 = Frequently
   4 = Often
   5 = Always

(Continues)

Are You Addicted to the Internet?—*continued*

10. How often do you block out disturbing thoughts about your life with soothing thoughts about the Internet?
    1 = Rarely
    2 = Occasionally
    3 = Frequently
    4 = Often
    5 = Always

11. How often do you find yourself anticipating when you will go online again?
    1 = Rarely
    2 = Occasionally
    3 = Frequently
    4 = Often
    5 = Always

12. How often do you fear that life without the Internet would be boring, empty, and joyless?
    1 = Rarely
    2 = Occasionally
    3 = Frequently
    4 = Often
    5 = Always

13. How often do you snap, yell, or act annoyed if someone bothers you while you are online?
    1 = Rarely
    2 = Occasionally
    3 = Frequently
    4 = Often
    5 = Always

14. How often do you lose sleep to late-night log-ons?
    1 = Rarely
    2 = Occasionally
    3 = Frequently
    4 = Often
    5 = Always

15. How often do you feel preoccupied with the Internet when off-line, or fantasize about being online?
    1 = Rarely
    2 = Occasionally
    3 = Frequently
    4 = Often
    5 = Always

16. How often do you find yourself saying "just a few more minutes" when online?
    1 = Rarely
    2 = Occasionally
    3 = Frequently
    4 = Often
    5 = Always

17. How often do you try to cut down the amount of time you spend online and fail?
    1 = Rarely
    2 = Occasionally
    3 = Frequently
    4 = Often
    5 = Always

18. How often do you try to hide how long you've been online?
    1 = Rarely
    2 = Occasionally
    3 = Frequently
    4 = Often
    5 = Always

19. How often do you choose to spend more time online over going out with others?
    1 = Rarely
    2 = Occasionally
    3 = Frequently
    4 = Often
    5 = Always

20. How often do you feel depressed, moody, or nervous when you are off-line, which goes away once you are back online? Do these feelings go away once you are back online?
    1 = Rarely
    2 = Occasionally
    3 = Frequently
    4 = Often
    5 = Always

After you have answered all the questions, add the numbers you selected for each response to obtain a final score. The higher your score, the greater your level of addiction and the problems your Internet usage causes.

20–49 points: You are an average Internet user. You may surf the Web a bit too long at times, but you have control over your usage.

50–79 points: You are experiencing occasional or frequent problems because of the Internet. You should consider the Internet's full impact on your life.

80–100 points: Your Internet usage is causing significant problems in your life. You should evaluate the impact of the Internet on your life and address the problems directly caused by your Internet usage.

Source: Reprinted by permission of Dr. Kimberly S. Young, director of Center for Online Addiction, 2002 (see http://www.netaddiction.com).

watching erotica. They may participate in a wide range of sexual activities, including affairs, sex with strangers, prostitution, voyeurism, exhibitionism, cross-dressing, rape, incest, and pedophilia.

People addicted to sex frequently experience crushing episodes of depression and anxiety, fueled by the fear of discovery. Suicide is high among people who have problems with sexual control. The toll that these addictions exacts is most clearly seen in loss of intimacy with loved ones, which frequently leads to family disintegration.

No group of people is more or less likely than another to become involved in sexual addictions. They affect men and women of all ages, including married and single people, and people of any sexual preference. Most people with sexual addictions share a similar background: a dysfunctional childhood family, often characterized by chemical dependency or other addictions. Many were physically and emotionally abused. People addicted to sex tend to have a history of sexual abuse.

Multiple Addictions

Treatment centers for addiction often find that addicts depend on more than one chemical and/or behavior. Though they tend to have a "drug of choice" or a "behavior of choice," one that they prefer because it is more effective at meeting their needs, as many as 60 percent of people in treatment have problems with more than one addiction. The figure may be as high as 75 percent for people addicted to chemicals. For example, alcohol addiction and eating disorders are commonly paired in women. Both chemically dependent women and men frequently resort to compulsive eating to keep themselves abstinent from drugs. One study showed that 49 percent of compulsive gamblers are also alcoholics.[23] While multiple addictions certainly complicate recovery, they do not make it impossible. As with single addictions, recovery begins with the recognition that there is a problem.

> WHAT DO YOU THINK? *We have used a broad definition of the concept of addiction in this text. Do you think any behavior can be addictive? Can one be a chocolate addict or a study addict? What potential dangers lie in using the term addiction too loosely?*

How Addiction Affects Family and Friends

The family and friends of an addicted person also suffer many negative consequences. Often they struggle with **codependence,** a self-defeating relationship pattern in which a person is "addicted to the addict." It is the primary outcome of dysfunctional relationships or families. Codependence is not accurately defined by isolated incidents but rather by a pattern of behavior. Codependents find it hard to set healthy boundaries and often live in the chaotic, crisis-oriented mode that naturally occurs around addicts. They assume responsibility for meeting others' needs to the point that they subordinate or even cease being aware of their own needs. They may be unable to perceive their needs because they have repeatedly been taught that their needs are inappropriate or less important than someone else's. Their behavior goes far beyond performing kind services for another person. Codependents feel less than human if they fail to respond to the needs of someone else, even when their help was not requested. Although the term *codependent* is used less frequently today, treatment professionals still recognize the importance of helping addicts recognize how their behavior affects those around them and working with family and friends to establish healthier relationships and boundaries.

Family and friends can play an important role in getting an addict to seek treatment. They are most helpful when they refuse to be enablers. **Enablers** are people who knowingly or unknowingly protect addicts from the natural consequences of their behavior. If they don't have to deal with the consequences, addicts cannot see the

codependence A self-defeating relationship pattern in which a person is "addicted to the addict."

enablers People who knowingly or unknowingly protect addicts from the natural consequences of their behavior.

self-destructive nature of their behavior and will therefore continue it. Codependents are the primary enablers of their addicted loved ones, although anyone who has contact with an addict can be an enabler and thus contribute (perhaps powerfully) to continuation of the addictive behavior. Enablers are generally unaware that their behavior has this effect. In fact, enabling is rarely conscious and certainly not intentional.

> **WHAT DO YOU THINK?** *Why do we tend to protect others from the natural consequences of their destructive behaviors? Have you ever confronted someone you were concerned about? If so, was the confrontation successful? What tips would you give someone who wants to confront a loved one about an addiction?*

Treatment for and Recovery from Addiction

A key step in the recovery process is to recognize the addiction. This can be difficult because of the power of denial. Denial—the inability to see the truth—is the hallmark of addiction. It can be so powerful that intervention is sometimes necessary to break down the addict's denial system.

Intervention

Intervention is a planned process of confrontation by people who are important to the addict, including spouse, parents, children, boss, and friends. Its purpose is to break down the denial compassionately so that the addict can see the destructive nature of the addiction. It is not enough to get the person to admit that he or she is addicted. The addict must come to perceive that the addiction is destructive and requires treatment.

Individual confrontation is difficult and often futile. However, an addict's defenses generally crumble when significant others collectively share their observations and concerns about the addict's behavior. It is critical that those involved in the intervention clarify how they plan to end their enabling. For example, a wife may state that she will no longer cover bounced checks or make excuses for her money-addicted husband's antisocial behavior. She may even close their joint account and open a personal account so she will not be legally responsible for his irresponsible acts. All parties involved in the intervention must choose consequences they are ready to follow through with, in the event that the addict refuses treatment. Significant others must also be ready to give support if the addict is willing to begin a recovery program. Components of effective intervention include the following:

intervention A planned process of confronting an addict, carried out by significant others.

- Emphasizing care and concern for the addicted person.

- Describing the behavior that is the cause for concern.

- Expressing how the behavior affects the addict, each person taking part in the intervention, and others.

- Outlining specifically what you would like to see happen.

Intervention is a serious step toward helping someone who probably does not want help. It should therefore be well planned and rehearsed. Most addiction treatment centers have specialists on staff who can help plan an intervention. In addition, books on the subject are available

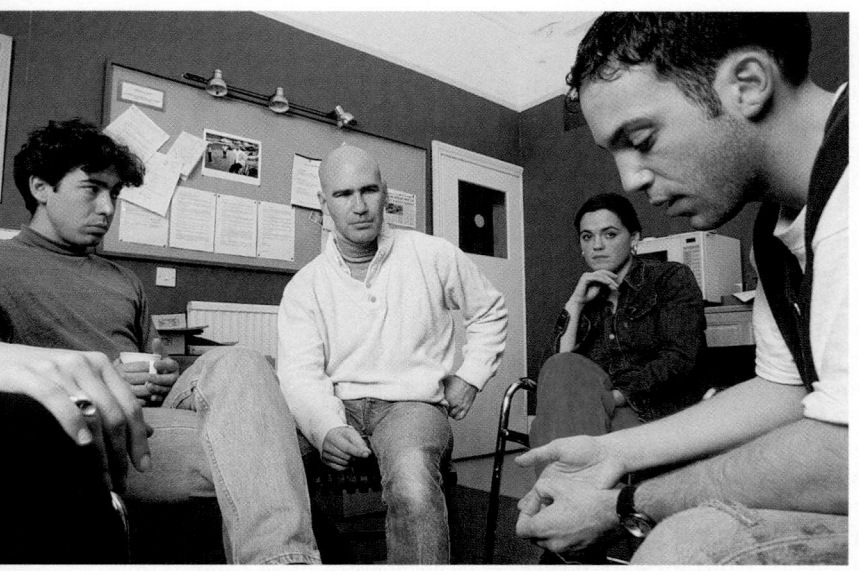

Group therapy provides a safe environment for people to learn how to be honest with themselves and others about the reality and consequences of their addictions.

HEALTH ETHICS

Conflict and Controversy: Abstinence or Moderation?

When Bill Wilson founded Alcoholics Anonymous in 1935, complete abstinence from alcohol was the foundation of his program. Most modern, mainstream addiction treatments are still based on abstinence as the key to success. However, over the past 10 years, offshoot treatment programs focusing on moderate use of alcohol have gained a foothold among the general public. Although the moderation philosophy has never been accepted by most treatment centers, a group called Moderation Management, founded by Audrey Kishline, has been gaining popularity, primarily through an extensive Internet presence.

Proponents of the moderation movement say that alcohol addiction should be seen as a continuum, similar to the way other health conditions, such as high blood pressure, are viewed. They claim that just as not everyone with high blood pressure needs the most extreme form of treatment, not all problem drinkers need to stop drinking completely to avoid further problems. They believe that a strict abstinence approach may just turn off people who could benefit from treatment.

Recently, however, the moderation movement took a huge blow when Kishline was sentenced to four and a half years in prison for killing two people while driving under the influence of alcohol. Kishline, whose blood alcohol concentration was .26, crossed the centerline, killing a 38-year-old man and his 12-year-old daughter. A few weeks before, Kishline had posted a message on the Moderation Management website, saying she could no longer moderate her own alcohol use and, although she still believed in the movement, would be seeking 12-step, abstinence-based treatment for herself. Just after Kishline's accident, the director of a leading treatment center in New York resigned after failing to gain his staff's support for offering moderation-based treatment to some clients.

Critics of the moderation movement cite these incidents as poignant evidence that the approach is flawed and simply another way for alcoholics to deny their problem and delay recovery. According to those in the traditional treatment industry, telling alcoholics they can get better while drinking is simply setting them up for failure.

With over 700,000 people in the United States seeking some form of treatment for alcohol problems daily, it is certain that the moderation/abstinence debate will continue for years to come.

Sources: From "License to Drink," by E. Rivera, *Time*, July 31, 2000; and "10th Special Report to the U.S. Congress on Alcohol and Health," by the National Institute on Alcohol Abuse and Alcoholism, July 2000.

---

for families and friends who are concerned about someone who may be addicted. Once the problem has been recognized, recovery can begin.

Treatment

Treatment and recovery for any addiction generally begin with **abstinence**— refraining from the addictive behavior. While literal abstinence is possible for people addicted to chemicals, it obviously is not for people addicted to behaviors like work and sex. For these addicts, abstinence means restoring balance to their lives through noncompulsive engagement in the behaviors, such as avoiding certain activities.

Over the years, a movement toward moderation-based treatments has emerged. This approach proposes that many addicts can learn to moderate their use of substances and activities without stopping entirely. However, this movement has not been without detractors. See the Health Ethics box for more information.

Detoxification refers to the early abstinence period during which an addict adjusts physically and cognitively to being free from the influence of the addiction. It occurs in virtually every recovering addict, and whereas it is uncomfortable for them all, it can be dangerous for some. This is primarily true for those addicted to chemicals, especially alcohol, heroin, and tranquilizers such as Valium. For these people, early abstinence may involve profound withdrawal symptoms that require medical supervision. Therefore, most inpatient treatment programs provide a pretreatment component of supervised detoxification to achieve abstinence safely before treatment begins.

abstinence Refraining from an addictive behavior.

detoxification The early abstinence period during which an addict adjusts physically and cognitively to being free from the influences of the addiction.

MEN'S HEALTH

WOMEN'S HEALTH

Addiction Treatment for Women: Still Confronting Barriers

The addiction treatment industry as a whole was built using a "male model" and has only recently begun to address the unique needs of women. Unfortunately, significant barriers remain for women seeking addiction treatment.

Although women entering treatment generally have fewer addiction-related legal problems (arrests for public intoxication or drug dealing, for example) than men do, they face more psychological issues and family, financial, and medical problems. Studies consistently indicate that the two primary barriers women face in successfully completing treatment are child care and transportation. One study found that women who were able to bring their children to inpatient treatment were more likely to remain healthy at six months after treatment. Additional barriers for women seeking addiction treatment include the following:

INDIVIDUAL

- Lack of insurance or inadequate coverage.
- Fear of losing child custody.
- Low self-esteem.
- Low feelings of self-efficacy.

FAMILY

- Too many responsibilities.

- Lack of family support for treatment.
- Abuse in the family environment.

COMMUNITY

- Lack of support from employer.
- Lack of gender-sensitive treatment options.

A "women-friendly" treatment center should offer the following:

- Educational programs on self-worth, assertiveness, family issues, parenting, and anger management.
- Women-only groups, especially for addressing issues of rape, incest, and abuse.
- Networking with and support from other women in recovery.
- Housing and day care.

Women clearly have different treatment needs than men do. Finding a program that addresses these needs improves the likelihood of long-term success and recovery.

Sources: From "How Are Women Who Enter Substance Abuse Treatment Different Than Men? A Gender Comparison from the Drug Abuse Treatment Outcome Study," by W. Weschberg, S. Craddock, and R. Hubbard. In *Women and Substance Abuse: Gender Transparency,* edited by S. Stevens and H. Wexler (New York: Haworth, 1998).

Abstinence alone does little to change the psychological, biological, and environmental dynamics that underlie the addictive behavior. Without recovery, an addict is apt to relapse time and again or simply to change addictions. Recovery involves learning new ways of looking at oneself, others, and the world. It may require exploring a traumatic past so that psychological wounds can be healed. It also involves learning *interdependence* with significant others and new ways of taking care of oneself, physically and emotionally. And involves developing communication skills and new ways of having fun.

Recovery programs are the fuel that gives addicts the energy to resist relapsing. For a large number of addicts, recovery begins with a period of formal treatment. A good treatment program includes the following characteristics:

- Professional staff familiar with the specific addictive disorder for which help is being sought.
- A flexible schedule of both inpatient and outpatient services.
- Access to medical personnel who can assess the addict's health and treat all medical concerns as needed.
- Medical supervision of addicts who are at high risk for a complicated detoxification.
- Involvement of family members in the treatment process.

- A team approach to treating addictive disorders (e.g., medical personnel, counselors, psychotherapists, social workers, clergy, educators, dietitians, and fitness counselors).

- Both group and individual therapy options.

- Peer-led support groups that encourage the addict to continue involvement after treatment ends.

- Structured after-care and relapse-prevention programs.

- Accreditation by the Joint Commission for the Accreditation of Healthcare Organizations (JCAHO) and a license from the state in which it operates.

Most programs apply a combination of family, individual, and group counseling, supplemented with attendance at a 12-step support group. Individuals may also wish to explore alternatives to 12-step groups. Organizations such as Rational Recovery and the Secular Organization for Sobriety provide support without the spiritual emphasis of 12-step groups such as Alcoholics Anonymous.

Choosing a Treatment

The National Institute on Alcohol Abuse and Alcoholism (NIAAA) recently completed Project MATCH (Matching Alcoholism Treatment to Client Heterogeneity), a large-scale study designed to determine if certain types of patients respond better to particular treatments.

The investigators studied three strategies: cognitive-behavioral therapy, motivational psychology, and a facilitated 12-step program with sessions run by a therapist. Results showed that patients did equally well in each of the treatment approaches. This outcome was somewhat surprising, given that it has been common practice for treatment professionals to match patients to certain approaches. Researchers concluded that the focus, therefore, should simply be on selecting a competently run treatment program. Large-scale studies on other addictions have yet to occur.[24]

The Women's Health/Men's Health box describes factors that are important to address when treating female addicts.

Relapse

Relapse is an isolated occurrence of or full return to addictive behavior. It is one of the defining characteristics of addiction. A person who does not relapse or have powerful urges to do so was probably not addicted in the first place. Relapse is proof that a person is addicted and has abandoned the practice of an ongoing recovery program. Addicts are set up to relapse long before they actually do so because of their tendency to meet change and other forms of stress in their lives with the same kind of denial they once used to justify their addictive behavior (e.g., "I don't have a problem, I can handle this"). This sets off a series of events involving immediate or gradual abandonment of structured recovery plans. For example, the addict may quit attending support group meetings and slip into situations that previously triggered the addictive behavior.

Because treatment programs recognize this strong tendency to relapse, they routinely teach clients and significant others concepts of relapse prevention. Relapse prevention teaches people to recognize the signs of imminent relapse and to develop a plan for responding to these signs. Without such a plan, recovering addicts are likely to relapse more frequently, more completely, and perhaps more permanently.

Relapse should not be interpreted as failure to change or lack of desire to stay well. The appropriate response to relapse is to remind addicts that they are addicted and to redirect them to the recovery strategies that have previously worked for them.

In addition to teaching skills, relapse prevention may involve after-care planning such as connecting the recovering person with support groups, career counselors, or community services.

WHAT DO YOU THINK? *Why do you think people with addictions resist seeking treatment, even when they may admit they have a problem? What factors need to be considered in helping addicted individuals prevent relapse?*

TAKING CHARGE

CONFRONTING ADDICTIVE BEHAVIORS

After reading this chapter, you know that addictions can be devastating not only to addicts, but to their families and friends as well. Addictions usually progress gradually, and it is difficult to know for certain when a person crosses the line from habit to addiction. Keep in mind that a behavior or chemical is problematic when it causes a person to incur negative consequences. If a person continues to perform the behavior or use the chemical despite these negative consequences, chances are that he or she is addicted.

Stop and think about your own behaviors for a minute. Do you have any of the habits discussed in this chapter? If you or someone you know lives with an addiction or is heading in that direction, the following checklists may provide some constructive strategies to help.

Checklist for Change

Making Personal Choices

- Are you ready to change or modify your behavior or substance use? Who can help support your decision?

- Have you thought about what impact your decision will have on your lifestyle? Are you ready to give up friends, activities, and environments that do not support your efforts?

- Rehearse things you may say or do if you find yourself in a situation that makes it difficult to stick with your behavior change.

- Remember that your motivation will decrease. During the times you are tempted, think about the reasons you decided to give up the behavior or substance.

- Realize that relapses happen. If you relapse, do not let the relapse serve as an excuse to slip back into old patterns of addiction. Talk with someone you trust, and start again. Recovery is difficult—give yourself a break.

- Join a self-help group. There are lots of 12-step groups that are free and confidential. Your university or college counseling service is another place to seek help.

Making Community Choices

- Do you sometimes participate or look the other way when someone you know engages in a behavior that may lead to addiction?

- Do you support policies, such as laws against drunk driving, that protect the community from the effects of addictive behaviors?

- Are you aware of what's happening in your own environment regarding identification of and help for addicts? Do you discuss alternatives or solutions to unhealthy behavior?

CHAPTER SUMMARY

- Addiction is the continued involvement with a substance or activity despite ongoing negative consequences.

- Habits are repeated behaviors whereas addiction is behavior resulting from compulsion; without the behavior, the addict experiences withdrawal. All addictions share four common symptoms: compulsion, loss of control, negative consequences, and denial.

- Addiction is a process, evolving over time through a pattern known as nurturing through avoidance. Mood-altering substances and experiences produce biochemical reactions that make the body feel good; when absent, the person feels a withdrawal effect. The biopsychosocial model of addiction takes into account biological (genetic) factors as well as psychological and environmental influences in understanding the addiction process.

- Addictions include money addictions (compulsive gambling, spending, and borrowing), work addiction, exercise addiction, sexual addiction, Internet addiction, and codependence. Codependents are "addicted to the addict." These behaviors are all addictive because they are mood-altering.

- Treatment begins with abstinence from the addictive behavior or substance, usually instituted through intervention by significant others. Treatment programs may include individual, group, or family therapy, as well as 12-step programs.

QUESTIONS FOR DISCUSSION AND REFLECTION

1. What factors distinguish a habit from an addiction? Is it possible for you to tell whether someone else is really addicted?

2. Explain why the biopsychosocial model is a more effective model for treatment than a single-factor model.

3. Explain the potential genetic, environmental, and psychological risk factors for addiction.

4. Discuss how addiction affects family and friends. What role do family and friends play in helping the addict get help and maintain recovery?

5. What are some key components of an effective treatment program? Do the components vary for men and women? Why or why not?

APPLICATION EXERCISES

Reread the What Do You Think? scenarios at the beginning of the chapter and answer the following questions.

1. If Evan decides to cut down on gambling, what will he need to do to ensure he doesn't relapse? Knowing he will still be in an environment with many gambling opportunities, what would you suggest he include in a relapse prevention plan?

2. How can Evan's roommate support him in dealing with his gambling problem? What steps should his roommate take to confront Evan effectively? What might his roommate try if his intervention fails?

3. How can Kelly approach her father and mother about her father's drinking?

4. What risk factors for developing addiction does Kelly face because of her family history and environment? How can she prevent such problems?

ACCESSING YOUR HEALTH ON THE INTERNET

Visit the following Internet sites to explore further topics and issues related to various forms of addiction and treatment. Many offer self-assessment profiles designed to give you more information about your own health practices. To visit an organization's website, go to the Companion Website for Access to Health, Eighth Edition at www.aw.com/donatelle, click on the book image, and select "Accessing Your Health on the Internet" from the navigation menu on the left.

1. ***Behavioral Health Online.*** A comprehensive addiction site with information on Internet, gambling, eating, and other addiction issues. Includes news briefs, features, and Ask an Expert.

2. ***Center for Online Addiction.*** Information and assistance for those dealing with Internet addiction.

3. ***The Wager.*** A weekly research report on compulsive gambling. Summarizes current research and resources pertaining to gambling.

4. ***Web of Addiction.*** A comprehensive listing of various resources related to self-help, treatment, and policy.

FURTHER READING

Elster, J. (ed.). *Addiction: Entries and Exits.* New York: Russell Sage Foundation, 2000.
Addresses current addiction controversies from an international perspective, with authors from the United States and Norway. Topics include whether addicts have a choice in their behavior and current addiction theories.

Hurley, J. (ed.). *Addiction: Opposing Viewpoints.* San Diego: Greenhaven Press, 2000.
Part of the Opposing Viewpoints series; addresses addiction theories, treatment approaches, and risk factors, among other topics.

Nakken, C. *The Addictive Personality.* Center City, MN: Hazelden, 1996.
A very down-to-earth overview of addiction, including nonsubstance addictions.

Peele, S. *The Meaning of Addiction: An Unconventional View.* San Francisco: Jossey-Bass, 1998.
One of the leading critics of the disease-view of addictions provides an alternative model of addiction.

Stevens, S., and H. Wexler (eds.). *Women and Substance Abuse: Gender Transparency.* New York: Haworth, 1998.
A collection of the most current research pertaining to women and substance abuse.

REFERENCES

1. H. F. Doweiko, *Concepts of Chemical Dependency* (Pacific Grove, CA: Brooks/Cole, 1993), 9.
2. C. Nakken, *The Addictive Personality* (Center City, MN: Hazelden, 1996), 24.
3. K. Blum and J. E. Payne, *Alcohol and the Addictive Brain* (New York: The Free Press, 1991), 186.
4. S. Peele, *Diseasing of America: How We Allowed Recovery Zealots and the Treatment Industry to Convince Us We Are Out of Control* (Lexington, MA: Lexington Books, 1995), 61.
5. V. Fox, *Addiction, Change, and Choice: The New View of Alcoholism* (Tucson, AZ: See Sharp Press, 1998), 11.
6. G. Hansen and P. Venturelli, *Drugs and Society,* 5th ed. (Boston: Jones and Bartlett, 1998), 47.
7. Ibid., 40.
8. Ibid.
9. L. Kurtz, *Self Help and Support Groups: A Handbook for Practitioners* (Thousand Oaks, CA: Sage, 1997), 12.
10. J. R. Wilson and J. A. Wilson, *Addictionary* (New York: Simon & Schuster, 1992), 166.
11. Nakken, op. cit, 24.
12. D. Gerstein et al., "Gambling Impact and Behavior Study: Report to the National Gambling Impact Study Commission," April 1999, National Opinion Research Center at the University of Chicago (see http://www.norc.uchicago.edu/new/pdf/gamble.pdf.
13. Ibid., 28.
14. A. Washton and D. Boundy, *Willpower's Not Enough: Recovering from Addictions of Every Kind* (New York: HarperCollins, 1990), 14.
15. Performance Resource Press, "Health Sentry Newsletter" 15 (1) (2002) (see http://www.prponline.net).
16. B. Yoder, *The Resource Recovery Book* (New York: Simon & Schuster, 1992), 259.
17. R. Olivardia, H. Pope, and J. Hudson, "Muscle Dysmorphia in Male Weightlifters: A Case-Control Study," *American Journal of Psychiatry* 157 (2000): 1291–1296.
18. M. Maine, *Body Wars: Making Peace with Women's Bodies* (Carlsbad, CA: Gurze, 2000), 282.
19. K. Young, M. Pistner, J. O'Mara, and J. Buchanan, "Cyber-Disorders: The Mental Health Concern for the New Millennium," paper presented at 107th APA convention, August 20, 1999 (see http://www.netaddiction.com/articles/cyberdisorders.htm).
20. K. Young, "Net Compulsions: The Latest Trends in the Area of Internet Addiction," 1999 (see http://www.netaddiction.com/net_compulsions.htm).
21. Ibid.
22. Nakken, op. cit., 16.
23. Wilson and Wilson, op. cit., 167.
24. National Institute on Alcohol Abuse and Alcoholism, Alcohol Alert Number 36, *Patient-Treatment Matching,* April 1997.

CHAPTER 17

TEST YOURSELF TRUE OR FALSE?

1. A person can become addicted to a behavior. **T or F**
2. Preventing an addiction is much easier than treating it. **T or F**
3. Most college students binge drink at least once a week. **T or F**
4. Nicotine is the addictive substance found in tobacco products. **T or F**
5. Anabolic steroids promote the development of male sexual characteristics in both males and females. **T or F**

Test Yourself answers can be found after the Chapter Summary.

Total Fitness: Addiction and Substance Abuse

have you smoked a cigarette, drunk alcohol to the point of intoxication, or gotten "high" sometime in the last month? If so, you may not think of yourself as addicted to these substances, and you may be right. However, regular use of substances such as these can lead to abuse of the substance, such that it affects a person's life and relationships. If you've ever had to skip class or call in sick at work because of a hangover, or if you've experienced a "blackout" where you were unable to remember what you did, said, or had done to you while you were drinking or using drugs, you have engaged in substance abuse. Many people think that such behaviors are a regular part of college life, but the reality is that not all college-aged individuals engage in these behaviors.

For those who do use and abuse alcohol, drugs, or tobacco, the short- and long-term consequences can directly affect health and, in some cases, can be deadly. In this chapter, we will discuss the nature of substance abuse and addiction, as well as specific, commonly used psychoactive drugs. We will also discuss strategies to avoid substance abuse. We begin by exploring the nature of addiction.

Taken from: *Total Fitness Update, Media Update,* Fifth Edition, by Scott K. Powers and Melinda Manore

What Is Addiction?

The term **addiction** refers to a habitual psychological and physical dependence on a substance or practice that is beyond voluntary control (1). Specific addictive behaviors are often associated with the following traits (2):

- *Reinforcement leading to craving.* Repeated behaviors that produce pleasurable emotional states reinforce the behavior. This repeated reinforcement can lead to a craving to engage in a particular behavior.

- *Loss of control.* Addictive behaviors lead to a loss of self-control, and the individual loses the ability to resist engaging in the activity.

- *Escalation.* Many addictive behaviors are associated with an increased need for the behavior. That is, as the person repeats the addictive behavior, higher levels of the substance or activity are required to provide the same level of satisfaction.

- *Negative outcomes.* In all cases, addictive unhealthy behavior is associated with negative consequences, such as impairment in physical or mental health.

Because **denial** is often a characteristic of addiction, many people won't see their behaviors as destructive or seek treatment on their own. Family members, friends, or co-workers may need to persuade the user to undergo screening for addiction. In all cases, preventing an addiction is much easier than treating it.

addiction Habitual psychological and physical dependence on a substance or practice that is beyond voluntary control.

denial An unconscious defense mechanism used to control anxiety by denying the existence of important troublesome information.

Addiction Can Involve a Substance or Behavior

Almost anything can be addicting. In addition to substances such as drugs, alcohol, and tobacco (which we will discuss at length in the next section), people can become addicted to behaviors such as gambling, Internet usage, pornography, sex, gaming, eating, and exercising. The key is an inability to control their behavior. People addicted to exercise, for example, may struggle with guilt and anxiety if they miss a workout. Many compulsive exercisers do so to feel more in control of their lives.

Another potentially addictive behavior that has come under scrutiny in recent years is playing video games. Spending a lot of time playing video games does not necessarily qualify as an addiction, but an individual who cannot control the impulse for gaming has become addicted. Gaming becomes an escape from real-life problems, and the individual withdraws from other activities and social networks. The isolation that the person experiences can jeopardize jobs and relationships as he or she spends more and more time gaming.

An estimated 2 million American adults become compulsive gamblers at some point in their lifetime. Compulsive gambling is technically classified as an impulse-control disorder (3), but it is similar to gaming and other addictive behaviors because the individual cannot resist the temptation or drive to gamble. In men, compulsive gambling typically starts in adolescence, whereas women tend to start later in life (3).

Compulsive shoppers and spenders share the same characteristics as compulsive gamblers. They shop to feel better, but often the compulsive spending makes them feel worse. Women with this compulsive disorder often have clothing and possessions that they have never used, with the price tags still attached. They are often in denial about the problem, and if family or friends complain about their purchases, they hide the things they buy.

The emotional and psychological dependence on these impulses will affect relationships, finances, and possibly even one's career. Avoiding

Not being able to control the amount of time spent playing video games or surfing the Internet can indicate an addiction to these behaviors.

these behaviors is the best strategy for preventing addiction, but because this may not always be possible, anyone who experiences the first sign of a problem needs to seek help.

Addiction Can Be Physical and/or Psychological

Addictions to substances such as drugs or alcohol often begin when an individual experiences a problem, discomfort, or some form of emotional or physical pain and looks for something to make him or her feel better. For example, moving away from home to attend college may cause you to miss your friends and family. Establishing new friendships on campus takes time and may involve an occasional rejection. Someone who feels like an outsider in a new environment or has been rejected by a group he or she wishes to join may turn to drugs or alcohol to ease the loneliness or the sting of rejection. At first, the drugs or alcohol seem to work because they dull the pain the person is trying to escape. As the person continues taking the substance, the drugs or alcohol may feel like the solution to their discomfort. Soon, a **dependence** on the substance is the individual's coping strategy for other painful or uncomfortable situations.

When drugs or alcohol are used on a regular basis, the body builds up a **tolerance** to them and needs more of the substance to achieve the same effects. Eventually, addiction results as the body cannot feel "normal" (physically and/or psychologically) without the substance. Because addiction can be a chronic relapsing disorder, meaning you tend to fall back into old addictive behaviors even after treatment, it is important to seek help and break the cycle as soon as possible.

The most serious forms of addiction involve **chemical dependence** to drugs or alcohol. Such a dependence means the body will experience physical **withdrawal symptoms** once the substance is no longer being taken. By the time a user develops a physical dependence on a drug, his or her body craves the drug and needs it to maintain equilibrium. When the user ceases to take the drug, withdrawal symptoms may include restlessness, bone and muscle pain, vomiting, and diarrhea. Such symptoms peak between 24 and 48 hours of stopping intake and may last a week or several months. The severity of withdrawal symptoms depends on the health of the person. Drugs that are known to cause a high amount of physical dependence in users include nicotine, cocaine, and alcohol.

Causes of Addiction

Addictions often result from numerous causes. With substance addiction, the type of drug can also play a role. Drugs vary in their potential for dependence, and some drugs, such as alcohol, heroin, and cocaine, can result in an addiction more quickly than others. Similarly, using tobacco products poses a great risk for dependence, because nicotine is a highly addictive drug (Table 17.1). By contrast, drugs such as marijuana and codeine are relatively less addictive. Cocaine and morphine also affect how the brain communicates with the nerve cells (4). In some cases, addictive behaviors such as drug abuse or gambling trigger the release of chemicals (neurotransmitters such as dopamine) in the brain, leading to a psychological "rush," or the sensation of pleasure (5).

In addition to the type of drug used, genetics, psychological makeup, and social factors also influence the risk of developing drug dependence. Research indicates that differences in brain chemistry and metabolism make some individuals more vulnerable to drug dependence (5). At present, the precise differences in brain chemistry and metabolism that contribute to increased risk of drug dependence remain unclear, and this topic remains an active area of research.

Personal characteristics such as poor coping skills, social environment (spending time with people who use drugs), and heredity can also play a role in the development of an addiction. Psychological risk factors for drug dependence include an inability to cope with stress or rejection, a strong need for excitement, and a tendency toward impulsive behavior. In this regard, people may turn to drugs to avoid coping with stress, rejection, or depression. Social risk factors such as easy access to

dependence The condition of being influenced by or subservient to a substance or practice.

tolerance The ability to endure the action of a drug continuously or in large doses without injurious effects.

chemical dependence A physical and psychological habituation to a mood- or mind-altering drug, such as alcohol or cocaine.

withdrawal symptoms Substance-specific symptoms that follow the cessation of, or reduction in, intake of a substance previously used regularly.

TABLE 17.1 Specific Drugs and Their Potential for Dependence

Drug	Potential for Physical Dependence	Potential for Psychological Dependence
Morphine	High	High
Codeine	Moderate	Moderate
Heroin	High	High
Methadone	High	High
Barbiturates	High	Moderate
Cocaine	Possible	High
Amphetamines	Possible	High
Methamphetamine	Possible	High
LSD	None	Unknown
Mescaline, peyote	None	Unknown
Ecstasy	Unknown	Unknown
Marijuana	Unknown	Moderate
Alcohol	Possible	Possible
Steroids	Possible	Possible
Nicotine	High	High

Source: U.S. Department of Health and Human Services and SAMHSA's National Clearinghouse for Alcohol and Drug Information. http://ncadi.samhsa.gov/govpubs/rpo926.

drugs, strong peer pressure to use drugs, drug use in your family, and a low education level increase your risk of developing a dependence on drugs.

Drug use and abuse occurs in people of all ages, education and income levels, and ethnic groups. However, research shows that some people are more likely to try illegal drugs and are consequently at greater risk for drug abuse. For example, young men with risk-taking personalities and a strong apathy toward school are at high risk for experimenting with drugs (6). In contrast, drug use is less common in individuals who are independent thinkers and are not easily influenced by their peers. Further, compared to individuals who are uninterested in schoolwork, individuals who attend school regularly and earn good grades are less likely to try illegal drugs.

Although brain chemistry, personality traits, and social factors do play a role in the development of some addictions, people are ultimately responsible for their own behavior, particularly in the early stages of experimentation with drugs, and must therefore take ownership of any addictive behaviors they exhibit. Making personal decisions not to experiment with potentially addictive substances or behaviors is the key to prevention. Further, recognizing the difference between a healthy habit and an addictive, unhealthy behavior is important to prevent addiction.

Substance Use versus Substance Abuse

substance abuse The use of illegal drugs, the inappropriate use of legal drugs, and/or the repeated use of drugs to produce pleasure, to alleviate stress, or to alter or avoid reality.

An individual can abuse a substance even if there is no full-blown addiction. There are many substances that are misused and abused without necessarily leading to addiction. In fact, you can think of the levels of drug use as a continuum, with complete abstinence at one end, progressing to occasional use, then to abuse, and leading eventually to addiction. **Substance abuse** occurs when use of a drug interferes with other areas of one's life, for example, grades, work, relationships, or legal issues.

The American Psychiatric Association defines substance abuse as one or more of the following traits (2):

- Recurrent drug use, resulting in failure to perform major responsibilities at work, home, or school
- Continued drug use despite social or personal problems caused by the effects of the drug
- Recurrent drug use in a situation where the drug imposes physical danger to the individual (e.g., drug use before driving a car)
- Recurrent legal problems associated with drug use

Many people who engage in intermittent use of drugs may not exhibit any of the above traits on a regular basis. However, intermittent drug use has been shown to lead to drug abuse and is a warning sign to stop this type of behavior before the problem escalates.

Make sure you know . . .

- Addiction is a compulsive psychological need for a drug or other behaviors.
- In addition to drugs, alcohol, and tobacco, people can become addicted to video games, gambling, shopping, using the Internet, and other behaviors.
- Drugs vary in their potential for dependence. Highly addictive drugs include nicotine, cocaine, alcohol, and heroin.
- Addictions are often the result of several causes, including characteristics such as poor coping skills, environment, and heredity. Factors that determine risk for drug addiction are the type of drug used, genetics, psychological makeup, and social factors.
- Recognizing the difference between a healthy habit and an addictive, unhealthy behavior is important in preventing addiction.

What Substances Are Commonly Abused?

Alcohol abuse and the use of **illicit drugs** are two of the biggest substance problems in the United States today. Millions of Americans abuse alcohol and use illicit drugs, which include marijuana, cocaine, heroin, hallucinogens, inhalants, and prescription-type pain relievers, tranquilizers, stimulants, and sedatives (7). In addition to the psychological and/or physical dependence, abuse of alcohol or recreational drugs increases your risk of accidents and may damage your health.

Psychoactive Drugs

Any drug that causes a user to experience an altered state of consciousness— that is, to feel "high"—is a **psychoactive drug**. Soon after ingestion, injection, or inhalation, psychoactive drugs cross the blood–brain barrier. Users typically report feeling a surge of pleasurable sensation — a "rush." The intensity of the rush depends on how much drug is taken and how rapidly the drug enters the brain. Drugs that enter the brain rapidly, such as opiates (including heroin and morphine), can be particularly potent. Alcohol, nicotine, opiates, marijuana, hallucinogens (such as LSD and Ecstasy), and numerous other drugs are all psychoactive drugs (Table 17.2).

Examples of Psychoactive Drugs

The most commonly abused drugs in the United States among individuals aged 18–25 are marijuana, prescription medications, cocaine, Ecstasy, alcohol, and tobacco (7). The physical effects associated with a **marijuana** "high" are produced by the chemical tetrahydrocannabinol (THC). The higher the THC concentration, the

illicit drugs Illegal drugs belonging to one of nine categories, including marijuana, cocaine, heroin, hallucinogens, inhalants; and the nonmedical use of prescription-type pain relievers, tranquilizers, stimulants, and sedatives.

psychoactive drugs Pharmacological agents that alter mood, anxiety, behavior, cognitive processes, or mental tension.

marijuana A psychoactive plant mixture (stems, leaves, or seeds) from either the *Cannabis sativa* or *Cannabis indica* (hemp) plants.

TABLE 17.2   Commonly Abused Drugs and Their Effects

Drug (Classification)	How Administered	Intoxication Effects	Health Effects
Heroin (opiate)	Injected, smoked, snorted	Pain relief, euphoria, drowsiness, staggering gait	Nausea, constipation, confusion, sedation, respiratory depression and arrest, tolerance, addiction, unconsciousness, coma, death
Opium (opiate)	Swallowed, smoked	Same as for heroin	Same as for heroin
Cocaine (stimulant)	Injected, smoked, snorted	Increased heart rate, blood pressure, metabolism; feelings of exhilaration, energy; increased mental alertness; increased temperature	Rapid or irregular heart beat, reduced appetite, weight loss, heart failure, nervousness, insomnia
Methamphetamine (stimulant)	Injected, swallowed, smoked, snorted	Same as for cocaine, plus: aggression, violence, psychotic behavior	Same as for cocaine, plus: memory loss, cardiac and neurological damage; impaired memory and learning; tolerance, addiction
Nicotine (stimulant)	Smoked, snorted, taken in snuff and spit tobacco	Same as for cocaine	Same as for cocaine, plus: adverse pregnancy outcomes, chronic lung disease, cardiovascular disease, stroke, cancer, tolerance, addiction
Marijuana (cannabinoid)	Swallowed or smoked	Euphoria, slowed thinking and reaction time, confusion, impaired balance and coordination	Cough, frequent respiratory infections, impaired memory and learning, increased heart rate, anxiety, panic attacks, tolerance, addiction
Lysergic acid diethylamide, also known as LSD (hallucinogen)	Swallowed, absorbed through mouth tissues	Altered state of perception and feeling	Persisting perception disorder (flashbacks); increased body temperature, heart rate, and blood pressure; loss of appetite; sleeplessness; numbness, weakness, tremors
Dextromethorphan, also known as DXM (narcotic)	Swallowed (found in some cough and cold medications)	Distorted visual perceptions to complete dissociative effects	At high doses, memory loss, numbness, nausea/vomiting
Anabolic steroids (hormones)	Injected, swallowed, applied to the skin	No intoxication	Hypertension, blood clotting, and cholesterol changes; liver cysts and cancer; kidney cancer; hostility and aggression; acne; in adolescents: premature stoppage of growth; in men: prostate cancer, reduced sperm production, shrunken testicles, breast enlargement; in women: menstrual irregularities, development of beard and other masculine characteristics
Laughing gas, whippets (inhalants)	Inhaled through nose or mouth	Stimulation, loss of inhibition; headache, nausea/vomiting, slurred speech, loss of motor coordination	Unconsciousness, cramps, weight loss, muscle weakness, depression, memory impairment, damage to cardiovascular and nervous systems, sudden death
Ecstasy, also known as MDMA (methylene dioxymethamphetamine) (stimulant)	Taken orally in tablet form	Feelings of well-being, mental stimulation; distortion in time and other sensory perceptions	Increase in body temperature, leading to kidney failure; increase in heart rate and blood pressure; heart wall stress

Source: Adapted from National Institute on Drug Abuse, Commonly abused drugs. www.drugabuse.gov/drugpages/dRugsofabuse.html.

greater the effect. The THC content varies between 0.5% and 3%, with the average percentage of THC in marijuana sold in the United States at about 1% (8). Marijuana is most often smoked in pipes or in hand-rolled cigarettes (joints) or cigars (blunts). Effects are generally felt within 15 to 30 minutes and usually disappear within 2 to 3 hours.

Marijuana is classified as a stimulant, and its immediate effects are increased heart rate and blood pressure, bloodshot eyes, and dry mouth and throat. Evidence suggests that acute use of marijuana increases the risk of stroke in male adolescent users (9). Use of marijuana also impairs motor coordination and may increase your risk of accidents. Further, acute use of marijuana alters the normal function of memory centers in the brain. This memory loss resembles that observed in normal aging. However, whether these changes in function put long-term marijuana users at risk for early mental disorders is not clear.

Psychoactive drugs can be ingested, smoked, injected, or inhaled using a variety of devices. Drugs that are injected or inhaled enter the blood more quickly than drugs that are ingested, and therefore their effects are felt more quickly.

The use of **cocaine** ("coke") in the United States increased dramatically during the 1980s, and today more than 5 million Americans use the drug annually. Between 1990 and 2000, Americans spent $35 billion to $70 billion yearly on cocaine (10). One survey suggests that as many as 6% of college students have experimented with cocaine, which makes cocaine the third most widely used drug by college students (1).

Cocaine is a powerful stimulant derived from the leaves of the coca shrub, which grows primarily in the Andes Mountains in South America. Cocaine is extracted from the coca leaves and produces a white powder that looks similar to sugar. Varying the extraction process can produce several different forms of cocaine, such as crack cocaine, rock cocaine, or freebase cocaine.

Common methods of taking cocaine include snorting, smoking, and intravenous injection. All routes of administration result in a rapid and short-lived high that generally lasts from 5 to 20 minutes. Cocaine is a highly addictive drug; when the cocaine high disappears, the user wants more. Spending over $1500 per day for cocaine is not uncommon for an addict. Cocaine addicts often suffer psychological damage, which eventually contributes to loss of jobs and financial ruin.

Cocaine is both an anesthetic and a central nervous system stimulant that increases heart rate and blood pressure. Other effects include a feeling of euphoria, heightened self-confidence, and increased alertness (11). In large doses, cocaine is extremely dangerous, and many people have died as a result of an overdose.

Another group of psychoactive drugs that have widespread popularity—the "club drugs"—includes several substances that young adults use at all-night dance parties ("raves" or "trances"), such as Ecstasy, gamma-hydroxybutyrate (GHB), ketamine, Rohypnol, methamphetamine, and LSD. The use of these drugs can cause serious health problems and in some cases can be fatal. Moreover, when club drugs are taken in combination with alcohol, the dangers are multiplied.

One particular club drug, methamphetamine, is a very addictive stimulant and is chemically related to amphetamines, but it is longer lasting, more potent, and more harmful to the central nervous system (CNS) (6). Methamphetamine is legally available only through a prescription that cannot be refilled. It has been manufactured in small, illegal laboratories, where its production endangers not only the people in the labs, but also neighbors and the environment. Short-term effects of methamphetamine include increased wakefulness, increased physical activity, decreased appetite, increased respiration, rapid heart beat, increased blood pressure, and hyperthermia. Cardiovascular collapse and death can occur from a single dose.

In addition to the "street drugs" that we often associate with drug abuse, there are numerous prescription medications that can also be highly addictive, on which people can become both psychologically and physically dependent. One example is the prescription painkiller OxyContin. The illegal use of this habit-forming drug, which was developed to ease the suffering of patients with painful diseases such as

cocaine A powerful stimulant derived from the leaves of the South American coca shrub.

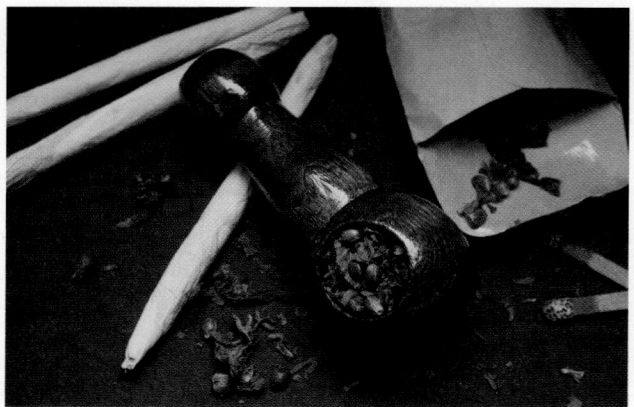

Marijuana leaves are usually smoked in a joint or pipe.

cancer, has grown markedly across the United States. Its addictive qualities have led to abuse among some recreational users; many have overdosed on this powerful painkiller, and others have turned to crime to feed their expensive habits.

Some people also misuse over-the-counter drugs to get a cheap high. Items such as cough suppressants and expectorants (which can contain as much as 40% alcohol) are sometimes ingested to achieve the same effects as derived from drinking alcohol. Cough and cold medications often contain dextromethorphan (DXM), a synthetic drug that is chemically similar to morphine. These medications are usually used successfully to treat cold symptoms and do not lead to addiction, but they can be misused to achieve other purposes. Chronic misuse of these substances may lead to dependence and have long-term adverse health effects.

Recovery from addiction to any psychoactive drug often requires professional help. For information on drug treatment programs, consult the National Institute on Drug Abuse website, www.nida.nih.gov.

Health Effects of Psychoactive Drug Use

Long-term use of marijuana can result in psychological dependence, and regular smoking of it causes lung damage similar to that caused by smoking tobacco (8). In fact, marijuana users usually inhale more deeply and hold their breath longer than tobacco smokers do, thereby increasing the lungs' exposure to carcinogenic smoke. The effect of long-term marijuana use on the heart is not well known; however, many investigators believe that marijuana increases the workload on the heart, which may eventually result in damage.

Some of the long-term complications from cocaine use are cardiovascular effects, including disturbances in heart rhythm and heart attacks; respiratory effects, such as chest pain and respiratory failure; neurological effects, including strokes, seizures, and headaches; and gastrointestinal complications, including abdominal pain and nausea. Long-term use of methamphetamines can result in paranoia, aggressiveness, extreme anorexia, memory loss, visual and auditory hallucinations, delusions, and severe dental problems.

Drug use by pregnant women can have serious health effects on the developing fetus. Prenatal exposure to marijuana results in the baby having weak responses to visual stimuli, increased tremulousness, and a high-pitched cry, which may indicate problems with neurological development. Many scientific studies have documented that babies born to mothers who abuse cocaine during pregnancy (so called "crack babies") are often delivered prematurely, have low birth weight, have smaller head circumference, and are shorter in length. Crack babies were once believed to suffer from severe, irreversible damage, such as reduced intelligence and social skills. Later research found that to be an exaggeration; however, crack babies do exhibit subtle, yet significant, deficits in cognitive performance, attention to tasks, and information processing. Babies born to women who used heroin and were treated with methadone while pregnant require treatment for withdrawal symptoms after birth.

Alcohol

Alcohol (ethyl alcohol) is the most widely used recreational drug in the United States, and the most popular drug on college campuses—it's used three times as much as marijuana and 20 times as much as cocaine (7). An estimated 64% of college students in the United States use alcohol, and some 38–44% abuse it (7). Full-time college students are more likely to use alcohol, binge drink, and drink heavily than are part-time college students and people of the same age who do not attend college (7).

Although many people consume alcohol to "get high," alcohol is actually a central nervous system depressant that slows down the function of the brain. This depressive effect results in impaired vision, slowed reaction time, and impaired motor coordination (12). Overconsumption of alcohol also impairs judgment. By decreasing the

CONSIDER THIS!
An estimated 1700 college students between 18 and 24 die each year from alcohol-related unintentional injuries, including motor vehicle crashes.

fear of danger, it can encourage risk-taking behaviors (such as driving too fast), which increases the likelihood of accidents (12). Drinking too much can also increase the risk of poor judgment in social situations and in making decisions concerning sexual behavior.

The blood level of alcohol determines the magnitude of central nervous system depression by the drug. The **blood alcohol concentration (BAC)** is determined by the amount of alcohol consumed, body weight, and the rate of alcohol metabolism by the body. For example, if two men of different weights (e.g., 200 pounds versus 150 pounds) consume the same amount of alcohol, the smaller individual will have the higher BAC. This is also the reason that women feel the effects of alcohol sooner than men do. Their lighter body weights and higher percentages of body fat lead to greater concentrations of alcohol in their nervous systems.

Alcohol is metabolized in the liver, and, in general, the body can remove 0.3 ounce of alcohol per hour. In practical terms, this rate of removal is approximately half of one drink (FIGURE 17.1) per hour. An individual who drinks slowly, that is, less than one drink per hour, can maintain a relatively low BAC. In contrast, someone who drinks rapidly, consuming more than two drinks per hour, will increase his or her BAC to higher levels, leading toward intoxication.

Even low doses of alcohol can have significant behavioral and physical effects (Table 17.3). For instance, relatively small amounts of alcohol in your blood can decrease your level of alertness and increase your risk of injury (12). Higher doses can lead to impaired motor skills and slowed reaction times (13). These negative physical effects are the reason that state laws specify the legal level of blood alcohol for driving. Because 0.05–0.10% BAC results in significant impairment in reaction times and motor skills, all states have established 0.08% BAC as the legal definition for alcohol intoxication (13, 14).

Alcohol Abuse versus Alcohol Addiction

Not everyone who uses alcohol will abuse it or become addicted to it, and many Americans drink moderate amounts of alcohol occasionally, or on a regular basis, without suffering any ill health effects. However, because alcohol is widely available

FIGURE 17.1 Ethyl alcohol is the psychoactive ingredient of all alcoholic beverages. A standard drink is defined as a 12-ounce beer, a 1.5-ounce cocktail drink, or a 5-ounce glass of wine. Each of these contains approximately 0.6 ounces of ethyl alcohol.

blood alcohol concentration (BAC) The concentration of alcohol in the blood measured as a percentage by mass, by mass per volume, or a combination of both. A BAC of 0.20% can mean 2 grams of alcohol per 1000 grams of an individual's blood, or it can mean 0.2 gram of alcohol per 100 milliliters of blood.

TABLE 17.3 Behavioral and Physiological Effects of Alcohol

Blood Alcohol Concentration (BAC)	Behavioral and Physiological Effects	Hours Required to Metabolize Alcohol
0.0–0.5%	Increased relaxation, feeling of euphoria, and decreased alertness.	2–3
0.05–0.10%	Reduced social inhibition and impairment in reaction time and motor skills. This level of alcohol may significantly impact driving skills. Many states define legally drunk as a BAC of 0.08% or higher.	4–6
0.10–0.15%	Increased impairment in reaction time and motor skills. Loss of peripheral vision.	6–10
0.15–0.30%	Difficulty walking, slurred speech, impaired pain perception, and impairment in other sensory perceptions.	10–24
More than 0.30%	Can result in unconsciousness. Death possible at BAC levels of 0.35% or more. These levels of BAC are generally achieved by binge drinking.	More than 24

Source: Data from Ogden, E., and H. Moskowitz. Effects of alcohol and other drugs on driver performance. *Traffic Injury Prevention* 5(3):185–198, September 2004.

Drinking games, such as those played at many college parties, contribute to the incidence of binge drinking among this population.

CONSIDER THIS!
In a national study, 91% of women and 78% of men who were frequent binge drinkers considered themselves to be moderate or light drinkers.

alcoholism A chronic, progressive behavioral disorder characterized by a strong urge to consume alcohol and an inability to limit the amount of drinking despite adverse consequences.

binge drinking Drinking 5 or more drinks (for men) or 4 or more drinks (for women) at the same time or within a couple of hours of each other on at least 1 day in the past 30 days.

and affordable, it is one of the most significant drug problems in our society. Alcohol addiction is a very real problem for many people, and it can happen to anyone.

Alcohol abuse is a difficult phrase to define, because the abuse tends to be in the eye of the beholder. On the one hand, for many individuals whose religion requires abstinence, simply tasting an alcoholic beverage constitutes alcohol abuse. Similarly, anyone who drinks any amount of alcohol without being of legal drinking age is abusing it. On the other hand, some college students may believe that heavy drinking is simply a way of having a good time.

The American Psychiatric Association has defined *alcohol abuse* according to the following four abuse criteria: alcohol use in hazardous situations, alcohol-related school or work problems, recurrent interpersonal problems, and recurrent legal problems (2). Drinking too much and/or drinking too often are major contributors to alcohol abuse.

Alcohol abuse is particularly harmful when it prevents the drinker from meeting work, school, or family responsibilities, and it can also be deadly. Approximately 1700 college students between the ages of 18 and 24 die each year as a result of alcohol abuse (15). In addition, consuming alcohol during pregnancy has been linked to alcohol-related birth defects, such as mental retardation.

Alcoholism, also known as *alcohol dependence*, is a disease that involves craving alcohol and not being able to control the impulse to drink — in other words, an addiction. Alcoholics develop a physical dependence on the alcohol as their tolerance to the drug increases over time. Addiction to alcohol may have hereditary, psychological, and environmental components. Treatment for alcoholism involves medication and counseling to help a person stop drinking. Three oral medications, disulfiram (Antabuse), naltrexone (Depade, ReVia), and acamprosate (Campral) are currently approved to treat alcohol dependence. These medications have been shown to help alcohol-dependent people reduce their drinking, avoid relapse, and achieve and maintain abstinence. They are not a "magic bullet," because no single medication works in every case and for every person. There is no cure for alcoholism, and once a person has stopped drinking, he must avoid all alcohol for life or suffer the possibility of a relapse with the next drink.

Unfortunately, alcohol abuse and alcohol addiction are not unknown among college students. A 2002 survey of more than 14,000 students at 119 four-year colleges showed that 31 percent of college students met the criteria for a diagnosis of alcohol abuse, and 6 percent for a diagnosis of alcohol dependence (16). Nearly 10% of college men under age 24 and nearly 5% of college women under age 24 met a 12-month diagnosis of alcohol dependence. Despite the prevalence of alcohol disorders on college campuses, few students reported having sought treatment for alcohol dependence.

Binge Drinking

One common type of alcohol abuse among college students is **binge drinking**. Binge drinking often begins around age 13, peaks between 18 and 22, and then gradually decreases over time (17). Binge drinking is associated with a wide array of social, emotional, behavioral, and health problems. Bars and alcohol distributors in college towns often provide easy access to cheap alcohol, which promotes binge drinking. In one study, binge drinking among college students aged 18–22 was reported to be around 44%, compared to 38% in people of the same age who were not enrolled full time in college (7). Students who live in fraternity or sorority houses tend to be the heaviest drinkers on campus, perhaps in response to the number of social events they host that include alcohol. Drinking games and tournaments, such as beer pong, encourage consumption of excessive amounts of alcohol over a short time period.

Alcohol poisoning, a severe and potentially fatal physical reaction to an alcohol overdose, is the most serious consequence of binge drinking. Approximately 300 deaths annually are due to alcohol-related injuries that include alcohol poisoning (16). A BAC of 0.35% or above can result in alcohol poisoning and death. Anyone who drinks to the point of unconsciousness may vomit and inhale the vomit, leading to asphyxiation, or may stop breathing. An individual whose breathing becomes too shallow (fewer than eight breaths per minute) or who cannot be awakened with shouting or shaking should be treated immediately by medical personnel, because this is a life-threatening medical emergency.

Most people who binge drink are not alcohol dependent; however, a consistent pattern of alcohol abuse can result in a need to drink more in order to feel the effects of the drug, which can lead to dependence on the drug.

Use the Steps for Behavior Change box below to get a sense of your drinking habits and to determine whether you may be abusing alcohol. You can do a more detailed assessment of your drinking habits by answering the questions in Laboratory 17.1. If you feel that you might be drinking too much, seek professional help from your health care provider or an organization such as Alcoholics Anonymous.

Children born with fetal alcohol syndrome exhibit several physical and mental effects.

STEPS FOR BEHAVIOR CHANGE

Do You Regularly Abuse Alcohol?

Take the following quiz to get a sense of your alcohol habits.

Y   N

❏ ❏ Do you find it difficult to get through a week without drinking?

❏ ❏ Is going out with friends for the purpose of drinking a regular weekend event?

❏ ❏ Do you and/or your friends engage in foolish or dangerous behavior while intoxicated?

❏ ❏ Would your grades or class attendance be better if you drank less alcohol?

❏ ❏ Do you regularly "black out" from drinking too much, such that you don't remember periods of time?

If you answered yes to any of the above, you've engaged in at least one episode of alcohol abuse. Although this doesn't necessarily mean you will become addicted to alcohol, it does mean you should take measures to modify your behavior.

Tips to Gain Control Over Your Drinking Habits

☑ Know your limits, and stay within them. If you are at a party and feel that you are drinking too much, learn to say no, dilute your drinks, or switch to a nonalcoholic beverage.

☑ When drinking, stick to the rule of less than 0.3 ounce (one drink) of alcohol per hour. This will reduce the likelihood that you will become physically or mentally impaired by alcohol.

☑ Wine, beer, and mixed drinks are less intoxicating than straight liquor. Stick to these more dilute drinks instead of the higher-alcohol beverages.

☑ Eating and drinking at the same time will slow the rate of alcohol absorption and reduce your chance of becoming impaired. Never drink on an empty stomach.

☑ When leaving a party or bar after drinking, don't drive; instead, call a cab, or have someone else—who is sober—drive you home.

Health Effects of Alcohol Abuse

Chronic abuse of alcohol over a period of years can result in liver disease (e.g., cirrhosis), damage to the nervous system, and an increased risk of certain cancers (18). Development of liver disease due to years of drinking may eventually result in total liver failure and death. The damage to the nervous system that results from alcohol abuse is often localized to the left side of the brain, which is responsible for written and spoken language, logic, and mathematical skills. The degree of brain damage that occurs appears to be directly related to the amount of alcohol consumed (18). Further, repeated irritation of the gastrointestinal system by alcohol has been linked to cancers of the esophagus, pancreas, stomach, mouth, tongue, and liver. Another and often overlooked problem linked to chronic consumption of alcohol is **malnutrition** (see the Closer Look box below).

Women who drink during pregnancy are subjecting the fetus to a wide range of preventable birth defects, including **fetal alcohol syndrome.** An estimated 1% of all live births show some alcohol-related prenatal damage, such as physical, behavioral, and learning problems. Babies born with fetal alcohol syndrome may have mild to severe learning disabilities and abnormal facial features (19). To prevent the effects of FAS, any woman who is pregnant, or thinks she may become pregnant, should abstain from consuming alcohol.

malnutrition Poor nutrition due to an insufficient or poorly balanced diet or to faulty digestion or utilization of foods; can include *undernutrition,* or lack of sufficient nutrients, and *overnutrition,* or intake of too many calories.

fetal alcohol syndrome A cluster of birth defects, which may include facial abnormalities, mental retardation, and growth problems, caused by alcohol consumption during pregnancy.

nicotine The addictive and psychoactive drug in tobacco plants.

Tobacco

Nicotine, contained in tobacco products, is the most heavily used addictive drug in the United States. In 2006, 20.8% of all adults (45.3 million people) in the United States smoked cigarettes (20). Individuals aged 18–24 comprise an estimated 23.9% of all smokers (slightly more than 11 million people) (20). Cigarette smoking was found to be more common among men (23.9%) than women (18.0%). The good news is that smoking rates for young Americans are no longer climbing and have declined slightly from the peaks reached in the late 1990s. Nonetheless, a large number of Americans still use tobacco products.

A CLOSER LOOK

Alcohol Abuse and Malnutrition

Malnutrition is commonly associated with chronic alcohol abuse because the frequent presence of alcohol irritates the gastrointestinal system. An irritated gastric lining can result in impaired appetite, which in turn decreases food intake. A lowered food intake forces the body to function on a diet that is deficient in both calories and in essential nutrients such as protein and vitamins. In extreme cases, the resulting *undernutrition* can promote a loss of muscle mass and abnormal functioning of many body organs. Lack of vitamin A may contribute to liver disease and other serious alcohol-related health problems. Lack of thiamin (vitamin B$_1$) has been associated with a degenerative brain disorder called Wernicke-Korsakoff syndrome. Alcohol abuse can also lead to *overnutrition*—and therefore contribute to overweight and obesity—because of its high calorie content.

Remember, alcohol is not calorie-free, and mixed drinks in particular can approach the calorie levels of snacks and even desserts.

The best approach to dealing with alcohol-related malnutrition is to seek professional help for alcoholism. In many cases, the cessation of alcohol abuse eliminates the alcohol-induced reduction in appetite, and the individual's return to normal eating habits provides the calories and nutrients needed for improved health. In severe cases of alcohol-related undernutrition, the advice of a physician and/or a nutritionist is required.

Source: National Institute of Neurological Disorders and Stroke. www.ninds.nih.gov; National Institute on Alcohol Abuse and Alcoholism (NIAAA). FAQs for the general public. www.niaaa.nih.gov/FAQs/General-English.

Cigarette smoking has been the most popular method of nicotine use since the beginning of the 20th century (21). In 2007, cigarettes were by far the preferred tobacco product among youths aged 12–17, with 2.5 million (9.8%) having used cigarettes in the past month. Other tobacco usage included cigars (4.2%), smokeless tobacco (2.4%), and pipe tobacco (0.7%) (7). An average dose of nicotine is 1.8 mg per cigarette, compared to 3.6 mg in snuff, and 4.6 mg in chewing tobacco. A single cigar can contain nicotine levels ranging from the equivalent of one cigarette to an entire pack of cigarettes (22).

Cigarettes and other forms of tobacco, such as those found in snuff, chewing tobacco, pipes, and cigars, are associated with major health risks.

Peer influence is one common reason that young people take up smoking.

Nicotine Addiction

Nicotine provides an almost immediate "psychological kick" to the body because it causes the release of epinephrine from the adrenal cortex (located in an endocrine gland near the kidneys). This stimulates the central nervous system and increases both heart rate and blood pressure. This stimulation is lost rapidly, which leads to both depression and fatigue and causes the user to seek more nicotine.

Nicotine is absorbed readily from tobacco smoke in the lungs, and it does not matter whether the smoke comes from cigarettes, cigars, or pipes (21). Nicotine is also absorbed in the mouth when tobacco is chewed. With regular use of tobacco, nicotine can accumulate in the body and remain for several hours (21).

Clove cigarettes have been used as an alternative to tobacco products; however, clove cigarettes contain about 60–70% tobacco and equal amounts of nicotine as do cigarettes (23). Exposure to tar, nicotine, and carbon monoxide is higher for smokers of clove cigarettes than for smokers of traditional tobacco cigarettes.

Addiction to nicotine results in withdrawal symptoms when a person tries to stop smoking. For example, studies indicate that when chronic smokers were deprived of cigarettes for 24 hours, they showed more anger, hostility, and aggression and less social cooperation (21). Further, people suffering from nicotine withdrawal take longer to regain emotional equilibrium following exposure to stress. Moreover, during periods of abstinence from smoking, smokers show a wide range of physical and mental impairments, such as impaired psychomotor skills (movement coordination) and impaired cognitive functions (21).

Studies have shown that some of the most successful long-term smoking cessation programs involve not only behavioral treatment but also pharmacological treatment (21). Most pharmacological treatments involve nicotine gum or transdermal patches (placed on the skin) to deliver nicotine during the initial stages of smoking cessation. The success of smoking cessation treatment varies widely across studies. Generally, the rates of relapse for smoking cessation are highest in the first few weeks after smoking cessation and diminish greatly after about 3 months (21). So, if you smoke, it is possible to stop.

Secondhand Smoke

Secondhand smoke is a mixture of gases and particles from both burning tobacco products (also known as *sidestream smoke*) and smoke exhaled by smokers (also known as *mainstream smoke*). Secondhand smoke lingers in the air hours after cigarettes have been extinguished and contains toxic chemicals, more than 50 of which are known to cause cancer. In addition to the absorption of nicotine from secondhand smoke, breathing secondhand smoke has immediate harmful effects on the cardiovascular system and can cause respiratory symptoms and slow lung growth in children. An estimated 150,000 to 300,000 new cases of bronchitis and pneumonia due to exposure to secondhand smoke have been diagnosed in American children under the age of 18 months (24). Additionally, secondhand smoke causes an estimated 3400 lung cancer deaths and 46,000 heart disease deaths in adult nonsmokers in the United States annually (25).

secondhand smoke The combination of smoke that comes from the burning end of a cigarette, cigar, or pipe and the smoke exhaled by the smoker.

New legislation is being passed in almost every community in the United States to curb the exposure to secondhand smoke for all citizens. Smoking is banned in almost all government buildings, and many cities and states have passed legislation banning smoking in restaurants as well as bars. Because of these new laws, exposure rates to secondhand smoke have declined (20).

Health Effects of Tobacco Use

Tobacco smoking is the leading preventable cause of death in the United States and accounts for approximately one in every five deaths (438,000) per year (20). Cigarette smoking causes coronary heart disease, the leading cause of death in the United States, and doubles a person's chance for stroke (20). Regular tobacco use increases the risk of several forms of cancer, including cancers of the lung, larynx, esophagus, pancreas, bladder, and kidney (21). Compared to nonsmokers, men who smoke are 23 times more likely to develop lung cancer, and women who smoke are 13 times more likely (20). Tobacco use results in an annual cost of more than $96 billion in direct medical costs and $97 billion from loss of productivity (20).

Pregnant women who smoke are more likely to lose the baby during pregnancy or deliver the baby prematurely, before the lungs are fully developed. Children born to women who smoke are lower in birth weight and tend to develop more illnesses. The nicotine and other harmful chemicals in tobacco products are absorbed in the mother's bloodstream and pass through the placenta to the unborn child. Several of these chemicals may interfere with the developing baby's ability to get enough oxygen and nutrients in the womb, thus contributing to the low birth weight.

Caffeine

Caffeine is a bitter substance found in coffee, tea, soft drinks, chocolate, and certain medicines. Caffeine enters the bloodstream through the stomach and small intestine and can stimulate the central nervous system as soon as 15 minutes after it is consumed. For most people, the amount of caffeine in two to four cups of coffee a day is not harmful. When consumed in moderate doses, caffeine can increase alertness and give you an energy boost; however, too much caffeine can make you restless and irritable. Caffeine has also been associated with insomnia, headaches, and abnormal heart rhythms. Caffeine is eliminated slowly from the body and can remain in the body for hours. If you have trouble sleeping at night, try to avoid ingesting any product containing caffeine after 2:00 PM.

Some studies have shown that caffeine causes psychological dependence. However, there is no agreement on how much caffeine you would have to consume daily to become physically dependent on it. Even if you consume caffeine in moderate doses, you could get withdrawal symptoms when you stop using it. Typical withdrawal symptoms include headache, muscle pain, and fatigue. Some people may find that they are more sensitive to the effects of caffeine than others and should limit their use of caffeine. In addition, certain drugs and supplements may interact with caffeine. If you have questions about whether caffeine is safe for you, talk with your health care provider. See also the following Closer Look box.

Make sure you know...

- Psychoactive drugs are those that cause a state of intoxication. Effects range from feelings of euphoria to increased heart rate, shallow breathing, a change in body temperature, and hallucinations.

- Commonly used psychoactive drugs include marijuana, cocaine, club drugs, alcohol, and tobacco. Common club drugs include Ecstasy, GHB, Rohypnol, ketamine, methamphetamine, and LSD.

- The most common recreational drug in the United States is alcohol, and it is estimated that over 85% of college students drink alcohol. Relatively low levels of blood alcohol (i.e., 0.05–0.10%) can impair both reaction time and motor skills, resulting in a diminished ability to drive.

caffeine A stimulant found in a wide variety of common foods such as coffee, tea, and chocolate.

A CLOSER LOOK

The Effects of Caffeine

Caffeine is a stimulant found in a wide variety of common foods, including coffee, tea, and cocoa (see the table), and it is one of the most frequently ingested psychoactive drugs in the world (29). Caffeine affects the central nervous system by stimulating a variety of brain centers, increasing alertness and decreasing drowsiness (30). In fact, caffeine has been shown to reduce fatigue and improve performance during prolonged endurance exercise (e.g., running a marathon) (31, 32). Evidence that caffeine may improve endurance exercise performance has prompted the International Olympic Committee to consider banning high blood levels of caffeine during performance in the Olympic games.

As with other habit-forming drugs, chronic use of caffeine can lead to addiction (29, 30). Abrupt discontinuation of caffeine intake can result in severe headache, fatigue, irritability, and gastrointestinal distress. Nonetheless, cessation of caffeine use has been shown to be considerably easier than cessation of other stimulants, such as nicotine (28).

There is no consensus whether long-term use of caffeine poses a significant health risk. However, one review concluded that moderate daily intake of caffeine (less than 400 mg/day) is not associated with adverse health effects (29). Nonetheless, high doses of caffeine (500 mg or more) can increase both heart rate and blood pressure, and in some people, caffeine increases the risk of abnormal heart rhythms (30). Further, for people unaccustomed to caffeine or who consume caffeine in large doses, it can produce tremors, nervousness, restlessness, and insomnia. Therefore, people who consume caffeine should do so only in moderation.

Caffeine may have health effects during pregnancy. Some studies suggest that higher intake of caffeine (about three or more 8-ounce cups of coffee a day) may increase the risk of miscarriage and of low birth weight in the infant (33). However, small amounts of caffeine (about one to two 8-ounce cups of coffee a day) appear to be safe during pregnancy.

Caffeine Content of Popular Foods and Nonprescription Drugs

Food or Nonprescription Drug	Serving Size	Caffeine (mg)
Coffee (drip method)	8 fluid ounces	85
Coffee (instant)	8 fluid ounces	62
Coffee (decaffeinated)	8 fluid ounces	3
Espresso coffee (brewed)	8 fluid ounces	502
Tea (bag or loose)	8 fluid ounces	47
Tea (decaffeinated)	8 fluid ounces	3
Tea (herbal)	8 fluid ounces	0
Cocoa	8 fluid ounces	5
Chocolate milk	8 fluid ounces	5
Mountain Dew (soft drink)	12 fluid ounces	54
Coca Cola (soft drink)	12 fluid ounces	46
Dr. Pepper (soft drink)	12 fluid ounces	40
Pepsi Cola (soft drink)	12 fluid ounces	38
Root beer, ginger ale (soft drink)	12 fluid ounces	0
Red Bull (energy drink)	8.3 fluid ounces	80
SoBe No Fear (energy drink)	8 fluid ounces	83
Full Throttle (energy drink)	16 fluid ounces	144
Milk chocolate	1 ounce serving	6
Dark chocolate	1.45 ounce serving	31
NoDoz (Maximum Strength)	1 tablet or capsule	200
Vivarin	1 tablet or capsule	200
Excedrin (Extra Strength)	2 tablets	130

Sources: U.S. Department of Agriculture National Nutrient Database for Standard Reference, Release 18. November 2005; American Beverage Association, www.ameribev.org., accessed August 2007.

- Nicotine, the psychoactive drug in tobacco products, is one of the most addictive drugs available. Prolonged use of tobacco products can lead to numerous health problems, including an increased risk of heart disease and cancer. Babies born to mothers who smoked during pregnancy are at higher risk of having a low birth weight and developing more illnesses.

Anabolic Steroids

Anabolic steroids are the familiar name for synthetic substances related to male sex hormones (e.g., testosterone). Steroids are a class of drugs that are legally available only by prescription and are used primarily to treat conditions that occur when the body does not produce enough testosterone, such as in delayed puberty and some types of impotence. Anabolic steroids can be taken orally in tablet or capsule form, injected directly into the muscle, or rubbed into the skin from ointment preparations.

During the 1930s, scientists discovered that anabolic steroids facilitated the growth of skeletal muscle in laboratory animals by mimicking the effect of naturally produced testosterone. This discovery led to abuse of these compounds first by bodybuilders and weight lifters and then by athletes in other sports. Doses taken by abusers for sports-related purposes can typically be 100 times more than the dosage used for treating legitimate medical conditions.

Long-term steroid use can have serious psychological side effects. Users become aggressive, developing extreme, uncontrolled bouts of anger known as "roid rage." Depression often results when the drugs are stopped and may contribute to dependence on anabolic steroids.

Anabolic steroids have been found to cause potentially fatal liver cysts and liver cancer, increased blood cholesterol levels, increased blood clotting, and increased hypertension, which can promote heart attack and stroke in both men and women. In boys and men, anabolic steroid abuse can reduce sperm production, shrink the testicles, lead to impotence, and cause baldness and irreversible breast enlargement (gynecomastia) (26). In girls and women, anabolic steroid abuse causes the development of masculine characteristics such as decreased body fat and breast size, deepened voice, excessive body hair growth, acne, male-pattern baldness, changes in the menstrual cycle, and enlargement of the clitoris (26).

About 3 million people use anabolic steroids, and one in four of these users started as a teenager (27). Some research has shown that 5% of teen boys and 2.5% of teen girls have used some form of anabolic steroids. Teenaged boys are more likely to use steroids to build muscle in the hopes that they will improve their athletic performance. Teenaged girls are more likely to use anabolic steroids as body-shaping drugs to increase their lean body mass (27). Regardless of the motive behind anabolic steroid use, these drugs are illegal and can do permanent damage to a person's health and negatively affect the reproductive system.

Make sure you know . . .

- Anabolic steroids are a class of synthetic substances related to the male sex hormone .

- Although there are legitimate medical uses of anabolic steroids, abuse of them for bodybuilding or for improving sport performance can lead to harmful health effects, including psychological problems (e.g., rage and aggression) and physical side effects (e.g., changes in sexual characteristics and an impaired reproductive system).

Strategies to Avoid Drug Abuse

Avoiding drug use requires self discipline and control. Several steps can help protect you from the temptation to use drugs (28):

1. *Increase your self-esteem.* Take pride in yourself and your achievements. This will boost your confidence and improve your ability to say no to drugs.

anabolic steroids Synthetic hormones related to the male sex hormone testosterone.

2. *Learn how to cope with stress.* When you are stressed, use one or more of the stress management techniques discussed in Chapter 14 (such as exercise or progressive relaxation).

3. *Develop numerous interests.* Find and participate in new hobbies or sports that you enjoy.

4. *Practice assertiveness.* Becoming assertive is an important key to being able to decline drug use.

CHAPTER SUMMARY

1. Alcohol, nicotine (tobacco products), marijuana, and cocaine are the most widely used and abused drugs in the United States. Alcohol is the single most common recreational drug used in the United States.

2. Use of alcohol, marijuana, and cocaine increases your risk of accidents, and prolonged use of these substances may result in psychological dependence, physical addiction, and damaged health.

3. Chronic abuse of alcohol can result in liver disease, damage to the nervous system, increased risk of certain cancers, and malnutrition. Blood alcohol concentrations of 0.05–0.10% can significantly reduce reaction time and impair motor skills.

4. Long-term use of marijuana may result in psychological dependence and may increase your risk of cardiopulmonary diseases.

5. Cocaine is a highly addictive drug that, when taken in large doses, can be lethal.

6. Use of tobacco can lead to an addiction to nicotine, and prolonged use of tobacco products can lead to numerous health problems, including increased risk of heart attack, stroke, and cancer.

7. Caffeine is a central nervous system stimulant found in numerous common foods and beverages. Whether chronic consumption of caffeine is a significant health risk is currently unclear.

8. Long-term use of anabolic steroids can cause psychological side effects, such as aggression and uncontrolled bouts of anger. In men, anabolic steroids also lead to shrunken testicles, reduced sperm count, breast development, infertility, and increased risk of prostate cancer. In women, use of anabolic steroids can cause the growth of facial hair, male-pattern baldness, changes in the menstrual cycle, enlargement of the clitoris, and a deepened voice.

9. You can decrease your risk of using drugs by increasing your self-esteem, learning how to cope with stress, developing numerous interests, and practicing assertiveness.

TEST YOURSELF ANSWERS

1. **True.** Addiction is a state in which a person cannot control his or her actions. It is possible for a person to become addicted to behaviors such as gambling, shopping, or even playing video games.

2. **True.** Whether the addiction is to alcohol, tobacco, or gambling, abstaining in the first place is easier than treating the symptoms of physical and psychological dependence.

3. **False.** Although many people assume that all college students overindulge in alcohol, only about 20–28%—less than a third—of college students engage in binge drinking at all.

4. **True.** Nicotine, found in cigarettes, cigars, pipes, and other tobacco products, is a highly addictive substance that is absorbed in the lungs from the tobacco smoke or in the mouth from chewed tobacco.

5. **True.** Anabolic steroids are synthetic versions of the male sex hormone testosterone. For men, anabolic steroids can cause the testicles to shrink, reduce sperm count, increase the risk of prostate cancer, and lead to infertility, baldness, and the development of breasts. For women, anabolic steroids can cause the growth of facial hair, baldness, changes in or cessation of the menstrual cycle, enlargement of the clitoris, and a deepened voice.

STUDY QUESTIONS

1. A key factor in preventing drug addiction is to
   a. know when to quit.
   b. use the drug only in a social setting.
   c. control the amount of drug you use.
   d. abstain from drug use.
   e. seek counseling.

2. Identify one trait that is not associated with addictive behavior.
   a. escalation of drug use
   b. loss of control
   c. craving the drug
   d. denying that there is a problem
   e. All of the above traits are associated with addictive behavior

3. Complete this sentence: One key factor that determines your risk for drug addiction is
   a. the type of drug used.
   b. how the drug enters your body.
   c. the cost of the drug.
   d. the time of day the drug is used.

4. Babies born to mothers who drink alcohol while pregnant tend to have
   a. autism.
   b. low birth weight.
   c. vision and hearing problems.
   d. respiratory problems.
   e. None of the above

5. Secondhand smoke is derived from
   a. exhaled smoke.
   b. smoke from burning tobacco products.
   c. smoke from industrial chimneys.
   d. smoke from wood-burning fireplaces.
   e. Both (a) and (b) are correct.
   f. Both (c) and (d) are correct.

6. Define and discuss the terms *substance abuse* and *addiction.*

7. Outline factors that determine the risk of developing an addiction to drugs.

8. Discuss the health effects of alcohol use.

9. Describe the changes in behavior and physical function that occur as blood alcohol levels increase.

10. What is the most widely used recreational drug in the United States?

11. List four steps that can help you feel less tempted to use drugs.

12. Discuss the health effects of marijuana use.

13. Describe the health effects of using anabolic steroids.

SUGGESTED READINGS

Donatelle, R. *Access to Health,* Green Edition. San Francisco: Benjamin Cummings, 2010.

Fields, R. *Drugs in Perspective,* 7th ed. St. Louis: McGraw-Hill, 2010.

Wilson, H. *Annual Editions: Drugs, Society, and Behavior,* 24th ed. St. Louis: McGraw-Hill, 2010.

WEB LINKS

For links to the organizations and websites listed below, visit The Total Fitness and Wellness Website at www.pearsonhighered.com/powers.

American Medical Association
Contains many sources of information about a wide variety of medical problems, including alcohol, tobacco, and drug use.

WebMD
Contains information about a wide variety of diseases and medical problems, including alcohol, tobacco, and drug use.

Higher Education Center for Alcohol and Other Drug Prevention
Presents information about alcohol and drug abuse on college campuses; also contains links to other related organizations.

National Institute on Drug Abuse
This comprehensive site contains information about commonly abused drugs, the incidence of drug abuse in the United States, and where to find help with rehabilitation from drug dependence.

REFERENCES

1. *Stedman's Medical Dictionary for the Health Professions and Nursing,* 5th ed. Philadelphia: Lippincott Williams & Wilkins, 2005.
2. American Psychiatric Association. *Diagnostic and Statistical Manual of Mental Disorders,* 4th ed., Text revision. Washington, DC: American Psychiatric Association, 2000.
3. MayoClinic.com. Compulsive gambling. January 2009. www.mayoclinic.com/health/compulsive-gambling/DS00443.
4. MayoClinic.com. Drug addiction. October 2007. www.mayoclinic.com/health/drug-addiction/DS00183.
5. Cannon, C., and M. Bseikri. Is dopamine required for natural reward? *Physiology of Behavior* 81:741–748, 2004.
6. National Institute on Drug Abuse. Research Report Series. Updated July 2009. www.drugabuse.gov/ResearchReports.

7. Department of Health and Human Services. *Results from the 2007 National Survey on Drug Use and Health: National Findings,* Rockville, MD: Substance Abuse and Mental Health Services Administration, Office of Applied Studies, 2008.

8. Liska, K. *Drugs and the Human Body*, Englewood Cliffs, NJ: Prentice Hall, 2000.

9. Geller T., L. Loftis, and D. Brink. Cerebellar infarction in adolescent males associated with acute marijuana use. *Pediatrics* 113:e365–370, 2004.

10. Office of National Drug Control Policy. *National Drug Control Strategy Data Supplement 2009,* Washington, DC: Office of National Drug Control Policy, 2009.

11. White, S., and C. Lambe. The pathophysiology of cocaine abuse. *Journal of Clinical Forensic Medicine* 10:27–39, 2003.

12. Sindelar, H., N. Barnett, and A. Spirito. Adolescent alcohol use and injury: A summary and critical review of the literature. *Minerva Pediatrics* 56:291–309, 2004.

13. Ogden, E., and H. Moskowitz. Effects of alcohol and other drugs on driver performance. *Traffic Injury Prevention* 5:185–198, 2004.

14. MADD. .08 per se, 2004. www.MADD.org/Drunk-Driving/Drunk-Driving/laws/law.aspx?law=11.

15. Hingson, R., T. Heeren, M. Winter, and H. Wechsler. Magnitude of alcohol-related mortality and morbidity among U.S. college students ages 18–24: Changes from 1998 to 2001. *Annual Review of Public Health* 26: 259–279, 2005.

16. Knight, J. R., et al. Alcohol abuse and dependence among U.S. college students. *Journal of Studies on Alcohol* 63:263–270, May 2002.

17. National Institute on Alcohol Abuse and Alcoholism. *Trends in Underage Drinking in the United States, 1991–2007*. Surveillance Report no. 86. Bethesda, MD: U.S. Department of Health and Human Services, 2009.

18. Robbins, S., and M. Angell. *Basic Pathology*. Philadelphia: W. B. Saunders, 1997.

19. National Institute on Alcohol Abuse and Alcoholism. Frequently asked questions for the general public. Bethesda, MD: U.S. Department of Health and Human Services, February 2007. www.niaaa.nih.gov/FAQs/General-English.

20. Centers for Disease Control and Prevention, National Center for Chronic Disease Prevention and Health Promotion. Smoking and tobacco use: Fact sheets. 2009. www.cdc.gov/tobacco/data_statistics/fact_sheets/index.htm.

21. National Institute on Drug Abuse. NIDA Info Facts: Cigarettes and other tobacco products. 2009. www.drugabuse.gov/Infofacts/tobacco.html.

22. American Cancer Society. Secondhand smoke. www.cancer.org/docroot/PED/content/PED_10_2X_Secondhand_Smoke-Clean_Indoor_Air.asp. Revised May 2009.

23. Centers for Disease Control and Prevention. Epidemiologic notes and reports of illnesses possibly associated with smoking clove cigarettes. *Morbidity and Mortality Weekly Report*, May 1985. Available from www.cdc.gov/mmwr.

24. U.S. Department of Health and Human Services. The health consequences of involuntary exposure to tobacco smoke: A report of the Surgeon General. Atlanta, GA: U.S. Department of Health and Human Services, 2006. www.surgeongeneral.gov/library/secondhandsmoke/report.

25. American Lung Association. Quit smoking: Secondhand smoke fact sheet. www.lungusa.org. Updated 2009.

26. National Institute on Drug Abuse. Research Report Series—Anabolic Steroid Abuse. September 2006. www.drugabuse.gov/ResearchReports/Steroids.

27. Medline Plus. Many teen girls use steroids, June 2007. www.nlm.nih.gov/medlineplus.

28. Glantz, M., and C. Hartel (eds.). *Drug Abuse: Origins and Interventions*. Washington, DC: APA Publications, 1999.

29. Nawrot, P., S. Jordan, J. Eastwood, J. Rotstein, A. Hugenholtz, and M. Feeley. Effects of caffeine on human health. *Food Additives and Contamination* 20:1–30, 2003.

30. Maughan, R. Dietary supplements. *Journal of Sports Sciences* 22:95–113, 2004.

31. Powers, S., and S. Dodd. Caffeine and endurance performance: A review. *Sports Medicine* 2:165–174, 1985.

32. Dodd, S., R. Herb, and S. Powers. Caffeine and exercise performance: An update. *Sports Medicine* 15:14–23, 1993.

33. American College of Obstetricians and Gynecologists (ACOG). *Your Pregnancy and Birth,* 4th ed. Washington, DC: American College of Obstetricians and Gynecologists, 2005.

VIDEOS

Log on to www.pearsonhighered.com/powers to view these chapter-related videos.

Addictions and Addictive Behavior

Kick Your Habit—Soft Addictions

Treating Addiction with Virtual Reality

Illicit Drugs

Eliminating Meth

Campus Drug Dealers

Alcohol

Spring Break Nightmare

Teen Drinking Test

Tobacco

Smash the Ash!

Second Hand Smoke

The Mitchell Report on Steroids in Baseball

CHAPTER 18

CHAPTER OBJECTIVES

After reading this chapter you will be able to:

1. Identify the types of microorganisms involved in food-borne illness, pp. 661–665.

2. Describe strategies for preventing food-borne illness at home, while eating out, and when traveling to other countries, pp. 667–675.

3. Explain the advantages and disadvantages of canning, pasteurization, use of preservatives, aseptic packaging, and irradiation to preserve foods, pp. 676–679.

4. Describe the process of genetic modification and discuss the potential risks and benefits associated with genetically modified organisms, pp. 679–681 and 695–697.

5. Identify at least five categories of food additives and explain why they are used, pp. 681–683.

6. Describe the process by which persistent organic pollutants accumulate in foods, pp. 684–685.

7. Discuss the benefits and safety concerns related to pesticides, pp. 685–687.

8. Explain the current system of labeling for organic foods, p. 688.

TEST YOURSELF TRUE OR FALSE?

1. Each year, about 100,000 Americans are sickened and about 500 die as a direct result of eating food contaminated with germs or their toxins. T or F

2. Freezing destroys any microorganisms that might be lurking in your food. T or F

3. Mold is the most common cause of food poisoning. T or F

4. Research has failed to show any nutritional advantage of organic foods. T or F

5. Every food additive approved for use by food companies in the United States has been tested and proven safe. T or F

Test Yourself answers can be found after the Chapter Summary.

Food Safety and Technology: Impact on Consumers

t he fall of 2006 was not a good season for produce. In September, more than 200 people became ill and three died after consuming raw spinach contaminated with a type of bacteria called *E. coli*. This was quickly followed by an outbreak of salmonellosis, another food-borne bacterial illness, in more than 150 people who consumed fresh tomatoes. In November, *E. coli* struck again, this time contaminating shredded iceberg lettuce consumed in Taco Bell restaurants in New York, New Jersey, and Pennsylvania and causing illness in more than 400 people.[1] The outbreaks prompted a national debate on food safety, with many experts calling for greater oversight by the United States Food and Drug Administration (FDA), the agency charged with protecting American produce. But fresh fruits and vegetables are not the only source of contamination in our food supply. For example, *E. coli* is a common resident of raw meats: in 1993, it caused more than 500 cases of severe illness and three deaths in peo-

ple who consumed undercooked hamburgers in a restaurant chain in Washington State. *Salmonella* bacteria are routinely found in raw poultry and eggs, and in early 2007 showed up in two national brands of peanut butter. Mercury, a toxic metal, can collect in the tissues of fish swimming in polluted waters, and microbes and pollutants can even contaminate drinking water.

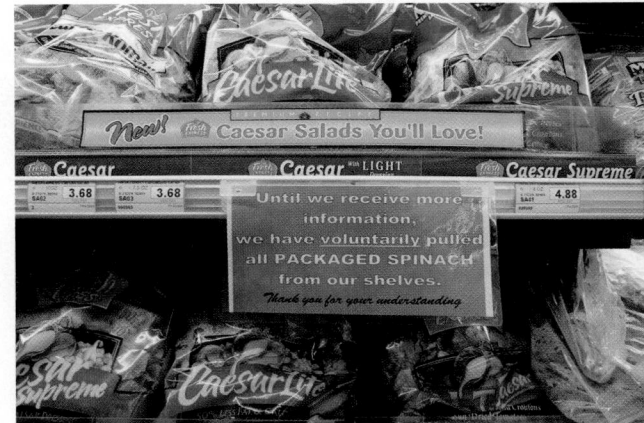

Spinach was pulled from supermarket shelves during an *E. coli* outbreak in 2006.

Food-borne illness is a term generally used to encompass any symptom or illness that arises from ingesting food or water that contains an infectious agent or toxic substance. Food-borne illness is commonly called *food poisoning*. According to the Centers for Disease Control and Prevention, approximately 76 million Americans report experiencing food-borne illness each year. It is estimated that over half the population of the United States have had symptoms of food-borne illness without ever knowing or reporting it. Of those afflicted by food-borne illness, 300,000 are hospitalized and 5,000 die each year.[2]

Although these statistics may seem frightening, most experts consider our food supply safe. That's partly because not all cases of food contamination make all people sick. For example, many strains of *E. coli* are harmless, and even virulent strains cause illness in only a small percentage of people. In the Taco Bell case, only about 400 people became ill out of the several thousands who ate at a Taco Bell restaurant in the three-state area affected during the contamination period. Moreover, modern science and technology have given us a wide array of techniques to decontaminate and preserve foods. We discuss these later in this chapter. Finally, food safety in the United States is monitored by several government agencies. In addition to the FDA, the United States Department of Agriculture (USDA), the Centers for Disease Control and Prevention (CDC), and the Environmental Protection Agency (EPA) monitor and regulate food production and preservation. Together, these agencies help to set standards to ensure the safety of our food supply. Information about these agencies and how to access them is in Table 18.1.

Despite these safeguards, food safety is emerging as a major global public health issue, as foods are produced farther and farther away from the regions in which they are consumed, and contamination can occur at any point from farm to table. In this chapter, we discuss how contaminants enter our food supply and describe some simple ways to protect yourself from getting sick. We also provide information about food spoilage and food preservation, including information on new techniques such as aseptic packaging and irradiation that increase the shelf life of many foods. Finally, we discuss the effect of various chemicals commonly used in food production, from food additives to pesticides to growth hormones. Whether your food comes from South America, a corporate farm, a local organic grower, or your own backyard, you'll learn about the safeguards that must be in place at every step from field to table to ensure food safety.

food-borne illness An illness transmitted through food or water by an infectious agent, a poisonous substance, or a protein that causes an immune reaction.

TABLE 18.1   Government Agencies That Regulate Food Safety

Name of Agency	Year Established	Role in Food Regulations	Web Site
U.S. Department of Agriculture (USDA)	1785	Oversees safety of meat, poultry, and eggs sold across state lines. Also regulates which drugs can be used to treat sick cattle and poultry.	www.usda.gov
Centers for Disease Control and Prevention (CDC)	1946	Works with public health officials to promote and educate the public about health and safety. Able to track information needed in identifying food-borne illness outbreaks.	www.cdc.gov
Environmental Protection Agency (EPA)	1970	Regulates use of pesticides and which crops they can be applied to. Establishes standards for water quality.	www.epa.gov
U.S. Food and Drug Administration (FDA)	1862	Regulates food standards of all food products (except meat, poultry, and eggs) and bottled water. Regulates food labeling and enforces pesticide use as established by EPA.	www.fda.gov

What Causes Food-Borne Illness **?**

Microbes or their toxic by-products cause most cases of food-borne illness. However, as discussed later in the chapter (page 684), chemical residues in foods can also cause illness.

Food-Borne Illness Is Commonly Caused by Microorganisms or Their Toxins

Two types of food-borne illness are common: *food infections* result from the consumption of food containing living microorganisms, whereas *food intoxications* result from consuming food in which microbes have secreted poisonous substances called *toxins*.[3]

FIGURE 18.1 The bacteria called *Campylobacter jejuni* causes more than 2 million cases of food infection each year in the United States.

Several Types of Microbes Contaminate Foods

The microbes that most commonly cause food infections are bacteria and viruses; however, helminths, fungi, and prions also contaminate foods.

According to the CDC, the majority of food infections are caused by **bacteria** (Table 18.2).[2] Bacteria are microorganisms that lack a true nucleus and have a chemical called peptidoglycan in their cell walls. Of the several species involved, *Campylobacter jejuni, Salmonella,* and *E. coli (Escherichia coli)* are thought to be the most common culprits, causing millions of cases each year in the United States (FIGURE 18.1). Most cases result from eating foods or drinking milk or water contaminated with infected animal feces. Infection with *Campylobacter jejuni* causes fever, pain, and bloody and frequent diarrhea.[3] Salmonellosis, the disease caused by eating food contaminated by certain strains of *Salmonella*, causes diarrhea, nausea, and vomiting, and cells of some strains of *Salmonella* can perforate the intestines and infect the blood. Certain virulent strains of *E. coli* can cause diarrhea and lead to kidney failure and death.

A strain of *Salmonella* called *S. typhi* causes the food-borne disease *typhoid fever.* The Highlight box on page 664 discusses this disease and its most famous host.

Although bacteria are the primary cause of food infections, some food-borne **viruses** also cause disease. Viruses are infectious agents that are much smaller than bacteria, lack independent metabolism, and are incapable of growth or reproduction apart from living cells. The hepatitis A virus can contaminate raw produce and cause liver damage. Hepatitis E also damages the liver and is fatal in about 20% of pregnant women. The hepatitis A and E viruses typically contaminate foods during harvesting, production, or preparation if work areas are unclean or workers have poor personal hygiene. In terms of sheer numbers, the rotaviruses are among the most serious: in the United States, they cause about 50,000 cases of severe diarrhea in children each year, and, in developing nations, they are responsible for about 1 million childhood deaths. The Norwalk virus, which was identified after an epidemic in Norwalk, Ohio, can contaminate water supplies and food in contact with the contaminated water, causing diarrhea, nausea, and vomiting.

Helminths, commonly called worms, include tapeworms, flukes, and roundworms (FIGURE 18.2). These microbes release their eggs into the environment, such as in vegetation or water. Animals, most commonly cattle, pigs, or fish, then consume the contaminated matter. The eggs hatch inside their host, and larvae develop in the host's tissue. The larvae can survive in the flesh long after the host is killed for food. Thoroughly cooking beef, pork, or fish destroys the larvae. In contrast, people who eat either raw or undercooked contaminated meat or fish consume living larvae, which then mature into adult worms in their small intestine. Some worms cause mild symptoms such as nausea and diarrhea, but others can grow large enough to cause

Hooks   Sucker

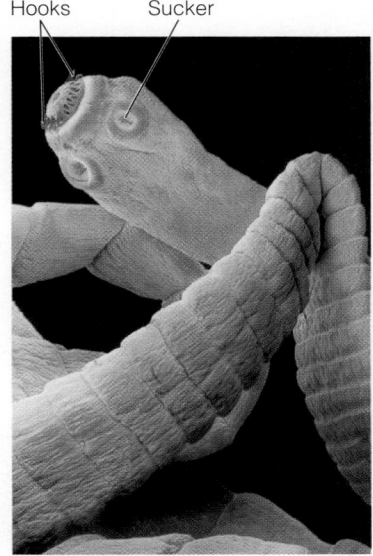

FIGURE 18.2 Tapeworms have long, wormlike bodies and hooks and suckers, which help them to attach to human tissues.

bacteria Microorganisms that lack a true nucleus and have a chemical called peptidoglycan in their cell walls.

viruses A group of infectious agents that are much smaller than bacteria, lack independent metabolism, and are incapable of growth or reproduction apart from living cells.

helminth A multicellular microscopic worm.

TABLE 18.2 Common Bacterial Causes of Food-Borne Illness

Bacteria	Incubation Period	Duration	Symptoms	Foods Most Commonly Affected	Usual Source of Contamination	Steps for Prevention
Campylobacter jejuni	1–7 days	7–10 days	Fever Headache and muscle pain followed by diarrhea (sometimes bloody) Nausea Abdominal cramps	Raw and undercooked meat, poultry or shellfish Raw eggs Cake icing Untreated water Unpasteurized milk	Intestinal tracts of animals and birds Raw milk Untreated water and sewage sludge	Do not drink unpasteurized milk Cook foods properly Avoid cross contamination
Salmonella (more than 2,300 types)	12–24 hours	4–7 days	Diarrhea Abdominal pain Chills Fever Vomiting Dehydration	Raw or undercooked eggs Undercooked poultry and meat Raw milk and dairy products Seafood Fruits and vegetables	Intestinal tract and feces of poultry *Salmonella enteritidis* in raw eggs	Cook thoroughly Avoid cross contamination Use sanitary practices
Escherichia coli (O157:H7 and other strains that can cause human illness)	2–4 days	5–10 days	Diarrhea (may be bloody) Abdominal cramps Nausea Can lead to kidney and blood complications	Contaminated water Raw milk Raw or rare ground beef, sausages Unpasteurized apple juice or cider Uncooked fruits and vegetables	Intestinal tracts of cattle Raw milk Unchlorinated water	Thoroughly cook meat Avoid cross contamination
Clostridium botulinum	12–36 hours	1–8 days	Nausea Vomiting Diarrhea Fatigue Headache Dry mouth Double vision Muscle paralysis (droopy eyelids) Difficulty speaking and swallowing Difficulty breathing	Improperly canned or vacuum-packed food Meats Sausage Fish Garlic in oil Honey	Widely distributed in nature Soil, water, on plants and intestinal tracts of animals and fish Grows only in little or no oxygen	Properly can foods following recommended procedures Cook foods properly Children under 16 months should not consume raw honey

(continued)

TABLE 18.2   Common Bacterial Causes of Food-Borne Illness (*continued*)

Bacteria	Incubation Period	Duration	Symptoms	Foods Most Commonly Affected	Usual Source of Contamination	Steps for Prevention
Staphylococcus	1–6 hours	2–3 days	Severe nausea and vomiting Abdominal cramps Diarrhea	Custard- or cream-filled baked goods Ham Poultry Dressing Gravy Eggs Mayonnaise-based salads and sandwiches Cream sauces	Human skin Infected cuts Pimples Noses and throats	Refrigerate foods Use sanitary practices
Shigella (more than 30 types)	12–50 hours	2 days–2 weeks	Bloody and mucus-containing diarrhea Fever Abdominal cramps Chills Vomiting	Contaminated water Salads Milk and dairy products	Human intestinal tract Rarely found in other animals	Use sanitary practices
Listeria monocytogenes	2 days–3 weeks	None reported	Fever Muscle aches Nausea Diarrhea Headache, stiff neck, confusion, loss of balance, or convulsions can occur if infection spreads to nervous system Infections during pregnancy can lead to miscarriage or stillbirth, premature delivery, or infection of newborn	Uncooked meats and vegetables Soft cheeses Lunch meats and hot dogs Unpasteurized milk	Intestinal tract and feces of animals Soil and manure used as fertilizer Raw milk	Thoroughly cook all meats Wash raw vegetables before eating Keep uncooked meats separate from vegetables and cooked foods Avoid unpasteurized milk or foods made from unpasteurized milk People at high risk should not eat hot dogs or lunch meats unless they are reheated until steaming hot

Source: Iowa State University Extension, Food Safety and Quality Project. 2000. Safe food: It's your job too! U.S. Food and Drug Administration (FDA). How can I prevent foodborne illness? *www.cfsan.fda.gov/~dms/qa-fdb1.html,* accessed August 2007; Centers for Disease Control and Prevention (CDC), Division of Bacterial and Mycotic Diseases. Disease Listing, Foodborne Illness.

HIGHLIGHT

How Typhoid Mary Earned Her Place in History

"Typhoid Mary" is a name commonly given to someone who has a contagious disease, but not many people know much about the real Typhoid Mary, an Irish immigrant named Mary Mallon. In 1868, Mallon came to the United States and found work as a cook. She first came to the attention of health officials after working for the Warren family at their summer home on Oyster Bay, Long Island. Soon after settling in for a summer vacation, one of the children became ill with typhoid fever, followed by her mother, a sister, and three of the hired help.

Typhoid fever's symptoms include a high fever (104°F) and continuous headaches, followed by diarrhea. It is caused by *Salmonella typhi* and is passed through food and water contaminated by an infected person's feces. An examination of the Warren family's outbreaks caused the public health investigator to stumble across Mary Mallon's employment history, which revealed that she had worked at seven previous jobs in which twenty-two people had contracted typhoid fever, with one death, after Mary began cooking for them.[4] Mary was apprehended and taken to a local hospital where samples from her stool and gallbladder tested positive for *S. typhi*. She had no symptoms, and so she became the United States' first "healthy carrier," a person who seems healthy but carries a contagious form of a disease that can infect others. Indeed, some people can have such a weak case of typhoid fever that they never know they were infected. Unfortunately, no one ever explained to Mary how she could be a "healthy carrier," and all her life she resisted the designation.

Mary was then sent to North Brother Island, part of the Riverside Hospital's facilities, in the East River to live in isolation. Mary believed she was unfairly persecuted and sued the health department. The judgment was found in favor of the health department, and Mary stayed on North Brother Island for another year, until a new health commissioner decided to release Mary on the condition that she never work as a cook again. Now using the pseudonym Mrs. Brown, Mary violated the conditions of her parole and returned to employment as a cook. Five years after her release from North Brother Island, she caused another out-

Working as a cook, Mary Mallon, also known as Typhoid Mary, caused more than 50 outbreaks of typhoid.

break of typhoid fever at the Sloan Maternity Hospital in Manhattan. This time, twenty-five people became ill, two of whom died. When it was discovered that Mrs. Brown was really Mary Mallon, she was immediately sent back to confinement where she lived out the remainder of her life. In all, it is believed that Typhoid Mary was the cause of fifty-three outbreaks, including the 1903 Ithaca, New York, epidemic in which 1,400 people were infected, including three deaths.[5]

---

giardiasis A diarrheal illness caused by the intestinal parasite *Giardia intestinalis* (or *Giardia lamblia*).

intestinal obstruction. Some spread beyond the gastrointestinal tract to damage other organs, such as the liver, bladder, or lungs. Some helminths can cause death.

A parasite known as *Giardia intestinalis* (or *Giardia lamblia*) causes a diarrheal illness called **giardiasis.** *Giardia* lives in the intestines of infected animals and humans, and it is passed into the environment from their stool. It is one of the most common causes of waterborne disease in humans in the United States. People typically consume *Giardia* by putting something in their mouth that has come in contact with the stool of an infected person or animal, by swallowing contaminated water, or by eating uncooked food contaminated with *Giardia*. Symptoms include diarrhea, loose or watery stools, stomach cramps, and upset stomach, but some people show no symptoms.

Fungi are plantlike spore-forming organisms that can grow either as single cells or as multicellular colonies. Two types of fungi are yeasts, which are globular, and molds, which are long and thin. Growths of these microbes on foods rarely cause food infection. This is due in part to the fact that very few species of fungi cause serious disease in people with healthy immune systems, and those that do cause disease in humans are not typically food-borne.[3] In addition, unlike bacterial growth, which is invisible and often tasteless, fungal growth typically makes food look and taste so unappealing that we immediately discard it (FIGURE 18.3).

FIGURE 18.3 Molds rarely cause human illness, in part because they look so unappealing that we throw the food away.

A food-borne illness that has had front-page exposure in recent years is mad cow disease, or *bovine spongiform encephalopathy* (*BSE*). Cattle contract this disease from eating feed contaminated with tissue and blood from other infected animals. First discovered in the early 1980s in Britain, this neurological disorder is caused by a **prion,** a proteinaceous infectious particle that is self-replicating. Prions are normal proteins of animal tissues that can misfold and become infectious. When they do, they can transform other normal proteins into abnormally shaped prions until they eventually cause illness.[6] The first reported case in the United States was in December of 2003 in Washington State, when an animal tested positive for the disease after it was slaughtered. Prions are not destroyed with cooking and are found only in the tissue of the central nervous system, retina, and lower intestines—not in the milk or muscle meats. BSE can be passed to humans who consume contaminated meat or tissue that has been ground into items such as sausages or burgers. For more information on mad cow disease, check out the Highlight box: Mad Cow Disease—What's the Beef?, on page 237.

Some Microbes Release Toxins

The microbes just discussed cause illness by directly infecting and destroying body cells. In contrast, other bacteria and fungi secrete chemicals called **toxins** that are responsible for serious and even life-threatening illnesses. These toxins bind to body cells and can cause a variety of symptoms such as diarrhea, vomiting, organ damage, convulsions, and paralysis. Toxins can be categorized depending on the type of cell they bind to; the two primary types of toxins associated with food-borne illness are **neurotoxins** and **enterotoxins.** Neurotoxins damage the nervous system, usually causing paralysis, while enterotoxins target the gastrointestinal system and generally cause severe diarrhea and vomiting.

One of the most common and deadly toxins is produced by the bacteria *Clostridium botulinum*. The botulism toxin blocks nerve transmission to muscle cells and causes paralysis, including paralysis of the muscles required for breathing. Common sources of contamination are split or pierced bulging cans, foods improperly canned at home, and raw honey.

Some fungi produce poisonous chemicals called *mycotoxins*. (The prefix *myco-* means "fungus.") These toxins are typically found in grains stored in moist environments. In some instances, moist conditions in the field encourage fungi to reproduce and release their toxins on the surface of growing crops. Long-term consumption of mycotoxins can cause organ damage or cancer, and they can be fatal if consumed in large doses. A mycotoxin called *aflatoxin* is produced by the mold *Aspergillus flavus*. Aflatoxin has been associated with peanuts and other crops and, if ingested, can cause illness in livestock and humans.

A highly visible fungus that causes food intoxication is the poisonous mushroom. Most mushrooms are not toxic, but a few, such as the deathcap mushroom (*Amanita*

fungi Plantlike spore-forming organisms that can grow either as single cells or as multicellular colonies.

prion An infectious, self-replicating protein.

toxin Any harmful substance; specifically, a chemical produced by a microorganism that harms tissues or causes harmful immune responses.

neurotoxins A type of toxin that targets the nervous system cells.

enterotoxins A type of toxin that targets the gastrointestinal tract cells.

FIGURE 18.4 Some mushrooms, such as this fly agaric, contain toxins that can cause illness or even death.

phalloides), can be fatal. Some poisonous mushrooms are quite colorful (FIGURE 18.4), a fact which helps to explain why the victims of mushroom poisoning are often children.[3]

Potatoes that have turned green contain the toxin solanine, which forms during the greening process. The green color is actually due to the pigment chlorophyll, which is harmless, and forms when the potatoes are exposed to light. Although the production of solanine occurs simultaneously with the production of chlorophyll, the two processes are separate and unrelated.[7] There is the potential for toxicity from consuming potatoes with a very high solanine content. Since solanine formation occurs near the potato's skin, the green areas can be cut away to remove any toxins. A good guide is to taste a small piece of the potato after the green areas have been removed. If the potato tastes bitter, then throw it away. If in doubt, or if serving the potato to someone with allergies or compromised immunity, you should also discard the potato. You can avoid the greening of potatoes by storing them for only short periods in a dark cupboard or brown paper bag in a cool area.

The Body Responds to Food-Borne Microbes and Toxins with Acute Illness

Many food-borne microbes are killed in the mouth by antimicrobial enzymes in saliva or in the stomach by hydrochloric acid. Any microbe that survives these chemical assaults will usually trigger vomiting and/or diarrhea as the gastrointestinal tract attempts to expel the offender. Simultaneously, the white blood cells of the immune system will be activated, and a generalized inflammatory response will cause the person to experience nausea, fatigue, fever, and muscle cramps. Refer back to Table 18.2 to identify the many possible symptoms resulting from food infection with various bacteria.

People most affected by food-borne illnesses are those with compromised immune systems. This group includes people with HIV, which reduces the number of healthy immune cells, and people undergoing chemotherapy, which destroys immune cells along with cancer cells. Since immune function declines somewhat with aging, the elderly are also at increased risk, as are children under the age of 10, whose immune responses are not yet mature. Pregnant women are also at increased risk, since immune function is somewhat reduced during pregnancy. However, food-borne illness can affect anyone. Depending on the state of one's health, the precise microbe involved, and the number of microbes ingested, the symptoms can range from mild to severe, including double vision, loss of muscle control, and excessive or bloody diarrhea. As noted earlier, some cases, if left untreated, can result in death.

To diagnose a food-borne illness, a specimen must be obtained and cultured. This means that the specimen is analyzed in a laboratory setting in which the offending microorganisms are grown in a specific chemical medium. Stool (fecal) cultures are usually analyzed, especially if diarrhea is a symptom. Blood is cultured if the patient has a high fever. A physician who suspects that a patient is suffering from a food-borne illness will take a detailed history including a 24-hour dietary recall. Treatment usually involves keeping the person hydrated and comfortable, as most food-borne illness tends to be self-limiting; the person's vomiting and/or diarrhea, though unpleasant, serve to rid the body of the offending microbe. In severe illnesses such as botulism, the patient's intestinal tract will be repeatedly treated to remove the microbe, and antibodies will be injected to neutralize its deadly toxin.

In the United States, all confirmed cases of food-borne illness must be reported to the state health department, which in turn reports these illnesses to the CDC in Atlanta, Georgia. The CDC monitors its reports for indications of epidemics of food-borne illness and assists local and state agencies in controlling such outbreaks.

Certain Environmental Conditions Help Microbes Multiply in Foods

Given the correct conditions, microbes can thrive and multiply in many types of food. These growth-favoring conditions include a precise range of temperature, humidity, acidity, and oxygen content. For example, many bacteria are destroyed by normal heating, and many cannot reproduce in a food that is refrigerated or frozen. Many microbes require a high level of moisture, and thus foods like boxed dried pasta do not make suitable microbial homes, though cooked pasta left at room temperature might prove hospitable.

Some microbes cannot tolerate acidic foods. For example, *Clostridium botulinum* cannot grow or produce its toxin in an acidic environment, so the risk of botulism is decreased in citrus fruits, pickles, wine, yogurt, tomato juice, soup, sauce, and other acidic foods. In contrast, more alkaline foods such as eggs, carrot juice, asparagus, green beans, beets, corn, and olives are a magnet for *C. botulinum*.

In addition, microbes need an entryway into a food. Just as skin protects the body from microbial invasion, the peels, rinds, and shells of many foods seal off access to microbes. Once such barriers are pierced or removed, however, the food loses its primary defense against contamination.

> RECAP: *Food infections result from the consumption of food containing living microorganisms, such as bacteria, whereas food intoxications result from consuming food in which microbes have secreted toxins. Food infections can be caused by bacteria, viruses, fungi, helminths, and prions. The body has several defense mechanisms, such as saliva, stomach acid, vomiting, diarrhea, and the inflammatory response, which help rid us of offending microorganisms or their toxins. In order to reproduce in foods, microbes require a precise range of temperature, humidity, acidity, and oxygen content.*

Peels protect foods against microbes.

How Can Food-Borne Illness Be Prevented?

Foods of animal origin are most commonly associated with food-borne illness. These include not only raw meat, poultry, and fish, but also eggs, shellfish, and unpasteurized milk. Foods that may be the product of several animals (such as ground beef) can be especially hazardous. In addition, a bacteria or virus present in one animal has the potential to contaminate the entire herd.

As we discussed at the beginning of this chapter, fruits and vegetables can also cause problems when they are consumed unwashed and raw. Washing decreases, but cannot eliminate, all contaminants, and the quality of the water used in washing is sometimes a factor. Unpasteurized fruit or vegetable juices may also be contaminated if the produce used to make these juices contained pathogens.[2]

When Preparing Foods at Home

When preparing foods at home, food-borne illness can be prevented by following four basic rules, each discussed in detail below (FIGURE 18.5):

1. Wash your hands and kitchen surfaces often.

2. Separate foods to prevent **cross contamination,** that is, the spread of bacteria or other microbes from one food to another. This commonly occurs when raw, unwashed foods are cut on the same cutting board or served together on the same plate.

3. Chill foods to prevent microbes from growing.

4. Cook foods to their proper temperatures (discussed on pages 671–673).

Wash Your Hands and Kitchen Surfaces Often

One of the easiest and most effective ways to prevent food-borne illness is to wash your hands both before and after preparing food. Scrub for at least 20 seconds with gentle soap under warm running water (sing "Happy Birthday" or recite the ABC's to time yourself). Hot water is too harsh: it causes the surface layer of the skin to break

cross contamination
Contamination of one food by another via the unintended transfer of microbes through physical contact.

FIGURE 18.5 The FightBAC! logo is the food safety logo of the U.S. Department of Agriculture.

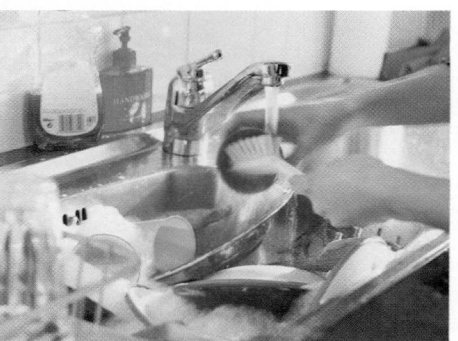

Washing dishes, utensils, and cutting boards with warm, soapy water reduces the chances for food contamination.

down, increasing the risk that microbes will be able to penetrate your skin. Pay special attention to the areas underneath your fingernails and between your fingers. Also, it's a good idea to remove rings and bracelets while cooking, as they can harbor bacteria. To prevent cross contamination, always wash your hands after working with each raw food and before progressing to the next one.

A clean area and tools are also essential in reducing cross contamination. Wash utensils, containers, and cutting boards in the dishwasher or with warm soapy water before and after contact with food. If a cutting board, plate, countertop, or other surface has held raw meat, poultry, or seafood, sanitize it with a solution of 1 teaspoon of chlorine bleach to 1 quart of water, or use a commercial kitchen cleaning agent.[8] It's also important to wash utensils, faucets, cabinet knobs, countertops, or other areas you have touched. Rinse, then air dry or dry with fresh paper towels. For cutting foods, use a nonporous, smooth plastic or stone cutting board because porous wood and scratched plastic can hold juices and harbor bacteria.

Dishtowels, cloths, and aprons should be washed in hot water often. It's a good idea to wash sponges in the dishwasher each time you run it and to replace them regularly. If you don't have a dishwasher, put sponges in boiling water for 3 minutes to sterilize them on a routine basis.

Separate Foods to Prevent Cross Contamination

Raw meat, poultry, and seafood harbor an array of microbes and can easily contaminate other foods through direct contact, as well as by the juices they leave behind on surfaces (including hands). Avoid contact between foods that have already been cooked or that won't be cooked, like salad ingredients, and these foods or their juices. Also avoid placing cooked or ready-to-eat foods on a plate or other surface that previously held raw meat, seafood, or poultry. When preparing meals with a marinade, reserve some of the fresh marinade in a clean container, then add the raw ingredients to the remainder. In this way, some noncontaminated marinade will be available if needed later in the cooking process. Raw food should always be marinated in the refrigerator.

Store Foods in the Refrigerator or Freezer

Different microbes thrive in different environmental temperatures. The majority of bacteria that cause food-borne illness prefer temperatures between 60 and 130°F (15 to 50°C); thus, the temperature range between 40 and 140°F (4.4 to 60°C) is referred to as the "danger zone" for food-borne illness.[9] Refrigeration (storage between 32 and 39°F) and freezing (storage below 32°F) are two of the most reliable methods of diminishing bacteria's ability to cause illness. Not all bacteria in cool environments are killed, but the rate at which they reproduce is drastically reduced. Also, naturally occurring enzymes that cause food decomposition are stopped at freezing temperatures.

Shopping for Perishable Foods. When shopping for food, purchase refrigerated and frozen foods last. Many grocery stores are actually designed so that these foods are in the last aisles. Put packaged meat, poultry, or fish into a plastic bag before placing it in your shopping cart.[10] This prevents drippings from the food from coming into contact with other foods in your cart.

When buying perishable foods, look for the "sell by" or "use by" date on their packaging. The "sell by" date indicates the last day a product can be sold and still maintain its quality during normal home storage and consumption. It is generally best to purchase foods prior to this date. The "use by" date indicates how long a product will maintain optimum quality.[11] It is best to avoid consuming foods after the "use by" date, even though they are generally still safe to eat. For nonperishable foods such as cereal and baking mixes, the "best if used by (or before)" dates indicate the shelf life of the product or the date at which the product is no longer at peak flavor, texture, and appearance. These foods can be safely eaten past the listed date if they have been stored properly, but they may not taste as good as they did or be as nutritious as they were before this date. Proper storage for nonperishable items includes storage in a dry, clean, cool (less than 85°F) cabinet or pantry.

Do not purchase foods with punctured or otherwise damaged packaging. Dented or bulging cans are especially dangerous, as they could harbor potentially deadly bacteria. Report any damaged packaging to the store manager.

Watch for unsanitary practices and conditions inside the store. For example, the unsafe displaying of food products, such as cooked shrimp on the same bed of ice as raw seafood, is illegal, as is trimming raw meat with the same knife used to slice cold cuts. Report such unsanitary practices or conditions to your local health authorities.[10]

After purchase, perishable foods should be taken home and put into the refrigerator or freezer within 1 hour. If the trip home will be longer than an hour, a cooler should be brought along to transport them in.

Refrigerating Foods. Once you get home, put meat, poultry, and seafood in the coldest part of the refrigerator. Keep them wrapped in plastic so their juices do not drip onto any other foods. If you are not going to use meat, poultry, or seafood within 48 hours of purchase, store them in the freezer.[11] Remember that eggs are also perishable and should be kept refrigerated. Avoid overstocking your refrigerator or freezer, as air needs to circulate around food to cool it quickly and discourage microbial growth. Purchase a refrigerator thermometer and check it regularly to ensure your refrigerator is below 40° F (4.4°C) to optimize the safety of foods stored there.

After a meal, leftovers should be promptly refrigerated—even if still hot—to discourage microbial growth. The standard rule for storing leftovers is *2 hours / 2 inches / 4 days*. Food should be refrigerated *within 2 hours* of serving. If the environmental temperature is 90°F or higher, such as at a picnic, then foods should be refrigerated within 1 hour.[12] Because a larger quantity of food takes longer to cool and will allow more microbes to thrive, food should be stored at a depth of no greater than *2 inches*. The interior of deeper containers of foods can remain warm long enough to allow bacteria to multiply rapidly even when the surface of the food has cooled. Leftovers should be refrigerated for only *up to 4 days*. If you don't plan on using the food within 4 days, freeze it. A guide for storing foods in your refrigerator is provided in FIGURE 18.6.

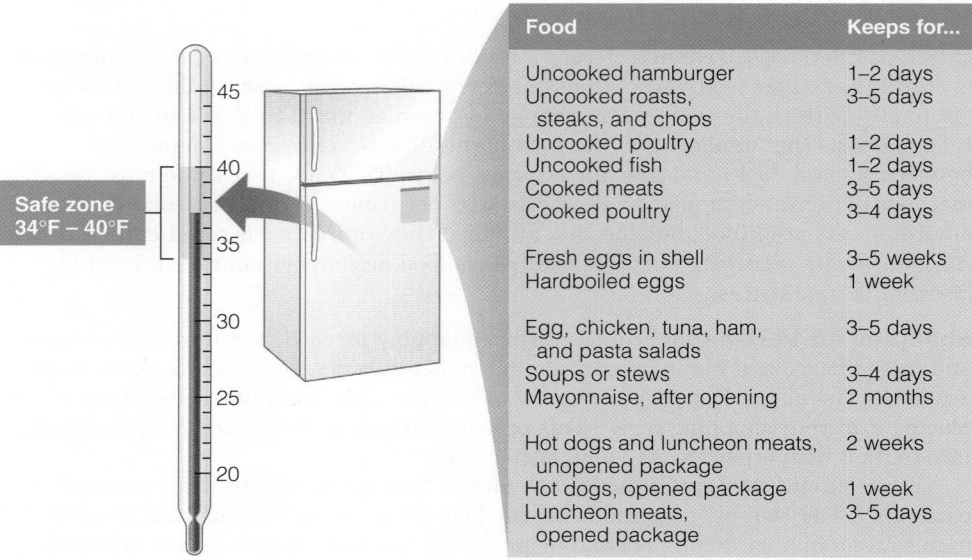

Food	Keeps for...
Uncooked hamburger	1–2 days
Uncooked roasts, steaks, and chops	3–5 days
Uncooked poultry	1–2 days
Uncooked fish	1–2 days
Cooked meats	3–5 days
Cooked poultry	3–4 days
Fresh eggs in shell	3–5 weeks
Hardboiled eggs	1 week
Egg, chicken, tuna, ham, and pasta salads	3–5 days
Soups or stews	3–4 days
Mayonnaise, after opening	2 months
Hot dogs and luncheon meats, unopened package	2 weeks
Hot dogs, opened package	1 week
Luncheon meats, opened package	3–5 days

FIGURE 18.6 While it's important to keep a well-stocked refrigerator, it's also important to know how long foods will keep. (From U.S. Department of Agriculture, Food Safety and Inspection Service, November 2005, Fact Sheets. Safe Food Handling. Refrigeration and Food Safety, www.fsis.usda.gov/Fact_Sheets/Refrigeration_&_Food_Safety/index.asp)

Freezing and Thawing Foods. The temperature in your freezer should not exceed 32°F (0°C). Use a thermometer to check periodically that a freezing temperature is being maintained. If your electricity goes out, avoid opening the freezer until the power is restored. When the power does come back on, check to make sure that the temperature on the top shelf of the freezer compartment is no warmer than 40°F (5°C). If it is warmer, you should inspect your freezer's contents and discard any items that are not firmly frozen.

When freezing items, remember that smaller packages will freeze more quickly. So rather than attempting to freeze an entire casserole or a whole batch of homemade spaghetti sauce, divide the food into multiple portions in freezer-safe containers, then freeze.

Sufficient thawing will ensure adequate cooking throughout, which is essential to preventing food-borne illness. Raw poultry is a good example of a food item that needs to be carefully contained as it thaws, so its juices don't contaminate other foods. The perfect place to thaw poultry is on the bottom shelf of the refrigerator in a large bowl to catch any of its juices. Table 18.3 shows recommended poultry thawing times based on weight. Never thaw frozen meat, poultry, or seafood on a kitchen counter or in a basin of warm water. Room temperatures allow growth of bacteria on the surface of food, although the inside may still be frozen.[11] A microwave is also useful for thawing, but be sure to follow your microwave's instructions carefully. Thaw with a microwave only if the food is to be cooked immediately afterward.

Molds in Refrigerated Foods. Have you ever taken cheese out of the refrigerator and noticed that it had a fuzzy blue or white growth on it? This is mold, one of the two types of fungus. Interestingly, cool temperatures and high acidity do not slow the growth of some molds; in fact, some prefer these conditions. For instance, when acidic foods such as applesauce, yogurt, and spaghetti sauce are refrigerated, they readily support the growth of mold. But how does mold get into a closed, refrigerated container? Mold spores are common in the atmosphere, and they randomly land on food either in the processing plant or in open containers at your home. If the temperature and acidity of the food are hospitable, they will grow.

TABLE 18.3 A Guide to Thawing Poultry

Method Needed	Size of Poultry	Approximate Length of Time
Refrigerator	1–3 pounds, small chickens, pieces	1 day
	3–6 pounds, large chickens, ducks, small turkeys	2 days
	6–12 pounds, large turkeys	3 days
	12–16 pounds, whole turkey	3–4 days
	16–20 pounds, whole turkey	4–5 days
Microwave (read instructions)	1–3 pounds, small chickens, pieces	8–15 minutes* (standing time 10 minutes)
	3–6 pounds, large chickens, ducks, small turkeys	15–30 minutes* (standing time 20 minutes)

*Approximate; read microwave's instructions.
Note: Turkeys purchased stuffed and frozen with the USDA or state mark of inspection on the packaging are safe because they have been processed under controlled conditions. These turkeys *should not* be thawed before cooking. Follow package directions for handling.
Sources: Lacey, R. W. 1994. *Hard to Swallow: A Brief History of Food*, pp. 85–187. Cambridge: Cambridge University Press; U.S. Department of Agriculture, Food Safety and Inspection Service. 2000. Turkey basics: Safe thawing. www.fsis.usda.gov/Fact_Sheets/Poultry_Preparation_Fact_Sheets/index.asp#talk_turkey.

Most people throw away moldy foods because they are so unappealing, but as we noted earlier, food-borne illnesses aren't commonly caused by fungi. If the surface of a small portion of a solid food such as hard cheese becomes moldy, it is generally safe to cut off that section down to about an inch and eat the unspoiled portion. If soft cheese, sour cream, yogurt, tomato sauce, apple sauce, or another soft or fluid product becomes moldy, discard it.

Some fungi are actually used in the food industry to create popular foods and beverages. The distinct flavor of Roquefort and blue cheeses can be attributed to the molds used in their ripening process. Yeast, the globular form of fungi, gives a distinct flavor to fermented foods such as sourdough bread, miso, soy sauce, beer, wine, and distilled spirits. Even the production of chocolate requires the help of yeasts, which ferment the cacao seeds, causing them to lose their bitter taste.

Cook Foods Thoroughly

Thoroughly cooking food is a sure way to kill the intestinal worms discussed earlier and many other microbes. The proper internal temperatures for doneness of meat, poultry, seafood, and eggs vary, as shown in FIGURE 18.7.

The color of cooked meat can be deceiving. Grilled meat and poultry often brown very quickly on the outside but may not be thoroughly cooked on the inside. The only way to be sure that meat is thoroughly cooked is with a food thermometer. Test the food in several places to be sure it's cooked evenly, and remember to wash the thermometer after each use. If you don't have a thermometer available, do not eat hamburger that is still pink inside.[12] For more information on safe grilling or barbecuing, see the Highlight box: Food Safety Tips for Your Next Barbecue on page 673.

Microwave cooking is convenient, but you need to be sure that your food is thoroughly cooked and there are no cold spots in the food where bacteria can thrive. For best results when microwaving, remember to cover food, stir often, and rotate for even cooking.[12] If you are microwaving meat or poultry, use a thermometer to check internal temperatures in several spots, since temperatures vary in different parts of food more in microwave cooking than in conventional ovens.[11] The U.S. Department of Agriculture has published a helpful fact sheet describing how to cook safely using the microwave; see the Web links at the end of this chapter.

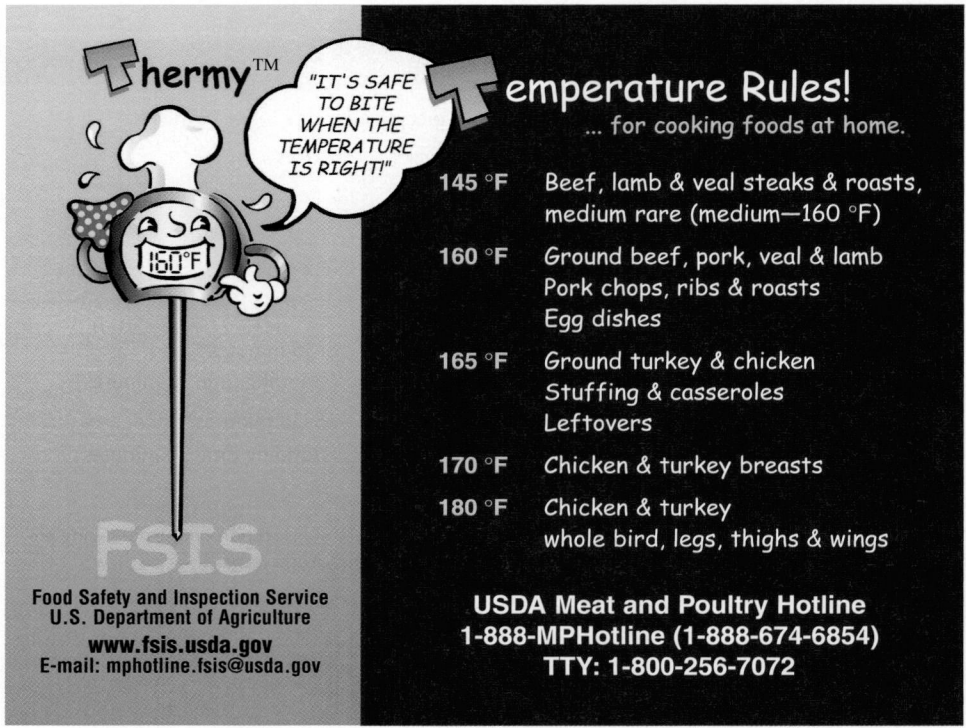

FIGURE 18.7 The U.S. Department of Agriculture's "Thermy" provides temperature rules for safely cooking foods at home.

Raw and semi-raw (such as marinated or partly cooked) fish delicacies, including sushi and sashimi, may be tempting, but their safety cannot be guaranteed. Always cook fish thoroughly. When done, fish should be opaque and flake easily with a fork. It is important to recognize that sushi restaurants cannot guarantee the safety of their food. All fish to be used for sushi must be flash frozen at $-31°$ F ($-35°$C) or below for 15 hours, or be regularly frozen to $-4°$ F ($-20°$ C) or below for 7 days.[13] Although this effectively kills any parasites that might be in the fish, it does not kill bacteria or viruses. Thus, eating raw seafood remains risky, and the FDA advises that people with compromised immunity, children, pregnant women, and the elderly avoid it.[10]

You may have memories of licking the cake batter off a spoon when you were a kid, but such practices are no longer considered safe. That's because most cake batters contain raw eggs, and an estimated one-third of chicken eggs in the United States are contaminated with *Salmonella*. For this reason, the USDA recommends that you cook eggs until the yolk and whites are firm. For example, hard-boiled eggs should be boiled for 7 minutes, and fried eggs should be cooked for 3 minutes on one side, 1 minute on the other. Scrambled eggs should not be runny. If you are using eggs in a casserole or custard, make sure that the internal temperature reaches at least 160°F.[14] Homemade mayonnaise is made with raw egg yolks; thus, it is more likely to cause food-borne illnesses than commercial mayonnaise, which contains pasteurized eggs. In addition, commercial mayonnaise has a consistently high level of acidity, produced by the addition of either vinegar or lemon juice, which inhibits bacterial growth.

Killing microorganisms with heat is an important step in keeping food safe, but it won't protect people against their toxins. That's because toxins are unaffected by heat and are capable of causing severe illness even when the microbes that produced them have been destroyed. For example, let's say you prepare a casserole for a team picnic. Unfortunately, you forget to wash your hands before serving it to your teammates, and you contaminate the casserole with the bacteria *Staphylococcus aureus*, which is commonly found on moist skin folds.[3] At the picnic, you and your friends go off and play soccer, leaving the food in the sun, and a few hours later, you take the

HIGHLIGHT

Food Safety Tips for Your Next Barbecue

It's the end of the term, and you and your friends are planning a lakeside barbecue to celebrate! Here are some tips from the Center for Food Safety and Applied Nutrition at the U.S. Food and Drug Administration for preventing food-borne illness at any outdoor gathering.

1. **Wash your hands, utensils, and food preparation surfaces.** Even in outdoor settings, food safety begins with hand washing. Bring along a water jug, some soap, and paper towels, or a box of moist disposable towelettes. Keep all utensils and platters clean when preparing foods.

2. **Keep foods cold during transport.** Use coolers with ice or frozen gel packs to keep food at or below 40°F. It's easier to maintain a cold temperature in small coolers. Consider packing three: put beverages in one cooler; washed fruits and vegetables and containers of potato salad, chicken salad, and so forth, in another; and meat, poultry, and seafood in another. Meat, poultry, and seafood may be packed while still frozen so that they stay colder longer. Be sure they are wrapped securely so that juices don't leak inside the cooler. Keep coolers in the air-conditioned passenger compartment of your car rather than in a hot trunk.

3. **Grill foods thoroughly.** Use a food thermometer to be sure the food has reached an adequate internal temperature before serving. For example:

   - Steaks should reach 145°F for medium rare, 160°F for medium, and 170°F for well done.
   - Ground beef should reach 160°F.
   - Poultry breasts should reach 170°F.
   - Fish should reach 145°F, or be cooked until the flesh is opaque and separates easily with a fork.

   When bringing food from the grill to the table, never use the same platter or utensils that previously held raw meat or seafood!

4. **Keep hot foods hot and cold foods cold.** Keep grilled food hot until it is served by moving it to the side of the grill, just away from the coals, so that it stays at or above 140°F. If grilled food isn't going to be eaten right away, wrap it well and place it in an insulated container. Cold foods like chicken salad should be kept in a bowl of ice during your barbecue. Drain off water as the ice melts and replace the ice frequently. Don't let any perishable food sit out longer than 2 hours. In temperatures above 90°F, don't let food sit out for more than 1 hour.

Source: U.S. Department of Agriculture, Food Safety and Inspection Service. 2003. Fact Sheets. Safe Food Handling. Barbecue and Food Safety. *www.fsis.usda.gov/fact_ sheets/ Barbecue_Food_Safety/index.asp.*

rest of the casserole home. At supper, you heat the leftovers thoroughly, thinking as you do so that this will kill any bacteria that might have multiplied while the casserole was left out. That night you wake up with nausea, severe vomiting, and abdominal pain. What happened? While your food was left out, the bacteria from your hands multiplied in the casserole and produced a toxin (FIGURE 18.8). When the food was reheated, the microorganisms were killed, but their toxin was unaffected by the heat. When you then ate the food, the toxin made you sick. Fortunately, in the case of *S. aureus,* symptoms typically resolve on their own in healthy people in about 24 hours.

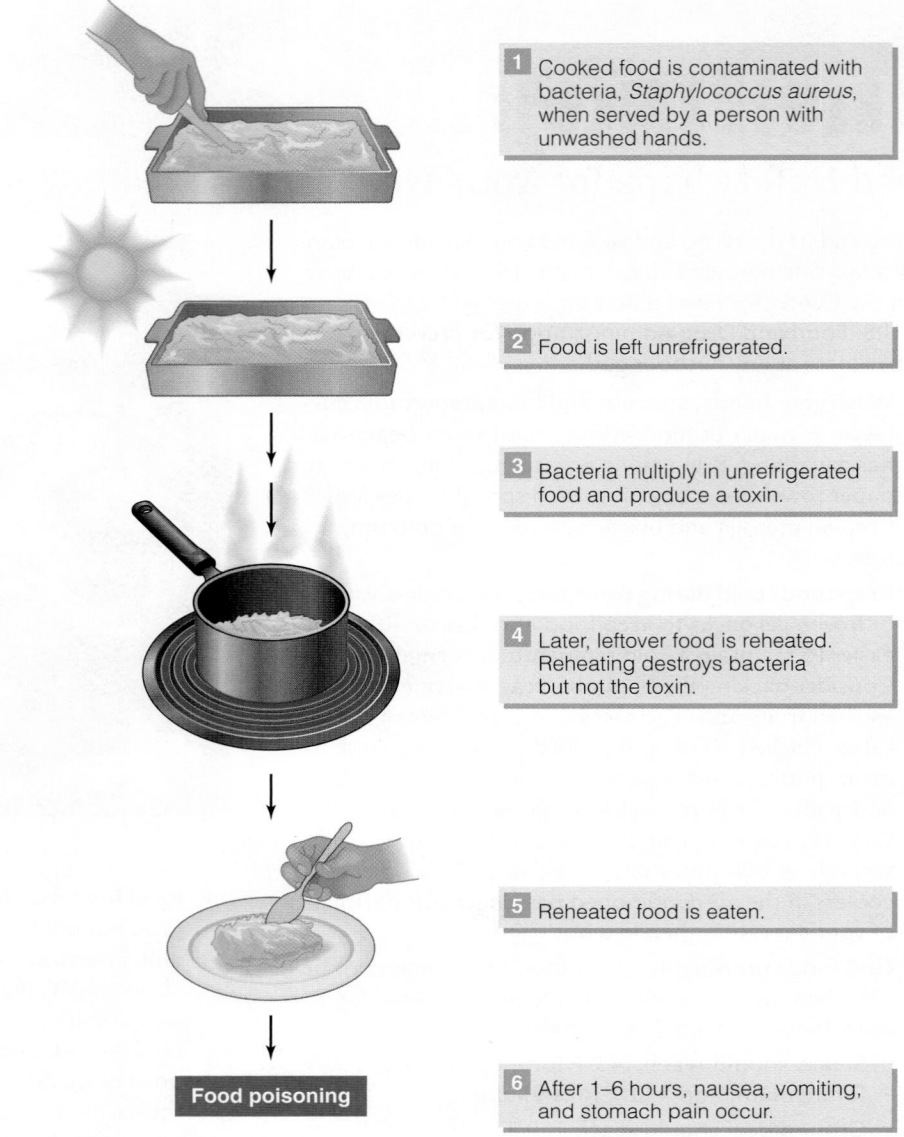

1 Cooked food is contaminated with bacteria, *Staphylococcus aureus*, when served by a person with unwashed hands.

2 Food is left unrefrigerated.

3 Bacteria multiply in unrefrigerated food and produce a toxin.

4 Later, leftover food is reheated. Reheating destroys bacteria but not the toxin.

5 Reheated food is eaten.

Food poisoning

6 After 1–6 hours, nausea, vomiting, and stomach pain occur.

FIGURE 18.8   Food intoxication can occur long after the microbe itself has been destroyed.

When Eating Out

When choosing a place to eat out, avoid restaurants that don't look clean. Grimy tabletops and dirty restrooms indicate indifference to hygiene. On the other hand, cleanliness of areas used by the public doesn't guarantee that the kitchen is clean. That is why health inspections are important. Public health inspectors randomly visit and inspect the food preparation areas of all businesses that serve food, whether eaten in or taken out. The results of these inspections can usually be found in the local newspaper, by contacting your local health department, or by checking the inspection results posted in the restaurant.

Another way to protect yourself when dining out is by ordering foods to be cooked thoroughly. If you order a hamburger that arrives pink in the middle or scrambled eggs that arrive runny, send the food back and ask for it to be cooked longer. Also request that it be returned on a clean plate, with clean silverware.

When Traveling to Other Countries

When planning your trip, tell your physician your travel plans and ask about vaccinations needed or any medications that should be taken along in case you get sick. Also pack a waterless antibacterial hand cleanser, and use it frequently during the trip. When dining, select foods and beverages carefully. All raw food has the potential for contamination, especially in areas where hygiene and sanitation are inadequate. All travelers are cautioned to avoid salads, uncooked fruits and vegetables, and unpasteurized dairy products. Fruits and vegetables are safe to eat if they are first washed thoroughly in bottled water or water that has been boiled for 1 minute and then allowed to cool. Peeling washed fruits and vegetables also reduces the likelihood of contamination. If fish is a local delicacy, be aware that many tropical species from the insular areas of the Caribbean and the Pacific and Indian Oceans can contain poisonous **biotoxins,** even when well cooked.[15] Biotoxins are naturally occurring poisonous chemicals.

Tap water is seldom a safe option, even if chlorinated, as chlorine doesn't kill all organisms that can cause disease. In regions where hygiene and sanitation are suspect, drink only the following: canned or bottled carbonated beverages such as bottled water and soft drinks, beverages made with boiled water such as tea, and fermented drinks such as beer and wine, as their processing will neutralize any potential pathogens. Also, remember to ask for drinks without ice, as freezing contaminated water does not kill microbes and parasites. If you think the water may be contaminated, don't even brush your teeth with it: use bottled water or boil the water for 1 minute, then allow the water to return to room temperature before brushing. You can find more information about food and water safety when traveling by visiting the CDC's Web site (see the Web links at the end of this chapter) or by contacting your local health department.

> RECAP: *Food-borne illness can be prevented at home by following these tips: wash your hands and kitchen surfaces often, separate foods to prevent cross contamination, store foods in the refrigerator or freezer, thaw frozen foods in the refrigerator, and heat foods long enough and at temperatures high enough to ensure proper cooking. When traveling, avoid all raw foods unless thoroughly washed in bottled or boiled water, and choose beverages that are boiled, bottled, or canned, without ice.*

biotoxins Naturally occurring poisonous chemicals.

NUTRI-CASE THEO

" I got really sick yesterday after eating lunch in the cafeteria. I had a turkey sandwich, potato salad, and a cola. I remember thinking that the potato salad looked a little off, as if it had been sitting around too long, but I was late for lunch and the cafeteria was about to close, so I had to make my choices fast. Anyway, around 5:00, in the middle of basketball practice, I started to shake and sweat. I got really nauseated, and barely made it to the bathroom before vomiting. Then I went back to my dorm room and crawled into bed. This morning I still feel a little nauseated and sort of weak. I asked some of my friends who ate in the cafeteria yesterday if they got sick, and none of them did, but I still think it was the food. I'm going off-campus for lunch from now on!"

Do you think that Theo's illness was food-borne? If so, what food and/or ingredient(s) do you most suspect, and why? What microbe? (Hint: See Table 18.2.) What do you think of his plan to go off-campus for lunch from now on? And what other actions might you advise Theo to take?

How Is Food Spoilage Prevented?

The majority of our food is derived from living plants and animals. Because living cells gradually die and decompose after being separated from their nutrient source, it makes sense that foods start to spoil over time. The breakdown of food is due to both enzymes naturally found in the food and microorganisms that colonize the food.

Spoilage alters food in several ways. Both fruits and meats turn brown, vegetables wilt, and milk starts to curdle and sometimes takes on a yellow tinge. The texture of foods also changes as components that give food their fibrous structure begin to break down. Think of the difference between a perfectly ripe tomato and one that has turned to "mush." The chemical reactions involved in spoilage also change the taste and smell of foods. Most importantly, spoiled food is no longer safe to eat: since decomposition of foods is accomplished in part by microbes, if someone eats a food that has spoiled, he or she risks developing a food-borne illness.

Food spoilage is certainly a concern for fresh foods such as meats, fruits, and vegetables, but if you're like many people who live in developed countries, a large part of your daily diet consists of processed foods. Do they spoil, too? **Processed foods** are created by mechanical or chemical manipulation of whole foods. For example, milk is manipulated to produce cheese, which is further manipulated to become the topping for your favorite frozen pizza. Although they are often very different in appearance from their original ingredients, many processed foods actually have the same potential for spoiling as unprocessed foods. They may not change in color as they age, but their flavor, texture, and smell typically degrade, and they begin to support microbial growth. Of course, some processed foods, such as dry pasta or canned soups, resist spoilage.

Oxygen, heat, and light are the three factors most often responsible for spoilage of foods. That is why air-tight packaging and cool, dark storage are so important in keeping foods safe to eat and enjoy. Here, we look at some techniques that people have used for centuries to preserve food, as well as more modern techniques used in the food industry today.

Natural Methods of Preserving Foods

Some methods of preserving foods have been used for thousands of years and employ naturally derived substances such as salt, sugars, and smoke or techniques such as drying and cooling.

Salting and Sugaring

processed foods Foods that are manipulated mechanically or chemically during their production or packaging. Processed foods may or may not resemble the original ingredients in their final form.

Both salt and sugar preserve food by drawing water out of the plant or animal cells by *osmosis,* as discussed in Chapter 7 (see FIGURE 7.4, page 271). Salting or sugaring essentially dehydrates the food, making it inhospitable to microbes, especially bacteria. Dehydration also dramatically slows the action of enzymes that would otherwise degrade the food.

Salt, one of the oldest and most effective preservatives, is especially good at drawing water from food. Because of current concerns about sodium intake and hypertension, this method is not used as much as it was in the past, but some pork products still rely on salting. A good example is Parma ham from Italy, which is dry-salted with sea salt for about a month.[16]

Foods preserved with sugar retain much of their shape, color, and texture because some of the sugar is absorbed into the cells, replacing the water drawn out. Nevertheless, molds tend to flourish in sweet, acidic environments such as jams. Sugar also adds calories and can contribute to dental caries (cavities).

Drying

A worker salting a Parma ham.

Drying is an ancient method of preserving food, used by many cultures in a variety of climates. There is evidence that the Egyptians dried fish and poultry in the hot desert sun as early as 12,000 BC.[16] Beans, peas, and fruits are also commonly preserved by drying.

By removing water, drying makes a food inhospitable to many microorganisms and slows its chemical deterioration. However, depending on the method used, the food's color, texture, and flavor may change, and the vitamin content can be decreased.

A modern technique for drying food is called *freeze-drying*. The food is first flash-frozen: any water is rapidly converted to fine ice crystals, which are evaporated in a vacuum. The product is then immediately packaged and sealed to ensure no penetration of moisture occurs. Freeze-drying preserves flavor, color, and texture and allows a shelf life of several years as long as the seal is not broken. Food manufacturers use freeze-drying for products such as coffee, tea, dried milk, gravy, and soup powders.

Smoking

Smoking has been used for centuries for preservation of meats, poultry, and fish. If food was not drying well, it would be hung near the campfire or chimney so the smoke of the fire would permeate the food, further drying it.

Unfortunately, smoking does not guarantee that a food is safe to eat. Reports of bacterial and helminth contamination in smoked fish, for example, are common.

Cooling

As mentioned earlier, in a cool environment bacteria's metabolism is slowed, and it becomes less able to multiply or produce toxins. So what did people use to cool and store foods before they had electric refrigerators?

For thousands of years, people have stored foods in underground cellars, caves, running streams, and even "cold pantries," north-facing rooms of the house that were kept dark and unheated and often were stocked with ice. The forerunner of our refrigerator, the miniature icehouse, was developed in the early 1800s, and in cities and towns, the local iceman would make rounds delivering ice to homes.

Before the modern refrigerator, an "iceman" would deliver ice to homes and businesses.

> RECAP: *Natural food preservation techniques include salting, sugaring, drying, and smoking, all of which draw water out of foods, making them inhospitable to microbes. Storage in ice houses, cold pantries, cellars, running streams, and other cold areas has been used for centuries to preserve food.*

Synthetic Preservative Techniques Improve Food Safety

To be successful, food producers have had to find ways to preserve the integrity of their products during the days, weeks, or months between harvesting and consumption. Until the latter part of the 20th century, industrial techniques for food preservation were limited to drying, canning, pasteurization, and the addition of certain preservative chemicals. However, in the last few decades, the modern techniques of aseptic packaging, irradiation, and genetic modification have greatly expanded our food choices.

Industrial Canning

The French inventor Nicolas-François Appert first developed the canning process in the late 1700s, and modern techniques have contributed to the retention of flavor, texture, and nutrients in canned foods. In the United States, 20 million canned foods are consumed per day.[16]

Producers of canned foods are required by law to ensure that all endospores of *Clostridium botulinum* be eliminated from their goods. As you recall, if the spores of this bacteria were to germinate inside a can of food, the food would soon become saturated with the deadly botulism toxin. The same process that destroys *C. botulinum* endospores also kills other microorganisms that could contaminate the food. This process involves several steps:

1. The food to be canned is sorted, and any spoiled food is removed.

2. The food is washed.

Canning food involves several steps to ensure all microorganisms in the food are killed.

Louis Pasteur.

FIGURE 18.9 Aseptic packaging allows foods to be stored unrefrigerated for several months without spoilage.

pasteurization A form of sterilization using high temperatures for short periods of time.

aseptic packaging Sterile packaging that does not require refrigeration or preservatives while the seal is maintained.

food preservatives Chemicals that help prevent microbial spoilage and enzymatic deterioration.

3. The food is parboiled or scalded to stop enzymatic processes and kill microorganisms on the food's surface.

4. Cans are filled and heated, air is siphoned out, and they are sealed.

5. The sealed cans are heated to a very high temperature by steam under pressure and then cooled in a water bath.

Canned food has an average shelf life of at least 2 years from the date of purchase. The U.S. Army has found canned meats, vegetables, and jam in "excellent states of preservation" after 46 years. Nevertheless, long storage of canned foods is not recommended. For high quality (versus safety), the broadest guideline given by the USDA is to use high-acid canned foods (fruits, tomatoes, and pickled products) within 18 to 24 months and low-acid foods (meats and vegetables) within 2 to 5 years.

Pasteurization

Pasteurization was developed in 1864 by Louis Pasteur to destroy microorganisms that spoiled wine. Its quick use of heat to eliminate pathogens without altering the taste or quality of the food product makes it a particularly useful and important process in the dairy and juice industry. Heating to 162°F (72°C) for 15 seconds pasteurizes milk, while ice cream, which is higher in fat, requires pasteurization at 180°F (82°C) for 20 seconds. Pasteurization does not eliminate all microbes but significantly decreases the numbers of heat-sensitive microorganisms, which tend to be the most harmful.

Aseptic Packaging

Many different packaging techniques have arisen over the past several decades. The newest and most environmentally sound one is **aseptic packaging,** which is probably most easily recognized as "juice boxes" (FIGURE 18.9). Food and beverages that are packaged in aseptic containers are first sterilized in a flash-heating and cooling process, then placed in the sterile container. Nutrient quality, as well as overall food quality, remains high as long as the package seals are not broken. The process uses less energy than traditional canning and less packaging material than any comparable container.[17] Aseptic cartons also require less energy to manufacture, fill, ship, and store, and by eliminating the need for refrigeration, they reduce consumer energy use.[17]

Addition of Preservatives

Food preservatives are substances added to a variety of foods to prevent or slow food spoilage. There are many natural and synthetically derived preservatives used in our food supply. One of the most commonly used natural preservatives is vitamin C. This powerful antioxidant helps protect foods from damage due to oxygen exposure. EDTA (ethylenediaminetetraacetic acid) is a commonly used synthetic preservative. It is used to trap trace amounts of metal impurities that can get into foods from containers and processing machinery.

Most processed foods contain preservatives, unless the package touts that it is "preservative free." All preservatives must be listed in the ingredients, but a person must know their chemical names to recognize them. Table 18.4 on page 682 identifies some common preservatives and the types of foods in which they are typically found. A few of these are discussed in more detail here.

BHT/BHA.   BHT **(butylated hydroxytoluene)** and BHA **(butylated hydroxyanisole)** are antioxidants that keep oils and fats in packaged foods from going rancid.

Propyl gallate, another antioxidant, works synergistically with both BHA and BHT to enhance their effectiveness.

Propionic Acid.   The bread you bought, left on the counter, and finally got around to eating a week later would have become moldy if it hadn't been treated with mold inhibitors such as propionic acid, calcium propionate, or sodium propionate. *Propionic acid* occurs naturally in apples, strawberries, and tea and is used to prevent mold growth in baked goods and processed cheese. *Sodium propionate* and *calcium* *propionate* are salts synthesized from propionic acid and are used as mold inhibitors in a variety of foods.

Sulfites.   **Sulfites** such as sodium bisulfite and sulfur dioxide are effective preservatives, antioxidants, bleaching agents, and antibrowning agents. Sulfites also have antibacterial and antifungal properties. They are widely used in the beer and wine industry as well as in dehydrated foods, maraschino cherries, and processed potatoes. Sulfites are not used in enriched grain products because of their capacity to bind with thiamin (vitamin B$_1$), making it unavailable for absorption.

Sulfur dioxide is used to control mold growth on fresh fruits and vegetables. For example, it has become standard commercial practice to fumigate stored grapes every 10 days with this chemical. Because of such procedures, it's important to remember to wash all fresh fruit and vegetables before eating.

The FDA has banned the use of sulfites as a preservative in salad bars because some people have had adverse asthmatic reactions. All foods that contain added sulfites must be labeled to warn those with sensitivities.

Nitrates and Nitrites.   **Nitrates** and **nitrites** have been used in the processed meat industry for many years as antibacterial agents and color enhancers. They give ham, hot dogs, and bologna their familiar pink color. They also inhibit microbial growth and rancidity. However, nitrites can easily be converted to *nitrosamines* during the cooking process. Nitrosamines have been found to be carcinogenic in animals, so the FDA has required all foods with nitrites to contain additional antioxidants to decrease the formation of nitrosamines.

Irradiation

Irradiation eliminates harmful food-borne bacteria in meats and poultry, and inhibits spoilage by fungus. In the United States, the process typically involves exposing food and its packaging to the energy of gamma rays from radioactive metals. Most of this energy simply passes through the food, leaving no residue. While the food remains relatively unchanged, bacteria and fungi are killed or left unable to reproduce.

Irradiation has been approved for use by fifty countries and endorsed by the World Health Organization (WHO) and the International Atomic Energy Agency (IAEA). In the United States, many foods are preserved using irradiation; among them are spices, grains, fruits, pork products, beef, and poultry. The National Aeronautics and Space Administration (NASA) uses irradiated foods for space flights.[18] Although irradiation rids foods of most pathogenic microbes, frozen foods remain frozen and raw foods stay raw through the process. While many foods can be safely irradiated without any noticeable changes, a recent consumer report on irradiated meat did note that the flavor of both beef and chicken had a subtle off-taste and smell, but one that many consumers might not notice.[19] Only a few nutrients, including vitamins A, E, and K and thiamin, seem to be affected by irradiation. Losses of these nutrients are comparable to what would be lost in conventional processing and preparation.

Although irradiated food has been shown to be safe to consume, the FDA requires that all irradiated foods be labeled with a "radura" symbol. The words "treated by irradiation, do not irradiate again" or "treated with radiation, do not irradiate again" must accompany the symbol (FIGURE 18.10). Irradiated food can be contaminated by improper handling and preparation, so consumers still need to store, clean, prepare, and cook them appropriately.

Genetic Modification

In **genetic modification,** also referred to as *genetic engineering,* the genetic material, or DNA, of an organism is altered to bring about specific changes in its seeds or offspring. Selective breeding is one example of genetic modification; for example, Brahman cattle that have poor-quality meat but high resistance to heat and humidity are bred with English shorthorn cattle that have good meat but low resistance to heat and humidity. The outcome of this selective breeding process is Santa Gertrudis

FIGURE 18.10   Radura—the international symbol of irradiated food—is required by the Food and Drug Administration to be displayed on all irradiated food sold in the United States.

BHT (butylated hydroxytoluene) An antioxidant used primarily to stop rancidity in fats and oils.

BHA (butylated hydroxyanisole) An antioxidant used primarily to stop rancidity in fats and oils.

sulfites Agents that are effective as preservatives and antioxidants and prevent browning. Sulfites also have antibacterial properties, are used to bleach flour, and inhibit mold growth in grapes, wine, and other foods.

nitrates Chemicals used in meat curing to develop and stabilize the pink color associated with cured meat; also function as antibacterial agents.

nitrites Chemicals used in meat curing to develop and stabilize the pink color associated with cured meat; also function as antibacterial agents.

irradiation A sterilization process utilizing gamma rays or other forms of radiation, but that does not impart any radiation to the food being treated.

genetic modification Changing an organism by manipulating its genetic material.

cattle, which have the desired characteristics of higher-quality meat and resistance to heat and humidity. Although selective breeding is effective and has helped increase crop yields and improve the quality and quantity of our food supply, it is a relatively slow and imprecise process, as a great deal of trial and error typically occurs before the desired characteristics are achieved.

Recently, technical advances have moved genetic modification beyond selective breeding. These advances include the manipulation of the DNA of living cells of one organism to produce the desired characteristics of a different organism. Called **recombinant DNA technology,** the process commonly begins when scientists isolate from an animal, plant, or microbial cell a particular segment of DNA that codes for a protein conferring a desirable trait, such as salt tolerance. Scientists extract and copy the DNA segment, then splice copies into cells of organisms normally lacking that trait, such as traditional tomato plants. The modified DNA causes the plant's cells to build the protein of interest, and the plant expresses the desired trait (FIGURE 18.11).

The term **genetically modified organism (GMO)** refers to an organism in which the DNA has been altered using recombinant DNA technology. A common use of this technology is to induce resistance to herbicides and pesticides. For example, genetically modified soybean, corn, and cotton crops can be sprayed with chemicals that kill weeds without harming the plants. Another use is to increase the nutritional value of a crop. For instance, researchers have modified soybeans and canola to increase their content of monounsaturated fatty acids. Scientists have also inserted a gene for salt tolerance into tomato and canola plants, enabling these GMOs to grow in soil so salty it would poison normal crops.[3] In addition, these crops remove salt from the soil, making it hospitable to unmodified plants. A **genetically modified food** is a food product derived from a GMO. The most common genetically modified foods currently on the market contain genetically modified soybeans and corn.

The relative benefits and harm of genetic modification have been debated worldwide. For instance, some environmentalists have raised the concern that seeds from genetically modified crops disrupt other crops through cross-pollination, even those many miles from where the altered ones are growing. Another concern is the long-term effect of genetically modified crops on the plants, insects, and animals that con-

recombinant DNA technology Type of genetic modification in which scientists combine DNA from different sources to produce a transgenic organism that expresses a desired trait.

genetically modified organism (GMO) An organism in which the genetic material, or DNA, has been altered using recombinant DNA technology.

genetically modified food A food product derived from a genetically modified organism.

DNA of host cell

Desired gene

1 Gene that expresses desired trait is extracted from cell.

2 Gene is combined with DNA of host cell that lacks this gene.

3 Host cell containing recombinant DNA is cultured, resulting in many copies of the gene.

4 Gene is extracted and inserted into DNA of cells of an organism that lacks this gene.

5 Genetically modified organism

5 Cells produce organism that expresses the desired trait.

FIGURE 18.11 Recombinant DNA technology involves producing plants and other organisms that contain modified DNA that enables them to express desirable traits that are not present in the original organism.

sume them or use them for their habitat. For more information about the debate surrounding genetic modification, see the Nutrition Debate at the end of this chapter.

> RECAP: *The canning process was developed in the late 18th century. Pasteurization has been in use for more than 100 years; this process destroys microbes using high heat for short durations on liquids such as milk and juice. Aseptic packaging is a relatively new form of packaging in which sterilized foods can be stored for long periods of time without refrigeration. Preservatives such as vitamin C, sulfites, and nitrates are often added to keep foods fresher longer. In the United States, irradiation typically involves the use of gamma rays to destroy the microbes in foods. The DNA of plants and animals can be genetically modified to enhance certain qualities of the food, such as its ability to resist pests.*

What Are Food Additives, and Are They Safe?

Have you ever picked up a loaf of bread and started reading its ingredients? You'd expect to see flour, yeast, water, and sugar, but what are all those other items? And why does it seem as if you need a degree in chemistry to understand what they are? They are collectively called **food additives,** and they are in almost every processed food. Food additives are not foods themselves, but are substances added to foods to enhance them in some way. For instance, food dyes make cheddar cheese orange, high-fructose corn syrup makes processed peanut butter taste sweet, and calcium increases the nutrient value of orange juice. Food preservatives, discussed earlier, are one category of food additives.

Although their use is regulated by the FDA, food additives have been a source of controversy for the past 50 years. Nevertheless, their use has steadily increased, allowing food producers to offer consumers a greater variety of foods at lower costs.

Additives Can Enhance a Food's Taste, Appearance, Safety, or Nutrition

It's estimated that more than 3,000 different additives are currently used in the United States. A few of these are identified in Table 18.4, and this section discusses some of the most common.

Additives Can Be Natural or Synthetic

Many of the additives used by the food industry come from natural sources. Beet juice, a natural food coloring, salt, and citric acid are common, naturally derived food additives, but in cases when supply or cost would prohibit using naturally derived additives, additives are synthesized. For instance, vanillin, the main flavoring substance in vanilla beans, is synthesized at a cost considerably lower than the cost of extracting it from the natural beans.

Flavorings

Flavoring agents can be obtained from natural or synthetic sources. Essential oils, extracts, and spices supply most of the naturally derived flavorings.

Flavor enhancers are also widely used. These additives have little or no flavor of their own but accentuate the natural flavor of foods. They are often added when very little of a natural ingredient is used.[20] The most common flavor enhancers used are maltol and MSG (monosodium glutamate). MSG is the sodium salt of glutamic acid, one of the nonessential amino acids, which also serves as a neurotransmitter. The glutamate portion of MSG can cross the blood–brain barrier and cause symptoms such as headaches, difficulty breathing, and heart palpitations in some people. A review of the research conducted in this area indicates that most individuals who report sensitivity to MSG do not show adverse reactions when they are fed MSG in controlled studies, particularly when MSG is given with food.[21]

food additives A substance or mixture of substances intentionally put into food to enhance its appearance, palatability, or quality.

flavoring agents Obtained from either natural or synthetic sources; allow manufacturers to maintain a consistent flavor from batch to batch.

TABLE 18.4 Examples of Common Food Additives

Food Additive	Foods Found In
Coloring Agents	
Beet extract	Beverages, candies, ice cream
Beta carotene	Beverages, sauces, soups, baked goods, candies, macaroni and cheese mixes
Caramel	Beverages, sauces, soups, baked goods
Tartrazine	Beverages, cakes and cookies, ice cream
Preservatives	
Alpha-tocopherol (vitamin E)	Vegetable oils
Ascorbic acid (vitamin C)	Breakfast cereals, cured meats, fruit drinks
BHA	Breakfast cereals, chewing gum, oils, potato chips
BHT	Breakfast cereals, chewing gum, oils, potato chips
Calcium propionate/ Sodium propionate	Bread, cakes, pies, rolls
EDTA	Beverages, canned shellfish, margarine, mayonnaise, processed fruits and vegetables, sandwich spreads
Propyl gallate	Mayonnaise, chewing gum, chicken soup base, vegetable oils, meat products, potato products, fruits, ice cream
Sodium benzoate	Carbonated beverages, fruit juice, pickles, preserves
Sodium chloride (salt)	Most processed foods
Sodium nitrate/Sodium nitrite	Bacon, corned beef, luncheon meats, smoked fish
Sorbic acid/Potassium sorbate	Cakes, cheese, dried fruits, jellies, syrups, wine
Sulfites (sodium bisulfite, sulfur dioxide)	Dried fruits, processed potatoes, wine
Texturizers, Emulsifiers, and Stabilizers	
Calcium chloride	Canned fruits and vegetables
Carageenan/Pectin	Ice cream, chocolate milk, soy milk, frostings, jams, jellies, cheese, salad dressings, sour cream, puddings, syrups
Cellulose gum/Guar gum/ Gum arabic/Locust gum/ Xanthan gum	Soups and sauces, gravies, sour cream, ricotta cheese, ice cream, syrups
Gelatin	Desserts, canned meats
Lecithin	Mayonnaise, ice cream
Humectants	
Glycerin	Chewing gum, marshmallows, shredded coconut
Propylene glycol	Chewing gum, gummy candies

Many foods, such as ice cream, contain colorings.

coaltar A food additive made from thick or semisolid tar derived from bituminous coal, the by-products of which have been found to cause cancer in animals.

Colorings

Food colorings, derived from both natural and synthetic sources, are used extensively in processed foods. In the past, many food colorings were made from **coaltar,** a thick or semisolid tar derived from bituminous coal. Derivatives of coaltar have been found to cause cancer in animals, and most have been banned by the FDA from use in foods. Natural colorings such as beet juice (which gives a red color), beta-carotene (which gives a yellow color), and caramel (which adds a brown color) are now used instead and do not need to be tested for safety. The coloring tartrazine (FD&C Yellow #5) causes an allergic reaction in some people, and its use must be indicated on the product packaging.

Vitamins and Other Nutrients

Vitamin E is usually added to fat-based products to keep them from going rancid, and vitamin C (or ascorbic acid) is commonly added as an antioxidant. Iodine is added to table salt to help decrease the incidence of goiter, a condition that causes the thyroid gland to enlarge. Calcium and vitamin D are added to beverages to promote bone health. Folate is added to many breads and ready-to-eat cereals to decrease the incidence of neural tube defects during fetal development.

Texturizers, Stabilizers, and Emulsifiers

Texturizers such as calcium chloride are added to foods to improve their texture. For instance, they are added to canned tomatoes and potatoes so they don't fall apart. **Stabilizers** are added to products to give them "body" and help them maintain a desired texture or color. **Thickening agents** are used to absorb water and keep the complex mixtures of oils, water, acids, and solids in foods balanced.[20] **Emulsifiers,** like thickening agents and stabilizers, help to keep fats evenly dispersed within foods.

Humectants and Desiccants

Moisture content is a critical component of food, and **humectants** and **desiccants** are added to maintain the correct moisture levels. Humectants keep foods like marshmallows, chewing gum, and shredded coconut soft and stretchy. Desiccants prevent moisture absorption from the air; for example, they are used to prevent table salt from forming clumps.

Bleaching Agents

Bleaching agents are used primarily in baked goods. Fresh ground flour is pale yellow, and when stored it slowly becomes white. Bleaching agents speed this whitening and decrease the possibility of spoilage or insect infestation.

Are Food Additives Considered Safe?

Federal legislation was passed in 1958 to regulate food additives. The Delaney Clause, also enacted in 1958, states that "No additive may be permitted in any amount if tests show that it produces cancer when fed to man or animals or by other appropriate tests." Before a new food additive can be marketed or used in food, the producer of the additive must submit data on its reasonable safety to the FDA. The FDA then makes a determination of the additive's safety based on these data.

During this same year, the U.S. Congress recognized that many substances added to foods would not require a formal safety review by the FDA prior to marketing and use, as their safety had already been established through long-term use or recognized by qualified experts through scientific studies. These substances are exempt from the more stringent testing criteria for new food additives, and are referred to as substances that are **Generally Recognized as Safe (GRAS).** The GRAS list identifies substances that either have been tested in the past and determined by the FDA to be safe and approved for use in the food industry, or are deemed safe as a result of consensus among experts qualified by scientific training and experience.

In 1985, the FDA established the Adverse Reaction Monitoring System (ARMS). Under this system, the FDA investigates complaints from consumers, physicians, or food companies. Many of the complaints are about sulfite preservatives causing headaches, asthmatic reactions, and in some cases anaphylactic shock. Because of these complaints and the investigations that followed, the FDA has banned the use of sulfites on many fruit and vegetables, while continuing to monitor sulfite use on other foods.

Mayonnaise contains emulsifiers to prevent separation of fats.

texturizers Chemicals used to improve the texture of various foods.

stabilizers Chemicals that help maintain smooth texture and uniform color and flavor in some foods.

thickening agents Natural or chemically modified carbohydrates that absorb some of the water present in food, making the food thicker while keeping food components balanced.

emulsifiers Chemicals that improve texture and smoothness in foods; stabilize oil–water mixtures.

humectants Chemicals that help retain moisture in foods, keeping them soft and pliable.

desiccants Chemicals that prevent foods from absorbing moisture from the air.

bleaching agents Chemicals used to speed the natural process of ground flour changing from pale yellow to white.

Generally Recognized as Safe (GRAS) list A list established by Congress that identifies several hundred substances that either have been tested and found to be safe and approved by the FDA for use in the food industry, or are deemed safe as a result of consensus among experts qualified by scientific training and experience.

> RECAP: *Food additives are chemicals intentionally added to foods to enhance their color, flavor, texture, nutrient density, moisture level, or shelf life. Although there is continuing controversy over food additives, they are considered safe based on testing and use in the food industry or as a result of consensus among experts qualified by scientific training and experience.*

Do Residues Harm Our Food Supply?

Food **residues** are chemicals that remain in foods despite cleaning and processing. Two residues of global concern are pollutants and pesticides.

Persistent Organic Pollutants Can Cause Illness

residues Chemicals that remain in the foods we eat despite cleaning and processing.

persistent organic pollutants (POPs) Chemicals released into the environment as a result of industry, agriculture, or improper waste disposal; automobile emissions also are considered POPs.

Many different organic chemicals are released into the atmosphere as a result of industry, agriculture, automobile emissions, and improper waste disposal. These chemicals, collectively referred to as **persistent organic pollutants (POPs),** eventually enter the food supply through the soil or water. If a pollutant gets into the soil, a plant can absorb the chemical into its structure and can pass it on as part of the food chain. Animals can also absorb the pollutants into their tissues or can consume them when feeding on plants growing in the polluted soil. Fat-soluble pollutants are especially problematic, as they tend to accumulate in the animal's body tissues and are then absorbed by humans when the animal is used as a food source (FIGURE 18.12).

POP residues have been found in virtually all categories of foods, including baked goods, fruits, vegetables, meat, poultry, and dairy products. The chemicals can travel long distances in trade winds and water currents, moving from tropical and

1 Industrial wastes are released into water.

2 Plant and animal plankton become contaminated.

3 Contaminated plankton are consumed by small fish.

4 Large fish such as tuna and swordfish regularly consume smaller, contaminated fish.

5 Consumer purchases contaminated fish at market and consumes pollutants in fish.

Plankton   Contaminant

FIGURE 18.12 Bioaccumulation of persistent organic pollutants in the food supply.

temperate regions to concentrate in the northern latitudes. It is believed that all living organisms on Earth carry a measurable level of POPs in their tissues.[22]

Mercury and Lead Are Nerve Toxins Found in the Environment

Mercury, a naturally occurring element, is found in soil, rocks, lakes, streams, and oceans. It is also released into the environment by pulp and paper processing and the burning of garbage and fossil fuels. As mercury is released into the environment, it falls from the air, eventually finding its way to streams, lakes, and the ocean, where it accumulates. Fish absorb mercury as they feed on aquatic organisms. This mercury is passed on to humans when they consume the fish. As mercury accumulates in the body, it has a toxic effect on the nervous system.

Large predatory fish, such as swordfish, shark, king mackerel, and tilefish tend to contain the highest levels of mercury.[23] Because mercury is especially toxic to the developing nervous system of fetuses and growing children, pregnant and breast-feeding women and young children are advised to avoid eating these types of fish. Canned tuna, salmon, cod, pollock, sole, shrimp, mussels and scallops do not contain high levels of mercury and are safe to consume; however, the FDA advises against eating any one type of fish more often than once a week.[23] Freshwater fish caught in local lakes and rivers have variable levels of mercury; thus, local and state governments routinely monitor mercury levels and post advisories when levels are too high. To learn more about the risks of mercury in seafood, visit the FDA's food safety Web site (see the Web links at the end of this chapter) or call their 24-hour information line (at 1-888-SAFEFOOD).

Lead, another naturally occurring element, can be found in the soil, water, and even the air. It also occurs as industrial waste from leaded gasoline, lead-based paints, and lead-soldered cans, now outlawed but decomposing in landfills. Some ceramic mugs and other dishes are fired with lead-based glaze. Thus, residues can build up in foods. Excessive lead exposure can cause learning and behavioral impediments in children and cardiovascular and kidney disease in adults. It is impossible to avoid lead residues completely, but because of lead's health implications, everyone should try to limit their exposure. To find out how to limit lead exposure, visit the Environmental Protection Agency's Web site (see the Web links at the end of this chapter).

Industrial Pollutants Also Create Residues

Polychlorinated biphenyls (PCBs) and **dioxins** are two industrial pollutants that enter the soil and can persist in the environment for years, easily accumulating in fatty tissues of animals. They have been found in food worldwide. Dioxins (by-products of waste incineration) and PCBs (from discarded transformers) enter the soil and can persist in the environment for years, easily accumulating in fatty tissues. In several studies done in Belgium, chicken, pork, and eggs were found to have concentrations of these chemicals in excess of international standards.[24] PCBs and dioxins, along with other POPs, have been linked to cancer, learning disorders, impaired immune function, and infertility.[22]

> RECAP: *Persistent organic pollutants (POPs) have been found in virtually all categories of foods. Mercury contaminates certain fish, and lead contaminates many foods. Both are toxic to the nervous system. Polychlorinated biphenyls (PCBs) and dioxins are two industrial pollutants that have been found in food worldwide.*

Pesticides Protect Against Crop Losses

Pesticides are a family of chemicals used in both the field and storage areas to help protects crops from weeds, insects, fungi, and other organisms, including birds and mammals. Rodents, for example, in addition to consuming food, also contaminate large quantities of food with their excreta. Pesticides also help reduce the potential of disease by decreasing the number of microorganisms on crops. They increase overall

One of the ways mercury is released into the environment is by pulp mills.

Antique porcelain is often coated with lead-based glaze.

polychlorinated biphenyls (PCBs) An industrial pollutant most commonly attributed to discarded transformers.

dioxins An industrial pollutant most commonly attributed to waste incineration.

pesticides Chemicals used either in the field or in storage to destroy plant, fungal, and animal pests.

Bt bacteria produces crystals, shown here, that are a widely used microbial biopesticide.

crop yield and crop diversity. The three most common types of pesticides used in food production are insecticides, herbicides, and fungicides. Insecticides are used to control insects that can infest crops; herbicides are used to control weeds and other unwanted plant growth; and fungicides are used to control plant-destroying fungal growth. It is estimated that 65% of all pesticides produced in the United States are herbicides.

Pesticides Can Be Natural or Synthetic

Many pesticides used today are **biopesticides,** species-specific chemicals or microorganisms that work to suppress a pest's population, not eliminate it. Biopesticides do not leave residues on crops—most degrade rapidly and are easily washed away with water. Synthetic pheromones are a type of chemical biopesticide. In nature, insects use pheromones, chemicals that act as signals, to attract mates. Synthetic pheromones are used to disrupt insect mating by attracting males into traps. Microbial biopesticides are derived from naturally occurring or genetically altered bacteria, viruses, or fungi. A widely used microbial biopesticide is *Bacillus thuringiensis,* or *Bt*. This is a common soil bacterium that is genetically altered to be toxic to several species of insects.

Aside from biopesticides, many natural products such as salt, boric acid, dried blood, crushed egg shells, and diatomaceous earth (soil made up of a type of algae called diatoms) are used as pesticides. Ladybugs are bred and sold commercially to reduce aphids, and marigolds, mint, sage, garlic, chives, onion, and other strong-smelling plants can be placed among crops to deter a variety of insect pests.

Many synthetic pesticides are made from petroleum-based products. Examples of commonly used synthetic pesticides include thiabendazole (a fungicide used on potatoes) and fungicides commonly used to prevent apple diseases (such as dithane, manzate, and polyram).

Synthetic Pesticides Are Potential Toxins

Years of studies show that synthetic pesticides can remain on food and pose a risk to human health. The liver is responsible for detoxifying chemicals that enter the body; however, if diseases such as cancer or AIDS or toxins such as alcohol already stress the liver, it may be unable to effectively remove pesticide residues. When pesticide residues are not effectively removed, they can build up and damage body tissues. The health effects depend on the type of pesticide. Some affect the nervous system, others the endocrine system, and still others may be carcinogens.[25] These effects depend on how toxic the pesticide is and how much of it is consumed.[26]

Children may be especially sensitive to pesticides for several reasons.[27] First, their internal organs are still developing and maturing. Second, they consume more food and water per unit of body weight than adults, possibly increasing their exposure. If a child's excretory system is not fully developed, the child may have a limited ability to remove pesticide residues. Also, pesticides may harm a developing fetus or child by blocking the absorption of important food nutrients necessary for normal healthy growth.[27] Because of the potential risks from pesticides to a developing child, pregnant and breastfeeding women should peel fruit and vegetable rinds to decrease their exposure to residues. This is also a sensible precaution when preparing fruits or vegetables for small children.

Government Regulations Control the Use of Pesticides

The Environmental Protection Agency is the government agency responsible for regulating the labeling, sale, distribution, use, and disposal of all pesticides in the United States. The EPA also sets a tolerance level, which is the maximum residue level of a pesticide permitted in or on food or feed grown in the United States or imported into the United States from other countries.[28] The EPA reviews every registered pesticide on a 15-year cycle.[28]

Before a pesticide can be accepted by the EPA for use, it must be determined that it performs its intended function with minimal impact to the environment. Once the EPA has certified a pesticide, states may set their own regulations for its use.

biopesticides Primarily insecticides, these chemicals use natural methods to reduce damage to crops.

Canadian regulation of pesticides closely resembles U.S. laws, with provinces and territories given free range to limit pesticide use.

The EPA provides these food-related tips to reduce exposure to pesticides:[29]

- Wash and scrub all fresh fruits and vegetables thoroughly under running water. Using running water instead of soaking fruits and vegetables is more effective in removing pesticides, as running water is more abrasive than soaking. It is important to understand that all pesticide residues cannot be removed by washing.

- Peel fruits and vegetables whenever possible, and discard the outer leaves of leafy vegetables such as cabbage and lettuce. Trim the excess fat from meat and remove the skin from poultry and fish because some pesticide residues collect in the fat.

- Eat a variety of foods from various sources, as this can reduce the risk of exposure to a single pesticide.

- Consume more organically grown foods.

> RECAP: *Pesticides are substances used to prevent or reduce food crop losses due to weeds, insects, fungi, and other organisms, including birds and mammals. Biopesticides may be chemical or microbial. Many synthetic pesticides are petroleum-based products. Pesticides are potential toxins; therefore, it is essential to wash all produce carefully. Pregnant and breastfeeding women and young children should eat produce without the peel. The Environmental Protection Agency (EPA) regulates the labeling, sale, distribution, use, and disposal of all pesticides in the United States.*

NUTRI-CASE GUSTAVO

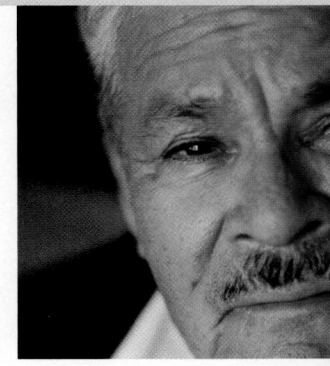

" My wife used to make her own corn tortillas from scratch. They were so good! But since she had her fall, she's been using more store-bought foods. Last night we ate tortillas made in New Jersey! Just like I thought, they tasted funny, so I checked the package to see what was in them besides corn. Well, I couldn't read it! I asked my daughter what all the words meant, and even she didn't know. There were three different kinds of acid, but why should tortillas need acid? Then there were cellulose gum and guar gum, whatever those are, and dextrose, and something called amylase. I can't wait for my wife to start home-cooking again, before all those chemicals make us sick."

What do you think of Gustavo's suspicion that the strange chemicals in the foods he eats will make him and his family sick? Dextrose is a sweetener, and amylase is used in baking to break down starches. But what do you think the "three different kinds of acid" might be? Explain why the food manufacturer might have included cellulose gum and guar gum in its brand of packaged tortillas. (Hint: See Table 18.4.)

Growth Hormones Are Injected into Cows to Increase Production of Meat and Milk

Introduced into the United States food supply in 1994, **recombinant bovine growth hormone (rBGH),** also known as *recombinant bovine somatotropin (rBST),* is a genetically engineered growth hormone. It is used in beef herds to induce animals to grow

recombinant bovine growth hormone (rBGH) A genetically engineered hormone injected into dairy cows to enhance their milk output.

more muscle tissue and less fat. It is also injected into a third of U.S. dairy cows to increase milk output. Currently, there are no labeling requirements for products containing rBGH.

Although the FDA has allowed the use of rBGH in the United States, both Canada and the European Union have banned its use because of studies showing an increased risk of mastitis (inflamed udders), infertility, and lameness in dairy cows injected with rBGH.[30] In addition, the milk of cows receiving this hormone has higher levels of insulin-like growth factor (IGF-1). This protein can pass into the bloodstream of humans who drink milk from cows who receive rBGH, and some studies have shown that an elevated level of IGF-1 in humans may increase the risk of breast and prostate cancers.[31,32] However, there are no studies directly linking increased risk of these cancers with eating products from animals injected with rBGH.

As just noted, dairy cows subject to this chemical have an increased tendency to develop mastitis, which is treated via administration of antibiotics. These antibiotics enter the cow's milk, and many researchers are concerned that consumption of antibiotic residues in milk may foster the development of antibiotic-resistant strains of bacteria.

Advocates of rBGH say that its use allows farmers to use less feed for the same yield, reducing resource use by each ranch or farm. In addition, they argue that approximately 90% of the hormone in milk is destroyed during pasteurization and that the remaining percentage is destroyed during digestion in the human gastrointestinal tract.

> RECAP: *Recombinant bovine growth hormone (rBGH) is a genetically engineered growth hormone injected into meat and dairy cows to increase meat production and milk output. Concerns about rBGH include possible immune system impairment, increased risk of prostate and breast cancers, and increased administration of antibiotics to dairy cows receiving the hormone.*

Are Organic Foods More Healthful?

The term *organic* is commonly used to describe foods that are grown without the use of synthetic pesticides. Recent national surveys indicate that approximately 27% of U.S. consumers use organic foods on a daily or weekly basis, and it is predicted that by 2025, 14% of the average household budget in the United States will be spent on organic products.[33,34]

To Be Labeled Organic, Foods Must Meet Federal Standards

The National Organic Program (NOP) of the USDA came into law in October of 2002. It established uniform definitions for all organic products. Any label or product claiming to be organic must comply with the following definitions:

- *100% organic:* Products containing only organically produced ingredients, excluding water and salt.

- *Organic:* Products containing 95% organically produced ingredients by weight, excluding water and salt; with the remaining ingredients consisting of those products not commercially available in organic form.

- *Made with organic ingredients:* A product containing more than 70% organic ingredients.

If a processed product contains less than 70% organically produced ingredients, then those products cannot use the term *organic* in the principal display panel, but ingredients that are organically produced can be specified on the ingredients statement on the information panel.

Products that are "100% organic" and "organic" may display the USDA seal (FIGURE 18.13) or mark of certifying agents. Any product that is labeled as organic must identify each organically produced item in the ingredient statement of the label. The name and address of the certifying agency must also be on the label.

FIGURE 18.13 The USDA organic seal identifies foods that are at least 95% organic.

The USDA Regulates Organic Farming

The USDA regulates organic farming standards, and farms must be certified as organic by a government-approved certifier who inspects the farm and verifies that the farmer is following all USDA organic standards. Companies that handle or process organic food before it arrives at your local supermarket or restaurant must also be certified.[35] Organic farming methods are strict and require farmers to find natural alternatives to many common problems, such as weeds and insects. Contrary to common belief, organic farmers can use pesticides as a final option for pest control when all other methods have failed or are known to be ineffective, but they are restricted to a limited number that have been approved for use based on their origin, environmental impact, and potential to persist as residues.[36] Organic farmers emphasize the use of renewable resources and the conservation of soil and water. Once a crop is harvested, a winter crop (usually of a legume origin) is planted to help fix nitrogen in the soil and decrease erosion, which also lessens the need for fertilizers.

Organic meat, poultry, eggs, and dairy products come from animals fed only organic feed, and if the animals become ill, they are removed from the others until well again. None of these animals are given growth hormones to increase their size or ability to produce milk. Irradiation is also prohibited in organic production.

Studies Comparing Organic and Conventionally Grown Foods Are Limited

Recent studies at the University of California, Davis and other institutions indicate that some organically grown foods are higher in vitamins E and C and in certain antioxidant phytochemicals than their non-organic counterparts.[37–39] Although these studies appear promising, they do not prove that organic foods are more nutritious than non-organic foods. To date there are very few studies that have assessed the nutritional content of organically grown foods and compared them to the same foods grown non-organically. Thus, no consensus can be reached as to whether organic foods are more healthful than conventionally grown foods.

> RECAP: *Organic standards enacted in 2002 established uniform definitions for all organic products sold in the United States. The USDA regulates organic farming standards and inspects and certifies farms that follow all USDA organic standards. Although a few recent studies indicate that some organic foods have higher levels of some nutrients than non-organic foods, there is insufficient evidence to support the claim that organic foods are more nutritious than non-organic foods.*

CHAPTER SUMMARY

- Approximately 76 million Americans report experiencing food-borne illness each year.
- Food infections result from the consumption of food containing living microorganisms, such as bacteria, whereas food intoxications result from consuming food in which microbes have secreted toxins.
- Food infections can be caused by bacteria, viruses, fungi, helminths, and prions.
- The body has several defense mechanisms, such as saliva, stomach acid, vomiting, diarrhea, and the inflammatory response, which help rid us of offending microorganisms and toxins.
- In order to reproduce in foods, microbes require a precise range of temperature, humidity, acidity, and oxygen content.

- You can prevent food-borne illness at home by following these tips: Wash your hands and kitchen surfaces often. Separate foods to prevent cross contamination. Cook foods to their proper temperatures. Store foods in the refrigerator or freezer. Thaw frozen foods in the refrigerator, and heat them long enough and at the required temperature to ensure proper cooking.

- When traveling, avoid all raw foods unless thoroughly washed in bottled or boiled water, and choose beverages that are boiled, bottled, or canned, without ice.

- Food spoilage affects a food's appearance, texture, taste, smell, and safety. Both fresh and processed foods are vulnerable to spoilage.

- Some natural techniques for food preservation include salting, sugaring, drying, smoking, and cooling.

- Synthetic food preservation techniques include canning, pasteurization, aseptic packaging, addition of preservatives, irradiation, and genetic modification.

- Food additives are natural or synthetic ingredients added to foods during processing to enhance them in some way. They include flavorings, colorings, nutrients, and texturizers.

- The GRAS list identifies several hundred substances that either have been tested and found to be safe and approved for use in the food industry, or are deemed safe as a result of consensus among experts qualified by scientific training and experience.

- Persistent organic pollutants (POPs) are chemicals released into the atmosphere as a result of industry, agriculture, automobile emissions, and improper waste disposal. Plants, animals, and fish absorb the chemicals from contaminated soil or water and pass them on as part of the food chain.

- Large predatory fish, such as swordfish, shark, king mackerel, and tilefish, tend to contain high levels of mercury, which is especially toxic to the developing nervous system.

- Although pesticides prevent or reduce crop losses, they are potential toxins; thus, their use is regulated by the Environmental Protection Agency.

- All produce should be washed carefully before eating. Produce prepared for pregnant women, breastfeeding women, and young children should be peeled whenever possible.

- Recombinant bovine growth hormone (rBGH) is injected into beef and dairy cows to increase their yield. Although the hormone is largely destroyed by pasteurization of milk and by human digestion, concerns remain about residues.

- Cows injected with rBGH have a higher rate of antibiotic use: the residue from these antibiotics may be contributing to the increased development of antibiotic-resistant strains of microorganisms.

- Organic standards established in 2002 established uniform definitions for all organic products sold in the United States.

- The USDA regulates organic farming standards and inspects and certifies farms that follow all USDA organic standards.

- A few recent research studies indicate that some organic foods may have higher levels of some nutrients than non-organic foods, but there is insufficient evidence to claim that organic foods are generally more nutritious than non-organic foods.

TEST YOURSELF ANSWERS

1. **False.** The actual number is much larger: each year, about 76 million Americans are sickened and about 5,000 die as a direct result of eating food contaminated with germs or their toxins.

2. **False.** Freezing inhibits the ability of most microbes to reproduce, but when the food is thawed, reproduction can resume.

3. **False.** Bacteria cause the vast majority of cases of food-borne illness.

4. **False.** Some recent studies have found higher levels of some micronutrients and antioxidant phytochemicals in organic foods than in non-organic foods. However, there are not enough studies published on this topic to state with confidence that organic foods are consistently more nutritious than non-organic foods.

5. **True.** Before a new food additive can be used in food, the producer of the additive must demonstrate its safety to the FDA. The producer of the additive is required to submit data on its reasonable safety prior to the marketing or use of the additive, and the FDA makes a determination of the additive's safety based on these data. The Delaney Clause, enacted in 1958, states that "No additive may be permitted in any amount if tests show that it produces cancer when fed to man or animals or by other appropriate tests."

REVIEW QUESTIONS

1. The three factors most often responsible for spoilage of foods are
   a. oxygen, heat, and light.
   b. carbon dioxide, heat, and light.
   c. moisture, heat, and cold.
   d. oxygen, cold, and light.

2. Yeasts are
   a. a type of mold used to make bread rise.
   b. a type of bacteria that can cause food intoxication.
   c. a type of fungus used to ferment foods.
   d. a type of mold inhibitor used as a food preservative.

3. Monosodium glutamate (MSG) is

    a. a thickening agent used in baby foods.

    b. a flavor enhancer used in a variety of foods.

    c. a mold inhibitor used on grapes and other foods.

    d. an amino acid added as a nutrient to some foods.

4. Foods that are labeled *100% organic*

    a. contain only organically produced ingredients, excluding water and salt.

    b. may display the EPA's organic seal.

    c. were produced without the use of pesticides.

    d. contain no discernible level of toxic metals.

5. Leftovers from a meal should be refrigerated within

    a. 30 minutes of serving.

    b. 2 hours of serving.

    c. 4 hours of serving.

    d. 24 hours of serving.

6. True or false? Heating foods to at least 160°F guarantees that a food will not cause food-borne illness.

7. True or false? The *E. coli* microbe commonly implicated in food-borne illness is a type of helminth.

8. True or false? In the United States, farms certified as organic are allowed to use pesticides under certain conditions.

9. True or false? Recombinant bovine growth hormone (rBGH) is used to increase the amount and quality of meat in beef herds and milk production in dairy cows.

10. True or false? Some colorings used as food additives do not need to be tested for safety.

11. A box of macaroni and cheese has the words *Certified Organic* on the front and the following ingredients listed on the side: "Organic durum semolina pasta (organic durum semolina, water), organic cheddar cheese (organic cultured pasteurized milk, salt, enzymes), whey, salt." Is this food 100% organic? Why or why not? Does it contain any food additives? If so, identify them.

12. Steven and Dante go to a convenience store after a tennis match looking for something to quench their thirst. Steven chooses a national brand of orange juice, and Dante chooses a bottle of locally produced, organic, unpasteurized apple juice. Steven points out to Dante that his juice is not pasteurized, but he shrugs and

FIND THE QUACK

You visit your cousin Lori, who has three school-age children. You take out a pack of chewing gum and offer a piece to each of the kids. "No way!" Lori says. "You need to check with me before offering food to the kids. Most foods sold in the United States are full of harmful additives! And that includes chewing gum!" Lori takes out a leaflet advertising a new book on food additives. It's called *Stealth Ingredients: The Dangerous Additives in Your Food*. You read the front of the leaflet. It states:

- Additives in your food destroy your health and may even cause cancer!

- Many of the most harmful ingredients in packaged foods are not listed on the label.

- Powerful food manufacturers' lobbies influence Congress to pass laws allowing food companies to add cancer-causing ingredients to your food.

- The Food and Drug Administration does not protect you against dangerous ingredients in your food.

The leaflet then offers a solution: a new book identifying and describing every ingredient added to foods. It suggests purchasing the book and taking it to the grocery

store so that you can check the ingredients panels of foods to make sure the foods you buy are safe.

The leaflet closes with three testimonials from individuals who state that, prior to reading the book, they were very ill, and now that they avoid all harmful food additives, their health has returned.

"See what I mean?" Lori asks you. "I bet you wish you knew what was *really* in that chewing gum!"

1. Evaluate the leaflet's statement that "Additives in your food destroy your health and may even cause cancer."

2. Comment on the statement that the FDA "does not protect you against dangerous ingredients in your food."

3. Look again at the leaflet's argument that "Many of the most harmful ingredients in packaged foods are not listed on the label." Identify the flaw in the argument that purchasing the book will protect you.

4. Discuss the value of the three testimonials at the end of the leaflet.

Answers can be found at www.aw-bc.com/thompson.

says, "I'm more afraid of the pesticides they used on the oranges in your juice than I am about microorganisms in mine!" Which juice would *you* choose, and why?

13. Pickling is a food-preservation technique that involves soaking foods such as cucumbers in a solution containing vinegar (acetic acid). Why would pickling be effective in preventing food spoilage?

14. In the 1950s and 1960s in Minamata, Japan, more than 100 cases of a similar illness were recorded: patients, many of whom were infants or young children, suffered irreversible damage to the nervous system. A total of 46 people died. Adults with the disease and mothers of afflicted young children had one thing in common: they had frequently eaten fish caught in Minamata Bay. What do you think might have been the cause of this disease? Using key words from this description, research the event on the Internet and identify the culprit(s).

15. Your sister Joy, who attends a culinary arts school, is visiting you for dinner. You want to impress her, so you've decided to make chicken marsala. You begin that afternoon by removing two chicken breasts from the freezer and putting them in a bowl in the refrigerator to thaw. Then you go shopping for fresh salad ingredients. When you get home from the market, you take the chicken breasts from the refrigerator and set them on a clean cutting board. You then take the lettuce, red pepper, and scallions you just bought, put them in a colander, and rinse them. Next, you slice them with a clean knife on your marble countertop and toss them together in a salad. You put the chicken breasts in a frying pan and cook them until they lose their pink color. In a separate pan, you prepare the sauce. Finally, using a clean knife, you slice some freshly baked bread on the countertop. You then wash the knives and the cutting board you used for the chicken. Joy arrives and admires your skill in cooking. Later that night, you both wake up vomiting. Identify *at least two* aspects of your food preparation that might have contributed to your illness.

WEB LINKS

www.cdc.gov/travel/contentSafeFoodWater.aspx
Centers for Disease Control and Prevention

Check out this Web page before your next trip for information on food safety when traveling.

www.foodsafety.gov
Foodsafety.gov

Use this Web site as a gateway to government food safety information; it contains news and safety alerts, an area to report illnesses and product complaints, information on food-borne pathogens, and much more.

www.fsis.usda.gov
The USDA Food Safety and Inspection Service

A comprehensive site providing information on all aspects of food safety. Click on Food Safety Education for links to information about food preparation, storage, handling, and other specific safety issues.

www.fsis.usda.gov/Fact_Sheets/Cooking_Safely_in_the_Microwave/index.asp
USDA Food Fact Sheet on Cooking Safely in the Microwave

This fact sheet provides information on safe cooking and reheating of foods using a microwave oven.

www.cspinet.org/foodsafety/index.html
Center for Science in the Public Interest: Food Safety

Visit this Web site for summaries of food additives and their safety, alerts and other information, and interactive quizzes.

www.consumerreports.org
Consumer Reports: Food

Click on Food at the top right or use the search index to find topics such as irradiated meat, produce washes, poultry safety, and mad cow disease.

www.cfsan.fda.gov
The USDA Center for Food Safety and Applied Nutrition

This site contains thorough information on topics such as national food safety programs, recent news, and food labeling. It also contains links to special program areas, such as regulation of mercury levels in fish, food colorings, and biotechnology.

www.extension.iastate.edu/foodsafety
Food Safety Project

The Food Safety Project compiles educational materials about food safety for consumer use. Provided on the site are links for food safety from farm to table.

www.gotmercury.org
Mercury Calculator

If you eat fish, visit this site to find out how much mercury you are consuming. Enter your weight, type of fish eaten, and amount per week, and the calculator does the rest.

www.epa.gov/pesticides
The U.S. Environmental Protection Agency: Pesticides

This site provides information about agricultural and home-use pesticides, pesticide health and safety issues, environmental effects, and government regulation.

www.epa.gov/lead/pubs/leadinfo.htm#protect
The U.S. Environmental Protection Agency: Lead

Visit this Web page to learn more about lead pollution and what you can do to prevent lead poisoning for yourself and your family.

www.ams.usda.gov/nop/indexIE.htm

The USDA National Organic Program (NOP)

This Web site describes the NOP's standards and labeling program, consumer information, and publications.

www.ota.com

The Organic Trade Association

Visit this industry site to learn about consumer use of organic foods, sales of organic foods, and recent research into conventional versus organic farming and their effects on foods and the environment.

REFERENCES

1. Food and Drug Administration (FDA). December 2006. Questions & Answers: Taco Bell *E. Coli* 0157:H7 Lettuce Outbreak. December 14, 2006. www.cfsan.fda.gov/~dms/tacobqa.html#cause. (Accessed August 2007.)
2. Centers for Disease Control and Prevention (CDC). 2005. Division of Bacterial and Mycotic Diseases. Disease Listing. Foodborne Illness. www.cdc.gov/ncidod/dbmd/diseaseinfo/foodborneinfections_g.html. (Accessed August 2007.)
3. Bauman, R. W. 2004. *Microbiology*. San Francisco: Pearson Benjamin Cummings.
4. Leavitt, J. W. 1996. *Typhoid Mary: Captive to the Public's Health*. Boston: Beacon Press.
5. Cunningham, A. (ed.). 2002. *Guinness World Records 2002*. Guinness World Records, Ltd. New York: Bantam.
6. Food and Drug Administration (FDA). 2005. Prions and Transmissible Spongiform Encephalopathies. www.cfsan.fda.gov/~mow/prion.html. (Accessed August 2007.)
7. Pavlista, A. D. 2001. Green potatoes: the problem and solution. NebGuide. The University of Nebraska-Lincoln Cooperative Extension. http://ianrpubs.unl.edu/horticulture/g1437.html. (Accessed August 2007.)
8. Food and Drug Administration (FDA). 2000. FDA Consumer. The unwelcome dinner guest: Preventing foodborne illness, Jan–Feb 1991. www.cfsan.fda.gov/~dms/qa-prp6.html (accessed August 2007).
9. National Digestive Diseases Information Clearinghouse (NDDIC). 2003. Bacteria and foodborne illness. NIH Publication No. 04-4730. http://digestive.niddk.nih.gov/ddiseases/pubs/bacteria/index.html. (Accessed August 2007.)
10. Food and Drug Administration (FDA). 2005. Eating defensively: Food safety advice for persons with AIDS. www.cfsan.fda.gov/~dms/aidseat.html.
11. Food Marketing Institute. 2003. A Consumer Guide to Food Quality and Safe Handling: Meat, Poultry, Seafood, Eggs. 2003 pamphlet, pp. 1–5.
12. U.S. Department of Agriculture (USDA). 2003. Safe Food Handling. Barbecue and Food Safety. www.fsis.usda.gov/Fact_Sheets/Barbecue_Food_Safety/index.asp. (Accessed August 2007.)
13. Food and Drug Administration (FDA). 2003. *Anisakis simplex* and Related Worms. Foodborne Pathogenic Microorganisms and Natural Toxins Handbook. www.cfsan.fda.gov/~mow/chap25.html. (Accessed August 2007.)
14. Center for Science in the Public Interest (CSPI). 2006. CSPI's "Eggspert" Egg Advice. www.cspinet.org/foodsafety/eggspert_advice.html. (Accessed August 2007.)
15. Centers for Disease Control and Prevention (CDC). 2005. Traveler's Health. Safe Food and Water. www.cdc.gov/travel/contentSafeFoodWater.aspx. (Accessed August 2007.)
16. Shephard, S. 2000. *Pickled, Potted and Canned: The Story of Food Preserving*. London: Headline Publishing.
17. Aseptic Packaging Council. 2005. The Award-Winning, Earth Smart Packaging for a Healthy Lifestyle. www.aseptic.org/main.shtml. (Accessed August 2007.)
18. Loaharanu, P. 2003. *Irradiated Foods*. New York: American Council on Science & Health Booklets.
19. Consumer Reports. 2003. The Truth about Irradiated Meat. www.consumerreports.org/cro/food/irradiated-meat-803/overview.htm. (Accessed August 2007.)
20. Center for Science in the Public Interest (CSPI). 2006. Food Additives. www.cspinet.org/reports/chemcuisine.html. (Accessed August 2007.)
21. Geha, R. S., A. Beiser, C. Ren, R. Patterson, P. A. Greenberger, L. C. Grammer, A. M. Ditto, K. E. Harris, M. A. Shaughnessy, P. R. Yarnold, J. Corren, and A. Saxon. 2000. Review of alleged reaction to monosodium glutamate and outcome of a multicenter double-blind placebo-controlled study. *J Nutr*. 130(suppl. 4):1058S–1062S.
22. Schafer, K. S., and S. E. Kegley. 2002. Persistent toxic chemicals in the US food supply. *J. Epidemiol. Community Health* 56:813–817.
23. Food and Drug Administration (FDA). 2004. What You Need to Know About Mercury in Fish and Shellfish. www.cfsan.fda.gov/~dms/admehg3.html. (Accessed August 2007.)
24. Larenbeke, N. Van, A. Covaci, P. Schepens, and L. Hens. 2002. Food contamination with polychlorinated biphenyls and dioxins in Belgium. Effects of the body burden. *Epidemiol. Community Health* 56(11): 828–830.
25. Environmental Protection Agency (EPA). 2005. Pesticides: Health and Safety: Human Health Issues. www.epa.gov/pesticides/health/human.html. (Accessed August 2007.)
26. Environmental Protection Agency (EPA). 2005. Pesticides: Health and Safety Pesticides and Food: Health Problems Pesticides May Pose. www.epa.gov/pesticides/food/risks.html.
27. Environmental Protection Agency (EPA). 2005. Pesticides: Health and Safety Pesticides and Food: Why Children May Be Especially Sensitive to Pesticides. www.epa.gov/pesticides/food/pest.html. (Accessed August 2007.)
28. Environmental Protection Agency (EPA). 2005. About Pesticides. www.epa.gov/pesticides/about/index.htm (accessed August 2007.)
29. Environmental Protection Agency (EPA). 2005. Pesticides and Food: Healthy, Sensible Food Practices. www.epa.gov/pesticides/food/tips.html. (Accessed August 2007.)
30. LeSage, L. 1999. News Release, January 14. Health Canada rejects bovine growth hormone in Canada. Health Canada Online. www.hc-sc.gc.ca/ahc-asc/media/nr-cp/1999/1999_03_e.html. (Accessed August 2007.)
31. Hankinson, S. E., W. C. Willett, G. A. Colditz, D. J. Hunter, D. S. Michaud, B. Deroo, B. Rosner, F. E. Speizer, and M. Pollak. 1998. Circulating concentrations of insulin-like growth factor-I and risk of breast cancer. *Lancet* 351(9113): 1393–1396.
32. Chan, J. M., M. J. Stampfer, E. Giovannucci, P. H. Gann, J. Ma, P. Wilkinson, C. H. Hennekens, and M. Pollak. 1998. Plasma insulin-like growth factor-I and prostate cancer risk: a prospective study. *Science* 279(5350):563–566.
33. Organic Trade Association. 2004. OTA Survey: U.S. organic sales reach $10.8 billion. *What's News in Organic*. Issue 28, Summer. www.ota.com/pics/documents/WhatsNews28.pdf. (Accessed August 2007.)
34. Organic Trade Association. 2005. News Release. Trends: Organic Trade Association Envisions Organic Industry of the Future. www.ota.com/news/press/183.html. (Accessed August 2007.)
35. Aiyana, J. 2002. What consumers should know about the new USDA organic labeling standard. The pulse of oriental medicine. www.pulsemed.org/usdaorganic.html. (Accessed August 2007.)

36. Heaton, S. 2003. *Organic Farming, Food Quality and Human Health: A Review of the Evidence.* Soil Association. Bristol: Briston House.

37. Asami, D. K., Y. J. Hong, D. M. Barrett, and A. E. Mitchell. 2003. Comparison of the total phenolic and ascorbic acid content of freeze-dried and air-dried marionberry, strawberry, and corn grown using conventional, organic, and sustainable agricultural practices. *J. Agric. Food Chem.* 51(5):1237–1241.

38. Carbonaro, M., M. Mattera, S. Nicoli, P. Bergamo, and M. Cappelloni. 2002. Modulation of antioxidant compounds in organic vs conventional fruit (peach, *Prunus persica L.,* and pear, *Pyrus communis L.*). *J. Agric Food Chem.* 50(19):5458–5462.

39. Grinder-Pedersen, L., S. E. Rasmussen, S. Bügel, L. V. Jørgensen, L. O. Dragsted, Gundersen, and B. Sandström. 2003. Effect of diets based on foods from conventional versus organic production on intake and excretion of flavonoids and markers of antioxidative defense in humans. *Agric. Food Chem.* 51(19):5671–5676.

40. U.S. Department of Agriculture (USDA). 2005. Economic Research Service. Data. Adoption of Genetically Engineered Crops in the U.S. www.ers.usda.gov/Data/BiotechCrops/. (Accessed August 2007.)

41. McHughen, A. 2000. *Pandora's Picnic Basket: The Potential and Hazards of Genetically Modified Foods,* pp. 17–45. Oxford: Oxford University Press.

42. James, C. 2004. Preview: Global Status of Commercialized Biotech/GM Crops: 2004. *ISAAA Briefs* No. 32. ISAAA: Ithaca, NY.

NUTRITION DEBATE

Genetically Modified Organisms: A Blessing or a Curse?

Current advances in biotechnology have opened the door to one of the most controversial topics in food science, genetically modified organisms (GMOs). GMOs are organisms that are created through *genetic engineering*, the standard U.S. term for a process in which foreign genes are spliced into a nonrelated species, creating an entirely new *(transgenic)* organism. Biotech foods, gene foods, bioengineered food, gene-altered foods, and transgenic foods are other terms used to describe foods that have been created through genetic engineering.

Developing GMOs is a lengthy, tedious, and costly process requiring years of research and testing. After carefully selecting and cultivating cells from an organism with a desired trait, the DNA is removed and scientists identify, isolate, and extract individual genes that code for the desired functions. Using bacteria to transfer these genes, scientists incorporate them into new cells where the introduced genes trigger the synthesis of proteins that accomplish the chosen functions. By using bacteria as the selected medium, DNA can be easily and efficiently produced and incorporated into any cell. Any plant, animal, or microorganism (such as bacteria or yeast) that has had its DNA altered in a laboratory to enhance or change certain characteristics is considered genetically engineered. For example, *Bacillus thuringiensis* is a genetically engineered bacterium that is used as a pesticide.

Since 1994, hundreds of plants and animals have been genetically modified and incorporated into our current food market. In the United States, soy, corn, canola, and cotton crops make up the majority of the genetically modified crop acreage. The U.S. Department of Agriculture reports that 52% of all corn crops, 79% of all cotton crops, and 87% of all soybean crops grown in the United States are genetically engineered varieties.[40] In addition, several important medical therapeutics have been developed using this process, including human insulin, human growth factor, and factor VIII (a protein needed for blood clotting in people with hemophilia). Many scientists are working on *gene therapy,* that is, replacing defective genes in patients with genetic diseases such as sickle cell anemia with genes from people without the disease. Currently, research labs around the world are devoted to expanding the capabilities and applications of genetic engineering.

However, in genetic engineering, commercial success is not guaranteed. In 1994, the FlavrSavr tomato became

Genetically modified corn is widely cultivated in the United States.

the first commercially sold GMO. Developing this tomato involved identifying the gene that codes for an enzyme called polygalacturonase, which causes ripening in the tomato. This gene was removed and inserted back in reverse orientation. As a result, polygalacturonase was not synthesized, and ripening slowed dramatically—making the tomato appear "fresh" longer and enabling it to maintain a longer shelf life.[41] Unfortunately, consumers felt the FlavrSavr tomato had poor flavor, and it was taken off the market in 1997.

Many people envision an ever-expanding role for genetic engineering in food production. They base their support on the numerous potential benefits resulting from the application of this technology. These benefits include:

- Enhanced taste and nutritional quality of food
- Crops that grow faster, have higher yields, can be grown in inhospitable soils, and have increased resistance to pests, disease, herbicides, and spoilage
- Increased production of high-quality meat, eggs, and milk

Golden rice (on right) is genetically engineered variety of rice that synthesizes precursors of beta-carotene. It was originally developed as a fortified food to be consumed in geographic regions where vitamin A food sources are inadequate. Due to controversy surrounding its use, it is currently not available for human consumption.

- Improved animal health due to increased disease resistance and overall hardiness
- Environmentally responsible outcomes such as use of less harmful herbicides and insecticides; conservation of soil, water, and energy; and more efficient food processing
- Increased food security for countries struggling with food insecurity and starvation

Despite these benefits, there is significant opposition to genetic engineering due to concerns related to environmental hazards, human health risks, and economic concerns. The concerns and potential problems of genetic engineering include:

- Gene transfer to nontarget species through cross-pollination, which could result in undesirable plants such as a super weed that is tolerant to herbicides and thus requires newer and stronger chemicals to destroy it
- Loss of biodiversity of plants and animals
- Increased risk of allergens, by either creating a new allergen or causing an allergic reaction in susceptible individuals
- Development of new diseases that can attack plants, animals, and humans
- Production of bacteria that are resistant to all antibiotics
- Potential for only a few food companies and countries to control the majority of world food production
- Inadequate or nonexistent labeling laws that prevent consumers from knowing whether they are consuming foods that are genetically modified
- Creation of biological weapons and increased risk of bioterrorism

Some who oppose genetic engineering believe that it is unnatural and unethical to alter the genes of any organism. Most opponents base their concern on the fact that the potential long-term risks and dangers are unknown and may far outweigh the potential short-term benefits.

Genetically modified organisms are welcomed in some countries and outlawed in others. Six countries grow almost 100% of the world's genetically modified crops—the United States (59%), Argentina (20%), Canada (6%), Brazil (6%), China (5%), and Paraguay (2%).[42] Even though the United States and Canada are among the top global producers of genetically modified crops, there is a movement within these countries to ban the production of GMOs. Some counties in California, including Mendocino,

Many oppose the genetic engineering of foods for environmental, health, or economic reasons.

Trinity, and Marin, have banned the production of GMOs, and the Canadian province of Prince Edward Island has also proposed a ban on GMOs.

The European Union (EU) has strict regulations regarding GMOs, including having mechanisms in place for the tracking of GMO products through production and distribution chains and also monitoring any effect of GMOs on the environment. All foods produced for human consumption and all animal feed products that contain GMOs must be clearly labeled. In addition, any foods that are produced from GMO ingredients must be clearly labeled, even if the final food product does not contain DNA or protein of the original GMO. Currently only 18 GMOs and 15 genetically modified foods are marketed in the EU. Companies who wish to market GMOs and genetically modified foods in the EU must submit an application that includes a full environmental risk assessment for GMOs and a safety assessment of genetically modified foods. This report is then reviewed by the designated government agencies and a decision made regarding the application.

As GMOs and genetically modified foods have been available for only a few years, it will take more time to understand their impact on the world. Based on your current knowledge of GMOs and genetically modified foods, do you support their use and mass distribution both within the United States and around the world? Do you feel that genetically modified foods should be clearly labeled for consumers?

In the United States, companies are not required to list whether ingredients are genetically modified. This label from England indicates the genetically modified content of the food.

CHAPTER 19

CHAPTER OBJECTIVES

After reading this chapter you will be able to:

1. Explain why maintaining a nutritious diet is important for prospective parents even before conception, p. 700.

2. Explore the relationship between fetal development, changes in the mother, and increasing nutrient requirements during the course of a pregnancy, pp. 700–703.

3. Identify the range of optimal weight gain for a pregnant woman in the first, second, and third trimesters, pp. 703–706.

4. Describe the physiologic events that lead to lactation, pp. 717–718.

5. Compare and contrast the nutrient requirements of pregnant and lactating women, pp. 706–710 and 719–720.

6. Identify the primary advantages and most common challenges of breastfeeding, pp. 720–723.

7. Relate the growth and activity patterns of infants to their nutrient needs, pp. 724–730.

8. Discuss some common nutrition-related concerns for infants, pp. 730–731.

TEST YOURSELF TRUE OR FALSE?

1. A pregnant woman needs to consume twice as many calories as she did prior to the pregnancy. T or F

2. Despite popular belief, very few pregnant women actually experience morning sickness, food cravings, or food aversions. T or F

3. Breast-fed infants tend to have fewer infections and allergies than formula-fed infants. T or F

4. When a breastfeeding woman drinks caffeinated beverages such as coffee, the caffeine enters the breast milk. T or F

5. Most infants begin to require solid foods by about 3 months (12 weeks) of age. T or F

Test Yourself answers can be found after the Chapter Summary.

Nutrition Through the Life Cycle: Pregnancy and the First Year of Life

When she was a baby, Theresa showed poor coordination, was slow to walk and start talking, and was what her grandmother called "a real handful." Now an energetic 12-year-old, she still struggles every day to learn new information and keep up with her classmates physically and academically. Even though she tries hard, Theresa has a poor attention span and is often in trouble for misbehaving in class. Unfortunately, Theresa's physical, mental, and behavioral problems will persist for the rest of her life, and new ones may develop. That's because, shortly after birth, Theresa was diagnosed with fetal alcohol syndrome (FAS). During her pregnancy, Theresa's mother consumed beer and liquor several times a week, causing lifelong health problems for her daughter.

What role does prenatal diet play in determining the future health and well-being of the child? What is the link between alcohol and birth defects? Why is inadequate iron or folate intake especially dangerous to a pregnant woman and her fetus? What roles do protein, zinc, calcium, and other nutrients play in maternal and fetal health? In this chapter, we discuss how adequate nutrition supports fetal development, maintains the pregnant woman's health, and contributes to lactation. We then explore the nutrient needs of breast-feeding and formula-feeding infants.

Starting Out Right: Healthful Nutrition in Pregnancy

At no stage of life is nutrition more crucial than during fetal development and infancy. From conception through the end of the first year of life, adequate nutrition is essential for tissue formation, neurological development, and bone growth, modeling, and remodeling. The ability to reach peak physical and intellectual potential in adult life is in part determined by the nutrition received during the earliest years of development.

Is Nutrition Important Before Conception?

Several factors make adequate nutrition important even before **conception,** the point at which a woman's ovum (egg) is fertilized with a man's sperm. First, some deficiency-related problems develop extremely early in the pregnancy, typically before the mother even realizes she is pregnant. An adequate and varied preconception diet reduces the risk of such problems, providing "insurance" during those first few weeks of life. For example, failure of the spinal cord to close results in *neural tube defects*; these defects are closely related to inadequate levels of folate during the first few weeks following conception. For this reason, all women capable of becoming pregnant are encouraged to consume 400 µg of folic acid daily, whether or not they plan to become pregnant.

Second, adopting a healthful diet prior to conception includes the avoidance of alcohol, illegal drugs, and other known **teratogens** (substances that cause birth defects). Women should also consult their healthcare provider about their consumption of caffeine, medications, herbs, and supplements, and if they smoke, they should attempt to quit.

Third, a healthful diet and appropriate level of physical activity can help women achieve and maintain an optimal body weight prior to pregnancy. Women with a pre-pregnancy body mass index (BMI) between 19.8 and 26.0 kg/m^2 have the best chance of a successful pregnancy.[1] As we will discuss shortly, women with a BMI above or below this range are at greater risk for pregnancy-related complications.

Finally, maintaining a balanced and nourishing diet before conception reduces a woman's risk of developing a nutrition-related disorder during her pregnancy. These disorders, which we discuss later in the chapter, include gestational diabetes and hypertensive disorders. Although genetic and metabolic abnormalities are beyond the woman's control, following a healthful diet prior to conception is something a woman can do to help her fetus develop into a healthy baby.

The man's nutrition prior to pregnancy is important as well, since malnutrition contributes to abnormalities in sperm.[2] Both sperm number and motility (ability to move) are reduced by alcohol consumption, as well as by the use of certain prescription and illegal drugs. Finally, infections accompanied by a high fever can destroy sperm; so, to the extent that adequate nutrition keeps the immune system strong, it also promotes a man's fertility.

Why Is Nutrition Important During Pregnancy?

A balanced, nourishing diet is important throughout pregnancy to provide the nutrients needed to support fetal development without depriving the mother of nutrients she needs to maintain her own health. It also minimizes the risk of excess energy intake. A full-term pregnancy lasts 38 to 42 weeks and is divided into three **trimesters,** with each trimester lasting about 13 to 14 weeks.

The First Trimester

About once each month, a non-pregnant woman of childbearing age experiences **ovulation**, the release of an ovum (egg cell) from an ovary. The ovum is then drawn into the uterine tube. The first trimester of pregnancy begins when the ovum and sperm unite to form a single, fertilized cell called a **zygote.** As the zygote travels through

During conception, a sperm fertilizes an egg, creating a zygote.

conception (also called *fertilization*) The uniting of an ovum (egg) and sperm to create a fertilized egg, or zygote.

teratogen Any substance that can cause a birth defect.

trimester Any one of three stages of pregnancy, each lasting 13 to 14 weeks.

ovulation The release of an ovum (egg) from a woman's ovary.

zygote A fertilized egg (ovum) consisting of a single cell.

the uterine tube, it divides into a ball of 12 to 16 cells, which, at about day 4, arrives in the uterus (**FIGURE 19.1**). By day 10, the inner portion of the zygote, called the *blastocyst,* implants into the uterine lining. The outer portion becomes part of the placenta, which is discussed shortly.

Further cell growth, multiplication, and differentiation occur, resulting in the formation of an **embryo.** Over the next 6 weeks, embryonic tissues continue to differentiate and fold into a primitive tubelike structure with limb buds, organs, and facial features recognizable as human (**FIGURE 19.2**). It isn't surprising, then, that the embryo

embryo Human growth and developmental stage lasting from the third week to the end of the eighth week after fertilization.

FIGURE 19.1 Ovulation, conception, and implantation.

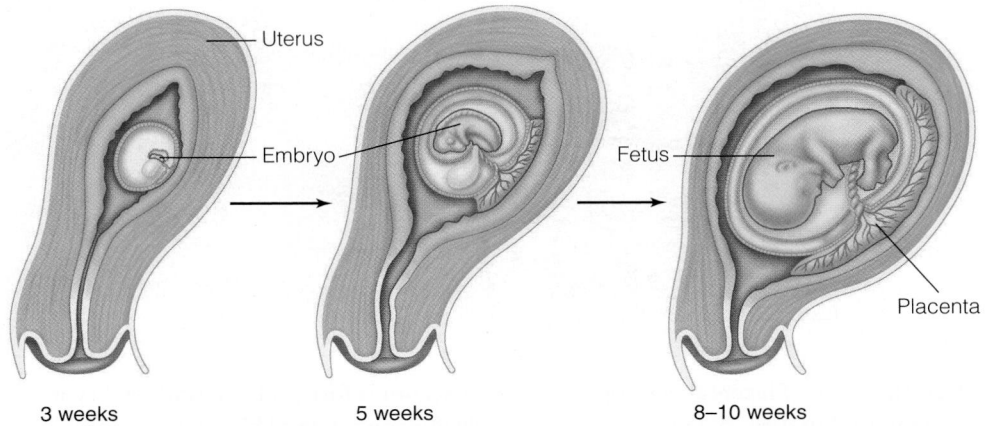

3 weeks   5 weeks   8–10 weeks

FIGURE 19.2 Human embryonic development during the first 10 weeks. Organ systems are most vulnerable to teratogens during this time, when cells are dividing and differentiating.

is most vulnerable to teratogens during this time. Not only alcohol and illegal drugs, but also prescription and over-the-counter medications, megadoses of supplements such as vitamin A, certain herbs, viruses, cigarette smoking, and radiation can interfere with embryonic development and cause birth defects.[2] In some cases, the damage is so severe that the pregnancy is naturally terminated in a **spontaneous abortion** (*miscarriage*), most of which occur in the first trimester.

During the first weeks of pregnancy, the embryo obtains its nutrients from cells lining the uterus. But by the fourth week, a primitive **placenta** has formed in the uterus from both embryonic and maternal tissue. Within a few more weeks, the placenta will be a fully functioning organ through which the mother will provide nutrients and remove fetal wastes (FIGURE 19.3).

By the end of the embryonic stage, about 8 weeks postconception, the embryo's tissues and organs have differentiated dramatically. A primitive skeleton, including fingers and toes, has formed. Muscles have begun to develop in the trunk and limbs, and some movement is possible. A primitive heart has begun to beat, and the digestive system is differentiating into distinct organs. The brain has differentiated, and the head has a mouth, eyespots with eyelids, and primitive ears.[2]

The third month of pregnancy marks the transition from embryo to **fetus.** To support its dramatic growth, the fetus requires abundant nutrients from the placenta. It is connected to the fetal circulatory system via the **umbilical cord,** an extension of fetal blood vessels emerging from the fetus's navel (called the *umbilicus*). Blood rich in oxygen and nutrients flows through the placenta and into the umbilical vein (see FIGURE 19.3). Wastes are excreted in blood returning from the fetus to the placenta via the umbilical arteries. Although many people think there is a mixing of blood from the fetus and the mother, the two blood supplies remain separate. Nutrients move from the maternal blood into the fetal blood and waste products are transferred out of the fetal blood into the maternal blood.

spontaneous abortion (also called *miscarriage*) Natural termination of a pregnancy and expulsion of pregnancy tissues because of a genetic, developmental, or physiologic abnormality that is so severe that the pregnancy cannot be maintained.

placenta A pregnancy-specific organ formed from both maternal and embryonic tissues. It is responsible for oxygen, nutrient, and waste exchange between mother and fetus.

fetus Human growth and developmental stage lasting from the beginning of the ninth week after conception to birth.

umbilical cord The cord containing arteries and veins that connect the baby (from the navel) to the mother via the placenta.

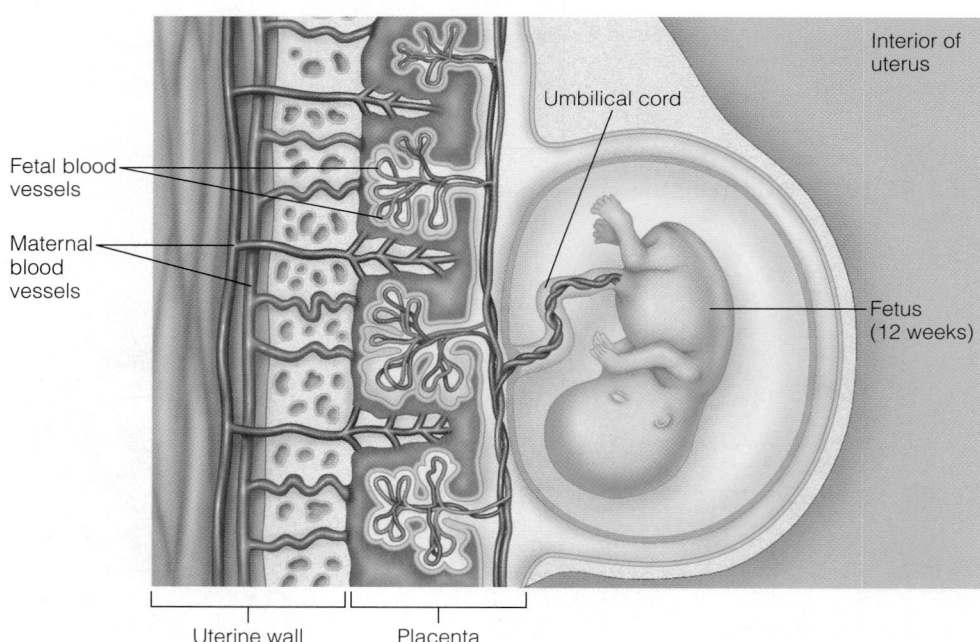

FIGURE 19.3 Placental development. The placenta is formed from both embryonic and maternal tissues. When the placenta is fully functional, fetal blood vessels and maternal blood vessels are intimately intertwined, allowing the exchange of nutrients and wastes between the two. The mother transfers nutrients and oxygen to the fetus, and the fetus transfers wastes to the mother for disposal.

The Second Trimester

During the second trimester (weeks 14 to 27 of pregnancy), the fetus continues to grow and mature. During this period, the fetus can suck its thumb, its ears begin to hear, and its eyes can open and close and react to light. At the beginning of the second trimester, the fetus is about 3 inches long and weighs about 1.5 pounds. By the end of this trimester, the fetus is generally over a foot long and weighs more than 2 pounds. Some babies born prematurely in the last weeks of the second trimester survive with intensive **neonatal** care.

The Third Trimester

During the third trimester (weeks 28 to birth), the fetus gains nearly half its body length and three-quarters of its body weight! At birth, an average baby will be approximately 18 to 22 inches long and about 7.5 pounds in weight (FIGURE 19.4). Brain growth (which continues to be rapid for the first 2 years of life) is also quite remarkable and the lungs become fully mature. The fetus acquires eyebrows, eyelashes, and hair on the head. Because of the intense growth and maturation of the fetus during the third trimester, it continues to be critical that the mother eat an adequate and balanced diet.

Impact of Nutrition on Maturity and Birth Weight

An adequate, nourishing diet is one of the most important variables under a woman's control for increasing the chances for birth of a mature newborn (at 38 to 42 weeks of **gestation**). Proper nutrition also increases the likelihood that the newborn's weight will be appropriate for his or her gestational age. Generally, a birth weight of at least 5.5 pounds is considered a marker of a successful pregnancy.

An undernourished mother is likely to give birth to a **low-birth-weight** baby.[3] Any infant weighing less than 5.5 pounds at birth is considered to be of low birth weight and is at increased risk of infection, learning disabilities, impaired physical development, and death in the first year of life (FIGURE 19.5). Many low-birth-weight babies are born **preterm,** that is, before 38 weeks gestation. Others are born at term but weigh less than would be expected for their gestational age; this is termed **small for gestational age**. While nutrition is not the only factor contributing to maturity and birth weight, its role cannot be overstated.

> RECAP: *A full-term pregnancy lasts from 38 to 42 weeks and is traditionally divided into trimesters lasting 13 to 14 weeks. During the first trimester, cells differentiate and divide rapidly to form the various tissues of the human body. The fetus is especially susceptible to nutrient deficiencies, toxicities, and teratogens during this time. The second and third trimesters are characterized by continued growth and maturation of organ systems and body structures. Nutrition is important before and throughout pregnancy to support fetal development without depleting the mother's reserves. An adequate, nourishing diet increases the chance that a baby will be born after 37 weeks and will weigh at least 5.5 pounds.*

How Much Weight Should a Pregnant Woman Gain?

Recommendations for weight gain vary according to a woman's weight *before* she became pregnant and whether she is expecting a single or multiple birth (Table 19.1). The average recommended weight gain for women of normal pre-pregnancy weight is 25 to 35 pounds; underweight women should gain a little more than this amount, and overweight and obese women should gain less. Adolescents, who may still be growing, should gain at the upper end of the ranges, and small women (5'2" or shorter) should aim for a total weight gain at the lower end of the ranges. Women who are expecting twins are advised to gain 35 to 45 pounds, and those with triplets should aim for a gain of 50 to 60 pounds, although recent evidence suggests that these guidelines should be adjusted based upon the mother's pre-pregnancy BMI.[4]

Women who have a low pre-pregnancy BMI (<19.8 kg/m^2) or gain too little weight increase their risk of having a preterm or low-birth-weight baby and of dangerously

neonatal Referring to a newborn.

gestation The period of intrauterine development from conception to birth.

low birth weight Having a weight of less than 5.5 pounds at birth.

preterm Birth of a baby prior to 38 weeks gestation.

small for gestational age (SGA) Term for infants whose birth weight for gestational age falls below the 10th percentile.

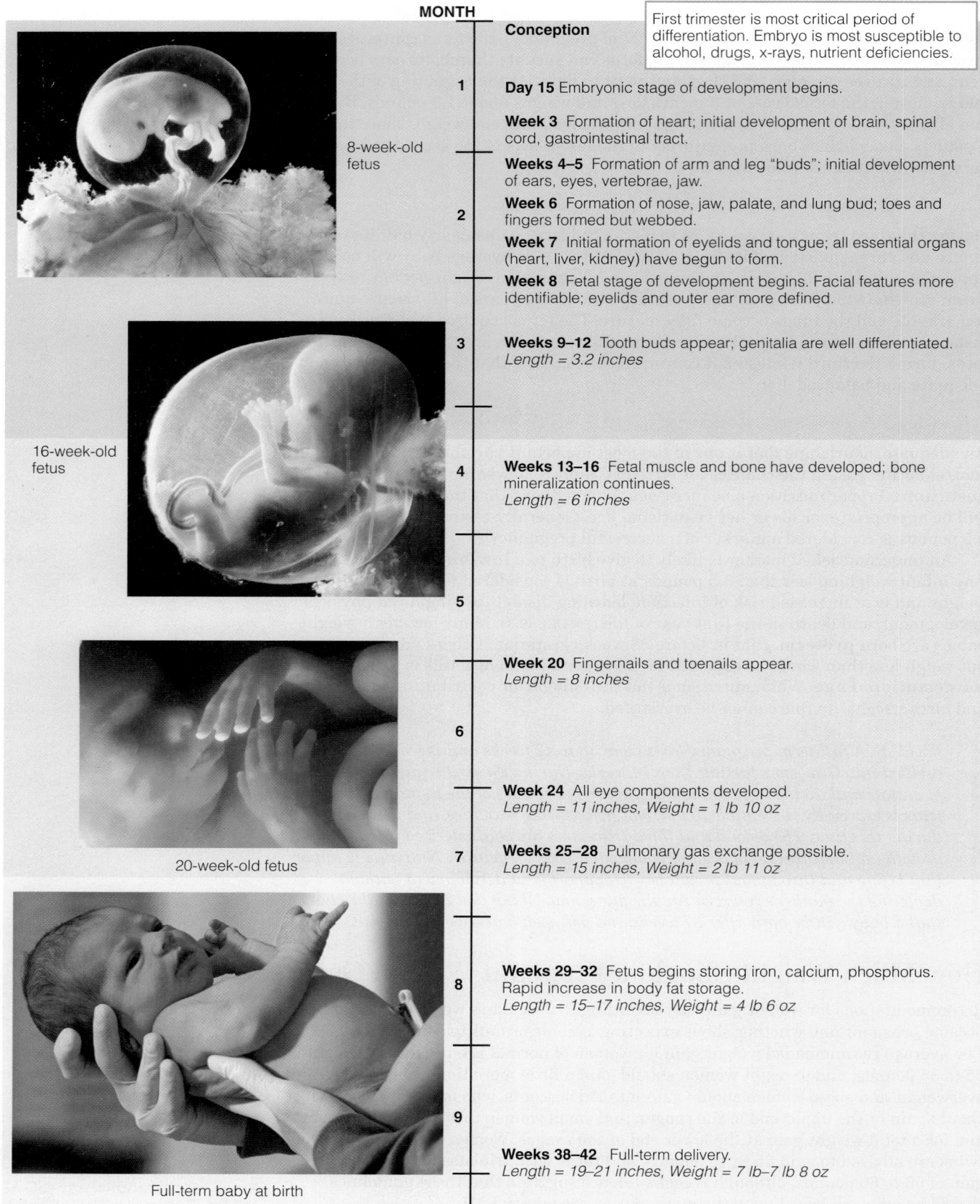

MONTH

Conception

First trimester is most critical period of differentiation. Embryo is most susceptible to alcohol, drugs, x-rays, nutrient deficiencies.

1

Day 15 Embryonic stage of development begins.

Week 3 Formation of heart; initial development of brain, spinal cord, gastrointestinal tract.

Weeks 4–5 Formation of arm and leg "buds"; initial development of ears, eyes, vertebrae, jaw.

8-week-old fetus

2

Week 6 Formation of nose, jaw, palate, and lung bud; toes and fingers formed but webbed.

Week 7 Initial formation of eyelids and tongue; all essential organs (heart, liver, kidney) have begun to form.

Week 8 Fetal stage of development begins. Facial features more identifiable; eyelids and outer ear more defined.

3

Weeks 9–12 Tooth buds appear; genitalia are well differentiated. *Length = 3.2 inches*

16-week-old fetus

4

Weeks 13–16 Fetal muscle and bone have developed; bone mineralization continues. *Length = 6 inches*

5

Week 20 Fingernails and toenails appear. *Length = 8 inches*

6

Week 24 All eye components developed. *Length = 11 inches, Weight = 1 lb 10 oz*

20-week-old fetus

7

Weeks 25–28 Pulmonary gas exchange possible. *Length = 15 inches, Weight = 2 lb 11 oz*

8

Weeks 29–32 Fetus begins storing iron, calcium, phosphorus. Rapid increase in body fat storage. *Length = 15–17 inches, Weight = 4 lb 6 oz*

9

Weeks 38–42 Full-term delivery. *Length = 19–21 inches, Weight = 7 lb–7 lb 8 oz*

Full-term baby at birth

FIGURE 19.4 A timeline of embryonic and fetal development.

FIGURE 19.5   A healthy 2-day-old infant (right) compared with two low-birth-weight infants.

TABLE 19.1   Recommended Weight Gain for Women During Pregnancy

Pre-Pregnancy Weight Status	Body Mass Index (kg/m^2)	Recommended Weight Gain (lb)
Normal	18.5–25.0	25–35
Underweight	<18.5	28–40
Overweight	25.1–29.9	15–25
Obese	≥30.0	No more than 15

depleting their own nutrient reserves. Gaining *too* much weight or being overweight (BMI >25 kg/m^2) or obese (BMI ≥30 kg/m^2) prior to conception is also risky. Excessive pre-pregnancy weight or prenatal weight gain increases the risk that the fetus will be large for gestational age, increasing the likelihood of trauma during vaginal delivery and of cesarean birth. Children born to overweight or obese mothers have higher rates of childhood obesity, and a high birth weight has been linked to increased risk of adolescent obesity.[5,6] In addition, the more weight a woman gains during pregnancy, the more difficult it will be for her to return to pre-pregnancy weight and the more likely it is that her weight gain will be permanent.

In addition to amount of weight, the *pattern* of weight gain is important. During the first trimester, a woman of normal weight should gain no more than 3 to 5 pounds. During the second and third trimester, about 1 pound a week is considered healthful. If weight gain is excessive in a single week, month, or trimester, the woman should not attempt to lose weight. Instead, the woman should merely attempt to slow the rate of weight gain. In short, weight gain throughout pregnancy should be slow and steady.

In a society obsessed with thinness, it is easy for pregnant women to worry about weight gain. Focusing on the quality of food consumed, rather than the quantity, can help women feel more in control. In addition, following a physician-approved exercise program helps women maintain a positive body image and prevent excessive weight gain.

A pregnant woman may also feel less anxious about her weight gain if she understands how that weight is distributed. Of the total weight gained in pregnancy, 10 to 12 pounds are accounted for by the fetus itself, the amniotic fluid, and the placenta

Following a physician-approved exercise program helps pregnant women maintain a positive body image and prevent excess weight gain.

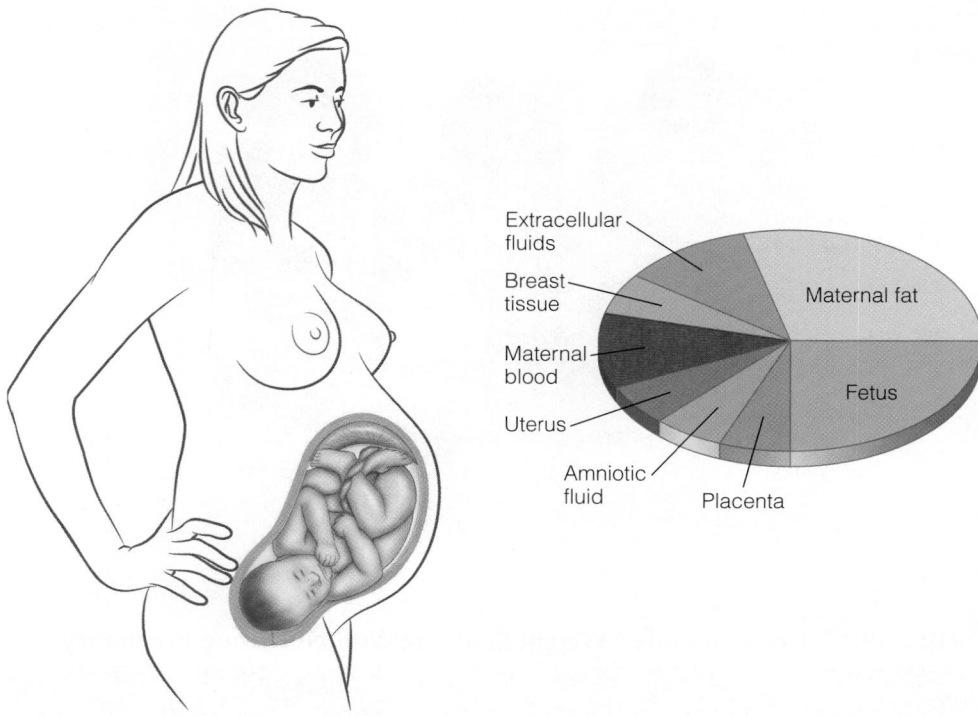

FIGURE 19.6 The weight gained during pregnancy is distributed between the mother's own tissues and the pregnancy-specific tissues.

(FIGURE 19.6). In addition, the woman's blood volume increases 40–50%, accounting for another 3 to 4 pounds. A woman can expect to be about 10 to 12 pounds lighter immediately after the birth and, within about 2 weeks, another 5 to 8 pounds lighter because of fluid loss. After that, losing the remainder of pregnancy weight depends on more energy being expended than is taken in. Although the production of breast milk requires significant energy, the effect of breastfeeding on postpartum weight loss varies.[7] We discuss breastfeeding on pages 716–723.

What Are a Pregnant Woman's Nutrient Needs?

The requirement for nearly all nutrients increases during pregnancy to accommodate the growth and development of the fetus without depriving the mother of the nutrients she needs to maintain her own health. With the exception of iron, most of these increased needs can be met by carefully selecting foods high in nutrient density.

Macronutrient Needs of Pregnant Women

During pregnancy, macronutrients provide necessary energy for building tissue. They are also the building blocks for the physical form and structure of the fetus, as well as for other pregnancy-associated tissues.

Energy.   Energy requirements increase only modestly during pregnancy. In fact, during the first trimester, a woman should consume approximately the same number of calories daily as during her non-pregnant days. Instead of eating more, she should attempt to maximize the nutrient density of what she eats. For example, drinking low-fat milk is preferable to drinking soft drinks. Low-fat milk provides valuable protein, vitamins, and minerals to feed the fetus's rapidly dividing cells, while soft drinks provide nutritionally empty calories.

During the last two trimesters of pregnancy, caloric needs increase by about 350 to 450 kcal/day. For a woman consuming 2,000 kcal/day, an extra 400 kcal represents only a 20% increase in calorie intake. For example, 1 cup of low-fat yogurt and a graham cracker with jam is about 400 kcal. At the same time, some vitamin and mineral needs increase by as much as 50%, so again, the key for getting adequate micronutrients while not consuming too many extra calories is choosing nutrient-dense foods.

Protein and Carbohydrate.   During pregnancy, protein needs increase to 1.1 g/day/kg body weight (an additional 25 g or so of protein per day). Many women already eat this much protein each day. Dairy products, meats, eggs, and soy products are all rich sources of protein, as are legumes, nuts, and seeds.

Carbohydrate intake should be at least 175 g/day. The majority of carbohydrate intake should come from whole-grain breads and cereals, brown rice, fruits, vegetables, and legumes. Not only are these carbohydrate-rich foods good sources of the B vitamins and other nutrients, but they also contain a lot of fiber. Fiber-rich foods contribute to one's sense of fullness, helping to avoid excess weight gain, and may lower risk of constipation.

Fat.   The guideline for the percentage of daily calories that comes from fat does not change during pregnancy. Pregnant women should be aware that, because new tissues and cells are being built, some fat in the diet is essential. In addition, the fetus stores most of its own body fat during the third trimester; these fat stores serve as a critical source of fuel in the newborn period and allow newborns to effectively regulate their body temperature.

Moderation in the amount of dietary fat and consumption of the right kinds of fats are important. Like anyone else, pregnant women should limit their intakes of saturated and *trans* fats because of their negative impact on cardiovascular health (as discussed in Chapter 5). An omega-3 polyunsaturated fatty acid known as *docosahexaenoic acid (DHA)* has been found to be uniquely critical for both brain growth and eye development. Because the fetal brain grows dramatically during the third trimester, DHA is especially important in the maternal diet. Women who breastfeed also need to choose good dietary sources of DHA because of the rapid brain growth that occurs during the first 3 months of life. Good sources of DHA are oily fish such as anchovies, mackerel, salmon, and sardines. It is also found in lesser amounts in tuna, chicken, and eggs (some eggs are DHA-enhanced by feeding hens a DHA-rich diet).

Pregnant women who eat fish should be aware of the potential for mercury contamination, as even a limited intake of mercury during pregnancy can impair a fetus's developing nervous system. While pregnant women should avoid large fish like swordfish, shark, tile fish, and king mackerel, they can safely consume up to 12 oz of most other types of fish per week, as long as it is cooked.

Micronutrient Needs of Pregnant Women

During pregnancy, expansion of the mother's blood supply and growth of the uterus, placenta, breasts, body fat levels, and the fetus itself all contribute to an increased need for micronutrients. In addition, the increased need for energy during pregnancy correlates with an increased need for micronutrients involved in the metabolism of macronutrients and ATP production. Discussions of the micronutrients that are most critical during pregnancy follow. Refer to Table 19.2 for an overview of the changes in micronutrient needs with pregnancy.

Folate.   Since folate is necessary for cell division, it follows that during a time when both maternal and fetal cells are dividing rapidly, the requirement for this vitamin would be increased. Adequate folate is especially critical during the first 28 days after conception, when it is required for the formation and closure of the **neural tube,** an embryonic structure that eventually becomes the brain and spinal cord. Folate deficiency is associated with neural tube defects such as **anencephaly,** a fatal defect in which there is partial absence of brain tissue, and **spina bifida**, in which a portion of the spinal cord protrudes through the spinal vertebrae, causing varying degrees of paralysis (FIGURE 19.7). Adequate folate intake does not guarantee normal neural tube development, as the precise cause of neural tube defects is unknown, and there is a genetic component in some cases. Still, it is estimated that 70% of all neural tube defects could be prevented by simply consuming enough folate or folic acid.[8]

To reduce the risk of a neural tube defect, all women capable of becoming pregnant are encouraged to consume 400 μg of folate per day. Of course, folate remains

neural tube Embryonic tissue that forms a tube, which eventually becomes the brain and spinal cord.

anencephaly A fatal neural tube defect in which there is partial absence of brain tissue most likely caused by failure of the neural tube to close.

spina bifida Embryotic neural tube defect that occurs when the spinal vertebrae fail to completely enclose the spinal cord, allowing it to protrude.

TABLE 19.2   Changes in Nutrient Recommendations with Pregnancy for Adult Women

Micronutrient	Pre-Pregnancy	Pregnancy	% Increase
Folate	400 µg/day	600 µg/day	50
Vitamin B$_{12}$	2.4 µg/day	2.6 µg/day	8
Vitamin C	75 mg/day	85 mg/day	13
Vitamin A	700 µg/day	770 µg/day	10
Vitamin D	5 µg/day	5 µg/day	0
Calcium	1,000 mg/day	1,000 mg/day	0
Iron	18 mg/day	27 mg/day	50
Zinc	8 mg/day	11 mg/day	38
Sodium	1,500 mg/day	1,500 mg/day	0
Iodine	150 µg/day	220 µg/day	47

(a)

(b)

FIGURE 19.7   Spina bifida, a common neural tube defect. **(a)** An external view of an infant with spina bifida. **(b)** An internal view of the protruding spinal membrane and fluid-filled sac.

Spinach is an excellent source of folate.

very important even after the neural tube has closed. The RDA for folate for pregnant women is therefore 600 µg/day, a full 50% increase over the RDA for a non-pregnant female.[9] A deficiency of folate during pregnancy can result in macrocytic anemia (a condition in which blood cells do not mature properly) and has been associated with low birth weight, preterm delivery, and failure of the fetus to grow properly. Sources of folate are discussed on page 412 and include fortified cereals and grains, spinach, and lentils.

Vitamin B$_{12}$.   Vitamin B$_{12}$ (cobalamin) is vital during pregnancy because it regenerates the active form of folate. Not surprisingly, deficiencies of vitamin B$_{12}$ can also result in macrocytic anemia. Yet the RDA for vitamin B$_{12}$ for pregnant women is only 2.6 µg/day, a mere 8% increase over the RDA of 2.4 µg/day for non-pregnant women. How can this be? One reason is that during pregnancy, absorption of vitamin B$_{12}$ is more efficient. The required amount of vitamin B$_{12}$ can easily be obtained from animal food sources. However, deficiencies have been observed in women who follow a vegan diet. Fortified foods or supplementation provides these women with the needed B_{12}.

Vitamin C.   Vitamin C is necessary for the synthesis of collagen, a component of connective tissue (including skin, blood vessels, and tendons) and part of the organic matrix of bones. The RDA for vitamin C during pregnancy is increased by a little more than 10% over the RDA for non-pregnant women (from 75 to 85 mg/day). A deficiency of vitamin C during pregnancy increases the risk for preterm birth, preeclampsia, and premature rupture of placental membranes. As described on pages 314–316, vitamin C is found abundantly in many food sources, such as citrus fruits and juices and numerous other fruits and vegetables.

Vitamin A.   Vitamin A needs increase during pregnancy by about 10%, to 770 µg/day. However, excess preformed vitamin A can cause fetal abnormalities, particularly in the kidneys and nervous system. Since an adequate diet supplies sufficient vitamin A, supplementation is not recommended. Beta-carotene (which is converted to vitamin A in the body) has not been associated with birth defects.

Vitamin D.   Despite the role of vitamin D in calcium absorption, the AI for this nutrient does not increase during pregnancy. Pregnant women who receive adequate exposure to sunlight do not need vitamin D supplements. However, pregnant women with limited sun exposure who do not regularly drink milk will benefit from vitamin D supplementation. Most prenatal vitamin supplements contain 10 µg/day of vitamin D, which is considered safe and acceptable.[10] Pregnant women should be cautious and avoid consuming excessive vitamin D from supplements, as toxicity can cause developmental disability in the newborn.

Calcium.   Growth of the fetal skeleton requires a significant amount of calcium. However, the AI for adult pregnant women is the same as that for non-pregnant adult women, 1,000 mg/day, for two reasons. First, pregnant women absorb calcium from the diet more efficiently than do non-pregnant women. Second, the extra demand for calcium has not been found to cause demineralization of the mother's bones or to increase fracture risk.[10] Sources of calcium are discussed on pages 369–371 and include milk, yogurt, and cheese and non-dairy foods such as kale, collard greens, and broccoli and calcium-fortified soy milk, juices, and cereals.

Iron.   Recall from Chapter 10 the importance of iron in the formation of red blood cells, which transport oxygen throughout the body. During pregnancy, the demand for red blood cells increases to accommodate the needs of the expanded maternal blood volume, growing uterus, placenta, and the fetus itself. Thus, more iron is needed. Fetal demand for iron increases even further during the last trimester, when the fetus stores iron in the liver for use during the first few months of life.

Severely inadequate iron intake has the potential to harm the fetus, resulting in an increased risk of low birth weight, preterm birth, stillbirth, and death of the newborn in the first weeks after birth. However, in most cases the fetus builds adequate stores by "robbing" maternal iron, prompting iron-deficiency anemia in the mother. During pregnancy, maternal iron deficiency causes pallor and exhaustion, but at birth, it endangers her life: anemic women are more likely to die during or shortly following childbirth because they are less able to tolerate blood loss and fight infection.

The RDA for iron for pregnant women is 27 mg/day, compared with 18 mg/day for non-pregnant women. This represents a 50% increase, despite the fact that iron loss is minimized during pregnancy because menstruation ceases. Typically, women of childbearing age have poor iron stores, and the demands of pregnancy are likely to produce a deficiency. To ensure adequate iron stores during pregnancy, an iron supplement (as part of, or distinct from, a total prenatal supplement) is routinely prescribed during the last two trimesters. Vitamin C enhances iron absorption, as do dietary sources of heme iron, whereas substances in coffee, tea, milk, bran, and oxalates decrease iron absorption. Therefore, many healthcare providers recommend taking iron supplements with foods high in vitamin C and/or heme iron. Sources of iron are discussed on pages 427–428.

Meats provide protein and heme iron that are important for maternal and fetal nutrition.

It is important that pregnant women drink about 10 cups of fluid a day.

Zinc.   The RDA for zinc for adult pregnant women increases by about 38% over the RDA for non-pregnant adult women, from 8 mg/day to 11 mg/day. Zinc is critical in DNA, RNA, and protein synthesis, and inadequate intake can lead to malformations in the fetus, premature delivery, and extended labor. It should be noted that the absorption of zinc is inhibited by high intakes of non-heme iron, such as high potency iron supplements, when these two minerals are taken with water. However, when food sources of iron and zinc are consumed together in a meal, absorption of zinc is not affected.[11] In addition, the heme form of iron does not appear to inhibit zinc absorption.

Sodium and Iodine.   During pregnancy, the AI for sodium is the same as for a non-pregnant adult woman, or 1,500 mg (1.5 g) per day.[12] Although too much sodium is associated with fluid retention, bloating, and high blood pressure, an increase in body fluids is a normal and necessary part of pregnancy, so some sodium is necessary to maintain fluid balance.

Iodine needs increase significantly during pregnancy, but the RDA of 220 μg/day is easy to achieve by using a modest amount of iodized salt (sodium chloride) during cooking.

Do Pregnant Women Need Supplements?

Prenatal multivitamin and mineral supplements are not strictly necessary during pregnancy, but most healthcare providers recommend them. Meeting all the nutrient needs would otherwise take careful and somewhat complex dietary planning. Prenatal supplements are especially good insurance for special populations such as vegans, adolescents, and others whose diet might normally be low in one or more micronutrients. It is important that pregnant women understand, however, that supplements are to be taken *in addition to,* not as a substitute for, a nutrient-rich diet.

Fluid Needs of Pregnant Women

Fluid allows for the necessary increase in the mother's blood volume, aids in regulating body temperature, and helps maintain the **amniotic fluid** that surrounds, cushions, and protects the fetus in the uterus. The AI for total fluid intake, which includes drinking water, beverages, and food, is 3 liters/day (or about 12.7 cups). This recommendation includes approximately 2.3 liters (10 cups) of fluid as total beverages, including drinking water.[12]

Drinking adequate fluid also helps combat two common discomforts of pregnancy, fluid retention and, possibly, constipation. Drinking lots of fluids may also lower risk of **urinary tract infections,** which are very common in pregnancy. Fluids also combat dehydration, which can develop if a woman has frequent bouts of vomiting. For these women, fluids such as soups, juices, and sports beverages are usually well tolerated.

amniotic fluid The watery fluid contained within the innermost membrane of the sac containing the fetus. It cushions and protects the growing fetus.

urinary tract infection A bacterial infection of the urethra, the tube leading from the bladder to the body exterior.

> RECAP: *Sufficient calories should be consumed so that a pregnant woman gains an appropriate amount of weight, typically 25 to 35 pounds, to ensure adequate growth of the fetus. The calories consumed during pregnancy should be nutrient-dense. Protein, carbohydrates, and fats provide the building blocks for fetal growth. Folate deficiency has been associated with neural tube defects. Most healthcare providers recommend prenatal supplements for pregnant women to ensure that sufficient micronutrients are consumed. Fluid provides for increased maternal blood volume and amniotic fluid.*

Nutrition-Related Concerns for Pregnant Women

Pregnancy-related conditions involving a particular nutrient, such as iron-deficiency anemia, have already been discussed. The following sections describe some of the most common discomforts and disorders of pregnant women that are related to their general nutrition.

Morning Sickness

Morning sickness, or *nausea and vomiting of pregnancy (NVP),* is a potentially serious medical condition.[13] The symptoms vary in severity, from occasional mild queasiness to constant nausea with bouts of vomiting. In truth, "morning sickness" is not an appropriate name because the nausea and vomiting can begin at any time of the day and may last all day. NVP usually resolves by week 12 to 16, but some women experience it throughout the pregnancy. Usually, the mother and fetus do not suffer lasting harm. However, some women experience such frequent vomiting that they are unable to nourish or hydrate themselves or their fetus adequately, and may require hospitalization or in-home intravenous (IV) therapy.

There is no cure for morning sickness. However, here are some practical tips for reducing its severity:

- An empty stomach can trigger nausea, so eating small, frequent meals and snacks is usually helpful. Many women find that once they start eating, they begin to feel better.

- Some women find it helpful to keep snacks such as dry cereal or crackers at their bedside to ease nighttime queasiness. A small snack before rising in the morning helps some women, as does rising from bed slowly.

- Prenatal supplements should be taken at a time of day when vomiting is least likely.

- Some women find it more comfortable to consume most of their fluids between meals and limit mealtime beverages. Frozen ice pops, watermelon, gelatin desserts, and mild broths are often well-tolerated sources of fluid.

- Women should avoid sights, sounds, smells, and tastes that bring on or worsen queasiness. Cold or room-temperature foods are often better tolerated than hot foods.

- For some women, alternative therapies such as acupuncture, acupressure wrist bands, biofeedback, meditation, and hypnosis help. Women should always check with their healthcare provider that the therapy they are using is safe and does not interact with other treatments, medications, or supplements.

Cravings and Aversions

It seems like nothing is more stereotypical about pregnancy than the image of a frazzled husband getting up in the middle of the night to run to the convenience store to get his pregnant wife some pickles and ice cream. This image, although humorous, is far from reality for most women. Although some women have specific cravings, most crave a particular type (such as "something sweet" or "something salty") rather than a particular food.

Why do pregnant women crave certain tastes? Does a desire for salty foods mean that the woman is experiencing a sodium deficit? While there may be some truth to the assertion that we crave what we need, scientific evidence for this claim is lacking. It is more likely that cravings during pregnancy are due to hormonal fluctuations or physiologic changes or have familial or cultural roots. In some cases, when a woman improves her diet after learning she is pregnant, she simply misses the "forbidden" foods that she used to eat.

Most cravings are, of course, for edible substances. But a surprising number of pregnant women crave nonfoods like laundry starch and clay. This craving, called **pica,** is the subject of the Highlight box on page 712.

Food aversions are also common during pregnancy but are by no means universal. For example, some pregnant women experience an aversion to fried foods, sweets, or coffee. Some food aversions originate from social, cultural, or religious beliefs. In some cultures, for example, pregnant women avoid shellfish ("causes allergies") or citrus fruits ("may increase risk of a miscarriage"). While these aversions may not be scientifically valid, they are often strongly woven into the family's belief system.

Deep-fried foods are often unappealing to pregnant women.

morning sickness Varying degrees of nausea and vomiting associated with pregnancy, most commonly in the first trimester.

pica An abnormal craving to eat something not fit for food, such as clay, paint, or chalk.

HIGHLIGHT

The Danger of Nonfood Cravings

For most of her life, Darcy had thoroughly enjoyed good food. Her husband even bragged about her being a "gourmet cook." But a few weeks after learning she was pregnant, her appetite seemed to disappear. She would wander through the aisles of the grocery store with an empty cart, knowing she should be choosing nutritious foods for her growing baby but feeling unable to find a single food that appealed to her. Eventually, she'd return home with a few things for her husband . . . and a large bag of ice. On weekends, she'd keep a cupful of ice with her almost constantly. She brought ice to work in a cold pack and ate it throughout the day, and she even kept a glass of ice by her bed at night. At her prenatal healthcare visits, her physician became concerned because she wasn't gaining weight. "I try to eat right," she confessed, "but nothing appeals to me." She was too embarrassed to admit to anyone, even her husband, that the only thing she really wanted to eat was ice.

Some people contend that a pregnant woman with unusual food cravings is intuitively seeking needed nutrients. Arguing against this claim is the phenomenon of *pica*—the craving and consumption of nonfood material during pregnancy or in children and non-pregnant women. A woman with pica may crave ice, freezer frost, clay, dirt, chalk, coffee grounds, baking soda, laundry starch, or many other substances. The cause of these nonfood cravings is not known, though cultural factors, socioeconomic status, emotional support, and family tendencies seem to contribute to the incidence. In the United States, pica is more common among pregnant African American women than women from other racial or ethnic groups.[14] The practice of eating clay has been traced to central Africa, and researchers theorize that people taken from central Africa and sent as slaves to the United States brought the practice with them. No matter what the cause, pica is dangerous. Consuming ice cubes or freezer frost can lead to inadequate weight gain if the substance substitutes for food. Ingestion of clay, starch, and other substances can cause deficiency of iron and other nutrients, as well as constipation, intestinal blockage, and even excessive weight gain.

Some women find it helpful to substitute food items for the craved nonfood. For instance, frozen juice bars can be substituted for ice, and nonfat powdered milk can replace starch.[2]

Heartburn

Heartburn, along with indigestion, is common during pregnancy. Heartburn occurs when the sphincter between the esophagus and the stomach relaxes, allowing acid and partially digested food from the stomach to well up and irritate the tissues of the esophagus. Hormones released during pregnancy relax smooth muscle, increasing the incidence of heartburn. During the last two trimesters, enlargement of the uterus pushes up on the stomach, worsening the problem. Practical tips for minimizing the distress of heartburn during pregnancy include the following:

- Avoid excessive weight gain.
- Eat small, frequent meals and chew food slowly.
- Don't wear tight clothing.
- Avoid foods that seem to trigger the problem.
- Wait for at least 1 hour after eating before lying down.
- Sleep with your head elevated.
- Ask your doctor and/or midwife for an antacid that is safe for use during pregnancy.

Constipation

Hormone production during pregnancy causes the smooth muscles to relax, including the muscles of the large intestine, slowing colonic movement of food residue. In addition, pressure exerted by the growing uterus on the colon can slow movement even further, making elimination difficult. Practical hints that may help a pregnant woman avoid constipation include the following:

- Include 25 to 35 g of fiber in the daily diet, concentrating on fresh fruits and vegetables, legumes, and whole grains.

- Keep fluid intake high as fiber intake increases. Drink plenty of water and eat water-rich fruits and vegetables such as melons, citrus, and lettuce.

- Keep physically active, as exercise is one of many factors that help increase motility of the large intestine.

Gestational Diabetes

Gestational diabetes, diagnosed in approximately 7% of U.S. pregnancies, is generally a temporary condition in which a pregnant woman is unable to produce sufficient insulin or becomes insulin resistant, resulting in elevated levels of blood glucose. Fortunately, gestational diabetes has no ill effects on either the mother or the fetus if blood glucose levels are strictly controlled through diet, exercise, and/or medication. Screening for gestational diabetes is routine for almost all healthcare practitioners and is necessary because the symptoms, which include frequent urination, fatigue, and an increase in thirst and appetite, can be indistinguishable from normal pregnancy symptoms. If uncontrolled, gestational diabetes can result in *preeclampsia,* which is discussed in greater detail below. It can also result in a baby who is too large as a result of receiving too much glucose across the placenta during fetal life. Infants who are overly large are at risk for early delivery and trauma during vaginal birth, and may need to be born by cesarean section. There is also evidence that exposing a fetus to maternal diabetes significantly increases the risk for type 2 diabetes during adolescence and adulthood.[15,16] Women who are obese, age 35 years or older, or of Native American, African American, or Hispanic origin have a greater risk of developing gestational diabetes. Any woman who develops gestational diabetes remains at greater risk of developing type 2 diabetes later in life—particularly if she is obese to begin with or fails to maintain normal body weight after pregnancy. As with any form of diabetes, attention to diet, weight control, and physical activity reduces the risk of gestational diabetes.

Foods high in fiber, such as dried fruits, reduce the chances of constipation.

NUTRI-CASE JUDY

" Back when I was pregnant with Hannah, the doctor told me I had gestational diabetes but I shouldn't worry about it. He said I didn't need any medication, and I don't remember changing my diet. In fact, I just kept eating whatever I wanted, and by the time Hannah was born, I had gained almost 60 pounds. I never did lose all that extra weight."

Review what you learned about diabetes in Chapter 4. What information would have been important for Judy to learn while she was pregnant? Is it common that women with gestational diabetes develop type 2 diabetes years later? What are some things Judy could have done to lower her risk of type 2 diabetes?

Hypertensive Disorders of Pregnancy

About 7–8% of U.S. pregnancies are complicated by some form of hypertension or high blood pressure. The term *hypertensive disorders of pregnancy* encompasses several different conditions.[17] A woman who develops high blood pressure, with no other symptoms, during her pregnancy is said to have *gestational hypertension.*

gestational diabetes Insufficient insulin production or insulin resistance that results in consistently high blood glucose levels, specifically during pregnancy; condition typically resolves after birth occurs.

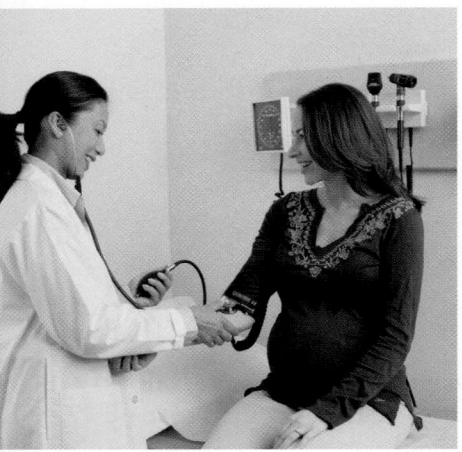

Pregnant women have their blood pressures taken to test for gestational hypertension.

Preeclampsia is characterized by sudden, high maternal blood pressure, swelling, excessive and rapid weight gain unrelated to food intake, and protein in the urine. If left untreated, it can progress to eclampsia, characterized by seizures, kidney failure, and, potentially, fetal and/or maternal death.

No one knows exactly what causes the various hypertensive disorders of pregnancy, but deficiencies in dietary protein, vitamin C, vitamin E, calcium, and magnesium seem to increase the risk. High levels of blood triglycerides (associated with high-sugar diets) have been correlated with preeclampsia.

Management of preeclampsia focuses mainly on blood pressure control. Typical treatment includes bed rest. Ultimately, the only thing that will cure the condition is childbirth. Today, with good prenatal care, gestational hypertension is nearly always detected early and can be appropriately managed, and prospects for both mother and fetus are usually very good. In nearly all women without prior chronic high blood pressure, maternal blood pressure returns to normal within about a day after the birth.

> RECAP: *About half of all pregnant women experience nausea and/or vomiting during pregnancy, called morning sickness, and many crave or feel aversions to specific types of foods. Pica is a craving for nonfood items experienced by some pregnant women. Heartburn and constipation in pregnancy are related to the relaxation of smooth muscles caused by certain pregnancy-related hormones. Gestational diabetes and hypertensive disorders in pregnancy are nutrition-related disorders that can seriously affect maternal and fetal health.*

Adolescent Pregnancy

Adolescents who become pregnant are subject to greater nutritional risks than adult women. Throughout the adolescent years, a woman's body is still changing and growing. Peak bone mass has not yet been reached. Full physical stature may not have been attained, and teens are more likely to be underweight than are young adult women. Thus, pregnant adolescents have higher needs for calories and calcium. In addition, many adolescents have not established healthful nutritional patterns; thus, the added burden of a pregnancy on an adolescent body creates a nutrient demand that can be very difficult to meet. Hence, adolescent mothers are more likely to have preterm births, low-birth-weight babies, and other complications related to nutritional deficiencies than are more mature women. With adequate and thorough prenatal care and close attention to proper nutrition and other healthful behaviors, the likelihood of a positive outcome for both the adolescent mother and infant is greatly increased.[18]

Vegetarianism

With the possible exception of iron and zinc, vegetarian women who consume dairy products and/or eggs (lacto-ovo-vegetarians) have no nutritional concerns beyond those encountered by every pregnant woman. In contrast, women who are totally vegetarian (vegan) need to be more vigilant than usual about their intake of nutrients that are derived primarily or wholly from animal products. These include vitamin D (unless exposed to adequate sunlight), vitamin B_6, vitamin B_{12}, calcium, iron, and zinc. Supplements containing these nutrients are usually necessary. A regular prenatal supplement will fully meet the vitamin and iron needs of a vegan woman but does not fulfill calcium needs, so a separate calcium supplement, or consumption of calcium-fortified soy milk or orange juice, might be required.

Dieting

Dieting to lose weight is not advisable during pregnancy. When calories are restricted, neither the woman nor the fetus obtains the nutrients necessary to grow and develop appropriately. Especially dangerous practices during pregnancy are fasting and abstaining from carbohydrates: recall from Chapter 4 that ketones are released when the body must rely on stored fats for fuel. These ketones are readily taken up and metabolized by the fetal brain, which could be detrimental to proper brain growth and development. Lack of glucose (carbohydrates) in the mother's diet

preeclampsia High blood pressure that is pregnancy specific and accompanied by protein in the urine, edema, and unexpected weight gain.

also has been shown to result in reduced fetal growth.[19] The best strategy during pregnancy to ensure health of mother and baby is a healthful balance of all nutrients.

Consumption of Caffeine

Caffeine is a stimulant found in several foods, including coffee, tea, soft drinks, and chocolate. Caffeine crosses the placenta and thus reaches the fetus. Current thinking holds that women who consume less than about 200 mg of caffeine per day (the equivalent of 1 to 2 cups of coffee) are very likely doing no harm to the fetus. Evidence suggests that consuming higher daily doses of caffeine (the higher the dose, the more compelling the evidence) may slightly increase the risk of miscarriage and low birth weight. It is sensible, then, for pregnant women to limit daily caffeine intake to no more than the equivalent of 2 cups of coffee.[20] Because coffee and colas have no nutritional value, drinking them can be especially detrimental during pregnancy because they can make one feel full and provide considerable calories (if sweetened) without contributing any nutrients at a time when nutrient intake is critical. Low- or nonfat lattes, known to Latinas as *café con leche*, offer a more healthful nutrient profile than coffee alone.

Consumption of Alcohol

Alcohol is a known teratogen that readily crosses the placenta and accumulates in the fetal bloodstream. The immature fetal liver cannot readily metabolize alcohol, and its presence in the fetal tissues is associated with a variety of birth defects. These effects are dose dependent: the more the mother drinks, the greater the potential harm to the fetus.

Heavy drinking (more than three to four drinks per day) throughout pregnancy can result in a condition called **fetal alcohol syndrome (FAS)** (see Figure 4 on page 167 of the *In Depth* on Alcohol). Babies born with FAS have characteristic malformations, particularly of the face, limbs, heart, and nervous system. They have a high mortality rate, and as we saw with Theresa in our opening vignette, those who survive typically have emotional, behavioral, social, learning, and developmental problems throughout life.

Frequent drinking (more than seven drinks per week) or occasional binge drinking (more than four to five drinks on one occasion) during pregnancy increases the risk for miscarriage, complications during delivery, preterm birth, and sudden infant death syndrome. Another consequence is **fetal alcohol effects (FAE),** a milder set of alcohol-related birth defects manifested in the child as developmental and behavioral problems (for example, hyperactivity and attention deficit disorder) and possibly physical abnormalities. Although some women do have the occasional alcoholic drink with no apparent ill effects, there is no amount of alcohol that is known to be safe. The best advice regarding alcohol during pregnancy is to abstain, if not from before conception, then as soon as pregnancy is suspected.[21]

Smoking

Although the dangers of smoking are well known, between 13% and 17% of pregnant women smoke, and the percentage is higher among pregnant adolescents. Maternal smoking exposes the fetus to toxins such as lead, cadmium, cyanide, nicotine, and carbon monoxide. Fetal blood flow is reduced, which limits the delivery of oxygen and nutrients, resulting in impaired fetal growth and development. Maternal smoking greatly increases risk of miscarriage, stillbirth, placental abnormalities, preterm delivery, and low birth weight.[4] Rates of sudden infant death, respiratory illness, and allergies are higher in the infants and children of smokers compared with nonsmokers. It has been estimated that every $1 spent on programs to help pregnant women stop smoking will save $3 in neonatal intensive care expenses.[22] Pregnant women can go to the Web site www.helppregnantsmokersquit.org or speak with their health-care provider to get the necessary assistance.

Illegal Drugs

Despite the fact that use of illegal drugs is unquestionably harmful to the fetus, as many as 3.7% of U.S. pregnant women report using illicit drugs.[23] Most drugs pass

fetal alcohol syndrome (FAS) A set of serious, irreversible alcohol-related birth defects characterized by certain physical and mental abnormalities.

fetal alcohol effects (FAE) A milder set of alcohol-related birth defects characterized by behavioral problems such as hyperactivity, attention deficit disorder, poor judgment, sleep disorders, and delayed learning.

through the placenta into fetal blood, where they accumulate in fetal tissues and organs, including the liver and brain. Prenatal use of illegal drugs such as marijuana, cocaine, heroin, ecstasy, and amphetamines poses similar risks: impaired placental blood flow (thus reduced transfer of nutrients to the fetus), higher risk of low birth weight and/or premature delivery, increased rate of miscarriage, and placental defects. Newborns suffer signs of withdrawal, including tremors, excessive crying, sleeplessness, and poor feeding. Even after several years, children born to women who used illicit drugs during pregnancy are at greater risk for developmental delays, impaired learning, and behavioral problems. All women are strongly advised to stop taking drugs before becoming pregnant. There is no safe level of use.

Food Safety

The U.S. Departments of Health and Human Services and of Agriculture recently recommended that pregnant women avoid unpasteurized milk, raw or partially cooked eggs, raw or undercooked meat/fish/poultry, unpasteurized juices, and raw sprouts.[24] Women who are or could become pregnant, as well as breastfeeding mothers, are advised to avoid eating large fish such as shark, swordfish, and king mackerel and to limit their intake of canned albacore tuna, because of their high mercury content.

Soft cheeses such as Brie, feta, Camembert, and Mexican-style cheeses, also called *queso blanco* or *queso fresco*, should be avoided unless the label specifically states the product is made with pasteurized milk. Unpasteurized milk and cheeses may be contaminated with the bacterium *Listeria monocytogenes*, which triggers miscarriage, premature birth, or fetal infection when consumed during pregnancy. All safe food-handling practices discussed in Chapter 18 should be rigorously followed by pregnant women to ensure a healthy pregnancy outcome.

Exercise

Physical activity during pregnancy is recommended for healthy women experiencing normal pregnancies.[25] Exercise can help keep a woman physically fit during pregnancy, enhance mood, and help women feel more in control of their changing bodies. Moreover, regular moderate exercise will help keep blood pressure down and confer all the cardiovascular benefits that it does for non-pregnant individuals.

If a woman was not active prior to pregnancy, she should begin an exercise program slowly and progress gradually under the guidance of her healthcare provider. If a woman was physically active before pregnancy, she can continue to be physically active during pregnancy, keeping track of heart rate and body temperature. The exercise should be comfortable for the woman. Low- or no-impact exercises are excellent choices for most women, although women who have been avid runners before pregnancy can often continue to run, although they may need to limit the distance and intensity of their runs.

During pregnancy, women should adjust their physical activity to comfortable low-impact exercises.

> **RECAP:** *As adolescents' bodies are still growing and developing, their nutrient needs during pregnancy become so high that adequate nourishment for the mother and baby becomes difficult. Women who follow a vegan diet usually need to consume multivitamin and mineral supplements, plus supplemental calcium, during pregnancy. Dieting during pregnancy is not advised, as it leads to inadequate nutrition for mother and fetus. Caffeine intake should not exceed 2 cups of coffee per day throughout pregnancy. Alcohol is a teratogen and should not be consumed in any amount during pregnancy. Smoking and use of illegal drugs threaten the health of both the mother and the child. Exercise (provided the mother has no contraindications) can enhance the health of a pregnant woman.*

Breastfeeding

Throughout most of human history, infants have thrived on only one food: breast milk. But during the first half of the 20th century, commercially prepared infant formulas slowly began to replace breast milk as the mother's preferred feeding method. Aggressive marketing campaigns convinced many families, even in developing nations, to switch. Soon formula-feeding had become a status symbol, proof of the family's wealth and modern thinking. In the 1970s, this trend began to reverse as the "back-to-the-land" movement led to a renewed appreciation for the natural simplicity of breastfeeding. At the same time, several international organizations, including the World Health Organization, UNICEF, and La Leche League, began to promote the nutritional, immunologic, financial, and emotional advantages of breastfeeding and developed programs to encourage and support breastfeeding worldwide. These efforts have paid off: in 2002, U.S. breastfeeding rates reached an all-time high with just over 70% of new mothers initiating breastfeeding in the hospital and over 33% of mothers still breastfeeding their babies at 6 months of age.[26]

How, exactly, does breastfeeding occur? What nutrients are important for breastfeeding mothers? Is breastfeeding painful and difficult? And what exactly are the advantages that everyone is talking about? The answers to these questions are presented in the following sections.

How Does Lactation Occur?

Lactation, the production of breast milk, is a process that is set in motion during pregnancy in response to several hormones. Once established, lactation can be sustained as long as the mammary glands continue to receive the proper stimuli.

The Body Prepares During Pregnancy

Throughout pregnancy, the placenta produces estrogen and progesterone. In addition to performing various functions to maintain the pregnancy, these hormones prepare the breasts physically for lactation. The breasts increase in size, and milk-producing glands (alveoli) and milk ducts are formed (FIGURE 19.8). Toward the end of pregnancy, the hormone *prolactin* increases. Prolactin is released by the anterior pituitary gland and is responsible for milk synthesis. However, estrogen and progesterone suppress the effects of prolactin during pregnancy.

What Happens After Childbirth

By the time a pregnancy has come to full term, the level of prolactin is about ten times higher than it was at the beginning of pregnancy. At birth, the suppressive

lactation The production of breast milk.

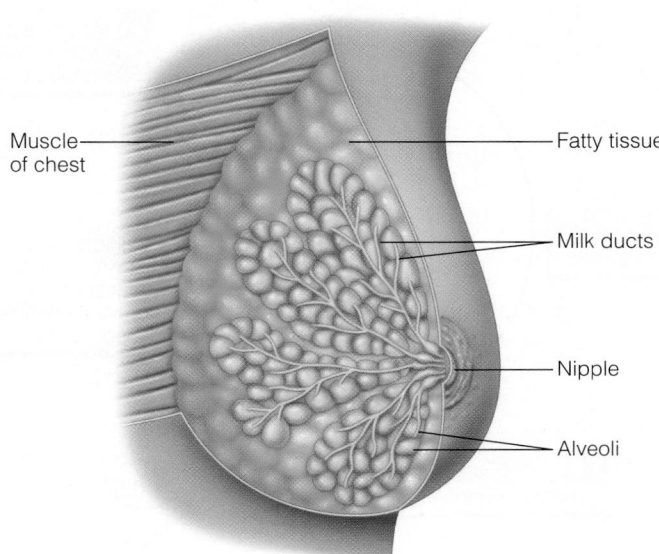

Muscle of chest

Fatty tissue

Milk ducts

Nipple

Alveoli

FIGURE 19.8 Anatomy of the breast. During pregnancy, estrogen and progesterone secreted by the placenta foster the preparation of breast tissue for lactation. This process includes breast enlargement and development of the milk-producing glands, or alveoli.

effect of estrogen and progesterone ends, and prolactin is free to stimulate milk production. The first substance to be released is **colostrum,** sometimes called pre-milk or first milk. It is thick, yellowish in color, and rich in protein and micronutrients, and includes antibodies that help protect the newborn from infection. Colostrum also contains a factor that fosters the growth of a particular species of "friendly" bacteria in the infant gastrointestinal tract. These bacteria in turn prevent the growth of other bacteria that could potentially be harmful. Finally, colostrum has a laxative effect in infants, helping the infant to expel *meconium,* the sticky "first stool."

Within 2 to 4 days in most women, colostrum is fully replaced by mature milk. Mature breast milk contains protein, fat, and carbohydrate (in the form of the sugar lactose). Much of the protein and fat are synthesized in the breast, while the rest enter the milk from the mother's bloodstream.

Mother–Infant Interaction Maintains Milk Production

Continued, sustained breast milk production depends entirely on infant suckling (or a similar stimulus like a mechanical pump). Infant suckling stimulates the continued production of prolactin, which in turn stimulates more milk production. The longer and more vigorous the feeding, the more milk will be produced. Thus even multiples (twins, triplets) can be successfully breastfed.

Prolactin allows for milk to be produced, but that milk has to move through the milk ducts to the nipple in order to reach the baby's mouth. The hormone responsible for this "let down" of milk is *oxytocin.* Like prolactin, oxytocin is produced by the pituitary gland, and its production is dependent on the suckling stimulus at the beginning of a feeding (FIGURE 19.9). This response usually occurs within 10 to 30 seconds but can be significantly inhibited by stress. Finding a relaxed environment in which to breastfeed is therefore important.

colostrum The first fluid made and secreted by the breasts from late in pregnancy to about a week after birth. It is rich in immune factors and protein.

3 Hypothalamus sends message to pituitary gland.

2 Nerves send message to hypothalamus.

4 Pituitary gland releases prolactin, which stimulates milk production, and oxytocin, which stimulates milk release.

1 Suckling stimulates nerves in nipple.

FIGURE 19.9 Sustained milk production depends on the mother–child interaction during breastfeeding, specifically the suckling of the infant. Suckling stimulates the continued production of prolactin, which is responsible for milk production, and oxytocin, which is responsible for the let-down response.

What Are a Breastfeeding Woman's Nutrient Needs?

You might be surprised to learn that breastfeeding requires even more energy than pregnancy! This is because breast milk has to supply an adequate amount of all of the nutrients an infant needs to grow and develop.

Nutrient Recommendations for Breastfeeding Women

It is estimated that milk production requires about 700 to 800 kcal/day. It is generally recommended that lactating women 19 years and above consume 330 kcal/day above their pre-pregnancy energy needs during the first 6 months of lactation and 400 additional kcal/day during the second 6 months. This additional energy is sufficient to support adequate milk production. The remaining energy deficit will assist in the gradual loss of excess fat and body weight gained during pregnancy. It is critical that lactating women avoid severe energy restriction, as this practice can result in decreased milk production.

The weight loss that occurs during breastfeeding should be gradual, approximately 1 to 4 pounds per month. Both breastfeeding and participating in regular physical activity can assist with weight loss. The 2005 Dietary Guidelines for Americans confirm that neither occasional nor regular exercise negatively affects a woman's ability to successfully breastfeed. Some active women, however, may lose too much weight during breastfeeding and must either increase their energy intake or reduce their activity level to maintain health.

Of the macronutrients, protein and carbohydrate needs are different from pregnancy requirements. An increase of 15 to 20 g of protein per day and 80 g of carbohydrate per day above pre-pregnancy requirements are recommended during lactation.

The needs of several vitamins and minerals increase over the requirements of pregnancy. These include vitamins A, C, E, riboflavin, vitamin B_{12}, biotin, and choline and the minerals copper, chromium, manganese, iodine, selenium, and zinc. The requirement for folate during lactation is 500 µg/day, which is decreased from the 600 µg/day required during pregnancy, but this requirement is higher than pre-pregnancy needs (400 µg/day).

Requirements for iron decrease significantly during lactation, to a mere 9 mg/day. This is because iron is not a significant component of breast milk, and in addition, breastfeeding usually suppresses menstruation for at least a few months, minimizing iron losses.

Calcium is a significant component of breast milk; but, as in pregnancy, calcium absorption is enhanced during lactation, and urinary loss of calcium is decreased. In addition, some calcium appears to come from the demineralization of the mother's bones, and increased dietary calcium does not prevent this. Thus, the recommended intake for calcium for a lactating woman is unchanged from pregnancy, that is, 1,000 mg/day. Because of their own continuing growth, however, teen mothers who are breastfeeding should continue to consume 1,300 mg/day. Typically, if calcium intake is adequate, a woman's bone density returns to normal shortly after lactation ends.

Do Breastfeeding Women Need Supplements?

If a breastfeeding woman appropriately increases her energy intake, and does so with nutrient-dense foods, her nutrient needs can usually be met without supplements. However, there is nothing wrong with taking a basic multivitamin for insurance, as long as it is not considered a substitute for proper nutrition. Lactating women should consume omega-3 fatty acids in either fish or supplements to support the infant's developing nervous system. Women who don't consume dairy products should monitor their calcium intake carefully.

Fluid Recommendations for Breastfeeding Women

Because extra fluid is expended with every feeding, lactating women need to consume about an extra quart (about 1 liter) of fluid per day. This extra fluid facilitates milk production and staves off dehydration. Many women report that, within a minute or two of beginning to nurse their baby, they become intensely thirsty. To prevent this thirst and achieve the recommended fluid intake, women are encouraged to

Breastfeeding has benefits for the mother and infant.

drink a nutritious beverage (for example, water, juice, or milk) each time they nurse their baby. However, it is not good practice to drink hot beverages while nursing because accidental spills could burn the infant.

> RECAP: *Lactation is the result of the coordinated effort of several hormones, including estrogen, progesterone, prolactin, and oxytocin. Breasts are prepared for lactation during pregnancy, and infant suckling provides the stimulus that sustains the production of prolactin and oxytocin needed to maintain the milk supply. It is recommended that lactating women consume an extra 300–400 kcal/day above pre-pregnancy energy intake, including increased protein, certain vitamins and minerals, and fluids. The requirements for folate and iron decrease from pregnancy levels, while the requirement for calcium remains the same.*

Getting Real About Breastfeeding: Pros and Cons

Breastfeeding is the perfect way to provide the best food for a baby's first 6 months of life.[27] However, the technique does require patience and practice, and teaching by an experienced mother or certified lactation consultant is important. For some women, illness, medication use, or other factors may make breastfeeding a difficult choice. The decision to breastfeed or use formula must be made independently by each family after careful consideration of all the factors that apply to their particular situation.

Advantages of Breastfeeding

As adept as formula manufacturers have been at simulating the components of breast milk, an exact replica has never been produced. In addition, there are other benefits that mother and baby can access only through breastfeeding.[28]

Nutritional Quality of Breast Milk. The amount and types of protein in breast milk are ideally suited to the human infant. The main protein in breast milk, lactalbumin, is easily digested in infants' immature gastrointestinal tracts, reducing the risk of gastric distress. Other proteins in breast milk bind iron and prevent the growth of harmful bacteria that require iron. Antibodies from the mother are additional proteins that help prevent infection while the infant's immune system is still immature. Certain proteins in human milk improve the absorption of iron; this is important since breast milk is low in iron. Cow's milk contains too much protein for infants, and the types of protein in cow's milk are harder for the infant to digest.

The primary carbohydrate in milk is lactose, a disaccharide composed of glucose and galactose. The galactose component is important in nervous system development. Lactose provides energy and prevents ketosis in the infant, promotes the growth of beneficial bacteria, and increases the absorption of calcium. Breast milk has more lactose than cow's milk, reinforcing the advantages of the breastfeeding process.

The amounts and types of fats in breast milk are ideally suited to the human infant. DHA and arachidonic acid (ARA) have been shown to be essential for growth and development of the infant's nervous system and for development of the retina of the eyes. Until 2002, these fatty acids were omitted from commercial infant formulas in the United States, although they have been available in formulas in other parts of the world for the better part of a decade. Interestingly, the concentration of DHA in breast milk varies considerably, is sensitive to maternal diet, and is highest in women who consume large quantities of fish.

The fat content of breast milk, which is higher than that of whole cow's milk, changes according to the gestational age of the infant and during the course of every feeding: The milk that is initially released (called *foremilk*) is watery and low in fat, somewhat like skim milk. This milk is thought to satisfy the infant's initial thirst. As the feeding progresses, the milk acquires more fat and becomes more like whole milk. Finally, the very last 5% or so of the milk produced during a feeding (called the *hindmilk*) is very high in fat, similar to cream. This milk is thought to satiate the infant. It is important to let infants suckle for at least 20 minutes at each feeding so that they get this hindmilk. Breast milk is also relatively high in cholesterol, which supports the rapid growth and development of the brain.

Another important aspect of breastfeeding (or any type of feeding) is the fluid it provides the infant. Because of their small size, infants are at risk of dehydration, which is one reason why feedings must be consistent and frequent. This topic will be discussed at greater length in the section on infant nutrition.

In terms of micronutrients, breast milk is a good source of readily absorbed calcium and magnesium. It is low in iron, but the iron it does contain is easily absorbed. Since healthy full-term infants store iron in preparation for the first few months of life, most experts agree that their iron needs can be met by breast milk alone for the first 6 months, after which iron-rich foods are needed. Although breast milk has some vitamin D, the American Academy of Pediatrics recommends that all breastfed infants be provided a vitamin D supplement.[1]

Breast milk composition continues to change as the infant grows and develops. Because of this ability to change as the baby changes, breast milk alone is entirely sufficient to sustain infant growth for the first 6 months of life. Throughout the next 6 months of infancy, as solid foods are gradually introduced, breast milk remains the baby's primary source of superior-quality nutrition. The American Academy of Pediatrics recommends exclusive breastfeeding for the first 6 months of life, continuing breastfeeding for at least the first year of life, and, if acceptable within the family, into the second year of life.[29]

Protection from Infections and Allergies.   Immune factors from the mother, including antibodies and immune cells, are passed directly from the mother to the newborn through breast milk. These factors provide important disease protection for the infant while its immune system is still immature. It has been shown that breastfed infants have a lower incidence of respiratory tract, gastrointestinal tract, and urinary tract infections than formula-fed infants. Even a few weeks of breastfeeding is beneficial, but the longer a child is breastfed, the greater the level of passive immunity from the mother. In the United States, infant mortality rates are reduced by 21% in breastfed infants.[29] A report from the United Nations Children's Fund estimates that, in part because of this immunologic protection, if every baby were exclusively breastfed from birth for 6 months, 1.3 million lives would be saved.[27]

In addition, breast milk is nonallergenic, and breastfeeding is associated with a reduced risk of allergies during childhood and adulthood. Breastfed babies also have fewer ear infections, die less frequently from **sudden infant death syndrome (SIDS),** and have a decreased chance of developing diabetes, overweight and obesity, and chronic digestive disorders.

Physiologic Benefits for Mother.   Breastfeeding causes uterine contractions that quicken the return of the uterus to pre-pregnancy size and reduce bleeding. Many women also find that breastfeeding helps them lose the weight they gained during pregnancy, particularly if it continues for more than 6 months. In addition, breastfeeding appears to be associated with a decreased risk for breast cancer.[30] The relationship between breastfeeding and osteoporosis is still unclear, and more research on this topic is needed.[31]

Breastfeeding also suppresses ovulation, lengthening the time between pregnancies and giving a mother's body the chance to recover before she conceives again. This benefit can be life-saving for malnourished women living in countries that discourage or outlaw the use of contraceptives. Ovulation may not cease completely, however, so it is still possible to become pregnant while breastfeeding. Healthcare providers typically recommend use of additional birth control methods while breastfeeding to avoid another conception occurring too soon to allow a mother's body to recover from the earlier pregnancy.

Mother–Infant Bonding.   Breastfeeding is among the most intimate of human interactions. Ideally, it is a quiet time away from distractions when mother and baby begin to develop an enduring bond of affection known as *attachment.* Breastfeeding enhances attachment by providing the opportunity for frequent, direct skin-to-skin contact, which stimulates the baby's sense of touch and is a

sudden infant death syndrome (SIDS) The sudden death of a previously healthy infant; the most common cause of death in infants over 1 month of age.

primary means of communication.[2] The cuddling and intense watching that occur during breastfeeding begin to teach the mother and baby about the other's behavioral cues. Breastfeeding also reassures the mother that she is providing the best possible nutrition for her baby.

Undoubtedly, bottle-feeding does not preclude parent–infant attachment! As long as attention is paid to closeness, cuddling, and skin and eye contact, bottle-feeding can foster bonding as well.

Convenience and Cost.   Breast milk is always ready, clean, at the right temperature, and available on demand, whenever and wherever it's needed. In the middle of the night, when the baby wakes up hungry, a breastfeeding mother can respond almost instantaneously, and both are soon back to sleep. In contrast, formula-feeding is a time-consuming process: parents have to continually wash and sterilize bottles, and each batch of formula must be mixed and heated to the proper temperature.

In addition, breastfeeding costs nothing other than the price of a modest amount of additional food for the mother. In contrast, formula can be relatively expensive, and there are the additional costs of bottles and other supplies, as well as the cost of energy used for washing and sterilization. A hidden cost of formula-feeding is its effect on the environment: the energy used and waste produced during formula manufacturing, marketing, shipping and distribution, preparation, and disposal of used packaging. In contrast, breastfeeding is environmentally responsible, using no external energy and producing no external wastes.

Challenges Associated with Breastfeeding

For some women and infants, breastfeeding is easy from the very first day. Others experience some initial difficulty, but with support from an experienced nurse, lactation consultant, or volunteer mother from La Leche League, the experience becomes successful and pleasurable. In contrast, some families encounter difficulties that make formula-feeding their best choice. This section discusses some challenges that may impede the success of breastfeeding.

Effects of Drugs and Other Substances on Breast Milk.   Many substances, including illegal, prescription, and over-the-counter drugs, pass into breast milk. Breastfeeding mothers should inform their physician that they are breastfeeding. If a safe and effective form of a necessary medication cannot be found, the mother will have to avoid breastfeeding while she is taking the drug. During this time, she can pump and discard her breast milk so that her milk supply will be adequate when she resumes breastfeeding.

Caffeine and alcohol also enter breast milk. Caffeine can make the baby agitated and fussy, whereas alcohol can make the baby sleepy, depress the central nervous system, and slow motor development, in addition to inhibiting the mother's milk supply. Women who are breastfeeding should abstain from alcohol since it easily passes into the breast milk at levels equal to blood alcohol concentrations. Nicotine also passes into breast milk; therefore, it is best for the woman to quit smoking altogether. Environmental contaminants, including pesticides, industrial solvents, and heavy metals such as lead and mercury, can pass into breast milk when breastfeeding mothers are exposed to these chemicals. Mothers can limit their infants' exposure to these harmful substances by controlling their own environments. Fresh fruits and vegetables should be thoroughly washed and peeled to minimize exposure to pesticides and fertilizer residues. Exposure to paint fumes, gasoline, solvents, and similar products should be greatly limited. Even with some exposure to these environmental contaminants, U.S. and international health agencies all agree that the benefits of breastfeeding almost always outweigh potential concerns.[32]

Food components that pass into the breast milk may seem innocuous; however, some substances, such as those found in garlic, onions, peppers, broccoli, and cabbage, are distasteful enough to the infant to prevent proper feeding. Some babies have allergic reactions to foods the mother ate, such as wheat, cow's milk, eggs, or citrus, and suffer gastrointestinal upset, diaper rash, or another reaction. The offending foods must then be identified and avoided.

Maternal HIV Infection.   HIV, which causes AIDS, can be transmitted from mother to baby through breast milk. Thus, HIV-positive women in the United States and Canada are encouraged to feed their infants formula.[33] This recommendation does not apply to all women worldwide, however, since the low cost and sanitary nature of breast milk, as compared to the potential for waterborne diseases with formula-feeding, often make breastfeeding the best choice for women in developing countries.

Conflict Between Breastfeeding and the Mother's Employment.   Breast milk is absorbed more readily than formula, making more frequent feedings necessary. Newborns commonly require breastfeedings every 1 to 3 hours versus every 2 to 4 hours for formula-feedings. Mothers who are exclusively breastfeeding and return to work within the first 6 months after the baby's birth must leave several bottles of pumped breast milk for others to feed the baby in their absence each day. This means that working women have to pump their breasts to express the breast milk during the work day. This can be a challenge in companies that do not provide the time, space, and privacy required.

Work-related travel is also a concern: if the mother needs to be away from home for longer than 24 to 48 hours, she can typically pump and freeze enough breast milk for others to give the baby in her absence. When longer business trips are required, some mothers bring the baby with them and arrange for childcare at their destination. Others resort to pumping, freezing, and shipping breast milk home via overnight mail. Understandably, many women cite returning to work as the reason they switch to formula-feeding.[34]

Some working women successfully combine breastfeeding with commercial formula. For example, a woman might breastfeed in the morning before she leaves for work, as soon as she returns home, and once again before retiring at night. The remainder of the feedings are formula given by the infant's father or a childcare provider. Women who choose supplemental formula feedings usually find that their bodies adapt quickly to the change and produce ample milk for the remaining breastfeedings.

Social Concerns.   In North America, women have been conditioned to keep their breasts covered in public even when feeding an infant. However, public places are beginning to be more accommodating for nursing mothers. For example, separate nursing rooms can often be found adjacent to, but not within, public restrooms. Some states have passed legislation preserving a woman's right to breastfeed in public (see the Nutrition Debate at the end of this chapter). Special nursing clothing or judicious placement of a scarf or shawl allows women to breastfeed discreetly. When women feel free to breastfeed in public, the baby's feeding schedule becomes much less confining.

What About Bonding for Fathers and Siblings?

With all the attention given to attachment between a breastfeeding mother and infant, it is easy for fathers and siblings to feel left out. One option that allows other family members to participate in infant feeding is to supplement breastfeedings with bottle-feedings of stored breast milk or formula. If a family decides to share infant feeding in this manner, bottle-feedings can begin as soon as breastfeeding has become well established. That way, the infant will not become confused by the artificial nipple. Fathers and other family members can also bond with the infant when bathing and/or clothing the infant as well as through everyday cuddling and play.

> RECAP: *Breastfeeding provides many benefits to both mother and newborn, including superior nutrition, heightened immunity, mother–infant bonding, convenience, and cost. However, breastfeeding may not be the best option for every family. The mother may need to use a medication that enters the breast milk and makes it unsafe for consumption. A mother's job may interfere with the baby's requirement for frequent feedings. The infant's father and siblings can participate in feedings using a bottle filled with either pumped breast milk or formula.*

Fathers and siblings can bond with infants through bottle-feeding.

NUTRI-CASE THEO

> I'm only 21, but my mom is already after me and my girlfriend, Tina, to get married and have babies. In Nigeria, where my folks grew up, people marry a lot younger than here, and they have kids right away. Tina and I talk about it, but we both want to finish school first. Besides, we like to stay out late at the clubs, and who'd be home watching the kids?"

Considering what you've learned so far in this chapter, do you think there is any ideal age at which to have children? If so, what would that age be, and why? What practical information could you suggest Theo offer his mom to justify his decision to wait a few years before starting a family?

Infant Nutrition: From Birth to 1 Year

Most first-time parents are amazed at how rapidly their infant grows. Optimal nutrition is extremely important during the first year, as the baby's organs and nervous system continue to develop and the baby grows physically. In fact, physicians use length and weight measurements as the main tools for assessing an infant's nutritional status. These measurements are plotted on growth charts (there are separate charts for boys and girls), which track an infant's growth over time (FIGURE 19.10). Although every infant is unique, in general, physicians look for a correlation between length and weight. In other words, an infant who is in the 60th percentile for length is usually in about the 50th to 70th percentile for weight. An infant who is in the 90th percentile for weight but is in the 20th percentile for length might be overfed. Consistency over time is also a consideration: for example, an infant who suddenly drops well below her established profile for weight might be underfed or ill.

Typical Infant Growth and Activity Patterns

Babies' basal metabolic rates are high, in part because their body surface area is large compared to their body size. Still, their limited physical activity keeps total energy expenditure relatively low. For the first few months of life, an infant's activities consist mainly of eating and sleeping. As the first year progresses, the repertoire of activity gradually expands to include rolling over, sitting up, crawling, standing, and finally taking the first few wobbly steps. Nevertheless, relatively few calories are expended in movement, and the primary use of energy during the first year of life is to support growth.

In the first year of life, an infant generally grows about 10 inches in length and triples in weight—a growth rate more rapid than will ever occur again. Not surprisingly, energy needs per unit body weight are also the highest they will ever be in order to support this phenomenal growth and metabolism.

Part of the rapid growth of an infant involves the brain, the growth of which is more rapid during the first year than at any other time. To accommodate such a large increase in brain size, infants' heads are typically quite large in proportion to the rest of their bodies. Pediatricians use head circumference as an additional tool for the assessment of growth and nutritional status. After around 18 months of age, the rate of brain growth slows, and gradually the body "catches up" to head size.

An infant's physical activity will progress beyond crawling before the first year of life is over.

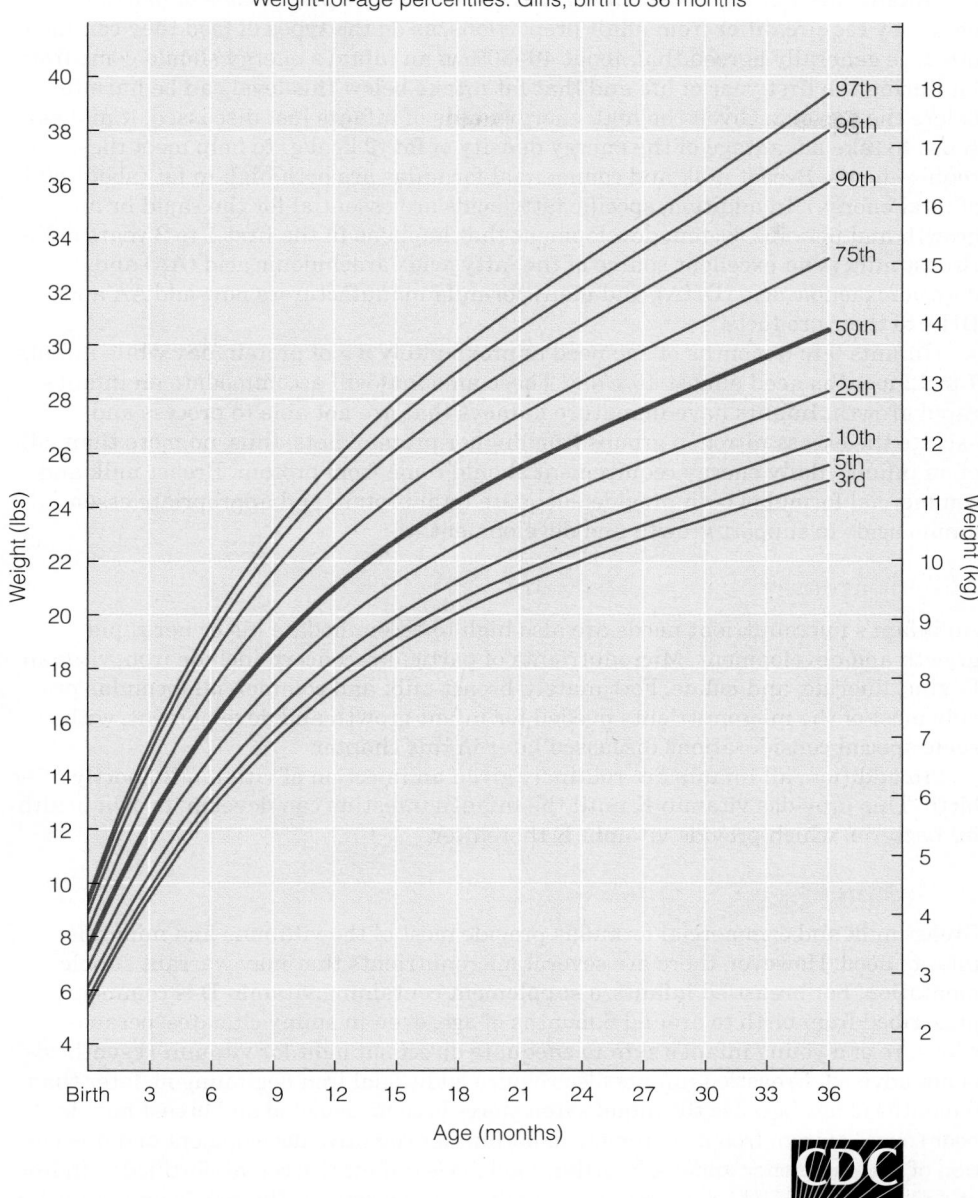

Weight-for-age percentiles: Girls, birth to 36 months

FIGURE 19.10 This weight-for-age growth chart is a much smaller version of charts used by healthcare practitioners to monitor and assess the growth of an infant/toddler from birth to 36 months. This example shows the growth curves of girls over time, each at different percentiles. (Developed by the National Center for Health Statistics in collaboration with the National Center for Chronic Disease Prevention and Health Promotion [2000].)

Nutrient Needs for Infants

Three characteristics of infants combine to make their nutritional needs unique. These are: 1) their high energy needs per unit body weight to support rapid growth; 2) their immature digestive tracts and kidneys; and 3) their small size.

Macronutrient Needs of Infants

An infant needs to consume about 40–50 kcal/lb of body weight per day. This amounts to about 600–700 kcal/day at around 6 months of age. Given the immature digestive tracts and kidneys of infants, as well as their high fluid needs, providing this much energy may seem difficult. Fortunately, breast milk and commercial formulas are energy dense, contributing about 650 kcal/quart of fluid. When solid foods are introduced after about 4 to 6 months of age, they provide even more energy in addition to the breast milk or formula.

Infants are not merely small versions of adults. The proportions of macronutrients they require differ from adult proportions, as do the types of food they can tolerate. It is generally agreed that about 40–50% of an infant's energy should come from fat during the first year of life and that fat intake below this level can be harmful before the age of 2. Given the high energy needs of infants just discussed, it makes sense to take advantage of the energy density of fat (9 kcal/g) to help meet these requirements. Breast milk and commercial formulas are both high in fat (about 50% of total energy). In addition, specific fatty acids are essential for the rapid brain growth and nervous system development that happens in the first 1 to 2 years of life. Breast milk is an excellent source of the fatty acids arachidonic acid (AA) and docosahexaenoic acid (DHA), and many formula manufacturers now add AA and DHA to their products.

Infants 0 to 6 months of age need approximately 9 g of protein/day while infants 7 to 12 months need almost 10 g/day. These amounts will accommodate an infant's rapid growth. Infants have immature kidneys that are not able to process and excrete the excess nitrogen groups from higher-protein diets; thus, no more than 20% of an infant's daily energy requirement should come from protein. Breast milk and commercial formulas both provide adequate total protein and appropriate essential amino acids to support growth and development.

Micronutrient Needs of Infants

An infant's micronutrient needs are also high to accommodate his or her rapid growth and development. Micronutrients of particular concern include iron, vitamin D, zinc, fluoride, and iodide. Fortunately, breast milk and commercial formulas provide most of the micronutrients needed for infant growth and development, with some special considerations discussed later in this chapter.

In addition, all infants are routinely given an injection of vitamin K shortly after birth. This provides vitamin K until the infant's intestine can develop its own healthful bacteria, which provide vitamin K thereafter.

Do Infants Need Supplements?

Breast milk and commercial formulas provide most of the vitamins and minerals infants need. However, there are several micronutrients that may warrant supplementation. For breastfed infants, a supplement containing vitamin D is commonly prescribed from birth to around 6 months of age, even in sunny climates, because exposure of a young infant's skin to adequate direct sunlight for vitamin D synthesis is not advised. Breastfed infants also require additional iron beginning no later than 6 months of age because the infant's iron stores become depleted and breast milk is a poor source of iron. Iron is extremely important for cognitive development and prevention of iron-deficiency anemia. Starting solid foods (infant rice cereal) fortified with iron at 4 to 6 months of age can serve as an additional iron source. Fluoride is important for strong tooth development, but fluoride supplementation is not recommended during the first 6 months of life. In addition, if the mother is a vegan, her breast milk may be low in vitamin B_{12}, and a supplement of this vitamin should be given to the baby.

For formula-fed infants, supplementation depends on the formula composition and the water supply used to make the formula. Many formulas are already fortified with iron, for example, and some municipal water supplies contain fluoride. If this is the case, and the baby is getting adequate vitamin D either in the formula or via sun exposure, then an extra supplement may not be necessary.

If a supplement is given, careful consideration should be given to dose. The supplement should be formulated specifically for infants, and the daily dose should not be exceeded. High doses of micronutrients can be dangerous. Too much iron can be fatal, too much fluoride can cause discoloration and pitting of the teeth, and too much vitamin D can lead to calcification of soft tissues such as the kidney.

Fluid Recommendations for Infants

Fluid is critical for everyone, but for infants the balance is more delicate for two reasons. First, because infants are so small, they proportionally lose more water through evaporation than adults. Second, their kidneys are immature and unable to concentrate urine. Hence, they are at even greater risk of dehydration. An infant needs about 2 oz of fluid per pound of body weight, and either breast milk or formula is almost always enough to provide this amount. Experts recently confirmed that "infants exclusively fed human milk do not require supplemental water."[12] However, there are certain conditions, such as diarrhea, vomiting, fever, or hot weather, which can greatly increase fluid loss. In these instances, supplemental fluid, ideally as water, may be necessary. Since too much fluid can be particularly dangerous for an infant, supplemental fluids (whether water or an infant electrolyte formula) should be given only under the advice of a physician. Generally, it is advised that supplemental fluids not exceed 4 oz per day and parents should avoid giving sugar water, fruit juices, or any sweetened beverage in a bottle. Parents can be reassured that their infant's fluid intake is appropriate if the infant produces six to eight wet diapers per day.

What Types of Formula Are Available?

We discussed the advantages of breastfeeding earlier in this chapter, and indeed both national and international healthcare organizations consider breastfeeding the best choice for infant nutrition, when possible. However, if breastfeeding is not feasible, several types of commercial formulas provide nutritious alternatives. By law, formula manufacturers must meet minimum and maximum standards for 29 different nutrients.

Most formulas are based on cow's milk proteins, casein and whey, that have been modified to make them more appropriate for human infants. The sugars lactose and sucrose, alone or in combination, provide carbohydrates, and vegetable oils and/or microbiologically produced fatty acids provide the fat component.[35] Recently, some manufacturers have added other nutrients to more closely mimic the nutrient profile of human milk. This chapter's Nutrition Label Activity gives you the opportunity to review some of these ingredients.

Soy-based formulas are a viable alternative for infants who are lactose intolerant (although this is rare in infants) or cannot tolerate the proteins in cow's milk–based formulas. Soy formulas may also satisfy the requirements of families who are strict vegans. However, soy-based formulas are not without controversy. Because soy contains isoflavones, or plant forms of estrogens, there is some concern over the effects these compounds have on growing infants. Babies can also have allergic reactions to soy-based formulas.[36] Soy-based formulas are not the same as soy milk, which is not suitable for infant feeding.

There are specialized formula preparations for specific conditions. Some contain proteins that have been predigested, for example, or have compositions designed to accommodate certain medical conditions. Some have been specially formulated for preterm infants, older infants, and toddlers. The final choice of formula should depend on infant tolerance, stage of infant development, cost, and the advice of the infant's pediatrician. Finally, the use of cow's milk (fresh, dried, evaporated, or condensed) is inappropriate for infants under the age of 1 year, as is the use of goat's milk.

When Do Infants Begin to Need Solid Foods?

Infants begin to need solid foods at around 6 months of age. Before this age, several factors make most infants unable to consume solid food.

One factor is the *extrusion reflex*. During infant feeding, the suckling response depends on a particular movement of the tongue that draws liquid out of breast or bottle. But when solid foods are introduced with a spoon, this tongue movement, known as the extrusion reflex, causes the baby to push most of the food back out of the mouth. The extrusion reflex begins to lessen around 4 to 5 months of age.

Another factor is muscle development. To minimize the risk of choking, the infant must have gained muscular control of the head and neck and be able to sit up (with or without support).

Still another part of being ready for solid foods is sufficient maturity of the digestive and kidney systems. While infants can digest and absorb lactose from birth,

The extrusion reflex will push solid food out of an infant's mouth.

NUTRITION LABEL ACTIVITY

Reading Infant Food Labels

Imagine that you are a new parent shopping for infant formula. **FIGURE 19.11** shows the label from a typical can of formula. As you can see, the ingredients list is long and has many technical terms. Even well-informed parents would probably be stumped by many of them. Fortunately, with the information you learned in previous chapters, you can probably answer the following questions.

- The first ingredient listed is a modified form of *whey protein*. What common food is the source of whey?
- The fourth ingredient listed is *lactose*. Is lactose a form of protein, fat, or carbohydrate? Why is it important for infants?
- The front label states the formula has a blend of *DHA* (docosahexaenoic acid) and *ARA* (arachidonic acid). Are DHA and ARA forms of protein, fat, or carbohydrate? Why are these thought to be important for infants?
- The label also claims that this formula is *"Our Closest Formula to Breast Milk."* Can you think of one or two differences between breast milk and this formula that still exist?

Look at the list of nutrients on the label. You'll notice that there is no "% Daily Value" column that you see on most food labels. Next time you are at the grocery store, look at other baby food items, such as baby cereal or pureed fruits. Do their labels simply list the nutrient content or is the "% Daily Value" column used? Why do you think infant formula has a different label format?

Let's say you are feeding a 6-month-old infant who needs about 500 kcal/day. Using the information from the nutrition section of the label, you can calculate the number of fluid ounces of formula the baby needs (this assumes that no cereal or other foods are eaten):

There are 100 kcal (calories) per 5 fl. oz

100 kcal ÷ 5 fl. oz = 20 kcal/fl. oz

500 kcal ÷ 20 kcal/fl. oz = 25 fl. oz of formula per day to meet the baby's energy needs.

A 6-month-old infant needs about 210 mg calcium per day. Based on an intake of 25 fl. oz of formula per day, as just calculated, you can use the label nutrition information to calculate the amount of calcium that is provided:

There are 78 mg calcium per 5 fl. oz serving of formula

78 mg ÷ 5 fl. oz = 15.6 mg calcium per fl. oz

15.6 mg calcium per fl. oz × 25 fl. oz = 390 mg of calcium per day

You can see that the infant's need for calcium is easily met by the formula alone.

the ability to digest starch does not fully develop until the age of 3 to 4 months. If an infant is fed cereal, for example, before he can digest the starch, diarrhea and discomfort may develop. In addition, early introduction of solid foods can lead to improper absorption of intact, undigested proteins, setting the stage for allergies. Finally, the kidneys must have matured so that they are better able to process nitrogen wastes from proteins and concentrate urine.

The need for solid foods is also related to nutrient needs. At about 6 months of age, infant iron stores become depleted; thus, iron-fortified infant cereals are often the first foods introduced. Rice cereal rarely provokes an allergic response and is easy to digest. Once a child reaches 6 months of age, other single-grain cereals, strained vegetables, fruits, and protein sources can gradually be incorporated into the diet.

Infant foods should be introduced one at a time, with no other new foods for about 1 week, so that parents can watch for signs of allergies such as a rash, gastrointestinal problems, a runny nose, or wheezing. Gradually, a variety of foods should be introduced by the end of the first year. Commercial baby foods are convenient, nutritious, and typically made without added salt or sugar; however, home-prepared baby foods are usually cheaper and reflect the cultural food patterns of the family. Throughout the first year, solid foods should only be a supplement to, not a substitute for, breast milk or iron-fortified formula. Infants still need the nutrient density and energy that breast milk and formula provide.

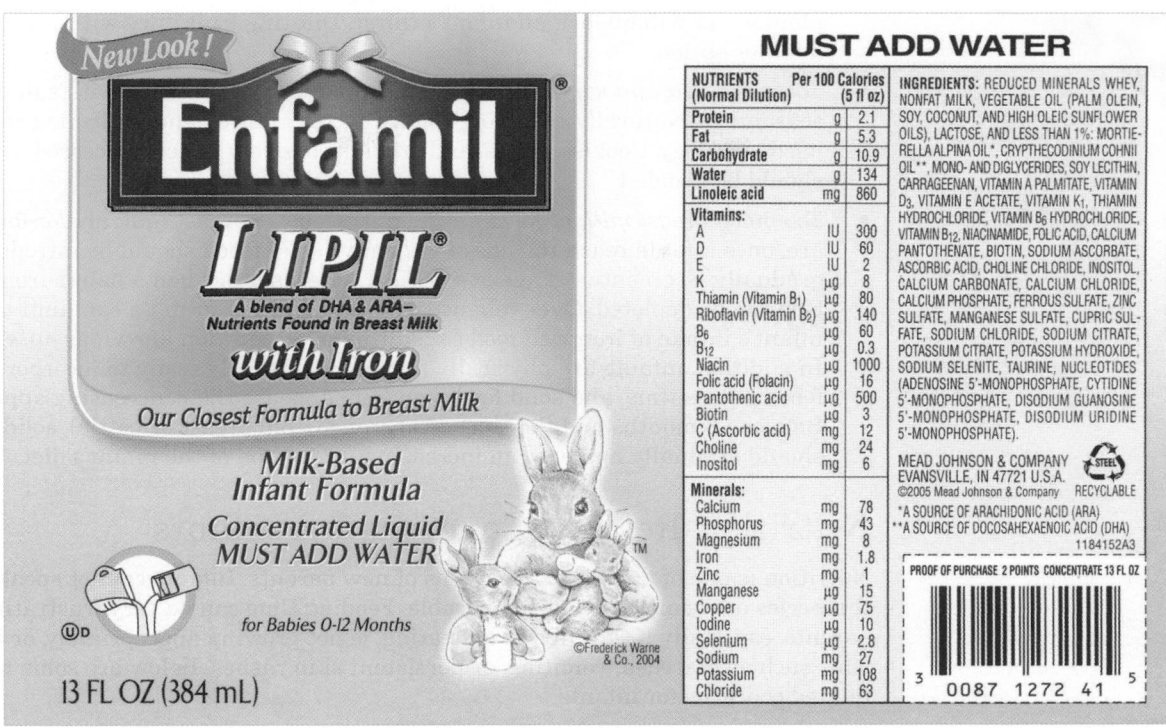

FIGURE 19.11 An infant formula label. Notice that there is a long list of ingredients and no % Daily Value.

What *Not* to Feed an Infant

The following foods should never be offered to an infant:

- *Foods that could cause choking.* Foods such as grapes, hot dogs, nuts, popcorn, raw carrots, raisins, and hard candies cannot be chewed adequately by infants and can cause choking.

- *Corn syrup and honey.* These may contain spores of the bacterium *Clostridium botulinum.* These spores can germinate and grow into viable bacteria in the immature digestive tracts of infants, whereupon they produce a potent toxin that can be fatal. Children older than 1 year can safely consume these substances because their digestive tracts are mature enough to kill any *C. botulinum* bacteria.

- *Goat's milk.* Goat's milk is notoriously low in many nutrients that infants need, such as folate, vitamin C, vitamin D, and iron.

- *Cow's milk.* For children under 1 year, cow's milk is too concentrated in minerals and protein and contains too few carbohydrates to meet infant energy needs. Infants can begin to consume whole cow's milk after the age of 1 year. Infants and toddlers should not be given reduced-fat cow's milk before the age of 2, as it does not contain enough fat and is too high in mineral content for the kidneys to handle effectively. Infants should not be given evaporated milk or sweetened condensed milk.

- *Large quantities of fruit juices.* Fruit juices are poorly absorbed in the infant digestive tract, causing diarrhea if consumed in excess. Large quantities of fruit juice can make an infant feel full and reject breast milk or formula at feeding time, thus causing him or her to miss out on essential nutrients. It is considered safe for infants older than 6 months to consume 4 to 8 oz of pure fruit juice (no sweeteners added) per day, with no more than 2 to 4 oz given at a time; however, plain water will quench an infant's thirst. Diluting fruit juice with water is another option.

- *Too much salt and sugar.* Infant foods should not be seasoned with salt or other seasonings. Naturally occurring sugars such as those found in fruits can provide needed energy. Cookies, cakes, and other excessively sweet, processed foods should be avoided.

- *Too much breast milk or formula.* As nutritious as breast milk and/or formula are, once infants reach the age of 6 months, solid foods should be introduced gradually. Six months of age is a critical time, as it is when a baby's iron stores begin to be depleted. Over-reliance on breast milk or formula can limit the infant's intake of iron-rich foods, resulting in a condition known as *milk anemia.* In addition, infants are physically and psychologically ready to incorporate solid foods at this time, and solid foods can help appease their increasing appetites. Between 6 months and the time of weaning (from breast or bottle), solid foods should gradually make up an increasing proportion of the infant's diet.

Nutrition-Related Concerns for Infants

Nutrition is one of the biggest concerns of new parents. Infants cannot speak, and their cries are sometimes indecipherable. Feeding time can be very frustrating for parents, especially if the child is not eating, is not growing appropriately, or has problems such as diarrhea, vomiting, or persistent skin rashes. Below are some nutrition-related concerns for infants.

Allergies

Many foods have the potential to stimulate an allergic reaction (see page 105). Breastfeeding helps deter allergy development, as does delaying introduction of solid foods until the age of 6 months. One of the most common allergies in infants is to the proteins in cow's milk–based formulas. Egg whites, peanuts, and wheat are other common triggers of food allergies. Symptoms vary but may include gastrointestinal distress such as diarrhea, constipation, bloating, blood in the stool, and vomiting. As stated above, every food should be introduced in isolation, so that any allergic reaction can be identified and the offending food avoided. While 85% of infants with cow's milk or egg allergies can safely tolerate these foods by age 5, only about 20% of infants allergic to peanuts can safely consume them by age 5.

Dehydration

Whether the cause is diarrhea, vomiting, or inadequate fluid intake, dehydration is extremely dangerous to infants, and if left untreated can quickly result in death. The factors behind infants' increased risk of dehydration were discussed on pages 726–727. Treatment includes providing fluids, a task that is difficult if vomiting is occurring. In some cases, the physician may recommend that a pediatric electrolyte solution be administered on a temporary basis. In more severe cases, hospitalization may be necessary. If possible, breastfeeding should continue throughout an illness. A physician should be consulted concerning formula-feeding and solid foods.

Colic

Perhaps nothing is more frustrating to new parents than the relentless crying spells of some infants, typically referred to as **colic.** In this condition, newborns and young infants who appear happy, healthy, and well-nourished suddenly begin to cry or even shriek, and continue no matter what their caregiver does to console them. The spells tend to occur at the same time of day, typically late in the afternoon or early in the

Colicky babies will begin crying for no apparent reason even if they otherwise appear well-nourished and happy.

colic Inconsolable infant crying that lasts for hours at a time.

evening, and often occur daily for a period of several weeks. Crying lasts for hours at a time. Overstimulation of the nervous system, feeding too rapidly, swallowing of air, and intestinal gas pain are considered possible culprits, but the precise cause is unknown.

As with allergies, if a colicky infant is breastfed, breastfeeding should be continued, but the mother should try to determine whether eating certain foods seems to prompt crying and, if so, eliminate the offending food(s) from her diet. Avoidance of spicy or other strongly flavored foods may also help. Formula-fed infants may benefit from a change in type of formula. In the worst cases of colic, a physician may prescribe medication. Fortunately, most cases disappear spontaneously, possibly because of maturity of the gastrointestinal tract, around 3 months of age.

Anemia

As stated earlier, full-term infants are born with sufficient iron stores to last for approximately the first 6 months of life. In older infants and toddlers, however, iron is the mineral most likely to be deficient. Iron-deficiency anemia causes pallor, lethargy, and impaired growth. Iron-fortified formula is a good source for formula-fed infants. Some pediatricians prescribe a supplement containing iron especially formulated for infants. Iron for older infants is typically supplied by iron-fortified rice cereal.

Nursing Bottle Syndrome

Infants should never be left alone with a bottle, whether lying down or sitting up. As infants manipulate the nipple of the bottle in their mouths, the high-carbohydrate fluid (whether breast milk, formula, or fruit juice) drips out, coming into prolonged contact with the developing teeth. This high-carbohydrate fluid provides an optimal food source for bacteria that are the underlying cause of **dental caries** (cavities). Severe tooth decay can result (FIGURE 19.12). Encouraging the use of a cup around the age of 8 months helps prevent nursing bottle syndrome, along with weaning the baby from a bottle entirely by the age of 15 to 18 months.

FIGURE 19.12 Leaving a baby alone with a bottle can result in the tooth decay of nursing bottle syndrome.

Lead Poisoning

Lead is especially toxic to infants and children because their brains and central nervous systems are still developing. Lead poisoning can result in decreased mental capacity, behavioral problems, impaired growth, impaired hearing, and other problems. Unfortunately, leaded pipes and lead paint can still be found in older homes and buildings. Measures to reduce lead exposure include:

- Allowing tap water to run for a minute or so before use, to clear the pipes of any lead-contaminated water

- Using only cold tap water for drinking and cooking, as hot tap water is more likely to leach lead.

- Professionally removing lead-based paint, or painting it over with latex paint.

> RECAP: *Infancy is characterized by the most rapid growth a human being will ever experience, and appropriate growth is the most reliable long-term indicator of adequate infant nutrition. Infants need large amounts of energy per unit body weight to keep up with growth. Breast milk or iron-fortified formula provides all necessary nutrients for the first 6 months of life. After that, solid foods can gradually be introduced into an infant's diet. Micronutrient supplements should be given only if prescribed. Infants must be monitored for allergies, dehydration, and other signs of distress.*

dental caries Dental erosion and decay caused by acid-secreting bacteria in the mouth and on the teeth. The acid produced is a by-product of bacterial metabolism of carbohydrates deposited on the teeth.

CHAPTER SUMMARY

- Nutrition is important before conception because critical stages of cell division, tissue differentiation, and organ development occur in the early weeks of pregnancy, often before a woman even knows she is pregnant.

- A plentiful, nourishing diet is important throughout pregnancy to provide the nutrients needed to support fetal development without depriving the mother of nutrients she needs to maintain her own health.

- A normal pregnancy progresses over the course of 38 to 42 weeks. This time is divided into three trimesters of 13 to 14 weeks. Each trimester is associated with particular developmental phases of the embryo/fetus.

- Pregnant women of normal weight should consume adequate energy to gain 25 to 35 pounds during pregnancy. Women who are underweight should gain slightly more, and women who are overweight or obese should gain less.

- Pregnant women need to be especially careful to consume adequate amounts of folate, vitamin B_{12}, vitamin C, vitamin D, calcium, iron, and zinc. A supplement is often prescribed to ensure adequate intake of these nutrients.

- A majority of pregnant women experience nausea and/or vomiting during pregnancy, called morning sickness, and many crave or feel aversions to specific types of foods and nonfood substances.

- Heartburn and constipation in pregnancy are related to the relaxation of smooth muscle caused by certain pregnancy-related hormones.

- Gestational diabetes and hypertensive disorders of pregnancy are nutrition-related conditions that can seriously affect maternal and fetal health.

- The bodies of adolescents are still growing and developing; thus, their nutrient needs during pregnancy are higher than those of adult pregnant women.

- Dieting during pregnancy leads to inadequate nutrition for mother and fetus.

- Alcohol, tobacco, and illegal drugs harm the fetus and should not be consumed in any amount during pregnancy. All women are strongly advised to stop drinking alcohol, smoking, and taking illegal drugs before becoming pregnant.

- Successful breastfeeding requires the coordination of several hormones, including estrogen, progesterone, prolactin, and oxytocin. These hormones govern the preparation of the breasts, as well as actual milk production and the let-down response.

- Breastfeeding women require more energy than they did during pregnancy. Protein needs increase, and an overall nutritious diet with plentiful fluids is important in maintaining milk quality and quantity, as well as preserving the mother's health.

- The advantages of breastfeeding include nutritional superiority of breast milk, protection from infections and allergies, promotion of attachment, convenience, and lower cost.

- Breastfeeding exclusively for at least the first 6 months of a baby's life is recommended by both North American and international healthcare organizations.

- Difficulties that might be encountered with breastfeeding include effect of medications on breast milk, scheduling conflicts for mothers who return to work, and social concerns.

- Infants are characterized by their extremely rapid growth and brain development.

- Physicians use length and weight measurements as the main tools for assessing an infant's nutritional status.

- An infant needs to consume about 40–50 kcal/lb of body weight/day.

- Because infant stores of iron become depleted after about 6 months, an iron supplement is sometimes prescribed for breastfeeding infants.

- Breast milk or formula is entirely sufficient for the first 6 months of life. After that, solid foods can be introduced (rice cereal fortified with iron at first) and expanded gradually, with breast milk or formula remaining very important throughout the first year.

- Infants need to be monitored carefully for appropriate growth and appropriate number of wet diapers every day to assess adequate nutrient intake and hydration.

- Nutrition-related concerns for infants include the potential for allergies, dehydration, colic, anemia, nursing bottle syndrome, and ingestion of lead.

TEST YOURSELF ANSWERS

1. **False.** Pregnant women need only 350–450 additional calories per day, and only during the second and third trimesters of pregnancy. This is an increase of only 20% or less, not a doubling of calories.

2. **False.** More than half of all pregnant women experience morning sickness, and food cravings or aversions are also common.

3. **True.** Breast milk contains various immune factors (antibodies and immune system cells) from the mother that protect the infant against infection. The nutrients in breast milk are structured to be easily digested by an infant, resulting in fewer symptoms of gastrointestinal distress and fewer allergies.

4. **True.** Caffeine quickly passes into breast milk, as do alcohol and most prescription and over-the-counter medications.

5. **False.** Most infants do not have a physiologic need for solid food until about 6 months of age.

REVIEW QUESTIONS

1. Folate deficiency in the first weeks after conception has been linked with which of the following problems in the newborn?
   a. anemia
   b. neural tube defects
   c. low birth weight
   d. preterm delivery

2. Which of the following hormones is responsible for the let-down response?
   a. progesterone
   b. estrogen
   c. oxytocin
   d. prolactin

3. Which of the following nutrients should be added to the diet of breast fed infants when they are around 6 months of age?
   a. fiber
   b. fat
   c. iron
   d. vitamin D

4. A pregnancy weight gain of 28 to 40 pounds is recommended for
   a. all women.
   b. women who begin their pregnancy underweight.
   c. women who begin their pregnancy overweight.
   d. women who begin their pregnancy at a normal weight.

5. The best solid food to introduce first to infants is
   a. cream of wheat cereal.
   b. applesauce.
   c. teething biscuits.
   d. iron-fortified rice cereal.

6. True or false? Major developmental errors and birth defects are most likely to occur in the third trimester of pregnancy.

7. True or false? Women who are breastfeeding require a higher energy intake than they needed when they were pregnant.

8. True or false? Growth is a key indicator of adequate infant nutrition.

9. True or false? Fetal alcohol effects can occur in children born to mothers who drink only two alcoholic beverages per day during pregnancy.

10. True or false? If gestational diabetes is uncontrolled, the fetus may not receive enough glucose and may be born small for gestational age.

11. Explain the relationship between the increased need for iron and the increased need for fluid in a pregnant woman.

12. Identify five advantages and five disadvantages of breastfeeding. Can you think of others?

13. Your cousin, who is pregnant with her first child, tells you that her physician prescribed supplemental iron tablets for her but that she decided not to take them. "You know me," she says, "I'm a natural food nut! I'm absolutely certain that my careful diet is providing all the nutrients my baby needs!" Is it possible that your cousin is partly right and partly wrong? Explain.

14. You visit your neighbors one afternoon to congratulate them on the birth of their new daughter, Katie. While you are there, 2-week-old Katie suddenly starts crying as if she is in terrible pain. "Oh, no," Katie's dad says to his wife. "Here we go again!" He turns to you and explains, "She's been like this every afternoon for the past week, and it goes on until sunset. I just wish we could figure out what we're doing wrong." What would you say?

15. You are on a picnic at a park with your friend Lila, who drapes a shawl over her shoulders and breastfeeds her 14-month-old son. A woman walking by stops and says, "Isn't that child getting too old for that?" What information could you share with her in response to her question?

FIND THE QUACK

Three weeks ago, Kaitlyn gave birth to her first child, Sean, whom she has been breastfeeding successfully. Or at least, she thinks so. But sometimes she finds herself wondering whether or not her breast milk is providing everything her son needs to grow up healthy and strong. This afternoon, while Sean naps, she leafs through a magazine and notices an ad for infant formula: it looks so thick and creamy in comparison to her breast milk, which looks thin and watery. On the next page, she sees another ad. "Are you breastfeeding?" it asks. "If so, congratulations on making this healthy choice. But how can you be sure you're meeting all of your infant's nutrient needs?" Attracted by the healthy-looking newborn in the photo, Kaitlyn reads the full-page ad, which promotes an infant vitamin supplement called First Days "ID" Drops. She reads:

- Mother's milk provides almost all of the nutrition a growing baby needs. But two vital nutrients are low in breast milk. These are iron and vitamin D.

- Both iron and vitamin D are low in breast milk. Both are critical to your baby's growth and health.

- Available without a prescription, First Days "ID" Drops will provide your baby with the level of iron and vitamin D he or she needs.

- For pennies a day, First Days "ID" Drops will safeguard your baby's growth and health.

1. Kaitlyn is consuming a diet rich in iron and vitamin D. Could her breast milk nevertheless be low in these two nutrients? Why or why not?

2. Kaitlyn's newborn Sean is 3 weeks old. Does Sean need to consume iron in either breast milk or a supplement? Why or why not? Does Sean need supplemental vitamin D? Why or why not?

3. The ad states that First Days "ID" Drops are "available without a prescription." Should Kaitlyn consult her healthcare provider before giving her baby these drops? Why or why not?

4. Does the ad for First Days "ID" Drops suggest that this is a legitimate product, or would you characterize it as an example of quackery? Defend your position.

Answers can be found at www.aw-bc.com/thompson.

WEB LINKS

http://aappolicy.aappublications.org
American Academy of Pediatrics

Visit this Web site for information on infants' and children's health. Searches can be performed for topics such as "neural tube defects" or "infant formulas."

http://fnic.nal.usda.gov
Food and Nutrition Information Center

Click on See Topics A–Z and then Child Nutrition and Health for a list of infant nutrition topics and a listing of child nutrition programs, links, and resources.

www.emedicine.com/ped
eMedicine: Pediatrics

Select Toxicology and then Toxicity, Iron to learn about accidental iron poisoning and its signs in children and infants.

www.marchofdimes.com/pnhec/pnhec.asp
March of Dimes

Click on During Your Pregnancy to find links on nutrition during pregnancy, exercise, and things to avoid.

www.diabetes.org
American Diabetes Association

Search for "gestational diabetes" to find information about diabetes that develops during pregnancy.

www.lalecheleague.org
La Leche League

Search this site to find multiple articles on the health effects of breastfeeding for mother and infant.

www.obgyn.net
OBGYN.net

Visit this site to learn about pregnancy health and nutrition, as well as breastfeeding and infant nutrition.

www.nofas.org
National Organization on Fetal Alcohol Syndrome

This site provides news and information relating to fetal alcohol syndrome.

www.helppregnantsmokersquit.org
The National Partnership for Smoke-Free Families

A site created for healthcare providers and smokers with the purpose of educating about the dangers of smoking while pregnant and providing tools to help pregnant smokers quit.

REFERENCES

1. Kleinman, R. E. (ed). 2004. *Pediatric Nutrition Handbook,* 5th edn. Elk Grove Village, IL: American Academy of Pediatrics.
2. Olds, S. B., M. L. London, P. W. Ladewig, and M. R. Davidson. 2003. *Maternal-Newborn Nursing and Women's Health Care,* 7th ed. Upper Saddle River, NJ: Prentice Hall Health.
3. Ramakrishnan, U. 2004. Nutrition and low birth weight: from research to practice. *Am. J. Clin. Nutr.* 79(1):17.

4. Luke, B., M. L. Hediger, C. Nugent, R. B. Newman, J. G. Mauldin, F. R. Witter, and M. J. O'Sullivan. 2003. Body mass index-specific weight gains associated with optimal birth weights in twin pregnancies. *J. Reprod. Med.* 48:217–224.

5. Oken, E., E. M. Taveras, K. P. Kleinman, J. W. Rich-Edwards, and M. W. Gillman. 2007. Gestational weight gain and child adiposity at age 3 years. *Am. J. Obstet. Gynecol.* 196(4):322.

6. Institute of Medicine, Food and Nutrition Board, Board on Children, Youth, and Families. 2006. *Influence of Pregnancy Weight on Maternal and Child Health: Workshop Report Influence of Pregnancy Weight on Maternal and Child Health.* Washington, DC: National Academies Press.

7. U.S. Department of Health & Human Services. 2007. Breastfeeding, Maternal & Infant Health Outcomes in Developed Countries. www.ahrq.gov/clinic/tp/brfouttp.htm. (Accessed August 2007.)

8. Centers for Disease Control and Prevention (CDC). 2003. Folic Acid Now. www.cdc.gov/ncbddd/fact/folicfaqs.htm. (Accessed August 2007.)

9. Institute of Medicine, Food and Nutrition Board. 1998. *Dietary Reference Intakes for Thiamin, Riboflavin, Niacin, Vitamin B_6, Folate, Vitamin B_{12}, Pantothenic Acid, Biotin, and Choline.* Washington, DC: National Academies Press.

10. Institute of Medicine, Food and Nutrition Board. 1997. *Dietary Reference Intakes for Calcium, Phosphorus, Magnesium, Vitamin D, and Fluoride.* Washington, DC: National Academies Press.

11. Whittaker, P. 1998. Iron and zinc interactions in humans. *Am. J. Clin. Nutr.* 68:442S–446S.

12. Institute of Medicine, Food and Nutrition Board. 2004. *Dietary Reference for Water, Potassium, Sodium, Chloride, and Sulfate.* Washington, DC: National Academies Press.

13. von Dadelszen, P. 2000. The etiology of nausea and vomiting in pregnancy. In: G. Koren, and R. Bishai, eds. *Nausea and Vomiting of Pregnancy.* First International Congress on NVP. www.nvp-volumes.org/index.htm. (Accessed August 2007.)

14. Kittler, P. G., and K. P. Sucher. 2003. *Food and Culture,* 4th edn. Belmont, CA: Brooks/Cole Publisher.

15. Benyshek, D. C., J. F. Martin, and C. S. Johnston. 2001. A reconsideration of the origins of type 2 diabetes epidemic among Native Americans and the implications for intervention policy. *Med. Anthropol.* 20(1):25–64.

16. Dabelea, D., R. L. Hanson, P. H. Bennett, J. Roumain, W. C. Knowler, and D. J. Pettitt. 1998. Increasing prevalence of type 2 diabetes in American Indian children. *Diabetologia* 41:904–910.

17. Roberts, C. L., C. S. Algert, J. M. Morris, J. B. Ford, and D. J. Henderson-Smart. 2005. Hypertensive disorders in pregnancy: a population-based study. *Med. J. Aust.* 182:332–335.

18. Barnet, B., A. K. Duggan, and M. Devoe. 2003. Reduced low birth weight for teenagers receiving prenatal care at a school-based health center: effect of access and comprehensive care. *J. Adolesc. Health* 33(5):349–358.

19. Harding, J. E. 2001. The nutritional basis of the fetal origins of adult disease. *Int. J. Epidemiol.* 30:15–23.

20. March of Dimes. 2005. Quick Reference: Fact Sheets: Caffeine in Pregnancy. Article R 4-07. www.marchofdimes.com (search on the term "coffee"). (Accessed August 2007.)

21. March of Dimes. 2005. Quick Reference: Fact Sheets: Drinking Alcohol During Pregnancy. Article 09-404-00. www.marchofdimes.com (search on the term "preconception risk reduction: drinking alcohol during pregnancy"). (Accessed August 2007.)

22. Centers for Disease Control and Prevention (CDC). 2007. Preventing smoking during pregnancy. www.cdc.gov/nccdphp/publications/factsheets/Prevention/smoking. (Accessed August 2007.)

23. Substance Abuse and Mental Health Services Administration. 2004. *Overview of Findings from the 2003 National Survey on Drug Use and Health.* NSDUH Series H-24, DHHS Publication No. 04-3963. Rockville, MD: Office of Applied Studies.

24. U.S. Department of Health and Human Services and U.S. Department of Agriculture. 2005. Dietary Guidelines for Americans 2005, 6th edn. Washington, DC: U.S. Government Printing Office. www.healthierus.gov/dietaryguidelines. (Accessed August 2007.)

25. Lumbers, E. R. 2002. Exercise in pregnancy: physiological basis of exercise prescription for the pregnant woman. *J. Sci. Med. Sport* 5(1):20–31.

26. U.S. Department of Health and Human Services, Health Resources and Services Administration. 2005. *Women's Health USA 2005: Health Status: Maternal Health: Breastfeeding.* Rockville, MD: U.S. Department of Health and Human Services. http://mchb.hrsa.gov/whusa_05/pages/0428breastfeed.htm. (Accessed August 2007.)

27. UNICEF (United Nations Children's Fund). 2003. Protecting, Promoting and Supporting Breastfeeding. www.unicef.org/nutrition/index_breastfeeding.html. (Accessed August 2007.)

28. Porter, D. V. 2003. Breastfeeding: Impact on Health, Employment, and Society. CRS Report for Congress. Congressional Research Service. The Library of Congress. www.breastfeeding.org/law/CRS1.pdf. (Accessed August 2007.)

29. American Academy of Pediatrics (AAP), Section on Breast Feeding. 2005. Breast feeding and the use of human milk policy statement. *Pediatrics* 115:496–506.

30. Collaborative Group on Hormonal Factors in Breast Cancer. 2003. Breast cancer and breastfeeding: collaborative reanalysis of individual data from 47 epidemiological studies in 30 countries, including 50,302 women with breast cancer and 96,973 women without the disease. *Lancet* 360:187–195.

31. Grimes, J. P., and S. J. Wimalawansa. 2003. Breastfeeding and postmenopausal osteoporosis. *Curr. Women's Health Rep.* 3(3):193–198.

32. Bauchner, E. 2004. Environmental contaminants and human milk. *LEAVEN* 39:123–125.

33. Jackson, D. J., M. Chopra, C. Witten, and M. J. Sengwana. 2003. HIV and infant feeding: Issues in developed and developing countries. *J. Obstet. Gynecol. Neonatal Nurs.* 32(1):117–127.

34. Adams, C., R. Berger, P. Conning, L. Cruikshank, and K. Dore. 2001. Breastfeeding trends at a community breastfeeding center: an evaluative survey. *J. Obstet. Gynecol. Neonatal Nurs.* 30(4):392–400.

35. Uauy, R., and P. Mena. 1999. Requirements for long-chain polyunsaturated fatty acids in the preterm infant. *Curr. Opin. Pediatr.* 11(2):115–120.

36. American Academy of Pediatrics (AAP). 2000. Policy Statement, Committee on Nutrition. Hypoallergenic Infant Formulas (RE0005). www.aap.org/policy/re0005.html. (Accessed August 2007.)

37. U.S. Department of Health & Human Services: *Healthy People 2010: With Understanding and Improving Health and Objectives for Improving Health.* 2 vols. 2000. Washington, DC: U.S. Government Printing Office. www.healthypeople.gov/document/HTML/Volume2/16MICH.htm. (Accessed August 2007.)

38. Weimer, D. R. 2003. Summary of state breastfeeding laws. CRS Report for Congress. Congressional Research Service. The Library of Congress. www.breastfeeding.org/law/CRS2.pdf. (Accessed August 2007.)

39. Oliver, L., and H. G. A. Park. 2004. *Maternal and Child Health: A Snapshot for State Legislatures.* Denver, CO: National Conference of State Legislators.

40. Baldwin, E. N., and K. A. Friedman. 2004. A current summary of breastfeeding legislation in the U.S. La Leche League International. www.lalecheleague.org/Law/Bills4.html. (Accessed August 2007.)

41. Eichna, C. 2007. Lactation legislation on the move. *City Hall News* January 2007. http://cityhallnews.com/012207/news3_012207.html. (Accessed August 2007.)

NUTRITION DEBATE

Should Breastfeeding Be Allowed in Public and in the Workplace?

a woman sitting at the food court at the mall is openly breastfeeding. A colleague excuses herself from an important meeting to pump her breast milk in the restroom. How do you feel about these two scenarios? Do they make you uncomfortable? How do you feel about a woman being excused from jury duty because she is breastfeeding, or a guard removing a woman from a public legislative session because she was breastfeeding her infant during the proceedings? Should maternity leave benefits be extended for women who are exclusively breastfeeding? Should a working woman be allowed paid break time to breastfeed, or should this time away from her work be unpaid? What rights do you feel a breastfeeding mother should have?

The benefits of breastfeeding for infant health are well established. One of the objectives of the U.S. Public Health Service is to increase the number of women who breast-feed their infants for at least the first 6 months of life.[37] Despite this and other endorsements, there remain a number of social and workplace restrictions on breastfeeding.

For example, some Americans feel that breastfeeding in public is indecent, and some public places, including restaurants, bookstores, and retail stores, have asked breastfeeding women to leave or stop nursing.[38] In fact, only sixteen states have legislation that specifically

exempts breastfeeding from being classified as indecent exposure. Thus, although breastfeeding in public is more common than it was 20 years ago, there is still a great deal of pressure for mothers to breastfeed only in private settings. Unfortunately, because breastfed babies require far more frequent feedings than formula-fed babies, and many breastfed babies refuse artificial nipples, this pressure to breastfeed in private can severely restrict the ability of these mothers to feed their babies when their babies show they want to be fed.

What about jury duty? Although it doesn't at first seem fair that breastfeeding women should be allowed an exemption, consider the consequences if exclusively breastfeeding women were forced to serve. Bringing the baby to court would inevitably cause disruptions whenever the baby fussed, cried, or needed diaper changes. In fact, many courtrooms have policies banning children outright. Leaving the baby behind would be equally unacceptable, as babies who are exclusively breastfed are unlikely to suddenly accept an artificial nipple and thus would go without food and hydration.

As you have learned in this chapter, breastfeeding mothers who work outside the home face additional challenges, including lack of privacy and time to pump breast milk at the worksite. Some of this lack of support for breastfeeding at worksites most likely stems from the historical facts that, throughout much of the 20th century, most mothers of young children stayed home, and worksite environments were designed for men. Although millions of mothers now work outside of the home, the social norms are relatively slow to change. Think of how challenging it must be for a female police officer to find

Some breastfed babies refuse to take a bottle.

Although breastfeeding is a much more common practice today than in the past, many people still consider it inappropriate to breastfeed in public.

the time and opportunity to pump breast milk. Most of her colleagues are males, and the work environment is typically fast-paced and demanding. Women returning to work in these types of environments are more likely to give up breastfeeding.

Numerous incidences of outright harassment of working women who breastfeed include the following:

- Not allowing women to pump breast milk during lunch or other sanctioned work breaks.
- Withholding pay from women who use work time to pump breast milk.
- Assigning women to less desirable work shifts as punishment for breastfeeding.
- Laying off or firing women who request time to express milk during standard working hours.

Ironically, working women who continue to breastfeed despite such harassment actually have less absenteeism due to infant-related illnesses as compared to working mothers who do not breastfeed.[39]

Because of these instances of social and worksite harassment, breastfeeding legislation has been enacted in over half of the states in the United States. It is important to emphasize that breastfeeding is not illegal, and legislation is not necessary to legalize this natural act. The primary purpose of legislation is to clarify that women have a right to breastfeed in public, and they should not be harassed or shunned if they do so.[40] Weimer reports that as of 2005, thirty-nine states, as well as Puerto Rico, had enacted legislation related to breastfeeding.[38] Many states have legislation stating that breastfeeding in public is not illegal, and twenty-five states permit women to breastfeed in any public or private location where children and mothers are authorized to be. Seven states exempt women from jury duty if they are breastfeeding, and ten states and Puerto Rico have laws related to the accommodation of breastfeeding mothers who return to work.[38] U.S. Congresswoman Carolyn Maloney (NY) has worked since the late 1990s to enact federal legislation that goes much further in supporting

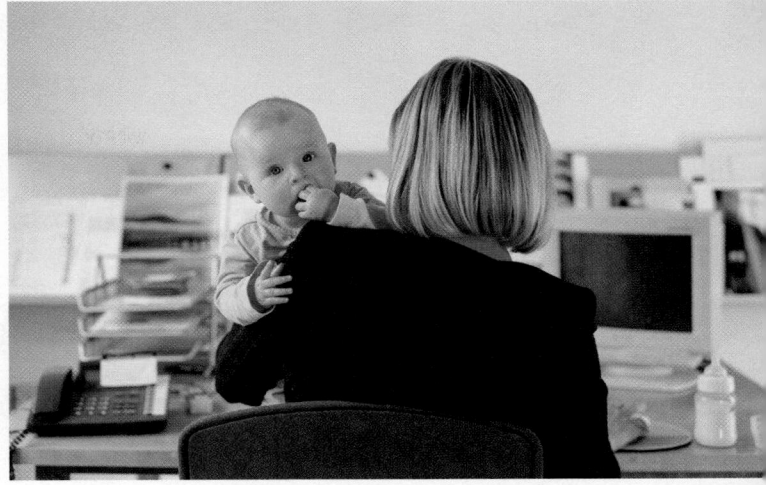

Working moms can be discouraged from breastfeeding.

breastfeeding mothers who go back to work.[41] If passed, this bill would:[40]

- Provide a tax credit to employers who set up a lactation location, purchase or rent lactation equipment, hire a health professional, or take other actions to promote a lactation-friendly environment.
- Ensure that breastfeeding is protected under civil rights law.
- Require the FDA to develop minimum quality standards for breast pumps.

What do you think of this legislation? Is it necessary? Does it go far enough? Does it go too far? What rights do you feel breastfeeding women should have? And what about infants—do they have a right to breastfeed? This debate will likely continue as both national and international healthcare organizations continue to urge policy makers, healthcare providers, and business leaders to support breastfeeding.

CHAPTER OBJECTIVES

After reading this chapter you should be able to:

1. Compare and contrast the growth and activity patterns of toddlers and children, pp. 740–746.

2. List at least three nutrients of concern when feeding a vegan diet to young children, pp. 744–746.

3. List at least two factors that can increase risk of obesity during childhood and adolescence, pp. 750–752 and 756–757.

4. Define puberty and describe how it influences changes in body composition, pp. 753–754.

5. Explain why adequate intakes of calcium and vitamin D are particularly important during the adolescent years, p. 755.

6. Identify at least three physiologic changes that occur with aging and describe how these changes affect nutrient needs of older adults, pp. 759–765.

7. Give two reasons why older adults may not be able to drink adequate amounts of fluid, p. 765.

8. Discuss several changes in health that can contribute to inadequate nutrient intake in older adults, pp. 765–769.

TEST YOURSELF TRUE OR FALSE?

1. Toddlers should be fed nonfat milk products to reduce their risk for obesity. T or F

2. The average girl reaches almost full height by the onset of menstruation. T or F

3. It is now believed that diet has virtually no role in the development of acne. T or F

4. Participating in regular physical activity can delay or reduce some of the loss of muscle mass that occurs with aging. T or F

5. Experts agree that, within the next 20–30 years, the human life span will exceed 150 years. T or F

Test Yourself answers can be found after the Chapter Summary.

Nutrition Through the Life Cycle:
Childhood to Late Adulthood

O n Sunday afternoons, the Sophat family gathers for dinner at the Long Beach apartment of their 88-year-old matriarch, Leng. Only 5 feet tall, Leng is as thin as a rail, as is her 70-year-old daughter and 67-year-old son. But when her granddaughters, who are cooking the family meal, send everyone to the table, a change becomes evident. Almost all of Leng's grandchildren and their spouses are overweight, as are most of her great-grandchildren. Even her "darling," 4-year-old great-great-granddaughter Jewel, is chubby. Leng worries about everyone's weight. Back home in Cambodia, overweight was rare and a sign of health, but here in America, it seems to bring illness. One of her grandsons has had a heart attack, and many in her family have been diagnosed with type 2 diabetes. Leng's family isn't alone in their weight problems: more than 17% of American children and adolescents (age 6 to 19 years) are overweight, along with more than 66% of American adults.[1] And type 2 diabetes, which afflicts about 10% of Asian Americans, occurs in about 6% of all Americans.[2]

Why have rates of obesity and its associated chronic diseases skyrocketed in the past 10 years, and what can be done to promote weight management across the life span? How do our nutrient needs change as we grow and age, and what other nutrition-related concerns develop in each life stage? This chapter will help you answer these questions.

Toddlers expend significant amounts of energy actively exploring their world.

Nutrition for Toddlers, Ages 1–3 Years

As babies begin to walk and explore, they transition out of infancy and into the active world of toddlers. During the second and third years of life, a toddler will grow a total of about 5.5 to 7.5 inches and gain an average of 9 to 11 pounds. Toddlers need to consume a lot of energy to fuel their increasing levels of activity as they explore their ever-expanding world and develop new skills. But feeding a toddler raises new challenges for parents and caregivers.

What Are a Toddler's Nutrient Needs?

Nutrient needs increase as a child progresses from infancy to toddlerhood. Although toddlers' rate of growth has slowed, their increased nutrient needs reflect their larger body size and increased activity. Refer to Table 20.1 for a review of specific nutrient recommendations.

Energy and Macronutrient Recommendations for Toddlers

Although the energy requirement per kilogram of body weight for toddlers is just slightly less than for infants, *total* energy requirements are higher because toddlers

TABLE 20.1 Nutrient Recommendations for Children and Adolescents

Nutrient	Toddlers (1–3 years)	Children (4–8 years)	Children (9–13 years)	Adolescents (14–18 years)
Fat	No DRI	No DRI	No DRI	No DRI
Protein	1.10 g/kg body weight per day	0.95 g/kg body weight per day	0.95 g/kg body weight per day	0.85 g/kg body weight per day
Carbohydrate	130 g/day	130 g/day	130 g/day	130 g/day
Vitamin A	300 μg/day	400 μg/day	600 μg/day	Boys = 900 μg/day Girls = 700 μg/day
Vitamin C	15 mg/day	25 mg/day	45 mg/day	Boys = 75 mg/day Girls = 65 mg/day
Vitamin E	6 mg/day	7 mg/day	11 mg/day	15 mg/day
Calcium	500 mg/day	800 mg/day	1,300 mg/day	1,300 mg/day
Iron	7 mg/day	10 mg/day	8 mg/day	Boys = 11 mg/day Girls = 15 mg/day
Zinc	3 mg/day	5 mg/day	8 mg/day	Boys = 11 mg/day Girls = 9 mg/day
Fluid	1.3 liters/day	1.7 liters/day	Boys = 2.4 liters/day Girls = 2.1 liters/day	Boys = 3.3 liters/day Girls = 2.3 liters/day

are larger and much more active than infants. The estimated energy requirements (EERs) vary according to the toddler's age, body weight, and level of activity.[3] In general, toddlers should consume a diet that provides energy to sustain a healthy and appropriate rate of growth.

Although there is currently insufficient evidence to set a DRI for fat for toddlers, healthy toddlers of appropriate body weight should consume 30–40% of their total daily energy intake as fat.[3] We know that fat provides a concentrated source of energy in a relatively small amount of food, and this is important for toddlers, especially those who are fussy eaters or have little appetite. Fat is also necessary during the toddler years to support the continuously developing nervous system.

Toddlers' protein needs increase modestly because they weigh more than infants and are still growing rapidly. The RDA for protein for toddlers is 1.10 g/kg body weight per day, or approximately 13 g of protein daily.[3] Remember that 2 cups of milk alone provide 16 g of protein; thus, most toddlers have little trouble meeting their protein needs.

The RDA for carbohydrate for toddlers is 130 g/day, and carbohydrate intake should be about 45–65% of total energy intake.[3] As is the case for older children and adults, most of the carbohydrates eaten should be complex, and refined carbohydrates from high-fat/high-sugar items such as desserts and snack foods should be kept to a minimum. Fruits and fruit juices are nutritious sources of simple carbohydrates that can also be included. Keep in mind, however, that too much fruit juice can displace other foods and can cause diarrhea. The American Academy of Pediatrics recommends that the intake of fruit juice be limited to 4–6 fl.oz/day for children 1 to 6 years of age.[4]

Adequate fiber is important for toddlers to maintain regularity. The AI is 14 g of fiber per 1,000 kcal of energy, or, on average, 19 g/day.[3] Whole-grain cereals, fresh fruits and vegetables, and whole-grain breads are healthful choices for toddlers. Too much fiber, however, can inhibit the absorption of iron, zinc, and other essential nutrients, harm the toddler's small digestive tract, and cause satiation before the toddler has consumed adequate nutrients.

Determining the macronutrient requirements of toddlers can be challenging. See the You Do the Math box for analysis of the macronutrient levels in one toddler's daily diet.

Micronutrient Recommendations for Toddlers

As toddlers grow, their micronutrient needs increase (Table 20.1). Of particular concern with toddlers is adequate intake of the minerals calcium and iron.

Calcium is necessary for children to promote optimal bone mass, which continues to accumulate until early adulthood. For toddlers, the AI for calcium is 500 mg/day.[5] Dairy products are excellent sources of calcium. When a child reaches the age of 1 year, whole cow's milk can be given; however, reduced-fat milk (2% or less) should *not* be given until age 2 due to the relatively high need for total energy. If dairy products are not feasible, calcium-fortified orange juice or soy milk can supply calcium, or children's calcium supplements can be given. Toddlers generally cannot consume enough food to depend on alternate calcium sources such as dark-green vegetables.

Iron-deficiency anemia is the most common nutrient deficiency in young children in the United States and around the world. Iron-deficiency anemia can affect a child's energy level, attention span, and mood. The RDA for iron for toddlers is 7 mg/day.[6] Good sources of well-absorbed heme iron include lean meats, fish, and poultry; non-heme iron is provided by eggs, legumes, greens, and fortified foods such as breakfast cereals. When toddlers consume non-heme sources of iron, a source of vitamin C at the same meal will enhance the absorption of iron from these sources.

Fluid Recommendations for Toddlers

Toddlers lose less fluid from evaporation than infants, and their more mature kidneys are able to concentrate urine, thereby sparing fluid. However, as toddlers become active, they start to lose significant fluid through sweat, especially in hot weather. Parents need to make sure an active toddler is drinking adequately. The

YOU DO THE MATH %=+>

Is This Menu Good for a Toddler?

A dedicated mother and father want to provide the best nutrition for their young son, Ethan, who is now 1½ years old and has just been completely weaned from breast milk. Ethan weighs about 26 pounds (or 11.8 kg). Below is a typical day's menu for Ethan. Grams of protein, fat, and carbohydrate are given for each food. The day's total energy intake is 1,168 kcal. Calculate the percentage of Ethan's calories that come from protein, fat, and carbohydrate (the numbers may not add up to exactly 100% because of rounding). In what areas are Ethan's parents doing well, and where could they use some advice for improvement?

Note: This activity focuses on the macronutrients. It does not ask you to consider Ethan's intake of micronutrients or fluids.

Meal	Foods	Protein (g)	Fat (g)	Carbo-hydrate (g)
Breakfast	Oatmeal (½ cup, cooked)	2.5	1.5	13.5
	Brown sugar (1 tsp.)	0	0	4
	Milk (1%, 4 fl. oz)	4	1.25	5.5
	Grape juice (4 fl. oz)	0	0	20
Mid-morning Snack	Banana slices (1 small banana)	0	0	16
	Yogurt (nonfat, fruit flavored, 3 fl. oz)	5.5	0	15.5
	Orange juice (4 fl. oz)	1	0	13
Lunch	Whole-wheat bread (1 slice)	1.5	0.5	10
	Peanut butter (1 tbsp.)	4	8	3.5
	Strawberry jam (1 tbsp.)	0	0	13
	Carrots (cooked, ⅛ cup)	0	0	2
	Applesauce (sweetened, ¼ cup)	0	0	12
	Milk (1%, 4 fl. oz)	4	1.25	5.5
Afternoon Snack	Bagel (½)	3	1	20
	American cheese product (1 slice)	3	5	1
	Water	0	0	0
Dinner	Scrambled egg (1)	11	5	1
	Baby food spinach (3 oz.)	2	0.5	5.5
	Whole-wheat toast (1 slice)	1.5	0.5	10
	Mandarin orange slices (¼ cup)	0.5	0	10
	Milk (1%, 4 fl. oz)	4	1.25	5.5

Calculations:

There is a total of 47.5 g protein in Ethan's menu.

47.5 g × 4 kcal/g = 190 kcal
190 kcal protein/1,168 total kcal × 100 = 16% protein

There is a total of 25.75 g fat in Ethan's menu.

25.75 g × 9 kcal/g = 232 kcal
232 kcal fat/1,168 total kcal × 100 = 20% fat

There is a total of 186.5 g carbohydrate in Ethan's menu.

186.5 g × 4 kcal/g = 746 kcal
746 kcal carbohydrate/1,168 total kcal × 100 = 64% carbohydrate

Analysis: Ethan's parents are doing very well at offering a wide variety of foods from various food groups; they are especially doing well with fruits and vegetables. Also, according to his estimated energy requirement, Ethan requires about 970 kcal/day, and he is consuming 1,168 kcal/day, thus meeting his energy needs.

Ethan's total carbohydrate intake for the day is 186.5 g, which is higher than the RDA of 130 g/day; however, this value falls within the recommended 45–65% of total energy intake that should come from carbohydrates. Thus, high carbohydrate intake is adequate to meet his energy needs.

However, Ethan is being offered far more than enough protein. The DRI for protein for toddlers is about 13 g/day, and Ethan is being offered more than three times that much!

It is also readily apparent that Ethan is being offered too little fat for his age. Toddlers need at least 30–40% of their total energy intake from fat, and Ethan is only consuming about 20% of his calories from fat. He should be drinking whole milk, not 1% milk. He should occasionally be offered higher-fat foods like cheese for his snacks or macaroni and cheese for a meal. Yogurt is fine, but it shouldn't be nonfat at Ethan's age.

In conclusion, Ethan's parents should be commended for offering a variety of nutritious foods but should be counseled that a little more fat is critical for toddlers' growth and development. Some of the energy currently being consumed as protein and carbohydrate should be shifted to fat.

recommended fluid intake for toddlers is listed in Table 20.1, and includes about 4 cups as beverages, including drinking water.[7] Suggested beverages include plain water, milk and soy milk, diluted fruit juice, and foods high in water content, such as vegetables and fruits.

Do Toddlers Need Nutritional Supplements?

Toddlers can be well nourished by consuming a balanced, varied diet. But given their typically erratic eating habits, the child's physician may recommend a multivitamin and mineral supplement as a precaution against deficiencies. The toddler's physician or dentist may also prescribe a fluoride supplement, if the community water supply is not fluoridated. Supplements should be considered for any child at risk for deficiency of one or more nutrients. These may include children in vegan families, children from families who cannot afford adequate amounts of nourishing foods, children with certain medical conditions or dietary restrictions, or very picky or erratic eaters.

As always, if a supplement is given, it should be formulated especially for toddlers and the recommended dose should not be exceeded. A supplement should not contain more than 100% of the Daily Value of any nutrient per dose.

> RECAP: *Growth during toddlerhood is slower than during infancy; however, toddlers are highly active and need to consume enough energy to fuel growth and activity. Total energy, fat, and protein requirements are higher for toddlers than for infants. While all forms of milk can be used to meet calcium requirements, until age 2, toddlers should drink energy-rich whole milk rather than reduced-fat (2% or lower) milk. Iron deficiency is a concern in the toddler years and can be avoided by feeding toddlers lean meats / fish / poultry, eggs, and iron-fortified foods. Toddlers need to drink about 4 cups of water or other beverages per day.*

Encouraging Nutritious Food Choices with Toddlers

Parents and pediatricians have long known that toddlers tend to be choosy about what they eat. Some avoid entire food groups, such as all meats or vegetables. Others will refuse all but one or two favorite foods (such as peanut butter on crackers) for several days or longer. Still others eat in extremely small amounts, seemingly satisfied by a single slice of apple or two bites of toast. These behaviors frustrate and worry many parents, but in fact, as long as a variety of healthful food is available, toddlers have the ability to match their intake with their needs. A toddler will most likely make up for one day's deficiency later on in the week. Parents who offer only nutritious foods can feel confident that their children are being well fed, even if a child's choices seem odd or erratic on any particular day. Food should never be "forced" on a child, as doing so sets the stage for eating and control issues later in life.

It is also important to recognize that toddlers' stomachs are still very small, and they cannot consume all of the calories they need in three meals. Toddlers need small meals, interspersed with nutritious snacks, every 2 to 3 hours. A successful technique is to create a snack tray filled with small portions of nutritious food choices, such as one-third of a banana, two pieces of cheese, and two whole-grain biscuits, and leave it within reach of the child's play area. The child can then "graze" on these healthful foods while he or she plays. A snack tray plus a spill-proof cup of milk or water is particularly useful on car trips.

Foods prepared for toddlers should be developmentally appropriate. Nuts, carrots, grapes, raisins, and cherry tomatoes are difficult for a toddler to chew and pose a choking hazard. Foods should be soft and sliced into strips or wedges that are easy for children to grasp. As the child develops more teeth and becomes more coordinated, the range of food can become more varied.

Foods prepared for toddlers should also be fun (FIGURE 20.1). Parents can use cookie cutters to turn a peanut butter sandwich into a pumpkin face, or arrange cooked peas or carrot slices to look like a smiling face on top of mashed potatoes. Juice and low-fat yogurt can be frozen into "popsicles" or blended into "milkshakes."

FIGURE 20.1 Most toddlers are delighted by food prepared in a fun way.

FIGURE 20.2   Portion sizes for preschoolers are much smaller than those for older children. Use the following guideline: 1 tbsp. of the food for each year of age equals 1 serving. For example, the meal shown here—2 tbsp. of rice, 2 tbsp. of black beans, and 2 tbsp. of chopped tomatoes—is appropriate for a 2-year-old toddler.

A positive environment helps toddlers develop good mealtime habits as well. Parents should consistently seat the toddler in the same place at the table and make sure that the child is served first. Television and other distractions should be turned off, and pleasant conversation should include the toddler, even if the toddler hasn't begun to speak. Toddlers should not be forced to sit still until they finish every bite as they still have short attention spans.

Even at mealtime, portion sizes should be small. One tablespoon of a food for each year of age constitutes a serving throughout the toddler and preschool years (FIGURE 20.2). Realistic portion sizes can give toddlers a sense of accomplishment when they "eat it all up" and minimize parents' fears that their child is not eating enough.

New foods should be introduced gradually. Most toddlers are leery of new foods, spicy foods, hot (temperature) foods, mixed foods such as casseroles, and foods with strange textures. A helpful rule is to encourage the child to eat at least one bite of a new food: if the child does not want the rest, nothing negative should be said and the child should be praised just for the willingness to try. The food should be reintroduced a few weeks later. Eventually, after several tries, the child might accept the food. Some foods, however, won't be accepted until well into adulthood as tastes expand and develop. Parents should never bribe with food, for example, promising dessert if the child finishes her squash. Bribing teaches children that food can be used to reward and manipulate. Instead, parents can try to positively reinforce good behaviors, for example, "Wow! You ate every bite of your squash! That's going to help you grow big and strong!"

Role modeling is important since toddlers emulate older children and adults: if they see their parents eating a variety of healthful foods, they will be likely to do so as well. Providing limited healthful alternatives will also help toddlers make nutritious food choices. For example, parents might say, "It's snack time! Would you like apples and cheese or bananas and yogurt?" Finally, toddlers are more likely to eat food they help prepare: encourage them to assist in the preparation of simple foods, such as helping pour a bowl of cereal or helping to arrange the raw vegetables on a plate.

Nutrition-Related Concerns for Toddlers

Just as toddlers have their own specific nutrient needs, they also have toddler-specific nutrition concerns, while others continue from infancy.

Continued Allergy Watch

As during infancy, new foods should be presented one at a time, and the toddler should be monitored for allergic reactions for a week before additional new foods are introduced. To prevent the development of food allergies, even foods that are established in the diet should be rotated, rather than served every day.

Overweight: A Concern Now?

Believe it or not, signs indicating a tendency toward overweight can occur as early as the toddler years. Toddlers should *not* be denied nutritious food; however, they should not be forced or encouraged to eat when they are full. In the toddler years, a child who is above the 80th percentile for weight (one who weighs more than 80% of children of the same age and height) should be monitored. These children should be encouraged and supported in increasing their physical activity, and, as for all children, intake of foods with low nutritional value should be limited.

Foods that may cause allergies, such as peanuts and citrus fruits, should be introduced to toddlers one at a time.

Vegetarian Families

For toddlers, a lacto-ovo-vegetarian diet in which dairy foods and eggs are included can be as wholesome as a diet including meats and fish. However, because red meat is an excellent source of zinc and heme iron, families who do not serve red meat must be careful to include enough zinc and iron from other sources in their child's diet.

In contrast, a vegan diet, in which no foods of animal origin are consumed, poses several potential nutritional risks for toddlers:

NUTRITION MYTH OR FACT?

Are Vegan Diets Appropriate for Young Children?

A glance at the headlines reveals that feeding a vegan diet to young children is a controversial issue. Strong proponents of veganism state that any consumption of animal products is wrong and that feeding animal products to children is forcing them into a life of obesity, clogged arteries, and chronic diet-related diseases. In addition, many people who consume a vegan diet feel that consumption of animal products wastes natural resources and contributes to environmental damage and is therefore morally wrong. In contrast, strong antagonists of veganism emphasize that feeding a vegan diet to young children deprives them of essential nutrients that can only be found in animal products. Some people even suggest that veganism for young children is, in essence, a form of child abuse.

As with many controversies, there are truths on both sides. For example, there have been documented cases of children failing to thrive, and even dying, on extreme vegan diets.[8–11] Cases have been cited of protein deficiency as well as vitamin B_{12} and other micronutrient deficiencies in vegan children. The nutrients of concern are found primarily or almost exclusively in animal products, and deficiencies can have serious and lifelong consequences. For example, not all of the neurologic impairments caused by vitamin B_{12} deficiency can be reversed by timely B_{12} supplement intervention. In addition, inadequate zinc, calcium, and vitamin D can result in impaired bone growth and strength, failure to reach peak bone mass, and retarded growth in general.

However, close inspection of the cases of nutrition-related illness in children that cite veganism as the culprit reveals that lack of education, fanaticism, and/or extremism is usually at the root of the problem. Informed parents following a responsible vegan diet are rarely involved. On the other hand, such cases do point to the importance of education in the challenges of this diet. Specifically, parents need to know which nutrients are not available in plant products and therefore must be supplemented. They also need to understand that typical vegan diets are high in fiber and low in fat, a combination that can be dangerous for very young children.[12] Moreover, certain staples of the vegan diet, such as wheat, soy, and nuts, commonly provoke aller-

gic reactions in children; when this happens, finding a plant-based substitute that contains adequate nutrients can be challenging.

Both the American Dietetic Association and the American Academy of Pediatrics have stated that a vegan diet can promote normal growth and development—provided that adequate supplements and/or fortified foods are consumed to account for the nutrients that are normally found in animal products. However, most healthcare organizations stop short of outright endorsement of a vegan diet for young children. Instead, many advocate a more moderate approach during the early childhood years. Reasons for this level of caution include acknowledgment of several factors:

- Some vegan parents are not adequately educated on the planning of meals, the balancing of foods, and the inclusion of supplements to ensure adequate levels of all nutrients.
- Most young children are picky eaters and are hesitant to eat certain food groups, particularly vegetables, a staple in the vegan diet.
- The high fiber content of vegan diets may not be appropriate for very young children.
- Young children have small stomachs, and they are not able to consume enough plant-based foods to ensure adequate intakes of all nutrients and energy.

Because of these concerns, most nutrition experts advise parents to take a more moderate dietary approach, one that emphasizes plant foods but also includes some animal-based foods, such as fish, dairy, and/or eggs.

Once children reach school age, the low fat, abundant fiber, antioxidants, and many micronutrients in a vegan diet will promote their health as they progress into adulthood. However, those who consume animal products can also live a healthful life and reduce their risk for chronic diseases by choosing low-fat, nutrient-dense foods such as lean meats, nonfat dairy products, whole grains, and fruits and vegetables. When a varied diet is consumed, there are fewer worries about consuming adequate amounts of all nutrients.

- Protein—Vegan diets can be too low in protein for toddlers, who need protein for growth and increasing activity. Few toddlers can consume enough legumes and whole grains to provide sufficient protein. The high fiber content of legumes and whole grains results in a rapid sense of fullness for toddlers, decreasing their total food intake.

Enriched foods such as fortified soy milk should be given to toddlers consuming vegan diets.

- Calcium, zinc, and iron—Calcium is a concern because of the avoidance of milk, yogurt, and cheese. As with protein, few children can consume enough calcium from plant sources to meet their daily requirement, and supplementation is advised. Zinc and iron are also commonly low in vegan diets due to the absence of meat, poultry, and seafood.

- Vitamins D and B_{12}—Both vitamins are typically lower in strict vegan diets. Vitamin B_{12} is not available in any amount from plant foods and must be supplemented.

- Fiber—Vegan diets often contain a higher amount of fiber than is recommended for toddlers, resulting in lowered absorption of iron and zinc as well as the early onset of fullness or satiety.

Although adults following a vegan diet have the ability to choose alternative foods and/or supplements to meet the demands for these nutrients, toddlers must depend on their parents to make appropriate food choices for them. If parents are very dedicated to maintaining a vegan diet for their toddler, choices such as fortified juices, soy milk, and other soy products, along with judicious supplement use, should be employed to ensure adequate nutrition.

The practice of feeding a vegan diet to infants and young children is highly controversial. See the Nutrition Myth or Fact? box on page 745 for more information about this controversy.

RECAP: *Toddlers require small, frequent, nutritious meals and snacks, and food should be cut in small pieces so it is easy to handle, mash, and swallow. Because toddlers are becoming more independent and can self-feed, parents need to be alert for choking and should watch for allergies and monitor weight gain. Role modeling by parents and access to ample healthful foods can help toddlers make nutritious choices. Feeding vegan diets to toddlers is controversial and poses potential deficiencies for protein, calcium, zinc, iron, vitamin D, and vitamin B_{12}.*

Nutrition for Children, Ages 4–13 Years

Children develop increased language fluency, enhanced decision-making skills, and improved physical coordination and dexterity. During the preschool and school-age years, growth rate slows. Children grow an average of 2 to 4 inches per year at a slow and steady pace, the "calm before the storm" of adolescence, when growth rates again become very rapid. For children age 6–11, the USDA has produced a MyPyramid for Kids poster (FIGURE 20.3) advising children to "Eat Right. Exercise. Have Fun." The nutrient requirements and nutrition issues of importance to preschool and school-aged children are discussed in this section.

Children grow an average of 2 to 4 inches per year.

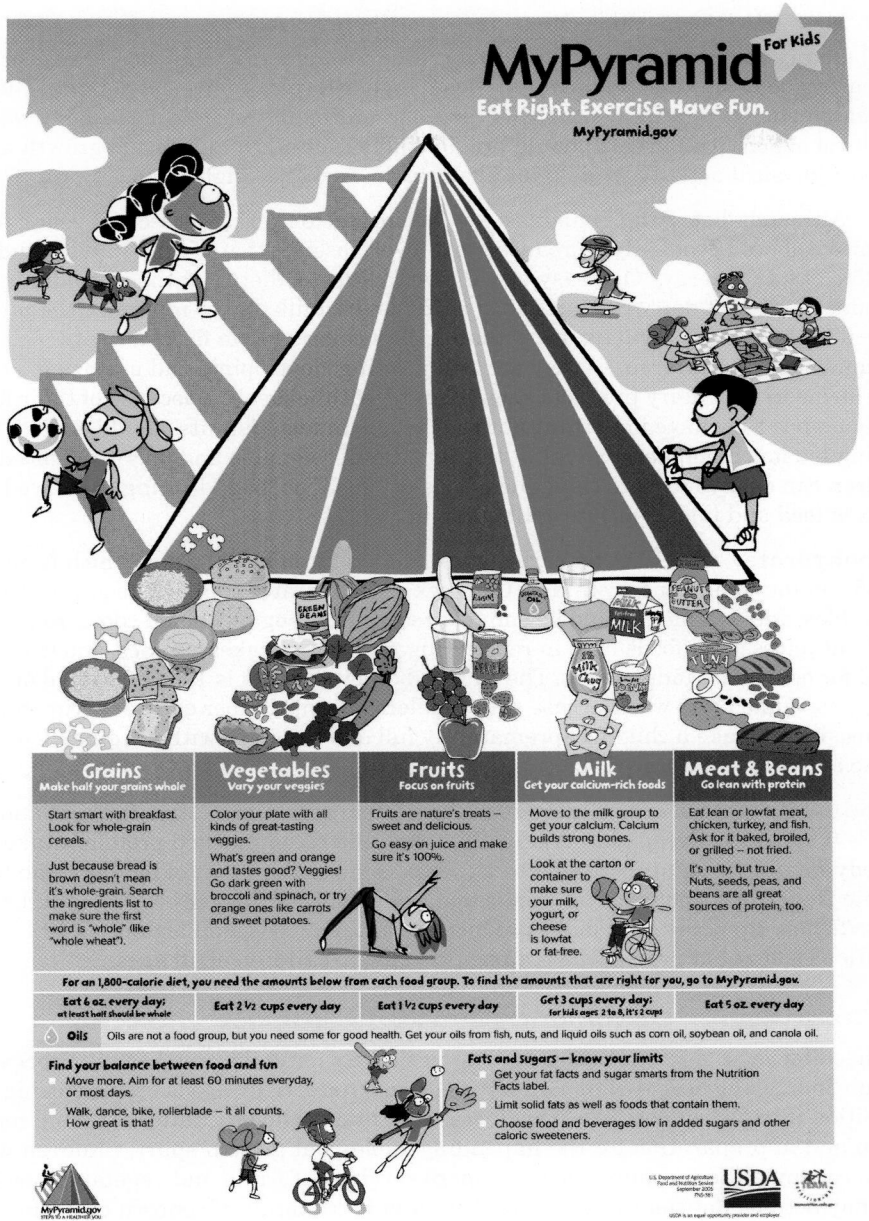

FIGURE 20.3 MyPyramid for Kids. This symbol modifies the MyPyramid graphic for the nutrition needs of children, and teaches them to "Eat Right. Exercise. Have Fun."

What Are a Child's Nutrient Needs?

Until the age of 8 or 9 years, the nutrient needs of young boys and girls do not differ; because of this, the DRI values for the macronutrients, fiber, and micronutrients are grouped together for children aged 4 to 8. The beginning of sexual maturation, however, is an important phenomenon that has a dramatic impact on the nutrient needs of children. Boys' and girls' bodies develop differently in response to gender-specific hormones. These changes in sexual maturation can begin subtly between the ages of 8 and 9 years; thus, the DRI values are separately defined for boys and girls age 9 to 13 years.[3] Table 20.1 (page 740) identifies the nutrient needs of children and adolescents.

Energy and Macronutrient Recommendations for Children

Total energy requirements continue to increase throughout childhood because of increasing body size and, for some children, higher levels of physical activity. The estimated energy requirement (EER) varies according to the child's age, body weight, and level of activity. Parents should provide diets that allow for normal growth and support physical activity while minimizing risk of excess weight gain.

Fat. Although dietary fat remains a key macronutrient in the preschool years, total fat intake should gradually be reduced to a level closer to that of an adult, around 25–35% of total energy.[3] One easy way to start reducing dietary fat is to gradually introduce lower-fat dairy products such as 2% or 1% milk and to minimize the intake of fried foods. A diet providing fewer than 25% of calories from fat is not recommended for children, as they are still growing, developing, and maturing. Foods such as meats and dairy products should not be withheld solely because of their fat content since they have important nutrient value. In fact, parents should avoid putting too much emphasis on fat at this age. Impressionable and peer-influenced children can easily be led to categorize foods as "good" or "bad," leading to skewed views of food and inappropriate eating habits.

Carbohydrate. The RDA for carbohydrate for children is 130 g/day, which is about 45–65% of total daily energy intake. Complex carbohydrates from whole grains, fruits, vegetables, and legumes should be emphasized. Simple sugars should come from fruits and fruit juices, with foods high in refined sugars, such as cakes, cookies, and candies, saved for occasional indulgences. The AI for fiber for children is 14 g/1,000 kcal of energy consumed.[3] As was the case with toddlers, too much fiber can be detrimental because it can make a child feel prematurely full and interfere with adequate food intake and nutrient absorption.

Children's multivitamins often appear in shapes or bright colors.

Protein. As you can see in Table 20.1, the protein recommendation for boys and girls is 0.95 g/kg body weight per day.[3] Although the recommended protein intake per kg body weight for children aged 4 to 13 years is lower than that of toddlers, the total protein intake of school-age children is higher due to their higher body weight. Lean meats/fish/poultry, lower-fat dairy products, soy-based foods, and legumes are nutritious sources of protein that can be provided to children of all ages.

Micronutrient Recommendations for Children

The need for most micronutrients increases slightly for children up to age 8 because of their increasing size. A sharper increase in micronutrient needs occurs during the transition into full adolescence; this increase is due to the beginning of sexual maturation and in preparation for the impending adolescent growth spurt. Children who fail to consume the recommended 5 or more servings of fruits and vegetables each day may become deficient in vitamins A, C, and E. Minerals of concern continue to be calcium, iron, and zinc, which come primarily from animal-based foods.[5] Notice that the RDA for iron is based on the assumption that most girls do not begin menstruation until after age 13.[6] Refer to Table 20.1 for a review of the nutrient needs of children.

If there is any concern that a child's nutrient needs are not being met for any reason (for instance, breakfasts are skipped, lunches are traded, parents lack money for nourishing food), a vitamin/mineral supplement that provides no more than 100% of the daily value for the micronutrients may help to correct any existing deficit.

Fluid Recommendations for Children

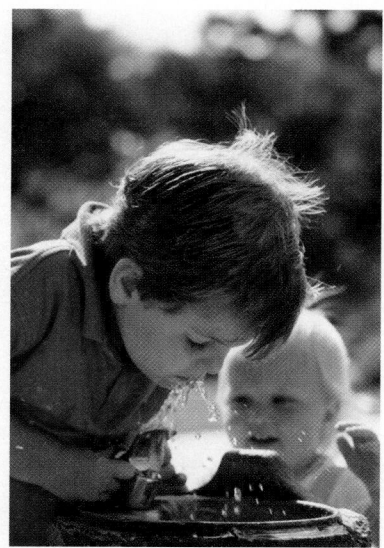

Fluid intake is important for children, who may become so involved in their play that they ignore the sensation of thirst.

The fluid recommendations for children are listed in Table 20.1 and include about 5–8 cups as beverages, including drinking water. The exact amount of fluid needed varies according to a child's level of physical activity and weather conditions. At this point in life, children are mostly in control of their own fluid intake. However, as they engage in physical activity at school and in sports and play, young children in particular may need reminders to drink in order to stay properly hydrated, especially if the weather is hot.

RECAP: *Total protein and energy needs are higher for children due to their larger size and higher activity levels. Dietary fat should be gradually reduced to the level of 25–35% of total energy. Calcium, iron, and zinc requirements are higher for children than toddlers. Children need to drink from 5 to 8 cups of water and other beverages throughout the day.*

Encouraging Nutritious Food Choices with Children

Peer pressure can be extremely difficult for both parents and their children to deal with during this life stage. Most children want to feel as if they "belong," and they admire and like to emulate children they believe to be popular. If the popular children at school are eating chips and drinking sugared soft drinks, it may be hard for a child to eat a peanut butter on whole wheat sandwich, apple, and low-fat milk without embarrassment.

Parents and children can work together, using age-appropriate language and concepts, to find compromises by regularly communicating about healthful nutrition. One strategy that parents might consider is to introduce their kids to "cool" role models such as star athletes or popular entertainers who follow nutritious diets. Continuing to involve children in family food choices and in meal preparation is also a good idea. If they have input into what is going into their bodies, children may be more likely to take an active role in their health. In addition, parents should continue to act as healthful role models to maintain consistent messages and images that children can rely upon when establishing their own eating and physical activity patterns.

What Is the Effect of School Attendance on Nutrition?

A child's school attendance can affect his or her nutrition in several ways. First, in the hectic time between waking and getting out the door, many children minimize or skip breakfast completely. If the entire morning is spent in a state of hunger, they are more likely to do poorly on schoolwork, have decreased attention spans, and have more behavioral problems than their peers who do eat breakfast.[13,14] For this reason, public schools now offer low- or no-cost school breakfasts. These breakfasts help children to optimize their nutrient intake and avoid the behavioral and learning problems associated with hunger in the classroom.

Another consequence of attending school is that, with little or no supervision of what they eat, children do not always consume appropriate types or amounts of food. They may spend their lunch time conversing or playing with friends rather than eating. If they purchase a school lunch, they might not like the foods being served, or their peers might influence them to skip certain foods with comments such as "This broccoli is yucky!" Even homemade lunches that contain nutritious foods may be left uneaten or traded for less nutritious fare.

Finally, some schools continue to advertise and sell soft drinks and snack foods in exchange for additional revenues to maintain school programs. Also, despite recent legislation and industry-sponsored initiatives, some schools still provide vending machines offering snacks that are high in energy, sugar, and fat. Eating too many of these foods, either in place of or in addition to lunch, can lead to overweight and potential nutrient deficiencies.

Are School Lunches Nutritious?

On the surface, the answer to this question is "yes." Although based on old (1989) nutrient standards, all school lunches must meet certain nutrition requirements set forth by federal guidelines. Every lunch must provide one-third of the 1989 RDAs for protein, vitamin A, vitamin C, iron, calcium, and energy.[15] No more than 10% and 30% of the total energy in a meal should come from saturated fat and total fat, respectively.

However, when examining this question in more detail, the answer is not so clear. This is because the actual nutrients a student *gets* depends on what the student actually *eats*. School lunch programs do not have to meet the federal guidelines

School-age children may receive a standard school lunch, but many young people choose to eat less healthful foods when given the opportunity.

every day, but only over the course of a week's meals.[16] As a result, the school lunches that students actually eat tend to be higher in fat than the guideline because students tend to favor pizza, hamburgers, hot dogs, and French fries over the more nutritious entrees and side dishes offered. Some schools actually have fast-food restaurants selling their food in competition with the school lunch program! Thus, even though school lunches as *planned* are considered a healthful choice, children may not be getting the benefit of these meals.

The good news is that many schools are working to ensure a more healthful food environment. This change in environment is due to the efforts of nutrition experts, school administrators and lunch program personnel, parents, and even former U.S. President Bill Clinton. Working with the beverage industry, he helped develop a series of voluntary industry guidelines in order to limit school-based sales of soft drinks and other high-sugar, low-nutrient beverages. The Institute of Medicine developed a set of related nutrition standards for foods and beverages in schools.[17] Competitive foods providing at least one serving of fruit, vegetables, and/or whole-grain or low-/no-fat dairy products, such as low-fat fruit granola bars or skim milk, would have the fewest restrictions, while foods of lower nutrient value would be either banned or tightly restricted in terms of when and where they could be sold. At the local level, attention to nutrition is resulting in the offering of healthful alternatives such as salad bars and is changing how foods are bought and prepared by food service staff. One school-based obesity prevention study in Native American schools found that by educating food service staff about healthful food purchasing and preparation, the fat content of school breakfasts and lunches could be reduced without sacrificing nutritional quality.[18,19]

RECAP: *Peer pressure has a strong influence on nutritional choices in children. Involving children in food purchasing and meal planning and preparation can help them make more healthful food choices. Skipping breakfast can reduce a child's school performance. School lunches are nutritious as planned and must meet federal guidelines, but the foods that children choose to eat at school can be high in fat, sugar, and energy and low in complex carbohydrates and micronutrients. Recent efforts, including state, federal, and industry guidelines, represent a shift toward a more healthful profile of school-based sales of competitive foods.*

Nutrition-Related Concerns for Children

In addition to potential nutrient deficiencies that have already been discussed, new concerns arise during childhood.

Childhood Overweight: Encouraging an Active Lifestyle

Overweight in children is now epidemic in the United States. Using the CDC classification system, children are **at risk for overweight** when their BMI is at or above the 85th percentile, that is, the child's body mass index is higher than that of 85% of U.S. children of the same age and gender. A child is considered by the CDC to be **overweight** if his or her BMI is above the 95th percentile. These classifications do not precisely align with the terminology used with adults (see Chapter 11), but regardless of the terminology, children in the United States are experiencing the same trends of inappropriate weight gain seen in the adult population: as noted in the introduction to this chapter, more than 17% of children age 6 to 19 are overweight.[1]

Overweight children are at higher risk of becoming overweight adults than are normal weight children, so preventing childhood overweight is important for the long-term health and happiness of the child. It is also important for the child's current health and happiness: even in early childhood, significant overweight can worsen asthma, cause sleep apnea, impair the child's mobility, and lead to intense teasing, low self-esteem, and social isolation. Children and adolescents who are overweight are at greater risk for type 2 diabetes, elevated blood pressure, and other medical problems. Parents should not be offended if the child's pediatrician, school nurse, or other healthcare provider expresses concern over the child's weight status; early intervention is often the most effective measure against lifelong obesity.

at risk for overweight (childhood) Having a body mass index (BMI) at or above the 85th percentile.

overweight (childhood) Having a body mass index (BMI) at or above the 95th percentile.

In the past decade, the skyrocketing rate of childhood overweight has become a concern of nutritionists, physicians, educators, policy makers, and parents across the United States. Experts agree that the main culprits are the same as those implicated in adult overweight and obesity: eating too much and moving too little. Establishing and maintaining healthful eating and physical activity behaviors is very important throughout childhood. Parental overweight, low parental concern about the child's weight, and tantrums over food are additional factors contributing to childhood overweight.[20] Rather than placing children on restrictive diets, however, experts advise encouraging physical activity and establishing more healthful eating patterns.[21]

The Institute of Medicine now recommends that children participate in physical activity and exercise for at least an hour each day.[3] For younger children, this can be divided into two or three shorter sessions, allowing them to regroup, recoup, and refocus between activity sessions. Older children may be able to be active for an hour without stopping. To encourage activity throughout the day, parents should limit their own and their children's television watching to no more than 2 hours per day. Electronic games, use of computers, and other sedentary activities should also be restricted. Studies have linked higher rates of television watching to higher rates of obesity in children and to less healthful food choices.[22–24]

In the past, children played freely outdoors and were relatively active indoors in times of bad weather or during the evening hours. In recent years, however, several factors have prompted childhood activities to become increasingly sedentary. One such factor is simply the availability of entertainment technologies, including television, video games, and computer games. Another factor is that the number of households in which no adult is home after school has risen in recent decades, either because of single-parent families or because both parents work to support their families. Safety concerns cause many working parents to forbid their children to venture out of the house when they are home alone after school.

Concerns about after-school isolation and inactivity are causing some communities to take action. Parents, schools, and community organizations such as Boys and Girls Clubs and the YMCA are banding together to develop after-school programs to encourage children to participate in running, hiking, bicycling, roller skating, karate, gymnastics, soccer, basketball, swimming, rock climbing, or other activities. Involvement in these activities helps children acquire new motor skills, strengthen muscles, make new friends, and develop self-esteem as they feel themselves becoming faster, stronger, and more skilled.

The ACTIVATE/Kidnetic.com Program is another approach aimed at encouraging children and their families to communicate and work together to be more physically active and to eat a more healthful diet. This is done through an interactive computer-based program (FIGURE 20.4). This program was developed through a partnership of many organizations that are committed to improving the nutritional status and physical activity levels of children and families, including the International Food Information Council, the American Academy of Family Physicians, and the American College of Sports Medicine. See the Web links at the end of this chapter.

VERB "It's What You Do" is a youth media campaign targeting "tweens," school-age children between the ages of 9 and 13 years. It is coordinated by the Centers for Disease Control and Prevention and the Department of Health and Human Services. This national, multicultural, social marketing campaign encourages children to be more active and to stay active. The message is relayed through paid advertising, marketing strategies, and partnership efforts. See the Web links for more information.

While increased activity is an important factor in maintaining a healthy weight, parents should also strive to consistently provide nutritious food choices, including a

Active, healthy-weight children are less likely to become overweight adults.

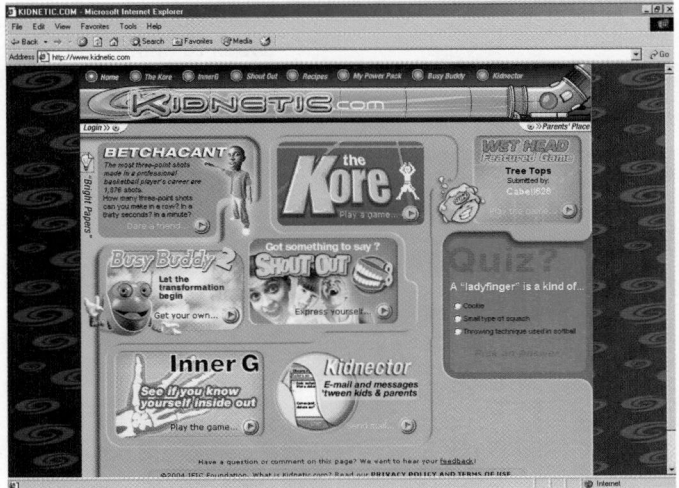

FIGURE 20.4   Kidnetic.com is an online program focused on increasing physical activity levels and promoting healthful eating among children and their families. (Reprinted from the International Food Information Council Foundation, 2007.)

FIGURE 20.5 "Eat Better, Eat Together" promotes family mealtimes as a way to improve children's diets. (Source: © Washington State University, Cooperative Extension, the Nutrition Education Network of Washington, and USDA Food and Nutrition Service.)

healthful breakfast and sitting down together to a shared family meal each evening (FIGURE 20.5).[25] (See the Web links for information on the "Eat Better, Eat Together" nutrition education program for families.) Large food corporations, including Kellogg's, have adopted voluntary nutrient standards for "kid-friendly" foods, such as snacks and cold cereals, to limit calories, saturated and trans fats, sodium, and added sugars. Their efforts will also make it easier for parents and children to locate nutrient information through the use of easy-to-read graphics on product labels. Parents can also keep a selection of fruits, vegetables, whole-grain products, and low-fat dairy foods readily available as healthful alternatives to high-fat, high-sugar snacks. For children "on the run," parents can keep a supply of nonperishable snacks such as granola bars, dried fruits, and nuts, along with kid-friendly fruits such as apples, bananas, and oranges, to grab as everyone dashes out the door. Mealtimes, especially dinner, should offer a colorful variety of foods with the emphasis on green, yellow, orange, and red vegetables and deep-brown grains.

Over time, overweight children who are offered nutritious foods and encouraged to be active can "catch up" to their weight as they grow taller without restricting food (and thus nutrient) intake.

Dental Caries

As discussed in Chapter 4, *dental caries,* or cavities, occur when bacteria in the mouth feed on carbohydrates deposited on teeth. As a result of metabolizing the carbohydrates, the bacteria then secrete acid that begins to erode tooth enamel, leading to tooth decay. The occurrence of dental caries can be minimized by limiting sugary sweets, especially those that stick to teeth, like jelly beans. Frequent brushing helps to eliminate the sugars on teeth, as well as the bacteria that feed on them.

Fluoride, through a municipal water supply, through fluoridated toothpaste or mouthwash, or through supplements, will also help deter the development of dental caries. Even though the teeth of a young child will be replaced by permanent teeth in several years, it is critical to keep them healthy and strong. This is because they make room for and guide the permanent teeth into position. Children should start having regular dental visits at the age of 3.

Inadequate Calcium Intake

Another nutrition-related concern for children is an inadequate intake of calcium. Adequate calcium is necessary to achieve peak bone mass, as well as for numerous other critical body and cell functions. As you learned in Chapter 9, peak bone mass is achieved in the late teens or early 20s, and childhood and adolescence are critical times to ensure adequate deposition of bone tissue. Inadequate calcium intake during childhood and adolescence leads to poor bone health and potential osteoporosis in later years.

Encouraging physical play with friends is a good way to maintain self-confidence and a positive body image.

Dairy products are the most common source of calcium for children in the United States.[5] During the infant, toddler, and preschool years, milk consumption can largely be monitored by parents or caregivers. However, once children begin to attend school, they may choose to spend the money intended for milk on soft drinks, if available. This "milk displacement" is a recognized factor in low calcium intake and poor bone health.[26] Diets that are low in calcium also tend to be low in other nutrients, so attention to calcium intake can help ensure a more healthful overall diet for children.

Body Image Concerns

As children, particularly females, approach puberty, appearance and body image play increasingly important roles in food choice. Concerns about appearance and body image are not necessarily detrimental to health, particularly if they result in children making more healthful food choices, such as eating more whole grains, fruits, and vegetables. However, it is important for children to understand that being thin does not guarantee health, popularity, or happiness and that a healthy body image includes accepting our own individual body type and recognizing that we can be physically fit and healthy at a variety of weights, shapes, and sizes. Children who are physically active may be more confident and accepting of their body image; thus, it is important to encourage daily participation in organized sports or unorganized playtime activities. Excessive concern with thinness can lead children to experiment with fad diets, food restriction, and other behaviors that can result in undernutrition and perhaps even trigger a clinical eating disorder. (Refer to Chapter 15 to learn more about disordered eating and eating disorders and how they can be prevented and treated.)

> **RECAP:** *Parents can communicate effectively with children to encourage healthful eating and can act as role models in regard to food choices and level of physical activity. Overweight and obesity are potential concerns for many children; their risk can be lowered with a healthful diet and regular physical activity. To prevent dental caries, children should brush their teeth regularly, limit sweets, and visit the dentist regularly beginning at age 3. Consuming adequate calcium to support the development of peak bone mass is also a primary concern for school-age children. Appearance and body image play increasingly important roles in children as they grow older, and disordered eating behaviors can result from these concerns.*

NUTRI-CASE HANNAH

"Today at school I got picked last for kickball, and I heard some boys on the other team laughing at me. Our phys. ed. teacher keeps telling me I should eat less, so this morning I didn't eat any breakfast at all, and I didn't eat all of my hamburger and French fries at lunch. I'm still sad though, because nobody wants to be my friend, except for Julia. She's chubby too, and we're going to try to help each other lose weight. We're going to watch TV together after school today, and we promised each other we're only going to drink the diet soda my mom has in the fridge."

What do you think of Hannah and her friend Julia's strategy for "helping each other lose weight"? How might you use Hannah's interest in science to help her and her friend achieve a more healthful body weight? How could her mother, Judy, help? How might her school and community participate in helping Hannah, Julia, and other children like them to achieve and maintain a healthful body weight?

Nutrition for Adolescents, Ages 14–18 Years

The adolescent years begin with the onset of **puberty,** the period in life in which secondary sexual characteristics develop and we become capable of reproducing. This is a physically and emotionally tumultuous time for adolescents and their families. The nutritional needs of adolescents are influenced by their rapid growth in height, increased weight, changes in body composition, and individual levels of physical activity.

puberty The period in life in which secondary sexual characteristics develop and people are biologically capable of reproducing.

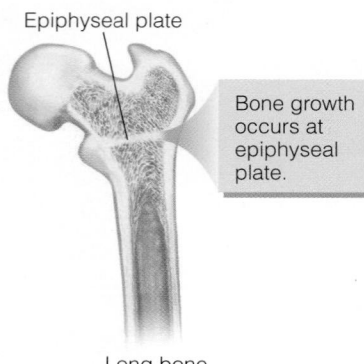

FIGURE 20.6 Skeletal growth ceases once closure of the epiphyseal plates occurs.

Adolescent Growth and Activity Patterns

Growth during adolescence is primarily driven by hormonal changes, including increased levels of testosterone for boys and estrogen for girls. Both boys and girls experience *growth spurts,* or periods of accelerated growth, during later childhood and adolescence. Growth spurts for girls tend to begin around 10 to 11 years of age, while growth spurts for boys begin around 12 to 13 years of age. These growth periods last about 2 years.

Adolescents experience an average 20–25% increase in height during the pubertal years. On average, girls tend to grow 2 to 8 inches and boys tend to grow 4 to 12 inches.[27] The average girl reaches almost full height by the onset of menstruation (called **menarche**). Boys typically experience continual growth throughout adolescence, and some may even grow slightly taller during early adulthood.

Skeletal growth ceases once closure of the *epiphyseal plates* occurs (FIGURE 20.6). The **epiphyseal plates** are plates of cartilage located toward the end of the long bones that provide for growth in length of the long bones. In some circumstances the epiphyseal plates can close early in adolescents and result in a failure to reach full stature. The most common causes of this failure are malnutrition during childhood and adolescence or use of anabolic steroids during this critical growth period.

Weight and body composition also change dramatically during adolescence. Weight gain is extremely variable during this time and reflects the adolescent's energy intake, physical activity level, and genetics. The average weight gained by girls and boys during this time is 35 and 45 pounds, respectively. The weight gained by girls and boys is dramatically different in terms of its composition. Girls tend to gain significantly more body fat than boys, with this fat accumulating around the buttocks, hips, breasts, thighs, and upper arms. Although many girls are uncomfortable or embarrassed by these changes, they are a natural result of maturation. Boys gain significantly more muscle mass than girls, and they experience an increase in muscle definition. Both girls and boys experience significant growth of their internal organs, including the liver, kidneys, heart, lungs, and sexual organs. Other changes that occur with sexual maturation include a deepening of the voice in boys and growth of pubic hair in both boys and girls.

The physical activity levels of adolescents are highly variable. Many are physically active in sports or other organized physical activities, whereas others become less interested in sports and more interested in intellectual or artistic pursuits. This variability in activity levels of adolescents results in highly individual energy needs. Although the rapid growth and sexual maturation that occur during puberty require a significant amount of energy, adolescence is often a time in which overweight begins. The following section discusses the unique nutrient needs of adolescents.

What Are an Adolescent's Nutrient Needs?

The nutrient needs of adolescents are influenced by rapid growth, weight gain, and sexual maturation, in addition to the demands of physical activity (see Table 20.1).

Energy and Macronutrient Recommendations for Adolescents

Adequate energy intake is necessary to maintain adolescents' health, support their dramatic growth and maturation, and fuel their physical activity. Because of these competing demands, the energy needs of adolescents can be quite high. While it is possible to calculate estimated energy requirements of an adolescent by using a published equation, it is more practical to monitor the growth pattern of the adolescent to ensure that weight remains in proportion to height.[3]

Fat. As with the younger age groups, there is no DRI for fat for adolescents. However, adolescents are at risk for the same chronic diseases as adults, including type 2 diabetes, obesity, coronary heart disease, and various cancers. Thus, it is prudent for adolescents to consume no more than 25–35% of total energy from fat and no more than 10% of total energy from saturated fat sources.

menarche The beginning of menstruation, or the menstrual period.

epiphyseal plates Plates of cartilage located toward the end of long bones that provide for growth in the length of long bones.

Carbohydrate. The RDA for carbohydrate for adolescents is 130 g/day. As with adults, this amount of carbohydrate covers what is needed to supply adequate glucose to the brain, but it does not cover the amount of carbohydrate needed to support daily activities. Thus, it is recommended that adolescents consume more than the RDA, or about 45–65% of their total energy as carbohydrate, and most should come from complex carbohydrate sources. The AI for fiber for adolescents is 26 g/day, which is similar to adult values.

Protein. The RDA for protein for adolescents is similar to that of adults at 0.85 g of protein per kg body weight per day. This value was selected because data are not available to determine protein maintenance requirements for this age group, and the amount of nitrogen needed to maintain protein balance in children is similar to that of adults.[3] This amount is assumed to be sufficient to support health and to cover the additional needs of growth and development during the adolescent stage.

Micronutrient Recommendations for Adolescents

Micronutrients of particular concern for adolescents include calcium, iron, and vitamins A and D.

Calcium and Vitamin D. Adequate calcium and vitamin D intakes are critical to achieve peak bone density. The AI for calcium from age 9 through adolescence is 1,300 mg/day. This amount of calcium can be difficult for many adolescents to consume because the quality of foods they select is often less than optimal to meet their nutrient needs. However, this level of calcium intake is easily achieved by eating at least 3 servings of dairy foods or calcium-fortified products daily.

The AI for vitamin D for adolescents is 5 μg/day. Most foods are naturally low in vitamin D; thus, fortified foods such as milk and cereals are important sources of this vitamin. If an adolescent is not consuming adequate milk and does not get adequate sunlight year round, he or she may need to take a supplement providing both calcium and vitamin D.

Iron. The iron needs of adolescents are relatively high; this is because iron is needed to replace the blood lost during menstruation in girls and to support the growth of muscle mass in boys. The RDA for iron for boys is 11 mg/day, while the RDA for girls is 15 mg/day. If energy intake is adequate and adolescents consume food sources of heme iron such as lean meat/fish/poultry each day, they should be able to meet the RDA for iron. However, many young people adopt a vegetarian lifestyle during this life stage, or they consume foods that have limited amounts of iron. Both of these situations can prevent adolescents from meeting the RDA for iron and, particularly in females, can increase their risk of iron-deficiency anemia.

Vitamin A. Vitamin A is critical to support the rapid growth and development that occur during adolescence. The RDA for vitamin A is 900 μg/day for boys and 700 μg/day for girls. The RDA can be met by consuming at least 5 servings of dark-green, yellow, and orange fruits and vegetables each day. As with iron and calcium, meeting the RDA for vitamin A can be a challenging goal if the adolescent fails to make healthful food choices. In such cases, a multivitamin and mineral supplement that provides no more than 100% of the Daily Value for the micronutrients could be beneficial as a safety net. As with younger children and adults, a supplement should not be considered a substitute for a balanced, healthful diet.

Fluid Recommendations for Adolescents

The fluid needs of adolescents are higher than those for children because of their higher physical activity levels and the extensive growth and development that occur during this phase of life. The AI for total fluid for adolescent girls and boys is listed in Table 20.1; it includes about 8 and 11 cups, respectively, as beverages, including drinking water. Boys require a higher fluid intake because they are generally more active than girls and have more lean tissue. Highly active adolescents who are exercising in the heat may have higher fluid needs than the AI, and these individuals should be encouraged to drink often to quench their thirst and avoid dehydration.

RECAP: *Puberty is the period in life in which secondary sexual characteristics develop and the physical ability to reproduce begins. Adolescents experience rapid increases in height, weight, and lean body mass and fat mass. Energy needs for adolescents can be very high. Fat intake should be 25–35% of total energy, and carbohydrate intake should be 45–65%. Because many adolescents fail to eat a variety of nutrient-dense foods, intakes of many nutrients such as calcium, iron, and vitamin A may be deficient. Calcium is needed to optimize bone growth and to achieve peak bone density, and iron needs are increased due to increased muscle mass in boys and to menstruation in girls. Adolescents need to drink about 8 cups (girls) and 11 cups (boys) of water or other beverages daily.*

Encouraging Nutritious Food Choices with Adolescents

At this point in their lives, adolescents are making most of their own food choices, and many are also buying and preparing a significant amount of the foods they consume. Although parents can still be effective role models, adolescents are generally strongly influenced by their peers, their preferences, and their own developing sense of what foods comprise a healthful and adequate diet. Adolescents are anxious to develop their own identity and establish a more self-reliant lifestyle. The decision to adopt a vegetarian diet, for example, may represent an adolescent's effort to establish some distance from the family unit. Although many teens become resistant to parental guidance, the importance of parental role modeling remains strong.

One particular area of concern in most adolescents' diet is a lack of vegetables, fruits, and whole grains. Many teens eat on the run, skip meals, and select fast foods and convenience foods because they are inexpensive, are accessible, and taste good. High school students are often allowed to leave campus for lunch, increasing their opportunities for high-fat, low-nutrient fast foods. Parents, caretakers, and school food service programs can capitalize on adolescents' preferences for pizza, burgers, spaghetti, and sandwiches by providing more healthful meat and cheese alternatives, whole-grain breads, and plenty of appealing vegetable-based sides or additions to these foods. In addition, keeping healthful snacks at home, such as fruits and vegetables that are already cleaned and prepared in easy-to-eat pieces, may encourage adolescents to consume more of these foods as between-meal snacks. Teens should also be encouraged to consume adequate milk and other calcium-enriched beverages while minimizing sodas, sports drinks, and other high-sugar beverages.

Nutrition-Related Concerns for Adolescents

Nutrition-related concerns for adolescents continue to include weight concerns and body image issues. Additional concerns include cigarette smoking and the use of alcohol and illegal drugs.

Obesity Watch: Balancing Food and Physical Activity to Encourage Healthful Weight Gain

Although expected and desirable, weight gain during adolescence can become excessive if increased energy intake is not balanced with adequate physical activity. Overweight and obesity are on the rise among adolescents. Many overweight and obese adolescents already have at least one risk factor for heart disease such as high blood pressure, elevated blood cholesterol, or type 2 diabetes.

As with younger children, a reduction in regular physical activity is a significant factor in adolescent overweight and obesity. Nearly half of all youth ages 12 to 21 years in the United States are not vigorously active on a regular basis, and about 14% of young people report doing no physical activity; physical inactivity is more common in females (14%) than in males (7%).[28] In one 10-year study, physically inactive female adolescents gained an average of 10 to 15 pounds more than active girls. This study supports a strong correlation between physical inactivity and increased fatness and body mass index (BMI). Minority adolescents are more likely to be physi-

Regular physical activity is good for adolescents.

cally inactive compared to Caucasian teens, and adolescent inactivity is a strong predictor of adult inactivity.[29]

By offering daily physical education in school and by providing more opportunities and encouragement for adolescents to participate in regular physical activity outside of school, the prevalence of overweight and obesity among adolescents can be reduced.

Disordered Eating and Eating Disorders

An initially healthful concern about body image and weight can turn into a dangerous obsession during this emotionally challenging life stage. Clinical eating disorders frequently begin during adolescence and can occur in boys as well as girls. Parents, teachers, and friends should be aware of the warning signs, which include rapid and excessive weight loss, a preoccupation with weight and body image, going to the bathroom regularly after meals, and signs of frequent vomiting or laxative use. Refer to Chapter 15 for a full discussion of eating disorders.

Adolescent Acne

The hormonal changes of puberty are largely responsible for the acne flare-ups that plague many adolescents. Emotional stress, genetic factors, and personal hygiene are secondary contributors. But what about foods? For decades, chocolate, fried foods, fatty foods, and other foods have been wrongfully linked to acne; it is now believed that diet has virtually no role in its development. On the other hand, a healthful diet, rich in fruits, vegetables, whole grains, and lean meats, can provide vitamin A, vitamin C, zinc, and other nutrients to optimize skin health and maintain an effective immune system.

Prescription medications, including the vitamin A derivative 13-*cis*-retinoic acid (Accutane), effectively control severe forms of acne. Prescription topical creams, applied directly to the skin, may also be used under the guidance of a physician. Neither Accutane nor any other prescription vitamin A derivative should be used by women who are pregnant, are planning a pregnancy, or may become pregnant. Accutane is a known teratogen, causing severe fetal malformations. Adolescent females who treat their acne with vitamin A-derivative prescription drugs must protect themselves against pregnancy and immediately contact their physician if they discover or believe they are pregnant. Incidentally, vitamin A taken in supplement form is not effective in acne treatment and, due to its own risk for toxicity, should not be used in amounts that exceed 100% of the Daily Value.

Use of Supplements

There are certain times when use of nutrient supplements by adolescents is desirable and appropriate. Pregnant adolescents, iron-deficient adolescent females, vegans, and dangerously underweight teens would all benefit from a multivitamin, multimineral supplement. Many teens who opt to use nutritional supplements, however, have unrealistic expectations.

Teenage athletes often turn to supplements to improve their performance, even though there is little evidence to suggest that "andro," ephedra, protein powders, and other highly promoted ergogenic aids actually produce beneficial results (see Chapter 13). In fact, some of these products can actually result in short- and long-term problems.

Some adolescents, particularly females, may purchase "beauty supplement" pills and capsules promoted as improving the look, feel, and health of the hair and skin. Although these products are probably not harmful, they tend to be expensive, and scientific research on their effectiveness is very limited.

Use of Tobacco, Alcohol, and Illegal Drugs

Cigarette smoking, alcohol consumption, and illegal drug use are additional concerns that face adolescents. Adolescents are naturally curious and most are open to experimenting with tobacco, alcohol, and illegal drugs. Cigarette smoking diminishes appetite and can interfere with nutrient metabolism. Indeed, it is frequently used by adolescent girls to maintain a low body weight. The effects of smoking were described in detail in Chapter 8. Among adolescents, smoking is also associated with an increased incidence of participation in other risky behaviors such as alcohol and drug abuse, fighting, and engaging in unprotected sex.

Alcohol and drug use can start at early ages, even in school-age children. The primary cause of death among high school–age youth is a motor vehicle accident; the risk of being involved in an accident is greatly increased by using alcohol and illegal drugs. Alcohol can also interfere with proper nutrient absorption and metabolism, and it can take the place of foods in an adolescent's diet; these adverse effects of alcohol put adolescents at risk for various nutrient deficiencies. Alcohol consumption and use of many illegal drugs are also associated with "the munchies," a feeling of food craving that usually results in the intake of large quantities of high-fat, high-sugar, nutrient-poor foods. This behavior can result in overweight or obesity, and also increases the risk of nutrient imbalance. Teens who use drugs and alcohol are typically in poor physical condition, are either underweight or overweight, have poor appetites, and perform poorly in school.

> RECAP: *Adolescents' food choices are influenced by peer pressure, personal preferences, and their own developing sense of what foods are healthful. Adolescents are at risk for skipping meals and selecting fast foods and snack foods in place of whole grains, fruits, and vegetables. Milk is commonly replaced with sugared soft drinks. Obesity can occur during adolescence because of increased appetite and food intake and decreased physical activity. Disordered eating behaviors, eating disorders, acne, inappropriate use of supplements, cigarette smoking, and use of alcohol and illegal drugs are also concerns for this age group.*

Nutrition for Older Adults, Age 65 Years and Older

The U.S. population is getting older each year. Consider the following statistics:

- In 2001, average life expectancy reached 77.2 years.[30]

- In 2003, almost 36 million people aged 65 and older lived in the United States, representing about 12% of the population.[31] It is estimated that by the year 2030, about 20% of Americans will be 65 years of age and older.[30]

- People 85 years of age and older currently represent the fastest growing U.S. population subgroup, projected to grow from 4.2 million in 2000 to over 20 million by the year 2050.

- The number of *centenarians,* persons over the age of 100 years, and *super-centenarians,* over 110 years, continues to grow as well. It has been estimated that there is one super-centenarian per million in the population, for a total of approximately 260 in the United States today.[32] These so-called "very elderly" or "oldest old" account for the majority of healthcare expenditures and nursing home admissions in the United States.[33]

These statistics have important nutrition-related implications even for younger adults, since a nutritious diet and regular physical activity throughout life can help prevent or delay the onset of chronic diseases and keep adults happy and productive in their later years. Throughout this book, our exploration of nutrition and physical activity has focused mainly on young and middle-age adults. In the following section, we discuss the unique nutritional needs and concerns of older adults, and identify ways in which diet and lifestyle affect the aging process.

Older adults have unique nutritional needs.

What Physiologic Changes Accompany Aging?

Older adulthood is a time in which growth is complete and body systems begin to slow and degenerate. If the following discussion of this degeneration seems disturbing or depressing, remember that the changes described are at least partly within an individual's control. For instance, some of the decrease seen in muscle mass, bone mass, and muscle strength is due to low physical activity levels.

Age-Related Changes in Sensory Perception

For most individuals, eating is a social and pleasurable process; the sights, sounds, odors, and textures associated with food stimulate and enhance one's appetite. Odor, taste, tactile, and visual perception all decline with age and negatively affect the food intake and nutritional status of older adults.

It has been estimated that over half of older adults experience a significant impairment in their sense of smell. The nerve receptors for taste and smell are complementary; thus, enjoyment of food relies heavily on the sense of smell. Older adults who cannot adequately appreciate the appealing aromas of food may be unable to fully enjoy the foods offered in a meal. While often a simple consequence of aging, loss of odor perception can also be caused by zinc deficiency or a medication side effect. If this is the case, a zinc supplement or change of medication may be a simple solution.

With increasing age, taste perception dims as well, especially the ability to detect salt and bitter tastes.[34] The ability to perceive sweetness and sourness also declines, but to a lesser extent. Some elderly experience *dysgeusia,* or abnormal taste perception. With this condition, an elderly person might experience the sensation of bitterness from a freshly cooked piece of chicken that others would find perfectly enjoyable.

Loss of visual acuity has unexpected consequences for the nutritional health of older adults. Many have difficulty reading food labels, including nutrient information and "pull dates" for perishable foods. Driving skills decline, limiting the ability of some older Americans to acquire healthy, affordable foods. Older adults with vision loss may not be able to see the temperature knobs on stoves or the controls on microwave ovens, and may therefore choose cold meals, such as sandwiches, rather than meals that require heating. Also, the visual appeal of a colorful, attractively arranged plate of food is lost to visually impaired elderly, further reducing their desire to eat healthful meals.

Age-Related Changes in Gastrointestinal Function

Significant changes in the mouth, stomach, intestinal tract, and related organs occur with aging.[35] Some of these changes have the potential to increase the risk of nutrient deficiency.

With increasing age, salivary production declines. In older adults with *xerostomia,* or dry mouth, teeth are more susceptible to decay, chewing and swallowing become more difficult, and taste perception declines. These elderly benefit from a diet rich in moist foods including fruits and vegetables, sauces or gravies on meats, and high-fluid desserts such as puddings.

A variety of gastrointestinal and other physiologic changes can lead to weight loss in older adults.

Some older adults experience *dysphagia* (difficulty swallowing foods), often as a result of a stroke or a condition such as Parkinsonism. Smooth, thick foods such as cream soups, applesauce, milkshakes, fruit nectars, and puddings are usually well tolerated. Dysphagia requires professional assessment and treatment, drawing upon the expertise of an occupational therapist, physician, and dietitian. If not accurately diagnosed and treated, it could lead to malnutrition, inappropriate weight loss, and aspiration of food or fluid into the lungs.

Older adults are also at risk for a reduced secretion of gastric acid, which limits the absorption of minerals such as calcium, iron, and zinc and food sources of folic acid and vitamin B_{12}.[36] Lack of intrinsic factor greatly reduces the absorption of vitamin B_{12} (see Chapter 10). These elderly, therefore, benefit from vitamin B_{12} supplements and/or B_{12} shots.

Age-Related Changes in Body Composition

With aging, body fat increases and muscle mass declines. It has been estimated that women and men lose 20–25% of their lean body mass, respectively, as they age from 35 to 70 years.[37] Decreased production of certain hormones, including testosterone and growth hormone, and chronic diseases contribute to this loss of muscle, as does poor diet and an inactive lifestyle. Older adults with *sarcopenia,* a severe loss of muscle mass and strength, are often so weak that they are unable to rise from a seated position, climb stairs, or carry a bag of groceries. Along with adequate dietary intake, regular physical activity, including strength or resistance training, can help older adults maintain their muscle mass and strength, delaying or preventing the need for institutionalization.

Body fat increases from young adulthood through middle age, peaking at approximately 55–65 years of age, then declining in persons over the age of 70 years. With aging, body fat shifts from subcutaneous stores, just below the skin, to internal or visceral fat stores. Older women tend to deposit more fat in their abdominal region compared to younger women; this shift in body fat stores is most dramatic after the onset of menopause and coincides with an increased risk for heart disease, diabetes, and metabolic syndrome.

Bone mineral density declines with age and may eventually drop to the critical fracture zone. Among older women, the onset of menopause leads to a sudden and dramatic loss of bone due to the lack of estrogen. Although it is less dramatic, elderly males also experience this loss of bone due in part to decreasing levels of testosterone. In addition to the well-known benefits of calcium and vitamin D, intakes of vitamins A, C, and K, phosphorus, magnesium, boron, fluoride, and protein are now recognized as influencing bone density as well. As noted in the accompanying Highlight: Seniors on the Move, bone health can be promoted through regular weight-bearing activity in adults well into their 90s and beyond.

> RECAP: *The physiologic changes that can occur with aging include sensory declines; impaired ability to chew, swallow, absorb, and metabolize various nutrients; loss of muscle mass and lean tissue; increased fat mass; and decreased bone density. These age-related changes influence the nutritional needs of older adults and their ability to consume a healthful diet.*

What Are an Older Adult's Nutrient Needs?

The requirements for many nutrients are the same for older adults as for young and middle-aged adults. A few nutrient requirements increase, and a few are actually lower. Table 20.2 identifies nutrient recommendations that do change, as well as the physiologic reasons behind these changes.

Energy and Macronutrient Recommendations for Older Adults

The energy needs of older adults are lower than those of younger adults. This decrease is due to loss of muscle mass and lean tissue, a reduction in thyroid hormones, and a less physically active lifestyle. It is estimated that total daily energy

HIGHLIGHT

Seniors on the Move

Recent information from the Centers for Disease Control and Prevention confirms that relatively few older adults participate in regular leisure-time physical activity.[38] On average, only 27% of adults 65–74 years of age and 16% of those 75 years and older maintain a routine of voluntary physical activity. Participation in vigorous activity is even less common among older adults: fewer than 20% of "young elderly" (65–74 years) and fewer than 10% of "older elderly" (75 years and above) devote even 10 minutes a week to vigorous exercise.[30]

For a minor investment of time and energy, older adults reap benefits worth literally thousands of dollars in reduced healthcare costs. A regular program of physical activity lowers the risk of heart disease, hypertension, type 2 diabetes, obesity, depression, and cognitive decline or dementia. The complications of arthritis can also be reduced with appropriate exercise, as can the risk of falls and bone fractures. The need for healthcare visits, diagnostics, medication, and other treatments to control blood glucose, serum cholesterol, blood pressure, and other factors in chronic illness can be reduced or eliminated with regular exercise.

Physically active elders live longer and enjoy better health while they live. Adults who maintain a regular schedule of physical activity live an average of 1 to 3 years longer than adults who are sedentary.[39] Also, men and women who were physically active in their 50s and beyond lived 1 to 3 more years without cardiovascular disease compared to inactive adults.[39]

Older adults should plan an activity program that includes four basic types of exercises:

- *Flexibility exercises:* These activities "set the stage" for other forms of exercise by stretching the muscles and improving range of motion. Gentle arm swings, ankle circles, and torso twists are examples of moves that can slowly increase flexibility. Such exercises can be done while sitting in a chair, standing, or even while in a shallow pool. Ideally, older adults should stretch every day of the week.
- *Balance exercises:* Balance is important in reducing the risk of falls. Older adults should also have confidence in their ability to maintain balance before starting strength or endurance exercises. Toe raises, side leg raises, and rear leg swings are examples of balance activities; Tai Chi is another popular way to improve balance. Fitness experts advise adults to start balance exercises by holding a table or large chair with both hands; with practice, the person can progress to using one hand only, then grasping with fingers only, and finally they may feel secure enough to try some balance activities with no handholds at all. Older adults should practice balance activities daily.

- *Strength or resistance training:* This type of activity can increase muscle mass and strength as well as enhance bone density, preserving the ability of older adults to maintain an independent lifestyle.[40] Gains in muscle strength also improve balance and provide the foundation for endurance exercise. A growing number of retirement communities and long-term care centers offer "weight rooms" where strength training equipment is available. Community centers, including congregate meal sites, offer strength training using cans of food, gallon bottles of water, and other common items; the exercises are designed for mobile and chair-bound elders. Ideally, older adults should engage in resistance training 2 to 3 days a week.

- *Endurance or aerobic exercise:* Activities such as brisk walking, bicycle riding, swimming, and dancing increase heart rate and improve cardiorespiratory function. These activities should be low impact (no jump ropes or high-impact aerobics classes!) to minimize risk to aging bones, joints, and muscles. Older adults should aim for an intensity perceived as "fairly light" to "somewhat hard"—a level that is challenging but not exhausting. As with resistance training, older adults should check with their healthcare provider before starting on a program of endurance exercise. Once given approval, they should try to take part in aerobic activities at least 3 days each week for 30 or more minutes a day.

Some seniors may be vulnerable to exercise-related complications such as dehydration, heat stress, fractures, or falls. Exercise rooms should offer appropriate temperature, ventilation, and lighting; participants should wear appropriate clothing and comfortable shoes; and supervised warm-up and cool-down periods should be incorporated into each activity. As always, a thorough medical exam is advised prior to the start of programmed exercise.

The benefits of regular physical activity by older adults almost always far outweigh potential risks—the payoff is better health, more independence, less disability, and a longer, happier life!

TABLE 20.2   Nutrient Recommendations That Change with Increased Age

Changes in Nutrient Recommendations	Rationale for Changes
Vitamin D Increased need for vitamin D from 5 μg/day for young adults to 10 μg/day for adults 51 to 70 years and to 15 μg/day for adults over age 70 years	Decreased bone density Decreased ability to synthesize vitamin D in our skin Decreased absorption of dietary calcium
Calcium Increased need for calcium from 1,000 mg/day for young adults to 1,200 mg/day for adults 51 years of age and older	Decreased bone density Decreased absorption of dietary calcium
Fiber Decreased need for fiber from 38 g/day for young men to 30 g/day for men 51 years and older. Decreases for women from 25 g/day for young women to 21 g/day for women 51 years and older	Decreased energy intake
B Vitamins Increased need for vitamin B_6 and need for vitamin B_{12} as a supplement or from fortified foods	Lower levels of stomach acid Decreased absorption of food B_{12} from gastrointestinal tract Increased need to reduce homocysteine levels and to optimize immune function

A less physically active lifestyle will lead to lower total energy requirements in older adults.

expenditure decreases approximately 10 kcal each year for men and 7 kcal each year for women ages 19 and older.[3] This means that a woman who needs 2,000 kcal at age 20 needs just 1,650 at age 70. Some of this decrease in energy expenditure is an inevitable response to aging, but some of the decrease can be delayed or minimized by staying physically active. Because their total daily energy needs are lower, older adults need to pay particularly close attention to consuming a diet high in nutrient-dense foods but not too high in energy in order to avoid weight gain. Refer to the Nutrition Debate at the end of this chapter to learn more about the theory of caloric restriction, which proposes that low-energy diets may significantly prolong our lives.

Fat. As with other age groups, there is no DRI for total fat intake for older adults. However, to reduce their risk for heart disease and other chronic diseases, it is recommended that total fat intake remain within 20–35% of total daily energy intake, with no more than 10% of total energy intake coming from saturated fat.

Carbohydrate. The RDA for carbohydrate for older adults is 130 g/day. As with all other age groups, this level of carbohydrate is sufficient to support brain glucose utilization. Complex carbohydrates should be emphasized over simple sugars: it is recommended that older individuals consume a diet that contains no more than 30% of total energy intake as sugars.[3] The fiber recommendations are slightly lower for older adults than for younger adults because older adults eat less energy. After age 50, 30 g of fiber per day for men and 21 g for women is assumed sufficient to reduce the risks for constipation and diverticular disease, maintain healthful blood levels of glucose and lipids, and provide good sources of nutrient-dense, low-energy foods.

Protein. The DRI for protein is the same for adults of all ages: 0.80 g protein/kg body weight per day.[3] Some researchers, however, have argued for a protein allowance of 1.0 to 1.2 g protein/kg body weight for older adults in order to optimize protein status.[41] Protein is critically important to help minimize the loss of muscle and lean tissue, optimize healing after injury or disease, maintain immunity, and help prevent excessive loss of bone. Many protein-rich foods are also important sources of vitamins and minerals that are typically low in the diets of older adults; thus, protein is an important nutrient for this age group.

Micronutrient Recommendations for Older Adults

The vitamins and minerals of particular concern for older adults are identified in Table 20.2.

Calcium and Vitamin D.   Preventing or minimizing the consequences of osteoporosis is a top priority for older adults. The requirements for both calcium and vitamin D are higher because of a reduced absorption of calcium from the gut, along with reduced production of vitamin D in our skin as a result of aging. Many older adults are at risk for vitamin D deficiency because they are institutionalized and are not exposed to adequate amounts of sunlight. Others may limit their intake of milk and dairy products due to lactose intolerance or perceived concerns over the fat content of these foods. The widespread use of sunscreen has lowered risk of skin cancer among older adults; however, these products also block the sunlight needed for vitamin D synthesis in the skin. It is critical that older adults consume foods that are high in calcium and vitamin D and, when needed, use supplements. The Tufts modified food pyramid for mature adults (FIGURE 20.7)

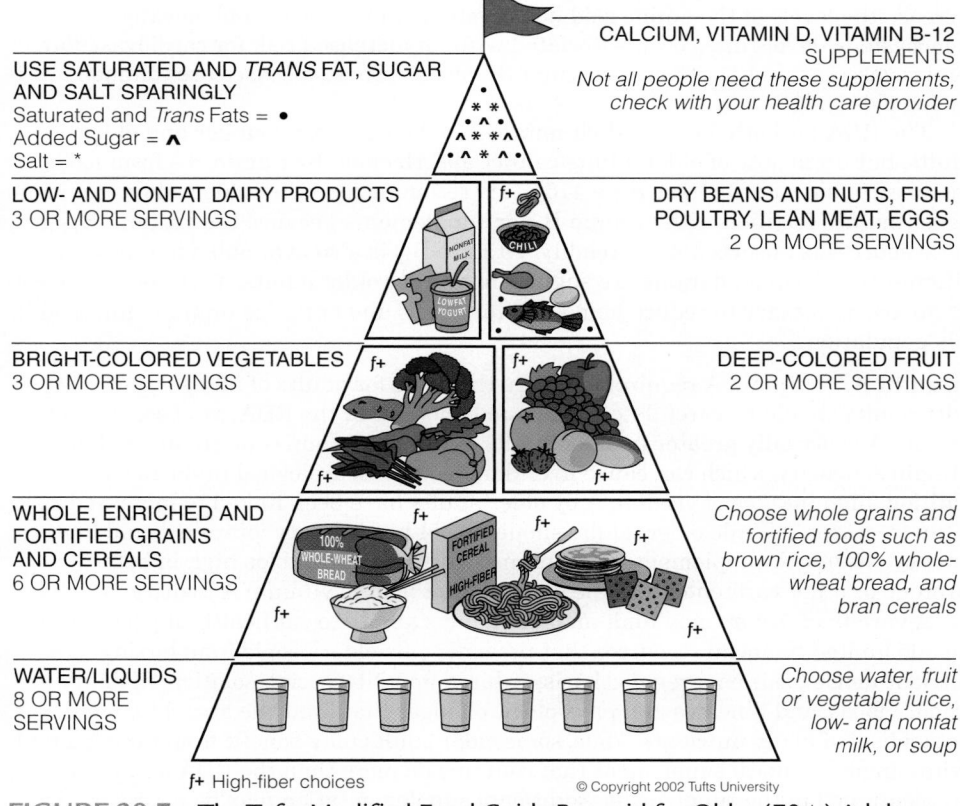

TUFTS
Food Guide Pyramid for Older Adults

CALCIUM, VITAMIN D, VITAMIN B-12
SUPPLEMENTS
Not all people need these supplements, check with your health care provider

USE SATURATED AND *TRANS* FAT, SUGAR AND SALT SPARINGLY
Saturated and *Trans* Fats = •
Added Sugar = ∧
Salt = *

LOW- AND NONFAT DAIRY PRODUCTS
3 OR MORE SERVINGS

DRY BEANS AND NUTS, FISH, POULTRY, LEAN MEAT, EGGS
2 OR MORE SERVINGS

BRIGHT-COLORED VEGETABLES
3 OR MORE SERVINGS

DEEP-COLORED FRUIT
2 OR MORE SERVINGS

WHOLE, ENRICHED AND FORTIFIED GRAINS AND CEREALS
6 OR MORE SERVINGS

Choose whole grains and fortified foods such as brown rice, 100% whole-wheat bread, and bran cereals

WATER/LIQUIDS
8 OR MORE SERVINGS

Choose water, fruit or vegetable juice, low- and nonfat milk, or soup

f+ High-fiber choices

© Copyright 2002 Tufts University

FIGURE 20.7   The Tufts Modified Food Guide Pyramid for Older (70+) Adults highlights the need for fluids and supplemental vitamins B_{12} and D by the elderly. (© 2002 Tufts University.)

recommends calcium and vitamin D supplements along with routine use of vitamin B_{12} supplements.

Iron. Iron needs decrease with aging. This decrease is primarily due to reduced muscle and lean tissue in both men and women and the cessation of menstruation in women. The decreased need for iron in older men is not significant enough to change the recommendations for iron intake in this group, thus the RDA for iron is the same for older men as for younger, 8 mg/day. However, the RDA for iron in older women is 8 mg/day, which is 10 mg/day lower than the RDA for younger women. Heme iron from meat, fish, and poultry represents the most available source of dietary iron; however, some older adults reduce their intake of these foods due to cost and possibly to difficulties in chewing and swallowing. Fortified grains and cereals, as well as legumes, greens, and dried fruits, can provide additional iron to the diet.

Zinc. Although zinc recommendations are the same for all adults, it is important to emphasize that zinc is a critical nutrient for optimizing immune function and wound healing in older adults. Zinc intake can be inadequate in older adults for the same reasons that heme iron intake may be deficient: red meats, poultry, and fish are relatively expensive and older adults may have a difficult time chewing meats due to loss of teeth and/or use of dentures.

Vitamins C and E. Although it is speculated that older adults have increased oxidative stress, the recommendations for the antioxidant vitamins C and E are the same as for younger adults. While some research suggests that intake of supplements containing vitamins C and E can lower the risk of cataracts and age-related macular degeneration, it is not possible to reach a conclusion regarding the benefits of antioxidant supplementation (see Chapter 8).

B-Complex Vitamins. Older adults need to pay close attention to consuming adequate amounts of the B-complex vitamins, specifically vitamin B_{12}, vitamin B_6, and folate. As discussed in detail in Chapter 10, inadequate intakes of these nutrients increase the levels of the amino acid homocysteine in the blood, and elevated homocysteine levels have been associated with an increased risk for cardiovascular, cerebrovascular, and peripheral vascular diseases.[42] These diseases are common among older adults.

The RDA for both folate and vitamin B_{12} is the same for younger and older adults, but up to 30% of older adults cannot absorb enough vitamin B_{12} from foods due to atrophic gastritis (see page 415). It is recommended that older adults consume foods that are fortified with vitamin B_{12} or supplements because the vitamin B_{12} in these sources is absorbed more readily. Vitamin B_{12} is also available via injection. Vitamin B_6 recommendations are slightly higher for older adults, as these higher levels appear necessary to reduce homocysteine levels and optimize immune function in this population.[43]

Vitamin A. Vitamin A requirements are the same for adults of all ages; however, older adults should be careful not to consume more than the RDA, as absorption of vitamin A is actually greater in older adults. Thus, this group is at greater risk for vitamin A toxicity, which can cause liver damage and neurological problems. In addition, high intakes of vitamin A by older adults have been linked to increased risk of hip fractures.[44] While older adults should avoid high dietary vitamin A and high-potency vitamin A supplements, consuming fruits and vegetables high in beta-carotene or other carotenoids is safe and does not lead to vitamin A toxicity.

A variety of factors may limit an older adult's ability to eat healthfully. These include limited financial resources that prevent some older people from buying nutrient-dense foods on a regular basis, reduced appetite, social isolation, inability to prepare foods, and illnesses and physiologic changes that limit the absorption and metabolism of many nutrients. Thus, some older adults may benefit from taking a multivitamin and mineral supplement that contains no more than the RDA for all nutrients contained in the supplement. Additional supplementation may be necessary for nutrients such as calcium, vitamin D, and vitamin B_{12}. However, supplementation with individual nutrients should be done only under the supervision of the individual's primary healthcare provider, as the risk of nutrient toxicity is high in this population.

NUTRI-CASE GUSTAVO

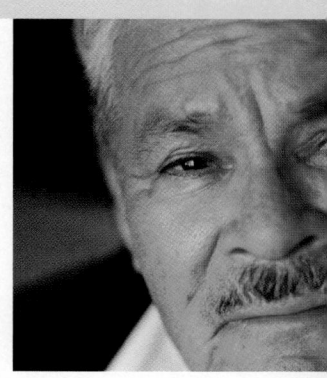

" I don't believe in taking vitamins. If you eat good food, you get everything you need and it's the way nature intended it. My daughter kept nagging at my wife and me to start taking B vitamins. She said when people get to be our age they have problems with their nerves and their blood pressure if they don't. I didn't fall for it, but my wife did, and then her doctor told her she needed calcium pills and vitamin D, too. The kitchen counter is starting to look like a medicine chest! You know what I think? I think this whole vitamin thing is just a hoax to get you to empty your wallet."

Would you support Gustavo's decision to avoid taking B-complex vitamin supplements? Given what you have learned in previous Nutri-Cases about Gustavo's wife, would you support or oppose her taking a B-complex vitamin, calcium, or vitamin D supplement? Explain your choices.

Fluid Recommendations for Older Adults

The AI for fluid is the same for older and younger adults. Men should consume 3.7 liters of total water per day, which includes 3.0 liters (about 13 cups) as beverages, including drinking water. Women should consume 2.7 liters of total water per day, which includes 2.2 liters (about 9 cups) as beverages. It is important to emphasize that kidney function changes with age, and the thirst mechanism of older people can be impaired. These changes can result in chronic dehydration and hypernatremia (elevated blood sodium levels) in this population. Some older adults will intentionally limit their beverage intake because they have urinary incontinence or don't want to be awakened for nighttime urination. This practice can endanger their health, so it is important for these individuals to seek treatment for the incontinence and continue to drink plenty of fluids.

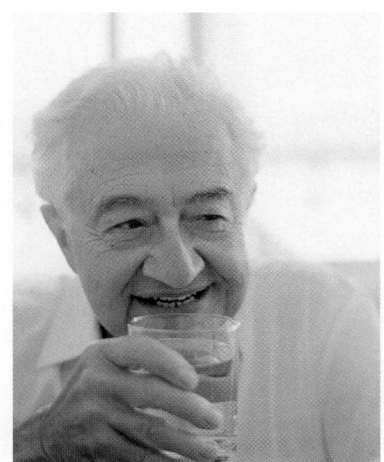

Older adults need the same amount of fluid as other adults.

> RECAP: *Older adults have lower energy needs due to their loss of lean tissue and lower physical activity levels. Older adults should consume 20–35% of total energy as fat and 45–65% of their energy as carbohydrate. Protein recommendations are the same as for younger adults. Micronutrients of concern include calcium, vitamin D, iron, zinc, vitamin B$_{12}$, vitamin B$_6$, and folate. Older adults need to carefully select nutrient-dense foods to meet their micronutrient needs, and supplementation may be necessary. Older adults are at risk for chronic dehydration. Men need to drink about 13 cups of water and other beverages per day, and women need about 9 cups.*

Nutrition-Related Concerns for Older Adults

Older adults have a number of unique nutritional concerns. In addition to overweight and underweight, they commonly face dental problems and potential interactions between nutrients and medications. Some older adults abuse alcohol, and some face financial difficulties that affect their nutritional choices. Each of these concerns is discussed briefly in the following sections.

Overweight and Underweight: A Delicate Balancing Act

Not surprisingly, overweight and obesity are also a concern for older adults. While adults 75 years and older are less likely to be obese compared to other age groups (FIGURE 20.8), it is estimated that the number of obese elderly will increase to as high

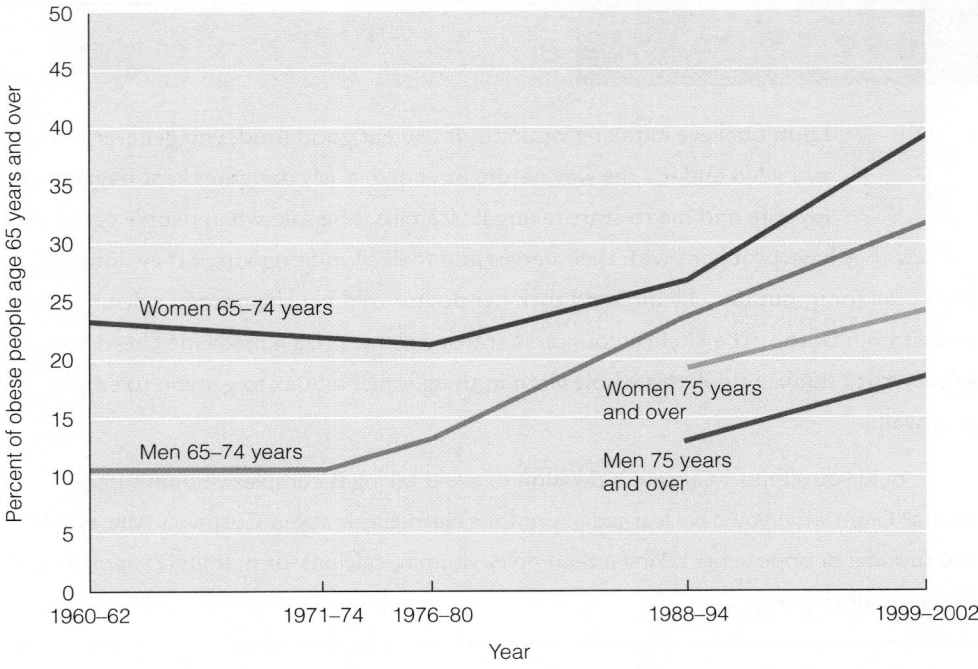

FIGURE 20.8 Obesity is becoming more common in the U.S. elderly population. (Source: Flegal, K. M., M. D. Carroll, C. L. Ogden, and C. L. Johnson. 2002. Prevalence and trends in obesity among US adults, 1999–2000. *J. Am. Med. Assoc.* 288:1723–1727. © 2002 American Medical Association. Used with permission.)

as 22 million, or 37.4% of all older adults, by the year 2010.[45] This population has a high risk for heart disease, hypertension, type 2 diabetes, and cancer, and these diseases are more prevalent in people who are overweight or obese. Obesity also increases the severity and consequences of osteoarthritis, limits the mobility of older adults, and is associated with a reduced ability to successfully perform routine activities of daily living.[46] In contrast, overweight can be protective against osteoporosis and fall-related fractures in older adults.

Underweight is also risky for older adults; as indicated in FIGURE 20.9, mortality rates are actually higher in underweight elderly than in overweight elderly.[47] Significantly underweight older adults have fewer protein reserves to call upon during periods of catabolic stress, such as post-surgery or trauma, and are more susceptible to infection. Inappropriate weight loss suggests inadequate energy intake, which also implies inadequate nutrient intake. Chronic deficiencies of protein, vitamins, and minerals leave older adults at risk for poor wound healing and a depressed immune response.

Gerontologists have identified "nine Ds" that account for most cases of geriatric weight loss (FIGURE 20.10). Several of these factors promote weight loss by reducing energy intake, others by increasing energy expenditure or loss of nutrients.

Dental Health Issues

Diet plays an important role in the maintenance of dental health in the elderly. Vitamin B-complex deficiencies contribute to irritation, inflammation, and cracking of the lips and tongue, whereas vitamin C deficiency increases risk of periodontal (gum) disease. A lack of adequate calcium, vitamin D, and protein contributes to the loss of bone in the oral cavity, which increases risk of tooth loss. Frequent intake of fermentable carbohydrates, which includes virtually every sugar and many starches, increases oral bacterial production of acid and demineralization of teeth. Chewing sugarless gum after a meal or snack helps neutralize the acids produced by oral bacteria; ending a meal with an apple or a similar highly textured food may effectively

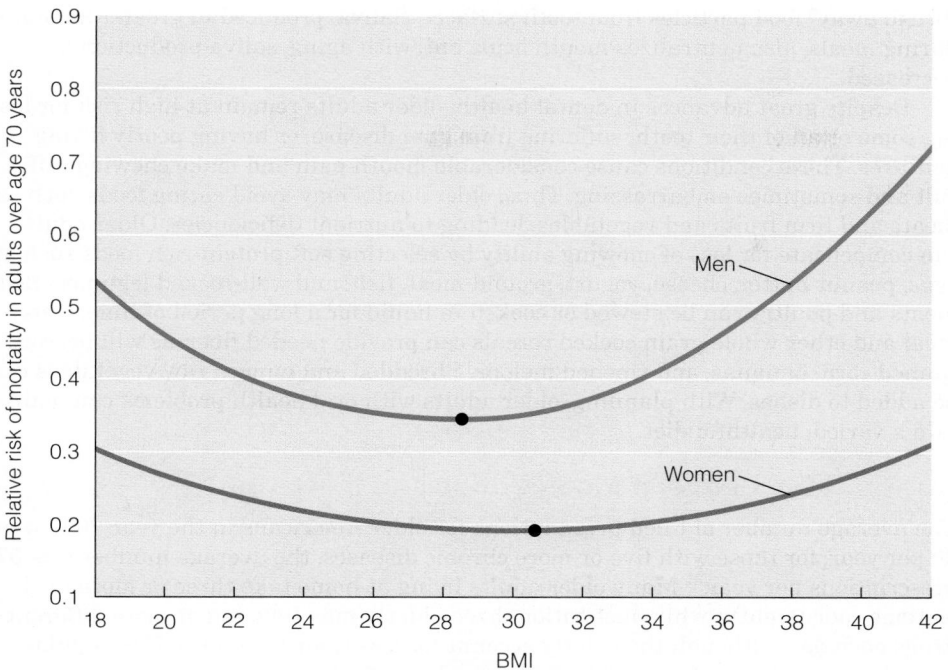

FIGURE 20.9 The effects of underweight and overweight on mortality in the elderly. The relationship between risk of mortality and BMI is U-shaped. For adults over the age of 70 years, the point of lowest mortality is a BMI of 30.2 for women and 28.4 for men. Mortality increases as BMI decreases from this point. (Source: Berg, F. M. 1996. New study finds higher weight protects elderly. *Healthy Weight J.* 10:1–7. Reprinted with permission from Frances M. Berg, MS, Healthy Weight Network (www.healthyweight.net).)

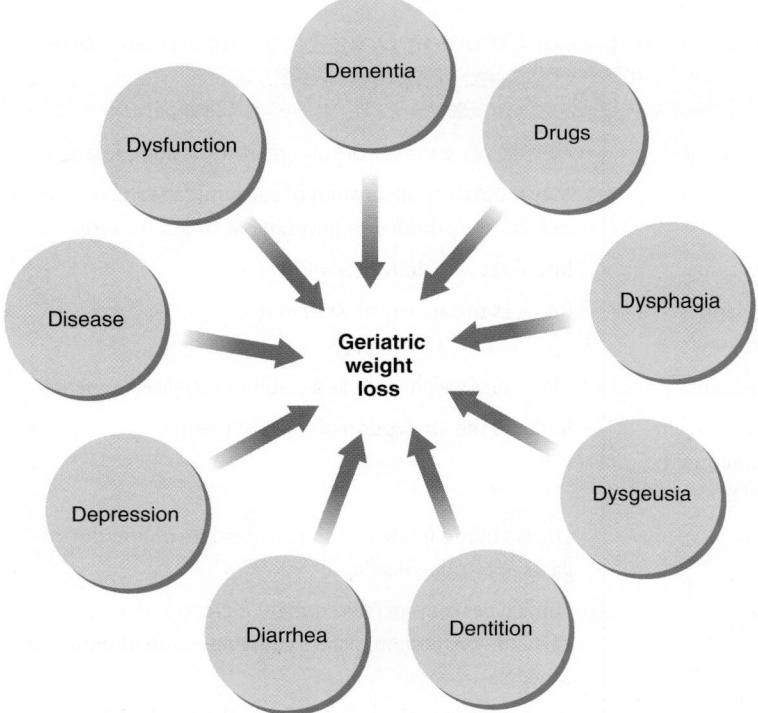

FIGURE 20.10 The nine Ds of geriatric weight loss: Many factors contribute to inappropriate weight loss in the elderly.

"brush away" food particles from tooth surfaces. Saliva, produced in greater amounts during meals, also neutralizes mouth acids but, with aging, saliva production is decreased.

Despite great advances in dental health, older adults remain at high risk for losing some or all of their teeth, suffering from gum disease, or having poorly fitting dentures. These conditions cause considerable mouth pain and make chewing difficult and sometimes embarrassing. Thus, older adults may avoid eating foods such as meats and firm fruits and vegetables, leading to nutrient deficiencies. Older adults can compensate for loss of chewing ability by selecting soft protein-rich foods such as eggs, peanut butter, cheese, yogurt, ground meat, fish, and well-cooked legumes. Red meats and poultry can be stewed or cooked in liquid for a long period of time. Oatmeal and other whole-grain cooked cereals can provide needed fiber, as will berries, canned corn, bananas, and ripened melons. Shredded and minced raw vegetables can be added to dishes. With planning, older adults with oral health problems can maintain a varied, healthful diet.

Interactions Between Medications and Nutrition

The average number of filled prescriptions for older Americans in the year 2000 was 30 per year; for those with five or more chronic diseases, the average number was 57 prescriptions per year.[31] Many older adults living at home take three or more medications concurrently, while institutionalized elderly may take ten or more different drugs each day. Although the elderly account for less than 15% of the U.S. population, they experience almost 40% of adverse drug effects, in part because of this *polypharmacy,* or use of multiple drugs.

Prescription drugs interact not only with each other, but also with nutrients and other food components. Some medications increase or decrease food intake, while others alter nutrient digestion, absorption, or excretion. Several drugs negatively affect the metabolism of nutrients such as vitamin D, folate, and vitamin B_6. Table 20.3 summarizes some of the more common drug–nutrient interactions.

TABLE 20.3 Examples of Common Drug–Nutrient Interactions

Category of Drug	Common Drug–Nutrient Interactions
Antacids	May decrease the absorption of iron, calcium, folate, vitamin B_{12}
Antibiotics	May reduce the absorption of calcium, fat-soluble vitamins; reduces the production of vitamin K by gut bacteria
Anticonvulsants	Interferes with activation of vitamin D
Anticoagulants ("blood thinners")	Reduces the activity of vitamin K
Antidepressants	May cause weight gain as a result of increased appetite
Antiretroviral agents (used in treatment of HIV/AIDS)	Reduces the absorption of most nutrients
Aspirin	Lowers blood folate levels; increases loss of iron due to gastrointestinal bleeding
Diuretics	Some types may increase urinary excretion of potassium, sodium, calcium, magnesium; others cause retention of potassium and other electrolytes
Laxatives	Increases fecal excretion of dietary fat, fat-soluble vitamins, calcium and other minerals

Alcohol Abuse Among Older Adults

While alcoholism is often thought of as a problem among young adults, there is growing concern over the prevalence of alcohol-related problems among older adults. One national survey reported that 9% of older adults reported binge drinking (five or more drinks on the same occasion) at least once in the past month and 2% reported heavy drinking (five or more binges in the past month).[48] About one-third of older alcoholics are defined as "late-onset," having developed the alcohol abuse after the age of 60 years. Stressors such as spousal death, divorce, loss of employment, physical disability, and isolation are common triggers for inappropriate use of alcohol.[49]

Alcohol is less efficiently metabolized by older adults, meaning that blood levels of alcohol rise higher and the physiologic effects of alcohol are more serious compared to those of a younger adult with the same alcohol intake. Some healthcare providers recommend a limit of one drink per day for older adult males compared to the more common definition of "moderate drinking" as no more than two drinks per day for young men.[50] Older adults are more susceptible to alcohol-induced increases in blood pressure, decreases in immune function, impairment of liver function, and irritation to the gastrointestinal tract. Alcohol abuse by the elderly is more likely to result in major depression and suicide compared to younger adults.

It is often difficult to diagnose alcohol abuse in older adults since they tend to be more secretive about it and the common signs of alcoholism overlap certain signs of aging, including poor balance, slurred speech, impaired memory, poor food intake, and loss of motor control. Once diagnosed, older adults can often be successfully treated with outpatient or community-based groups and/or medication.[51] If detoxification is required, hospitalization may be needed since older adults tend to suffer more severe and prolonged withdrawal symptoms compared to younger adults.[52] Once the alcohol abuse has been controlled, the need for a healthful diet is more important than ever.

Financial Problems

The U.S. Department of Agriculture reports that approximately 6–7% of households with older Americans experience food insecurity.[53] This means that they are unable to obtain enough food to meet their physical needs every day. In response, the federal government has developed a network of food and nutrition services for older Americans. Some, such as the Food Stamp and Commodity Supplemental Food programs, are open to people of all ages, whereas others fall under the Nutrition Services Incentive Program, previously called the Nutrition Program for the Elderly, which is restricted to people 60 years of age and older. These services are typically coordinated with state and local governments as well as non-profit or community organizations. They include the following:

- **Food Stamp Program:** This USDA program serves as the primary food assistance program for low-income households. It is designed to meet the basic nutritional needs of eligible households or individuals. Participants are provided with a monthly allotment, typically in the form of a pre-paid debit card or food coupons. There are very few restrictions on the foods that can be purchased under this plan.

- **Child and Adult Care Program:** This program provides healthy meals and snacks to older and functionally impaired adults in qualified adult day-care settings. While only 2% of program funds are in support of adult care programs, they are a valuable source of revenue for the religious and community agencies who run the programs.

- **Commodity Supplemental Food Program:** This program targets low-income pregnant women, infants and young children, and older adults. Income guidelines must be met. Specific commodity foods are distributed, including cereals, peanut butter, dry beans, rice or pasta, and canned juice, fruits, vegetables, meat, poultry, and tuna. Unlike food stamps, this program is not intended to provide a complete array of foods.

- **Senior Farmers' Market Nutrition Program:** This program is sponsored by the USDA and provides coupons to low-income seniors so they can buy eligible foods at farmers' markets and roadside stands. Seniors enjoy the nutritional benefits of fresh produce and the opportunity to increase the variety of foods within their meals.

- **Nutrition Services Incentive Program:** The Department of Health and Human Services provides cash and USDA commodity foods to individual state agencies for meals for senior citizens. There is no income criteria; any person 60 years or older (plus his or her spouse, even if younger) can take part in this program. Meals, designed to provide one-third of the RDA for key nutrients, are served at senior centers located in community complexes, public housing units, religious centers, schools, or similar locations. Some centers provide "bag dinners" for evening meals and others send home meals on Fridays for consumption over the weekend. For qualified elders, meals can be delivered to their homes through the Meals on Wheels program. While free, participants are encouraged to contribute what they can to cover the cost of each meal. The Congregate Meal program also provides nutrition and health education, offers social activities, and provides referrals to social service agencies.

For homebound disabled and older adults, community programs such as Meals on Wheels provide nourishing, balanced meals as well as vital social contact.

A major review by the federal government confirmed that participation in the Nutrition Services Incentive Program improved the dietary quality and nutrient intakes of older adults.[54] Unfortunately, Congregate Meal and Meals on Wheels programs may have long waiting lists and be unable to meet the current demands of their communities.

> RECAP: *Overweight and obesity are important concerns for older adults, as they increase the risk for chronic diseases. Underweight is also a concern, as it can lead to increased illness and injury. Older adults may lose their sense of smell and taste, and dental problems can limit intake of meats, fruits, and vegetables, leading to nutrient deficiencies. Medications and certain nutrients can have adverse interactions, and alcohol abuse remains an underdiagnosed problem. Several government and community programs are available for older adults in need of food assistance.*

CHAPTER SUMMARY

- Energy, fat, and protein requirements are higher for toddlers than for infants. Until age 2, toddlers should drink whole milk rather than reduced-fat milk to meet calcium requirements. Iron deficiency is a concern in the toddler years and can be minimized by the consumption of foods naturally high in iron and iron-fortified foods.

- Toddlers are still at risk for choking, and parents should watch for allergies and monitor weight gain.

- For toddlers and preschoolers, a serving of food equals 1 tbsp. for each year of age. For example, 4 tbsp. of yogurt is a full serving for a 4-year-old child.

- Feeding vegan diets to toddlers is controversial and poses potential deficiencies for protein, iron, calcium, zinc, vitamin D, and vitamin B_{12}.

- Children need less fat, as a percent of total calories, than toddlers but slightly more than adults. Protein and energy needs are higher for children due to their larger size and higher activity levels. Calcium, iron, and zinc are nutrients of concern for children.

- Overweight and obesity are concerns for children of all ages and can be avoided by regular physical activity and eating a healthful diet.

- Calcium needs increase as children mature, while iron needs decrease slightly.

- Many children skip breakfast and do not choose healthful foods during school lunch. Peer pressure and popularity are strong influences on food choices. School lunches are nutritious as planned and meet federal guidelines, but the foods that children choose to eat at school, both during and outside of the lunch break, can be high in fat, sugar, and energy and low in nutrients.

- Disordered eating behaviors and eating disorders can result throughout childhood and adolescence from concerns about body image.

- Puberty results in rapid increases in height, weight, lean body mass, and fat mass; adequate energy is needed to support the growth, maturation, and physical activity of adolescents.

- Many adolescents replace whole grains, fruits, and vegetables with fast foods and snack foods, placing them at risk for deficiencies for calcium, iron, and vitamin A. Calcium is needed to optimize bone growth and to achieve peak bone density, and iron needs are increased because of increased muscle mass in adolescent boys and menstruation in girls.

- Obesity can occur during adolescence if food intake increases and physical activity decreases. Disordered eating behaviors, cigarette smoking, and use of alcohol and illegal drugs are also concerns for this age group.

- Growth is complete in older adults, and their body systems begin to degenerate as part of the normal aging process. Some of the physiologic changes that occur with aging include sensory deficits, loss of muscle mass and lean tissue, increased fat mass, decreased bone density, decreased immune function, and impaired ability to absorb and metabolize various nutrients. A nutritious diet and regular physical activity can reduce the rate of some of these changes.

- Older adults have lower energy needs due to their loss of lean tissue and lower physical activity levels. Older adults should consume 20–35% of total energy as fat and 45–65% of their energy as carbohydrate. Protein recommendations are the same as for younger adults.

- Micronutrients of concern for older adults include calcium, vitamin D, iron, zinc, vitamin B_{12}, vitamin B_6, and folate. Older adults need to carefully select nutrient-dense foods to meet their micronutrient needs, and supplementation may be necessary. Older

adults are at risk for chronic dehydration, so ample fluid intake should be encouraged.

- Overweight and obesity are important concerns for older adults, as they increase the risk for chronic diseases. A variety of factors also increase the older adult's risk for underweight, which then increases risk for death.

- Dental problems can affect an older adult's nutritional status. Medications can interfere with nutrient absorption and metabolism, and nutrients can also interfere with the actions of medications. Alcohol abuse is underdiagnosed in older adults and can have serious effects on health and nutritional status.

- Many older adults struggle to make ends meet. Several government and community programs are available for older adults in need of food assistance.

TEST YOURSELF ANSWERS

1. **False.** Toddlers have a higher need for fat than do older children or adults, so they should consume foods, including dairy products, that are higher in fat.

2. **True.** Girls may grow only a few more inches after menstruation begins, while boys continue to grow throughout adolescence and even into early adulthood.

3. **True.** Experts agree that food choices, including consumption of fried foods, chocolate, and sodas, have virtually no impact on the development of acne.

4. **True.** Although a reduction of muscle mass and lean tissue is inevitable with aging, some of this loss can be attenuated with regular physical activity.

5. **False.** It is unlikely that the human life span will exceed 125 years.

REVIEW QUESTIONS

1. Which of the following nutrients is needed in increased amounts in older adulthood?
   a. fiber
   b. vitamin D
   c. iron
   d. vitamin A

2. Carbohydrate should make up what percentage of total energy for children?
   a. 25–40%
   b. 35–50%
   c. 45–65%
   d. 65–85%

3. Which of the following is a major nutrition-related concern for toddlers?

   a. lacto-ovo-vegetarianism

   b. skipping breakfast

   c. botulism

   d. allergies

FIND THE QUACK

Sal is having lunch at the golf club with his friend Donald. Normally, they spend most of their time discussing their game, which Sal usually wins, and Donald usually complains that he's lost because of his painful joints. But today is different. Donald shows Sal something he's just received free in the mail: *Longevity Today* magazine. He says there are articles in it that prove that most of the problems of aging can be cured by a remedy containing a substance called procaine. Sal shakes his head. "Sounds like a scam to me!"

"But these articles are written by doctors," his friend insists. "And scientists. And one is even written by a former nutrition consultant for the Olympics! For instance," he continues, stabbing his finger at a particular page, "here's an article written by an M.D. that says that this procaine stuff 'reverses the physical and cognitive effects of aging, including hypertension, enlarged prostate, joint pain, constipation, and even depression!' That's a quote!"

Sal laughs. "One pill is supposed to do all that?"

"They cite studies!" Donald exclaims. "Listen: 'Clinical trials in Europe, Asia, and the United States have consistently demonstrated the benefits of procaine as an anti-aging wonder drug.' It's only twenty bucks for a month's supply. I say it's worth a try."

Sal shrugs. "Listen, Donald, if you want to throw away your money, go ahead. But I'd rather save my twenty bucks and take Doris out for a walk on the beach at sunset. That's my anti-aging remedy!"

1. Look up procaine in a reputable online encyclopedia or another source. What is it, and what is behind the claims for its anti-aging properties?

2. Donald is impressed by the authorship of the articles he read in *Longevity Today* magazine—physicians, scientists, and a nutrition consultant— and by the fact that the articles "cite studies." Are you? Why or why not?

3. Comment on the fact that Donald received *Longevity Today* magazine free in the mail.

4. What do you think of Sal's "anti-aging remedy"?

Answers can be found at www.aw-bc.com / thompson.

4. Which of the following breakfasts would be most appropriate to serve a 20-month-old child?

   a. ½ cup of iron-fortified cooked oat cereal, 2 tbsp. of mashed pineapple, and 1 cup of whole milk

   b. 2 tbsp. of nonfat yogurt, 2 tbsp. of applesauce, one slice of melba toast spread with strawberry preserves, and 1 cup of calcium-fortified orange juice

   c. ½ cup of iron-fortified cooked oat cereal, 1/4 cup of cubed pineapple, and 1 cup of low-fat milk

   d. two small link sausages cut in 1-inch pieces, 2 tbsp. of scrambled egg, one slice of whole-wheat toast, four cherry tomatoes, 2 tbsp. of applesauce, and 1 cup of whole milk

5. Which of the following statements about cigarette smoking is true?

   a. Cigarette smoking can interfere with the metabolism of nutrients.

   b. Cigarette smoking commonly causes food cravings, known as "getting the munchies."

   c. Cigarette smoking is the number one cause of death in adolescents.

   d. All of the above statements are true.

6. True or False? Preschool children are too young to understand and be influenced by their parents' examples.

7. True or False? The food choice patterns of children are heavily influenced by circumstances at school.

8. True or false? High-potency vitamin A supplements are an effective treatment for acne.

9. True or false? Older adult males are advised to consume two alcoholic drinks per day to lower their risk of heart disease.

10. True or false? Older adults who regularly participate in strengthening and aerobic exercises have a reduced risk for fractures.

11. Identify some advantages and disadvantages of modern technology (such as television and computers) in terms of their impact on the lifestyle and nutritional status of children and adolescents.

12. Explain why a toddler in a vegan family might be at risk for protein deficiency.

13. Imagine that you are taking care of a small group of 5-year-old children for an afternoon. Design a menu for the children's lunch that is nutritious and that will be fun for them to eat.

14. Imagine that you manage a college cafeteria. Design a menu with three lunch choices that are nutritious and that are likely to be popular with 18- to 21-year-old students.

15. Imagine that you and your parents live in Dallas, where you attend college and your parents are employed as architects. A year ago, your grandmother,

who lives in Boston, stayed with you for several weeks following the death of your grandfather. She seemed fit at the time, going for walks with you and your dog, and cooking large meals for your family throughout her stay. Last night your mother received a phone call from a Boston hospital saying that your grandmother had been admitted following a hip fracture suffered in a fall at home and was battling significant dehydration as well. Identify several factors that might have contributed to your grandmother's condition.

WEB LINKS

www.kidnetic.com
Kidnetic.com

A fun Web site developed to help children and families get active, providing instructions and ideas for physical games and challenges, recipes for kids to make, and information about nutrition and the body.

www.verbnow.com
VERB

Create a character, write a story, or select a game and get out there and play. A hip activity-promoting site for kids age 9–13, from the CDC.

www.kidsnutrition.org
USDA/ARS Children's Nutrition Research Center at Baylor College of Medicine

This site provides information about current research projects, nutrition Web links, and consumer and nutrition news.

www.keepkidshealthy.com
Keep Kids Healthy.com

Find information about nutrition and health for toddlers, children, and adolescents on this Web site.

www.cdc.gov
The Centers for Disease Control and Prevention

Click on Life Stages & Populations, then you can select topics such as Adolescents & Teens, Older Adults & Seniors, Men, or Women, plus many others.

www.vrg.org
The Vegetarian Resource Group

Visit this Web site to learn more about vegetarianism for all ages. Included on the site are special sections for teens and kids, as well as recipes and guides for vegetarian and vegan eating in all kinds of situations.

www.health.gov/dietaryguidelines
Dietary Guidelines for Americans

Visit this site to read the current edition of Dietary Guidelines for Americans and to learn about their development.

www.nichd.nih.gov/milk
Milk Matters

Need ideas on how to increase milk and dairy foods intakes? This Web site provides practical tips and menus for children and adolescents.

http://nutrition.wsu.edu/ebet/toolkit.html
Eat Better, Eat Together

This Web site offers educational materials for strengthening family meal time. Suggestions for community events, media interviews, and educational materials are available.

www.fns.usda.gov
USDA Food & Nutrition Service

Read about governmental programs to provide food to all ages, including school meals programs, the Child and Adult Care Food Program, and the Women, Infants, and Children Program.

www.nlm.nih.gov/medlineplus/dentalhealth.html
MedlinePlus Dental Health

Contained on this site are links to articles about dental health for all ages.

www.eatright.org
American Dietetic Association

Visit this Web site to learn about healthy eating habits for all stages of life.

www.nia.nih.gov
The National Institute on Aging

The National Institute on Aging provides information about how older adults can benefit from physical activity and good diet.

www.nihseniorhealth.gov
NIH Senior Health

This Web site, written in large print, was developed for older adults, and offers up-to-date information on popular health topics for older Americans.

www.aarp.org
AARP

A national advocacy group for the elderly, AARP, an organization of 35 million older Americans, can be joined by adults 50 years and older. Their Web site has links to articles focusing on all aspects of health, finances, housing, and legal issues that are of importance to the elderly.

www.aoa.gov
Administration on Aging

Follow legislative updates on this Web site for information related to the Congregate Meal and Meals on Wheels programs. Also provided are resources on Alzheimer's, elder rights and resources, housing, and elder nutrition.

www.healthandage.com
Health and Age

This site lists comprehensive information about nutrition, exercise, and preventative medicine with relation to aging. Features include a section for caregivers and a newsletter.

REFERENCES

1. Centers for Disease Control and Prevention (CDC). 2007. National Center for Health Statistics. Fast Stats. Overweight. www.cdc.gov/nchs/fastats/overwt.htm. (Accessed August 2007.)
2. National Diabetes Information Clearinghouse (NDIC). 2005. National Diabetes Statistics. National Institutes of Health Publication No. 06–3892. http://diabetes.niddk.nih.gov/dm/pubs/statistics/index.htm. (Accessed August 2007.)
3. Institute of Medicine, Food and Nutrition Board. 2002. *Dietary Reference Intakes for Energy, Carbohydrates, Fiber, Fat, Protein and Amino Acids (Macronutrients)*. Washington, DC: National Academies Press.
4. Kleinman, R. E. (ed.) 2004. *Pediatric Nutrition Handbook*, 5th edn. Elk Grove Village, IL: American Academy of Pediatrics.
5. Institute of Medicine, Food and Nutrition Board. 1997. *Dietary Reference Intakes for Calcium, Phosphorus, Magnesium, Vitamin D, and Fluoride*. Washington, DC: National Academies Press.
6. Institute of Medicine, Food and Nutrition Board. 2001. *Dietary Reference Intakes for Vitamin A, Vitamin K, Arsenic, Boron, Chromium, Copper, Iodine, Iron, Manganese, Molybdenum, Nickel, Silicon, Vanadium, and Zinc*. Washington, DC: National Academies Press.
7. Institute of Medicine, Food and Nutrition Board. 2004. *Dietary Reference Intakes for Water, Potassium, Sodium, Chloride, and Sulfate*. Washington, DC: National Academies Press.
8. Bailey, I. 2001. Daughters, 9 and 5, starving on a vegan diet, father claims. *National Post*. http://fact.on.ca/news/news0103/np010305.htm. (Accessed August 2007.)
9. Centers for Disease Control and Prevention (CDC). 2001. Neurologic impairment in children associated with maternal dietary deficiency of cobalamin. *Morbid. Mortal. Wkly. Rep.* 52(04):61–64.
10. Second Opinions. 2002. Child Abuse by Vegan Parents. www.second-opinions.co.uk/child_abuse.html. (Accessed August 2007.)
11. Stern, R. 2007. Diet from hell. *Phoenix New Times*, May 10, 2007. www.phoenixnewtimes.com/2007-05-10/news/diet-from-hell/. (Accessed August 2007.)
12. Mangels, R. 2001. The Vegetarian Resource Group. Vegetarianism in a Nutshell. Feeding Vegan Kids. www.vrg.org/nutshell/kids.htm. (Accessed August 2007.)
13. USDA. Food and Nutrition Service. 2003. School Breakfast Program. Healthy Eating Helps You Make the Grade. www.fns.usda.gov/cnd/Breakfast/SchoolBfastCampaign/theresearch.html. (Accessed August 2007.)
14. Kleinman, R. E., S. Hall, H. Green, D. Korzec-Ramirez, K. Patton, M. E. Pagano, and J. M. Murphy. 2002. Diet, breakfast, and academic performance in children. *Ann. Nutr. Metab.* 46:24–30.
15. Food and Nutrition Board. Institute of Medicine. 1989. *Recommended Dietary Allowances*, 10th edn. Washington, DC: National Academies Press.
16. USDA. Food and Nutrition Service. 2003. National School Lunch Program. www.fns.usda.gov/cnd/Lunch/AboutLunch/NSLPFactSheet.pdf. (Accessed August 2007.)
17. Stallings, V. A., and A. L. Yaktine (eds.) 2007. *Nutrition Standards for Foods in Schools: Leading the Way Toward Healthier Youth*. Washington, DC: National Academies Press.
18. Cunningham-Sabo, L., M. P. Snyder, J. Anliker, J. Thompson, J. L. Weber, O. Thomas, K. Ring, D. Stewart, H. Platero, and L. Nielsen. 2003. Impact of the Pathways food service intervention on breakfast served in American-Indian schools. *Prevent. Med.* 37:S46–S54.
19. Himes, J. H., K. Ring, J. Gittelsohn, L. Cunningham-Sabo, J. Weber, J. Thompson, L. Harnack, and C. Suchinidran. 2003. Impact of the Pathways intervention on the dietary intakes of American Indian schoolchildren. *Prevent. Med.* 37:S55–S61.
20. Agras, W. S., L. D. Hammer, F. McNicholas, et al. 2004. Risk factors for childhood overweight: a prospective study from birth to 9.5 years. *J. Ped.* 145:19–24.
21. Zeller, M., and S. Daniels. 2004. The obesity epidemic: family matters. *J. Ped.* 145:3–4.
22. Jago, R., T. Baranowski, J. C. Baranowski, D. Thompson, and K. A. Greaves. 2005. BMI from 3–6 y of age is predicted by TV viewing and physical activity, not diet. *International Journal of Obesity*. 29: 557–565.
23. Taveras, E. M., T. J. Sandora, M. C. Shih, D. Ross-Degnan, D. A. Goldmann, and M. W. Gillman. 2006. The association of television and video viewing with fast food intake by preschool-age children. *Obesity* 14:2034–2041.
24. Salmon, J., K. J. Campbell, and D. A. Crawford. 2006. Television viewing habits associated with obesity risk factors: a survey of Melbourne schoolchildren. *Med. J. Aust.* 184:64–67.
25. Ritchie, L. D., G. Welk, D. Styne, D. E. Gerstein, and P. B. Crawford. 2005. Family environment and pediatric overweight: what is a parent to do? *J. Am. Diet. Assoc.* 105:S70–S79.
26. Heaney, R. P., and K. Rafferty. 2001. Carbonated beverages and urinary calcium excretion. *Am. J. Clin. Nutr.* 74:343–347.
27. Polan, E. U., and D. R. Taylor. 2003. *Journey Across the Lifespan*, 2nd edn. Philadelphia: F. A. Davis.
28. Centers for Disease Control and Prevention (CDC). 1999. National Center for Chronic Disease Prevention and Health Promotion. Physical Activity and Health. A Report of the Surgeon General. Adolescents and Young Adults. www.cdc.gov/nccdphp/sgr/adoles.htm. (Accessed August 2007.)
29. Gordon-Larsen, P., M. C. Nelson, and B. M. Popkin. 2004. Longitudinal physical activity and sedentary behavior trends: adolescence to adulthood. *Am. J. Prevent. Med.* 27:277–283.
30. Centers for Disease Control and Prevention (CDC). 2004. National Center for Chronic Disease Prevention and Health Promotion. Healthy Aging. Healthy Aging for Older Adults. www.cdc.gov/aging/. (Accessed August 2007.)
31. Federal Interagency Forum on Aging-Related Statistics. 2004. *Older Americans 2004: Key Indicators of Well-Being*. Washington, DC: U.S. Government Printing Office.
32. Geiser, M. 2006. Living a longer life—do you want to live to 100? *MEG Fitness Health News*. http://megfithealthnews.blogspot.com/2006_08_01_archive.html. (Accessed August 2007.)
33. Chernoff, R. 2006. Demographics of aging. *Geriatric Nutrition: The Health Professional's Handbook*, 3rd edn. Sudbury, MA: Jones and Bartlett Publishers.
34. Schiffman, S. S., M. O. Rogers, and J. Zervakis. 2004. Loss of taste, smell, and other senses with age. *Handbook of Clinical Nutrition and Aging*. Totowa, NJ: Humana Press.
35. Moskovitz, D. N., J. Saltzman, and Y. I. Kim. 2006. The aging gut. *Geriatric Nutrition, The Health Professional's Handbook*, 3rd edn. Sudbury, MA. Jones and Bartlett Publishers.
36. Dryden, G. W., and S. A. McClave. 2004. Gastrointestinal senescence and digestive diseases of the elderly. *Handbook of Clinical Nutrition and Aging*. Totowa, NJ: Humana Press.
37. National Institute on Aging. 2002.
38. Centers for Disease Control and Prevention. 2004. Summary health statistics for U. S. adults: National Health Interview Survey, 2002. Vital and Health Statistics, Series 10, No. 222.
39. Franco, O. H., C. de Laet, A. Peeters, J. Jonker, J. Mackenbach, and W. Nusselder. 2005. *Arch. Intern. Med.* 165:2355–2360.

40. Pu, C. T., M. T. Johnson, D. E. Forman, J. M. Hausdorff, R. Roubenoff, M. Foldvari, R. A. Fielding, and M. A. Fiatarone Singh. 2001. Randomized trial of progressive resistance training to counteract the myopathy of chronic heart failure. *J. Appl. Physiol.* 90:2341–2350.

41. Campbell, W. W., N. S. Carnell, and A. E. Thalacker. 2006. Protein metabolism and requirements. *Geriatric Nutrition: The Health Professional's Handbook*, 3rd edn. Sudbury, MA: Jones and Bartlett Publishers.

42. Hackam, D. G., and S. S. Anand. 2003. Emerging risk factors for atherosclerotic vascular disease: a critical review of the evidence. *J. Am. Med. Assoc.* 290:932–940.

43. Institute of Medicine, Food and Nutrition Board. 1998. *Dietary Reference Intakes for Thiamin, Riboflavin, Niacin, Vitamin B_6, Folate, Vitamin B_{12}, Pantothenic Acid, Biotin, and Choline*. Washington, DC: National Academies Press.

44. Feskanich, D., V. Singh, W. C. Willett, and G. A. Colditz. 2002. Vitamin A intake and hip fractures among postmenopausal women. *J. Am. Med. Assoc.* 287:47–54.

45. Arterburn, D. D., P. K. Crane, and S. D. Sullivan. 2004. The coming epidemic of obesity in elderly Americans. *J. Am. Ger. Soc.* 52:1907–1912.

46. Jensen, G. L., and J. M. Friedmann. 2002. Obesity is associated with functional decline among community dwelling rural older persons. *J. Am. Ger. Soc.* 102:918–923.

47. Dolan, C. M., H. Kraemer, W. Browner, K. Ensrud, and J. L. Kelsy. 2007. Associations between body composition, anthropometry, and mortality in women aged 65 years and older. *Am. J. Public Health* 97:913–918.

48. Sattar, S. P., F. Petty, and W. J. Burke. 2003. Diagnosis and treatment of alcohol dependence in older alcoholics. *Clin. Geriatr. Med.* 19:743–761.

49. Friedlander, A. H., and D. C. Norman. 2006. Geriatric alcoholism: pathophysiology and dental implications. *J. Am. Dental Assoc.* 137:330–338.

50. Dufour, M. C., L. Archer, and E. Gordis. 1992. Alcohol and the elderly. *Clin. Geriatr. Med.* 8:127–141.

51. Culbertson, J. W. 2006. Alcohol use in the elderly: beyond the CAGE. Part 2: screening instruments and treatment strategies. *Geriatrics*. 61:20–26.

52. Dufour, M., and R. K. Fuller. 1995. Alcohol in the elderly. *Annu. Rev. Med.* 46:123–132.

53. U. S. Department of Agriculture (USDA). 2006. Economic Research Service. Food Security in the United States: Conditions and Trends: 2005. www.ers.usda.gov/Briefing/FoodSecurity/trends.htm. (Accessed August 2007.)

54. Ponza, M., J. C. Ohls, and B. A. Millen. 1996. Serving Elders at Risk: The Older Americans Act Nutrition Programs—National Evaluation of the Elderly Nutrition Program, 1993–1995. Washington, DC: Mathetmatica Policy Research, Inc.

55. Dhahbi, J. M., H.-J. Kim, P. L. Mote, R. J. Beaver, and S. R. Spindler. 2004. Temporal linkage between the phenotypic and genomic responses to caloric restriction. *Proc. Natl. Acad. Sci. USA* 101(15):5524–5529.

56. Wang, C., R. Weindruch, J. R. Fernández, C. S. Coffey, P. Patel, and D. B. Allison. 2004. Caloric restriction and body weight independently affect longevity in Wistar rats. *Int. J. Obesity* 28(3):357–362.

57. Anderson, R. M., M. Latorre-Esteves, A. R. Neves, S. Lavu, O. Medvedik, C. Taylor, K. T. Howitz, H. Santos, and D. A. Sinclair. 2003. Yeast life-span extension by calorie restriction is independent of NAD fluctuation. *Science* 302(5653):2124–2126.

58. Fontana, L., and S. Klein. 2007. Aging, adiposity, and calorie restriction. *J. Am. Med. Assoc.* 297:986–994.

59. Masoro, E. J. 2005. Overview of caloric restriction and ageing. *Mech. Ageing Dev.* 126:913–922.

60. Heilbronn, L. K., and E. Ravussin. 2003. Calorie restriction and aging: review of the literature and implications for studies in humans. *Am. J. Clin. Nutr.* 78(3):361–369.

61. Kostoff, R. N. 2001. Energy restriction. *Am. J. Clin. Nutr.* 74(4):556–557.

NUTRITION DEBATE

Can We Live Longer by Eating a Low-Energy Diet?

how old do you want to live to be— 80 years, 100 years, 110 years? If you were to discover that you could live to be 125 years of age by eating a little more than half of your current energy intake and still be healthy as you age, would you do it? Believe it or not, a growing number of people are already doing this in response to studies indicating that low-energy diets can significantly increase the life span of animals.

Existing research shows that consuming low-energy diets, also referred to as *caloric restriction*, can significantly extend the life span of small species; most of this research has been done in rats, mice, fish, flies, and yeast cells.[55–57] Until recently, we did not know whether this same effect would be seen in nonhuman primates and in humans. But a recent summary of published articles suggests that caloric restriction can improve various metabolic, hormonal, and functional measures of health in humans as well.[58]

How can caloric restriction prolong life span? The answer to this question is not fully understood, but there are several proposed mechanisms, most based upon animal research.[59] For example, it is speculated that the reduction in metabolic rate that occurs with restricting energy intake results in a much lower production of free radicals, which in turn significantly reduces oxidative damage and can prolong life. Caloric restriction also causes marked improvements in insulin sensitivity and results in hormonal changes linked to a lower incidence of chronic diseases such as heart disease and diabetes. In fact, caloric restriction can alter gene expression, which can reduce the effects of aging and prevent diseases such as cancer.[55] Some of the effects of prolonged caloric restriction in *rodents* include:[60]

- Decreased insulin levels and improved insulin sensitivity
- Decreased body temperature
- Decreased energy expenditure
- Decreased oxidative stress
- Decreased fat mass and lean body mass
- Increased levels of voluntary physical activity

While no long-term studies have been conducted with humans, the effects of *short*-term caloric restriction in humans include:[58]

- Reduced blood pressure
- Improved blood lipid profile
- Increased insulin sensitivity
- Decreased plasma levels of inflammatory markers

It is important to emphasize that animal studies demonstrating the life-prolonging effects of caloric restriction are based on *highly nutritious* low-calorie diets. Unhealthful energy-restriction situations in humans such as starvation, wasting caused by diseases such as cancer,

Maintaining an energy-restricted diet that is also highly nutritious requires significant planning and preparing most of your own meals.

Nutrient-dense, low-calorie vegetables make up the bulk of a calorie-restricted diet.

and eating disorders such as anorexia nervosa do not result in prolonged life. In fact, these situations are associated with increased risks for illness and premature death.[61] In addition, a recent study found that older adults with the lowest BMI had the highest risk of death.[47] Figure 20.9 on page 767 illustrates what is termed the "U-shaped" relationship between BMI and risk of death among older adults. It seems clear then that caloric restriction would be inappropriate for adults in this age group if it prompted a reduction in BMI below about 26.

Although caloric restriction is successful in extending the lives of some animal species, there are no *long-term* studies suggesting that this same effect will occur in humans.[58] Such studies in humans might never be conducted because of ethical and logistical concerns. Finding enough people to participate in any research study over their entire lifetime would be extremely difficult. In addition, most people find it challenging to follow a caloric-restricted diet for just a few months; compliance to this type of diet over decades could be almost impossible. Institutional committees that review research studies are hesitant to approve caloric-restriction research in humans not only because of these logistical problems, but also because of the potential risks of malnutrition that could occur.

A calorie-restricted diet can make family meals challenging.

All food must be carefully measured and weighed in low-energy diets.

You may be wondering how much less energy you would have to consume to meet the caloric-restriction levels studied in animals. Most studies have found a significant extension of life span when animals are fed 30–40% less energy than control animals. If you are a woman who normally eats about 2,000 kcal/day, this level of reduction would result in an energy intake of about 1,200 to 1,400 kcal/day. While this amount of energy reduction does not seem excessive, it would be very difficult to achieve this reduction every day over a lifetime. You must also keep in mind that this diet must be of very high nutritional quality, which presents a huge number of challenges, including meticulous planning of meals, preparation of most, if not all, of your own foods, limited options for eating meals outside of your home, and the challenge of working the demands of your special diet around the eating behaviors of family members and friends.

Considering the potential benefits of caloric restriction, do you think it is worth following this type of diet? Are you willing to make the sacrifices necessary to try to significantly prolong your life, even though we are unsure whether this practice can prolong the lives of humans? If we do find that caloric restriction substantially improves the health of humans and in turn can prolong their lives, should caloric restriction be recommended for all people? This debate will continue as more research is conducted. In the meantime, some people are already consuming diets that are low in energy in the hope that they will live much longer, healthier lives.

Global Nutrition

READ ON.

in Malawi, a small country in southern Africa, a widowed mother of three risks death to pull the stems of water lilies from crocodile-infested waters. They are bitter and give her children diarrhea, but they are the only food she can find. She is not alone: across southern Africa, mismanagement, corruption, drought, lack of irrigation, and disease—especially infection with HIV—combine to cause recurring cycles of hunger for millions of people. And hunger contributes to early death: in Malawi, one in ten mothers dies in childbirth, and nearly one in five children dies before reaching age 5.[1]

The Food and Agriculture Organization of the United Nations (FAO) estimates that, worldwide, 850 million people are undernourished.[2] In parts of central Africa, more than 70% of the population goes hungry. Why is this so? Does malnutrition occur only in developing nations? And is there anything you can do to help? We explore these questions here.

Increasingly today, **malnutrition** is a fiend with two faces. In developing nations, it typically appears in the form of **undernutrition**, that is, people simply don't have enough to eat. Undernutrition most often kills its victims by making them vulnerable to infectious diseases. But for about the past decade, all over the world, another form of malnutrition has been emerging: **overnutrition**, or consumption of more energy than the body expends. Overnutrition causes overweight and obesity, and threatens its victims with chronic diseases such as heart disease and diabetes. It is increasingly seen not only in developed areas like North America and Western Europe, but also in nations transitioning from the very poorest to the middle range of gross national income, including Brazil, India, and China. Here, we explore *In Depth* these two forms of malnutrition and explain how they're linked. And if what you read and see on the next few pages spurs you to action, we'll give you plenty of suggestions about how you can fight malnutrition, both globally and in your community.

Malnutrition in the Developing World

The FAO estimates that one in five people in the developing world is chronically hungry.[3] The problem is greatest in sub-Saharan Africa and Southeast Asia, in countries ranging from Ethiopia to Sudan and India to Uzbekistan (see FIGURE 1). Chronic hunger results in **wasting**, a condition of very low body weight for height. Children who are chronically undernourished also suffer from **stunting**; that is, they are shorter than expected for their age. People who are undernourished are highly susceptible to infectious diseases such as tuberculosis, infectious diarrhea, and pneumonia. Indeed, in some developing nations, undernutrition is estimated to contribute to 60% of childhood deaths each year, largely due to this decreased resistance to infection.[4]

What Causes Hunger in Developing Nations?

Hunger exists in every nation of the world; however, the causes vary. In wealthy nations, it is usually caused by unequal distribution of abundant food to people who are poor. In developing nations, unequal distribution can be a factor, but the most common causes are natural disasters, war, overpopulation, poor farming practices, lack of infrastructure, and disease.

Natural Disasters

In the summer of 2004, a drought in western Africa brought life-threatening undernutrition to about 20% of the population of Niger and Mali.[5] Such natural disasters often result in widespread hunger because they destroy substantial amounts of local crops in a short time. Drought and other natural disasters, including floods, tsunamis, high winds, hurricanes, frosts, and infestations by insects, worms, or microbes can even result in **famine,** a severe food shortage affecting a large percentage of the population in a limited geographic area at a particular time.

An Indian farmer inspects what is left of his crop during a drought.

War

Unfortunately, famine is often a human-made disaster. In 2003, a rebellion against the Sudanese government led to violent repression in the Darfur region of Sudan.[6] Tens of thousands of people either were killed outright or died of starvation when crops and food supplies were burned. Hundreds of thousands more were relocated to camps where, because of governmental obstacles to international aid, they too faced starvation.[7]

Wars also induce famine when they interfere with planting or harvest times, or when farmlands

malnutrition A state of poor nutritional health that can be improved by adjustments in nutrient intake.

undernutrition Malnutrition defined by an absolute lack of adequate energy leading to underweight.

overnutrition Malnutrition defined by an absolute excess of calories leading to overweight. Diet may be high quality or poor quality.

wasting Very low weight for height.

stunting Low height for age.

famine A widespread severe food shortage that causes starvation and death in a large portion of a population in a region.

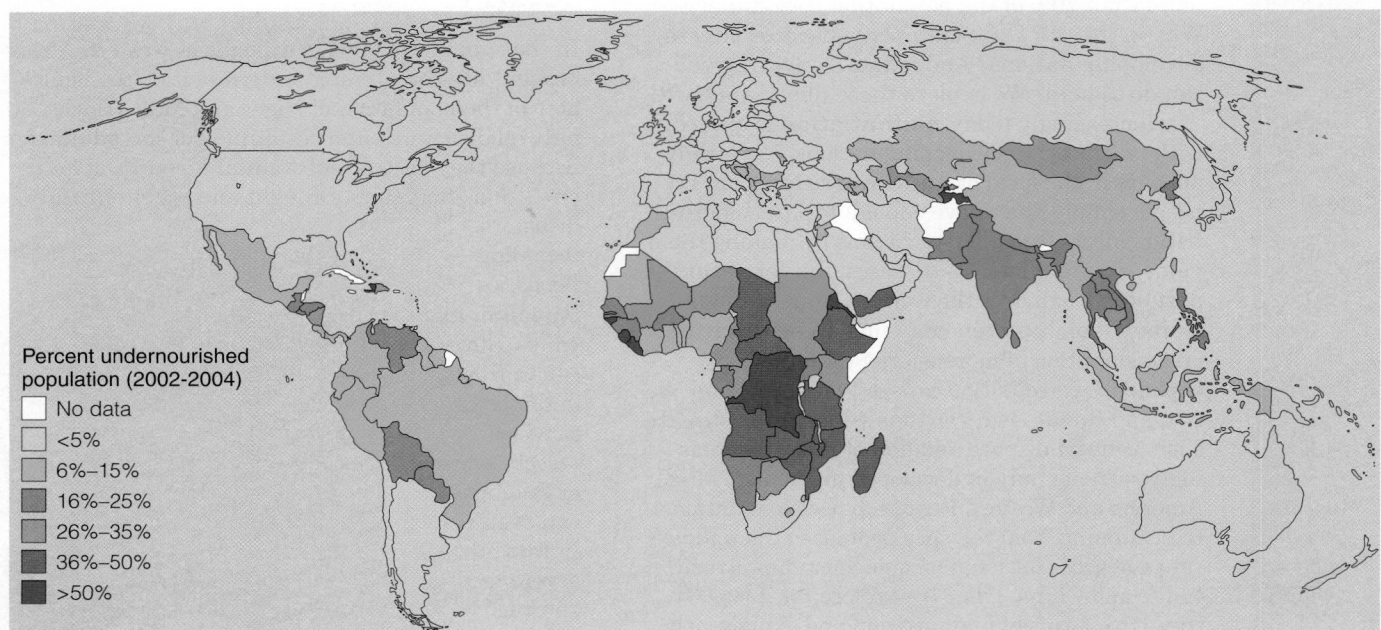

FIGURE 1 Undernutrition is most prevalent in parts of sub-Saharan Africa and Southeast Asia. (*Source:* © Food and Agriculture Organization of the United Nations 2004. Undernourished Population (2002–2004). http://www.fao.org/es/ess/faostat/ foodsecurity/FS%20Map/ map14.htm. Used with permission.).

are taken over by military forces. Explosives may destroy roads, bridges, or rail lines needed for distribution of food, and fear of military activity may keep markets closed.

Overpopulation

An area is said to be **overpopulated** when its resources are insufficient to support the number of people living there. In parts of the world with fertile land and adequate rainfall or irrigation systems to support abundant harvests, food shortages are rare. In more arid climates, especially in areas with high fertility rates and poor access to imported foods, food shortages are common.

One way of improving the food/population ratio is to increase food production and importation. Another strategy is to focus on slowing population growth. One of the most effective ways to do this is to improve the education of women and girls.[8] Their increased earning potential, access to information about contraception, and better health practices lead to smaller, healthier, more economically stable families.

Yet another way of slowing population growth is through improved public health measures such as immunization programs that reduce the spread of infectious

disease. When parents feel confident that their children will survive to adulthood, they have fewer children.

Poor Farming Practices

Some traditional farming practices have the potential to destroy useable land. Deforestation and overgrazing pastures and croplands destroy the trees and grass roots that preserve soils from wind and water erosion. Growing the same crop year after year on the same plot of ground can deplete the soil of nutrients and reduce crop yield. Use of agricultural land for **cash crops** such as cotton, coffee, and tobacco may replace land use for local food crops such as sorghum and corn. The end result may be less food available for local consumption.

Lack of Infrastructure

Many developing countries lack roads and transportation into rural areas. This limits available food to whatever can be produced locally. Lack of electricity and refrigeration can limit storage and enhance spoilage of even local foods before they can be used. Other crucial aspects of infrastructure are irrigation systems, sanitation services, communication systems, an adequate healthcare delivery system, and adequate public education.

Impact of Disease

Disease reduces the work capacity of individuals, and this in turn reduces their ability to ward off poverty and malnutrition. This vicious cycle is demonstrated by the AIDS epidemic. In some African nations, more than one

overpopulated Characteristic used to describe a region that has insufficient resources to support the number of people living there.

cash crops Crops grown to be sold rather than eaten, such as cotton, tobacco, jute, and sugar cane.

in four adults are believed to be infected with HIV, and 3 million died from AIDS in 2005.[9] Because AIDS most commonly strikes young adults who are the primary wage earners in their families, their illness or death orphans their children, impoverishes their elderly parents, and devastates their communities. By creating populations in which children and the elderly predominate, the AIDS epidemic has exacerbated the risk of undernutrition in many developing countries.

Unequal Distribution

In the developing world, more than three-fourths of malnourished children live in countries with food surpluses.[10] The major cause of unequal distribution of food within a community is, of course, poverty. The most at risk are people who do not own enough land to grow their own food and must work to buy food in areas where employment opportunities are scarce.

Unequal distribution also occurs because of cultural biases. In many countries, limited food is distributed first to men and boys and only secondarily to women and girls.[10] Food distribution to the elderly is also sometimes limited. Access to food also can differ by ethnicity and religion. For example, higher mortality was documented in some ethnic and religious groups during the drought-induced famine in northern Ethiopia in the 1980s.[11]

What Health Problems Result from Undernutrition?

Undernutrition can cause a wide variety of health problems. The most common are discussed here.

Increased Infant and Child Mortality

Undernutrition increases by close to 50% the likelihood that a child will die between birth and age 5.[12] The infant mortality rate in industrialized countries was only 5 per 1,000 in 2005, whereas in countries where malnutrition is endemic, the average was 98 per 1,000.[13]

Increased Vulnerability to Infection

The most common way that undernutrition kills infants and children is by making them more vulnerable to infection. In impoverished nations, pneumonia and infectious diarrhea are the leading causes of death among children under 5 years of age.[14] By decreasing a child's general health, malnutrition increases the likelihood that the child will not survive infection. Moreover, infection exacerbates malnutrition by decreasing appetite, causing vomiting and diarrhea, and generally weakening the immune system. A vicious cycle of malnutrition, infection, worsening malnutrition, and increased vulnerability to infection develops.

Macronutrient Deficiencies

Marasmus is a disease of children that results from grossly inadequate intakes of energy. As we explained in Chapter 6, it commonly occurs when chronic food short-

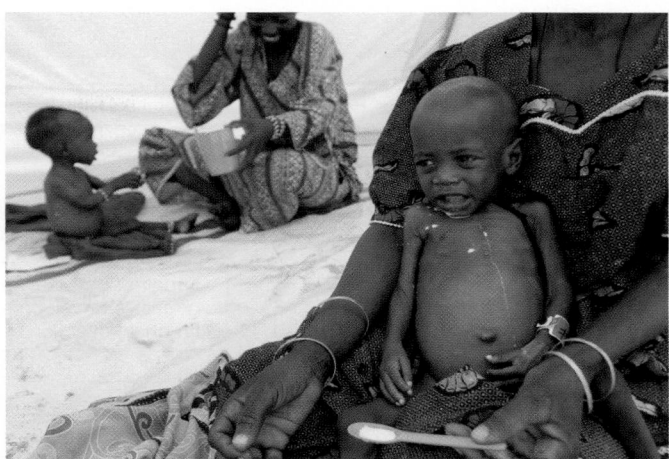

Malnourished children often suffer impaired growth and development.

ages reduce children's total energy intake. As a result, the children slowly starve to death. Typically, their weakened immune system makes them highly vulnerable to infection; thus, they often die from pneumonia or from dehydration caused by diarrhea. Alternatively, they suffer heart failure from a weakened heart muscle.

Kwashiorkor is a disease of toddlers who have recently been weaned from breast milk, which is replaced with a watery porridge that has inadequate and poor-quality protein. The lack of dietary protein causes edema because the level of protein in the blood is inadequate to keep fluids from seeping into the tissue spaces. Edema swells the child's belly and makes the face and limbs appear adequately nourished. The child experiences severe wasting of muscle tissue and easily succumbs to infection.

Micronutrient Deficiencies

Undernourished people are at risk for a variety of micronutrient deficiencies. Iron deficiency is the world's most common nutrient deficiency. It increases the risk of infection, premature birth, low birth weight, and maternal death during or immediately following childbirth. It also impairs children's ability to learn and adults' ability to work. Iodine deficiency is responsible for mental impairment in children and goiter in adults. Zinc deficiency reduces growth and immune function. Deficiency of vitamin B_{12} can result in severe cognitive impairment. Lack of sufficient vitamin A in the diet is a preventable cause of night blindness in children.

Poor Work Capacity in Adults

The debilitating weakness caused by undernutrition affects the productivity of adults in many developing nations. It is especially detrimental when manual labor involved in subsistence farming is the main source of food and income. Nutrient deficiency also contributes to poor work capacity. Iron-deficiency anemia is particularly debilitating because of iron's role in oxygen transport.

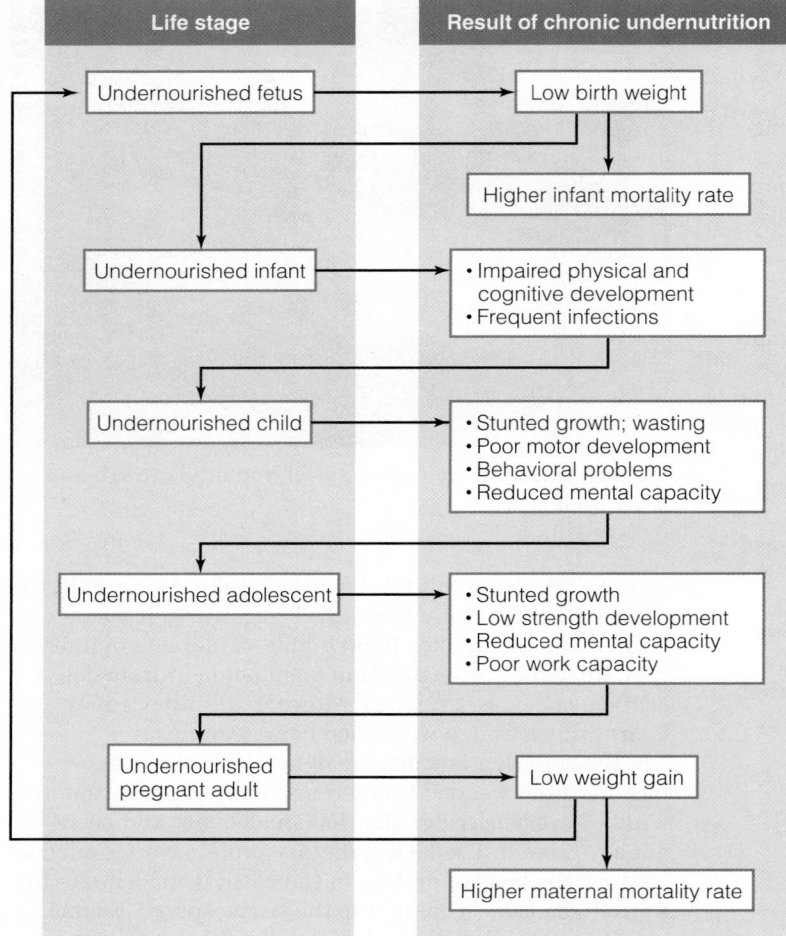

Life stage	Result of chronic undernutrition
Undernourished fetus	Low birth weight
	Higher infant mortality rate
Undernourished infant	• Impaired physical and cognitive development • Frequent infections
Undernourished child	• Stunted growth; wasting • Poor motor development • Behavioral problems • Reduced mental capacity
Undernourished adolescent	• Stunted growth • Low strength development • Reduced mental capacity • Poor work capacity
Undernourished pregnant adult	Low weight gain
	Higher maternal mortality rate

FIGURE 2 Acute and long-term effects of malnutrition throughout the life cycle.

FIGURE 2 illustrates the varied and cruel effects of chronic undernutrition throughout the life span. As you can see, the cycle is perpetuated across generations when undernourished women give birth to undernourished infants.

Why Is Obesity a Growing Problem in Developing Nations?

People living in countries with growing economies, such as Egypt, India, and China, enjoy increased food availability and variety. Unfortunately, their new diet usually includes more processed foods with high energy density due to added fat and sugar, including snack foods and fast foods. These foods are usually less expensive than traditional foods such as fish, fresh fruits, and vegetables.[15] This shift in dietary pattern as poverty is relieved is called the **nutrition transition.** And while the population is consuming more energy, greater access to motorized transportation and a decrease in manual labor are reducing their energy expenditure. The result of this equation is overnutrition.

In addition, there is now significant evidence linking undernutrition during fetal life to overnutrition in adulthood. The hypothesis known as "fetal origins of adult disease" states that fetal adaptations to poor maternal nutrition help the child during times of food shortages but make the child susceptible to obesity and chronic disease when food is plentiful.[16] For example, when a mother is malnourished during pregnancy, her newborn will tend to have a low birth weight but be relatively fat. This may occur because the fetal body has favored growth of the brain, which is more than 50% fat, at the expense of muscle tissue. Researchers theorize that this adaptation may prompt a permanent physiological tendency to gain fat tissue when food is plentiful.[17]

Given these factors, it is not surprising that transitioning countries have been experiencing an alarming increase in the prevalence of obesity and its associated diseases. These countries are challenged to support economic prosperity without promoting overnutrition.

Malnutrition in the United States

As we discussed in Chapter 11, overnutrition is becoming a national health crisis. A majority of Americans are now overweight or obese, and the prevalence of type 2 diabetes and other chronic diseases associated with obesity is increasing. But even in the United States, unequal distribution of abundant food leads to undernutrition among the nation's poorest citizens.

As shown in FIGURE 3, the U.S. Department of Agriculture (USDA) estimates that 11% of U.S. households (about 12.6 million families) suffer **food insecurity.**[18] This means that they are unable to obtain enough food to meet their physical needs every day. Of households with income below the official U.S. poverty level ($19,806 for a family of four in 2005), 36% experience food insecurity.

nutrition transition A shift in dietary pattern toward greater food security, greater variety of foods, and more foods with high energy density; associated with increased incidence of obesity and chronic disease.

food insecurity Situation in which households are uncertain of having, or unable to acquire, enough food to meet the needs of all their members because they have insufficient money or other resources for food.

FIGURE 3 Food security status of U.S. households in 2005. Note: Food-insecure households include those with low food security and very low food security. (Source: Calculated by the Economic Research Service (ERS) using data from the December 2005 Current Population Survey Food Security Supplement. www.ers.usda.gov/Briefing/FoodSecurity/trends.htm.)

Most at risk are families consisting of single mothers and their children.[18] In 2005, 30.8% of households with children headed by a single woman experienced food insecurity. In 2005, more than 600,000 children lived in homes with *very low food security,* meaning that the normal eating patterns of one or more household members were disrupted and food intake was reduced at times during the year. Other vulnerable groups are the homeless, the unemployed, migrant laborers, and other workers in minimum wage jobs.

What Can Be Done to Relieve Malnutrition?

To combat malnutrition and achieve global food security, long-term solutions are critical. We discuss some of the most effective here.

Global Solutions

Among the most important long-term solutions for improving the health and nutrition of children worldwide are programs that encourage breastfeeding. This is because breast milk provides optimal nutrition for healthy growth of the newborn and contains antibodies that protect against infections. In contrast, feeding infants with formula increases the infant's risk of diarrhea if the powder is mixed with unsanitary water. In developing countries, breastfeeding is considered to reduce diarrheal deaths in young children by 50–95%. The World Health Organization (WHO) sponsors programs to encourage breastfeeding throughout the developing world.

Strategies to increase immunization of children are helping to reduce the rate of infectious disease in children worldwide. At the same time, supplying local health agencies with oral rehydration therapy, a simple solution of fluids and electrolytes that can be administered to children with diarrhea, is helping to reduce deaths from dehydration.

Many international organizations help improve the nutrient status of the poor by enabling them to produce their own foods. For example, both USAID and the Peace Corps have agricultural education programs, the World Bank provides loans to fund small business ventures, and many non-profit and non-governmental organizations support community and family farms.

Another method for increasing local food production is **sustainable agriculture.** The goal of the sustainable agriculture movement is to develop local, site-specific farming methods that improve soil conservation, crop yields, and food security in a sustainable manner, minimizing the adverse environmental impact. For example, soil erosion can be controlled by terracing sloped land for the cultivation of crops (see FIGURE 4), by tillage that minimizes disturbance to the topsoil, and by the use of herbicides to remove weeds rather than hoeing. Another practice associated with sustainable agriculture is the use of **transgenic crops,** plant varieties that have had one or more genes altered to reduce the need for insecticides or permit the cultivation of marginally fertile land.

FIGURE 4 Terracing sloped land to avoid soil erosion is one practice of sustainable agriculture.

sustainable agriculture Techniques of food production that preserve the environment indefinitely.

transgenic crops Plant varieties that have had one or more genes altered by use of genetic technologies; also called genetically modified organisms, or GMOs.

Local Solutions

In the United States, several government programs help low-income citizens acquire food over extended periods of time. Among these programs are the Food Stamp Program, which helps low-income individuals of all ages, the Special Supplemental Nutrition Program for Women, Infants and Children (WIC), which helps pregnant women and children to age 5, the National School Lunch and National School Breakfast Programs, which help low-income schoolchildren, and the Summer Food Service Program, which helps low-income children in the summer. The U.S. Department of Agriculture also sponsors programs to distribute emergency foods and surplus commodity foods to qualifying families. Foods may be distributed through charitable organizations or local or county agencies.

Get Involved!

Several times each year, college students from hundreds of campuses all over the United States gather to fight hunger. Members of the National Student Campaign Against Hunger and Homelessness, they hold Hunger Clean-Ups, staff relief agencies, solicit donations of food and money, and promote community activism. Their organization is just one of dozens in which you can get involved. For more information, see the Web links at the end of this *In Depth* report. In addition, the accompanying Highlight box identifies steps you can take to fight hunger every day in your role as consumer, student, and citizen of the world.

If you still wonder whether or not your acts can make a difference, consider the advice of historian and civil rights activist Howard Zinn. He urges us to "just do something, to join with millions of others who will just do something, because all of those somethings, at certain points in history, come together and make the world better."[19]

NUTRI-CASE JUDY

"I never seem to be able to quite make ends meet. I keep thinking that next month will be different, but then I get my paycheck and, by the time I pay the rent and the utilities, it's almost all gone! I'm behind on my car payments, I owe the dentist for Hannah's last visit, and last night, the credit card company called and said that if I didn't pay them at least $100, they'd take me to court. So there goes a chunk of this month's grocery money! Maybe if I just buy some cans of soup and beans, powdered milk, the store brands of cereal and soda, and bread from the day-old bin, we'll be able to get by. Hannah won't like it, but I'll tell her it's just for this month. Next month will be different!"

What, if any, nutrients are missing from Judy's planned food choices for this month? If you had just $35 to spend on a week's groceries for yourself and a growing child, what would you buy? What options could Judy explore to help her get through this month, and to help increase her food security permanently?

HIGHLIGHT HIGHLIGHT HIGHLIGHT HIGHLIGHT HIGHLIGHT

HIGHLIGHT

What Can You Do to Combat Global Malnutrition?

Have you ever wondered whether or not your actions inadvertently contribute to the problem of global malnutrition? Or whether any efforts you make in your home or community can help feed people thousands of miles away? If so, you might want to reflect on your behaviors in each of three roles you play every day: consumer, student, and citizen of the world.

In your role as a consumer, ask yourself:

How can I use my food purchases to promote the production of more healthful, less processed foods?

Any grocery store manager will tell you that your purchases influence the types of foods that are manufactured and sold. If people become aware of the benefits of eating whole-grain bread and stop buying soft white bread, stores will stop carrying it and food companies will stop making it. In our global economy, the types of foods you choose can influence the types of foods produced nationally and by our trading partners. Also, purchasing less processed foods saves global energy.

1. Choose fresh, locally grown, organic foods more often to support local sustainability.
2. Choose whole or less-processed versions of packaged foods (for example, peanut butter made solely from ground peanuts, or plain yogurt from a local dairy) rather than versions of foods made with high-fructose corn syrup, dyes, and other additives. This encourages increased production of less-processed foods.
3. Limit purchases of nutrient-poor foods and beverages to discourage their profitability. This includes limiting nutrient-poor, high-calorie, highly processed fast-food meals.
4. Consider how much packaging is used for a given food or fast-food meal, and whether you will be able to recycle the package.

How often do I eat vegetarian?

Plant-based sources of protein can be produced with less energy cost than animal-based sources, so reducing your consumption of animal foods saves global energy.

1. Experiment with some recipes in a vegetarian cookbook. Try making at least one new vegetarian meal each week.
2. Introduce friends and family members to your new vegetarian dishes.

3. When eating out, choose restaurants that provide vegetarian menu choices. If the campus cafeteria or a favorite restaurant has no vegetarian choices, request that one or more be added to the menu.

How much do I eat?

Eating just the calories you need to maintain a healthy weight leaves more of the global harvest for others and will likely reduce your use of medical resources as well.

1. To raise your consciousness about the physical experience of hunger, consider fasting for 1 day. If health or other reasons prevent you from fasting safely, try keeping silent during each meal throughout 1 day so that you can more fully appreciate the food you're eating and reflect on those who do not enjoy food security.
2. For 1 week, keep track of how much food you throw away, and why. Do you put more food on your plate than you can eat? Do you allow foods stored in your refrigerator to spoil? Do you often buy new foods to "try" and then throw them away because you don't like them?
3. On a daily basis, check in with your body before and as you eat: are you really hungry, and if so, how much and what type of food does your body really need right now?

In your role as a student, ask yourself:

How can I use what I have learned about nutrition to combat malnutrition in my neighborhood?

1. Visit each of your local fast-food restaurants and ask for information about the nutritional value of their foods. Analyze the nutrition information, then summarize it in simple language. Offer to submit a series of articles about your findings to your school or local newspaper.
2. Research what local produce is available in each season. Write an article for your school newspaper listing what is in season each month of the year and include two healthful recipes using vegetables and fruits that are in season during the month your article will be published.
3. Create an entertaining skit or puppet show that encourages young children to eat healthful foods. Offer to entertain on Saturday at your local library, day-care center, or after-school community program.

(continued)

What Can You Do to Combat Global Malnutrition? (continued)

4. Begin or join a food cooperative, community garden, or shared farming program. Donate a portion of your produce each week to a local food pantry.

What careers could I consider to help combat global malnutrition?

You could become a member of the Peace Corps and serve in a developing country. If you want to teach, see the Feeding Minds, Fighting Hunger Web site listed in this chapter's Web links for information on teaching young people about global nutrition. If you are interested in science, you could have a career helping to develop more nutrient-dense or perennial crops, better food preservation methods, or projects to improve food or water safety.

If you plan a career in business, you could enter the food industry and work for the production and marketing of healthful products. If you pursue a career in healthcare, you could join an international medical corps to combat deficiency diseases. No matter what career you choose, use your unique talents to advocate global food security.

In your role as a world citizen, ask yourself:

How can I improve the lives of people in my own community?

1. You can volunteer at a local soup kitchen, homeless shelter, food bank, or community garden.

2. You can join a food cooperative, that is, a store or farm in which you work a number of hours each week in exchange for discounts on healthful foods.

3. Because obesity is likely to be a significant problem in your community, you can help increase opportunities for physical activity in your community. Start a walking group, or volunteer to teach or coach children in a favorite sport.

How can I improve the lives of people in developing nations?

1. Donate time or money to one of the international agencies that work to provide relief from famine or chronic hunger. Check out options for charitable contributions and volunteer efforts at www.charitynavigator.org.

2. Research the global effects of protectionist agricultural subsidies in the United States and Europe, then write letters to newspapers, elected officials, and political action groups expressing your concerns.

3. Join efforts to influence government foreign policies to support global food security.

4. Research the human rights records of international food companies whose products you buy. If you don't like what you find out, switch brands, and write to the company and tell them why you did.

WEB LINKS

www.actionagainsthunger.org
Action Against Hunger

This site explains the mission of an international organization that aids in food crises and promotes long-term food security, and explains how you can help.

www.secondharvest.org
America's Second Harvest

Check out this site for information on programs for fighting hunger in the United States.

www.bread.org
Bread for the World

Visit this site to learn about a faith-based effort to advocate local and global policies that help the poor obtain food.

www.care.org
CARE

This site links to CARE organizations in many countries working to improve economic conditions in over 70 developing nations.

www.feedingminds.org
Feeding Minds, Fighting Hunger

Visit this international electronic classroom to explore the problems of hunger, malnutrition, and food insecurity.

www.freedomfromhunger.org
Freedom from Hunger

This international organization works toward sustainable self-help against chronic hunger and poverty.

www.studentsagainsthunger.org
National Student Campaign Against Hunger and Homelessness

Visit this site to learn what students like you are doing to fight hunger, and how you can get involved.

www.oxfamamerica.org

Oxfam America

Oxfam International is a confederation of organizations in more than 100 countries working to build a better world.

www.hungerbanquet.org

Hunger Banquet

At this site, sponsored by Oxfam America, you can play a "hunger game" that confronts you with some of the same choices facing people in developing nations every day, or take a "hunger quiz" to find out how much you know about global hunger.

www.unicef.org

The United Nations Children's Fund

Visit this site to learn about international concerns affecting the world's children, including nutrient deficiencies and hunger.

www.who.int/nutrition/en

The World Health Organization Nutrition Site

Visit this site to learn about global malnutrition, micronutrient deficiencies, nutrition transition, and other issues of world hunger.

REFERENCES

1. Associated Press. 2005. Malawi drought highlights food shortage. *New York Times*, October 17.
2. Food and Agriculture Organization (FAO). 2006. World Food Day 2006 targets public and private investment. FAONewsroom, October 16. www.fao.org/newsroom/en/news/2006/1000424/index.html. (Accessed August 2007.)
3. Food and Agriculture Organization (FAO). 2005. The spectrum of malnutrition. www.fao.org/FOCUS/E/SOFI00/img/sofisum-e.pdf. (Accessed August 2007.)
4. World Health Organization (WHO). 2002. The World Health Report, 2002: Reducing Risks, Promoting Healthy Life. Geneva: World Health Organization.
5. National Aeronautics and Space Administration (NASA). 2005. Earth observatory: Famine in Niger and Mali. http://earthobservatory.nasa.gov/NaturalHazards/natural_hazards_v2.php3?img_id=13028. (Accessed August 2007.)
6. U.S. Agency for International Development (USAID). 2006. The Humanitarian Situation in Sudan. www.usaid.gov/locations/sub-saharan_africa/sudan/index.html. (Accessed August 2007.)
7. Stroehlein, A. 2004. Darfur starvation will be televised . . . eventually. *The Christian Science Monitor*, June 8. www.csmonitor.com/2004/0608/p09s02-coop.htm. (Accessed August 2007.)
8. Herz, B. 2004. The importance of educating girls. *Science* 305:1910–1911.
9. UNAIDS/WHO. 2005. AIDS Epidemic Update, 2005. www.unaids.org/epi/2005/index.asp. (Accessed August 2007.)
10. Struble, M. B., and L. L. Aomari. 2003. Position of the American Dietetic Association: addressing world hunger, malnutrition and food insecurity. *J. Am. Diet. Assoc.* 103:1046–1057.
11. Ezra, M., and G. E. Kiros. 2000. Household vulnerability to food crisis and mortality in the drought-prone areas of northern Ethiopia. *J. Biosoc. Sci.* 32:395–409.
12. Black, R. E., S. S. Morris, and J. Bryce. 2003. Where and why are 10 million children dying every year? *Lancet* 361:2226–2234.
13. UNICEF. 2004. *The State of the World's Children 2005*. UNICEF.
14. World Health Organization (WHO). 2003. *The World Health Report: Shaping the Future*. Geneva: WHO.
15. Drewnowski, A. 2004. Poverty and obesity. www.niehs.nih.gov/drcpt/beoconf/postconf/overview/drewnowski2.pdf. (Accessed August 2007.)
16. Adair, L. S., and A. M. Prentice. 2004. A critical evaluation of the fetal origins hypothesis and its implications for developing countries. *J. Nutr.* 134:191–193.
17. Yajnik, C. S. 2004. Early life origins of insulin resistance and type 2 diabetes in India and other Asian countries. *J. Nutr.* 134:205–210.
18. U.S. Department of Agriculture (USDA). 2006. Economic Research Service. Food Security in the United States: Conditions and Trends. www.ers.usda.gov/Briefing/FoodSecurity/trends.htm. (Accessed August 2007.)
19. Zinn, H. 2006. *Original Zinn*, p. 167. New York: Harper Perennial.

CHAPTER 21

CHAPTER OBJECTIVES

After reading this chapter you will be able to:

1. Differentiate between chronic illness and infectious illness, pp. 790–791.

2. Explain the natural history of a chronic illness, including the asymptomatic and symptomatic periods, pp. 791–792.

3. Relate lifestyle choices to the occurrence of chronic illness, p. 792.

4. Describe the risk factors associated with cardiovascular disease and determine your personal risk for cardiovascular disease, pp. 793–795.

5. Name several cardiovascular diseases and describe the symptoms and treatment modalities for each, pp. 795–796.

6. Describe the risk factors associated with cancer, pp. 798–799.

7. Name several types of cancer and describe the prevalence of each, pp. 799–801.

8. Explain the importance of early detection of cancer and name several screening procedures that can lead to early detection, p. 801.

9. Name and describe at least three chronic diseases other than heart disease and cancer, pp. 806–808.

10. Examine ways of helping individuals who have chronic illness, including psychological support, pp. 808–809.

TEST YOURSELF TRUE OR FALSE?

1. Cardiovascular disease accounts for more deaths in the United States than any other disease. T or F

2. The American Heart Association recommends that an electrocardiogram (ECG) test be taken annually after age forty in order to detect heart disease at an early stage. T or F

3. Early detection of cancer is successful because if tumors are detected when benign, they can be removed before they become malignant and spread. T or F

4. In the United States, lung cancer rates are in decline due to decreased tobacco use among men. T or F

5. The most prevalent chronic diseases affecting both children and adults are cancers. T or F

Test Yourself answers can be found after the Chapter Summary.

Reducing the Risk for Chronic Disease

a chronic problem is one that is marked by long duration or frequent recurrence. In fact, the term chronic comes from the Greek word chronos, which means "time." In a social sense, think of chronic unemployment, chronic homelessness, or chronic urban decay. It is not a pretty picture. So, too, it is not pleasant to think of chronic illnesses with their accompanying progressive pain and increasing disability. In some cases, however, there are ways to interrupt and even reverse the course of a chronic disease.

Everyone knows someone who suffers from heart disease, cancer, diabetes, arthritis, asthma, tooth decay and gum disease, or a host of other chronic conditions. Chronic diseases are the leading cause of death and disability in the United States and a major source of pain and discomfort.

Chronic diseases develop over a long period of time, in part as a result of lifestyle choices. Smoking alone is associated with an increased incidence of the leading chronic diseases—heart disease, cancer, and lung disease. Still other chronic diseases develop through the process of living in a highly industrialized country in the twenty-first century. Certain cancers and lung diseases, for example, are associated with polluted air and chemicals in the workplace. Another important factor associated with chronic diseases is that people are living longer and so are subject to diseases that usually do not present themselves until the later years of life, such as osteoporosis and Alzheimer's disease.

It may be difficult for young adults to appreciate the relevance of chronic diseases in their life because they may think it will be many years before they have symptoms of one. However, people of all ages are at risk for chronic conditions that can affect their quality of life.

Taken from: *Decisions for Healthy Living,* by B.E. Pruitt and Jane J. Stein

Characteristics of Chronic Illness

Chronic illness is a generic term for diseases such as atherosclerosis, cancer, asthma, diabetes, multiple sclerosis, schizophrenia, or arthritis. Chronic illness may result from a genetic condition, such as cystic fibrosis, or from poor hygiene, such as tooth decay. A chronic illness can affect the individual physically, mentally, or both. Sometimes, a chronic illness only minimally interferes with daily functioning; at other times, it requires round-the-clock medical attention.

Even given these differences, chronic illnesses have several common characteristics:

- They involve some degree of permanence.

- They result in some form of disability.

- They are progressive—that is, they get increasingly worse or become more debilitating.

- They require a long period of care or supervision.

Chronic Versus Infectious Diseases

Chronic diseases differ from infectious diseases in three key ways. First, the two disease groups differ in their causes. For the most part, infectious or communicable diseases are a result of microorganisms and are contagious. Chronic diseases, in contrast, are generally not contagious. They are mostly a result of inherited factors or lifestyle factors, such as diet, personal hygiene, tobacco use, or exposure to toxic chemicals. (Recent research shows that microorganisms may play a role in some chronic conditions, for example stomach ulcers.)

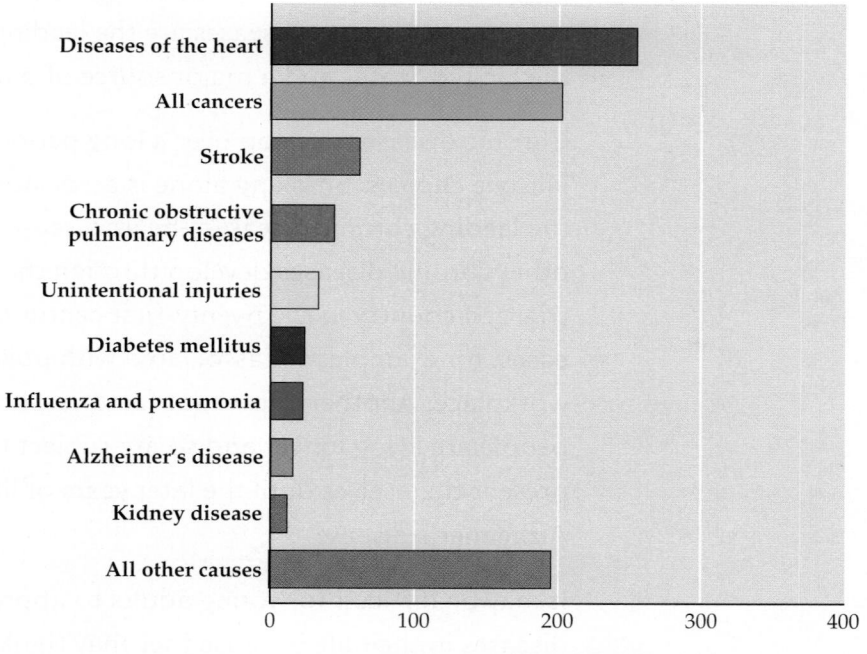

Most Common Causes of Death, United States, 2002

FIGURE 21.1   Most common causes of death, United States, 2002.
Chronic diseases are the leading cause of death in the United States, and are a major source of disability, pain, and discomfort.
Source: National Center for Health Statistics

Second, infectious diseases usually develop quickly and last for a comparatively brief period—sometimes only a matter of hours or days. Chronic diseases develop over a period of years and usually linger for a lifetime.

Third, chronic and infectious diseases differ concerning outcome. Persons who have infectious diseases may recover completely. Healthy people generally do not die of the common cold. As with many infectious diseases, they may feel miserable for a while, but in time, they usually recover completely. (There are exceptions to this role, including malaria, hepatitis, HIV, and other virulent infectious diseases.) It is just the opposite with chronic diseases. People who have chronic diseases tend to remain ill for a long period of time. Again, there are exceptions. People have recovered from cancer, heart disease, and other chronic conditions.

Changing Patterns of Mortality

At the beginning of the twentieth century, infectious diseases were the leading cause of death. Now at the beginning of the twenty-first century, with thanks to medical interventions and healthier lifestyles, infants, children, and young adults now survive what once were fatal illnesses and often live long enough to incur chronic illnesses. At a time when adults could anticipate living only about fifty or sixty years, chronic diseases were proportionately less common. But the proportion of population over age sixty-five is growing. In 1900, one out of every twenty-five Americans was sixty-five years old or older. As of 2000, one out of every eight Americans had celebrated his or her sixty-fifth birthday. And, according to the U.S. Administration on Aging, most older persons have at least one chronic condition and many have multiple conditions.

Natural History of Chronic Diseases

Chronic diseases occur over a long period of time, sometimes without initial outward signs or clinical symptoms. This is called the **asymptomatic period**. In most cases, people with asymptomatic chronic conditions live normal lives without knowing that they have a chronic disease.

In the case of cardiovascular disease, for example, the presence of **plaque**, or fatty deposits, in the arteries is a clear signal of disease. Yet until the symptoms of disease appear, most people do not know that they have been accumulating plaque in their arteries.

More dramatically, a college basketball player might not know that he or she has an enlarged heart until collapsing during a game, or an elderly woman might not know she has osteoporosis until she fails, compresses her spine, and is left crippled and in chronic pain.

At some point during the course of a disease, clinical symptoms appear. This is called the **symptomatic period**. These signs, such as a lump, lesion, or other abnormal growth, may be apparent to the trained eye or touch. But many of the symptoms of chronic diseases are nonvisual, such as an increase in blood pressure.

It is usually up to a physician to determine when signs and abnormalities suggest the presence of a disease. This determination is called the **diagnosis**. Given the complexity of medical practice, diagnosis has become an extensive focus of medical training. A lump in the breast, for example, may or may not indicate the presence of cancer. Only through a **biopsy** of the lump tissue, a medical diagnostic procedure, can the lump be evaluated properly to determine whether it is cancerous.

Most chronic diseases, if left unrecognized and untreated, eventually lead to major impairment or even death. For this reason, early detection is highly important. Early signs, although not proof, should be taken as serious warnings and reasons to see your physician. One consistent fact concerning nearly all chronic diseases is that early detection through recognition of signs and symptoms leads to an increased chance of survival and a higher quality of life.

asymptomatic period A period in which a disease exists without outward signs or clinical symptoms.

plaque A deposit of fatty material in a blood vessel wall.

symptomatic period A period during the course of a disease in which symptoms appear.

diagnosis A physician's opinion of the nature or cause of a disease based on observation and laboratory tests.

biopsy The removal of bits of living tissue and fluid from the body for diagnostic examination.

Eating a healthy diet is an important factor in preventing chronic diseases such as heart disease and some cancers.

Source: FPG International/
© Ralph Pleasant

Lifestyle Choices and Disease

Lifestyle choices are important factors not only in chronic disease but also in overall personal health. Many such behaviors are presented in greater detail in other chapters of this book. The most common lifestyle causes of chronic diseases are smoking, poor diet, failure to exercise, and heavy consumption of alcohol.

Other factors contribute to the occurrence of chronic disease: not taking advantage of available health screening techniques, such as **mammography** to detect breast cancer and **sigmoidoscopy** or **colonoscopy** to detect colon cancer, or not taking medication for hypertension. Genetic predisposition, gender, and advancing age are recognized factors that contribute to chronic and degenerative diseases over which you have little control.

Given the current state of knowledge about chronic diseases, it is important to control the modifiable factors about which you are aware, monitor those you cannot avoid, and take steps to minimize the negative health impact of all lifestyle choices. Although prevention does not guarantee that you will not develop a chronic disease, it could improve your odds in favor of better health.

Chronic diseases are far too numerous to provide complete information about each one in this chapter. Table 21.1 provides a brief overview of the common chronic diseases.

The remainder of this chapter focuses on two of the most common and most life-threatening chronic diseases: cardiovascular disease and cancer. Three other diseases are presented briefly: Type II diabetes, asthma, and dental disease.

Cardiovascular Disease: The Nation's Leading Cause of Death

Diseases of the heart and blood vessels—collectively called **cardiovascular diseases**—are the leading cause of death in the United States. They claimed the lives of nearly one million Americans in 1999, and nearly 62 million more have some form of cardiovascular disease, according to the American Heart Association. To illustrate how great a toll cardiovascular diseases take, the National Center for Health Statistics estimates that if all forms of cardiovascular disease were eliminated, life expectancy would rise by almost ten years. In contrast, if all forms of cancer were eliminated, the gain would be three years.

Heart disease remains the number one killer despite the fact that the death rate from cardiovascular disease has declined dramatically over the past several decades (see FIGURE 21.2). This decline is due in great part to better surgical techniques, improved drugs, more effective medical management, and a better understanding of the risk factors for heart disease.

Who Is at Risk?

The major risk factors associated with cardiovascular disease are related to lifestyle and include smoking, **hypertension**, elevated cholesterol, elevated iron in the blood, obesity or being overweight, adult-onset diabetes, and sedentary lifestyle. Risk factors for cardiovascular disease that are not related to lifestyle include family history of the disease, age, and sex.

Smoking is the single most important risk factor associated with heart disease. It is estimated that smoking accounts for more than 20 percent of all coronary heart disease deaths. The good news in this regard, however, is that smoking cessation can substantially reduce this death rate. According to the World Health Organization, after one year of not smoking, the risk of coronary heart disease drops by 50 percent. Quitting can also significantly reduce the risk for stroke.

Data from the Framingham Heart Study—the longest ongoing study in the United States of heart disease—show that people who have high blood pressure have three to four times the risk for developing coronary heart disease and as much as seven times the risk for a stroke as do those who have normal blood pressure.

mammography A screening technique used to detect breast cancer.

sigmoidoscopy A screening procedure in which a physician uses a hollow lighted tube to inspect the rectum and lower colon.

colonoscopy A screening procedure in which a physician uses a hollow lighted tube to inspect the entire bowel and some portions of the small intestines.

cardiovascular disease Disease of the heart and blood vessels.

hypertension High blood pressure; generally means the heart is working harder than normal.

TABLE 21.1   Common chronic diseases and risk factors

Disease	Nonbehavioral Risk Factors	Behavioral Risk Factors	Symptoms	Preventive Measures
Asthma	Allergies; family history; young age; viral infections; bronchitis	An attack may be triggered by cigarette smoking; perfumes; exercise; aspirin; industrial/occupational exposures to air pollution; emotional anxiety	Coughing; shortness of breath; tightness in chest; wheezing; itchy or sore throat; increased breathing rate	Stay away from triggers; take allergy medications; exercise; recognize and treat symptoms early
Breast cancer	Genetic predisposition; cancer in one breast; uterine cancer; age; Caucasian race; early menstruation—late menopause	Women who have delayed child-bearing; women over 35; increased use of alcohol; increased fat content in diet; never having given birth	Lump in breast; armpit; breast pain; nipple discharge; itching, enlargement, retraction of nipple; change in breast contour or symmetry	Self-examination of breast every month; mammography; physical examination by gynecologist annually
Cervical cancer	Genetic predisposition; age	Intercourse at early age; multiple partners; smoking; papilloma virus infection	Abnormal vaginal bleeding; abnormal Pap smear	Avoid early sexual intercourse; avoid multiple partners; avoid cigarette smoking; annual gynecological exam
Cirrhosis of the liver	Genetic predisposition	Heavy alcohol/drug consumption; hepatitis	Weakness, fatigue; weight loss; nausea; abdominal pain; jaundice; amenorrhea; impotence; male breast increase	Discontinue use of alcohol/drugs
Dental disease	Age; fluoride-deficient drinking water; poverty	Fear of professional care; excessive between-meal snacks; failure to brush and floss regularly	Stained teeth; bad breath; tooth cavities; tooth loss; painful gums and tongue	Well-balanced nutritious diet; limit between-meal snacks; brush and floss regularly; have regular professional dental care
Diabetes	Genetic predisposition	Obesity or being overweight; trauma to trigger onset	Increased urination; excessive thirst; rapid weight loss; high blood glucose levels; increased ketones in blood glucose	Well-balanced nutritious diet; maintain proper weight; exercise
Heart disease	Genetic predisposition; age; high blood pressure; diabetes	Poor physical exercise; cigarette smoking; obesity; poor stress management	Chest pain; breathing difficulty; spitting up blood; weight loss; lung collapse	Discontinuance of smoking; maintain low cholesterol levels; healthy diet (low in saturated fat, low amounts of junk food); regular exercise program; medical checkup
Lung cancer	Genetic predisposition; age	Cigarette smoking; environment (air, industrial pollution)	Cough; breathing difficulty; spitting up blood; weight loss; lung collapse	Discontinuance of smoking; elimination of environmental risks; education; medical checkup
Lung disease	Genetic predisposition; age	Environment (air, industrial pollution); cigarette smoking	Breathlessness; persistent cough; crowing sound during breathing; wheezing; spitting up blood; weight loss; lung collapse	Discontinuance of smoking; elimination of environmental risks; education; medical checkup
Stroke	Genetic predisposition; previous stroke; heart attack; age; high blood pressure	Cigarette smoking; heavy alcohol consumption; high-fat diet	Brief loss of vision; slurred speech; nausea; vomiting; sensory loss; weakness or paralysis	Discontinuance of smoking; control blood pressure; maintain low cholesterol levels; healthy diet (low in saturated fat, low amounts of junk food); regular exercise program; medical checkup

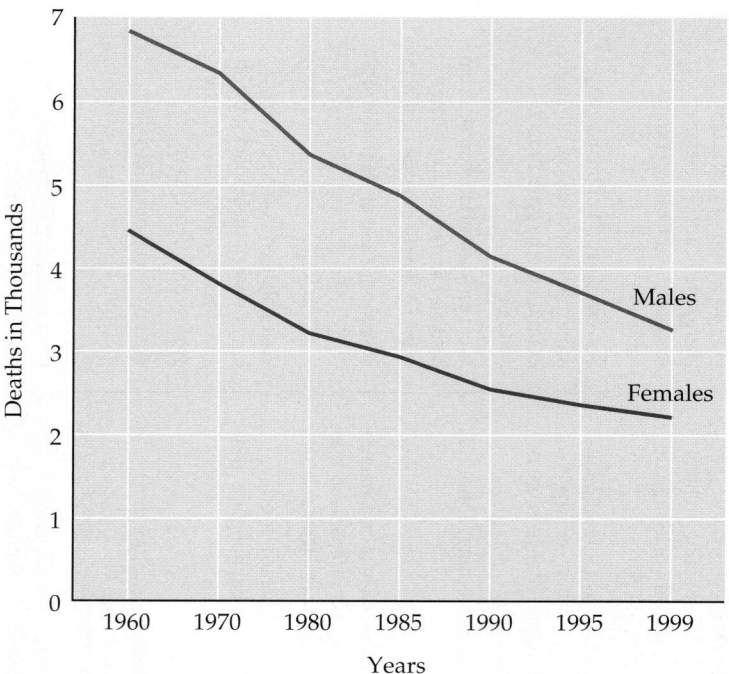

FIGURE 21.2   Cardiovascular mortality trends for men and women.
Even though the death rate from cardiovascular disease has dropped dramatically for
decades, it is the number one killer in the United States.
Source: National Center for Health Statistics

Obesity is a risk factor by itself, but it also contributes to high blood pressure levels.
Even a 10 percent weight loss in an overweight, hypertensive person can significantly reduce his or her blood pressure. Obesity also contributes to adult-onset diabetes, which in turn is a risk factor for heart disease because it may speed the rate at
which fat is deposited on the artery wall, thus clogging the flow of blood to the heart.

The Framingham Study has also found that the incidence of heart disease
increases as blood cholesterol levels rise. The Centers for Disease Control and Prevention (CDC), however, has found that a 10 percent decrease in total cholesterol
levels may result in an estimated 30 percent reduction in the incidence of coronary
heart disease.

Sedentary lifestyle is another major contributor to heart disease, and recent
data from the CDC show that people who are not physically active are twice as likely
as physically active people to die of coronary heart disease. Less active, less fit individuals have a 30 percent to 50 percent greater risk of developing high blood pressure. Much has been written about athletes who drop dead from heart disease while
competing, but it is important to note that healthy people usually do not die while
exercising. The athletes in the news tend to have either serious heart defects (which
are usually present from birth) or advanced but undetected coronary artery disease.

Diagnosing Heart Disease

screening Analysis of risk factors
done on a person thought to be
well, for the purpose of preventing
disease or making an early
diagnosis.

detection Medical procedures
(tests) done on individuals
suspected of having a disease, for
the purpose of confirming the
presence of the disease and, if
present, determining the progress
of the disease.

Heart disease is diagnosed in two ways: **screening** and **detection**. Screening for
heart disease involves an analysis of risk factors associated with the disease. Such
procedures are done on individuals assumed to be healthy. Although screening tests
do not provide absolute proof of the existence of an abnormal heart condition, so
much is known about the relationship of specific risk factors to the incidence of heart
disease that by identifying them early, a physician can prescribe the appropriate
behavior change—for example, stop smoking, adjust your diet, or begin blood pressure medication. Should a screening test or a combination of apparent risk factors

raise suspicion of the existence of heart disease, a physician is more likely to detect heart disease at a very early stage.

Detection of heart disease is done on individuals suspected of having some form of cardiovascular abnormality. In many cases, detection involves the same procedure as screening; the difference is mainly in the physician's purpose.

An **electrocardiogram (ECG)** is used for both screening for and detecting heart disease. To perform an ECG, a medical technician attaches electrodes to the body. As the heart beats, these electrodes transmit the electrical impulses that cause the heart to contract to a device that records them. After a series of impulses is recorded, a trained technician or physician interprets the ECG and can identify any abnormalities.

An ECG is the principal test for screening asymptomatic individuals, that is, those who have yet to experience chest pains or have a heart attack. The American Heart Association recommends that a baseline ECG be taken at age twenty, again at age forty, to forty-five, and then only as suggested by other risk factors. An ECG can

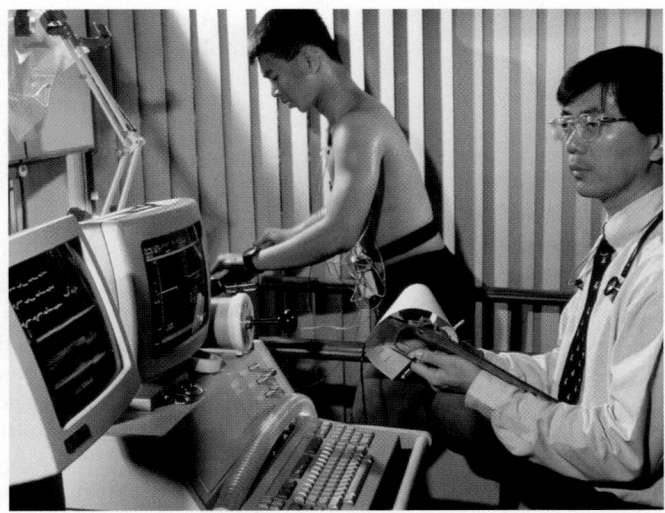

An electrocardiogram (ECG) can detect abnormalities in the heart at an early stage of disease. You should have a baseline ECG at age twenty and again at age forty to forty-five.

also detect heart disease at an early stage. When used for detecting heart disease, an ECG should not be the only diagnostic tool used.

Some people, in addition, undergo a stress electrocardiogram (stress ECG). A stress ECG is also known as a maximal exercise tolerance test or treadmill test, because a treadmill is used to produce an elevated heart rate. Reliable testing protocols have also been developed using walking, running, a stationary bicycle, or going up and down steps. The stress ECG might be compared with a high-speed road test of a car. The results reveal how the heart performs under pressure—more precisely, under high-intensity exercise. A stress ECG is a better diagnostic procedure than a resting ECG. It is also an effective means of determining fitness level.

Stress tests are recommended for people who have a history of cardiac risk factors and for sedentary individuals who wish to begin an exercise program. This is because strenuous exercise may result in severe heart problems and even death for at-risk persons. Stress tests are also required in certain occupations that involve unusual endurance and strength and that affect public safety, such as police work and fire fighting.

Forms of Heart Disease

The term *cardiovascular disease* actually refers to many diseases. Some are directly related to the heart; others are related to the circulatory system, including veins and arteries. **Atherosclerosis**, the most common form of hardening of the arteries (also called arteriosclerosis), is the single biggest cause of heart and blood vessel disease. It is a slow, progressive disease that may start in early life. Atherosclerosis is characterized by thick deposits of fatty substances (plaque) such as cholesterol on the inner walls of the arteries. As a result of these deposits, the internal channels of the arteries become narrow, and blood moves through them with great difficulty. This makes it easier for a clot to form, which can block the artery and thus deprive the heart, brain, or other organs of blood.

Heart attack (myocardial infarction), the number one killer in the nation (about 500,000 deaths a year), usually results from atherosclerosis. Heart attacks are fatal for about 36 percent of the people who have them, so there are far more people who have had a heart attack and lived to tell the story than there are people who have died of them. However, those who survive a heart attack are at a significantly increased risk of having a second heart attack and of developing angina and other heart-related conditions.

electrocardiogram (ECG) A screening procedure used to detect heart disease; a graphic record of the heart's action obtained from an instrument that records heart activity.

atherosclerosis A thickening and loss of elasticity of the inner walls of the arteries.

heart attack (myocardial infarction) A condition that occurs when the blood supply to part of the heart muscle (the myocardium) is severely reduced or stopped. Normally circulating blood brings oxygen and other nutrients to the heart.

Angina pectoris, a condition that results in a temporary reduction in the blood supply to the heart, can cause feelings of discomfort similar to but not as strong as those of a heart attack. Although an angina attack is not a heart attack, its symptoms should be taken seriously because they could be a forewarning of other heart problems. An angina attack usually takes place during physical activity or periods of emotional upset. Nitroglycerin or some other medication can prevent or reduce the pain of angina.

Arrhythmia is an erratic beating of the heart that can cause a heart attack. Nearly everyone experiences an occasional skip of a heartbeat due to too much excitement, too much caffeine, or for no reason at all. There is nothing dangerous about this. Arrhythmia becomes life threatening when a chain of beats is missed so that the heart muscle does not contract effectively. As a result of this, the brain does not get enough oxygen-containing blood and the victim loses consciousness and can go into cardiac arrest and die. Arrhythmias may be caused by a damaged heart muscle or by extreme emotional distress. Common forms of arrhythmia include **tachycardia** (excessively rapid heart rate), **bradycardia** (abnormally slow heart rate), and **fibrillation** (irregular, convulsive movements of the heart muscle resulting in a failure to pump blood).

Stroke, also called a cerebrovascular accident (CVA), is the third leading cause of death in the country. Each year, according to the American Stroke Association, about 600,000 Americans have a stroke and more than 160,000 die from it. A stroke results when the supply of blood pumped by the heart to the brain is cut off or when bleeding occurs in the brain. When the damage takes place in the right side of the brain, sensory and motor function is lost on the left side of the body. This is known as left **hemiplegia.** When the damage occurs on the left side of the brain, loss of function occurs on the right side of the body, affecting communication skills, including speaking, writing, reading, and listening. This condition is known as right hemiplegia.

Transient ischemic attacks (TIAs) are little strokes that cause minimal damage but are warning signals of the possibility of a more severe stroke. Men are more likely to suffer all kinds of strokes than are women, and African Americans are more likely to suffer strokes than are whites. Women who take oral contraceptives are more at risk for stroke than are those who do not. The risk for stroke increases with age for both sexes.

Hypertension (high blood pressure) is called the silent killer because it has few symptoms but affects about 50 million Americans and can lead to heart attack, stroke, and heart and kidney failure. High blood pressure adds to the workload of the heart and arteries and can cause them not to function as well as they should. Approximately 25 percent of adults have high blood pressure, defined as blood pressure greater than a **systolic pressure,** (contraction of the heart muscle) of 140 or a **diastolic pressure** (relaxation of the heart muscle) of 90. This is written as 140/90, and is referred to as 140 over 90. Normal blood pressure is about 120/80 for young adults.

Hypertension occurs more frequently after age thirty-five and among African Americans more often than among whites. It is associated with obesity, high-sodium diets, and other controllable risk factors, but by far the most important factor predicting hypertension is genetic predisposition. If one of your parents has or had hypertension, you have a 50 percent chance of having it too. This risk rises to 90 percent if both parents are or were affected. Blood pressure can be lowered successfully through salt restriction, weight control, and exercise. If these treatments fail to lower blood pressure, medication is indicated.

Repairing the Heart

From a good pair of walking shoes to a coronary artery bypass or a heart transplant, there are many ways to prevent and treat heart disease. Regular aerobic exercise, the kind that raises the heart rate and is done for 20 minutes three or more times a week, can help prevent and correct high blood pressure. As little as a five- to ten-pound weight loss can also help decrease blood volume and the amount of blood pumped by the heart, which in turn reduces pressure in the arteries.

angina pectoris Chest pain; a symptom of a condition in which the heart does not get as much blood as it needs.

arrhythmia An erratic heartbeat.

tachycardia Excessively rapid beating of the heart.

bradycardia Abnormally slow beating of the heart.

fibrillation Irregular convulsive movement of the heart muscle.

stroke A clot or break in a blood vessel in the brain that disrupts blood flow to the brain.

hemiplegia The loss of sensory and motor function on one side of the body.

transient ischemic attack (TIA) A stroke that causes minimal damage but signals the possibility of a more severe stroke.

systolic pressure The pressure measured in the arteries when the heart contracts.

diastolic pressure The pressure measured in the arteries when the heart relaxes.

Medications have proven successful in lowering blood pressure, stabilizing mild to moderate heart-beat irregularities, relieving angina, raising cardiac output, and lowering the heart's demand for blood. A class of cholesterol-lowering drugs called statins can reduce the risk of a heart attack or stroke by one third if taken daily. The cost: $2.50 a day. Another drug can reduce heart attack deaths by more than 25 percent if administered within the first few hours after the onset of heart attack symptoms and can cost more than $2,000 per dose.

Far cheaper is common aspirin. Extensive studies show that healthy men and women can cut their risk of a heart attack nearly in half by taking one low-dose or baby aspirin every day, a regimen recommended by the U.S. Prevention Services Task Force.

Drugs usually have side effects, and heart drugs are no different. Some side effects of heart drugs include fatigue, nausea, impotence in men, and depression. Even aspirin can cause stomach ulcers and internal bleeding when taken on a regular basis. If medications are successful in reducing the cardiac problem, however, more risky surgery can be avoided.

A low-cost lifesaving technique for heart attack victims is **cardiopulmonary resuscitation (CPR)**. CPR, which involves rescue breathing (mouth-to-mouth resuscitation) alternating with pressure applied to the chest, is a basic life skill that is used in emergency situations. It has been estimated that if one of every three Americans were trained in CPR, more than one hundred thousand lives a year could be saved.

For people who have severely clogged arteries, surgical options include **coronary angioplasty**, in which the coronary artery is widened with an inflated balloon catheter; **coronary artery bypass**, in which the blood flow is rerouted from the blocked part of the artery using a length of vein taken from another part of the body; and a **heart transplant**, in which a normally functioning heart from a person who has recently died is implanted in place of the diseased one. Each of these procedures has limited success, but collectively, they have improved the quality of life and in many cases have extended the lives of millions of heart patients.

Artificial hearts have been used to extend the lives of otherwise terminal patients until transplant donors can be found. The artificial heart gets its power to operate from a source outside the body, so it is not an effective long-term replacement for the original organ. Even with incredible advances such as an artificial heart, the best advice is to take care of the organs you have and not count on medicine to provide replacement parts when they malfunction.

Exercise is a good way to maintain a healthy heart. It is also cost-effective: You can buy a good bike for a couple hundred dollars; a heart transplant costs several hundred thousand.

Cancer: The Nation's Second Leading Cause of Death

One of the most feared of all diseases, cancer, strikes people of all ages—in childhood, adolescence, the prime of life, and old age. Cancer is the second leading cause of death in the United States. It accounts for about one of every four deaths from all causes in the United States, and it kills more children than any other disease. It is estimated that in 2002, 1.3 million Americans were diagnosed with cancer and approximately 555,500 died of it. Because of exposure to **carcinogens** (cancer-causing substances) in the environment, the longer a person lives, the greater the chance of developing cancer.

The incidence of cancer in the population is increasing, mainly because of increases in lung cancer. To illustrate this point, lung cancer recently replaced breast cancer as the leading cause of cancer death among women.

cardiopulmonary resuscitation (CPR) A combination of mouth-to-mouth breathing and chest compression used during cardiac arrest to keep blood flowing to the heart muscle and brain; an emergency procedure.

coronary angioplasty A surgical procedure to widen the coronary artery with an inflated balloon catheter.

coronary artery bypass A surgical procedure to reroute blood flow from the blocked part of an artery by using a length of vein taken from another part of the body.

heart transplant A surgical procedure in which a normally functioning heart from a person who has recently died is implanted into a person with a diseased heart.

carcinogen A cancer-causing agent or factor.

The Basics of Cancer

Cancer is not actually one disease. It is a group of more than 100 diseases, all characterized by uncontrolled growth and spread of abnormal cells. Normally, cells reproduce in an orderly manner following the genetic rules of growth. But some cells become abnormal and fail to follow these rules. They continue to divide and grow and eventually band together into **tumors**, or masses of tissue.

Not all tumors are cancerous. In fact, most are benign, or harmless. **Benign tumors** do not invade other cells or spread to other parts of the body. They are different from cancerous tumors in their very structure, and they cannot change into cancerous tumors. Benign tumors, however, can cause problems if they block some crucial part of the body and prevent it from functioning.

Only **malignant tumors** are cancerous. If left untreated, malignant tumors spread into nearby tissues and organs, crowding out healthy cells and replacing them with cancer cells. The most dangerous characteristic of malignant tumors is that they **metastasize**, or spread to other parts of the body through the bloodstream or lymph system. In this way, a single cancer cell can spread the disease throughout the entire body.

No one knows exactly what causes a normal cell to become a cancer cell. Scientists believe that most cancers develop through repeated or long-term contact with cancer-causing agents. There are two basic kinds of carcinogens: **initiators** and **promoters**. Initiators start the cell damage that can lead to cancer. Examples of initiators are cigarette smoking, X rays, and certain chemicals. Promoters do not actually cause cancers, but they help them to grow. Alcohol, for example, promotes mouth, throat, and possibly liver cancer when combined with an initiator such as tobacco.

Who Is at Risk?

Although the basic causes of cancer are unknown, scientists have discovered several conditions often connected with abnormal cell growth. In some—but not all—cases, you can do something to reduce your risk for getting cancer.

The single behavior that most often results in death from cancer is smoking. People who smoke two or more packs of cigarettes a day are fifteen to twenty-five times more likely to die of cancer than are nonsmokers. Smoking also increases the risk for developing other cancers, particularly those of the mouth, pharynx, larynx, esophagus, pancreas, and bladder. Studies also show that cancer can be caused by passive smoking in healthy nonsmokers, by smokeless tobacco, and by the tar produced by smoking marijuana.

Repeated exposure to sunlight over a long period of time is a major cause of skin cancer. The sun's ultraviolet rays harm the skin. Fair-skinned people have less of a pigment called **melanin** in their skin to block some of the sun's damaging rays, and they are at greater risk of getting skin cancer than are dark-skinned people. The amount of time spent in the sun or in a tanning booth determines the extent of damage.

Large doses of X rays or ionizing radiation can cause cancer, depending on both the dose and the duration of exposure. The most common sources of ionizing radiation for medical reasons are diagnostic procedures and radiation therapy. Medical equipment is now designed to deliver the lowest possible dose without sacrificing the beneficial effects. Most of the information about the effects of radiation comes from studies of survivors of the atomic bombs dropped in Japan in 1945. The studies show increased rates among survivors of several types of cancer, including breast, thyroid, lung, and stomach cancer and acute leukemia.

Excessive amounts of alcohol are linked to a number of cancers. Heavy drinking is associated with cancers of the mouth, throat, esophagus, and liver. The cancer risks of alcohol are increased even more in drinkers who also smoke cigarettes.

Foods are linked to the risk of certain cancers, both positively and negatively. On the down side, cancers of the esophagus and stomach are common where large quantities of smoked, salt-cured, and nitrite-cured foods are eaten. Salami, bologna, and ham are examples of these foods. A high-fat diet not only is full of calories but also

tumor A mass of tissue that accumulates in the body.

benign Not harmful.

benign tumor A noncancerous tumor that is usually harmless and does not invade other cells or spread to other parts of the body.

malignant tumor A cancerous tumor that spreads to nearby tissues and organs, crowding out healthy cells and replacing them with cancer cells.

metastasize To spread to other parts of the body through the bloodstream or lymph system.

initiator A carcinogen that starts cell damage that leads to cancer.

promoter A carcinogen that helps cancer to grow.

melanin Brownish-black skin pigment.

increases your risk for developing breast, colon, and prostate cancer. On the protective side, foods high in fiber—whole-grain breads, rice, broccoli, carrots, apples—appear to dilute intestinal contents and reduce the amount of time carcinogens spend in the intestine. A high-fiber diet may reduce your risk for developing colon cancer. Vitamin A protects against cancers of the esophagus, larynx, and lung, and vitamin C protects against cancer of the esophagus and stomach. Fresh fruits and vegetables are good sources of both of these vitamins.

Many occupations expose workers to toxic fumes, gases, airborne particles, and liquids. Occupational carcinogens include asbestos, vinyl chloride, formaldehyde, and arsenic. In addition to the worker being at risk, his or her family may also be in jeopardy. Some carcinogens such as asbestos attach themselves to workers' clothing, thus exposing family members who either wash the work clothes or include their own clothes in the same wash. Exposed workers and family members significantly multiply their risks if they smoke.

Certain families are no doubt cancer-prone, and up to 10 percent of all cancers may be hereditary. Specific examples of genetically linked cancers are retinoblastoma (an eye cancer that causes blindness) and familial polyps of the colon (which lead to colon cancer). Breast cancer in the family accounts for about 5 percent to 10 percent of all breast cancer.

Types of Cancer

Cancer comes in many shapes and forms. It can affect your lungs or your limbs. It can affect your bones or your skin. All of the body's tissues and organs are susceptible to cancer (see Table 21.2). The following descriptions of several common cancers include statistics on incidence, risk factors, symptoms, and survival rates.

TABLE 21.2   Where Cancer Strikes
Leading Sites of New Cancer Cases and Deaths—2002 Estimates*

	Cancer in Males New Cases	Deaths		Cancer in Females New Cases	Deaths
Prostate	189,000	30,200	Breast	203,500	39,600
Lung	90,200	89,200	Lung	79,200	65,700
Colon & rectum	72,600	27,800	Colon & rectum	75,700	28,800
Urinary bladder	41,500	8,600	Uterine corpus	39,300	6,600
Melanoma of the skin	30,100	4,700	Non-Hodgkin's lymphoma	25,700	11,700
Non-Hodgkin's lymphoma	28,200	12,700	Melanoma of the skin	23,500	
Kidney	19,100	7,200	Ovary	23,300	13,900
Oral cavity	18,900		Thyroid	15,800	
Leukemia	17,600	12,100	Pancreas	15,600	15,200
Pancreas	14,700	14,500	Urinary bladder	15,000	4,000
Liver	11,000	8,900	Leukemia	13,200	9,600
Esophagus	9,800	9,600	Brain	7,400	5,900
All sites	637,500	288,100	All sites	647,400	267,300

*Excluding basal and squamous cell skin cancer and in situ carcinomas except bladder. American Cancer Society Inc., Surveillance Research, 2002.
Source: Reprinted with the permission of the American Cancer Society, Inc., from *Cancer Facts and Figures* 2002.

Lung Cancer

Lung cancer is responsible for 28 percent of all deaths due to cancer. Since 1992, the number of new cases diagnosed has been declining, so eventually the rate of deaths will decline as well. The reduced rate of lung cancer is primarily a result of decreased tobacco use among men. Unfortunately, the rate of lung cancer in women continues to rise. The main risk factors for lung cancer are cigarette smoking, exposure to sidestream smoke, and occupational exposures to asbestos and other agents.

Symptoms include excessive coughing, chest pain, shortness of breath, chronic bronchitis, sputum containing blood, and difficulty in swallowing. Early detection may be difficult because these symptoms do not usually appear until the disease is at an advanced stage and has metastasized or spread.

The outlook for lung cancer patients is bleak: Most die within a year, and only 15 percent survive for five years after diagnosis.

Breast Cancer

Breast cancer is the second leading cause of death from cancer for women (after lung cancer). The incidence of breast cancer increased about 4.5 percent a year between 1982 and 1998 and has recently leveled off. The increase is due in great part to screening programs that can detect tumors before they become clinically apparent. (A small percentage of men get breast cancer, and about four hundred of them a year die from it.)

The main risk factors for women are being over age fifty, a family history of breast cancer, never being pregnant, or having a first pregnancy after age thirty and estrogen therapy. (Estrogen is taken by some post-menopausal women to treat discomforts sometimes associated with the cessation of menstruation. Studies suggest that it can protect against heart disease and osteoporosis but also that it can promote the growth of existing breast cancer and contribute to cancer of the uterus.)

Symptoms of breast cancer include a lump, thickening or swelling of the breast, discharge from the nipple, or retraction of the nipple. Early detection by breast self-examination or mammography can significantly increase survival rates.

When the disease is localized at the time of diagnosis, five-year survival rates are as high as 96 percent. If the cancer has spread regionally to adjacent lymph nodes, survival rates drop to 76 percent, and for distant metastases, to 20 percent.

Prostate Cancer

Prostate cancer is the second most common cause of cancer death in men (after lung cancer). The prostate is a small gland that surrounds the urethra and produces much of the liquid in semen. Risk factors are being over age fifty, workplace exposures to cadmium and other carcinogens, and a high-fat diet. The rate of prostate cancer in African American men is significantly higher than in whites. The increased incidence is thought to be due to lifestyle rather than to genetics, because this high rate developed in African Americans only in recent decades.

(a)

(b)

(c)

Photographs of skin cancers: (a) basal cell carcinoma. (b) squamous cell carcinoma, (c) melanoma.

Symptoms include problems with urination, blood in the urine, and persistent pain in the back, hips, and pelvis. Prostate cancer grows slowly, and in the early stages, there are often no symptoms. Early detection can increase survival rates.

The outlook is excellent when the disease is confined within the prostate. These men are just as likely to be alive fifteen years later as men in the general population. If the disease is still localized, the five-year survival rate approaches 100 percent.

Colon and Rectum (colorectal) Cancers

Colon and rectum (colorectal) cancers have declined in recent years, probably because of increased sigmoidoscopic and colonoscopic screening and polyp removal (which helps prevent progression of polyps to invasive cancers). This decline is seen largely among whites; the incidence rates for African Americans have stabilized but have not yet begun to decline. The colon is the last five or six feet of the digestive tract. Major risk factors are being over age forty, family history of polyps of the colon, inflammatory bowel disease, and a high-fat diet.

Symptoms include rectal bleeding, blood in the stool, change in bowel habits (constipation or diarrhea), and general abdominal discomfort. When colorectal cancer is detected at an early localized stage, the five-year survival rate is 81 percent for colon cancer and 61 percent for rectal cancer. However, only about one third of cases are discovered at this stage.

Skin Cancer

Skin cancer falls into two broad classes: **basal cell** and **squamous cell** cancers, which are more common and highly curable, and **melanomas**, which are relatively rare but more serious. The epidermis, or outer layer of the skin, contains both basal and squamous cells. Basal cells are small, round cells found in the lower part, or base, of the epidermis; squamous cells are flat cells that look like fish scales and make up most of the epidermis. More than 900,000 cases of basal and squamous cell cancers are diagnosed each year. Most are discovered so early and are so readily cured that few people die from basal or squamous cell cancers. Melanomas, in contrast, are far more fatal.

General risk factors associated with skin cancer are extensive exposure to the sun, fair complexion, and freckling (see the Developing Health Skills box). The incidence of skin cancer is very low among African Americans because of heavy skin pigmentation. For basal and squamous cell cancers specifically, additional risk factors include X-ray treatments for skin conditions, burn scars, occupational exposure to certain chemicals, and a precancerous change of the skin known as actinic **keratosis**. For melanomas, additional risk factors are brown moles and three or more blistering sunburns during adolescence.

Symptoms of skin cancer include a mole, birthmark, or beauty mark that changes color, size, or texture or an open sore that does not heal correctly. Early diagnosis is critical. For basal and squamous cell cancers, cure is likely if they are detected and treated early. Catching melanomas before they spread can result in an 89 percent five-year survival rate. About 80 percent of melanomas are diagnosed at the early stage.

Other common sites of cancer are the cervix, testicles, colon, and stomach. Some cancers are clearly linked to specific behaviors, such as oral cancer to smokeless tobacco use. Other cancers, such as leukemia (a cancer of the white blood cells), arise from unknown origins.

Screening for Cancer

As the statistics clearly illustrate, the best line of defense against a cancer spreading is early detection. Studies show that screening for cancer of the breast, cervix, colon, rectum, uterus, and other areas can significantly reduce cancer mortality.

A **Pap test** involves scraping and analyzing some cells from the cervix and is effective in reducing death from cancer of the cervix. The American Cancer Society recommends that women who are or have been sexually active or have reached age eighteen should have an annual Pap test and pelvic examination. After three consecutive normal annual examinations, the test may be performed less frequently.

basal cell A small, round cell in the lower part (base) of the epidermis.

squamous cell A flat cell that makes up most of the epidermis.

melanoma A skin cancer that often starts as a mole-like growth and grows in size and changes color; the most serious of the various types of skin cancer.

keratosis A rough patch or horny growth of the skin.

Pap test A test for identifying cervical cancer that involves scraping and analyzing cells from the cervix.

DEVELOPING HEALTH SKILLS

The Sun and Skin Cancer

The sun is the leading cause of cancer in the United States. One in six Americans can expect to develop some form of skin cancer, and for those who live in the Sunbelt states, the prediction is one in three. The most serious damage from overexposure to the sun occurs to children. Eighty percent of the skin damage that will eventually lead to cancer takes place when you are young. A bad burn before age eighteen heightens the chance of developing malignant melanoma later in life. But it is difficult to convince teenagers to wear sunscreen, and only one in five uses it.

The increased incidence of skin cancer is due in part to the gradual depletion of the ozone layer, which protects the earth from the sun's ultraviolet rays. As a result, the intensity of the sun's ultraviolet rays is greater than anything previous generations were exposed to.

Experts agree that the best way to combat the increased risk of cancer is to concentrate prevention efforts on the young. The good news is that nine out of ten women interviewed in a Gallup Poll said they were more careful with their children than they had been with themselves when they were younger. And in Hollywood, California, none of the celebrities has a tan, says a prominent dermatologist there. The same ultraviolet rays that cause skin cancer cause premature aging of the skin, and the actors and actresses know they will be ineligible for parts if they look old.

WHAT CAN YOU DO TO PROTECT YOURSELF?

- Avoid peak sun hours whenever possible. Peak hours are 10 A.M. to 2 P.M., or 11 A.M. to 3 P.M. during daylight saving time.
- Wear a wide-brimmed hat and other protective clothing if sun exposure will be prolonged or occur during peak hours.
- Be aware that sand, snow, water, and even concrete can reflect up to 85 percent of the sun's rays—so you are getting a double dose!
- Do not assume that a tan protects against the sun. It is a sign of skin damage. Keep using sunscreen to avoid further damage.
- Keep babies under six months old out of direct exposure to the sun; their delicate skin is especially vulnerable to damage.

- Remember that it is never too late to be careful. Adults who stay out of the sun or use sun protection will reduce their risk of cancer and reverse existing skin damage; skin will become smoother, sunspots will begin to fade, and wrinkling will be less obvious.
- Examine yourself monthly for any changes in your skin, especially a mole or beauty mark, and make sure that a physician looks at any spot that has changed in color, texture, or size.
- Research about the benefits and possible side effects of sunscreen is still being done. Proponents of sunscreen advise liberal application 20 minutes before going into the sun, and they suggest that you use about one ounce per whole body application, that the sunscreen have a sun protection factor (SPF) of 15 or greater, and that if you live in the Sunbelt, use a sunscreen daily, year-round.

The sun is the leading cause of cancer in the United States. Don't bask in the sun, and when you go out wear a wide-brimmed hat and a sunscreen with a sun protection factor (SPE) of at least 15.

Mammography, which is a low-dose breast X ray, along with a clinical breast examination can reduce death due to breast cancer. Women should get a baseline mammogram at age thirty-five to have for comparison, have a new one every year or every other year from age forty to age forty-nine, and then one every year thereafter. Based on studies reported in 2002, the U.S. Preventive Services Task Force found "fair evidence" that screening every 12 to 23 months significantly reduces mortality from breast cancer. Other studies, however, question the benefit of regular mammograms.

A yearly **prostate-specific antigen (PSA) test** is recommended by the American Cancer Society for men over age fifty. A higher level of PSA in the blood can be a sign of prostate cancer. Men over age forty who have a family history of prostate cancer or who are African American should also have this test every year. The value of early detection of prostate cancer is controversial. Many prostate tumors are slow growing and no rigorous study has demonstrated that men who are treated early with surgery and radiation survive longer.

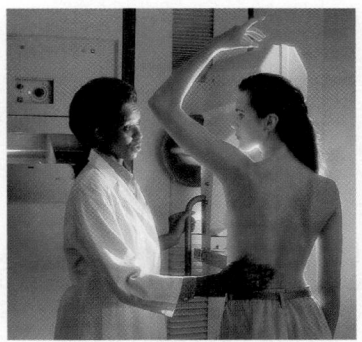

A mammogram—a low-dose breast X ray—and a clinical breast examination can detect breast cancer early and reduce death from this disease by 30 percent.
Source: FPG international/
© Jeff Kaufman

Self-Tests for Cancer

A free test, which is being done by a growing percentage of women, is **breast self-examination (BSE)**. The American Cancer Society recommends that all women over age twenty do a BSE every month. Because BSE is not nearly as effective as mammography or examination by a physician, women are encouraged not to depend solely on it for early detection. See the Developing Health Skills box to learn how to do a breast self-exam.

Although testicular cancer is relatively rare—it accounts for only one percent of all cancers among men—the risk for dying from it can be reduced with a self-examination. Adult men—particularly young men—should conduct this **testicular self-examination** monthly. Testicular cancer is the most common form of cancer among men between the ages of twenty and thirty-five. This procedure is especially important for men who have a history of undescended testicles. A testicular examination by a trained physician is recommended as a routine part of all periodic health examinations. See the Developing Health Skills box to learn how to do a testicular self-exam.

To check for colon and rectum cancers, the American Cancer Society recommends a digital rectal examination every year after age forty, a stool blood test every year after age fifty, and sigmoidoscopy or colonoscopy every three to five years after age fifty. A digital rectal examination is also recommended each year for men over forty as a means of detecting prostate cancer. In sigmoidoscopy, a physician uses a hollow lighted tube to inspect the rectum and lower colon. In colonoscopy, the physician looks at the entire bowel; along with some portions of the small intestines.

In addition, a cancer-related checkup is recommended every three years for people twenty to forty years of age and every year after age forty. This checkup includes looking for cancer of the thyroid, mouth, skin, lymph nodes, testes, prostate, and ovaries. Your physician should also review good health habits, including tips on eating a healthy diet, quitting smoking, and other lifestyle choices that relate to cancer. This is because an unhealthy lifestyle is the cause of two thirds of all cancers. Your dentist too, should check regularly for signs of oral cancer, most of which are associated with smoking and smokeless tobacco.

You should be aware of any changes in your own body and be alert to the American Cancer Society's seven caution signals:

- Change in bowel or bladder habits
- A sore that does not heal
- Unusual bleeding or discharge
- Thickening or lump in breast or elsewhere
- Indigestion or difficulty in swallowing
- Obvious change in wart or mole
- Nagging cough or hoarseness

The American Cancer Society recommends that you see your physician if you have any of these warning signals.

prostate-specific antigen (PSA) test A blood test that can identify signs of prostate cancer.

breast self-examination (BSE) An examination done by a woman to herself to identify abnormal breast tissue; a screening exam for the presence of breast cancer.

testicular self-examination An examination done by a man to himself to identify abnormal testicular tissue; a screening exam for the presence of testicular cancer.

DEVELOPING HEALTH SKILLS

How to Perform a Breast Self-Exam

The best time to do breast self-exam is right after your period, when breasts are not tender or swollen. If you do not have regular periods or sometimes skip a month, do it on the same day every month. Use the following procedure to perform your breast self-exam.

1. Lie down with a pillow under your right shoulder and place your right arm behind your head.

2. Use the finger pads of the three middle fingers on your left hand to feel for lumps in the right breast, Your finger pads are the top third of each finger.

3. Press firmly enough to know how your breast feels. A firm ridge in the lower curve of each breast is normal. If you're not sure how hard to press, ask your health care provider, or try to copy the way your health care provider uses the finger pads during a breast exam.

4. Move around the breast in a set way. You can choose either the up and down line, the circular pattern, or the wedge pattern. Do it the same way every time. It will help you to make sure that you've gone over the entire breast area, and to remember how your breast feels.

BSE Patterns

5. Now examine your left breast using the finger pads of your right hand. (Move the pillow to under your left shoulder.) If you find any changes, see your doctor right away.

For added safety, you should also visually check your breasts while standing in front of a mirror right after you do your breast self-exam each month. See if there are any changes in the way your breasts look: dimpling of the skin, changes in the nipple, or redness or swelling.

You might also want to do a breast self-exam while you're in the shower. Raise one arm above your head and press firmly in your preferred pattern. Then raise the other arm, and check your other breast. Your soapy hands will glide over wet skin, making it easy to check how your breasts feel.

Source: Reprinted by the permission of the American Cancer Society, Inc.

Benefits and Risks of Treatment

Surgery, radiation, and chemotherapy are the principal forms of cancer treatment. Although each carries risks, the benefits—as documented in survival rates—more often outweigh them.

The primary treatment for cancer is surgical removal of the malignant growth. This is particularly effective when the cancer has not metastasized. Over the years, surgical techniques have improved so that removal causes less bodily disfigurement. For example, in 1970, most mastectomies done in the United States involved the complete removal of the breast and the surrounding tissue, particularly the lymph nodes, This is called a **radical mastectomy**. Today, such radical surgery is very seldom done. Alternatives include **lumpectomy**, a procedure that involves removal of the cancerous lump only; **partial mastectomy**, which involves removal of only the part of the breast containing the lump; and **modified radical mastectomy**, which involves selective removal of the breast and surrounding tissue.

For some kinds of cancer—notably cancers of the blood and lymph system—radiation and chemotherapy are the primary forms of treatment. With those treatments, the survival rates for patients who have the lymph node cancer known as Hodgkin's

radical mastectomy The complete surgical removal of the breast and surrounding tissue, particularly the lymph nodes.

lumpectomy The surgical removal of only the cancerous lump from the breast.

partial mastectomy The surgical removal of only the part of the breast containing the cancerous lump.

modified radical mastectomy A selective removal of the breast and surrounding tissue.

DEVELOPING HEALTH SKILLS

How to Perform a Testicular Self-Exam

The best time to do a testicular self-exam is during or after a shower or bath, when the skin of the scrotum is relaxed and the testicles descend. Some doctors recommend that all men do this once a month. Use the following procedure to perform your testicular self-exam.

Stand in front of a mirror and hold the penis out of the way. Check for any swelling.

Examine each testicle with both hands. Hold the testicle between the thumbs and index and middle fingers, and roll it gently between the fingers.

Look and feel for any hard lumps or nodules (smooth rounded masses) or any change in the size, shape, or consistency of the testes. Cancerous lumps usually are found on the sides of the testicle, but they can show up on the front.

You will also feel a soft tubelike structure behind the testicle. This is the epididymis, which contains the blood vessels, tissues, and tubes that conduct sperm. If you know what this feels like, you won't mistake it for a suspicious lump. Lumps on the epididymis are not cancerous.

If you feel a lump—or if you have any doubts—consult your doctor immediately.

disease are around 83 percent. Men who have prostate cancer often choose radiation as the primary therapy because traditional prostate surgery can cause impotence.

For most other cancers, radiation and chemotherapy are used following surgery to prevent metastases, shrink growths that cannot be removed, and relieve pain. The side effects of radiation and chemotherapy are both dangerous and dramatic and may include anemia, severe nausea, uncontrollable infections, and baldness. In each case, the benefits of treatment, as documented in survival rates, need to be weighed against the risks and the resulting quality of life.

There are, in addition, alternative cancer treatments, most of which have proven to be ineffective. Alternative treatments include megavitamins, shark cartilage, and macrobiotic diets. These treatments may provide a ray of hope to the otherwise hopeless cancer patient, but a recent study by Harvard Medical School researchers found that these treatments had no effectiveness in delaying the effects of the disease, relief from the symptoms of cancer or treatments for it, and overall survival. Traditional medicine remains greatly concerned that patients who avail themselves of such ineffective approaches run the risk for greater suffering and may miss opportunities for treatment that could prolong life.

One form of alternative cancer treatment the Harvard researchers found to be beneficial is mind-body therapy, such as relaxation training, yoga, support groups and similar interventions that ease the stress of living with cancer. The field of mind-body therapy is officially called **psychoneuroimmunology**—*psycho* for the mind and emotions, *neuro* for the brain and central nervous system, and *immunology* for the body's natural defense against abnormal cells or external invaders such as bacteria or viruses. This chapter discusses mind-body treatments for cancer.

In one study of people treated for the early stages of colon cancer or malignant melanoma whose cancers were in remission, thirty patients received an eight-week course in relaxation and cognitive therapy, a technique that focuses on changing a person's self-defeating beliefs. Researchers found that patients who took the course had more active natural killer cells, which protect the body against tumor growth, than did patients who did not take the course.

Another example of a mind-body treatment for cancer is imagery. Clinical studies show that cancer patients can reduce their level of pain through imagery—for example, thinking of something pleasant. This helps promote relaxation, which, in turn, can ease the pain. A more controversial use of imaging is to shrink a cancer by focusing the mind on an image of it being attacked by the body and visualizing the cancer getting smaller. To learn more about mind-body treatments and cancer, see the Cultural View box.

The Harvard study of alternative cancer therapies also endorsed moderate exercise, soy supplementation for prostate cancer, and acupuncture for chemotherapy-related nausea and vomiting.

Other Chronic Conditions

Type 2 Diabetes

More than seven million Americans have diabetes and the incidence rate for this chronic disease is rising at an alarming pace. **Type 2 diabetes** is the most common form of diabetes. It has sometimes been called adult-onset diabetes because most cases are diagnosed in adulthood. Some children, however, are diagnosed with type 2 diabetes.

Type 2 diabetes has two possible causes: (1) either the body's cells ignore **insulin** that is produced (insulin resistance) or (2) the body does not produce enough insulin. Insulin is a substance produced by the pancreas that helps move glucose from the blood into the cells. Type 2 diabetes usually begins as insulin resistance. Then, as the need for insulin rises, the pancreas gradually loses its ability to produce insulin leading to an undersupply of insulin. If the body does not produce enough insulin, the body's cells may be starved for energy and, thus, fail to function. This condition, along with a build-up of glucose in the blood, may result in damage to the eyes, kidneys, nerves, or heart.

psychoneuroimmunology A mind-body approach to treatment. It involves the mind and emotions (psycho), the brain and central nervous system (neuro), and the body's natural defense system (immunology).

type 2 diabetes The most common form of diabetes; also called adult-onset diabetes.

insulin A substance produced by the pancreas that helps move glucose from the blood into cells; without enough insulin, the body's cells do not function properly.

CULTURAL VIEW

CULTURAL VIEW CULTURAL VIEW CULTURAL VIEW

Mind-Body Treatments for Chronic Conditions

Mainstream medicine is increasingly accepting some of the principles of mind-body treatment. Side by side with chemotherapy and radical surgery to remove tumors, doctors are "prescribing" meditation and mental exercises to breathe in good healthy air and exhale bad cancer cells. "The people who do the best are the people who say to themselves, 'I am going to beat this thing,' " says a California breast cancer patient who meditates, prays, and attends support groups.

Each year at just one Kaiser hospital in Sacramento, California, about eight hundred cancer and other patients listen to a tape while they are unconscious during surgery. What they hear is a soothing voice guiding their bodies through relaxation and then recovery. In addition to imagery, other techniques used in mind-body treatment include:

- Hypnosis: During a state that resembles sleep, the therapist can use the power of suggestion to help reduce perceptions of pain. Some studies show that hypnosis can prolong the lives of breast cancer patients; other studies do not confirm this.

- Meditation: Using this technique, a cancer patient can "breathe away" cancer, or "relax away" pain by relaxing all the muscles in the body, starting with the face and moving downward.

- Art therapy: Cancer patients use art therapy as a way to express themselves. The emotions that accompany a life-threatening disease such as cancer are sometimes difficult to express. Through art, however, a cancer patient can express emotions such as anger and fear without feeling that those expressions are a burden to his or her family, friends, and caregivers.

- Prayer: This is perhaps the oldest form of mind-body therapy. One study from a San Francisco hospital found that heart patients who knew they were being prayed for suffered fewer heart attacks and needed fewer drugs than did similar patients who were not being prayed for.

What is the science behind these treatments? Studies published in mainstream journals, including the *Journal of the American Medical Association* and the *Annals of Internal Medicine*, suggest that mind-body techniques reduce stress, which can hamper the response of the immune system. A more contro-versial theory considers mind-body techniques to be potent medicines in themselves. According to this theory, imagery, meditation, or prayer, for example, can trigger the body's endocrine or immune system to counterattack disease. Controlled clinical studies are under way to examine the effectiveness of several of the mind-body techniques being used.

So mind-body treatments may—or may not—cure cancer, but can they harm patients? Some doctors say yes. They are concerned that patients may rely more on their own healing powers and not seek traditional, proven treatments for cancer, such as chemotherapy.

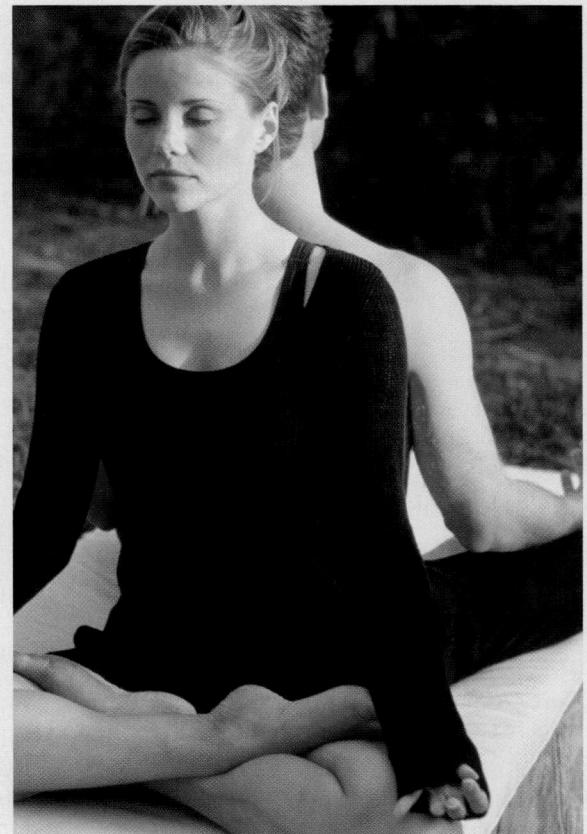

Mind-body treatments, which include meditation, can help patients boost their immune system.

With a good treatment plan, however, a person with diabetes can maintain blood sugar levels within a normal range. Treatment includes careful meal planning, exercise, weight loss, and, when necessary, either diabetes pills, insulin shots, or both.

Asthma

Asthma is a serious, chronic lung disease characterized by wheezing, shortness of breath, chest tightness and coughing. Since about 1980, the prevalence of asthma has increased substantially, especially among children. Recent studies suggest that exposure to dust mites, cockroaches, mold, pet dander, tobacco smoke, and other biological and chemical pollutants influences the occurrence and severity of asthma.

Asthma is treated according to the severity of the disease and the persistence of symptoms. Long-term medications are used to control asthma and to limit the underlying airway inflammation that contributes to asthma attacks. Quick-relief medications such as inhalers are used to treat acute symptoms and to prevent exercise-induced asthma. Since there is no cure for asthma, the goal of asthma therapy is to successfully manage the disease. With proper management and care, a person with asthma can live a long, healthy life—with few symptoms.

Dental Disease

Fortunately, the most prevalent of the chronic diseases affecting both children and adults is not life threatening, but it is often an overlooked source of discomfort, pain, and possible disfigurement: dental disease.

The two major families of dental disease are **dental caries**, or tooth decay, and **periodontal disease**, or gum disease. Tooth decay develops when the acids in plaque attack the teeth. **Dental plaque** is a colorless film of bacteria that forms on the teeth and gums. If not removed, dental plaque becomes concentrated colonies of bacteria. These colonies mix with sugars and starches to form acids that attack the enamel of the tooth, break it down, and lead to a cavity—a single location of decay in a tooth.

Plaque affects the gums as well, causing them to become red, tender, and swollen. This is called **gingivitis**, and it is the first stage of periodontal disease. If left untreated, periodontal disease can result in a degeneration of the gum tissue that holds the teeth in place. This is called **periodontitis**, or pyorrhea. Although this usually begins as a painless condition, it can result over time in painful loss of the supporting bone and ultimately in loss of teeth.

The good news about dental diseases is that they are preventable with routine brushing and flossing and regular professional dental care.

Living with a Chronic Disease

When you ask people how they feel, most respond, "Fine, thank you." But for people who have a chronic disease, and especially for those who have a degenerative disease such as arthritis, life can be difficult. Chronically ill people may never regain the full level of health they enjoyed before the onset of their illnesses, and they may face a continuing loss of function and the constant threat of even more serious medical problems as their illnesses progress. As medical advances help people who have chronic diseases live longer, they are left with the human challenge of coping with their disability. This may affect not only the person who has the disease but also his or her family and friends.

asthma A chronic lung disease characterized by wheezing, shortness of breath, chest tightness, and coughing.

dental caries Tooth decay.

periodontal disease Gum disease.

dental plaque Noncalcified accumulation of microorganisms that attach to the teeth.

gingivitis A condition in which the gums are red, tender, and swollen.

periodontitis Degeneration of the gum tissue that holds the teeth in place; also called pyorrhea.

Psychological Adjustment

One of the most difficult adjustments for someone who has a chronic disease to make is modifying the view of him- or herself from a healthy, fully abled person to one who is not fully able. Think of how sick you view yourself when you are fighting a bout of influenza or are weak from mononucleosis. Yet your role as a sick person is likely to last only a few weeks at most. For people who have chronic diseases, being sick or in pain becomes a lifelong state. There is assault on self-esteem, and a period of depression is not uncommon. In fact, psychiatrists find that depression—not the threat of another attack—is one of the most formidable problems in getting heart attack patients through convalescence and rehabilitation.

Realistic adjustments in lifestyle often need to be made at school or work to accommodate a chronic disease. A college student recently diagnosed as a diabetic, for example, might have to allow some extra time during the day for monitoring blood glucose or administering insulin. With the same diagnosis, someone who has an extremely strenuous job—a police officer or fire-fighter, for example—might need to consider some job or career modifications.

Similarly, leisure activities might change as a result of chronic disease. An avid rock climber newly diagnosed with diabetes may find at some point that rock climbing carries too high a risk for foot injury. (People who have diabetes are at high risk for serious foot injuries because the disease compromises the body's circulatory system.) A safer alternative for exercise might be swimming or riding a stationary bike.

As with other health conditions, positive steps can be taken. For example, cancer patients who believe that they have some control over their health status are less likely to experience severe depression than are patients who give up. In addition to using basic coping skills, there are specific things that researchers have identified that chronically ill patients and their families can do to help themselves cope with the illness:

- Learn as much as possible about the disease and treatment options.

- Accept and adjust to physical changes in the body.

- Learn how to express feelings about having the disease.

- Express a personal sense of empowerment and control, particularly as related to health care decisions.

- Seek out support groups and other resources in the community.

- Develop meaningful relationships with family, friends, and members of the health care team (physician, nurse, social worker, and others).

- Maintain a sense of hope.

Concluding Thoughts

The best medical advice concerning chronic diseases is to keep them in the proper perspective for your life. For the most part, they tend to act slowly and provide years of warning. Preventive measures—most particularly, not smoking and following a healthy diet—along with early detection and medical intervention have proven effective in the treatment and cure of many chronic diseases that only a few years ago were considered death sentences.

Case Study 21: Coping with Chronic Disease

Louise was in a state of panic. She had discovered what she thought could be a lump in her left breast. But her breasts were lumpy, so she wasn't sure. She had read a lot about breast cancer in the newspaper and in women's magazines, and the thought of it made her very anxious.

As the months went by, Louise's anxiety increased, and unfortunately, so did the size of the tumor. Eventually, she could no longer deny its existence. She went to a physician who, after running the proper tests, confirmed Louise's worst fears—the tumor was malignant. Because she had waited until the tumor had grown larger, Louise needed more extensive surgery than she might have had if she had seen her physician when she first detected the lump. In addition, there was concern that the cancer may have spread. Louise had a partial mastectomy, a course of chemotherapy, and a breast reconstruction. Five years later, she remains cancer-free and is happy to be alive.

When Mariana felt a lump in her breast, she, too, was in a state of panic. But she channeled that panic into swift action. She made an appointment to see her physician the next day, and her physician immediately ordered a mammogram and an ultrasound. When the results indicated the lump was malignant, she directed Mariana to a breast cancer specialist.

After a series of tests, including biopsies, and a second opinion from another breast cancer specialist, Mariana underwent a lumpectomy. Her doctors were confident that the cancer had been detected and treated early enough to prevent it from spreading to other tissue. Mariana's mental and physical scarring were minimal, but five years later, she remains vigilant and faithfully examines her breasts every month.

In Your Opinion

Louise avoided treatment; Mariana sought it immediately. Even so, both are living five years later.

- What health habits should Louise and Mariana have been practicing to detect breast cancer?
- Given that both women survived their breast cancer, how important is early detection and treatment?
- What advice would you give to a man or woman who had detected a lump or otherwise suspected that he or she had cancer?
- Would you respond differently if that person had early signs of heart disease?

CHAPTER SUMMARY

1. A chronic disease is marked by long duration or frequent recurrence.

2. A large percentage of the population has chronic diseases or disabilities, and the proportion of people who have to limit their activities due to chronic illness is increasing.

3. Over the past fifteen years, the death rate from diseases of the heart and blood vessels has declined dramatically due in great part to better surgical techniques, improved drugs, more effective medical management, and a better understanding of the risk factors for heart disease.

4. Smoking is the single most important risk factor associated with heart disease. Smokers have a 70 percent greater risk than nonsmokers for dying of heart disease.

5. Hypertension is called the silent killer because it has few symptoms but can lead to heart attack, stroke, and heart and kidney failure.

6. Cancer is a group of more than a hundred diseases, all characterized by uncontrolled growth and spread of abnormal cells.

7. Benign tumors do not invade other cells or spread to other parts of the body. Malignant tumors spread to nearby tissues and organs, crowding out healthy cells and replacing them with cancer cells.

8. Mammography, a low-dose breast X ray, and clinical breast examination reduce death from breast cancer by 30 percent.

9. The most prevalent chronic diseases are dental caries and periodontal disease—both preventable with brushing, flossing, and regular professional dental care.

10. Coping with a chronic illness includes making realistic adjustments in your lifestyle.

TEST YOURSELF ANSWERS

1. **True.** Heart disease takes such a toll that if it could be eliminated, life expectancy would increase by almost ten years.

2. **False.** The American Heart Association recommends that a baseline ECG be taken at age twenty, again at age forty to forty-five, and then only as suggested by other risk factors.

3. **False.** Benign tumors are not cancerous and cannot change into cancerous tumors. Thus, benign tumors cannot become malignant tumors. However, early detection of malignant tumors can help ensure that cancer is diagnosed at the earliest possible stage when there is the greatest chance of successful treatment.

4. **True.** True. Lung cancer rates among men are dropping because they are smoking less, but rates for women continue to rise.

5. **False.** Dental diseases are the most prevalent chronic diseases affecting both children and adults.

REVIEW QUESTIONS

1. Compare and contrast chronic illness and infectious illness.

2. List lifestyle choices that lead to chronic illness. List lifestyle choices that reduce the risk for chronic illness.

3. Describe controllable risk factors associated with cardiovascular disease. Describe noncontrollable risk factors that increase the potential for cardiovascular disease.

4. Identify the symptoms and treatment modalities for atherosclerosis, myocardial infarction, angina pectoris, arrhythmia, stroke, transient ischemic attacks, and hypertension.

5. Describe controllable risk factors associated with cancer. Describe noncontrollable risk factors that increase the potential for cancer.

6. Identify the symptoms and treatment modalities for lung cancer, breast cancer, prostate cancer, colon and rectum cancer, and skin cancer.

7. Explain the importance of early detection of cancer and name several screening procedures that can lead to early detection.

8. Explain the importance of good dental hygiene as a means of reducing the risk for dental disease.

9. List similarities and differences between cardiovascular disease, cancer, diabetes, asthma, and dental disease.

10. List specific strategies for coping with chronic illness and describe how you would help someone implement these strategies.

CRITICAL THINKING QUESTIONS

1. Two reasons cited for the rising mortality due to chronic disease are (1) medicine's success in dealing with infectious diseases and (2) medicine's success in extending life expectancy. Therefore, it could be said that successful medical intervention does not prevent death; it just changes the causes of death. Suppose

cures for cardiovascular disease and cancer were discovered. What chronic disorder might then emerge as the next leading cause of death?

2. The *Healthy People 2010* objectives include the following: "Increase the proportion of adults who have had their blood cholesterol checked within the preceding 5 years." The relationship between high cholesterol and cardiovascular disease is well established, yet most Americans don't even know their blood cholesterol level. How might this situation be changed? Do you think the entire U.S. population should be required to have cholesterol screening? Would such an extensive program be cost-effective?

3. The *Healthy People 2010* objectives include the following: "Increase the proportion of persons who use at least one of the following protective measures that may reduce the risk of skin cancer: avoid the sun between 10 A.M. and 4 P.M., wear sun-protective clothing when exposed to sunlight, use sunscreen with a sun protective factor (SPF) of 15 or higher, and avoid artificial sources of ultraviolet light." Currently, only about 30 percent of the U.S. population take such precautions. Given the clear evidence that associates sun exposure with cancer, why do you think so few Americans use sunscreens and protective clothing? If it took more than forty years to change public opinion about the hazards of smoking, how long do you think it will take to change public opinion about sun exposure?

4. The most common chronic disease is not heart disease, cancer, or diabetes. It is dental disease. Even though dental disease does not cause death, it is similar in some ways to the major killers of our time. How is dental caries similar to heart disease and cancer? How is it different? What prevention strategies are effective in reducing the occurrence of all three?

JOURNAL ACTIVITIES

1. Carefully review your family's health history, going back as far as you can to grandparents and great-grandparents and including blood relatives such as aunts and uncles. Document risk factors for chronic diseases that you think might affect you. For example, is there a pattern of heart disease, breast cancer, or diabetes in your family? Given this information, what can you do to reduce your risks of developing a chronic disease?

2. Think about someone you know who has a chronic disease. This might be a classmate your age, an older relative, or a professor nearing retirement. Write down your feelings about this person and how he or she copes with the disease. How do you think you would handle living with a chronic illness?

3. Observe people in your community and try to identify those at risk for heart disease. A good place for watching might be a fast-food restaurant. Notice what people eat, whether they put salt on their food, whether they smoke and whether they have other noticeable risk factors. Do your habits mirror theirs?

4. Survey twenty students about their dental care. Ask how often they brush and floss their teeth, and when they last went to a dentist. Do you expect to find that college-age men and women take good—or poor—care of their teeth? Compare your expectations with your findings.

SELECTED BIBLIOGRAPHY

A Breast Cancer Journey: Your Personal Guidebook from the Experts at the American Cancer Society. Atlanta, GA: American Cancer Society, 2001.

The Burden of Chronic Diseases and Their Risk Factors. Atlanta, GA: Centers for Disease Control and Prevention, National Center for Chronic Disease Prevention and Health Promotion, 2002.

Burt, V., et al. "Prevalence of Hypertension in the U.S. Adult Population." *Hypertension* 25 (1995): 305–313.

Cancer Facts and Figures. Atlanta, GA: American Cancer Society (updated annually).

Heart and Stroke Statistical Update. Dallas, TX: American Heart Association (updated annually).

Hoffman, C., et al. "Persons with Chronic Conditions: Their Prevalence and Costs." *Journal of the American Medical Association* 276, no. 18 (1996): 1473–1479.

Lenfant, C. *Benefits of Exercise and Lifestyle Modification.* Rockville, MD: National Heart, Lung, and Blood Institute, August, 2000.

Peeters, A., et al. "A Cardiovascular Life History: A Life-Course Analysis of the Original Framingham Heart Study Cohort." *European Heart Journal* 23, no. 6 (2002): 458–466.

Unrealized Prevention Opportunities: Reducing the Health and Economic Burden of Chronic Disease. Atlanta, GA: Centers for Disease Control and Prevention, National Center for Chronic Disease Prevention and Health Promotion, 2000.

Wilson, S., and Poulter, N. "Cardiovascular Risk: Its Assessment in Clinical Practice." *British Journal of Biomedical Science* 58, no. 4 (2001): 248–251.

HEALTHLINKS
Websites for Reducing the Risk of Chronic Diseases

You can access better health as it relates to this chapter by checking out some of the following sites on the Internet. These sites can be accessed directly from the *Decisions for Healthy Living* Website located at www.aw.com/pruitt.

CDC National Center for Chronic Disease Prevention and Health Promotion
The home page for the division of the Centers for Disease Control and Prevention dedicated to the prevention of chronic diseases and maternal and infant health. Access the latest information on cancer, cardiovascular disease, diabetes, oral diseases and conditions, and other serious chronic diseases and conditions and discover what is and can be done to prevent these disorders.

American Dental Association
A link with the leading private organization dedicated to dental health, containing pertinent information on research and clinical issues.

American Cancer Society
The leading private organization dedicated to cancer prevention, including information, statistics, and resources regarding cancer.

American Diabetes Association
Home page for the leading private organization on diabetes including patient and education information.

American Heart Association
The leading private organization dedicated to heart health, providing statistical data, and resources regarding cardiovascular care.

Asthma and Allergy Foundation of America
Home page for the leading private site for educational and clinical information on asthma and allergies, and links to other resources.

National Cancer Institute
Information about cancer diagnosis, treatment, and prevention, as well as trends related to the disease.

National Heart, Lung, and Blood Institute
Information about cardiovascular disease, lung and blood disorders, as well as the latest information on the Women's Health Initiative.

National Institute of Neurological Disorders and Stroke
Information about stroke and neurological disorders as well as trends related to them.

HEALTH HOTLINES
Reducing the Risk for Chronic Disease

American Cancer Society
(800) ACS-2345 (227-2345)
National Office
1599 Clifton Road NE
Atlanta, GA 30329

American Dental Association
(800) 621-8099
Public Information and Education
211 East Chicago Avenue
Chicago, IL 60611

American Diabetes Association
(800) 342-2383
1701 Beauregard Street
Alexandria, VA 22311

American Heart Association
(800) 242-8721
7272 Greenville Avenue
Dallas, TX 75231-4596

National Cancer Institute
Cancer Information Services
(800) 4-CANCER (422-6237)
6116 Executive Boulevard, MSC8322
Bethesda, MD 20892-8322

National Heart, Lung and Blood Institute
Education Programs Information Center
(800) 575-WELL (575-9355)
P.O. Box 30105
Bethesda, MD 20824-0105

National Institute of Neurological Disorders and Stroke
(800) 352-9424
P.O. Box 5801
Bethesda, MD 20892

CHAPTER OBJECTIVES

After reading this chapter you will be able to:

1. Describe complementary and alternative medicine (CAM), and identify its typical domains.

2. Explain major types of complementary and alternative medicine providers and common treatments they offer.

3. Discuss the various types of complementary and alternative medicines being used today, who is most likely to use them, their patterns of use, and their potential benefits and risks.

4. Understand how to evaluate testimonials and claims related to complementary and alternative products, services, and practitioners.

5. Summarize the challenges and opportunities related to complementary and alternative medicine in ensuring our health and wellness.

TEST YOURSELF

1. What makes alternative medicine different from conventional medicine?

2. How do I evaluate alternative medicine resources for reliability?

3. How does acupuncture work?

4. Do herbal remedies have any risks or side effects?

5. Will echinacea teas boost my immune system?

Complementary and Alternative Medicine: New Choices and Responsibilities for Healthwise Consumers

O ne of the newest movements toward self-care and health promotion focuses on **complementary and alternative medicine (CAM)**. These therapies are defined as a group of diverse medical and health care systems, practices, and products that are not presently considered part of conventional medicine.[1] Various products and services offer today's consumers a new range of health choices and an opportunity for greater control over their own health.

Taken from: *Access to Health,* Green Edition, by Rebecca J. Donatelle

Complementary and Alternative Medicine: What Is It and Who Uses It?

Although often used interchangeably, there is a distinction between the terms *complementary* and *alternative* when referring to therapies. **Complementary medicine** is used *together with* conventional medicine as part of the modern integrative-medicine approach. An example of complementary medicine would be using massage therapy along with prescription medicine to treat anxiety.[2] **Alternative medicine** has traditionally been used *in place of* conventional medicine, such as following a special diet or herbal remedy to treat cancer instead of using radiation, surgery, or other conventional treatments. However, as some alternative medical approaches have gained scientific credibility, they are being used along with conventional treatment. A survey conducted by the National Center for Complementary and Alternative Medicine revealed that 36 percent of adults used some form of CAM within the past 12 months, while almost 50 percent reported having used CAM at any time.[3] When prayer that is used specifically for health reasons is included in the definition of CAM, those numbers rise to 62 percent and 74 percent, respectively. FIGURE 22.1 shows more results from this study.

Complementary and alternative therapies vary widely in terms of nature of treatment, extent of therapy, and types of problems for which they offer help. Typically, CAM therapies are compared with conventional medicine. Conventional medicine is practiced by those with MD (medical doctor) or DO (doctors of osteopathy) degrees and by allied health professionals such as physical therapists, psychologists, and registered nurses. Other terms for conventional medicine include *allopathy, Western medicine, mainstream, orthodox,* and *biomedicine.* In general, practitioners of conventional medicine treat disease by using remedies that include pharmaceutical drugs or surgery. They have graduated from U.S.-sanctioned schools of medicine or nursing, or are licensed practitioners recognized by the American Medical Association (AMA), American Nurses Association (ANA), or other certification board. Some conventional medical practitioners are also CAM practitioners.

The list of practices that are considered CAM changes continually as therapies become accepted as mainstream. In general, CAM therapies serve as alternatives to an allopathic system that some people regard as too invasive, too high-tech, and too toxic in terms of laboratory-produced medications. CAM therapies incorporate a **holistic** approach to medicine that focuses on treating both the mind and body as opposed to an isolated part of the body. Often CAM users seek what they perceive as a natural, gentle approach to healing and believe that alternative practices will give them greater control over their own health care than conventional medicine. CAM therapies can vary, based on whether they have been scientifically studied and whether those studies have shown them to be beneficial. Scientific research has shown that many types

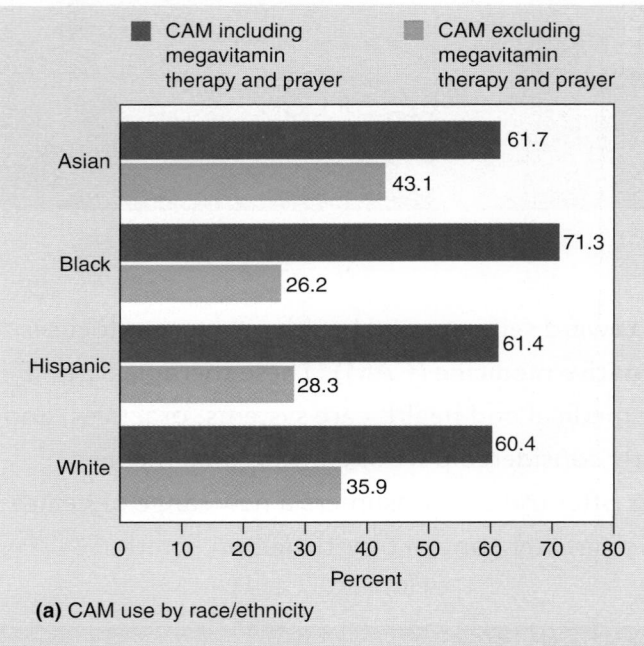

(a) CAM use by race/ethnicity

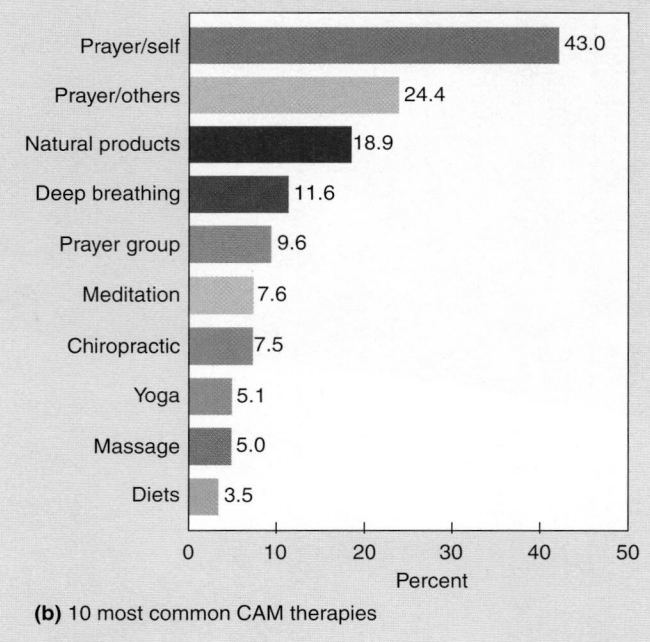

(b) 10 most common CAM therapies

FIGURE 22.1   Use of complementary and alternative medicine in the United States.
Source: National Center for Complementary and Alternative Medicine, "The Use of Complementary and Alternative Medicine in the United States," NCCAM Publication No. D234, 2007.

of CAM, including acupuncture and massage therapy, are beneficial in treating conditions such as chronic back pain and cancer.[4]

Comparing CAM with Conventional Medicine

As with traditional Western medicine, practitioners of most complementary and alternative therapies spend years learning their practice. Various forms of CAM are increasingly being taught in U.S. medical schools and are available to patients in some clinics and hospitals. Some, such as acupuncture, are even covered under many health insurance policies.

However, it is important to note that complementary and alternative therapies vary widely in terms of the nature of treatment, extent of therapy, and types of problems for which they offer help. There is no national training or licensure standard, and states differ in their practices (this is also true for conventional medicine). Whereas practitioners of conventional medicine have graduated from U.S. sanctioned schools of medicine or are licensed medical practitioners recognized by the AMA—the governing body for all physicians—each CAM domain has a different set of training standards, guidelines for practice, and licensure procedures. Although it is not possible to provide a detailed examination of each profession here, including the amount of training necessary, licensure, and continuing education requirements, a quick Internet search of each profession can provide you with detailed information. See the Spotlight on Your Health box for information on finding reliable Internet resources.

The History of CAM in the United States

Some variations of CAM have been influencing medicine in the United States throughout our history. For example, an estimated 25 percent of all modern pharmaceutical drugs are derived from herbs, including aspirin (white willow bark), the heart medication digitalis (foxglove), and the cancer treatment Taxol (Pacific yew tree). In addition, many of our recent pharmacological advances have their roots in the herbal remedies used in cultures throughout the world.

Although plant-based medicines were widely used in the United States until World War II, a new generation of FDA-tested pharmaceuticals took over in the later years of the twentieth century. Older treatments fell out of favor among all but a few segments of the U.S. population and became associated with the undeveloped and impoverished parts of the world. However, with the populace's growing dissatisfaction with the techno-wizardry of early twenty-first-century U.S. medicine, many of these earlier treatments have reemerged in treatment arsenals.

CAM in the United States Today

A survey of over 31,000 Americans revealed that 36 percent of adults use some form of CAM.[5] Why do so many people seek alternative therapy? Distinct patterns of CAM users emerge from this survey:

- More women than men
- People with higher educational levels
- People who had been hospitalized in the past year

DIDyouKNOW?

Aspirin is derived from salacin, a compound found in the bark of the white willow tree that was used for centuries before aspirin came on the market. Hippocrates, the Greek physician and father of modern medicine, prescribed the leaves and bark of the willow tree to relieve pain and fever in the 5th century B.C.!

What makes alternative medicine different from conventional medicine?

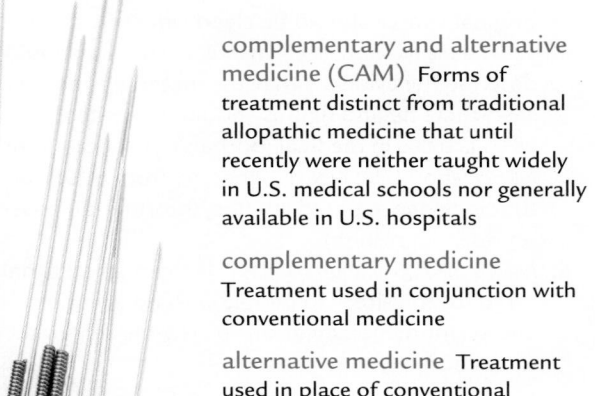

complementary and alternative medicine (CAM) Forms of treatment distinct from traditional allopathic medicine that until recently were neither taught widely in U.S. medical schools nor generally available in U.S. hospitals

complementary medicine Treatment used in conjunction with conventional medicine

alternative medicine Treatment used in place of conventional medicine

holistic Relating to or concerned with the whole body and the interactions of systems, rather than treatment of individual parts

SPOTLIGHT ON YOUR HEALTH

Evaluating CAM Resources on the Web

Planning to research CAM information online? The National Center for Complementary and Alternative Medicine recommends that you ask these questions about any website you visit:

1. *Who runs this site?* Any good health-related website should be clear about who is responsible for the site and its information, with the name of the site's sponsor and a link to its home page on every major page of the site.

2. *Who pays for the site?* How does the site pay for its existence? The source of its funding should be clearly stated or readily apparent. For example, Web addresses ending in ".gov" denote a federal government-sponsored site. Does the site sell advertising? Is it sponsored by a drug company? The source of funding can affect the choice of content, how the information is presented, and what the site owners want to accomplish.

How do I evaluate alternative medicine resources for reliability?

3. *What is the purpose of the site?* This question is related to who owns and pays for the site. An "About This Site" link appears on many sites; if it's there, use it. The site's purpose should be clearly stated and should help you evaluate the trustworthiness of the information.

4. *Where does the information come from?* Many health and medical sites post information collected from other websites or sources. If the person or organization in charge of the site did not create the information, the original source should be clearly identified.

5. *What is the basis of the information?* The site should describe the evidence that the material is based on. Medical facts and figures should have references (such as to articles in medical journals). Also, opinions or advice should be clearly set apart from information that is evidence based (that is, information based on research results).

6. *How is the information selected?* Is there an editorial board listed for the site? Do people with excellent professional and scientific qualifications review the material before it is posted?

7. *How current is the information?* Websites should be reviewed and updated on a regular basis. It is particularly important that medical information be current. The most recent update or review date should be clearly posted. Even if the information has not changed, you want to know whether the site owners have reviewed it recently to ensure that it is still valid.

8. *How does the site choose links to other sites?* Some websites take a conservative approach and don't link to any other sites. Some link to any site that asks—or pays—for a link. Others link only to sites that have met certain criteria.

9. *What information about you does the site collect, and why?* Websites routinely track the paths visitors take through their sites to determine which pages are being used. However, many health websites ask for you to "subscribe" or "become a member." In some cases, this may be so they can collect a user fee or select information that is relevant to your concerns. In all cases, this will give the site personal information about you. Any credible health site asking for this kind of information should tell you exactly what will and will not be done with it. Many commercial sites sell data about their users to other companies—information such as what percentage of their users are women with breast cancer, for example. In some cases, they may collect and reuse information that is "personally identifiable," such as your zip code, gender, and birth date. Be certain that you read and understand any privacy policy or similar language on the site, and don't sign up for anything that you do not fully understand.

10. *How does the site manage interactions with visitors?* There should always be a way for you to contact the site owner if you run across problems or have questions or feedback. If the site hosts chat rooms or other online discussions, it should inform visitors of its terms of using this service. Is it moderated? If so, by whom, and why? Spend time reading the discussion without joining in so that you feel comfortable with the environment before becoming a participant.

Source: National Center for Complementary and Alternative Medicine, "Ten Things to Know about Evaluating Medical Resources on the Web," 2006, http://nccam.nih.gov/health/webresources.

- Former smokers (compared with current smokers or those who have never smoked)

- People with back, neck, head, or joint aches or other painful conditions

- People with gastrointestinal disorders or sleeping problems

To better understand why Americans behave as they do when confronted with an illness or disorder, it is necessary to understand fears, concerns, and sources of hope for a positive outcome. Many of us have a powerful distrust of traditional medical practice. Through either direct experience or media portrayals of problems with today's health care system, many people believe that when they are sick, the worst place to be is in a hospital or health care setting. FIGURE 22.2 summarizes the reasons respondents to the NCCAM survey stated for deciding to use CAM.

Alternative Medical Systems

Alternative (whole) medical systems are built upon specific systems of theory and practice. There are many alternative systems of medicine that have been practiced by various cultures throughout the world. Some, such as traditional Chinese medicine and Ayurveda, have evolved from centuries-old Asian practices and are at the root of much of our CAM thinking today. Other newer alternative medical systems include homeopathy and naturopathy.

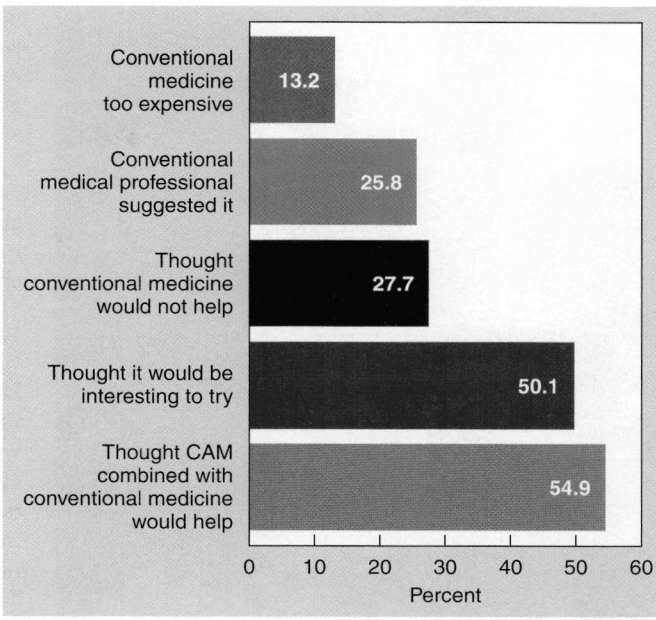

FIGURE 22.2   Reasons adults in the United States use CAM.

Survey respondents who reported having used CAM were asked to describe why they used it. People could select more than one reason.

Source: National Center for Complementary and Alternative Medicine, "The Use of Complementary and Alternative Medicine in the United States," NCCAM Publication No. D234, 2007.

Traditional Chinese Medicine

Traditional Chinese medicine (TCM) emphasizes the proper balance or disturbances of *qi* (pronounced "chee"), or vital energy in health and disease, respectively. Diagnosis is based on personal history; on observation of the body (especially the tongue); on palpation; and on pulse diagnosis, an elaborate procedure requiring considerable skill and experience of the practitioner. Techniques such as acupuncture, herbal medicine, massage, and *qigong* (a form of energy therapy) are among the TCM approaches to health and healing. These are discussed in more detail later in this chapter.

TCM practitioners within the United States must complete a graduate program at a college or university approved by the Accreditation Commission for Acupuncture and Oriental Medicine (ACAOM). Graduate programs vary based on the specific area of concentration within TCM but usually involve an extensive 3- or 4-year clinical internship. In addition, an examination by the National Commission for the Certification of Acupuncture and Oriental Medicine, a standard for licensing in the United States, must be completed.[6] Specific practices incorporated in TCM are discussed later in the chapter under the different CAM domains.

Ayurveda

Ayurveda (Ayurvedic medicine) relates to the "science of life," an alternative medical system that began and evolved over thousands of years in India. Ayurveda seeks to integrate and balance the body, mind, and spirit and restore harmony in the individual.[7] Ayurvedic practitioners use various techniques, including asking questions, observing, touching patients, and classifying patients into one of three body types (or *doshas*) before establishing a treatment plan. The goals of Ayurvedic treatment are to eliminate impurities in the body and reduce symptoms. Dietary

alternative (whole) medical systems   Complete systems of theory and practice that cross several CAM domains

traditional Chinese medicine (TCM)   Ancient comprehensive system of healing that uses herbs, acupuncture, and massage to bring the body into balance and to remove blockages of vital energy flow that lead to disease

qi   Element of traditional Chinese medicine that refers to the vital energy force that courses through the body; when *qi* is in balance, health is restored

Ayurveda (Ayurvedic medicine)   A comprehensive system of medicine, derived largely from ancient India, that places equal emphasis on the body, mind, and spirit, and strives to restore the body's innate harmony through diet, exercise, meditation, herbs, massage, exposure to sunlight, and controlled breathing

Shirodhara is a traditional Ayurvedic treatment in which warm medicated oil is steadily poured over the forehead in guided rhythmic patterns. This treatment is said to relieve stress and anxiety, treat insomnia and chronic headaches, and improve memory.

modification and herbal remedies drawn from the vast botanical wealth of the Indian subcontinent are common. Treatments may also include animal and mineral ingredients, powdered gemstones, yoga, stretching, meditation, massage, steam baths, sun exposure, and controlled breathing.[8]

Training of Ayurvedic practitioners varies; there is no national standard for certifying or training, although professional groups are working toward licensure. Specific practices incorporated in Ayurvedic medicine are discussed later in the chapter under the different CAM domains.

Homeopathy

Homeopathic medicine is an unconventional Western system based on the principle that "like cures like." In other words, the same substance that in large doses produces the symptoms of an illness will, in very small doses, cure the illness. It was developed in the late 1700s by Samuel Hahnemann, a German physician, as a medical approach that was not as harsh as other treatments of the time, such as bloodletting and blistering.[9] Homeopathic physicians use herbal medicine, minerals, and chemicals in extremely diluted forms to kill infectious agents or ward off illnesses that are caused by more potent forms or doses of those substances.

Homeopathic training varies considerably and is offered through diploma programs, certificate programs, short courses, and correspondence courses. Laws that detail requirements to practice vary from state to state.

Naturopathy

Naturopathic medicine views disease as a manifestation of an alteration in the processes by which the body naturally heals itself. Disease results from the body's effort to ward off impurities and harmful substances from the environment. Naturopathic physicians emphasize restoring health rather than curing disease. They employ an array of healing practices, including diet and clinical nutrition; homeopathy; acupuncture; herbal medicine; hydrotherapy (the use of water in a range of temperatures and methods of application); spinal and soft-tissue manipulation; physical therapies involving electrical currents, ultrasound, and light therapy; therapeutic counseling; and pharmacology.

Several major naturopathic schools in the United States and Canada provide training, conferring the *naturopathic doctor (ND)* degree on students who have completed a 4-year graduate program that emphasizes humanistically oriented family medicine.

Other Alternative Medical Systems

While these medical philosophies and patterns of treatment have exerted great influence on populations worldwide, other medical traditions are also noteworthy. American Indian, Aboriginal, African, Middle Eastern, and South American cultures also have their own alternative systems.

As the number of alternative therapists grows and systems become intertwined, so do the number of health care options available to consumers. Before considering any treatments, wise consumers will consult the most reliable resources to thoroughly evaluate risks, the scientific basis of claimed benefits, and any contraindications to using the CAM product or service. Avoid practitioners who promote their treatments as a cure-all for every health problem or who seem to

homeopathic medicine
Unconventional Western system of medicine based on the principle that "like cures like"

naturopathic medicine System of medicine originating from Europe that views disease as a manifestation of alterations in the body's natural self-healing processes, and that emphasizes health restoration as well as disease treatment promise remedies that have thus far defied the best scientific efforts of mainstream medicine. In short, apply the same strategies to researching CAM as you would to choosing allopathic care. See the Skills for Behavior Change box on page 823 for more information on choosing a CAM practitioner.

Major Domains of CAM

The U.S. government has created the National Center for Complementary and Alternative Medicine (NCCAM) within the National Institutes of Health (NIH) to provide a mechanism for reliable information about CAM practices. The NCCAM serves as a clearinghouse for CAM information and a focal point for research initiatives, policy development, and general recommendations. It has grouped the many varieties of CAM into four domains of practice (FIGURE 22.3), recognizing that the domains may overlap and aspects of them may be part of larger alternative medical systems:

*   *Manipulative and body-based practices* are based on manipulation or movement of one or more body parts. Examples include chiropractic or osteopathic manipulations and massage.

*   *Energy medicine* involves the use of energy fields, such as magnetic fields or biofields (energy fields that some believe surround and penetrate the body). Examples include Reiki and therapeutic touch.

*   *Mind–body medicine* uses a variety of techniques to enhance the mind's ability to affect bodily function and symptoms. Some examples include support groups, meditation, and the use of cognitive behavioral theory.

*   *Biologically based practices* use substances found in nature, such as herbs, special foods, or vitamins (in doses outside those used in conventional medicine). This includes the use of natural but unproven therapies, such as dietary supplements and herbal products.

Manipulative and Body-Based Practices

The CAM domain of **manipulative and body-based practices** includes methods that are based on manipulation or movement of the body. For example, chiropractors focus on the relationship between the body's structures (primarily the spine) and functions and on how that relationship affects the preservation and restoration of health. Massage therapists use various hand techniques to move muscles and soft tissues to increase the flow of blood and oxygen to these areas or to release muscular tension.

Chiropractic Medicine

Chiropractic medicine has been practiced for over 100 years and focuses on manipulation as a key therapy.[10] A century ago, allopathic medicine and chiropractic medicine were in direct competition. Today, however, many health care organizations work closely with chiropractors, and many insurance companies will pay for chiropractic

1. **Manipulative and body-based practices** are based on manipulation or movement of one or more body parts.

2. **Energy medicine** involves the use of energy fields, such as magnetic fields or biofields (energy fields that some believe surround and penetrate the human body).

3. **Mind–body medicine** uses a variety of techniques designed to enhance the mind's ability to affect bodily function and symptoms.

4. **Biologically based practices** use substances found in nature, such as herbs, special diets, or vitamins (in doses outside those used in conventional medicine).

Whole medical systems are built upon complete systems of theory and practice. Often, these systems have evolved apart from and earlier than the conventional medical approach used in the United States.

FIGURE 22.3 The domains of complementary and alternative medicine.
NCCAM groups CAM practices into four domains, recognizing there can be some overlap. In addition, NCCAM studies CAM whole medical systems, which cut across all domains.
Source: National Center for Complementary and Alternative Medicine, "The Use of Complementary and Alternative Medicine in the United States," NCCAM Publication No. D234, 2007.

manipulative and body-based practices Treatments involving manipulation or movement of one or more body parts

chiropractic medicine Manipulation of the spine to allow proper energy flow

A chiropractor treats a patient using a variety of techniques to manipulate the spine into proper alignment.

treatment, particularly if it is recommended by a medical doctor. More than 20 million Americans now visit chiropractors each year.

Chiropractic medicine is based on the idea that a life-giving energy flows through the spine via the nervous system. If the spine is subluxated (partly misaligned or dislocated), that force is disrupted. Chiropractors use a variety of techniques to manipulate the spine back into proper alignment, allowing the energy to flow unimpeded. Their treatment is often used for back pain, neck pain, and headaches.

The average chiropractic training program requires 4 years of intensive courses in biochemistry, anatomy, physiology, diagnostics, pathology, nutrition, and related topics, combined with hands-on clinical training. Many chiropractors continue their training to obtain specialized certification, for instance, in neurology, geriatrics, or pediatrics. There are currently 16 accredited programs and 2 chiropractic educational institutions in the United States. Most state boards require 2 years of undergraduate education, and more states are requiring a bachelor's degree in addition to the doctor of chiropractic degree for licensure. The practice of chiropractic medicine is licensed and regulated in all 50 states.[11]

Massage Therapy

Massage therapy is defined as soft-tissue manipulation by trained therapists for healing purposes.[12] References to massage have been found in ancient writings from many cultures, including those of Ancient Greece, Ancient Rome, Japan, China, Egypt, and the Indian subcontinent.[13] Today, massage therapy is being used as a means of treating painful conditions such as low back pain (see the Health Headlines box on page 825), relaxing tired and overworked muscles, reducing stress and anxiety, rehabilitating sports injuries, and promoting general health.[14] This is accomplished by manipulating soft tissues in order to improve the body's circulation and remove waste products from the muscles. There are many different types of massage therapy; some of the more popular include the following:[15]

- *Swedish massage.* Uses long strokes, kneading, and friction on the muscles and moves the joints to aid flexibility.

- *Deep-tissue massage.* Uses patterns of strokes and deep finger pressure on parts of the body where muscles are tight or knotted, focusing on layers of muscle deep under the skin.

- *Trigger-point massage (also called pressure-point massage).* Uses a variety of strokes but applies deeper, more focused pressure on myofascial trigger points— "knots" that can form in the muscles, are painful when pressed, and cause symptoms elsewhere in the body as well.

- *Shiatsu massage.* Uses varying, rhythmic pressure from the fingers on parts of the body that are believed to be important for the flow of vital energy.

Other varieties include massage of specific body parts, such as the feet or fingers, application of hot rocks, water massage, oil massage, or other techniques. Massage techniques are important aspects of both traditional Chinese medicine and Ayurvedic medicine.

There are about 1,300 massage therapy schools, college programs, and training programs in the United States. The course of study typically covers subjects such as anatomy, physiology, and kinesiology; therapeutic evaluation; massage techniques; first aid; business, ethical, and legal issues; and hands-on practice. These educational programs vary in respect to length, quality, and whether they are accredited. Many require 500 hours of training, which is the same number of hours that many states require for certification. Some therapists also pursue specialty or advanced training. Massage therapists work in an array of settings both private and public,

SKILLS FOR BEHAVIOR CHANGE

Selecting a CAM Provider

Before starting a CAM therapy or choosing a practitioner, talk with your primary health care provider(s) and others who are knowledgeable about CAM. Interview the potential CAM provider and investigate the recommended treatment. Here are some tips for going about these processes:

√ Ask your doctor or other health professional to recommend or refer you to a CAM therapist, or consult someone you trust who has used CAM.

√ If your therapy will be covered by insurance, ask your carrier for a list of approved CAM providers.

√ Contact a professional organization for the type of practitioner you are seeking. Often they have standards of practice and websites or publications that list recommended providers. If there is a regulatory or licensing board for this specialty, verify that your practitioner has the proper credentials.

√ Write down questions to ask at your first visit. You may want to bring a friend or family member who can help you ask questions and note answers.

√ Bring medical information with you, including any tests you've had, information about your health history, surgical history, allergies, and any medications (including prescription, over-the-counter, and herbal or other supplements) you are taking.

√ Ask if there are diseases or health conditions in which the practitioner specializes and how frequently he or she treats patients with conditions like yours.

√ Ask if there is any scientific research supporting the use of this treatment for your condition and find out about any potential risks or side effects. Be sure to ask whether the therapy will interfere with any conventional medical treatments you are undergoing.

√ Is the provider supportive of traditional medicine as well as CAM treatments? Does he or she have a good relationship with conventional practitioners in order to give referrals to them?

√ What are the charges and payment options? What percentage might you have to pay out of pocket?

including private offices, studios, hospitals, nursing homes, fitness centers, and sports medicine facilities.[16]

Bodywork

Bodywork actually consists of several forms of exercise. The *Feldenkrais Method* is a system of movements, floor exercises, and bodywork designed to retrain the central nervous system to find new pathways around areas of blockage or damage. It is gentle and effective in rehabilitating trauma victims. *Rolfing*, a more invasive form of bodywork, aims to restructure the musculoskeletal system by working on patterns of tension held in deep tissue. The therapist applies firm—sometimes painful—pressure to different areas of the body. Rolfing can release repressed emotions as well as dissipate muscle tension. *Shiatsu* is a traditional healing art from Japan that applies firm finger pressure to specified points on the body and is intended to increase the circulation of vital energy. *Trager bodywork* employs gentle shaking motions of the patient's limbs in a rhythmic fashion to induce states of deep, pleasant relaxation.[17]

Energy Medicine

Acupuncture has been found to be effective in treating many problems but should always be performed by a licensed practitioner.

Energy medicine therapies focus either on energy fields thought to originate within the body (biofields) or on fields from other sources (electromagnetic fields). Biofield therapies are intended to affect energy fields said to surround and penetrate the human body. The existence of these fields has not been experimentally proven. Some forms of energy therapy manipulate biofields by applying pressure or manipulating the body by placing the hands in, or through, these fields.[18]

Popular examples of biofield therapy include *qigong, Reiki,* and *therapeutic touch.*[19] Qigong, a component of traditional Chinese medicine, combines movement, meditation, and regulation of breathing to enhance the flow of vital energy (*qi*), improve blood circulation, and enhance immune function. *Reiki* (Japanese for "universal life energy") is based on the belief that by channeling spiritual energy through the practitioner, the spirit is healed, and it in turn heals the physical body. *Therapeutic touch* derives from the ancient technique of "laying on of hands" and is based on the premise that the therapist's healing force brings about the patient's recovery and that healing is promoted when the body's energies are in balance. By passing the hands over the body, the healer identifies bodily imbalances.

Bioelectromagnetic-based therapies involve the unconventional use of electromagnetic fields, such as pulsed fields, magnetic fields, or alternating current or direct current fields, to treat asthma, cancer, pain, migraines, and other conditions.

There is little scientific documentation to support claims for energy field techniques at this point. However, two derivatives of energy medicine have gained much wider acceptance in recent years: acupuncture and acupressure.

Acupuncture

How does acupuncture work? **?**

Acupuncture, one of the oldest forms of traditional Chinese medicine, and one of the most popular among Americans, is sought for a wide variety of health purposes, including healing musculoskeletal dysfunction, mood enhancement, and wellness promotion. It describes a family of procedures that involve stimulating anatomical points of the body with a series of precisely placed needles. The placement and manipulation of acupuncture needles is based on traditional Chinese theories of life-force energy (*qi*) flow through meridians, or energy pathways, in the body. Following acupuncture, most respondents and participants in clinical studies report high satisfaction with the treatment, improved quality of life, improvement in or cure of the condition, and reduced reliance on prescription drugs and surgery. In particular, results have been promising in the treatment of nausea associated with chemotherapy, dental pain, and knee pain.[20] Some Western researchers believe that acupuncture may work through stimulating or repressing the autonomic nervous system.[21]

Acupuncturists in the United States are state licensed, and each state has specific requirements regarding training programs. Most acupuncturists have either completed a 2- to 3-year postgraduate program to obtain a master of traditional Oriental medicine (MTOM) degree or attended a shorter certification program in North America or Asia. Some licensed MDs and chiropractors have trained in acupuncture and obtained certification to use this treatment.

Acupressure

Acupressure is similar to acupuncture but does not use needles. Instead, the practitioner applies pressure to points critical to balancing *yin* and *yang*, the two Chinese principles that interact to influence overall harmony (health) of the body. Practitioners must have the same basic understanding of energy pathways as do acupuncturists.

energy medicine Therapies using energy fields, such as magnetic fields or biofields

acupuncture Branch of traditional Chinese medicine that uses the insertion of long, thin needles to affect flow of energy (*qi*) along pathways (meridians) within the body

acupressure Branch of traditional Chinese medicine, related to acupuncture; uses application of pressure to selected body points to balance energy

HEALTH HEADLINES

The Benefits of Massage for Low Back Pain

With 39 million American adults per year getting massages, and 30 percent of those adults using massage therapy for medical purposes, recent American Massage Therapy Association (AMTA) consumer surveys show that massage therapy is a growing trend. Massage has been credited with alleviating a wide variety of ailments, including migraines, carpal tunnel syndrome, and anxiety. In particular, massage has been looked at as a useful treatment for low back pain (LBP). More than 100 million Americans suffer from LBP, and nearly $25 billion a year is spent in search of relief. In the CDC's thirtieth annual report on the nation's health status, *Health, United States, 2006,* LBP was the most commonly reported type of pain, the most common cause of job-related disability, and a leading contributor to missed work and reduced productivity.

Medication may still be the most common way to treat LBP, but increasing evidence suggests it is neither the most effective nor the safest treatment method. The need for more effective solutions to this problem has led many health care organizations to increase research for alternative treatments such as massage therapy. A recent study in the *Annals of Internal Medicine* showed that massage therapy produced better results and reduced the need for pain-killers by 36 percent when compared to other therapies, including acupuncture and spinal modification.

As evidence that massage therapy is increasingly on the public's mind, the AMTA reports that 9 million more people discussed massage therapy with their health care provider in 2006 than in 2001. Moreover, almost twice as many doctors recommended massage therapy to their patients in 2006 than in 2001. When patients inquire about massage therapy, physicians are more likely to recommend it (59 percent), while nearly half of all chiropractors (48 percent) and physical therapists (47 percent) also recommended it. Despite lingering pessimism from some in the conventional medical community, an impressive 25 million more Americans each year are getting massages today than they did 10 years ago, according to the 2006 AMTA study. Many people are coming to believe massage is not just a luxury but a medical necessity, but Medicare and Medicaid have not yet supported insurance coverage for massage as a remedy for LBP, and many insurance companies offer only limited coverage

for it. Because massage therapy, as with most CAM care, is paid for by the patients, it is not accessible to all Americans. Only those who can afford the out-of-pocket costs have access to broader choices in their health care.

To address the issues of cost, availability, and widespread acceptance, the AMTA and Integrative Healthcare Policy Consortium (IHPC) have proposed that the NIH hold a consensus conference on the use of massage for lower back pain. Both the AMTA and Associated Bodywork and Massage Professionals (ABMP) have pledged funds to this conference and to efforts to gain medical recognition of massage as a therapy for LBP. Through this conference, which is projected to take place within the next 2 years, these organizations hope to elicit a federal statement declaring that massage is effective for LBP. Historically, the conference panel's findings have triggered Medicare and Medicaid reimbursement policies that, in turn, have expanded insurance coverage policies. If the conference goal is reached, it is anticipated that massage for LBP will be widely accepted by the health care community.

Source: Adapted from M. Vivo, "Making a Statement About Massage," *Massage Today,* August 2007. Copyright © 2007 Used with permission. www.massagetoday.com.

Mind–Body Medicine

Mind–body medicine employs a variety of techniques designed to facilitate the mind's capacity to affect bodily functions and symptoms. Many therapies might fall into this category, but some areas, such as biofeedback and cognitive-behavioral techniques, have been so well investigated that they are no longer considered alternative. However, meditation, yoga, tai chi, certain uses of hypnosis, dance, music and art therapy, prayer and mental healing, and several others are still categorized as complementary and alternative. (See Chapter 12 for more on yoga and tai chi.)

Psychoneuroimmunology

Psychoneuroimmunology (PNI) is a relatively new field of study. It is defined as the "interaction of consciousness *(psycho)*, the brain and central nervous system *(neuro)*, and the body's defense against external infection and internal aberrant cell division *(immunology)*."[22] Many researchers have postulated over the years that excessive stress and maladaptive coping can lead to immune system dysfunction and increased risk of disease. Scientists are exploring ways in which relaxation, biofeedback, meditation, yoga, laughter, exercise, and activities that involve either conscious or unconscious mind "quieting" may counteract negative stressors.

A classic study of PNI and mind–body health attempted to assess the effects of relaxation and coping techniques on the immune system by studying nursing home patients. Participants were divided into three groups: those who were taught relaxation techniques, those who were provided with abundant social contact, and those who received no special techniques or contact. After 1 month, immune system function greatly improved in those who received stress management therapy as compared to the other groups.[23] Several studies have shown promising positive effects of mind–body techniques that encourage relaxation and other stress-reduction strategies for those with cancer or other health problems.

Buying herbal supplements can be confusing, because so many brands exist and their manufacture is not strictly regulated for potency or quality.

Biologically Based Practices

Biologically based practices are perhaps the most controversial domain of CAM therapies because of the sheer number of options available and the many claims that are made about their effects. Many of these claims have not been thoroughly investigated, and regulation of this aspect of CAM has been slow in coming. Biologically based practices include natural treatments, interventions, and products, many of which overlap with conventional medicine's use of dietary supplements. The FDA defines dietary supplements as "products (other than tobacco) that are intended to supplement or add to the diet; that contain one or more of the following ingredients: vitamins, minerals, amino acids, herbs, or other substances that increase total dietary intake; that are intended for ingestion in the form of a capsule, powder, soft gel, or gelcap; and are not represented as a conventional food."[24] Included are herbal remedies, special dietary supplements, individual biological therapies, and functional foods.[25] Typically, people take these supplements and remedies—often without guidance from any CAM practitioner—to improve health, prevent disease, or enhance mood.

mind–body medicine Techniques designed to enhance the mind's ability to affect bodily functions and symptoms

biologically based practices Treatments using substances found in nature, such as herbs, special diets, or vitamin megadoses

Herbal Remedies

Derived largely from Ayurvedic or traditional Chinese medicine, herbal medications are widely available in the United States. Fueled by mass advertising and promoted

GREEN GUIDE

GUIDE GREEN GR
GUID

As herbal supplement use

becomes increasingly common, environmentally-conscious health consumers can take steps toward supporting herbal supplement manufacturers who adhere to sustainable environmental practices. One way to promote sustainability is to purchase fair trade herbal supplement products.

In brief, fair trade advocates that manufacturers pay suppliers a fair price, purchasing as directly possible while supporting social and environmental standards. Fair trade certified sales commonly involve exports of coffee, cocoa, and sugar from developing nations to developed nations. As a multibillion-dollar industry, fair trade certified product sales continue to grow each year. Fair trade teas and herbs are a relatively new idea, with many products only becoming available during the last several years. Through purchasing fair trade herbal supplements, you can assist with supporting sustainable farming methods and providing a living wage to farmers and workers. Further, fair trade practices seek to enhance communities by providing funding for social and business development.

One U.S. organization, TransFair USA (www.transfairusa .org), is a third-party certifier of fair trade products, such as herbal teas, and allows consumers to search their website for companies that are devoted to fair trade. The company's parent organization, Fairtrade Labelling Organizations International (FLO; www.fairtrade.net), is a global network of fair trade organizations that offer the Fairtrade Certification Mark. Standards for a product to earn certification include buyers paying at least the fair trade price set by FLO, buyers paying a fair trade premium that is used for community development, and buyers establishing a long-term relationship with the seller.

as part of multiple vitamin and mineral regimens by major drug manufacturers, herbal supplements represent the hottest trend in the health market.

Herbal remedies are not to be taken lightly. Just because something is natural does not necessarily mean that it is safe. For example, in recent years, the FDA has warned that certain herbal products containing kava may be associated with severe liver damage.[26] Even rigorously tested products can be risky. Many plants are poisonous, and some can be toxic if ingested in high doses. Others may be dangerous when combined with prescription or over-the-counter drugs, they could disrupt the normal action of the drugs. They could cause unusual side effects.[27] Properly trained herbalists and homeopaths have received graduate-level training in special programs such as herbal nutrition or traditional Chinese medicine. These practitioners have been trained in diagnosis; in mixing herbs, titrations, and dosages; and in the follow-up care of patients.

Herbal remedies come in several different forms. **Tinctures** (extracts of fresh or dried plants) usually contain a high percentage of grain alcohol to prevent spoilage and are among the best herbal options. Freeze-dried extracts are very stable and offer good value for your money. Standardized extracts, often available in pill or capsule form, are also among the more reliable forms of herbal preparations. Increasingly, herb preparations of many forms are being made available through environmentally responsible means and companies (see the Green Guide for more information).

In general, herbal medicines tend to be milder than chemical drugs and produce their effects more slowly; they also are much less likely to cause toxicity, because they are diluted rather than concentrated forms of drugs. But diluted or not, and no matter how natural they are, herbs still contain many of the same chemicals as synthetic prescription drugs. Too much of any herb, particularly one from nonstandardized extracts, can cause problems. The following discussion gives an overview of some of the most common herbal supplements on the market.

Do herbal remedies have any risks or side effects?

WHAT DO YOU THINK? *Why do you think more and more people are opting for complementary and alternative treatments? What are the potential benefits of these treatments? What are the potential risks? • What types of controls are reasonable to regulate the quality and consistency of foreign-trained health care providers?*

tinctures Herbal extracts usually combined with grain alcohol to prevent spoilage

Ginkgo Biloba

Ginkgo biloba is an extract from the leaves of a deciduous tree that lives up to 1,000 years. Ginkgo leaves and seeds have been used in Chinese herbal medicine for centuries.[28] Today, ginkgo leaf extracts are widely prescribed in many countries and are gaining in popularity.

Ginkgo biloba is said to have many benefits and is used to treat depression, impotence, premenstrual syndrome, eye diseases (such as retinopathy and macular degeneration), and general vascular disease. Though there is no definitive verdict on the benefits of ginkgo, numerous studies have been carried out for a variety of conditions. Some promising results have been seen for Alzheimer's disease and dementia, and research continues to determine the effect on its ability to enhance memory, reduce the incidence of cardiovascular disease, and decrease the rate of premature death. NCCAM is also looking at potential interactions between ginkgo and prescription drugs.[29]

Most nutritional experts and physicians recommend that people who are considering using ginkgo take a 40-milligram tablet three times a day for a month or so to determine whether there is any improvement. If there is none, taking this supplement is largely unwarranted. It has been shown to cause gastric irritation, headache, nausea, dizziness, or allergic reactions. Also, remember that disturbing memory loss or difficulty thinking, regardless of age, should be checked with a physician to determine underlying causes. Ginkgo should not be taken by those on blood thinners or who are at risk for bleeding.

Today, much of what we know about ginkgo biloba remains controversial, even though extensive research on its effects has been conducted. Until the results of these tests are available, consumers should exercise caution in any use of ginkgo.

St. John's Wort

The bright yellow, star-shaped flowers of St. John's wort (SJW) have a rich and varied history of medicinal use in Europe, Asia, and Africa. In the United States, SJW grows in abundance in northern California and southern Oregon and is also called *Klamath weed*.

Today, SJW enjoys global popularity. It is the favored therapy for depression in many countries, including Germany, actually surpassing most standard antidepressants as the first mode of treatment for clinical depression. Research into the herb has yielded mixed results: some studies have indicated it is more effective than a placebo and has fewer side effects than prescription antidepressants, while others have found no effect on depression at all.[30]

NCCAM has published the following summary points about SJW:[31]

- There is some scientific evidence that SJW is useful for treating mild to moderate depression. However, two large studies, one sponsored by NCCAM, showed that the herb was no more effective than a placebo in treating major depression of moderate severity.

- Research shows that SJW interacts with some drugs, including antidepressants, anticoagulants, and birth control pills.

- It is important to remember that SJW is not a proven therapy for depression. If depression is not adequately treated, it can become severe. Anyone who may have depression should see a health care provider. There are effective proven therapies available.

Like other plants, SJW contains a number of different chemicals, many of which are not clearly understood. The herb also has several side effects. Most are more bothersome than severe and range from slight gastrointestinal upset to fatigue, dry mouth, anxiety, sexual dysfunction, dizziness, skin rashes, and itching. Some people develop extreme sensitivity to sunlight.

Due to conflicting news about SJW, consumers should proceed with caution. Since the herb is sold in the United States as a dietary supplement, not a drug, it has not been regulated by the FDA, and rigorous testing has not been done. Anyone suffering from clinical depression should be under a physician's and a psychologist's care. In addition, SJW should never be taken in combination with prescription anti-depressants. When combined with drugs such as Prozac and other serotonin reup-take inhibitors (SSRIs), SJW may result in serotonin overload, leading to tremors, agitation, or convulsions. Because the safety margins have not been established, SJW also should not be used by pregnant women or women who are nursing, by young children, or by the frail elderly.

Echinacea

Echinacea, or the *purple coneflower,* is found primarily in the Midwest and prairie regions of the United States. As the herb's popularity has increased, two of the nine species of echinacea in the United States are now on the federal endangered species list, a cause of growing concern for many environmentalists. Believed to be used extensively by Native Americans for centuries, echinacea eventually gained wide-spread acceptance in the United States before being shipped to Europe, where its use grew gradually over the eighteenth and nineteenth centuries.

Today, echinacea is the best-selling herb in the United States and is widely used throughout most of the world. It is said to stimulate the immune system and increase the effectiveness of the white blood cells that attack bacteria and viruses. Many people believe it helps prevent and treat the symptoms of a cold or flu.

However, echinacea remains controversial. While many studies in Europe have provided preliminary evidence of its effectiveness, a recent controlled study in the United States indicated that it is no more effective than a placebo in preventing or treating a cold.[32] As with many herbal treatments, little valid research has been conducted on the benefits and risks of echinacea. Because this herb can affect the immune system, people with autoimmune diseases such as rheumatoid arthritis should not take it. Other people who should avoid echinacea include pregnant women, those with diabetes or multiple sclerosis, and anyone allergic to the daisy family of plants. Some studies have also raised concerns about increased risks for people who take echinacea before organ transplants.[33]

Ginseng

Grown commercially throughout North America, ginseng is much prized for its reported sexual restorative value. It is believed that ginseng affects the pituitary gland, increasing resistance to stress, affecting metabolism, aiding skin and muscle tone, and providing the hormonal balance necessary for a healthy sex life. Other purported benefits include improvements in muscle endurance, muscle strength, recovery from exercise, oxygen metabolism during exercise, auditory and visual reaction time, and mental concentration. To date, these benefits have not been scientifically validated.[34]

However, studies have raised questions about the appropriate dosages. Because the potency of plants varies considerably, dosage is difficult to control and side effects are fairly common. Noteworthy side effects of high doses of ginseng include nervousness, insomnia, high blood pressure, headaches, skin eruptions, chest pain, depression, and abnormal vaginal bleeding.[35]

Green Tea

Although some studies have shown promising links between green and white tea consumption and cancer prevention, recent research questions the ability of tea to significantly reduce the risk of breast, lung, or prostate cancers.[36] At the same time, other research suggests green tea may lower cholesterol, protect the skin from sun damage, and bolster mental alertness.[37]

Some scientists suspect that green tea may boost heart health because it contains high levels of flavonoids. These plant compounds, which are also found in fruits, vegetables, and red wine, are thought to promote health by combating oxidation, a process in which cell-damaging free radicals accumulate. Oxidative damage can be caused by outside factors, such as cigarette smoking, or by factors on the cellular level. Oxidation is suspected of increasing the risk of heart disease,

Will echinacea teas boost my immune system?

stroke, and several other diseases. Although promising, more research on the role of green tea must be conducted to determine whether its perceived benefits are actually due to the tea or to some other characteristic that tea drinkers have in common.

Ephedra (Ma Huang)

An herbal ingredient formerly found in many weight-loss and fitness supplements, ephedra's active ingredient is ephedrine, which is similar to amphetamine. Comprehensive research has found that ephedra has only limited effects on weight loss and athletic performance but has numerous adverse effects, including heart attack, stroke, and death. Other side effects such as heart palpitations, psychiatric problems, upper-gastrointestinal effects, tremors, and insomnia also have been noted.[38] In 2004, the FDA banned the sale of all supplements containing ephedra. These products are no longer legally available for sale in the United States.

Special Supplements

Not all the supplements on the market today are directly derived from plant sources. In recent years, there have been increasing reports in the media on the health benefits of various vitamins, minerals, amino acids, and other specific biological compounds.

When taken to increase work output or the potential for it, dietary supplements are labeled as **ergogenic aids**. Examples include bee pollen, caffeine, glycine, carnitine, lecithin, brewer's yeast, and gelatin. In recent years, a new generation of performance-enhancing ergogenic aids has hit the market. Many of these claim to increase muscular strength and performance, boost energy, and enhance resistance to disease.

Muscle Enhancers

Androstenedione ("andro"), a substance that is found naturally in meat and some plants and is also produced in the human body by the adrenal glands and gonads, is a precursor to the human hormone testosterone. In other words, the body converts "andro" directly into testosterone, which enables an athlete to train harder and recover more quickly. Andro has a chemical structure similar to that of anabolic steroids. When taken over time and in sufficient quantities, andro may increase the risk of serious medical conditions. It is no longer available over the counter.

Creatine is a naturally occurring compound found primarily in skeletal muscle that helps to optimize the muscles' energy levels. In recent years, creatine use has increased dramatically because of claims that it increases muscle energy, allows a person to work harder with less muscle fatigue, and builds muscle mass with less effort. Reports of creatine's benefits, however, appear exaggerated. Over one-third of those taking creatine are unable to absorb it into their muscles and thus achieve no benefit. Side effects include muscle cramping, muscle strains, and possible liver and kidney damage.[39]

Glucosamine

Glucosamine is a substance the body produces that plays a key role in the growth and development of cartilage. When present in sufficient amounts, it stimulates the manufacture of substances necessary for proper joint function and joint repair. As a supplement, it is manufactured commercially and sold under a variety of different names, usually glucosamine sulfate.

Glucosamine has been shown to be effective for treating osteoarthritis and related degenerative joint diseases and appears to relieve swelling and decrease pain. Unlike many other herbal supplements, glucosamine sulfate has a good safety record with few noteworthy side effects. However, in recent years, questions have arisen as to its effectiveness. While results of meta-analysis reviews and industry-sponsored research have shown it to be moderately effective, smaller independent studies have shown no significant benefits. A large study called the Glucosamine

ergogenic aids Special dietary supplements taken to increase strength, energy, and the ability to work

Arthritis Intervention Trial was recently completed, and the results indicate that a combination of glucosamine and chondroitin sulfate (another substance the body needs for joint repair) appear to alleviate moderate to severe pain associated with osteoarthritis of the knee.[40]

SAMe

SAMe (pronounced "Sammy") is the nickname for S-adenosyl-L-methionine, a compound produced biochemically in all humans to help perform some 40 functions in the body, ranging from bone preservation to DNA replication.

SAMe has long been reported to have a significant effect on mild to moderate depression without many of the typical side effects of prescription medications, such as sexual dysfunction, weight gain, and sleep disturbance. Scientists speculate that SAMe somehow affects brain levels of the neurotransmitters noradrenaline, serotonin, and possibly dopamine, all of which are related to the human stress response and the origins of depression in the body. Questions still remain over how much SAMe a person should take, what form it should be administered in, and if there are long-term side effects such as liver toxicity or cancer.[41]

Antioxidants

Antioxidants are chemicals that combat free radicals and oxidative damage in cells. They are present in many plant foods (including green tea, discussed earlier). It should be noted here that antioxidants are among the most sought-after supplements on the market. Primary antioxidants include beta-carotene, selenium, vitamin C, and vitamin E.

See Table 22.1 for other popular supplements and herbal remedies and their associated risks and benefits.

Green tea has become popular in recent years for its antioxidant properties and for its purported value in preventing cancer.

Foods as Healing Agents

The term *functional foods* is used to describe foods or supplements believed or designed to improve some specific aspect of physical or mental functioning. Sometimes referred to as **nutraceuticals** for their combined nutritional and pharmaceutical benefit, several are believed to work in much the same way as pharmaceutical drugs in making a person well or bolstering the immune system.

Some of the most common functional foods and their purported benefits include the following:

- *Plant stanols/sterols.* Can lower "bad" (LDL) cholesterol.

- *Oat fiber.* Can lower "bad" (LDL) cholesterol; serves as a natural nerve soother; stabilizes blood sugar levels.

- *Sunflower.* Can lower risk of heart disease; may prevent angina.

- *Soy protein.* May lower heart disease risk by reducing LDL cholesterol and triglycerides.

- *Garlic.* Lowers cholesterol and reduces clotting tendency of blood; lowers blood pressure; may serve as a form of antibiotic.

- *Ginger.* Fights motion sickness and stomach pain and upset; discourages blood clots; may relieve rheumatism.

- *Yogurt.* Yogurt that contains "live active cultures" has active, friendly bacteria that can fight off infections.

nutraceuticals Term often used interchangeably with *functional foods;* refers to the combined nutritional and pharmaceutical benefit derived through use of foods or food supplements

TABLE 22.1 Common Herbal, Vitamin, and Mineral Supplements: Benefits versus Risks

Supplement	Claims of Benefits	Potential Risks
Chondroitin (protein found in animal cartilage)	Improves osteoporosis and arthritis by improving cartilage function	Fewer benefits than glucosamine; benefits still unproven
Dehydroepiandrosterone (DHEA) (hormone)	Fights aging, boosts immunity, strengthens bones, and improves brain functioning	No antiaging benefits proven; could increase cancer risk and lead to liver damage, even when taken briefly
Dieter's teas (e.g., herbal blends containing senna, aloe, rhubarb root, buckthorn, cascara, or castor oil)	Act as laxatives	Can disrupt potassium levels and cause heart arrhythmias; linked to diarrhea, vomiting, chronic constipation, fainting
Flaxseed and flaxseed oil (herb)	The seed is used as a laxative and for hot flashes and breast pain; the oil is used for arthritis; both flaxseed and flaxseed oil have been used for cholesterol level reduction and cancer prevention.	Delays absorption of medicine
Vitamin E (vitamin)	Antioxidant effect; reduces risk of heart disease; better survivability after heart attack	High dose causes bleeding when taking blood thinners
Kava (herb)	Relaxation; relief of anxiety, insomnia, and menopausal symptoms; sometimes used topically as a numbing agent	Increases the effect of alcohol and other drugs; causes drowsiness; associated with severe liver damage
L-Carnitine (amino acid derivative)	Improves metabolism in heart muscle, purported to increase fat-burning enzymes; also used to combat fatigue and aging	Nausea, vomiting, abdominal cramps, diarrhea, "fishy" body odor; more rarely, muscle weakness in uremic patients and seizures in those with seizure disorders; interacts with some medications
Licorice root (herb)	Reduces inflammation; used for stomach ulcers, bronchitis, and sore throat, as well as for infections caused by viruses	Speeds potassium loss; may contribute to high blood pressure
Melatonin (hormone)	Used to regulate circadian rhythms and sleep patterns; treats insomnia; claims of antiaging benefits	May cause nausea, headaches, dizziness, blood vessel constriction; possibly a danger for people with high blood pressure or other cardiovascular problems.
Valerian (herb)	Relaxation; used for sleep disorders and anxiety; also used for headaches, depression, irregular heartbeat, and trembling	Mild side effects, such as headaches, dizziness, upset stomach, and tiredness the morning after use
Zinc (mineral)	Supports immune system; used to lessen duration and severity of cold symptoms; aids wound healing	Excessive intake associated with reduced immune function, reduced levels of high-density lipoproteins (good cholesterol)

Sources: Office of Dietary Supplements, National Institutes of Health, "Dietary Supplement Fact Sheets," 2008, http://ods.od.nih.gov/Health_Information/Information_About_Individual_Dietary_Supplements.aspx; National Center for Complementary and Alternative Medicine, "Herbs at a Glance," 2008, http://nccam.nih.gov/health/herbsataglance.htm.

Protecting Consumers and Regulating Claims

Although many CAM procedures and products appear promising, be aware that most are not currently regulated in the United States as strictly as are foods, drugs, and Western medical procedures. Supplement regulation in the United States in particular, is in sharp contrast to nations such as Germany, where the government holds companies to strict standards for ingredients and manufacturing. In the United States, new FDA regulatory controls are just starting to appear. While FDA regulation of supplements are being phased in, and other regulations of CAM are not yet in place, it is important to have as much information as possible to make a smart decision when evaluating CAM options (FIGURE 22.4).

Strategies to Protect Supplement Consumers' Health

The burgeoning popularity of nutraceuticals and functional foods concerns many scientists. Though some alternative therapies, such as acupuncture, have been widely studied, there is little quality research to support the many claims in the area of nutraceuticals and supplements. If you are considering using herbal supplements or functional foods, start your own research at the websites for NCCAM (http://nccam.nih.gov) and the Cochrane Collaboration's review on complementary and alternative medicine (www.cochrane.org).

Herbal supplements and functional foods can currently be sold without FDA approval. This raises issues of consumer safety to new levels. Even when products are dispensed by CAM practitioners, the situation can be risky. Some homeopaths and herbalists who mix their own tonics may not use standardized measures. Lack of standard regulation means that some unskilled and untrained people may be treating patients without fully understanding the potential chemical interactions of their preparations.

> **WHAT DO YOU THINK?** *Why do you think the government has not acted more aggressively to regulate herbal and other dietary supplements?* • *Why are many CAM treatments not covered under typical insurance plans?*

Consumer groups, members of the scientific community, and government officials are calling for action. Pressure has mounted to establish consistent standards for herbal supplements and functional foods similar to those used in Germany and other countries. Many scientists have advocated a more stringent FDA-approval process for virtually all supplements sold in the United States. As a result, the FDA recently passed new regulations to oversee the manufacture of dietary supplements, including herbal supplements. These new regulations require manufacturers to evaluate the identity, purity, strength, and composition of the supplements to ensure they contain what the label claims. However, these regulations are in the process of being phased in over the next 3 years, and many supplements are currently not tested. The official public standards-setting authority for all medicines, supplements, and other health

MORE SAFE

May be safe; efficacy unclear
- **Treatment examples:** Acupuncture for chronic pain; homeopathy for seasonal allergies; low-fat diet for some cancers; massage therapy for low-back pain; mind–body techniques for cancer; self-hypnosis for cancer pain
- **Advice:** Physician monitoring recommended

Likely safe and effective
- **Treatment examples:** Chiropractic care for acute low-back pain; acupuncture for nausea from chemotherapy; acupuncture for dental pain; mind–body techniques for chronic pain and insomnia
- **Advice:** Treatment is reasonable; physician monitoring advisable

LESS EFFECTIVE ←————————————→ **MORE EFFECTIVE**

Dangerous or ineffective
- **Treatment examples:** Injections of unapproved substances; use of toxic herbs; delaying/replacing essential medical treatments; taking herbs that are known to interact dangerously with conventional medications (e.g., St. John's wort and indinavir)
- **Advice:** Avoid treatment

May work, but safety uncertain
- **Treatment examples:** St. John's wort for depression; saw palmetto for an enlarged prostate; chondroitin sulfate for osteoarthritis; ginkgo biloba for improving cognitive function in dementia
- **Advice:** Physician monitoring is important

LESS SAFE

FIGURE 22.4 Assessing the risks and benefits of CAM treatments. Medical experts devised this chart to gauge the potential liability of recommending alternative treatments, but it can also help patients and consumers choose treatments based on safety and effectiveness by determining how the treatment is categorized.
Source: M. H. Cohen and D. M. Eisenberg, "Potential Physician Malpractice Liability Associated with Complementary and Integrative Medical Therapies," *Annals of Internal Medicine* 136, no. 8 (2002): 596–603. Copyright © 2002 American College of Physicians. Used with permission.

SKILLS FOR BEHAVIOR CHANGE

CAM and Self-Care

Today, we are faced with an exciting array of possible health choices. To help you make the best decisions, consider these pointers:

√ Take charge of your health by being an informed consumer. Find out what scientific studies have been done on the safety and effectiveness of the CAM treatment in which you are interested. Consult only reliable sources—texts, journals, periodicals, and government resources. Start with the websites listed at the end of this and every chapter.

√ Remember that decisions about treatment should be made in consultation with your health care provider and based on your own condition and needs. If you use any CAM therapy, inform your primary health care provider. It is particularly important to talk with your provider if you are thinking about replacing your prescribed treatment with one or more supplements, are currently taking a prescription drug, have a chronic medical condition, are planning to have surgery, are pregnant or nursing, or are thinking about giving supplements to children or pets.

√ If you use a CAM therapy such as acupuncture, choose the practitioner with care. Check with your insurer to see if the services will be covered.

√ Remember that natural and safe are not necessarily synonymous. Many people have become seriously ill from seemingly harmless "natural" products. Be cautious about combining herbal medications, just as you should be cautious about combining other drugs. Seek help if you notice any unusual side effects.

√ Realize no one is closely monitoring the purity of herbal supplements and that dosage levels in many herbal products are in the process of getting regulated. Look for the word standardized or the "USP Dietary Supplement Verified" seal on any herbal product you buy, and look for reputable manufacturers. German manufacturers produce identical batches of herbal remedies as required by law.

care products manufactured and sold in the United States is the U.S. Pharmacopeia, which currently tests select products, including herbal supplements, to comply with safety and purity standards. Products that meet these standards display a "USP Dietary Supplement Verified" seal.[42]

Looking to Science for More Answers

Even as CAM treatments gain credibility, this credibility still must be tempered with good science. The NCCAM has established research centers at universities and other institutions throughout the United States, where many clinical trials are being conducted.[43] Numerous other studies into the effectiveness of alternative treatments, such as those using acupuncture, green tea, fish oil, flaxseed, and shark cartilage, among others, are taking place across the United States. One of the most promising aspects of this research is the enthusiastic support of professionals who have the training and laboratory expertise to evaluate the efficacy of market-driven claims.

Healthy Living in the New Millennium

Clearly, CAM appears to serve a very real need for consumers. But while consumers are making the adjustment to CAM in record numbers, members of the health care delivery system seem slow to act. Although progress has been noted, there is still a long way to go before CAM becomes fully accepted in mainstream medical practice.

Enlisting Support from Insurers and Providers

More and more insurers are hiring alternative practitioners as staff or are covering alternative care, at least to some degree. This is especially true as criticisms of managed care increase and government agencies get involved.

Today, nearly all health insurance providers cover at least one form of CAM, with acupuncture and massage therapy being the most common. However, the changing nature of HMOs and health care insurers makes it impossible to determine exactly how many companies cover CAM therapies. Many patients will continue to pay out of pocket for alternative therapies until scientific evidence supporting alternative medical care becomes impossible to ignore. What is known is that the numbers are increasing despite a reimbursement system that is biased in favor of traditional treatments.

Support from professional organizations such as the American Medical Association (AMA) is also increasing, as more physician training programs require or offer electives in alternative treatment modalities. In many cases, medical schools are educating a new generation of medical doctors to be better prepared to advise patients about the pros and cons of alternative treatments and how to follow integrative practices. Although alternative medicine is becoming increasingly integrated into today's health care programs and plans, there is still a long way to go. As we learn more, we will be better able to apply both traditional and alternative care to our efforts toward health and healing. See the Skills for Behavior Change box on page 834 for specific tips on how to ensure you get the best possible care.

Fill out this assessment online at
www.pearsonhighered.com/myhealthlab
or www.pearsonhighered.com/donatelle.

Are You a Savvy CAM Consumer?

If you are like millions of Americans, you've already tried one or more CAM therapies (including the use of supplements) or may be considering one. Take this quiz to assess your knowledge of complementary and alternative medicine. For each statement, indicate whether you believe the following items are true or false.

		True	False
1.	When considering a CAM technique, it is important to do some research and identify scientific findings of the specific CAM therapy.	❏	❏
2.	Researching the credentials of a CAM practitioner is an important step to take before receiving any type of CAM treatment.	❏	❏
3.	CAM therapies can be used with traditional medical treatments.	❏	❏
4.	You should inform new practitioners of all the treatments you are currently receiving, including all CAM and traditional therapies.	❏	❏
5.	If my friend or family member didn't have success with a CAM therapy, then it probably won't work for me either.	❏	❏
6.	I should ask if the CAM therapy is covered by insurance before receiving the treatment.	❏	❏
7.	Learning about CAM therapies can be a proactive way to maintain good health.	❏	❏
8.	Taking supplements is a good idea, because even if a product isn't helpful, it isn't likely to be harmful.	❏	❏
9.	The term *natural* on a supplement package means that the product is healthful and safe.	❏	❏
10.	When buying supplements, I should choose those with the USP (United States Pharmacopeia) seal on their labels.	❏	❏
11.	Any potentially dangerous supplement product is required to have cautionary information on the label.	❏	❏
12.	A recall of a harmful product guarantees that all such harmful products will be immediately and completely removed from the marketplace.	❏	❏
13.	There is no reason for me to consult a physician before taking a supplement.	❏	❏
14.	Fewer than 10 percent of Americans use dietary supplements.	❏	❏

Scoring Key

1. *True.* Finding out scientific evidence on a particular CAM therapy can help to identify its effectiveness.

2. *True.* CAM techniques require rigorous training, and it is important to receive treatment from only those practitioners who have received extensive training and are licensed for their particular CAM technique. Inadequate training can result in injury, transmission of disease, and improper balancing of energy.

3. *True.* CAM techniques can be used with traditional medical treatment and can provide additional benefits for a comprehensive treatment plan.

4. *True.* Any new practitioner, whether CAM or traditional, should be aware of all therapies you are receiving to prevent any complications if a new therapy is introduced and to allow all providers to communicate with one another to provide the best overall care.

5. *False.* Individuals respond differently to CAM therapies. You should consult your physician when considering CAM therapies.

6. *True.* Many CAM therapies are not covered by insurance. If the procedure is covered, you may still have to pay a percentage of the total amount. It is important to find this out before pursuing the treatment.

Are You a Savvy CAM Consumer?—*continued*

7. *True.* A recent study showed that those who inquired about CAM therapies were more health conscious than those who did not.

8. *False.* When consumed in high enough amounts, for a long enough time, or in combination with certain other substances, all chemicals can be toxic, including nutrients, plant components, and other biologically active ingredients.

9. *False.* The term *natural* on labels is not well defined and is sometimes used ambiguously to imply unsubstantiated benefits or safety. For example, many weight-loss products claim to be "natural" or "herbal," but this doesn't necessarily make them safe. Their ingredients may interact with drugs or may be dangerous for people with certain medical conditions.

10. *True.* Since FDA regulations are in the process of being implemented, the USP symbol is currently the best way to tell if the supplement has been tested and dissolves properly in the body.

11. *False.* Dietary supplement manufacturers may not necessarily include warnings about potential adverse effects on their product labels. If consumers want to know about the safety of a specific dietary supplement, they should contact the manufacturer of that brand directly.

12. *False.* A product recall of a dietary supplement is voluntary, and while many manufacturers do their best, a recall does not necessarily remove all harmful products from the marketplace.

13. *False.* Supplements can interact with prescription medications, so telling your doctor what you intend to take can help him or her check for such interactions.

14. *False.* National surveys indicate that about half of all Americans use dietary supplements. Research shows that people who take supplements tend to have better diets and generally healthier habits than those who don't. They also tend to have higher levels of both education and income.

Interpreting Your Score

Add up the number of items you got right. The higher your score, the better your knowledge of the potential risks and benefits of supplements and other CAM techniques. Any incorrect responses may indicate areas you need to learn more about in order to be an informed consumer. Ultimately, you are the one most responsible for your health and safety, so think about ways to increase your awareness and understanding of the CAM methods you consume.

Sources: Adapted from NCCAM, "Are You Considering Using CAM?" 2006 http://nccam.nih.gov/health/decisions; Council of Colleges of Acupuncture and Oriental Medicine, 2008, www.ccaom.org/aom.asp; NCCAM, "Selecting a CAM Practitioner," 2007, http://nccam.nih.gov/health/practitioner/index.htm; NCCAM, "CAM Use in America: Up Close," *CAM at the NIH: Focus on Complementary and Alternative Medicine* 15, no. 1 (2008), http://nccam.nih.gov/news/newsletter/2008_april/usacamuse.htm; D. Sinovic, "Choosing and Using Supplements," Meriter Healthy Living, Created for Wellness Library, 2006, http://meriter.staywellsolutionsonline.com/InteractiveTools/Quizzes/40,SupplementsVitaminsMQuiz; Council for Responsible Nutrition, "The Benefits of Nutritional Supplements Test Your Supplement Savvy," 2007, www.crnusa.org/benpdfs/CRN00benefits_quiz.pdf.

Make it Happen!

The Assess Yourself activity gave you the chance to evaluate your understanding of responsible use of CAM treatments. Depending on the results of the assessment, and your own interest in pursuing CAM therapies, you may consider investigating CAM further.

Today, you can:

- Take a few moments to close your eyes and think of a calm place or activity you enjoy. Perhaps you are lying on a tropical beach or are curled up in front of a fireplace. Clear your mind of everything else, and use relaxation to improve your health.

- Go to a credible website and look up information on a CAM therapy. What are the scientific findings? What are the benefits?

Within the next 2 weeks, you can:

- Check with your insurance provider and see what CAM therapies are covered. Ask what expenses you'll be responsible for, and if you are limited to a certain network of practitioners.

- Check with your college's health clinic and find out what types of alternative therapies it offers.

By the end of the semester, you can:

- Schedule an appointment with your current health care provider to discuss any CAM therapies you are considering.

- Make relaxation and mind–body stress reducing techniques a part of your everyday life. This can simply mean practicing meditation, deep breathing, or even taking long walks in nature. You don't need to visit a CAM practitioner or follow a specific therapeutic practice to benefit from methods of relaxation, meditation, and spiritual awakening.

TAKING CHARGE

CHAPTER SUMMARY

- Throughout the world, people are choosing complementary and alternative medicine options in increasing numbers. Much of the influence of these strategies may be traced to other cultures, particularly those that are part of alternative medical systems such as traditional Chinese medicine or Ayurvedic medicine, which are sources for acupuncture and yoga.

- The National Center for Complementary and Alternative Medicine (NCCAM) groups complementary and alternative medicine (CAM) practices into four major domains: (1) manipulative and body-based methods (manipulation or movement of one or more body parts); (2) energy medicine (use of biofields or energy fields); (3) mind–body medicine (techniques designed to enhance the mind's ability to affect bodily function and symptoms); and (4) biologically based practices (including substances found in nature, such as herbs and vitamin megadoses). Several alternative medical systems cut across all of these domains.

- Herbal remedies include ginkgo biloba, St. John's wort, echinacea, ginseng, and green tea. Special supplements include muscle enhancers, glucosamine, chromium picolinate, SAMe, and antioxidants. A number of functional foods may also serve as healing agents.

- Though many positive effects are associated with CAM, there are also many risks. The drive for profits and the lack of strict government regulation in the United States make the CAM market a free-for-all. As a consumer, you must be aware of the risks and check reputable sources to ensure that you are not being lured by false claims and promises.

- Health in the new millennium provides an interesting assortment of choices for health care consumers. By enlisting the support of health care professionals and health care services and by making informed decisions, you will reap positive rewards in your quest for health enhancement.

REVIEW QUESTIONS

1. Which of the following treatments is based on soft-tissue manipulation by trained therapists for healing purposes?
   a. Acupuncture
   b. Reiki
   c. Psychoneuroimmunology
   d. Massage therapy

2. What type of practitioner makes diagnoses by observation and touch, and assigns patients to one of three body types?
   a. Chiropractic practitioner
   b. Naturopathic practitioner
   c. Ayurvedic practitioner
   d. Homeopathic practitioner

3. The alternative system of medicine based on the principle that "like cures like" is
   a. naturopathic medicine.
   b. homeopathic medicine.
   c. Ayurvedic medicine.
   d. chiropractic medicine.

4. Chiropractic treatment is based on the theory that diseases can be caused by
   a. misalignment of the bones.
   b. poor eating habits.
   c. taking too many drugs.
   d. muscle atrophy.

5. The use of techniques to improve the psychoneuroimmunology of the human body is called
   a. acupressure.
   b. mind–body medicine.
   c. Reiki.
   d. bodywork.

6. What alternative medicine system focuses on restoring the proper flow of *qi* throughout the body?

    a. Ayurvedic medicine

    b. Homeopathic medicine

    c. Naturopathic medicine

    d. Traditional Chinese medicine

7. What is the best-selling herbal remedy in health and natural food stores in the United States?

    a. Green tea

    b. Ginkgo biloba

    c. St. John's wort

    d. Echinacea

8. Plant stanols/sterols, oat fiber, sunflower, and soy protein are examples of

    a. antioxidants.

    b. ergogenic aids.

    c. nutraceuticals.

    d. phytomedicines.

9. The energy therapy derived from the ancient technique of "laying on of hands" is

    a. Reiki.

    b. qigong.

    c. therapeutic touch.

    d. acupressure.

10. The food that may fight motion sickness and stomach pain and upset, and discourages blood clots is

    a. garlic.

    b. ginger.

    c. sunflower.

    d. oat fiber.

QUESTIONS FOR DISCUSSION AND REFLECTION

1. What are some of the potential benefits and risks of CAM? Why do you think these practices and products are becoming so popular?

2. What are some of the major domains of CAM treatments? Have you tried any of them? Would you feel comfortable trying any new ones? Why or why not?

3. What are the major herbal remedies? Special supplements? What are some of the risks and benefits associated with each?

4. What can you do to ensure that you are receiving accurate information regarding CAM treatments or medicines? Which federal agency oversees CAM in the United States?

5. What is being done in the United States to ensure continued growth of CAM?

ACCESSING YOUR HEALTH ON THE INTERNET

The following websites explore further topics and issues related to personal health. You'll also find links to each organization's website on the Companion Website for *Access to Health,* Green Edition, at www.pearsonhighered.com/donatelle.

1. *National Center for Complementary and Alternative Medicine (NCCAM).* A division of the National Institutes of Health dedicated to providing the latest information on complementary and alternative practices, including NCCAM-funded centers of research on alternative medicine. www.nccam.nih.gov

2. *ClinicalTrials.gov.* Includes the latest information on CAM research and clinical trials. Search for results from NCCAM and complementary and alternative medicine. http://clinicaltrials.gov

3. *Acupuncture.com.* Provides resources for consumers regarding traditional Asian therapies; geared toward students and practitioners. www.acupuncture.com

4. *National Institutes of Health, Office of Dietary Supplements.* An excellent resource for information on dietary supplements. Includes access to CARDS (Computer Access to Research on Dietary Supplements), a database of federally funded research projects pertaining to dietary supplements. http://dietary-supplements.info.nih.gov

FURTHER READING

D. Rakel, *Complementary Medicine in Practice* (Sudbury, MA: Jones and Bartlett, 2006).
Evidence-based overview of common CAM therapies, particularly those supported by research and accepted by physicians and consumers.

N. Cuellar, *Conversations in Complementary and Alternative Medicine: Insights and Perspectives from a Leading Practitioner* (Sudbury, MA: Jones and Bartlett, 2006).
Based on interviews with 27 leading experts in CAM, including acupuncturists, chiropractors, massage therapists, and herbalists. Includes questions about practice, education, and research.

REFERENCES

1. National Center for Complementary and Alternative Medicine, "What Is CAM?" NCCAM Publication No. D347, 2007, www.nccam.nih.gov/health/whatiscam.
2. Mayo Clinic Staff, "Complementary and Alternative Medicine: What Is It?" Mayo Clinic, 2007, www.mayoclinic.com/health/alternative-medicine/PN00001.
3. National Center for Complementary and Alternative Medicine, "The Use of Complementary and Alternative Medicine in the United States," NCCAM Publication No. D234, 2007, http://nccam.nih.gov/news/camsurvey_fs1.htm.
4. J. Tsao, "Effectiveness of Massage Therapy for Chronic, Non-malignant Pain: A Review," *Evidence Based Complementary and Alternative Medicine* 4, no. 2 (2007): 165–79; American Medical Student Association, "EDCAM: CAM and Medical Education Report," 2008, www.amsa.org/humed/CAM/mededreport.cfm; National Cancer Institute, "Acupuncture: Human/Clinical Studies," 2008, www.cancer.gov/cancertopics/pdq/cam/acupuncture/HealthProfessional/page6.
5. National Center for Complementary and Alternative Medicine, "The Use of Complementary and Alternative Medicine in the United States," 2007.
6. L. Huang, "Acupuncture and Oriental Medicine Education in the United States," Council of Colleges of Acupuncture and Oriental Medicine, 2008, www.ccaom.org/aom.asp.
7. National Center for Complementary and Alternative Medicine, "Ayurvedic Medicine: An Introduction," NCCAM Publication No. D287, 2008, http://nccam.nih.gov/health/ayurveda.
8. Ibid.
9. American Institute of Homeopathy, "Homeopathy: Efficacy and Evidence Base," 2007, http://homeopathyusa.org/homeopathy-now.html; Health Alternatives Online, "Homeopathy," 2008, www.healthalternativesonline.com/homeopathy.html.
10. National Center for Complimentary and Alternative Medicine, "An Introduction to Chiropractic," NCCAM Publication No. D403, 2007, http://nccam.nih.gov/health/chiropractic.
11. Bureau of Labor Statistics, U.S. Department of Labor, "Chiropractors," *Occupational Outlook Handbook, 2008–09 Edition,* www.bls.gov/oco/ocos071.htm.
12. J. Tsao, "Effectiveness of Massage Therapy for Chronic, Non-malignant Pain: A Review," 2007.
13. National Center for Complimentary and Alternative Medicine, "Massage Therapy as CAM," NCCAM Publication No. D327, 2006, http://nccam.nih.gov/health/massage.
14. Mayo Clinic Staff, "Massage: A Relaxing Method to Relieve Stress and Pain" Mayo Clinic, 2008, www.mayoclinic.com/health/massage/SA00082; National Center for Complimentary and Alternative Medicine, "Massage Therapy as CAM."
15. Ibid.
16. Bureau of Labor Statistics, U.S. Department of Labor, "Massage Therapists," *Occupational Outlook Handbook, 2008–09 Edition,* www.bls.gov/oco/ocos295.htm.
17. National Center for Complimentary and Alternative Medicine, "Manipulative and Body Based Practices: An Overview," NCCAM Publication no. D238, 2007, http://nccam.nih.gov/health/backgrounds/manipulative.htm; United States Trager Association, "The Trager Approach," 2008, www.trager-us.org/the_trager_approach.html.
18. National Center for Complimentary and Alternative Medicine, "Manipulative and Body Based Practices: An Overview."
19. Ibid.
20. American Cancer Society, "Acupuncture," 2007, www.cancer.org/docroot/ETO/content/ETO_5_3X_Acupuncture.asp.
21. National Center for Complementary and Alternative Medicine, "An Introduction to Acupuncture," NCCAM Publication no. D404, 2007, http://nccam.nih.gov/health/acupuncture.
22. B. Seaward, *Managing Stress.* 5th ed. (Sudbury, MA: Jones and Bartlett, 2006); D. Tosevski et al., "Stressful Life Events and Physical Health," *Current Opinions in Psychiatry* 19, no. 2 (2006): 184–89.
23. J. Robins et al., "Research in Psychoneuroimmunology: Tai Chi as a Stress Management Approach for Individuals with HIV Disease," *Applied Nursing Research* 19, no. 1 (2006): 2–9; M. Opp et al., "Sleep and Psychoneuroimmunology," *Neurology Clinician* 24, no. 3 (2006): 493–506; A. Starkweather et al., "Immune Function, Pain, and Psychological Stress in Patients Undergoing Spinal Surgery," *Spine* 31, no. 18 (2006): E641–E647.
24. Office of Dietary Supplements, National Institutes of Health, "Dietary Supplements: Background Information," 2006, http://ods.od.nih.gov/factsheets/dietarysupplements.asp.
25. National Center for Complementary and Alternative Medicine, "Biologically Based Practices: An Overview," NCCAM Publication no. D237, 2007, http://nccam.nih.gov/health/backgrounds/biobasedprac.htm.
26. National Center for Complementary and Alternative Medicine, "Consumer Advisory: Kava Linked to Liver Damage," modified October 2007, http://nccam.nih.gov/health/alerts/kava.
27. Mayo Clinic Staff, "Herbal Supplements: What to Know Before You Buy," 2007, www.mayoclinic.com/health/herbal-supplements/SA00044.
28. University of Maryland Medical Center, "Ginkgo Biloba," 2007, www.umm.edu/altmed/articles/ginkgo-biloba-000247.htm.
29. National Center for Complementary and Alternative Medicine, "Herbs at a Glance: Ginkgo," NCCAM Publication no. D290, 2008, http://nccam.nih.gov/health/ginkgo.
30. National Center for Complementary and Alternative Medicine, "Herbs at a Glance: St. John's Wort," NCCAM Publication no. D269, 2008, http://nccam.nih.gov/health/stjohnswort; National Center for Complementary and Alternative Medicine, "Get the Facts: St. John's Wort and Depression," NCCAM Publication no. D005, 2007, http://nccam.nih.gov/health/stjohnswort/sjwataglance.htm.
31. National Center for Complementary and Alternative Medicine, "St. John's Wort and Depression"; National Center for Complementary and Alternative Medicine, "St. John's Wort"; Mayo Clinic Staff, "St. John's Wort," 2008, www.mayoclinic.com/health/st-johns-wort/NS_patient-stjohnswort.
32. National Center for Complementary and Alternative Medicine, "Herbs at a Glance: Echinacea," NCCAM Publication no. D271, 2008, http://nccam.nih.gov/health/echinacea.
33. Ibid.
34. National Center for Complementary and Alternative Medicine, "Herbs at a Glance: Asian Ginseng," NCCAM Publication no. D284, 2008, http://nccam.nih.gov/health/asianginseng.
35. Ibid.
36. American Cancer Society, "Green Tea," 2007, www.cancer.org/docroot/ETO/content/ETO_5_3x_Green_Tea.asp.
37. Mayo Clinic Staff, "Green Tea," 2008, www.mayoclinic.com/health/green-tea/NS_patient-green_tea.
38. U.S. Food and Drug Administration, "FDA Statement on Tenth Circuit's Ruling to Uphold FDA Decision Banning Dietary Supplements Containing Ephedrine Alkaloids" 2006, www.fda.gov/bbs/topics/NEWS/2006/NEW01434.html.
39. Natural Standard Research Collaboration, "Creatine," Medline Plus, 2008, www.nlm.nih.gov/medlineplus/druginfo/natural/patient-creatine.html.
40. D. Clegg et al., "Glucosamine, Chondroitin Sulfate and the Two in Combination for Painful Knee Osteoarthritis," *New England Journal of Medicine* 354 (2006): 795–808.
41. PDRhealth, "S-Adenosyl-L-Methionine (SAMe)," 2008, www.pdrhealth.com/drugs/altmed/altmed-a-z.aspx.
42. Mayo Clinic Staff, "Herbal Supplements: What to Know Before You Buy," 2007.
43. National Center for Complementary and Alternative Medicine, "What Is CAM?" 2007.

CHAPTER 23

CHAPTER OBJECTIVES

After reading this chapter you will be able to:

1. Explain the nursing process as it relates to nutritional health.

2. Discuss various nursing functions related to nutrition in selected practice settings.

3. Describe the role of the registered dietitian in nutrition care.

4. Explain the components of medical nutrition therapy.

5. Describe under- and overnutrition and the potential effects on nutritional health.

6. Compare and contrast the nutrition screening and nutrition assessment process.

7. Recognize the signs of nutritional risk.

8. List the components of a nutrition assessment and how these are used to formulate a nutrition diagnosis.

TEST YOURSELF TRUE OR FALSE?

1. Nutrition plays a key role in health promotion and disease prevention, but is not usually a part of treatment of disease. T or F

2. Registered dietitians are responsible for integrating nutrition care plans into the larger patient treatment plan. T or F

3. Nutrition screening and assessment are typically performed by the nurse. T or F

4. The purpose of a nutrition assessment is to identify parameters that may indicate nutrition risk. T or F

5. A nutrition history may include a diet recall, food frequency questionnaire, food record, and the focused interview. T or F

Test Yourself answers can be found at the end of the chapter.

Nursing and Nutrition Care

nutrition is a basic human need that remains crucial throughout the lifespan, both during times of health and periods of illness. As providers of holistic care, nurses must have more than a passing understanding of the nutritional needs of both healthy individuals and those with chronic conditions or disease. The nutritional needs of an individual are based on life stage, health-illness considerations, cultural and religious preferences, and genetic influences.

There is increasing awareness among health professionals and the public that nutrition plays a key role in disease prevention and health promotion, and for some conditions, nutrition is also an integral component of disease treatment. Nurses are in a position to help identify nutrition risk factors and reinforce the benefits of a nutritionally sound diet. Working as part of a multidisciplinary health care team, nurses can help advocate for the nutritional needs of patients and clients in both hospital and community settings. In today's health care, there is increasing emphasis on wellness and the nurse must be prepared to participate in initiatives that are focused on prevention and treatment of problems that have a significant nutrition component. This chapter presents the role of nursing as part of the health care team to evaluate and promote nutritional health.

Excerpts taken from: *Nutrition and Diet Therapy for Nurses,* by Sheila Buckley Tucker and Vera Dauffenbach

Nursing Process and Nutritional Health

The nurse has a critical role in assessing and promoting nutritional health, which affects overall health. The nurse works closely with individuals, families, and groups to identify health needs and develops plans for addressing these needs. In doing so, the nurse can evaluate and provide basic nutrition services in various practice settings. See FIGURE 23.1 for examples of how nurses in a variety of settings integrate nutrition knowledge into their practices. Regardless of the practice setting, it is vital that the nurse carefully gathers accurate data about a client's nutritional health to aid in the development of a holistic plan of care for the client.

The **nursing process** is the systematic gathering of subjective and objective data, analyzing data for the purpose of establishing nursing diagnoses, planning realistic goals, implementing activities to achieve the goals, and evaluating goal accomplishment. (Refer to page 872 for a detailed representation of the nursing process). It is important to follow each step of the process to develop an optimum plan of care that is acceptable to the client and meets current standards of nursing practice. Each step of the nursing process as it relates to nutrition assessment is outlined in the following sections. An important component of this assessment is understanding how and when to consult with a registered dietitian (RD). It is paramount that nurses work in collaboration with the RD throughout the nursing process and consult with the RD early in the process for the best client outcomes.

Nursing Process

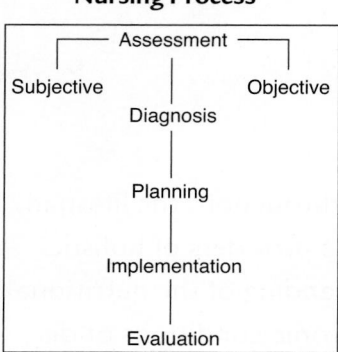

School nurse	• Classroom teaching about healthy eating, all grade levels • Work with teachers of children with food allergies (e.g., peanuts, eggs, wheat) • Review health forms for nutrition-related diagnoses and any treatments that occur during the school day (e.g., diabetes, use of liquid nutrition supplement)
Home health nurse	• Assess changing nutritional status (e.g., unintentional weight loss, change in appetite) • Assess the ability of the client and family to obtain and prepare foods for healthy eating • Make referrals to community resources for nutrition (e.g., Meals on Wheels) • Reinforce nutrition education or therapeutic diet principles prescribed • Collaborate with team members providing care for individuals on home nutrition support
Long-term care nurse	• Assess for changing nutritional status (e.g., weigh residents, check for properly fitting dentures, note appetite changes) • Monitor dietary intake and feeding practices • Provide pleasant environment to allow for a positive dining experience
Postsurgical care nurse	• Check clients for return of gag reflex • Assess for presence of nausea or other side effects • Advance diet as appropriate • Measure and record intake and output • Refer clients at risk for poor nutritional health to registered dietitian for evaluation

FIGURE 23.1 Sample nursing functions related to nutrition in selected practice settings.

RDs complete the following education and training to meet credentialing requirements:

- Complete a minimum of a bachelor's degree at a US regionally accredited university or college and course work approved by the Commission on Accreditation for Dietetics Education (CADE) of the American Dietetic Association.
- Complete a CADE-accredited, supervised practice program at a healthcare facility, community agency, or a foodservice corporation, or combined with undergraduate or graduate studies. Typically, a practice program will run six to twelve months in length.
- Pass a national examination administered by the Commission on Dietetic Registration (CDR).
- Complete continuing professional educational requirements to maintain registration.

Approximately 50% of RDs hold advanced degrees. Some RDs also hold additional certifications in specialized areas of practice, such as pediatric or renal nutrition, nutrition support, and diabetes education. Many states have licensure laws for dietitians. Frequently these state requirements are met through the same education and training required to become an RD.

FIGURE 23.2   Education and professional requirements for registered dietitians.

Role of the Registered Dietitian

RDs are part of the multidisciplinary health care team, responsible for integrating nutrition plans into the larger patient or client treatment plan. RDs provide **medical nutrition therapy** (MNT), which includes nutrition assessment, determining the nutrition diagnosis, determining and implementing a nutrition intervention, and then in subsequent visits monitoring and evaluating the patient's progress. Nutrition education for disease prevention and nutrition counseling for chronic conditions provided over a series of visits are essential components of a comprehensive health care program.

MNT provided by RDs can improve a client's health and well-being, and increase productivity and satisfaction levels through decreased doctor visits, hospitalizations and reduced prescription drug use (ADA, 2010). According to the Institute of Medicine (IOM) "the registered dietitian is currently the single identifiable group of health care professionals with standardized education, clinical training, continuing education, and national credentialing requirements necessary to be directly reimbursed as a provider of nutrition therapy" (IOM, 2000). RDs use MNT as a cost-effective means to achieve significant health benefits by preventing or altering the course of diabetes, obesity, hypertension, disorders of lipid metabolism, heart failure, osteoporosis, celiac disease, and chronic kidney disease, among other diseases (ADA, 2010). Chapter 24 will discuss application of MNT related to diet therapy and the Nutrition Care Process.

See FIGURE 23.2 for information on the education and professional requirements for registered dietitians.

Assessment

Assessment is the first step of the nursing process. This step is lengthy and involves recognition of factors that influence health, including nutrition, activity level, and lifestyle. Typically, assessment data are gathered directly from the client during the history, from measurements of the body called anthropometric data, and from laboratory data. In addition, the client's sociocultural and religious beliefs are important areas to be assessed prior to making a determination of the client's overall and nutritional health status. Occasionally, laboratory data may not be available, but the nurse should determine if they are required to formulate an accurate diagnosis.

Nutritional health is influenced by many factors and may be evident as undernutrition or overnutrition. **Undernutrition**, also called malnutrition, is a term used to describe compromised nutritional status that results from insufficient intake or low body stores of one or more nutrients. Most often, this term is synonymous with protein-calorie malnutrition, which is associated with poor wound healing, loss of muscle mass, functional decline, altered immune status, and in children, growth faltering (Norman, Pichard, Lochs, & Pirlich, 2008). **Overnutrition** is a term used to describe poor nutritional health that results from intake or stores of nutrients that exceed recommended amounts. Obesity, hypercholesterolemia, and toxic levels of stored vitamins from oversupplementation are examples of overnutrition. Both undernutrition and overnutrition are associated with negative health consequences. For example, an individual who abuses alcohol can be deficient in thiamine yet be overweight. An obese child who consumes excess fat but no fruits and vegetables can have both overnutrition and undernutrition. The presence of risk factors for overnutrition or undernutrition should become apparent during the nutrition screening and assessment process. The nurse should be aware of the risk factors for poor nutritional health before beginning the nutrition screening or assessment process. Table 23.1 outlines risk factors for undernutrition and overnutrition.

Nutrition Screening and Assessment

In most health care settings, a registered dietitian is responsible for performing a thorough nutrition assessment. However, the nurse can play an important role in screening for nutritional risk. Factors for nutritional risk vary depending on client

TABLE 23.1   Risk Factors for Poor Nutritional Health

Undernutrition
Medical:
- Chronic disease, acute illness, injury, or wounds
- Disease symptoms, including pain
- Treatment side effects such as nausea, anorexia
- Polypharmacy (multiple medications)
- Drug-nutrient interactions
- Gastrointestinal complaints, malabsorption
- Chewing or swallowing difficulties
- Poor dental health—loose or missing teeth, caries, poorly fitting dentures
- Alcohol and drug abuse
- Depression
- Anorexia/eating disorders

Altered functional status:
- Cognitive changes
- Inability to self-feed
- Visual impairment
- Poor muscle strength
- Diminished ability to perform activities of daily living or instrumental activities of daily living such as shopping and food preparation.

Diet:
- Poor quality intake
- Poor quantity intake—poor appetite, missed meals, restrictive eating (e.g., dieting, faddism, limited intake because of cultural or religious beliefs, disordered eating)

Socioeconomic:
- Food insecurity—limited access to food because of finances or living situation
- Sadness, bereavement, social isolation
- Limited knowledge or skills about food and health

Overnutrition
Excessive intake of one or more nutrients such as calories, saturated fats, vitamins, or minerals
Excessive intake of dietary supplements
Alcohol abuse
Sedentary activity level
Limited knowledge or skills about food and health

age and setting. For adults in acute care settings, screening criteria most often used include history of weight loss, poor intake prior to admission, nutrition support, chewing/swallowing issues, skin breakdown, medical diagnosis, visceral protein status, and specific diet orders (Chima et al., 2008). The nurse should collaborate with the dietitian throughout the nursing care process to provide seamless holistic nutritional care to the individual. In some practice settings, there may not be a registered dietitian on staff, such as in schools or home care settings. The nurse needs to be knowledgeable about the components of a nutrition screening and assessment in such circumstances and possible resources for referrals.

A **nutrition screening** is less comprehensive than an assessment and is done to identify the presence of risk factors for poor nutritional health, whereas assessment is used to determine nutritional status. The abbreviated evaluation process used in screening is not intended to diagnose nutritional problems, but rather serves as a basic initial step toward identifying individuals requiring further nutrition assessment. Generally, a nutrition screening is brief and noninvasive, containing just a few questions or parameters to be checked. Examples include current weight, weight history (i.e., unintentional weight loss), changes in appetite, and ability to take oral nutrition. In all health care settings, a nutrition screening is required within the first 24 hours of a client's admission (Charney, 2008). Most often, the nurse is responsible for this initial screening as part of the nursing assessment (Charney, 2008; Chima, Dietz-Seher, & Kushner-Benson, 2008).

Many screening and assessment tools exist and new tools are constantly being developed. No consensus exists on the most reliable parameters to measure in a nutrition screening or assessment. When choosing to use a screening or assessment tool, the nurse should choose one that is population specific and has research supporting it as both reliable and valid for its intended use. See FIGURE 23.3 for examples of nutrition screening and assessment tools.

A **nutrition assessment** serves as the foundation on which nutritional intervention goals are based. Although a registered dietitian is responsible for a comprehensive nutritional assessment in most health care facilities, the nurse can also complete a basic nutrition assessment and in some settings is the primary clinician gathering and evaluating nutritional data. In either situation, a nurse is ideally situated to help facilitate early nutrition intervention for clients with compromised nutritional health. A complete nutritional assessment is comprised of three major components:

- Nutrition history
- Physical assessment
- Laboratory measurements

No single assessment component or any one parameter provides the necessary scope of information needed for a complete assessment. Findings obtained during the physical assessment or from a single laboratory value are affected by factors other than nutrition, such as disease, the environment or medications. The nurse should gather as much data as possible when conducting a nutrition screening or assessment. Throughout the assessment, the nurse should be aware of cultural considerations. Relying on limited data, or worse, a single parameter, can lead to inaccurate or missed nutritional diagnoses. Poor nutritional health occurs along a continuum. The nurse should always be aware of any alteration in assessment parameters, such as weight changes, even if the findings remain within established normal limits. Sharp clinical judgment is a necessary adjunct to the available data when completing an assessment.

Nutrition History

The nutrition history portion of the nutritional assessment contains one or more components. Each of these components is subjective in nature, relying on self-reporting by the client. When time permits, the nurse should use more than one component to provide an information cross-check.

Malnutrition Universal Screening Tool (MUST)

The Malnutrition Universal Screening Tool (MUST) is a nutrition screening tool for use in adults. This instrument is supported by evidence-based research that validates its use (Anthony, 2008). Only three parameters are part of this quick screen: BMI, weight history, and the effect of disease on ability to take oral nutrition. Clients at risk of malnutrition are either monitored or referred to a dietitian, depending on level of risk. An on-line version of the tool is available that contains instructions and scoring.

MyPyramid

MyPyramid, the food guide pyramid that is based on the *Dietary Guidelines for Americans*, was not developed as a nutritional screening or assessment tool, but it can easily be used to provide a quick assessment of intake using a food record or diet recall. The nurse can compare an individual's intake to the quantity and distribution of food groups recommended within MyPyramid for a general assessment of the reported diet. MyPyramid can be used as a quick point of reference by the nurse conducting an estimate of dietary intake in adults and children.

In health care settings with access to the Internet, an interactive tool utilizing MyPyramid can be used by the nurse and as a teaching tool for the client seeking to improve intake.

Tools for Use in Older Adults

Older adults are at a disproportionate risk of malnutrition compared with other age groups. The aging process and medical conditions and treatments are among the reasons this disparity exists. Screening and assessment tools have been developed in an effort to address the incidence of undernutrition in this population.

Nutrition Screening Initiative

The Nutrition Screening Initiative (NSI) consists of three tools aimed at improving the routine nutrition screening and assessment of older adults in the community (NSI). This broad-based public health strategy was developed by the American Academy of Physicians, the American Dietetic Association, and the National Council on Aging. One of the three tools is a checklist using the mnemonic DETERMINE and is intended for exclusive use as a screening tool. Nine risk factors for undernutrition are surveyed in the checklist: Disease, Eating poorly, Tooth loss/mouth pain, Economic hardship, Reduced social contact, Multiple medications, Involuntary weight loss/gain, Needs assistance with self-care, Elder years above age 80 years. The *Determine Your Nutritional Health Checklist* can be filled out by the older adult or by those interacting with older adults in the community, such as at a congregate meal site. The checklist should not be used in the in-patient setting because it is not validated for that use (Sahyoun, Jacques, Dallal, & Russell, 1997). Individuals with high scores are encouraged to seek nutritional health advice.

Minimum Data Set

The Minimum Data Set (MDS) is used in all Medicare-certified health care institutions as a component of the Resident Assessment Instrument (Centers for Medicare and Medicaid Services [CMS], 2000). Nutritional parameters are included in the MDS and must be assessed on a regular basis as mandated. Additionally, any nutritional status change in a client warrants a full reassessment and response by the health care team (IOM, 2000).

Mini Nutrition Assessment

The Mini Nutrition Assessment (MNA) is an assessment tool validated for use with the older adult (Guigoz, 2006). The nurse working with older adults in a variety of health care and community settings can use the MNA as a routine and quick assessment tool to evaluate nutritional status. Anthropometric measurements and general physical and nutritional assessment questions comprise the tool. A Web-based version of the tool is available in many languages for use in settings with easy Internet access, such as an office, a clinic, or home care.

FIGURE 23.3 Nutrition screening and assessment tools.

Diet Recall

A **diet recall** is also called a 24-hour recall because it involves the client's recollection of everything consumed in a set 24-hour time span. The client should be prompted to recall in sequence all the food, liquids, and dietary supplements consumed at all meals and snacks throughout the day. The nurse should make note of the time and location of intake, portion sizes, food preparation methods, use of fortified versions of foods, and types and doses of dietary supplements. Hot Topic Box: Why Ask about Dietary Supplements? outlines the importance of including information about dietary supplements in an assessment.

Proper estimation of portion sizes is needed to accurately judge intake. Visual portion comparisons help a client estimate intake by providing a point of reference. Photographs and life-size food models can be helpful, especially if age- and culturally appropriate foods are depicted. Large-size portion models are available to represent customarily consumed portions because large portions tend to be underreported (Harnack, Steffen, Arnett, Gao, & Luepker, 2004). Portion analogies to common items like a deck of cards can universally be adapted to the recall process in any setting. Box 23.1 contains portion analogies for use in estimating intake. Clients responding to questions with statements such as "it depends" or "probably" should be asked further questions to clarify answers. Using visuals for portion estimates can be helpful for clarification.

Open-ended, nonjudgmental questions should be used during the interview. Open-ended questions allow the individual to answer with more than a simple *yes* or *no* and provide important details about intake. Nonjudgmental questions are essential to establish rapport with the client and to obtain valid and reliable information. Hinting at a correct answer, such as asking "what did you have for lunch?" when the person may have skipped lunch, or appearing to judge a client can lead to fabricated answers and other misreporting. Table 23.2 illustrates positive and negative examples of questions for a diet recall. The nurse should be aware that body language, word choice, and tone of voice can contribute to the client's responses (Livingstone & Black, 2003). An individual may overreport or underreport intake in order to avoid judgment or to gain approval by the nurse (Kristal, Andrilla, Koepsell, Diehr, & Cheadle 1998). Intake of alcohol tends to be underreported (Nevitt & Lundak, 2005; Walker & Cosden, 2007). Those who are obese or have a low socioeconomic or educational level are more likely to underreport overall intake than others (Scagliusi et al., 2008). Additionally, clients on a therapeutic diet may underreport foods that are restricted by the diet prescription (Foster & Leonard, 2004). Intake of fruits and vegetables tends to be overreported because of perceived social approval with such answers (Miller, Abdel-Maksoud, Crane, Marcus, & Byers, 2008). Conducting the diet recall in a nonjudgmental fashion helps establish an interview climate that fosters full answers by the client.

Because the diet recall provides only a snapshot view of intake, it cannot be exclusively used to generalize usual intake. The nurse can conduct a recall for several sample days to better assess intake. Asking for an example of a work and

hot Topic

Why Ask about Dietary Supplements?

Vitamins, minerals, weight loss and sports nutrition products, herbs, and other plant products are all regulated by the federal government as foods, yet many of these substances act like medications, interfere with medications, or have other health effects. Many consumers assume that dietary supplements have been tested for safety when, in fact, no premarket safety testing is required. Drug-supplement interactions, alterations in platelet activity, and product contamination are among the concerns with dietary supplements.

The use of dietary supplements by people of all ages is on the rise in the United States, while the reporting of this use to health care providers is poor. Estimates range as high as 75% of adults in the United States use dietary supplements at least intermittently when vitamins and minerals are included in the definition. Up to 20% of adults in the United States and Canada reported using nonvitamin/nonmineral types of supplements over a 12-month period (Kelly et al., 2005; Singh & Levine, 2006). Use of nonvitamin/nonmineral supplements by adults over age 65 years doubled between the years 1998 and 2002 (Kelly et al., 2005). Over half of all older adults who take prescription drugs also take at least one dietary supplement (Qato et al., 2008). The nurse should be aware that the prevalence of dietary supplement use is higher among children with a chronic disease or condition compared with healthy peers. Over 60% of chronically ill children use dietary supplements with almost one-third of those using a supplement that was not recommended by a health care provider (Ball, Kertesz, & Moyer-Mileur, 2005). Further, in 80% of the cases of supplement use, no communication occurred with the health care provider about the supplement, a dismal statistic that has been approximated by other studies in children and adults (Ball et al., 2005; Gardiner, Buettner, Davis, Phillips, & Kemper, 2008).

Given the increasing prevalence of dietary supplement use combined with the possibility of drug interactions and health consequences, the nurse should routinely ask clients, parents, or caregivers specifically about supplement use. It is a common practice to encourage new clients to bring all prescribed and over-the-counter medications to a first health care visit; the nurse should also encourage the client to include dietary supplements in that initial assessment.

BOX 23.1   Sample Portion Estimates for Use in a Nutrition History

It is not always practical to have food models or other portion facsimiles available in a health care or community setting. The following verbal analogies can be helpful when estimating intake.
1 cup dry weight (not volume) measure = small, clenched woman's fist
2 tbsp = a single golf ball
4 tbsp = 4 thumb's tips, from knuckle to fingertip
1 oz cubed cheese = small-sized wooden match box or 2 dominoes
3 oz cooked animal protein = deck of cards
Piece of fruit, small potato, or dinner roll = computer mouse
Small pancake, tortilla = compact disc

TABLE 23.2   Sample Diet Recall Questions

Question	Do Ask	Do Not Say
Beginning the recall	"When was the first time you had something to eat or drink (name the day)?"	"What did you have for breakfast?"
Clarifying meal or snack content	The nurse listens as the client lists what was consumed, gently prompting the client to remember by asking "Was there anything else with that?"	"So that was breakfast" when perhaps the client had more to eat at the meal but was slow or forgetful at reporting it.
Sequence of intake	"And then when was the next time you had something to eat or drink?"	"What did you have for lunch?" or "Did you have lunch?"
Food portions	"What portion of ice cream did you have compared to this container?" (Show picture, food model, or use Box 23.1 examples.)	"You said you had a cup of coffee?" The nurse then records the portion as 8 oz without clarifying the portion with the client.
Food preparation methods	"Who prepared the chicken? Can you tell me about how it was prepared?"	"Was that chicken baked or fried?"
Supplement use	"Dietary supplements include vitamins, minerals, herbs, and sports and weight loss products. Have you ever bought or taken any of these? Are you currently taking any dietary supplements? What was your reason for wanting a supplement? For how long have you been taking this? What is the dose? Where did you get the supplement?"	"Do you take any supplements?"

nonwork day would be an example. Food intake and habits can vary in an inconsistent manner that is not apparent in a diet recall. Significant alterations in intake occur occasionally and will be missed by a diet recall. For example, intake of alcohol or dietary supplements may not occur regularly, but each has significant effect on nutritional health. Table 23.3 outlines the strengths and weaknesses of the diet recall and other components of the nutrition history.

Food Frequency Questionnaire

A **food frequency questionnaire** is used to assess usual intake of a variety of foods or food groups over time. Specific foods or general food groups are listed on the questionnaire and frequency of intake by the day, week, month, or longer is recorded by the nurse or the client. Food frequency questionnaires will not provide information regarding the distribution or pattern of intake unless the nurse asks specifically about this intake when administering the tool. Food preparation methods generally

TABLE 23.3   Nutrition History Tools: Strengths and Weaknesses

Component	Strengths	Weaknesses
Diet Recall	Quick and easy	Relies on memory Subject to misreporting and reporting bias Portion size estimates difficult Not representative of overall intake since a snapshot in time
Food Frequency Questionnaire	Short versions are quick and easy Can be used with diet recall to fill information gaps	Relies on memory Needs to be population specific with familiar foods Does not represent eating patterns or food distribution
Food Record	May estimate usual intake over time Does not rely on memory	Cumbersome to maintain May erroneously be filled out retrospectively Subject to misreporting Some clients alter intake because of record Requires writing skills Portions size estimates may be difficult
Focused Interview	In-depth review of intake, habits, and beliefs Allows more time to establish rapport with client	Time consuming Misreporting possible

are not included, making this tool less detailed than the diet recall. Informational gaps from a diet recall can be filled when a food frequency questionnaire is conducted in combination with the recall. For example, an individual may report no dairy intake during a 24-hour recall, but the nurse may learn from the food frequency questionnaire that a gallon of milk is consumed per week. Formal food frequency tools exist that are often derived from epidemiological research. When using an existing formal questionnaire, care should be taken to choose a tool that is population specific. Long questionnaires can be a time burden to the client and the nurse. Brief questionnaires are quicker and can be administered verbally as part of the history. Table 23.4 illustrates a nutrition history form used in the college health setting with a food frequency questionnaire that is administered verbally.

Food Record

A food record is a diary of recorded intake that is filled out by the client in an ongoing fashion. Intake is reported for several days or more to estimate usual intake. Food records run the same risks of misreporting as the diet recall. The nurse should use a food record as an assessment tool in a limited fashion to avoid overburdening the client, which can cause the client to resort to retrospective recording of intake that will affect reliability of the information.

Focused Interview

Combining the diet recall and food frequency questionnaire with a focused interview provides a comprehensive view of intake. The diet recall process serves as the foundation of the interview, providing a base from which to ask further questions than is possible with the recall or questionnaire alone. Interview questions cover both present and past nutritional habits. For example, when assessing an overweight client, the nurse can inquire about weight history, past dieting attempts and successes, supplement use, sources of dieting information, and social support. When assessing a pregnant female, information regarding preconception nutritional health would be important historical data to include. Box 23.2 outlines nutrition history data to gather during the focused interview. Data specific to concerns across the lifespan are included in Lifespan Box: Lifespan Considerations with a Nutrition History.

TABLE 23.4 Sample Nutrition History Form (used in a college setting)

NUTRITION EVALUATION				
NAME: _____		DATE: _____		
SCHOOL ADDRESS/CLASS: _____		PHONE: _____		
		AGE: _____		
HOME ADDRESS: _____		REFERRED BY: _____		
_____		SIGNED CONSENT/DATE: _____		
HEIGHT	WEIGHT	RECENT WT CHANGE	MAX/MIN WEIGHTS	WEIGHT HISTORY
BODY COMPOSITION MEASUREMENTS	BODY FAT %	EXERCISE	EXERCISE FREQ/DURATION	OTHER ACTIVITIES
MEDICAL HISTORY	MEDICATION: RX,OTC	VITAMINS/MINERALS	HERBS	OTHER SUPPLEMENTS
PREVIOUS DIETS	FOOD ALLERGIES/ INTOLERANCES	DORM REFRIG/COOKING LIVING WITH?	RESTRICTIVE? BINGE? PURGE? LAXATIVES? OTHER?	CLIENT'S SELF-REPORTED NUTRITION GOAL
Diet History: M-F			Diet History: Weekends	

Food Frequency (note per week, day, month, or other)

Fruit: fresh other		Dairy:		Fluids: note type, include caffeine, water	
juice		Starches/grains:		Alcohol:	
Vegetables:		note type		Sugar/Sweets:	
green or orange		Animal Protein:		Fats: note type	
other		Plant Protein:		Supplements:	List above

Physical Assessment

The physical assessment component of the nutritional assessment includes both **anthropometric measurements** and a head-to-toe review of systems. Anthropometric measurements are any scientific measurement of the body, such as weight, height, and body fat. The nurse should routinely incorporate the nutritional aspects of a physical assessment into the nursing process. Not all physical assessment parameters can be practically evaluated in all health care situations. Some parameters are only population specific. A complete nutritional assessment should include as many assessment parameters as is feasible because no single physical parameter is specifically predictive of nutrition status.

Anthropometric Measurements

Assessment of body measurements ideally includes both current and historical values. The nurse should measure current weight and height and avoid simply asking the client for these values. The client or caregiver can be asked about weight history, but this information should be corroborated with documentation in medical records

BOX 23.2   Comprehensive Nutrition History Data

Food
- All meals and snacks: frequency, number, missed meals
- All liquids: volume, type including water, alcohol, caffeinated and sugary beverages
- Portion sizes
- Use of fortified foods
- Location of meals and snacks; e.g., restaurant, home, school, vending machine, car
- Food preparation methods
- Grocery habits
- Food allergies and intolerances
- Food idiosyncrasies, foods avoided, or aversions
- Therapeutic diet prescription

Beliefs and Practices
- Cultural and religious influences on diet
- Faddism—trendy beliefs and practices
- Lifestyle food choices; e.g., vegetarianism, organic, extremely low fat
- Pica—eating of nonfood substances like clay, ice, laundry starch
- Knowledge, skills relative to food and health
- Source of food and health knowledge

Medical/Physical
- Medical history, including symptoms, treatment
- Gastrointestinal complaints and remedies
- Substance abuse
- Appetite
- Chewing and swallowing ability
- Functional capacity, including strength, sensory evaluation, and activities of daily living
- Physical activity level including type, frequency, and duration of activity

Supplement and Medication Use
- Vitamin and mineral use, including dose
- Use of herbal products, including dose and source
- Use of other dietary supplements such as weight loss or sports nutrition products
- Over-the-counter medications
- Prescribed medications
- Folk or home remedies; e.g., baking soda as an antacid, cider vinegar for general health

Socioeconomic Factors
- Education and literacy level
- Social environment and support; e.g., isolated, preparing food for others or only self
- Food security—access to food and sufficient funds for food

Lifespan

Lifespan Considerations with a Nutrition History
In addition to the standard data included in a nutrition history in Box 23.2, the nurse should consider the following when assessing specific populations:

Infants
- Breastfed vs. bottle fed

Breastfed infant:
Number and lengths of feedings
Number of wet diapers
If mother is vegan, assess mother for synthetic source of vitamin B$_{12}$ intake

Bottle-fed infant:
Type and volume of feeding
- Iron source by age 4–6 months with concomitant vitamin C source to improve absorption
- Intake of solids: note age at introduction, appropriateness to developmental stage, types and amount, intolerances, food allergies
- Medical conditions that affect diet: therapeutic diet, medication side effects, feeding difficulties, nutrient–drug interactions

- Food beliefs and practices of caregiver
- Inappropriate food practices: early introduction of solids, cereal added to bottle, putting to bed with bottle, nonprescribed dietary supplements, cow's milk before age 1 year

Children and Adolescents
- Meal and snack pattern, including number and frequency of meals, missed meals or meals on the run
- Self-prescribed restrictive food habits or diets
- Body satisfaction in older children and adolescents
- Activity level

Adults
- Meal and snack pattern, including number and frequency of meals, missed meals, or meals on the run
- Self-prescribed restrictive food habits or diets
- Adequacy of calcium, iron, and folic acid intake in females of childbearing age
- Nutrition health promotion beliefs and practices
- Activity level

Pregnant/Lactating Female
- Folic acid, calcium, vitamin D, and iron intake
- Caffeine and alcohol intake
- Fluid intake

(continued)

Lifespan *(continued)*

- Mercury exposure from consuming fish
- Food aversions or cravings
- Cultural beliefs related to food during pregnancy and lactation
- Prescribed and self-prescribed dietary supplement use
- Dietary treatments of pregnancy-associated symptoms (e.g., heartburn, constipation, nausea)

Older Adults

- Therapeutic diet use
- Food intolerances
- Alcohol intake
- Meal pattern and setting (assess for dining alone or missed meals)
- Alterations in sense of taste, smell, vision, or hearing that affect intake
- Functional capacity to prepare and eat food, self-feed
- Food insecurity
- Drug-nutrient interactions

Each lifespan chapter in this text provides further detail on assessing the nutritional health of individuals across each stage of the lifespan.

where available. Omitting this portion of the assessment or simply relying on client-supplied values can lead to overlooked nutrition risk or poor reference values if nutrition health declines and historical comparison is needed.

Height

Accurate measurement of height is essential in both children and adults. In adults, accurate height is needed to properly assess weight status. Inaccurate height can lead to mistaken conclusions about overweight, underweight, or normal weight status. Height is monitored over time in children to assess growth. The nurse should compare the child's measured height to standard references. These references are classified by population percentiles, allowing the nurse to estimate how the child's anthropometric measurements compare to a large population of age and gender-matched peers. The best use of percentile classifications is in the monitoring of a child over time, being alert to any changes in the child's percentile channel. On-line training tools for using growth charts are available from the CDC.

Height is ideally measured in children and adults using a standing measure. Alternative measurements are indicated when the individual cannot stand freely without assistance or has altered posture because of kyphosis from osteoporosis or other conditions. Proper technique for obtaining a standing height is contained in FIGURE 23.4. Reliance on self-reported heights can overestimate true height as discussed in the Evidence-Based Practice Box: Are self-reported height and weight accurate enough for screening purposes with over-

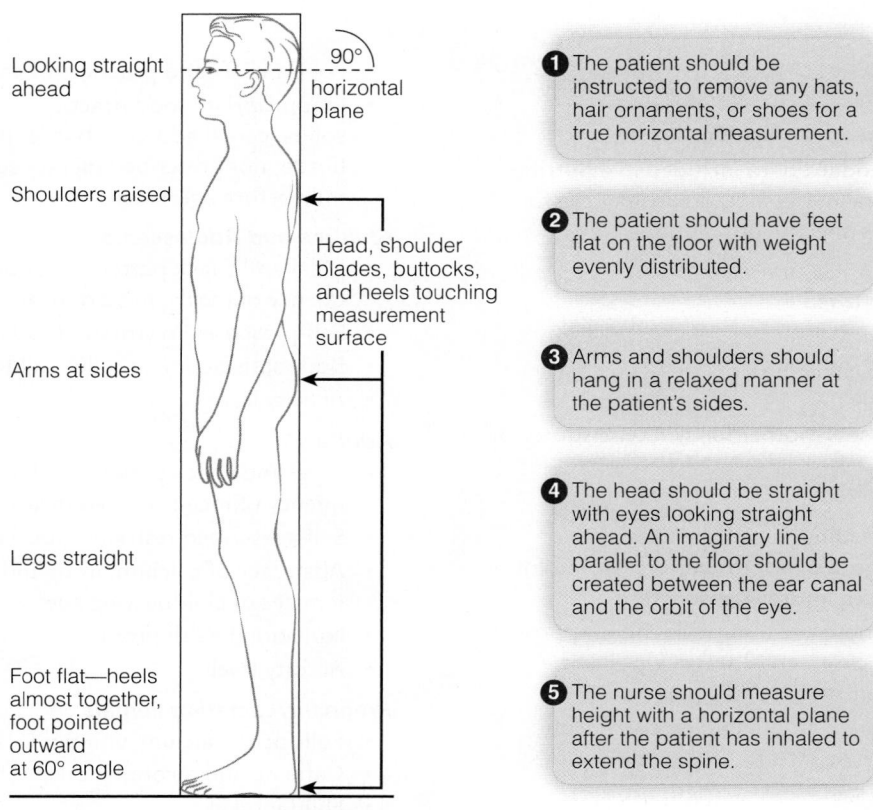

FIGURE 23.4 Measurement of standing height.

weight individuals? If self-reported height must be used, the nurse should document its use in the medical record.

Recumbent length is an alternative to standing height and is used in the measurement of young children or individuals who cannot stand freely, such as frail older adults or individuals who must stay in bed. The client must be able to lie flat for an accurate measurement. An **infantometer** is a formal tabletop device developed for recumbent length measurements in infants and young children. The child is placed

EVIDENCE-BASED PRACTICE RESEARCH BOX

Are self-reported height and weight accurate enough for screening purposes with overweight individuals?

Clinical Problem: Many people prefer not to get weighed when visiting a health care provider. This preference is particularly true for overweight and obese individuals. If an accurate body mass index (BMI) could be calculated from self-reported height and weight, the usefulness of screening programs could be increased.

Research Findings: Numerous studies have been conducted using children, adolescents, and adults to determine the accuracy of self-reported height and weight and, therefore, the accuracy of BMI. Because BMI is useful in classifying individuals as underweight, normal, overweight, or obese, knowledge of BMI can be used for determining individuals at risk for disease.

Studies of older schoolchildren and adolescents in several countries have shown that males and females are usually inaccurate in self-reporting height and weight. Most often, weight was underreported by both boys and girls and height was overreported. Girls underreported weight to a greater degree than boys, and boys overreported height to a greater degree than girls. Youth who were overweight consistently underreported weight to a greater extent than those who had normal weight. Interestingly, those who were underweight tended to overreport weight (Brener, McManus, Galuska, Lowry, & Wechsler, 2003; Goodman, Hinden, & Khandelwal, 2000; Hauck, White, Cao, Woolf, & Strauss, 1995; Jacobson & DeBock, 2001; Jansen, van de Looij-Jansen, Ferreira, de Wilde, & Brug, 2006; Morrissey, Whetstone, Cummings, & Owen, 2006; Tokmakidis, Christodoulos, & Mantzouranis, 2007; Tsigilis, 2006; Wang, Patterson, & Hills, 2002). When the BMI was calculated using self-report data and compared with measured height and weight, the data were less clear. The bias of self-report resulted in BMI values that ranged from 0.5 to 2.6 units higher in measured versus self-report data (Brener et al., 2003; Morrissey et al., 2006). The percentage of misclassification of overweight (BMI greater than 25) or obesity (BMI greater than 30) by self-report ranged from 4% to 31% (Goodman et al., 2001; Hauck et al., 1995; Morrissey et al., 2006; Tokmakidis et al., 2007; Wang et al., 2002).

One study of adolescents added an additional variable, body weight perception, in which students were asked if they perceived themselves as underweight, normal weight, or overweight. In the sample of 2,032 youth, 34.8% perceived themselves as underweight, 42.9% saw themselves as about right, and 22.3% perceived themselves as overweight. On the basis of BMI calculated from measured height and weight, only 1.5% of students were classified as underweight, whereas 51.2% were normal weight and 47.4% were overweight (Brener, Eaton, Lowry, & McManus, 2004).

Similar data exist for adults; women tend to understate weight and men tend to overstate height. Self-reported data also led to misclassification of BMI, especially in those who were already overweight or obese (Brunner-Huber, 2007; Engstrom, Paterson, Doherty, Trabulsi, & Speer, 2003; Kuczmarski, Kuczmarski, & Najjar, 2001; Nawaz, Chan, Abdulrahmann, Larson, & Katz, 2001; Nyholm et al., 2007; Rossouw, Senekal, & Stander, 2001; Spencer, Appleby, Davey, & Key, 2002; Taylor et al., 2006). There were no significant differences for African Americans or Hispanics compared to individuals of European descent (Avila-Funes, Gutierrez-Robledo, & Ponce De Leon Rosales, 2004; Brunner-Huber, 2007; Gillum & Sempos, 2005).

Nursing Implications: The current evidence is clear that individuals across the lifespan do not accurately report height and weight. Although the reasons for self-report inaccuracies were not explored, it is clear that discrepancies exist. Because the BMI is calculated to identify individuals at risk for disease and self-reported height and weight lead to inaccurate calculation of BMI, actual measurement should be performed by nurses to gather clinically accurate data.

CRITICAL THINKING QUESTIONS:

1. When a client who is on a weight reduction program asks why it is necessary to come to the clinic for a weight check, how should the nurse respond?

2. A community organization is planning to use a telephone survey to determine the prevalence of overweight and obesity in an area. How might the nurse respond when asked to volunteer time for such an effort?

on the table in a supine position with head and feet flat against the fixed headboard and sliding footboard. The child's arms should be at the side, eyes looking straight ahead, and knees straightened. The nurse may find it easier to perform an accurate measurement on a frightened child when a parent or caregiver assists by soothing the child and gently holding the head in position. FIGURE 23.5 shows an example of an infantometer.

Recumbent length measurement of older individuals is done at the bedside. The individual must lie flat in the same supine position as is used with the infantometer, with soles of the feet perpendicular to the bed. Any straightedge object, such as a book, is placed flat against the feet and then head to mark those positions lightly with a pencil on the bed linens. The client should not move until both positions are marked. A measuring tape is used to measure the distance between the marks. Recumbent length overestimates height by up to 2% because of spinal compression that occurs with standing (American Medical Directors Association, 2001). The use of a recumbent rather than standing measurement should be documented when recording height.

Individuals who cannot stand freely nor lie flat for recumbent measurements require indirect measurements of height. Direct measurements are preferred because indirect measurements are less accurate (Luft, Beghetto, Castro, & deMello, 2008).The nurse should choose the best indirect measurement suitable to a client's situation.

- *Knee height* measurements are used with clients who have the flexibility to keep one foot bent at a 90-degree angle to the leg but who cannot stand freely. A sliding knee-height caliper is used to measure the distance between the bottom of the foot and the knee. Using the measurements, age and gender-specific predictive equation estimates height.

- *Armspan* and *demi-armspan* indirectly measure height in individuals who can fully and comfortably extend one or both arms in a straight line out to the side at shoulder level. The armspan measurement is made from right-hand fingertips to left-hand fingertips using a flexible tape. Demi-armspan is calculated by doubling the distance from either hand fingertips to the sternal notch. Predictive equations for demi-armspan are also used, including the following equation recommended by the World Health Organization (WHO 1999, chap. 9, p. 37):

$$\text{Height (m)} = [0.73 \times < 2 \times \text{demi-armspan (m)}>] + 0.43$$

FIGURE 23.5   Infantometer.

Weight and Weight History

Obtaining and documenting the client's current weight is a vital component of a nutritional assessment and should be standard practice. Additionally, the use of body weight to determine medication and anesthesia dosing underscores the need for accurate measurement (Jensen et al., 2003). The client should be weighed with a minimum of clothing, no shoes, and after voiding. Any deviation from this standard, such as the presence of a leg brace or heavier clothing, should be noted when the weight is recorded. The nurse should also note and quantify the presence of any edema when recording body weight. Assessment of clients with renal failure and receiving dialysis treatment should be done using a dry weight that is obtained following a dialysis session. Clients with an eating disorder should be assessed for any hidden objects intended to weight the scale. Pockets and underwear can be used to conceal heavy items.

A variety of scales exist for measuring weight. Standing beam scales are used for individuals who can stand freely without grasping the scale, wall, cane, or other object to maintain balance. These types of scale have the advantage of movable weights and a balance to maintain accuracy with regular calibration. It is advisable to balance, or zero, the scale at the start of each clinical day (United States Department of Health and Human Services [USDHHS], n.d.). Other types of scales without balances, such as those intended for minimal home use, should be regularly cross-checked with a balanced scale if used in a clinical setting. Clients who cannot stand without assistance should be weighed in a chair scale. Bed scales are used to weigh the client who must remain in bed. FIGURE 23.6 depicts use of a bed scale. Some hospital beds include an integrated scale.

The nurse should obtain a weight history during the nutritional assessment. This information can be gathered during the focused interview and corroborated with any documentation in the medical record. Weight history is important in the assessment of children and the pregnant female especially but is also needed to assess for unplanned weight loss or weight gain patterns in adults and older adults. An unplanned weight loss of 5% of body weight or more in 1 month or 10% or more in 6 months is considered significant. Box 23.3 outlines a calculation of weight change.

FIGURE 23.6   Using a bed scale to obtain weight.

Body Mass Index

Body mass index (BMI) is used to assess weight status in both children and adults. Accurate height and weight are required for calculation of BMI using the following formula: BMI = weight (kg)/height^2 (m). The National Heart, Lung and Blood Institute (NHLBI) and the WHO have established parameters to categorize normal weight, overweight, obesity, and underweight in adults based on BMI. These classifications are illustrated in Table 23.5. Quick reference tables and nomograms are available to make the BMI calculations easier. If self-reported height or weight is used, BMI could be miscalculated because of underreporting of weight and overreporting of height.

The CDC has growth charts for children 2 to 20 years of age that outline BMI by percentile, and these are contained in Appendix E. In children over age 2 years, risk of overweight and overweight are defined as BMI-for-age of greater than the 85th percentile and 95th percentile, respectively (CDC, 2009). Underweight is defined as less than the 5th percentile. These parameters should be used as screening criteria for assessing weight status, but not as a diagnostic criterion (Cunningham, 2004). A child should be monitored for any change in percentile channel compared with prior measurements.

Use of BMI exclusively to determine weight status has limitations. Because the BMI equation factors in only height and weight, its use assumes that all persons of any given weight also have identical body composition. This assumption is false and

BOX 23.3 Weight Change Calculations

Weight change calculations are done by using present weight, prior weight, and weight loss amount. Unplanned weight loss of greater than 5% in 1 month or greater than 10% in 6 months is considered significant.

1. Subtract current weight from prior weight to calculate weight loss.
2. Divide weight loss amount by prior weight to calculate weight loss percentage.

Example A client seen in home care weighs 130 lb and the medical record reports a weight of 145 lb on admission to the hospital 2 months ago.

1. 145 lb prior weight − 130 lb current weight = 15 lb weight loss
2. 15 lb weight loss ÷ 145 lb prior weight = 0.10 or 10% weight loss

TABLE 23.5 Body Mass Index (BMI) Classifications for Adults

BMI	Classification
Less than 16	Severe malnutrition
16–16.99	Moderate malnutrition
17–18.49	Mild malnutrition
18.5–24.9	Normal
25–29.9	Overweight
30–34.9	Obese class 1
35–39.9	Obese class 2
Greater than or equal to 40	Obese class 3

Sources: Adapted from NHLBI Obesity Education Initiative Expert Panel, 1998; Willett, Dietz, & Colditz, 1999; World Health Organization (WHO), 1999 (Table 13, p. 38).

Measuring Waist Circumference

Place the client in front of a mirror when measuring waist circumference. Stand behind the client to locate the lateral border of the ileum by palpating the right hip. Place a mark at that location. Use the mirror to make sure that the measurement tape is kept horizontal to the floor. Hold the measuring tape taut but not tight (CDC, 2000).

limits use of BMI as a physical assessment parameter. Physically fit individuals with little body fat can be misclassified as overweight because of the contribution of ample muscle. Other individuals can have a normal weight status using BMI but have excess body fat and little muscle mass. Older adults typically lose muscle with age but can also gain fat, maintaining a steady weight; BMI masks this change in body composition. Racial and ethnic differences in body composition exist, but no population-specific BMI classifications are yet in existence (Lear, Humphries, Kohli, & Birmingham, 2007; Wen et al., 2009).

Waist Circumference

Excess adipose specifically situated along the waistline is considered an independent risk factor for type 2 diabetes, elevated blood lipids, hypertension, and cardiovascular disease in adults (NHLBI, n.d.; Zhang, Rexrode, van Dam, Li, & Hu, 2008). Inclusion of a waist circumference measurement in a nutritional assessment is recommended in the adult, especially when cardiovascular risk factors are present. The NHLBI advises that a waist circumference greater than 102 cm (40 in) in adult males and greater than 88 cm (35 in) in adult females is an indicator of cardiovascular risk (NHLBI, 1998). These cut points are for BMIs within the range of 25 to 34.9 only. Waist circumference in individuals with a BMI *greater than* 35 loses its predictive power of estimating health risk (NHLBI, n.d.).

The nurse should measure the waist circumference using a spring-loaded measuring tape to ensure even tension with each measurement. Establishment of a bony landmark to guide the measurement is best, though there is some disagreement as to the best landmark to use (CDC, 2000). The CDC recommends use of the lateral border of the ileum (CDC, 2000). Measurement should be done directly over the skin and not over clothing. Avoid measuring waist circumference using the umbilicus as a reference point because its position can be altered with obesity. Practice Pearl: Measuring Weight Circumference is used to perform a reliable waist circumference.

Waist circumference measurements are not a valid nutrition assessment tool for all adults. Pregnant females and clients with increased abdominal girth from medical conditions, such as ascites, edema, or an abdominal mass should not have waist circumference measured as part of a nutrition assessment. Additionally, not all increases in body fat are reflected by changes in waist circumference, limiting its use (Lean & Han, 2002). Waist circumference will not give an accurate assessment of abdominal adiposity in clients with pendulous abdominal fat when gravity causes the excess fat to no longer remain along the waistline.

Body Composition

Measurement of weight, waist circumference, or BMI does not give the nurse specific information about body composition. Muscle mass, also called skeletal protein, **somatic protein**, or lean body mass, cannot directly be determined by these simple measurements. Body fat, bone mass, total body water, and other components of body composition are not determined easily, yet are important. Measurement of body composition is done indirectly using varying techniques with different levels of reliability and sophistication. Simple analysis techniques, like skinfold measures, assess only lean body mass and body fat, whereas more sophisticated technology can differentiate among the lean components to calculate protein, bone mass, and water. Because of variability in accuracy between different methods, it is recommended that serial monitoring of body composition be assessed using the same method each time (Hetzler, Kimura, Haines, Labotz, & Smith, 2006).

Skinfold Measurements   Skinfold measurements are performed using a caliper on up to eight sites on the body. Measurements are then used to estimate subcutaneous body fat. The most common site for skinfold measurement is the tricep skinfold. Other sites include specific points on the chest, abdomen, medial calf, upper thigh, and subscapular, suprailiac, and midaxillary sites. Professional grade calipers should be used. Plastic calipers are available but quickly become unreliable with use. The nurse should become practiced at doing skinfold measurements before reliably performing them on clients because specific technique is essential. Subsequent skinfold measurements on an individual should be repeated by the same clinician. When different clinicians perform an assessment on the same client, there is individual variability in measurements that will affect reliability and the ability to detect changes (Woodrow, 2009). On-line tutorials exist that demonstrate skinfold and other anthropometric measurements. Box 23.4 and FIGURE 23.7 illustrate the tricep skinfold technique.

The best use of skinfold measurement results is in the monitoring of a client over time. Prior measurements serve as a self-reference against which client progress can be compared. The nurse should keep in mind that small and short-term changes are difficult to detect using skinfold measurements.

In addition to using serial skinfold measurements as a self-reference, measurements can be compared against reference values. Reference values exist for specific population groups and are age and gender specific. The nurse can compare the client's skinfold measurements with the reference value for the same measurement in a similar gender and age population group. These references are generally presented as percentiles. Age, fitness level, race, and gender each affect body composition and require specific reference values. Specific references for all groups do not exist, limiting the use of existing references. Older adults have loss of skin elasticity and changes in total body water, muscle mass, and fat distribution because of age; this change requires skinfold reference values that are unique to this population (Institute of Medicine [IOM], 2000; Kuczmarski, Kuczmarski, & Najjar, 2000; Woodrow, 2009). Lean muscle mass, fat distribution, and total body water are affected by disease states, such as renal failure or human immunodeficiency virus (HIV) infection (Aghdassi, Arendt, Salit, & Allard, 2007; DeLegge & Drake, 2007). Specific reference values should be used for these populations as well. More research is needed to develop additional reference values to represent the existing diverse population.

Circumference Measurements   Calf and midarm circumferences can be included in a body composition analysis. Measurements are done at the site of maximum calf width and the midpoint between the olecranon process and the acromium process, respectively. A spring-loaded measuring tape is used. Measurement values are felt to

BOX 23.4   Tricep Skinfold Technique

1. Instruct the individual to flex the right arm at a 90-degree angle for ease in finding the bony landmarks.
2. Measure length of the arm from the posterior edge of the acromium process to the olecranon process.
3. Establish and mark on the back of the arm the midpoint of that distance.
4. Instruct the individual to allow the arm to hang freely once marked.
5. Just above the marked site, grasp both the subcutaneous fat and skinfold layer between the thumb and forefinger, creating a fold parallel to the arm. Avoid grasping the underlying muscle by carefully pulling skinfold away from body.
6. Place the skinfold caliper perpendicular to the skinfold.
7. Grasp the skinfold with the caliper jaws while maintaining skinfold grasp with the other hand. Let go of the caliper's lever and read the measurement to the nearest 0.1 mm within few seconds.
8. Repeat the measurement at least once and average the results.

Source: Adapted from CDC, 2000 (Section 3.3.1.9 Skinfolds, pp. 3–34).

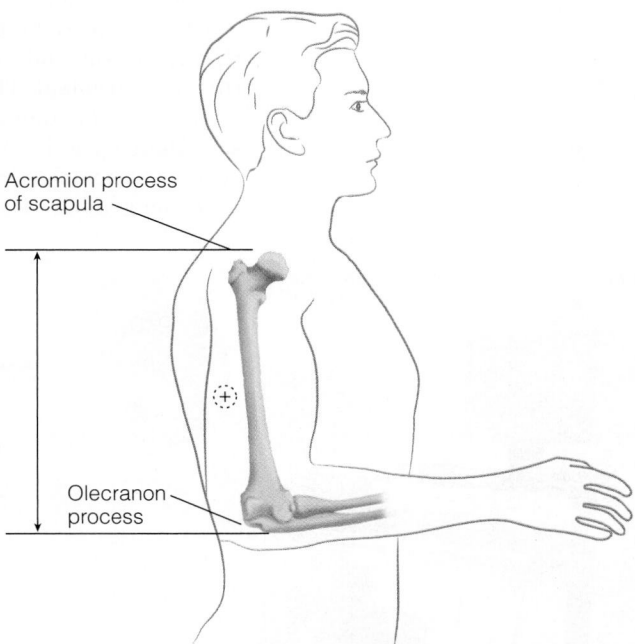

Acromion process of scapula

Olecranon process

FIGURE 23.7   Site of tricep skinfold measurement.

Lifespan

Anthropometric Measurements across the Lifespan

Anthropometric measurements are an important part of a nutritional assessment, but lose their reliability when used incorrectly. Measurements intended for use in the adult, such as waist circumference, have no merit when used to assess nutritional health in a child. Likewise, head circumference should be used only up to age 3 years. Age and gender-specific body composition references are needed when using skinfold calipers or more advanced technology such as bioelectrical impedance analysis (BIA). Body composition changes across the lifespan; using references that are intended for a young adult to instead assess an older adult who has altered skin elasticity and loss of muscle will yield incorrect results.

reflect the relationship between body volume and body mass (Wagner & Heyward, 1999). Predictive equations based on the midarm circumference and tricep skinfold are used to estimate body fat and fat-free mass while correcting for the underlying bone.

Head circumference is measured in children up to age 3 years. This measurement is not part of an assessment of body composition, but rather an indirect measurement of nutritional health, growth, and development. Lifespan Box: Anthropometric Measurement across the Lifespan discusses the topic of anthropometric measurements and age.

Technology and Body Composition Several noninvasive tools exist that measure body composition. Some require a laboratory setting and expensive equipment, whereas others are portable. Bioelectrical impedance analysis (BIA) is based on the principles of electroconduction. Electricity is conducted more easily through tissues with a high water and electrolyte content, such as muscle and body fluids, than through fat tissue. The original version of a BIA device used electrodes and a nonconductive table surface to measure conduction from foot to hand. There is less error associated with BIA than with skinfold measurements (Aghdassi et al., 2007). Newer handheld and standing versions are available that only measure conduction through the arm or leg segments. Hand-to-hand and leg-to-leg devices are not as accurate as traditional devices (Buchholz, Bartok, & Schoeller, 2004). The nurse working in sports medicine or wellness is likely to encounter these devices. Bathroom scales that measure body fat use this technology. Overhydration, including edema; dehydration; or altered skin temperature can cause measurement errors with BIA (DeLegge & Drake, 2007). The use of BIA is not recommended in individuals with a pacemaker because of the associated small electrical current (Lee & Gallagher, 2008).

Near-infrared interactance devices predict body fat by passing infrared light through tissue and measuring light reflection. The bicep is a common site used in this measurement. These devices are convenient handheld tools but have a greater standard error than BIA or skinfold measurements, especially in the overweight person (DeLegge & Drake, 2007). These devices are often used in the wellness setting, such as at health fairs. The nurse should use population-specific predictive equations based on gender, fitness level, height, and weight.

Other methods for measuring body composition include underwater weighing, dual x-ray absorptiometry (DEXA), and plethysmography. These methods are more commonly utilized in the research rather than clinical setting because of high cost. Underwater weighing measures water displacement when the individual is completely submerged beneath the water. Predictive equations calculate body composition based on known densities of fat and fat-free tissue. DEXA is capable of measuring all components of body composition, including bone and total body water, unlike most other methods and uses x-ray technology. Plethysmography measures the body's composition via air displacement in a chamber called a BOD POD. FIGURE 23.8 illustrates plethysmography being used on a client.

Body Fat Standards Reference values for body composition are used to compare an individual to existing data gathered for a similar specific population. For example, reference values for body fat exist for various types of athletes. Standards differ from references and should not be confused. A standard is a value that is believed to be a

FIGURE 23.8 Air plethysmography.

health target and is not the same as a population norm or reference value. Reference values for weight using BMI would reflect the distribution or underweight, normal weight, and overweight individuals in a population; this distribution differs from the recommended standard of "healthy" BMI of 20 to 24.9. Standards for total body fat specifically do not currently exist, but rather a range is recommended. The nurse should be careful not to recommend a specific body fat target to an individual. Individual differences in essential fat and the known measurement error associated with predicting body composition make too specific a recommendation unreliable. In adults, a total body fat of 12% to 20% in males and 20% to 30% in females is recommended, but more population-specific research is yet to be published (Gallagher et al., 2000).

Physical Findings

When conducting the physical assessment of any individual, the nurse should be aware of any physical findings that impact nutritional status or indicate altered nutritional health. A head-to-toe assessment and review of systems yields important information. Findings such as poor dental health, swallowing difficulties, gastrointestinal complaints, limited strength, and alterations in cognition or vision problems negatively affect intake. Medical conditions and treatment can lead to nutritional challenges. Any functional or physical findings that impact nutrition status or are suggestive of an existing nutrition problem should be documented.

Physical changes related to altered nutritional health do not occur acutely. Any physical findings that are present indicate a nutritional issue that has been occurring for weeks, months, or longer. Deficiency of a fat-soluble vitamin is slow to manifest itself physically because of the storage of these vitamins in adipose tissue and the liver. Deficiency of water-soluble nutrients is more likely to occur sooner than fat-soluble nutrients because of limited body pools of these nutrients. Initially, deficiencies occur subclinically and are difficult to detect upon physical examination. Many of the physical findings that occur with poor nutritional health can also occur because of medical conditions or environmental effects. For example, hair texture and amount is affected with protein-calorie malnutrition, medications, and harsh hair treatments. Therefore, the nurse should combine the physical assessment with other nutritional parameters for a broader assessment. Use of the examination alone will not provide complete data for an accurate assessment. Table 23.6 outlines a review of physical findings and the possible nutritional implications.

Laboratory Assessment

No one laboratory measurement can uniquely assess nutritional status. The nurse should consider confounding medical conditions and laboratory value limitations when completing this portion of the nutritional assessment.

Plasma Proteins

Plasma proteins are synthesized in the liver and are often called **visceral proteins** along with the proteins found in organs. Albumin, prealbumin, and transferrin are plasma proteins that are commonly used as part of a nutritional assessment. Each of these proteins has a different half-life, or time span over which half the body pool breaks down. The nurse should recall that the shorter the half-life of the protein, the more current the reflection of visceral protein status. Additionally, these proteins are acute-phase reactant proteins that provide substrate to the body for reacting to the physiological stresses of infection or inflammation, such as with trauma, burns, or sepsis. As a result, during infection or inflammatory responses, these plasma proteins decrease unrelated to nutritional status.

Albumin is a routine laboratory value commonly used in a nutritional assessment. Normal plasma albumin is 3.5 gm/L to 5 gm/L. It has a long half-life (14 days to 21 days) and a large body pool, which detracts from its sensitivity as a marker of current nutritional status despite its wide use. Decreased plasma levels can be indicative of altered nutrition status as outlined in Table 23.7. It has been suggested that a slightly higher threshold of 3.8 gm/L be used to mark low normal

TABLE 23.6   Overview of Nutritional Findings during Physical Assessment

System or Body Part	Clinical Finding	Examples	Potential Nutrient Deficiency
Hair	Dull, sparse, easily pluckable, brittle, **flag sign** (band of hair without pigment)	*Source:* Centers for Disease Control and Prevention (CDC)	Protein
	Alopecia		Protein, biotin, zinc
Eyes	Night blindness, blindness, foamy spots (**Bitot's spots**), dry and hard mucosa (**xerophthalmia**)	*Source:* Centers for Disease Control and Prevention (CDC)	Vitamin A
	Pale conjunctiva		Iron
Mouth	Cracks at corners of lips (angular stomatitis), inflamed lips (cheilosis)	*Source:* Centers for Disease Control and Prevention (CDC)	Riboflavin, niacin, pyridoxine
	Smooth, magenta or beefy red tongue (glossitis)	*Source:* Centers for Disease Control and Prevention (CDC)	Riboflavin, niacin, pyridoxine

TABLE 23.6   Overview of Nutritional Findings during Physical Assessment *(continued)*

System or Body Part	Clinical Finding	Examples	Potential Nutrient Deficiency
	Diminished taste buds (atrophic papillae)		Iron
	Complaint of diminished taste		Zinc
	Delayed eruption of teeth in children		Vitamin D
	Development of caries in infant or young child		Check if child is being put to bed with bottle (baby bottle tooth decay)
	Mottled enamel		Overexposure to fluoride
	Spongy, bleeding gums	 *Source:* Centers for Disease Control and Prevention (CDC)	Vitamin C
Head and Neck	Facial pallor		Iron
	Moon face		Protein
	Increased thyroid size		Iodine
	Increased parotid size		Protein and calories, assess for bulimia
Skeleton/Trunk	Ascites		Protein
	Growth stunting		Protein and calories, zinc
	Rickets (bowed legs), widened epiphyses, narrow chest, rachitic rosary (beading on ribs)	 *Source:* Centers for Disease Control and Prevention (CDC)	Vitamin D
	Muscle and fat wasting		Protein, calories
Limbs	Muscle and fat wasting		Protein, calories
	Edema of lower limbs	 *Source:* Centers for Disease Control and Prevention (CDC)	Protein

(continued)

TABLE 23.6 Overview of Nutritional Findings during Physical Assessment *(continued)*

System or Body Part	Clinical Finding	Examples	Potential Nutrient Deficiency
Nails	Koilonychia (spoon-shaped nails), ridges in nails		Iron
Skin	Bruising		Vitamins C and K
	Pinpoint hemorrhages (petechiae)		Vitamin C
	Dry scaly skin		Vitamin A, essential fatty acids
	Follicular hyperkeratosis (goosebump flesh)		Vitamins A and C
	Poor wound healing		Protein, calories, vitamin C, zinc
	Symmetrical rash on sun-exposed areas only	*Source:* Centers for Disease Control and Prevention (CDC)	Niacin
Genitalia	Hypogonadism		Zinc
Nervous system	Hyporeflexia, confabulation, neuropathy		Thiamine
	Neuropathy, confusion, ataxia		Vitamin B_{12}
	Tetany		Calcium, magnesium
Cardiac	Tachycardia		Iron, folic acid, vitamin B_{12}
	Arrhythmia		Magnesium, potassium

Source: CDC, Public Health Image Library. (1970). Retrieved March 20, 2009, from http://phil.cdc.gov/phil/home.asp

albumin in the assessment of older adults because of the risk of undernutrition in that population (IOM, 2000). Albumin less than 3.5 mg/dL is associated with increased risk of morbidity and mortality in the older adult following discharge from the hospital (Carriere et al., 2008; Sullivan, Roberson, & Bopp, 2005). The nurse should be aware that any condition leading to dehydration or fluid overload will result in hemoconcentration or dilution, respectively, and a false measurement of albumin status. Additionally, disease states such as liver disease or nephrotic syndrome can lead to decreased albumin unrelated to nutritional status. Because of the many confounding variables affecting albumin, there are many who believe it is more an indicator of morbidity and mortality risk than an exclusive indicator of current nutrition status in adults and children (DeLegge & Drake, 2007; Horowitz & Tai, 2007; Horwich, Kalantar-Zadeh, MacLellan, & Fonarow, 2008).

Prealbumin is also called thyroxine-binding prealbumin or transthyretin. Normal plasma prealbumin is 150 mg/L to 350 mg/L. Similar alterations occur during inflammation or infection but to a lesser extent than seen with albumin. Prealbumin is felt to be a better nutrition screening tool, reflecting a more current picture of visceral

TABLE 23.7   Common Laboratory Measurements Used in Nutritional Assessment

Laboratory	Normal Value	Mild Malnutrition	Moderate Malnutrition	Severe Malnutrition	Half-life (days)	Nonnutritional Causes of Altered Value
Albumin	3.5–5 gm/L	2.8–3.4 gm/L	2.1–2.7 gm/L	Less than 2.1 gm/L	14–20	Inflammation, infection, liver disease, renal losses
Transferrin	200–400 mg/L	180–200 mg/L	160–180 mg/L	Less than 160 mg/L	8–10	Inflammation, infection, iron deficiency, liver disease, renal losses
Prealbumin	150–350 mg/L	110–150 mg/L	50–109 mg/L	Less than 50 mg/L	2–3	Inflammation, infection, liver disease, renal losses
Total lymphocyte count (TLC)	2,000–3,500 cells/m^3	1,200–1,500 cells/m^3	800–1,200 cells/m^3	Less than 800 cells/m^3	N/A	Immune suppressive disease or treatment

Sources: Adapted from Beck & Rosenthal, 2002; Fuhrman, Charney, & Mueller, 2004; Omran & Morley, 2000; Shenkin, Cederblad, Ellia, & Isaksson, 1996.

protein status than albumin in part because of its shorter half-life of 2 to 3 days (Robinson et al., 2003). Like albumin, low prealbumin is associated with increased risk of morbidity and mortality in the older adult (Carriere et al., 2008).

Transferrin has a role in iron binding and transport in the body. Normal transferrin is above 200 mg/dL. The half-life of transferrin is 8 to 10 days, reflecting a more current picture of nutrition status than with albumin but less current than prealbumin. Transferrin levels are altered during physiological stress because of its role as an acute phase reactant protein, limiting its use as a true indicator of nutrition status under such conditions. Transferrin values derived in the laboratory from total iron-binding capacity value will be affected by low iron states.

Immunocompetence

An assessment of a client's immune status, or **immunocompetence**, can be included in a nutritional assessment. Undernutrition is associated with a decline in immune function, which can be reflected in laboratory assessments of the immune system. Many disease states and medications, such as HIV, autoimmune diseases, and chemotherapy also impact immune status, limiting the use of these parameters as nutritional indicators in these clients.

Total lymphocyte count (TLC) and delayed skin hypersensitivity testing are used to assess immunocompetence. Decreased TLC can indicate poor immunocompetence and potential malnutrition as outlined in Table 23.7. TLC is calculated using the white blood cell (WBC) count and lymphocyte percentage using the formula:

$$TLC = WBC \times \% \text{ lymphocytes}$$

Delayed skin hypersensitivity testing detects delayed or absent immune response to common antigens, such as streptococcus. An altered response can indicate poor immunocompetence, undernutrition, or simply lack of exposure to the antigen. Testing is done by administering intradermal injections of a panel of antigens while monitoring the injection sites for signs of hypersensitivity, such as induration and erythema, occurring within 48 hours. A positive reaction with induration of at least 0.5 cm is indicative of a good immune status. No response to the antigens despite known exposure is called **anergy** and indicates poor immune status.

Nitrogen Balance Assessment

A nitrogen balance assessment estimates the adequacy of dietary intake and is used in the monitoring of the nutrition status of an individual. A client is in nitrogen balance when nitrogen intake from protein equals nitrogen output by the body. Nitrogen output is measured with a 24-hour urine urea nitrogen; insensible nitrogen losses from hair, feces, and skin are accounted for in the nitrogen balance equation. Negative nitrogen balance arises when protein intake is low or nitrogen losses are high, or both. Negative nitrogen balance can occur with poor quantity or quality intake or **catabolism**, the breakdown of stored proteins by the body. **Anabolism**, or synthesis of tissue, requires a positive nitrogen balance. Box 23.5 outlines the nitrogen balance equation and a sample calculation that a nutrition support nurse or dietitian uses.

Laboratory Measures of Nutrient Status

Laboratory values of select nutrients can be included in a nutrition assessment where available. Indices that screen for nutritional anemias should be included in a nutritional assessment. Hemoglobin, hematocrit, red blood cell volume, and measures of folic acid and vitamin B_{12} status provide the nurse with useful information to include in the assessment.

Low serum cholesterol, defined as less than 160 mg/dL, is associated with frailty and risk of mortality in the older adult but debated by others as to its clinical use as a nutrition parameter (Okamura et al., 2008; Spada et al., 2007). Currently, the use of cholesterol-lowering medications limits the use of low serum cholesterol in many individuals as an independent indicator of undernutrition.

Plasma levels of many nutrients are not valid measures of nutrient status. For example, serum calcium accounts for only a small fraction of total body calcium and is not directly related to calcium intake. Although serum calcium is included in routine laboratory assays, it is evaluated for medical purposes and not as a routine part of a nutritional assessment. For other nutrients, measurement of the nutrients' total

BOX 23.5 Nitrogen Balance Calculations

Nitrogen balance studies can be used to estimate whether a client is receiving adequate nutrition. A client is said to be "in nitrogen balance" when nitrogen intake from protein and nitrogen output are equal. Negative nitrogen balance occurs when intake is too low or losses are too great and this leads to catabolism. Positive nitrogen balance occurs when intake exceeds losses, and tissue synthesis, or anabolism, is possible. Calculations will not be pertinent in clients with abnormal urine output, such as in renal failure.

Nitrogen balance = nitrogen in (from protein) − nitrogen losses (from urine and insensible loss)
Nitrogen in = calculation of 24-hour protein intake (gm) / 6.25 gm nitrogen per gram of protein
Nitrogen out = 24-hour urine urea nitrogen collection (UUN) + 4 gm nitrogen insensible loss

Example:
The nutrition support nurse suggests a nitrogen balance study for a client transitioning from a feeding tube to oral intake. The 24-hour intake from diet, liquids, and feeding formula is recorded by the nursing staff. A 24-hour urine collection is sent to the laboratory. The client is estimated to have consumed 120 gm protein. The 24-hour UUN reveals 10 gm nitrogen.

Nitrogen in = 120 gm protein / 6.25 gm nitrogen per gram protein = 19.2 gm nitrogen
Nitrogen out = 10 gm UUN + 4 gm insensible loss = 14 gm nitrogen
Nitrogen balance = 19.2 gm nitrogen in - 14 gm nitrogen out = positive nitrogen balance of 5.2 gm

body pool cannot be measured via the plasma, but blood levels do reflect overall stores. Plasma vitamin C levels are an example (Mosdol, Erens, & Brunner, 2008). Measurement of plasma and tissue levels of most nutrients is generally reserved for research and is not a routine nutrition assessment practice. Use of hair analysis to assess nutrient status is a controversial topic and is outlined in Hot Topic Box: Hair Analysis of Mineral Status.

Laboratory Measurements Associated with Overnutrition

Hypercholesterolemia, defined as a serum cholesterol greater than 200 mg/dL, is associated with risk of cardiovascular disease and overnutrition. Elevated fasting triglyceride levels are also considered a cardiac risk factor. Increased fasting glucose and hemoglobin A1C levels are associated with glucose intolerance and diabetes and should be noted. Medical nutrition therapy for hyperlipidemia and diabetes are discussed in detail in the respective chapters dedicated to those diagnoses.

Oversupplementation with some dietary supplements affects platelet function and clotting time, especially in the client taking medications that also alter blood clotting. Vitamin E, ginkgo biloba, feverfew, and ginseng are examples. Alterations in clotting time should be noted in an assessment and the client should be questioned about supplement use.

Cultural Considerations

Cultural competency is an important factor in providing effective health care. During the nutritional assessment, the nurse should be mindful of the influence that culture has on food and nutrition habits and also on the conduct of the assessment itself. During the focused interview, the nurse should ask specific questions about the influence of culture on food beliefs and practices. The nurse should not make assumptions about how an individual belonging to any cultural or religious population adheres to generalized beliefs. Food and health beliefs vary within and among ethnic groups and the nurse should inquire about how an individual interprets and practices these beliefs. Acculturation can influence nutrition practices of individuals who have immigrated to a new country and adopted some or many new food habits. Cultural Considerations Box: Cultural Considerations with a Nutrition Assessment outlines key points for the nurse to consider during the nutrition assessment.

Cultural and religious beliefs can influence the physical assessment portion of the nutritional assessment. Beliefs that discourage touch by members of the opposite gender or the removal of certain garments present obstacles to the gathering of anthropometric measurements and the physical examination. The nurse should ask the client or a translator about the presence of these issues and explain the physical assessment process before attempting to begin this portion of the nutritional assessment. In some cases, the nurse may need to seek assistance from another nurse of the same gender as the client; in other cases, certain portions of the assessment may need to be modified to accommodate the client's beliefs. The nurse should engage in decision making with the client about how to proceed when these issues are present.

hot Topic

Hair Analysis of Mineral Status

Laboratory Hair Analysis: Fact, Fiction, or Fraud?
Laboratory analysis of hair is used in forensic medicine to detect mineral or heavy metal contamination. The deaths of both President Andrew Jackson and Napoleon Bonaparte have been attributed by some to poisoning, supported by present-day analysis of hair strands indicating that they suffered from lead exposure and arsenic and cyanide poisoning, respectively (Deppisch, Centeno, Gemmel, & Torres, 1999; Kintz, Ginet, Marques, & Cirimele, 2007). Mercury poisoning can also be detected through hair analysis, though levels are not considered as accurate as those from blood or urine assays (Ng, Chan, Soo, & Lee, 2007). Many companies exist that will provide hair analysis and some sell vitamin and mineral supplements based on the laboratory findings. Almost $10 million is spent yearly on hair analysis in the United States (Seidel, Kreutzer, Smith, McNeel, & Gilliss, 2001). Should the use of laboratory hair analysis be a part of a comprehensive nutritional assessment?

The nurse should warn any individual considering hair analysis that ongoing evidence does not support its use as a part of a nutritional assessment (Barrett, 2001; Seidel et al., 2001; Steindel & Howanitz, 2001). A correlation between dietary intake of minerals and the amount found in hair is lacking (Gonzalez-Munoz, Pena, & Meseguer, 2008). Uniform standards for hair mineral content are not established. Environmental factors and hair treatment choices affect the analysis. Little research has been conducted about the relationship between mineral content of the hair and overall mineral status (Seidel et al., 2001). The American Medical Association (AMA) opposes the use of hair analysis in determining the need for medical therapy and believes the potential for health care fraud exists with this practice (AMA, 2004).

Cultural Considerations

Cultural Considerations with a Nutrition Assessment

Culture can influence food and health beliefs and practices. The nurse should take into consideration any of these influences when gathering data for a nutritional assessment.

Assess for:

- Core foods in the diet.
- Food preparation methods and types of ingredients used, such as type of fat for frying.
- Dietary laws observed such as kosher, vegetarian, or vegan practices or avoidance of other specific foods.
- Use of fasting as part of religious observation. Assess frequency and duration of fast.
- Foods consumed as part of traditional celebrations or religious observations.
- Foods believed to have health or curative powers (such as consuming "hot" foods to balance "cold" health conditions, yin and yang foods, or foods felt to assist with childbirth).
- Use of dietary supplements, including herbs and other plant products.
- Influence of family on reinforcing cultural practices.
- Changes in diet because of acculturation; note healthful and unhealthful changes like addition of fats, processed foods, extra sugar, and elimination of traditional healthy foods.

Establishing Diagnoses

It is important to carefully review the assessment data prior to establishing the nursing diagnoses. NANDA (2007) lists criteria that should be met prior to identification of any specific diagnosis. A diagnosis that is inaccurate, incomplete, or vague will lead to inappropriate goals and ineffective planning.

Setting Goals

Setting realistic, achievable, and measurable nutritional goals is important for clients. When clients have short-term goals that can be readily achieved, they are more likely to develop confidence in their ability to set long-term goals that can have a lasting impact on their nutritional status.

Nursing Diagnosis

The second step in the nursing process is the identification of the nursing diagnosis or diagnoses. A nursing diagnosis is based on analysis of the subjective and objective data obtained from the nursing assessment. Depending on the client situation, there are numerous nursing diagnoses that have a nutritional focus or may be related to nutrient intake or absence (NANDA International, 2007). These diagnoses are published by the North American Nursing Diagnosis Association (NANDA). Box 23.6 lists many of the NANDA nursing diagnoses that relate to nutrition. Selection of the appropriate diagnosis will depend on the cause of the alteration in nutritional status. For example, *Imbalanced nutrition: Less than body requirements* may be related to decreased nutrient intake, excess energy expenditure, or prolonged anorexia. When stating the nursing diagnosis, the nurse should always include a "related to" statement to link the diagnosis to the assessment data. In addition, the nurse should include the relevant evidence. For example, *Imbalanced nutrition: Less than body requirements* related to decreased nutrient intake as evidenced by unplanned weight loss of 10 pounds in the past 6 weeks. See the Practice Pearl "Establishing Diagnoses" for a discussion of how to formulate a nursing diagnosis.

Planning

Following the establishment of appropriate nursing diagnoses, the third step of the nursing process is to develop a plan of care for the client. Goals, or outcomes, are established jointly by the client and the nurse. Goals must be realistic, achievable, and measurable. They must also arise from the nursing diagnoses and be congruent with them. Goals should also be prioritized by those that require immediate attention and those that are less urgent. Goals may be short term (a few days or less) or long term (a week or longer). For example, a realistic goal for a client with a nursing diagnosis of *Imbalanced nutrition: Less than body requirements* related to decreased nutrient intake evidenced by unplanned weight loss of 10 pounds in 6 weeks may be to increase caloric intake by 200 calories per day within 1 week. A long-term goal may be to regain the weight within 2 months. A goal that the nurse may consider realistic is "consultation with a dietitian by the client." The planning phase of the nursing process is very important because it sets the stage for the implementation of measures that will assist the client to achieve goals. Practice Pearl "Setting Goals" serves as a reminder when developing goals.

Implementation

The fourth step of the nursing process is the implementation phase. The goals listed in the plan guide the interventions performed by the nurse and/or the client. This is the action step for the plan. While implementing various nursing interventions, the nurse should carefully reflect on what is being done and monitor progress toward goal achievement. It is a challenging step because it

BOX 23.6   Nursing Diagnoses Related to Nutritional Status

The following nursing diagnoses with a nutritional focus approved by NANDA (2007–2008) are frequently used as part of the nursing process. This is not an exclusive list, but these are the diagnoses most frequently used by nursing students when planning client care. Please note that registered dietitians also follow the Nutrition Care Process and have specific language for nutrition diagnoses.

Aspiration, risk for

Blood Glucose, risk for Unstable

Body Image, Disturbed

Breastfeeding,
   Effective
   Ineffective
   Interrupted

Constipation, risk for

Dentition
   Impaired

Development
   Delayed, risk for

Diarrhea

Failure to Thrive
   Adult

Fluid Balance
   Readiness for Enhanced

Fluid volume
   Deficient,
   Excess, risk for Deficient
   Imbalanced, risk for

Infant Feeding Pattern
   Ineffective

Knowledge
   Deficient
   Readiness for Enhanced

Mucous Membrane
   Impaired Oral

Nausea

Nutrition, Imbalanced
   Less than Body Requirements,
   More than Body Requirements,
   Risk for More than Body Requirements

Nutrition,
   Readiness for Enhanced

Sedentary Lifestyle

Self-care Deficit
   Feeding

Swallowing
   Impaired

Source: NANDA, 2007.

often involves considerable effort on the part of the nurse to help motivate a client to make changes in dietary choices or nutritional behavior. The nurse should brainstorm with the client about factors that may assist with achievement of goals as well as those that may be barriers to success. Discussing these factors and any needed solutions early in the process helps improve the collaboration between the nurse and the client when determining the steps needed to achieve a goal. For example, if an overweight client decides that increased exercise is a goal and that it will occur before work every day, the nurse can explore if there have been prior attempts at exercise in the past and if early morning exercise is likely to occur. If rising early to exercise was a barrier to success in the past, the nurse can revisit that goal with the client and formulate one that is more likely to be successful. The initial response of the client to interventions should be monitored. It is appropriate for the nurse to make early corrections to the interventions based on initial client response or the plan may never be fully implemented. During the implementation phase the nurse should carefully document the interventions and the client response.

Evaluation

Evaluation is the final phase of the nursing process. It is related to the planning phase because it focuses on the goals that were established with the client. Assuming the diagnoses were accurate and the goals were realistic, evaluation answers the question, "Were the goals achieved?" It should examine where the client stands in relation to goal achievement. Any changes that occurred that caused the plan to be unworkable must be evaluated and the plan modified. It must further determine if the interventions that were implemented were appropriate and correct. A final part of the evaluation should lead to further assessment of the client and any refinement of the care plan. This provides for the cyclical nature of the nursing process.

Nursing Care Plan: Nutrition for Weight Loss

Case Study

Kay is a 50-year-old school teacher who has come to the clinic for a routine checkup. She has been a regular client for the past 10 years and has had no significant health concerns during that time. She tells the nurse how proud she is of her daughter who has decided to study nutrition science in college. Kay informs the nurse that, given her daughter's major, she feels the need to improve her own nutritional health by losing weight and getting in better shape. She notes that she has developed what she calls "middle-age spread" and wants to keep it from getting worse. She has no other health concerns at this time. FIGURE 23.10 outlines the nursing process for this case.

Applying the Nursing Process

ASSESSMENT
Height: 5 feet 7 inches, Weight: 176 pounds, BMI: 27.7
BP 128/76, P 76, R 14, Lab Data: Within normal limits
Waist: 39 inches, Hips: 46 inches, Waist-Hip Ratio: 0.9

DIAGNOSIS
Nutrition: Readiness for enhanced related to stated goals as evidenced by willingness to make lifestyle changes

EXPECTED OUTCOMES
Weight loss averaging 1 pound per week for 20 weeks
Increase activity level to 30 minutes a day, four times a week

INTERVENTIONS
24-hour food recall
Food diary for 1 week
Use MyPyramid to introduce a balanced nutritional plan
Collaborate with the client to develop a plan for increased activity with daily and weekly goals
Introduce the "rule of 500" to aid in planning for weight loss where a caloric deficit of 500 kcalories/day leads to a weekly deficit of 3,500 kcalories to foster a 1-pound weight loss. A combination of decreased intake and increased activity can achieve this goal

EVALUATION
After 6 weeks, Kay is excited about the changes in her life. She has been sharing her new knowledge with her daughter, who has also been eager to share what she has learned with her mother. She has started to do some small things like use the steps more at work and park in a more distant parking spot. She has lost 5 pounds and likes using the "rule of 500" because she feels she can make small changes everyday to make progress toward her goal. She plans to stay with her diet and increase her activity by joining the YWCA near her home.

Critical Thinking in the Nursing Process

1. What are some strategies that the nurse can use to assist a client who is otherwise in good health to improve nutritional status?

Nutrition for Weight Loss *(continued)*

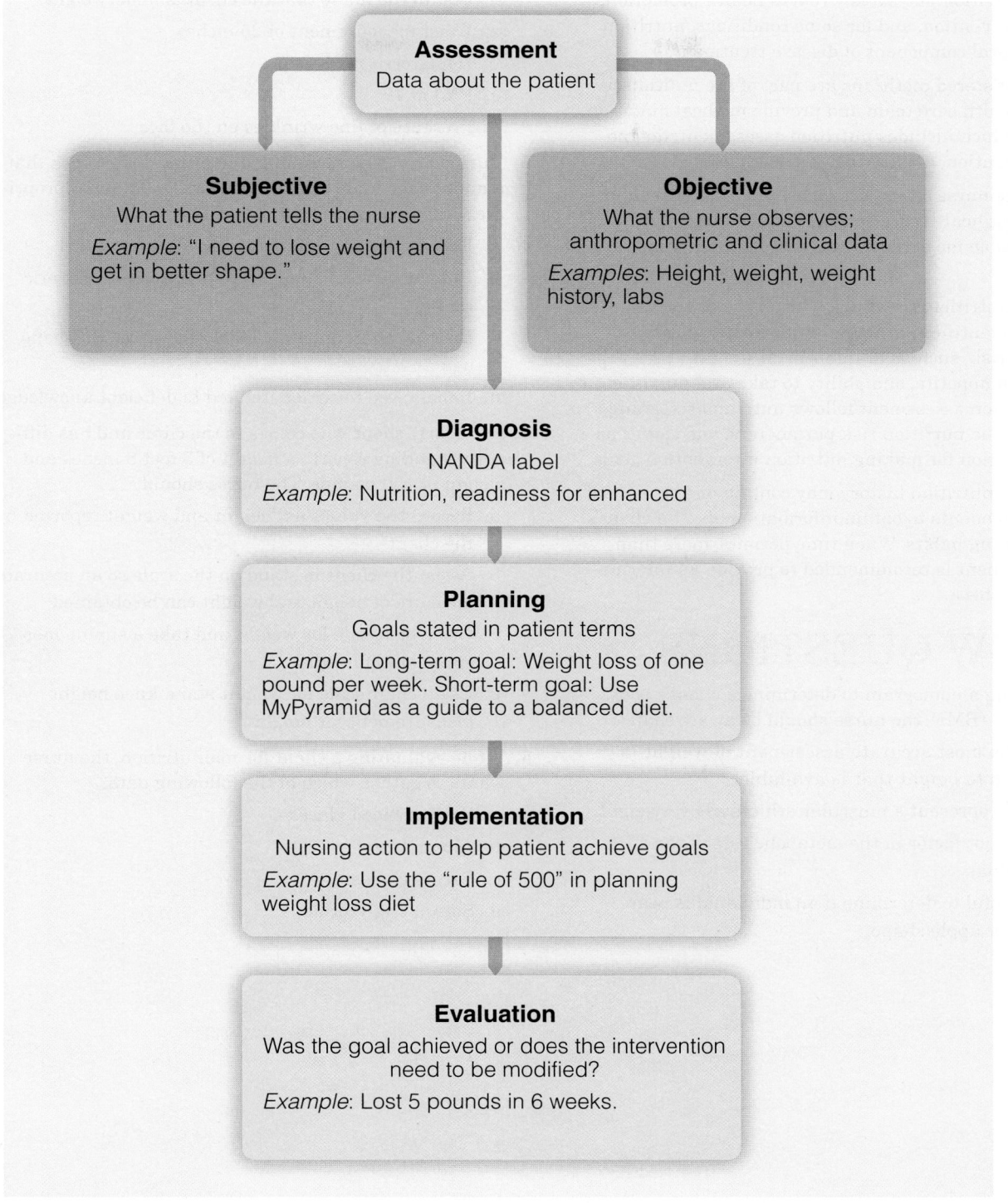

Assessment
Data about the patient

Subjective
What the patient tells the nurse
Example: "I need to lose weight and get in better shape."

Objective
What the nurse observes; anthropometric and clinical data
Examples: Height, weight, weight history, labs

Diagnosis
NANDA label
Example: Nutrition, readiness for enhanced

Planning
Goals stated in patient terms
Example: Long-term goal: Weight loss of one pound per week. Short-term goal: Use MyPyramid as a guide to a balanced diet.

Implementation
Nursing action to help patient achieve goals
Example: Use the "rule of 500" in planning weight loss diet

Evaluation
Was the goal achieved or does the intervention need to be modified?
Example: Lost 5 pounds in 6 weeks.

FIGURE 23.9   Nursing Care Plan process: Nutrition for weight loss.

TEST YOURSELF ANSWERS

1. **False.** Nutrition plays a key role in health promotion, disease prevention, and for some conditions, nutrition is an integral component of disease treatment.

2. **True.** Registered dietitians are part of the multidisciplinary health care team and provide medical nutrition therapy, which includes nutrition assessment, diagnosis, intervention, monitoring, and evaluation.

3. **False.** The nurse often performs a nutrition screening, but in most health care settings, a registered dietitian is responsible for performing a thorough nutrition assessment.

4. **False.** A nutrition screening, which is brief and noninvasive, identifies parameters that may indicate nutrition risk, such as unintentional weight loss, changes in appetite, and ability to take oral nutrition. The nutrition assessment follows nutrition screening, evaluates the nutrition risk parameters, and serves as the foundation for making nutrition intervention goals.

5. **True.** The nutrition history may contain one or more of these components to obtain information about a client's typical eating habits. When time permits, more than one component is recommended to provide an information cross-check.

REVIEW QUESTIONS

1. When using a nomogram to determine a client's body mass index (BMI), the nurse should be aware that:
   a. It is the most accurate assessment of weight in relation to height that is available.
   b. It may represent a muscular athlete as overweight.
   c. It does not factor in the metabolic rate of the individual.
   d. It is useful to determine if an individual is pear shape or apple shape.

2. When analyzing data from a nutritional assessment of a middle-age female client, which of the following would suggest to the nurse that the client is underweight?
   a. Waist measurement of 25 inches
   b. Hematocrit of 39
   c. BMI of 19
   d. Presence of fine wrinkles on the face

3. During a routine screening, the nurse determines that a middle-age male client has a BMI of 33. An appropriate nursing diagnosis for this client would be:
   a. Risk for obesity, related to above-normal BMI
   b. Imbalanced nutrition, related to excessive caloric intake
   c. Risk for altered metabolism, related to advancing age
   d. Imbalanced nutrition, related to deficient knowledge

4. An elderly client who comes to the clinic and has difficulty standing reports a height of 5 feet 8 inches and weight of 150 pounds. The nurse should:
   a. Record the values as "height and weight reported by the client"
   b. Assist the client to stand on the scale so an accurate measure of height and weight can be obtained
   c. Use a bed scale for weight and take a supine measurement of height
   d. Use a chair scale for weight and a knee height measurement for height

5. While evaluating a client for malnutrition, the nurse wants to gather which of the following data?
   a. Fasting blood glucose
   b. Albumin
   c. Serum cholesterol
   d. Serum triglyceride

REFERENCES

Adachi-Mejia, A. M., Longacre, M. R., Gibson, J. J., Beach, M. L., Titus-Ernstoff, L. T., & Dalton, M. A. (2007). Children with a TV in their bedroom at a higher risk for being overweight. *International Journal of Obesity (London), 31*(4), 644–651.

Aghdassi, E., Arendt, B., Salit, I. E., & Allard, J. P. (2007). Estimation of body fat mass using dual-energy x-ray absorptiometry, bioelectrical impedance analysis, and anthropometry in HIV-positive male subjects receiving highly active retroviral therapy. *Journal of Parenteral and Enteral Nutrition, 31*, 135–141.

American Dietetic Association. (2010). Position of the American Dietetic Association: Integration of medical nutrition therapy and pharmacotherapy. *Journal of the American Dietetic Association, 110*, 950–956.

American Dietetic Association. (2002). Position of the American Dietetic Association: Weight management. *Journal of the American Dietetic Association, 102*, 1145–1148.

American Dietetic Association, Council on Practice Quality Management Team. (1994). Identifying patient at risk: ADA's definitions for nutrition screening and nutrition assessment. *Journal of the American Dietetic Association*, 94, 838–839.

American Medical Association (AMA). (2004). *Policy H-175.955 Hair analysis—a potential for medical abuse.* Retrieved March 20, 2009, from http:www.ama-assn.org

American Medical Directors Association (2001). *Altered nutritional status: Clinical practice guideline.* Washington, DC: Author.

Anderson, B. (2005). Nutrition and wound healing: The necessity of assessment. *British Journal of Nursing (Tissue Viability Supplement), 14*(9), S30–S38.

Anthony, P. S. (2008). Nutrition screening tools for hospitalized patients. *Nutrition in Clinical Practice, 23*, 373–382.

Avila-Funes, J. A., Gutierrez-Robledo, L. M., & Ponce De Leon Rosales, S. (2004). Validity of height and weight self-report in Mexican adults: Results from the national health and aging study. *The Journal of Nutrition, Health & Aging, 8*, 355–361.

Ball, S. D., Kertesz, D., & Moyer-Mileur, L. J. (2005). Dietary supplement use is prevalent among children with chronic illness. *Journal of the American Dietetic Association,105*, 78–84.

Barrett, S. (2001). *Commercial hair analysis: A cardinal sign of quackery.* Retrieved March 21, 2009, from http://www.quackwatch.org/01QuackeryRelatedTopics/hair.html

Beck, F. K., & Rosenthal, T. C. (2002). Prealbumin: A marker for nutritional evaluation. *American Family Physician, 65*, 1575–1578.

Brener, N. D., Eaton, D. K., Lowry, R., & McManus, T. (2004). The association between weight perception and BMI among high school students. *Obesity Research, 12*, 1866–1874.

Brener, N. D., McManus, T., Galuska, D. A., Lowry, R., & Wechsler, H. (2003). Reliability and validity of self-reported height and weight among high school students. *Journal of Adolescent Health, 32*, 281–287.

Brunner-Huber, L. R. (2007). Validity of self-reported height and weight in women of reproductive age. *Maternal and Child Health Journal, 11*, 137–144.

Buchholz, A. C., Bartok, C., & Schoeller, D. A. (2004). The validity of bioelectrical impedance models in clinical populations. *Nutrition in Clinical Practice, 19*, 433–446.

Burdette, H. L., & Whitaker, R. C. (2005). A national study of neighborhood safety, outdoor play, television viewing, and obesity in preschool children. *Pediatrics, 116*(3), 657–662.

Carriere, I., Dupuy, A. M., Lacroux, A., Cristol, J. P., Delcourt, C., & Pathologies oculaires liees a l'age study group. (2008). Biomarkers of inflammation and malnutrition associated with early death in healthy elderly people. *Journal of the American Geriatric Society, 56*, 840–846.

Centers for Disease Control and Prevention (CDC), National Center for Health Statistics. (2000). *Anthropometry procedures manual.* Retrieved March 21, 2009, from http://www.cdc.gov/nchs/data/nhanes/nhanes_01_02/body_measures_year_3.pdf

Centers for Disease Control and Prevention (CDC). (2009). *Defining childhood overweight and obesity.* Retrieved March 21, 2009, from http://www.cdc.gov/obesity/childhood/defining.html

Centers for Medicare and Medicaid Services (CMS). (2000). *Minimum data set (version 2.0).* Retrieved March 21, 2009, from http://www.cms.hhs.gov/medicaid/mds20/mds0900b.pdf

Charney, P. (2008). Nutrition screening vs. nutrition assessment: How do they differ? *Nutrition in Clinical Practice, 23*, 366–372.

Chima, C. S., Dietz-Seher, C., & Kushner-Benson, S. (2008). Nutrition risk screening in acute care: A survey of practice. *Nutrition in Clinical Practice, 23*, 417–423.

Cunningham, E. (2004). Is body mass index for children and adolescents assessed differently than for adults? *Journal of the American Dietetic Association, 104*, 694.

DeLegge, M. H., & Drake, L. M. (2007). Nutritional assessment. *Gastroenterology Clinics of North America, 36*, 1–22.

Delville, C. L. (2008). Are your patients at nutritional risk? *Nurse Practitioner, 33*(2), 36–39.

Dennison, B. A., Erb, T. A., & Jenkins, P. L. (2002). Television viewing and television in bedroom associated with overweight risk among low-income preschool children. *Pediatrics, 109*(6), 1028–1035.

Deppisch, L. M., Centeno, J. A., Gemmel, D. J., & Torres, L. (1999). Andrew Jackson's exposure to mercury and lead: Poisoned president? *Journal of the American Medical Association, 282*, 569–571.

DiMaria-Ghalili, R. A., & Guenter, P. A. (2008). The Mini Nutritional Assessment. *American Journal of Nursing, 108*(2), 50–59.

Engstrom, J. L., Paterson, S. A., Doherty, A., Trabulsi, M., & Speer, K. L. (2003). Accuracy of self-reported height and weight in women: An integrative review of the literature. *Journal of Midwifery and Women's Health, 48*, 338–345.

Foster, B. J., & Leonard, M. B. (2004). Measuring nutritional status in children with chronic kidney disease. *American Journal of Clinical Nutrition, 80*, 801–814.

Francis, L. A., & Birch, L. L. (2006). Does eating during television viewing affect preschool children's intake? *Journal of the American Dietetic Association, 106*(4), 598–600.

Fuhrman, M. P., Charney, P., & Mueller, C. M. (2004). Hepatic proteins and nutrition assessment. *Journal of the American Dietetic Association, 104*, 1258–1264.

Gable, S., Chang, Y., & Krull, J. L. (2007). Television watching and frequency of family meals are predictive of overweight onset and persistence in a national sample of school-aged children. *Journal of the American Dietetic Association, 107*(1), 53–61.

Gallagher, D., Heymsfield, S. B., Heo, M., Jebb, S. A., Murgatroyd, P., & Sakamoto, Y. (2000). Healthy percentage body fat ranges: An approach for developing guidelines based on body mass index. *American Journal of Clinical Nutrition, 72*, 694–701.

Gans, K. M., Ross, E., Barner, C. W., Wylie-Rosett, J., McMurray, J., & Eaton, C. (2003). REAP and WAVE: New tools to rapidly assess/discuss nutrition with patients. *The Journal of Nutrition, 133*, 556S–562S.

Gardiner, P., Buettner, C., Davis, R. B., Phillips, R. S., & Kemper, K. J. (2008). Factors and common conditions associated with adolescent dietary supplement use: An analysis of the National Health and Nutrition Exam Survey (NHANES). *BMC Complementary and Alternative Medicine, 31*, 9.

Gillum, R. F., & Sempos, C. T. (2005). Ethnic variations in validity of classification of overweight and obesity using self-reported weight and height in American women and men: The Third National Health and Nutrition Examination Survey. *Nutrition Journal, 4*, 27.

Gonzalez-Munoz, M. J., Pena, A., & Meseguer, I. (2008). Monitoring heavy metal contents in food and hair sample of young Spanish subjects. *Food & Chemical Toxicology, 46*, 3048–3052.

Goodman, E., Hinden, B. R., & Khandelwal, S. (2000). Accuracy of teen and parental reports of obesity and body mass index. *Pediatrics, 106*, 52–58.

Guigoz, Y. (2006). The Mini Nutrition Assessment (MNA) review of the literature—what does it tell us? *Journal of Nutrition, Health & Aging, 10*, 466–485.

Harnack, L., Steffen, L., Arnett, D. K., Gao, S., & Luepker, R. V. (2004). Accuracy of estimation of large food portions. *Journal of the American Dietetic Association, 104*, 804–806.

Hauck, F. R., White, L., Cao, G., Woolf, N., & Strauss, K. (1995). Inaccuracy of self-reported weights and heights among American Indian adolescents. *Annals of Epidemiology, 5*(5), 386–392.

Hetzler, R. K., Kimura, I. F., Haines, K., Labotz, M., & Smith, J. (2006). A comparison of bioelectrical impedance and skinfold measurements in determining minimum wrestling weights in high school wrestlers. *Journal of Athletic Training, 41*, 46–51.

Hickson, M., & Frost, G. (2003). A comparison of three methods for estimating height in the acutely ill elderly population. *Journal of Human Nutrition and Dietetics, 16*(1), 13–20.

Horowitz, I. N., & Tai, K. (2007). Hypoalbuminemia in critically ill children. *Archives of Pediatric and Adolescent Medicine, 161*, 1048–1052.

Horwich, T. B., Kalantar-Zadeh, K., MacLellan, R. W., & Fonarow, G. C. (2008). Albumin levels predict survival in patients with systolic heart failure. *American Heart Journal, 155*, 883–889.

Institute of Medicine (IOM). (2000). *The role of nutrition in maintaining health in the nation's elderly: Evaluating coverage of nutrition services for the Medicare population*. Washington DC: National Academies Press.

Institute of Medicine, Committee on Nutrition Services for Medicare Beneficiaries, Food and Nutrition Board. (2000). *The Role of Nutrition in Maintaining Health in the Nation's Elderly: Evaluating Coverage of Nutrition Services for the Medicare Population*. Washington, DC: National Academy Press.

Jacobson, B. H., & DeBock, D. H. (2001). Comparison of body mass index by self-reported versus measured height and weight. *Perceptual and Motor Skills, 92*, 128–132.

Jansen, W., van de Looij-Jansen, P. M., Ferreira, I., de Wilde, E. J., & Brug, J. (2006). Differences in measured and self-reported height and weight in Dutch adolescents. *Annals of Nutrition & Metabolism, 50*, 339–346.

Jensen, G. L., Friedmann, J. M., Henry, D. K., Skipper, A., Beiler, E., Porter, C., et al. (2003). Noncompliance with body weight measurement in tertiary care teaching hospitals. *Journal of Parenteral and Enteral Nutrition, 27*, 89–90.

Kelly, J. P., Kaufman, D. W., Kelley, K., Rosenberg, L., Anderson, T. E., & Mitchell, A. A. (2005). Recent trends in use of herbal and other natural products. *Archives of Internal Medicine, 165*, 281–286.

Kintz, P., Ginet, M., Marques, N., & Cirimele, V. (2007). Arsenic speciation of two specimens of Napoleon's hair. *Forensic Science International, 170*, 204–206.

Kristal, A. R., Andrilla, H. A., Koepsell, T. D., Diehr, P. H., & Cheadle, A. (1998). Dietary assessment instruments are susceptible to intervention-associated response set bias. *Journal of the American Dietetic Association, 98*, 40–43.

Kuczmarski, M. F., Kuczmarski, R. J., & Najjar, M. (2000). Descriptive anthropometric reference data for older Americans. *Journal of the American Dietetic Association, 100*, 59–66.

Kuczmarski, M. F., Kuczmarski, R. J., & Najjar, M. (2001). Effects of age on validity of self-reported height, weight and body mass index: Findings from the Third National Health and Nutrition Examination Survey 1988–1994. *Journal of the American Dietetic Association, 101*, 28–34.

Lean, M. J., & Han, T. S. (2002). Waist worries. *American Journal of Clinical Nutrition, 76*, 699–700.

Lear, S. A., Humphries, K. H., Kohli, S., & Birmingham, C. L. (2007). The use of BMI and waist circumference as surrogates of body fat differs by ethnicity. *Obesity, 15*, 2817–2824.

Lee, S. Y., & Gallagher, D. (2008). Assessment methods in human body composition. *Current Opinion in Clinical Nutrition and Metabolic Care, 11*, 566–572.

Levin, S., Martin, M. W., & Riner, W. F. (2004). TV viewing habits and body mass index among South Carolina Head Start children. *Ethnicity & Disease, 14*(3), 336–339.

Livingstone, M. B., & Black, A. E. (2003). Markers of the validity of reported energy intake. *Journal of Nutrition, 133*, 895S–920S.

Luft, V. C., Beghetto, M. G., Castro, S. M., & deMello, E. D. (2008). Validation of a new method developed to measure the height of adult patients in bed. *Nutrition in Clinical Practice, 23*, 424–428.

Miller, S. A., Taveras, E. M., Rifas-Shiman, S. L., & Gillman, M. W. (2008). Association between television viewing and poor diet quality in young children. *International Journal of Pediatric Obesity, 4*, 1–9.

Miller, T. M., Abdel-Maksoud, M. F., Crane, L. A., Marcus, A. C., & Byers, T. E. (2008). Effects of social approval bias on self-reported fruit and vegetable consumption: A randomized controlled study. *Nutrition Journal, 27*, 18.

Morrissey, S. L., Whetstone, L. M., Cummings, D. M., & Owen, L. J. (2006). Comparison of self-reported and measured height and weight in eighth grade students. *Journal of School Health, 76*, 512–515.

Mosdol, A., Erens, B., & Brunner, E. J. (2008). Estimated prevalence and predictors of vitamin C deficiency within U.K.'s low-income population. *Journal of Public Health, 30*, 456–460.

NANDA International. (2007). *NANDA-I nursing diagnosis: Definitions & classification 2007–2008*. Philadelphia: Author.

National Center for Health Statistics. (2007). *Health, United States, 2007: With chartbook on trends in the health of Americans*. Hyattsville, MD: U.S. Department of Health and Human Services.

National Heart, Lung, and Blood Institute (NHLBI). (n.d). *Guidelines on overweight and obesity: Electronic textbook*. Retrieved March 17, 2009, from http://www.nhlbi.nih.gov/guidelines/obesity/e_txtbk/index.htm

National Heart, Lung, and Blood Institutes (NHLBI), Obesity Education Initiative Expert Panel (1998). *Clinical guidelines on the identification, evaluation and treatment of overweight and obesity in adults: The evidence report*. Retrieved March 21, 2009, from http://www.nhlbi.nih.gov/guidelines/obesity/ob_gdlns.pdf

Nawaz, H., Chan, W., Abdulrahmann, M., Larson, D., & Katz, D. L. (2001). Self-reported weight and height: Implications for obesity research. *American Journal of Preventative Medicine, 20*, 294–298.

Nevitt, J. R., & Lundak, J. (2005). Accuracy of self-reports of alcohol offenders in a rural midwestern county. *Psychology Reports, 96*, 511–514.

Ng, D. K., Chan, C. H., Soo, M. T., & Lee, R. S. (2007). Low-level chronic mercury exposure in children and adolescents: Meta-analysis. *Pediatrics International, 49*, 80–87.

Norman, K., Pichard, C., Lochs, H., & Pirlich, M. (2008). Prognostic impact of disease-related malnutrition. *Clinical Nutrition, 27*, 5–15.

Nyholm, M., Gullberg, B., Merlo, J., Lundqvist-Persson, C., Rastam, L., & Lindblad, U. (2007). The validity of obesity based on self-reported weight and height: Implications for population studies. *Obesity (Silver Spring), 15*, 198–208.

Okamura, T., Hayakawa, T., Hozawa, A., Kadowaki, T., Murakami, Y., Kita, Y., et al. (2008). Lower levels of serum albumin and total cholesterol associated with decline in activities of daily living and excess mortality in a 12-year cohort study of elderly Japanese. *Journal of the American Geriatric Society, 56,* 529–535.

Omran, M. L., & Morley, J. E. (2000). Assessment of protein-energy malnutrition in older persons, part II: Laboratory evaluation. *Nutrition, 16,* 131–140.

Osterkamp, L. K. (1995). Current perspective on assessment of human body proportions of relevance to amputees. *Journal of the American Dietetic Association, 95,* 215–218.

Qato, D. M., Alexander, G. D., Conti, R. M., Johnson, M., Schumm, P., & Lindau, S. T. (2008). Use of prescription and over-the-counter medications and dietary supplements among older adults in the United States. *Journal of the American Medical Association, 300,* 2867–2878.

Robinson, M. K., Trujillo, E. B., Mogensen, K. M., Rounds, J., McManus, K., & Jacobs, O. (2003). Improving nutritional screening of hospitalized patients: The role of prealbumin. *Journal of Parenteral and Enteral Nutrition, 27,* 389–395.

Rodriguez, L. (2004). Nutritional status: Assessing and understanding its value in the critical care setting. *Critical Care Nursing Clinics of North America, 16*(4), 509–514.

Rossouw, K., Senekal, M., & Stander, I. (2001). The accuracy of self-reported weight by overweight and obese women in an outpatient setting. *Public Health Nutrition, 4,* 19–26.

Sahyoun, N. R., Jacques, P. F., Dallal, G. E., & Russell, R. M. (1997). Nutrition Screening Initiative checklist may be a better awareness/educational tool than a screening one. *Journal of the American Dietetic Association, 97,* 760–764.

Scagliusi, F. B., Ferriolli, E., Pfrimer, K., Laureano, C., Sanita Cunha, C., Gualano, B., et al. (2008). Underreporting of energy intake in Brazilian women varies according to dietary assessment: A cross-sectional study using doubly labeled water. *Journal of the American Dietetic Association, 108,* 2031–2040.

Seidel, S., Kreutzer, R., Smith, D., McNeel, S., & Gilliss, D. (2001). Assessment of commercial laboratories performing hair analysis. *Journal of the American Medical Association, 285,* 67–72.

Shenkin, A., Cederblad, G., Ellia, M., & Isaksson, B. (1996). Laboratory assessment of protein energy status. *Clinica Chimica Acta, 253,* S5–S59.

Singh, S. R., & Levine, M. A. (2006). Natural health product use in Canada: Analysis of the National Population Health Survey. *Canadian Journal of Clinical Pharmacology, 13,* e240–e250.

Spada, R. S., Toscano, G., Cosentino, F. I., Iero, I., Lanuzza, B., Tripodi, M., et al. (2007). Low total cholesterol predicts mortality in the nondemented oldest old. *Archives of Gerontology & Geriatrics, 44,* 381–384.

Spencer, E. A., Appleby, P. N., Davey, G. K., & Key, T. J. (2002). Validity of self-reported height and weight in 4808 EPIC-Oxford participants. *Public Health Nutrition, 5,* 561–565.

Steindel, S. J., & Howanitz, P. J. (2001). The uncertainties of hair analysis for trace metals. *Journal of the American Medical Association, 285,* 83–85.

Sullivan, D. H., Roberson, P. K., & Bopp, M. M. (2005). Hypoalbuminemia 3 months after hospital discharge: Significance for long-term survival. *Journal of the American Geriatric Society, 53,* 1222–1226.

Taveras, E. M., Sandora, T. J., Shih, M. C., Ross-Degnan, D., Goldmann, D. A., & Gillman, M. W. (2006). The association of television and video viewing with fast food intake by preschool-age children. *Obesity (Silver Spring), 14*(11), 2034–2041.

Taylor, A. W., Dal Grande, E., Gill, T. K., Chittleborough, C. R., Wilson, D. H., Adams, RJ., et al. (2006). How valid are self-reported height and weight? A comparison between CATI self-report and clinic measurements using a large cohort study. *Australia and New Zealand Journal of Public Health, 30,* 238–246.

Tokmakidis, S. P., Christodoulos, A. D., & Mantzouranis, N. I. (2007). Validity of self-reported anthropometric values used to assess body mass index and estimate obesity in Greek school children. *Journal of Adolescent Health, 40,* 305–310.

Tsigilis, N. (2006). Can secondary school students' self-reported measures of height and weight be trusted? An effect size approach. *European Journal of Public Health, 16*(5), 532–535.

United States Department of Health and Human Services (USDHHS), Maternal Child Health Bureau. (n.d.). *Accurately weighing and measuring infants, children and adolescents: Equipment.* Retrieved March 21, 2009, from http://depts .washington.edu/growth/index.htm

U.S. Department of Agriculture (USDA). (2005). *Dietary guidelines for Americans 2005* (6th ed.). Washington, DC: Author. (www .healthierus.gov/dietaryguidelines)

U.S. Department of Agriculture (USDA), Center for Nutrition Policy and Promotion. (2005). *MyPyramid food guidance system.* Washington, DC: Author. (www.mypyramid.gov)

U.S. Department of Health and Human Services, Public Health Service. (2000). *Healthy people 2010: National health promotion and disease prevention objectives.* Washington, DC: Author.

Wagner, D. R. & Heyward, V.H. (1999). Techniques of body composition assessment: A review of laboratory and field methods. *Research Quarterly for Exercise and Sport, 70,* 135–149.

Walker, S., & Cosden, M. (2007). Reliability of college student self-reported drinking behavior. *Journal of Substance Abuse Treatment, 33,* 405–409.

Wang, Z., Patterson, C. M., & Hills, A. P., (2002). A comparison of self-reported and measured height, weight and BMI in Australian adolescents. *Australia and New Zealand Journal of Public Health, 26,* 473–478.

Wen, C. P., David Cheng, T. Y., Tsai, S. P., Chan, H. T., Hsu, H. L., Hsu, C. C., et al. (2009). Are Asians at greater mortality risk for being overweight than Caucasians? Redefining obesity for Asians. *Public Health Nutrition, 12,* 497–506.

Willett, W. C., Dietz, W. K., & Colditz, G. A. (1999). Guidelines for healthy weight. *New England Journal of Medicine, 341,* 427–434.

Williams, G., & Keir, B. (2008). MUST scoring—a 'must' or a waste of nursing time? *British Journal of Nursing (BJN), 17*(10), 622–624.

Woodrow, G. (2009). Body composition analysis techniques in the aged adult: Indications and limitations. *Current Opinion in Clinical Nutrition and Metabolic Care, 12,* 8–14.

World Health Organization (WHO). (1999). *Management of malnutrition: A manual for physicians and other senior healthcare workers.* Retrieved February 28, 2005, from http://www.who.int/ nutrition/publications/severemalnutrition/en/manage_severe_ malnutrition_eng.pdf

Zhang, C., Rexrode, K. M., van Dam, R. M., Li, T. Y., & Hu, F. B. (2008). Abdominal obesity and the risk of all-cause, cardiovascular, and cancer mortality: Sixteen years of follow-up on U.S. women. *Circulation, 117,* 1658–1667.

CHAPTER 24

CHAPTER OBJECTIVES

After reading this chapter you will be able to:

1. Define medical nutrition therapy and how it is used as part of comprehensive health care.

2. Describe the Nutrition Care Process and its four steps.

3. List the diseases and conditions for which medical nutrition therapy can be provided.

4. Explain how nursing plays a central role in overseeing nutrition care.

5. Describe the different types of texture-modified diets and the indications for their use.

6. Discuss the situations when oral nutrition supplements may be appropriate.

7. Describe when liberalizing a therapeutic diet may be warranted.

8. Identify key elements of diets used to treat disease, including purpose, indications for use, foods recommended and not allowed, and special considerations.

TEST YOURSELF TRUE OR FALSE?

1. Modifications to food and nutrient intake are among the least expensive and safest means to prevent and treat disease. T or F

2. Texture-modified diets are typically inadequate in nutrients. T or F

3. If a client has a chronic poor appetite, a therapeutic diet order can be liberalized to encourage improved intake. T or F

4. Sugar-containing foods should be strictly avoided in the diet for diabetes. T or F

5. In the treatment of hypertension, an eating plan reduced in saturated fat, total fat, cholesterol, and sodium with plenty of fruits, vegetables, and low-fat dairy products and nuts is recommended. T or F

Test Yourself answers can be found at the end of the chapter.

Diet Therapy in Disease Management

the process of nutrition care involves the assessment of an individual's nutrition status followed by the planning, implementation, and monitoring of customized goals and objectives that are targeted at optimizing health as outlined in the previous chapter. The nutrition care of a client in acute, subacute, long-term care, or community settings follows this same process and includes goals that are aimed at the role nutrition plays in any acute process occurring during hospitalization as well as long-term goals.

Nutrition care that encompasses the assessment and treatment of any disease, condition, or illness is referred to as **medical nutrition therapy** (MNT). MNT is an essential component of comprehensive health care, defined in the 2001 Medicare benefit legislation as "nutritional diagnositic, therapy, and counseling services for the purpose of disease management, which are furnished by a registered dietitian (RD) or nutrition professional" (Medicare, 2001). Thus, treatment may include nutrition therapy with a modified diet, nutrition education, and provision of specialized nutrition support with oral nutrition supplements, tube feedings, or intravenous nutrition. Nutrition intervention and counseling has been shown to significantly improve weight, body mass index, hemoglobin A1c, blood pressure, and serum lipid levels (ADA EAL). Because all individuals must ingest food and nutrients to survive, modifications to food and nutrient intake are among the least expensive and safest means to prevent and treat disease (ADA, 2010). In most health care settings, the nurse collaborates with the nutrition professional to ensure that optimal nutrition care is provided.

Excerpts taken from: *Nutrition and Diet Therapy for Nurses,* by Sheila Buckley Tucker and Vera Dauffenbach

The health and quality of life in individuals with a variety of conditions and illnesses can be improved when MNT is provided (ADA, 2010). Medical nutrition therapy includes:

1. Performing a comprehensive nutrition assessment to determine the nutrition diagnosis;

2. Planning and implementing a nutrition intervention using evidence-based nutrition practice guidelines;

3. Monitoring and evaluating an individual's progress over subsequent visits with a registered dietitian (RD).

Overview of the Nutrition Care Process

Similar to the Nursing Process, registered dietitians use the Nutrition Care Process (NCP), which is a systematic approach to provide high quality nutrition care. Medical nutrition therapy is a specific application of the NCP in clinical settings that is focused on the management of diseases. MNT involves in-depth individualized nutrition assessment and identifying duration and frequency of care using the NCP to manage disease. NCP also includes other forms of nutrition care, such as obtaining feeding assistance or referring to another practitioner. The NCP consists of four distinct, interrelated steps:

- **Nutrition Assessment:** This involves collection and documentation of information such as food or nutrition-related history; biochemical data, medical tests and procedures; anthropometric measurements, nutrition-focused physical findings and client history.

- **Diagnosis:** Data collected during the nutrition assessment guides the practitioner in selection of the appropriate nutrition diagnosis (i.e., naming the specific problem).

In 2002, MNT became a covered service through Medicare; however, coverage was limited to diabetes and renal disease until Congress could collect more data on other conditions that could benefit from nutrition counseling. In 2006, the Ryan White Treatment and Modernization Act included MNT as a core medical service. Also in 2006, the Older Americans Act (OAA) was enhanced by including nutrition screening, counseling and education for OAA meal recipients.

However, the current limitation on the MNT benefit in Medicare negatively impacts many of these and other government and private health-care programs. For example, home-health programs cannot reimburse for the services of a dietitian and the home-health company must pay for all administrative fees. In addition, coverage of intensive nutrition counseling could benefit millions of Americans by helping to prevent or delay onset of diseases such as type 2 diabetes and cardiovascular disease. This would not only improve the lives of Americans, but could potentially save the government millions of dollars. It is estimated that 57 million Americans are at risk for developing diabetes—a disease that costs the U.S. over $174 billion each year. These costs may be reduced with proper nutrition intervention programs.

MNT and other nutrition services can be provided for a variety of diseases and conditions including:

- Diabetes: Type 1, Type 2, Gestational
- Renal Disease: insufficiency, chronic failure, transplantation
- Cardiovascular Diseases: hypertension, dyslipidemia, congestive heart failure
- Pulmonary Disease: COPD
- Weight Management: overweight/obesity, bariatric surgery, eating disorders
- Oncology: optimize oral intake to improve treatment outcomes
- Women's Health: pregnancy, osteoporosis, anemia
- Immunocompromise: food allergy, HIV/AIDS
- Pediatrics: infant/child feeding, failure-to-thrive, inborn errors of metabolism
- Nutritional Support: oral, enteral, parenteral
- GI Disorders: celiac disease, cirrhosis, Crohn's disease
- Disease Prevention: general wellness

FIGURE 24.1 History and application of medical nutrition therapy.

Source: American Dietetic Association, www.eatright.org

- **Intervention:** The practitioner then selects the nutrition intervention that will be directed to the root cause (or etiology) of the nutrition problem and aimed at alleviating the signs and symptoms of the diagnosis.

- **Monitoring/Evaluation:** The final step of the process is monitoring and evaluation, which is used to determine if the patient/client has achieved, or is making progress toward, the planned goals.

Using the NCP, dietitians can individualize care, taking into account the patient's needs and values and using the best evidence available to make decisions. In 2003, the American Dietetic Association adopted the NCP to provide dietetics professionals with a framework for critical thinking and decision-making—leading to more efficient and effective care and greater recognition of the role of dietetic professionals in all care settings.

The Nutrition Care Process is represented as a circle in the Nutrition Care Model. This graphic visualization illustrates the steps of the Nutrition Care Process as well as internal and external factors that impact application of the NCP (see FIGURE 24.2). Although the Nutrition Care Process may seem like a linear approach, the circular depiction shows that new or changing information at any time can lead to re-assessment or re-diagnosis, with subsequent alterations in the intervention and monitoring.

The Nutrition Care Process

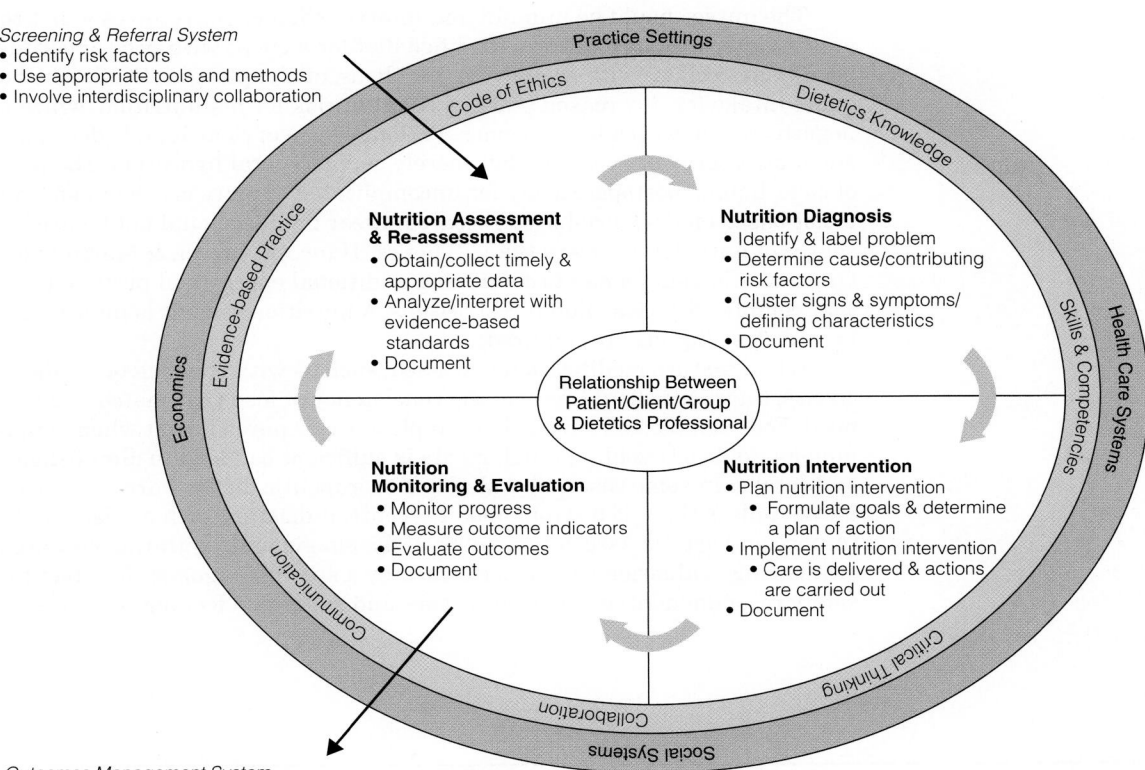

Courtesy of American Dietetic Association.

FIGURE 24.2 The central component of the Model is the relationship of the target patient, client, or group and the dietetics professional. The inner ring illustrates the four steps of the NCP, while the middle ring represents the skills and abilities of the RD along with application of evidence-based practice, Code of Ethics, and knowledge. The outer ring represents environmental factors such as healthcare systems, socioeconomics and practice settings that impact the ability of the target group or client to benefit from RD services. Screening and referral and outcomes management are also components of the model.

Therapeutic Diets

Nursing plays a central role in overseeing nutrition care because of the central nursing position on the health care team and the concentrated involvement of the nurse in direct client care. Nutrition care is part of the nursing process in all health care settings. Therefore, it is essential for nurses to understand the purpose, indications for use, specific foods allowed or not allowed, and special considerations for therapeutic diets. Therapeutic diets can include texture modified diets or diets that allow only specific foods based on disease or condition. Nurses also must be aware of special meal assistance needs of clients to help ensure optimal intake of meals (FIGURE 24.3).

A variety of normal and therapeutic diets are prescribed in health care settings. The diet order is typically placed during admission. The order may be written by the admitting physician, or a nurse or registered dietitian may place the initial diet order until a nutrition assessment is performed to determine if a modified diet is required. A regular or house diet does not restrict intake of any nutrient, food group, or consistency of food. Other types of diets can alter the texture and types of foods provided based on a client's nutritional or physical needs. An outline of nutrition services and detailed information on normal and therapeutic diets used in a health care setting is available in each institution's diet manual. Some may refer to the diet manual as a nutrition practice manual. Hospital protocols for nutrition practices, including specialized nutrition support, would be included in the manual. Table 24.1 outlines common acute and long-term care diets that are modified in texture or food consistency.

The nurse should be mindful and intervene if a client receives a diet that is not appropriate, such as an overly modified diet for a client with poor appetite or a regular diet for a client with swallowing problems, or **dysphagia.** Diminished or inadequate intake for any reason places a client at risk for malnutrition, which can negatively impact health outcomes. Prolonged use of clear liquids does not provide adequate energy or nutrients but merely serves as oral hydration. The prescription of clear liquids postoperatively for uncomplicated surgery is a common practice but is not based on evidence-based research. Clear liquids should not be used as the sole source of nutrition for more than 72 hours (Hancock, Cresci, & Martindale 2002). Oral nutrition supplements containing additional energy and protein are available that comply with clear liquid restrictions. A nutrition consult is indicated when prolonged clear liquids are required.

When texture modification is needed, such as with chewing or swallowing difficulties, the client should receive the consistency of food that matches their assessed need. For example, offering a client applesauce or pureed meat when simply chopping an apple or avoiding tough meats is sufficient can lead to diminished appetite and intake. In some cases, liberalizing a therapeutic diet is warranted to optimize intake unless there is a strong medical contraindication such as risk for choking (American Dietetic Association 2005). If dysphagia and aspiration risk are present, a swallowing evaluation can be performed by a speech language therapist to determine safety recommendations on food texture and suggested feeding practices.

Within health care institutions, the style of food service delivery varies. Services range from hotel-style room service to traditional predetermined meals served at specific times with minimal client choice. A selective menu is offered by many health care institutions, allowing the client to choose among foods permitted by the diet prescription. Selective menus help optimize intake by allowing the client to make food choices.

The nurse should assess whether a client has any barriers that could interfere with filling out this type of menu, such as vision difficulties, illiteracy, or inability to understand the language used on the menu. Cultural food practices could leave some clients unable to decipher unfamiliar foods offered. Appropriate assistance should be provided. Some food service departments have menus available in a variety of languages to assist in meal selection.

FIGURE 24.3 Food service styles and meal assistance.

TABLE 24.1   Common Texture-Modified Diets

Diet	Use	Foods Allowed	Foods Not Allowed	Nutritional Adequacy and Advice
Regular or House	General diet for those not requiring texture or nutrient modification	All	None	Adequate if consumed as offered.
Clear Liquids	Hydration Bowel preparation for some procedures Transition to solid food from nil per os (NPO)	See-through items liquid at room temperature Clear juices—cranberry, apple, grape Clear drinks—fruit punch, sodas (ginger ale, lemon-lime, etc.), plain tea, black coffee Broth, bouillon Gelatin Popsicles, ices Hard candy, honey	Opaque liquids Solid food	Inadequate in all nutrients and low in energy. Consider nutrition supplementation to diet in at-risk clients. Monitor length of time on diet and consult nutrition team if 5 days or more.
Full Liquids	Chewing or swallowing difficulties	Foods liquid or pourable at room temperature Juices Dairy or dairy alternative—beverages, ice cream, yogurt Custard, pudding Hot cereal Liquid oral nutrition supplements All clear liquid items	Solid foods Liquid at room temperature foods with added solids (e.g., ice cream w/nuts or fruit)	Nutritionally adequate when supplements consumed. If dysphagia and aspiration risk are present, consult speech language therapist for swallowing evaluation and safety recommendations on food texture. High lactose content can be lowered w/use of dairy alternatives. High-fat and low-fiber content for prolonged use.
Mechanical or Dental Soft	Chewing or swallowing difficulties	Liquids Minced, soft, chopped or ground food: Proteins—poultry, fish w/o bones, cooked beans, eggs, chopped or cut meats w/o casings or grizzle, sauces added for moisture as needed Grains—all except as noted Fruit and vegetables—soft, peeled, cooked, or canned as tolerated Desserts on full liquid diet or as tolerated	Whole nuts Seeds Meat with casings (hotdogs, sausage) Tough meats Hard crusted bread Fruits/vegetables with edible skin Raw vegetables	Nutritionally adequate if all food groups consumed; can be low fiber. Customize texture modification to minimum amount that meets client needs. Avoid overmodification. If dysphagia and aspiration risk are present, consult speech language therapist for swallowing evaluation and safety recommendations on food texture.
Pureed	Advanced chewing or swallowing difficulties	Blenderized or pureed foods Any food allowed that can be pureed to a custard-like consistency w/o solids remaining Liquids can be added to yield desired consistency	Whole nuts Seeds Hard bread/rolls Dried fruit Fruits/vegetable skin Any food that cannot be pureed to a smooth consistency	Nutritionally adequate. Customize texture modification to minimum amount that meets client needs. Avoid overmodification. Essential food is presented in attractive manner to stimulate appetite (e.g., molds, garnishes, parfait presentation). Refrain from commenting on unappealing appearance of diet if providing feeding assistance.

Low-Fat, Low-Cholesterol Diet (also known as Heart Healthy Diet, or TLC Diet)

Indications for Use

A low-fat, low-cholesterol diet may be prescribed for:

- hypercholesterolemia, or high levels of total blood cholesterol and/or LDL-cholesterol
- following myocardial infarction (heart attack)
- following coronary artery bypass graft (CABG) or angioplasty

Current nutrition guidelines maintain that dietary intervention be incorporated into both primary and secondary prevention of cardiovascular disease (CVD) through a multifactorial lifestyle approach termed therapeutic lifestyle changes (TLC) (NCEP 2002). Primary prevention refers to delaying or preventing onset of coronary heart disease and secondary prevention refers to preventing recurrant coronary events or death in those with existing heart disease.

Description of the Diet

The National Cholesterol Education Program (NCEP) of the National Heart, Lung, and Blood Institute (NHLBI) issues national guidelines for detecting, evaluating, and treating hypercholesterolemia. In the NCEP guidelines, dietary manipulation is considered to be the cornerstone of management of high levels of LDL ("bad") cholesterol (NCEP 2002). The TLC diet is recommended by NCEP and the American Heart Association, and replaces the previous Step I and Step II diets.

Because control of blood cholesterol is the primary target, the focus of the diet is on reducing intake of dietary saturated fats, trans fats, and cholesterol, and increasing intake of dietary fiber and omega-3 fats (heart healthy fats). Control of calories to achieve or maintain a healthy weight is also a component of the diet. Specific types of fats in food can affect levels of LDL cholesterol and HDL ("good") cholesterol in different ways (Table 24.2). Dietary goals for the TLC diet are presented in Table 24.3.

Overall recommendations for the TLC Diet (or Heart Healthy or Low-Fat/Low-Cholesterol Diet) are as follows (ADA Nutrition Care Manual, 2009). See Table 24.4 for specific food lists.

Limit saturated fats and trans fats.

- Foods high in saturated fats include fatty meat, poultry skin, bacon, sausage, whole milk, cream, and butter.
- Trans fats are found in stick margarine, shortening, some fried foods, and packaged foods made with hydrogenated oils.
- Replace butter or stick margarine with reduced-fat, whipped, or liquid spreads.

TABLE 24.2   Effects of Dietary Fats on LDL-Cholesterol and HDL-Cholesterol Levels

Fat	LDL Cholesterol	HDL Cholesterol
Saturated	↑	Modest ↑
Polyunsaturated	↓	Modest ↑ or No change
Cis-Monounsaturated	Modest ↓ or No change	Modest ↑ or No change
Trans-Monounsaturated	↑	↓

Sources: Mensink, 2005; NCEP ATP III, 2002; Woodside & Krombhout, 2005.

TABLE 24.3   Dietary Goals for the TLC Diet

Nutrient	Recommended Intake
Energy	Adequate calories to lose or maintain weight
Total Dietary Fat	25–35% of total calories
Saturated Fat	Less than 7% of total calories
Polyunsaturated Fat	Up to 10% of total calories
Monounsaturated Fat	Up to 20% of total calories
Carbohydrate	50–60% of total calories
Total Dietary Fiber	20–30 grams per day
Viscous fiber	10–25 grams per day
Protein	Approximately 15% of total calories
Dietary Cholesterol	Less than 200 mg per day

Source: NCEP Adult Treatment Panel III, 2002.

Limit the amount of cholesterol to less than 200 milligrams (mg) per day.

- Foods high in cholesterol include egg yolks (one egg yolk has about 212 mg of cholesterol), fatty meat, whole milk, cheese, shrimp, lobster, and crab.

Eat more omega-3 fats (heart-healthy fats):

- Good choices include salmon, tuna, mackerel, and sardines. Aim to eat fish twice a week.
- Other foods with omega-3 fats include walnuts and canola and soybean oils.
- Flaxseed is another source of omega-3 fats, include it as flaxseed oil or ground flaxseed.

Limit the total amount of fat (including heart-healthy fats) to 25% to 35% of total calories. For example, in a 2,000-calorie diet, fat intake can be between 50 grams (g) and 75 g per day.

Include 20 g to 30 g of dietary fiber per day:

- Fruits, vegetables, whole grains, and dried beans are good sources of fiber; aim for 5 cups of fruits and vegetables per day.
- Include at least 3 ounces (oz) of whole grain foods every day.

Eat more plant-based meals, using beans and soy foods for protein.

Set goals to reach and maintain a healthy weight.

Include at least 30 minutes of physical activity on most days.

Carbohydrate-Controlled Diet (also known as Diet for Diabetes)

Indications for Use

A carbohydrate-controlled diet may be prescribed for:

- Pre-diabetes
- Type 1 and type 2 diabetes
- Gestational diabetes (diabetes during pregnancy)
- Metabolic syndrome

TABLE 24.4   Food Lists for Low-Fat, Low-Cholesterol Diet

Food Group	Recommended Foods	Foods Not Recommended
Grains	Whole grain breads and cereals, including oats and barley	High-fat bakery products, such as doughnuts, biscuits, croissants, danish pastries, pies, cookies
	Pasta, especially whole wheat or other whole grain types	Snacks made with partially hydrogenated oils, including chips, cheese puffs, snack mixes, regular crackers, butter-flavored popcorn
	Brown rice	
	Low-fat crackers and pretzels	
Vegetables	Fresh, frozen, or canned vegetables without added fat or salt	Fried vegetables
		Vegetables prepared with butter, cheese, or cream sauce
Fruits	Fresh, frozen, canned, or dried fruit	Fried fruits
		Fruits served with butter or cream
Milk	Nonfat (skim), low-fat, or 1%-fat milk or buttermilk	Whole Milk
	Nonfat or low-fat yogurt or cottage cheese	2% fat milk
	Fat-free and low-fat cheese	Whole milk yogurt or ice cream
		Cream
		Half-&-half
		Cream cheese
		Sour cream
		Cheese
Meat and Other Protein Foods	Lean cuts of beef and pork (loin, leg, round, extra lean hamburger)	Higher-fat cuts of meats (ribs, t-bone steak, regular hamburger)
	Skinless poultry	Bacon
	Fish	Sausage
	Venison and other wild game	Cold cuts, such as salami or bologna
	Dried beans and peas	Corned beef
	Nuts and nut butters	Hot dogs
	Meat alternatives made with soy or textured vegetable protein	Organ meat (liver, brains, sweetbreads)
	Egg whites or egg substitute	Poultry with skin
	Cold cuts made with lean meat or soy protein	Fried meat, poultry, and fish
		Whole eggs, and egg yolks
Fats and Oils	Unsaturated oils (olive, peanut, soy, sunflower, canola)	Butter
	Soft or liquid margarines and vegetable oil spreads	Stick margarine
	Salad dressings	Shortening
	Seeds and nuts	Partially hydrogenated oils
	Avocado	Tropical oils (coconut, palm, palm kernel oils)

Source: ADA Nutrition Care Manual, 2009.

Treatment of diabetes involves a multifactorial approach to prevent complications associated with high and low levels of blood glucose. Diet is a cornerstone of treatment, along with weight loss as needed, a diet that follows recommendations for reducing risk for cardiovascular disease risk, and regular physical activity. The American Diabetes Association recommends a weight loss of 5% to 10% of body weight if overweight and at least 150 minutes/week of moderate activity (American Diabetes Association 2009).

Description of the Diet

The diet for diabetes is a general heart-healthy diet with emphasis on controlling intake of carbohydrates (CHO). CHO and mono-unsaturated fats should comprise 60% to 70% of the total calories in the diet (American Diabetes Association 2008). In the past, the term "ADA Diet" was used along with a specific calorie level to denote a set distribution of CHO, fat, and protein in the diet that was believed to be ideal for all people with diabetes (American Diabetes Association 2008). Current recommendations are individualized based on the client's needs. Monitoring CHO intake, whether by CHO counting, exchanges, or experience-based estimation, is a key strategy in achieving glycemic control. Sugar-containing foods are allowed in moderation and can be substituted for other carbohydrates in the meal plan, but care should be taken to avoid excess intake.

The first step in prescribing the diet is to calculate CHO recommendations. This involves estimating total energy needs and allotting half of the calories to CHO in the diet, calculated based on 1 gram of CHO having 4 calories. The CHOs are then divided between three meals and any snacks. FIGURE 24.4 outlines an example of these calculations.

An approach known as "carbohydrate counting" is most often used to determine food choices that contain CHO, which will have a direct effect on blood glucose levels. The amounts of CHOs consumed are balanced with insulin or oral medications to control blood glucose levels. Foods with CHOs include:

- Breads, crackers, and cereals
- Pasta, rice, and grains

A client with diabetes is estimated to need 2,400 calories/day. What is the recommendation for carbohydrate intake?

1. **Multiply calorie requirement by recommended range of carbohydrate intake:**

   2,400 calories × 50% carbohydrate calories = 1,200 total carbohydrate calories

2. **Divide total carbohydrate calories by calories/gm carbohydrate:**

   1,200 total carbohydrate calories ÷ 4 calories/ gm carbohydrate = 300 gm carbohydrate

3. **Divide carbohydrate intake over the day into the appropriate amount of meals and snacks:**

   300 gm of carbohydrate can be divided into three meals with 100 gm of carbohydrate each if no snacks are consumed.

   OR

   If two snacks with 30 gm of carbohydrate each are consumed, the amount of carbohydrate/meal is lowered to 80 gm each.

4. **For the client using the "carbohydrate choice," each set portion of food with 15 gm of carbohydrate is one choice. Divide total carbohydrate grams by 15 gm per carbohydrate choice:**

   300 gm total carbohydrate per day ÷ 15 gm carbohydrate per choice = 20 carbohydrate choices/day. These choices should be distributed over the day. The client must know correct portion that equals 15 gm of carbohydrate for each food.

FIGURE 24.4 Calculating carbohydrates.

- Starchy vegetables, such as potatoes, corn, and peas
- Beans and legumes
- Milk, soy milk, and yogurt
- Fruits and fruit juices
- Sweets, such as cakes, cookies, ice cream, jam, and jelly

In CHO counting, a defined serving of a food with CHO has about 15 grams of CHO. Table 24.5 lists the specific servings of foods that contain 15 grams of CHO, which are often referred to as a CHO serving or a "carbohydrate choice." A person

TABLE 24.5   Food Lists for Carbohydrate Counting

1 serving = about 15 grams of carbohydrate

Starches

- 1 slice bread (1 ounce)
- 1 tortilla (6-inch size)
- ¼ large bagel (1 ounce)
- 2 taco shells (5-inch size)
- ½ hamburger or hot dog bun (1 ounce)
- ¾ cup ready-to-eat cereal
- ½ cup cooked cereal
- 1 cup broth-based soup

- ⅓ cup pasta or rice (cooked)
- ½ cup beans, peas, corn, sweet potatoes, winter squash, or mashed or boiled potatoes (cooked)
- ¼ large baked potato (3 ounces)
- ¾ ounce pretzels, potato chips, or tortilla chips
- 3 cups popcorn (popped)
- 4–6 small crackers

Fruit

- 1 small fresh fruit (4 ounces)
- ½ cup canned fruit
- ¼ cup dried fruit (2 tablespoons)
- 17 small grapes (3 ounces)

- 1 cup melon or berries
- 2 tablespoons raisins
- ½ cup fruit juice

Milk

- 1 cup fat-free or reduced-fat milk
- 1 cup soy milk

- ⅔ cup (6 ounces) fat-free yogurt sweetened with sugar-free sweetener

Sweets and Desserts

- 2-inch square cake (unfrosted)
- 2 small cookies (⅔ ounce)
- ½ cup ice cream or frozen yogurt
- ¼ sherbet or sorbet

- 1 tablespoon syrup, jam, jelly, table sugar, or honey
- 2 tablespoons light syrup

Other Foods

- Count 1 cup raw vegetables or ½ cup cooked nonstarchy vegetables as zero carbohydrate serving or "free" foods. If you eat 3 or more servings at one meal, count them as 1 carbohydrate serving.

- Foods that have less than 20 calories in each serving also may be counted as zero carbohydrate servings or "free" foods.

- Count 1 cup of casserole or other mixed foods as 2 carbohydrate servings.

Source: ADA Nutrition Care Manual, 2009.

with diabetes is allowed a specific number of CHO servings per meal or snack, which allows for flexibility in making food selections. For many adults, eating 3 to 5 servings, or choices, of CHO foods at each meal and 1 or 2 CHO servings for each snack works well. The amount of 'total carbohydrates' on food labels can be used to determine the number of CHO servings consumed from packaged foods. In advanced CHO counting, an individual can learn to match insulin dosage to the total amount of CHOs consumed at a meal or snack, also referred to as insulin-to-carbohydrate ratio. However, this requires a high level of knowledge and motivation.

An alternative method of determining CHO intake utilizes a system of food exchanges. This involves calculating the total calories and grams of CHO per day and then establishing a recommended meal plan based on work habits, lifestyle, food preferences, medication scheduling, and other factors. The meal plan specifies the servings of food from each food group allowed at each meal. There is less flexibility with this system, but this approach works well for individuals who prefer an established meal plan that does not require counting CHOs.

In the exchange system, foods are divided into three groups based on the three major nutrients: carbohydrates, protein (meat and meat substitutes), and fats. Within the CHO group, the meal plan will designate the number of starches, fruits, milk, sweets and desserts, and non-starchy vegetables allowed per meal and snack. Specific food lists for each food grouping are then used by the client to select foods for each meal or snack. Each food list contains foods grouped together because they have similar nutrient content and serving sizes. Table 24.6 shows the amounts of nutrients in 1 serving from each list. Foods within each list can be "exchanged" to allow flexibility, but the number of servings from each group at meals and snacks must follow the established meal plan. Complete food lists are available in the education booklet, *Choose Your Foods: Exchanges Lists for Diabetes* (American Diabetes Association, American Dietetic Association 2008).

TABLE 24.6 Nutrients in Foods in the Exchange Lists for Diabetes

Food List	Carbohydrate (grams)	Protein (grams)	Fat (grams)	Calories
Carbohydrates				
Starch: breads, cereals and grains, starchy vegetables, crackers, snacks, and beans, peas, and lentils	15	0–3	0–1	80
Fruits	15	—	—	60
Milk				
Fat-free, low fat, 1%	12	8	0–3	100
Reduced-fat, 2%	12	8	5	120
Whole	12	8	8	160
Sweets, Desserts, and Other Carbohydrates	15	varies	varies	varies
Nonstarchy Vegetables	5	2	—	25
Meat and Meat Substitutes				
Lean	—	7	0–3	45
Medium-fat	—	7	4–7	75
High-fat	—	7	8+	100
Plant-based proteins	varies	7	varies	varies
Fats	—	—	5	45
Alcohol	varies	—	—	100

Source: Choose Your Foods: Exchanges Lists for Diabetes. American Diabetes Association, American Dietetic Association, 2008.

Sodium-Controlled Diet

Indications for Use

A sodium-controlled diet may be used for:

- Hypertension
- Heart failure
- Kidney disease
- Other conditions involving swelling or fluid retention

A sodium-controlled diet can help to prevent build up of fluid in the body and reduce blood pressure. The general recommendation for daily sodium intake is 2,400 milligrams per day, however, some experts recommend sodium intake as low as 1,500 mg for the general population. As a therapeutic diet to lower blood pressure or prevent fluid retention, sodium is typically reduced to a range of 1,500 to 2,000 mg per day. Lifestyle modifications, such as improving dietary quality, managing weight, and participating in physical activity, are recommended for the prevention and treatment of hypertension.

Description of the Diet

For treatment of hypertension, a specific type of sodium-controlled diet called the DASH Diet (Dietary Approaches to Stop Hypertension) may be prescribed. In the DASH clinical trial sponsored by NHLBI, an eating plan reduced in saturated fat, total fat, cholesterol, and sodium with plenty of fruits, vegetables, and low-fat dairy products and inclusion of nuts, was effective in reducing elevated blood pressure. In a follow-up trial, a DASH diet at two levels of sodium, 1,500 and 2,400 mg/day, were studied (Sacks et al. 2001). The greatest blood pressure reductions occurred on the DASH diet that was limited to 1,500 mg of sodium per day. Persons with pre-hypertension or hypertension had lower blood pressure while consuming this dietary pattern with reduced sodium levels.

The DASH Eating Plan incorporates reduction in sodium; inclusion of fruits, vegetables, and whole grains; and limitation of fats consistent with Therapeutic Lifestyle Changes (TLC) to lower blood cholesterol (NIH, NHLBI 2006). It provides an eating pattern that is high in potassium, calcium, magnesium, and fiber, while limiting sodium to levels between 1,500 mg and 2,400 mg per day. For a 2,000-calorie diet, the servings for the food groups are as follows:

- Seven to eight servings of grains daily, three of which are whole grains
- Four to five servings of fruits daily
- Four to five servings of vegetables daily
- Two to three servings of low-fat or nonfat dairy daily
- Two or fewer servings of lean meat, fish, or poultry daily
- Four to five servings of nuts, seeds, legumes weekly
- Limited fats and sweets

In addition to the DASH Eating Plan, the 7th Report of the Joint National Treatment of High Blood Pressure also provides the following lifestyle modification guidelines to manage hypertension (Chobanian et al. 2003):

- Maintain normal body weight (body mass index, 18.5 kg/m^2 to 24.9 kg/m^2). Weight loss of 10 kg can result in an approximate systolic blood pressure reduction of 5 mm Hg to 20 mm Hg.
- Engage in regular aerobic physical activity such as brisk walking (at least 30 minutes per day, most days of the week) to lower systolic blood pressure approximately 4 mm Hg to 9 mm Hg.
- Limit consumption of alcohol to no more than two drinks (1 oz, or 30 mL, of ethanol, for example, 24 oz of beer, 10 oz of wine, or 3 oz of 80-proof whiskey) per day in most men and to no more than one drink per day in women and lighter-weight persons

A diet that focuses solely on limiting sodium is based on understanding the following principles (ADA Nutrition Care Manual, 2009). Table 24.7 shows a meal plan with recommended foods and other foods to limit or avoid for following a 2,000 mg sodium diet.

TABLE 24.7   2,000 mg Sodium Diet

Food Groups	Best Choices	Limit or Avoid
Milk/Dairy (2 servings/day) • One serving has ~150 mg	Milk (1 cup) Yogurt (1 cup) Low sodium cheese (1 oz) Ice Cream (1 cup) Chocolate milk (1 cup) Cottage cheese, dry—non creamed Hard cheese like cheddar, Swiss, Monterey jack, mozzarella (1 oz—150-200 mg)	Buttermilk (1 cup—300 mg) no other dairy foods if you drink 1 cup buttermilk Cottage cheese (1/2 cup—450 mg); wash it under cold water in a sieve to remove most of the sodium Cheese spread (2 Tbs—600 mg) Processed cheese (1 oz—375 mg)
Meat/Protein (Servings/day: 1 egg and two 3-oz servings of meat) • One serving has 60 mg	Plain meats, fish, and poultry are very low in sodium (~60 mg for 3 oz cooked meat). However, many raw meats now have added broth with sodium salts that make the meat hold moisture and taste juicy and tender. Read all meat labels! Choose a product with less than 5% of the DV for sodium. Eggs (1 large—60 g sodium)	Lunch meat (1 oz bologna—300 mg) Sausage (1 oz—360 mg) Deli ham (1 oz—360 mg) *Bacon (1 medium strip—127 mg) Turkey dark meat (4 oz "basted"—350 mg)
Vegetables & Fruit • One serving has only about 10 mg	All unsalted fresh, frozen, or canned Tomato or vegetable juice canned without salt (6 oz—20 mg) Tomatoes, tomato sauce canned without salt Fresh, frozen, canned fruits Fruit juices	Tomato juice (6 oz —490 mg) Sauerkraut (1/2 cup—470 mg) Pickled vegetables No need to avoid any fruit—all are very low in sodium
Bread and Cereals (5 Servings/day) • One serving has ~150 mg	These foods have almost no sodium and do not need to be counted in the 5 servings per day: • shredded or puffed wheat, puffed rice • cooked cereals—regular or quick • plain rice or pasta • yeast bread made at home with no salt Other ready-to-eat cereals with more than 5% DV for sodium—serving size is ½ cup (1 cup = 2 of your 5 servings/day) 1 oz bread, roll, pita, tortilla, crackers	Instant hot cereals (1 cup cooked instant oatmeal—420 mg sodium) Ready-to-eat cereal (read label and choose less than 5% DV for sodium) Quick breads made with baking powder or baking soda (biscuit, pancake, waffle, muffin, etc.) Crackers with salted tops
Desserts and Others	Fruit (trace sodium) Ice cream (50 mg sodium in ½ cup) Sherbet (90 mg sodium in 1 cup) Homemade pie made without salt Homemade pudding (count as milk serving) Unsalted nuts Butter or margarine (30–50 mg/tsp); buy the unsalted kind as it has almost no sodium	Commercial dessert mixes Cake (1 slice white, chocolate or angel food—250 to 300 mg) Pie (varies—up to 350 mg) Instant pudding (4 oz—320 mg)

If you follow this diet strictly and avoid processed foods, the sodium content will be about 1500 mg/day. This will allow you to have about 1/8 tsp table salt to season your food. Use "lite" salt and you may have ¼ tsp.

Source: ADA Nutrition Care Manual, 2009.

TABLE 24.7 *2,000 mg Sodium Diet (continued)*

The following should be avoided on a 2,000 mg Sodium Diet:

Salt—¼ teaspoon of table salt has almost 600 milligrams sodium. This is over ¼ of the amount allowed each day. If the diet is followed *strictly*, ⅛ teaspoon may be used to season food.

Processed foods

Salt is added in large amounts to some regular foods. Examples are:

- canned foods: soups, stews, sauces, gravy mixes, and some vegetables
- frozen foods: dinners, entrees, vegetables with sauces
- snack foods: salted chips, popcorn, pretzels, pork rinds and crackers
- packaged starchy foods: seasoned noodle or rice dishes, stuffing mix, macaroni and cheese dinner
- instant cooking foods to which you add hot water and stir: potatoes, cereals, noodles, etc.
- mixes: cornbread, biscuit, cake, pudding
- meats and cheeses
  - deli or lunch meats: bologna, ham, turkey, roast beef, etc.
  - cured or smoked meats: corned beef, sausage of any kind (patty, link, Kielbasa, Italian, wieners or hot dogs), bacon
  - canned meats: potted meats, spreads, Vienna sausage, etc.
  - cheeses: avoid those with more than 140 mg sodium per serving

Condiments, sauces, and seasonings

The following are typically high in sodium:

- mustard, ketchup, salad dressings, bouillon cubes or granules
- sauces: Worcestershire, barbecue, pizza, chili, steak, soy, or horseradish
- meat tenderizer, monosodium glutamate
- any seasoning that has "salt" in the name or on the label, such as celery salt, garlic salt and onion salt; however, it is okay to have garlic or onion powder or flakes
- pickles and olives

Gluten-Free Diet

Indications for Use

A gluten-free diet is used for:

- Celiac disease

  Persons with celiac disease are advised to adhere to a lifelong, gluten-free nutrition prescription, strictly avoiding the **prolamins** of wheat, barley, and rye (termed gliadin, hordein, and secalin, respectively). Strict adherence to a gluten-free diet allows the intestine to heal, resolves the symptoms of malabsorption, and helps prevent the complications associated with long-term untreated celiac disease, which may include reduced bone mineral density and lymphoma (Janatuinen et al. 1995).

  Prolamins are proline-rich and glutamine-rich storage proteins found in the endosperm of grain (Kasarda, 1996). Although many grains contain prolamins, not all prolamins contain the specific amino acid sequences harmful to persons with celiac disease. The corn prolamin zein and the rice prolamin orzenin are considered safe to consume for persons with celiac disease.

Description of the Diet

A gluten-free diet is a general diet with strict avoidance of gluten found in the following grains. These ingredients are found in many food products, including flours, bread products, pasta, breakfast cereals, cakes, and cookies:

- Wheat
  - All varieties, including einkorn, emmer, spelt, and kamut
  - All forms, including wheat starch[1], wheat bran, wheat germ, cracked wheat, and hydrolyzed wheat protein
- Barley
- Rye
- Cross-bred varieties, such as triticale (a cross between wheat and rye)

Following are grains and plant foods **allowed** in a gluten-free diet:

- Rice
- Corn
- Amaranth
- Quinoa
- Teff (or Tef)
- Millet
- Finger Millet (Ragi)
- Sorghum
- Indian Rice Grass (Montina)
- Arrowroot
- Buckwheat
- Flax
- Job's Tears
- Sago
- Potato
- Soy
- Legumes
- Mesquite
- Tapioca
- Wild rice
- Cassava (Manioc)
- Yucca
- Nuts
- Seeds

The diet requires vigilance in reading ingredient labels to avoid all sources of gluten. Many processed foods contain ingredients derived from grains that are not allowed. Examples of processed foods that may contain wheat, barley, or rye include the following:

- Bouillon cubes
- Brown rice syrup
- Candy
- Cold cuts, hot dogs, salami, sausage
- French fries
- Gravy
- Imitation fish
- Licorice
- Matzo
- Rice mixes
- Sauces
- Seasoned snack foods (eg, tortilla chips, potato chips)
- Seitan
- Self-basting turkey
- Soups
- Soy sauce
- Vegetables in sauce

Until diagnosis of celiac disease occurs, damage to the small intestinal mucosa may result in varying degrees of malabsorption. There may be deficiencies of vitamins and minerals, including the following (ADA Nutrition Care Manual, 2009):

- Calcium
- Vitamin D
- Iron
- Folate

[1]The Food and Drug Administration is proposing that a food containing wheat starch may be labeled gluten-free if the final food product contains less than 20 ppm gluten.

Newly diagnosed patients may be prescribed vitamin and mineral supplements to correct any existing nutrient deficiencies. Because of reduced levels of the enzyme lactase, a (usually) temporary form of lactose intolerance also may affect some persons newly diagnosed with celiac disease. These patients generally are advised to follow a lactose-free or lactose-reduced diet while their intestine heals and the lactose intolerance naturally resolves. Vitamin D and calcium intakes should be carefully monitored in these patients.

High-Fiber Diet

Indications for Use

A high-fiber diet may be used for:

- Constipation
- Diverticular disease
- Irritable bowel syndrome
- Crohn's disease
- Cardiovascular disease
- Diabetes

A high-fiber diet containing 25–35 grams of fiber/day may be used to prevent and treat various gastrointestinal, cardiovascular, and metabolic diseases (ADA 2008). Most often, increasing fiber intake is used to promote regularity, treat and prevent constipation associated with various diseases, and can also help ease diarrhea. Certain types of fiber, including beta-glucan in oats and soluble fiber in legumes, are recommended to help normalize blood cholesterol levels. For people with diabetes, fiber can help to modulate the blood glucose response after meals. Adequate intakes of fiber may also help protect against certain types of cancer, and may play a role in weight management.

Description of the Diet

The high-fiber diet is a general diet with an emphasis on fiber-rich food sources, including fruits, legumes, vegetables, and whole-grain breads, cereals, and other products made with whole grains and/or bran. See Table 24.8 for a list of recommended fiber-rich foods. Increased fiber intake should come from a variety of food sources, rather than from fiber supplements to ensure adequate intake of vitamins, minerals, and other nutrients. Fiber intake should be increased gradually to minimize potential adverse side effects, such as abdominal distress, bloating, flatulence, cramps, and diarrhea. These effects are usually temporary and subside within several days. Fluid intake should be increased with the gradual increase in fiber.

Lactose-Controlled Diet

Indications for Use

A lactose-controlled diet may be used for:

- Lactose intolerance
- Lactose malabsorption

The lactose-controlled diet is used to prevent or reduce gastrointestinal symptoms of bloating, flatulence, cramping, nausea, and diarrhea associated with consumption of lactose in individuals with lactose malabsorption or lactose intolerance. Lactose is a disaccharide (sugar) found in milk that is hydrolyzed to galactose and glucose by the intestinal enzyme lactase. It is the principle carbohydrate found in human and animal milk.

Lactose malabsorption, also referred to as lactose nonpersistance, occurs when digestion of lactose is reduced due to low activity of lactase. Symptoms may not be present unless the amount of lactose consumed exceeds the available lactase. Lactose intolerance is the occurrence of gastrointestinal symptoms resulting from

TABLE 24.8 Recommended Foods for a High-Fiber Diet

Foods with at Least 4 g Fiber per Serving

Food Group	Choose
Grains	⅓–½ cup high-fiber cereal (check Nutritional Facts label and choose products with at least 4 g dietary fiber per serving)
Dried beans and peas	½ cup cooked red beans, kidney beans, large lima beans, navy beans, pinto beans, white beans, lentils, or black-eyed peas
Vegetables	1 artichoke (cooked)
Fruits	½ cup blackberries or raspberries 4 dried prunes

Foods with 1 to 3 g Fiber per Serving

Food Group	Choose
Grains	1 bagel (3.5-inch diameter) 1 slice whole wheat, cracked wheat, pumpernickel, or rye bread 2-inch square cornbread 4 whole wheat crackers 1 bran, blueberry, cornmeal, or English muffin ½ cup cereal with 1–3 g fiber per serving (check dietary fiber on the product's Nutrition Facts label) 2 tablespoons wheat germ or whole wheat flour
Fruits	1 apple (3-inch diameter) or ½ cup applesauce ½ cup apricots (canned) 1 banana ½ cup cherries (canned or fresh) ½ cup cranberries (fresh) 3 dates 2 medium figs (fresh) ½ cup fruit cocktail (canned) ½ grapefruit 1 kiwi fruit 1 orange (2½-inch diameter) 1 peach (fresh) or ½ cup peaches (canned) 1 pear (fresh) or ½ cup pears (canned) 1 plum (2-inch diameter) ¼ cup raisins ½ cup strawberries (fresh) 1 tangerine
Vegetables	½ cup bean sprouts (raw) ½ cup beets (diced, canned) ½ cup broccoli, brussels sprouts, or cabbage (cooked) ½ cup carrots ½ cup cauliflower ½ cup corn ½ cup eggplant ½ cup okra (boiled) ½ cup potatoes (baked or mashed) ½ cup spinach, kale, or turnip greens (cooked) ½ cup squash—winter, summer, or zucchini (cooked) ½ cup sweet potatoes or yams ½ cup tomatoes (canned)
Other	2 tablespoons almonds or peanuts 1 cup popcorn (popped)

Source: ADA Nutrition Care Manual, 2009.

incomplete digestion of lactose caused by a shortage of the enzyme lactase. There are three basic types:

- *Primary lactose intolerance* is the most common form and is genetically determined. Symptoms do not usually become apparent until late adolescence or early adulthood.

- *Secondary lactose intolerance* occurs as a result of disease, surgery, radiation, or medications. Lactase activity is restored when the underlying condition resolves.

- *Congenital lactose intolerance,* a lifelong complete absence of lactase, is a rare condition.

Lactose malabsorption can be diagnosed by having individuals ingest a standard dose of lactose after fasting and finding elevated levels of breath hydrogen, which is produced by bacterial fermentation of undigested lactose in the colon (NIH 2010). Other diagnostic tools include measuring the lactase activity in an intestinal biopsy sample or genetic testing. However, the demonstration of lactose malabsorption does not necessarily indicate that an individual will be symptomatic.

Description of the Diet

Many individuals with real or perceived lactose intolerance avoid dairy and ingest inadequate amounts of calcium and vitamin D, which may predispose them to decreased bone accrual, osteoporosis, and other adverse health outcomes (NIH 2010). In most cases, individuals do not need to eliminate dairy consumption completely. Therefore, the diet should be based on individual tolerance to lactose. Several factors influence tolerance—amount of lactose consumed at one time, whether it is consumed with a meal, the type of dairy food, and colonic adaptation. It is well-established that most people with lactose malabsorption or intolerance can tolerate 1–2 cups of milk daily with meals without discomfort (Saviano et al. 2006). Several strategies can be used to improve tolerance to lactose and ensure adequate intakes of dairy nutrients:

- Drink milk with food in small amounts throughout the day.
- Choose aged cheeses like Cheddar and Swiss, which are lower in lactose.
- If dairy has been avoided, re-introduce slowly, and gradually increase the amount.
- Try lactose-free milk and milk products, or lactose digestive aids (tablets, drops).
- Include yogurt, kefir, and other fermented dairy products, which contain live and active cultures that help to digest lactose.

Table 24.9 lists the relative amounts of lactose in a variety of dairy-based foods. Foods made from dairy products (such as pudding, cream soups, cream or cheese sauces, etc.) also contain lactose. The amount of lactose in a product will depend on the amount of dairy products used. Other foods such as baked items, instant mixes, salad dressings, etc., may also contain lactose. The following ingredients suggest that a product may contain lactose:

- Butter
- Caseinates
- Cheese
- Cream
- Curds
- Dry milk solids
- Lactose
- Milk
- Milk by-products
- Milk solids
- Milk sugar
- Non-fat dry milk powder
- Skim milk solids
- Whey
- Yogurt

Depending on individual choices, the diet can provide adequate amounts of all essential nutrients. When dairy products are limited, intake of calcium, phosphorus, vitamins A and D, and riboflavin may be inadequate.

TABLE 24.9   Lactose Content of Common Foods and Beverages

Product	Lactose (grams)
Milk (nonfat, 1%, 2%, whole, chocolate), 1 cup	11
Buttermilk, 1 cup	10
Acidophilus Milk, 1 cup	11
Evaporated Milk, 1 cup	24
Sweetened Condensed Milk, undiluted, 1 cup	40
Lactose-reduced milk, 1 cup	<1
Whipping Cream, ½ cup	3
Cream, light, ½ cup	4
Half-and-Half, ½ cup	5
Sour Cream, ½ cup	4
Ice cream, ½ cup	6
Ice milk, ½ cup	9
Sherbet, orange, ½ cup	2
Cottage cheese, creamed, ½ cup	3
Cream cheese, 1 ounce	1
Cheese, 1 ounce	
• American cheese	1
• Bleu cheese	2
• Cheddar cheese, sharp	0
• Parmesan cheese, grated	1
• Swiss cheese	1
Yogurt, low-fat, 1 cup	5
Margarine, 1 tsp	Trace
Butter, 1 tsp	Trace

Source: ADA Nutrition Care Manual, 2009.

High-Calorie, High-Protein Diet

Indications for Use

A high-calorie, high-protein diet may be used for:

- Conditions that increase calorie and/or protein requirements, such as HIV/AIDS, cancer, burns, wounds
- Maximizing calorie and protein consumption in persons with poor intake, associated with cancer treatment, malnutrition, trauma, chronic gastrointestinal problems, cystic fibrosis, etc.
- Weight gain

A high-calorie, high-protein diet is appropriate for individuals who are malnourished or at risk of becoming malnourished and can tolerate oral feedings.

Protein-energy malnutrition may occur as a result of inadequate intake, increased requirements, reduced retention or increased losses of nutrients. Assessment and identification of the underlying cause is necessary in determining appropriate use of the high-calorie, high-protein diet. In severe cases, the individual must be evaluated carefully for electrolyte and mineral deficiencies prior to starting this diet to avoid refeeding syndrome.

Description of the Diet

The high-calorie, high-protein diet consists of foods that are calorie-dense and protein-dense. Because fats are often added to increase calorie-density of foods, the diet often exceeds 30 percent of calories from fat. Generally, the diet should provide at least 120 to 150 percent of the recommended intakes for energy and protein. The actual amounts of calories and protein provided will depend on the individual's height, weight, medical status, and nutrition goals.

Small frequent feedings of at least 6 meals and snacks containing calorie-dense and protein-dense foods are encouraged in maximize intake. Supplement drinks may also help to increase intake. Overall recommendations are as follows (ADA Nutrition Care Manual, 2009):

Eat More Fat

- Fat is calorie dense; a tablespoon of oil, butter, or margarine has about 100 calories.
- Fry foods in oil, margarine, or butter.
- Add butter, margarine, or oil to bread, potatoes, vegetables, hot cereals, and soups.
- Use mayonnaise, salad dressing, and peanut butter freely.

Choose High-Calorie Drinks

- Choose drinks like whole milk, juice, fruit nectars, or soda made with sugar.
- Choose plain water, tea, and coffee less often.
- Mix 1 cup whole milk with ⅓ cup powdered milk; add chocolate or strawberry syrup and sugar. Make milkshakes and smoothies with ice cream, yogurt, heavy cream, fruit, and syrups. Add peanut butter or powdered milk to boost protein.

Boost Calories in Fruits and Vegetables

- Most fruits and vegetables are low in calories and protein. Get more calories and protein by adding cheese sauce, butter, margarine, gravy, oil, or salad dressing.
- Potatoes and corn have more calories than nonstarchy vegetables like green beans, zucchini, carrots, and tomatoes.
- Eat chips with bean dip or guacamole. Cooked dried beans like pinto beans and kidney beans are good choices for protein. Avocados are high in calories.
- Choose fruits canned in heavy syrup instead of water or juice; dried fruits are calorie dense.

Choose High-Protein Foods

- Eat milk, eggs, cheese, meat, fish, poultry, beans, and nuts for good sources of protein. Other options include protein powders and meal replacement shakes and bars.
- Choose higher-fat meats for more calories than lean meats.
- Choose whole milk instead of low-fat or skim milk.
- Pick high-fat cheeses instead of low-fat or nonfat ones. Add cheese to egg dishes, casseroles, pasta dishes, salads, stews, chilis, sauces, potatoes, hamburgers.
- Add powdered milk to foods to boost protein, such as casseroles, puddings, cereals, potatoes, cream soups, gravies, sauces, scrambled eggs, and meatloaf.
- Add extra eggs to pancake or cookie batter; hard-boiled eggs may be chopped and added to salads, vegetables, or casseroles.
- Add nuts to ice cream, pudding, muffins, cookies, salads, and pasta sauces.

Nursing Care Plan: Nutrition and Hyperlipidemia
Case Study

Horace, age 58 years, describes himself as a "meat and potatoes man." He works the day shift at an auto-parts assembly plant, a job he has had for 33 years. He is looking forward to retiring in 2 years, at which time he and his wife of 36 years plan to travel around the country and spend time with their adult children and grandchildren. When his insurance plan changed he had a blood screening that showed an elevated LDL cholesterol level and a mildly elevated blood glucose. He says he has not seen a physician for many years, feels fine, and that his parents are in their 80s and in generally good health. He says he knows he has "good genes" and there is no need to worry about cholesterol levels or anything else. He has come to the clinic as a follow-up to the screening because the insurance company sent him a letter strongly suggesting an appointment with a health care provider. He says he is here only because he does not want to risk getting in trouble with the insurance company because of the coverage it provides for his wife's arthritis.

Applying the Nursing Process

ASSESSMENT

> Height: 5 feet, 10 inches Weight: 212 pounds
> BMI: 30 BP 148/90 mm Hg P 76 bpm RR 16
> Fasting cholesterol (mg/dL): 290; LDL: 137; HDL: 38; Fasting serum glucose: 128 mg/dL

Horace has central obesity and loose flesh on his upper arms. His skin is smooth and dry with no obvious lesions. Teeth are in good condition. He says he eats "three squares" a day, one of which is the lunch he carries to work. He denies alcohol intake beyond one beer each Friday after work with his friends. He typically glances at the paper and watches TV after eating a dinner prepared by his wife.

DIAGNOSES

> *Imbalanced nutrition; more than body requirements* related to BMI of 30
> *Risk for cardiovascular disease* related to elevated LDL cholesterol and serum glucose, low HDL cholesterol, high blood pressure
> *Alteration in health maintenance* related to knowledge deficit as evidenced by belief in "good genes"
> *Sedentary lifestyle* related to lack of interest in physical activity

EXPECTED OUTCOMES

> Weight loss of 1 pound a week
> Knowledge of risk factors for cardiovascular disease and diabetes
> Participation in 30 minutes of physical activity three times a week
> Meal plans that include increased fruit, vegetables, and fiber; reduced sodium

PLANNING

24-hour food recall and 3 days (2 week days and 1 weekend day) of recording food and beverages

Involve his wife in diet teaching

Meet with a dietitian to develop acceptable strategy for weight reduction along with cholesterol, glucose, and blood pressure control

Discuss factors that contribute to the development of cardiovascular disease

Develop a plan for increasing physical activity

Monitor serum cholesterol, glucose, and blood pressure after 2 months

EVALUATION

Horace and his wife met with the dietitian and nurse. He expresses gratitude for finding out about his elevated cholesterol because he "wants to be around for the grandkids." Because family is so important, he and his wife are working hard to eat more whole grain products and more vegetables. His wife has begun preparing only the amount of food they will eat at each meal; she gives the example of making only one pork chop for each of them. She also heard about using smaller plates and is doing that as well. Vegetables are not a favorite but she makes sure they eat frozen green beans or a salad two or three times a week. Horace has begun taking turkey sandwiches in his lunch and using mustard instead of mayonnaise for flavoring. He says he is still hungry and cannot stand to give up an afternoon snack, so he tries to eat a few reduced sodium saltine crackers or pretzels instead of cookies. The activity is a challenge because he really feels tired at the end of his shift. In the nice weather he tries to walk around the block, but because his wife has arthritis she cannot always go with him and he does not like to walk alone. His weight is now 201 pounds and he feels that he can continue to work on lowering it. His cholesterol is 262 mg/dL with an LDL of 131 mg/dL and HDL of 40 mg/dL. His glucose is 123 mg. He will continue working on diet and activity and return in 2 months for additional laboratory work. FIGURE 24.5 outlines the nursing process for this case.

Critical Thinking in the Nursing Process

1. What are some of the immediate dietary steps a nurse can suggest to a client who presents with an elevated LDL cholesterol level?

2. What are some things a nurse can explain to a client who states that it is no longer necessary to follow dietary interventions because a cholesterol-lowering medication has been started?

Assessment
Data about the patient

Subjective
What the patient tells the nurse

Example: I am a meat and potatoes man; I don't worry about cholesterol because I have good genes.

Objective
What the nurse observes; anthropometric and clinical data

Examples: 212 pounds; BMI: 30; serum cholestrol: 290 mg/dL; blood glucose: 128 mg/dL

Diagnosis
NANDA label

Example: Imbalanced nutrition: more than body requirements related to excess nutrient intake

Planning
Goals stated in patient terms

Example: Long-term goal: weight loss of 1 pound per week; Short-term goal: identify foods high in fiber and low in saturated fat

Implementation
Nursing action to help patient achieve goals

Example: Refer to dietitian; discuss factors that contribute to development of heart disease

Evaluation
Was the goal achieved or does the intervention need to be modified?

Example: 11-pound weight loss in 2 months; cholesterol: 262 mg/dL; eating more whole grain bread

FIGURE 24.5 Nursing Care Plan process: Nutrition and hyperlipidemia.

TEST YOURSELF ANSWERS

1. **True.** All individuals must ingest food and nutrients to survive. Thus, modifications to food and nutrient intake are relatively inexpensive, safe, and effective means to prevent and treat disease. Nutrition intervention and counseling has been shown to significantly improve weight, body mass index, hemoglobin A1c, blood pressure, and serum lipid levels.

2. **False.** Depending on the type of texture modification, diets that provide foods with altered consistency, such as pureed or mechanical soft, can be nutritionally adequate. However, a clear liquid diet does not provide adequate nutrients and serves primarily as oral hydration.

3. **True.** Diminished or inadequate intake for any reason places a client at risk for malnutrition, which can negatively impact health outcomes. Liberalizing a therapeutic diet to allow greater variety of foods is warranted in some situations to optimize intake, unless there is a strong medical contraindication, such as risk for choking.

4. **False.** Sugar-containing foods are allowed in moderation and can be substituted for other carbohydrates in the meal plan, but care should be taken to avoid excess energy intake.

5. **True.** The DASH (Dietary Approaches to Stop Hypertension) has been shown to lower elevated blood pressure. It provides an eating pattern that is high in potassium, calcium, magnesium, and fiber, while limiting sodium to levels between 1,500 mg and 2,400 mg per day.

REVIEW QUESTIONS

1. A client is placed on a mechanical soft diet. The nurse knows the client understood dietary teaching when the client states which of the following foods should not be eaten?
   1. Hot dogs
   2. Apricot nectar
   3. Macaroni and cheese
   4. Canned tuna

2. A middle-age client with mildly elevated serum LDL cholesterol wants to use diet to lower his cholesterol level. The client asks the nurse about what foods, in addition to oatmeal, may help lower cholesterol. The nurse suggests which of the following?
   1. Whole wheat bread
   2. Apples
   3. Cabbage
   4. Corn

3. The nurse knows that teaching about a low-sodium diet has been effective when a client states which of the following food choices would be good to take to work for lunch?
   1. Salami sandwich with whole wheat bread
   2. Ham salad with low-sodium crackers
   3. Shrimp with lettuce and low-fat French dressing
   4. Roast turkey sandwich on white bread

4. The nurse knows that the client with type 2 diabetes mellitus understands teaching about carbohydrates in the diet when the client states:
   1. "I need to have about half of my daily calories come from carbohydrates."
   2. "I need to be on a low-carbohydrate diet for the rest of my life."
   3. "I should substitute artificial sweeteners for natural sugar when baking."
   4. "I need to learn carbohydrate counting if I want to be successful with my diet."

5. A child has been diagnosed with celiac disease. When teaching the family, what foods should the nurse be certain are eliminated from the diet plan?
   1. Puffed rice cereal
   2. Whole wheat bread
   3. Peanuts
   4. Yogurt

REFERENCES

American Diabetes Association (ADA). (2008). Nutrition recommendations and interventions for diabetes: A position statement of the American Diabetes Association. *Diabetes Care, 31*(Suppl. 1), S61–S78.

American Diabetes Association (ADA). (2009). Standards of medical care in diabetes—2009. *Diabetes Care, 32*, S13–S61.

American Dietetic Association. *Nutrition Care Manual* (online). 2009. http://www.nutritioncaremanual.org.

American Dietetic Association. (2008). Position of the American Dietetic Association: Health Implications of Dietary Fiber. *Journal of the American Dietetic Association*, 108, 1716–1731.

American Dietetic Association. (2010). Position of the American Dietetic Association: Integration of medical nutrition therapy and pharmacotherapy. *Journal of the American Dietetic Association*, 110, 950–956.

American Dietetic Association Evidence Analysis Library. Medical nutrition therapy effectiveness for specific diseases or condition. American Dietetic Association Evidence Analysis Library Web site. http://www.adaevidencelibrary.com/topic.cfm?cat=3586. Accessed June 7, 2010.

Chobanian AV, Bakris GL, Black HR, Cushman WC, Green LA, Izzo JL, Jones DW, Materson BJ, Oparil S, Wright JT, Rocella EJ. The Seventh Report of the Joint National Committee on Prevention, Detection, Evaluation, and Treatment of High Blood Pressure. The JNC 7 Report. *JAMA*. 2003;289:2560-2572.

Hancock, S., Cresci, G., & Martindale, R. (2002). The clear liquid diet: When is it appropriate? *Current Gastroenterology Reports*, 4, 324–331.

Janatuinen EK, Pikkarainen PH, Kemppainen TA, Kosma V-M, Jarvinen RMK, Uusitupa MIJ, Julkunen RJK. A comparison of diets with and without oats in adults with celiac disease. *N Engl J Med*. 1995;333:1033-1037.

Kasarda D. Gluten and gliadin: Precipitating factors in coeliac disease. In: Maki M, Collin P, Visakorpi JK, eds. *Coeliac Disease. Tampere, Finland: Proceedings of the Seventh International Symposium on Coeliac Disease*. 1996:195-212.

Institute of Medicine, Committee on Nutrition Services for Medicare Beneficiaries, Food and Nutrition Board. (2000). *The Role of Nutrition in Maintaining Health in the Nation's Elderly: Evaluating Coverage of Nutrition Services for the Medicare Population*. Washington, DC: National Academy Press.

Medicare Program; Revisions to Payment Policies and Five Year Review of and Adjustments to the Relative Values Units Under the Physician Fee Schedule for Calendar Year 2002; Final Rule. Subpart G—Medical nutrition therapy. 66 Federal Register 55331 (2001) (codified at 42 CFR 405, 410, 411, 414, and 415).

National Cholesterol Education Program (NCEP) Expert Panel on Detection, Evaluation and Treatment of High Blood Cholesterol in Adults (Adult Treatment Panel [ATP] III). (2002). Third report of the National Cholesterol Education Program (NCEP) expert panel on detection, evaluation and treatment of high blood cholesterol in adults (Adult Treatment Panel III) final report. *Circulation, 106*, 3143–3421.

National Institutes of Health Concensus Development Conference: Lactose Intolerance and Health, February 22–24, 2010. http://consensus.nih.gov/2010/lactosestatement.htm. Accessed June 23, 2010.

National Institutes of Health, National Heart, Lung, and Blood Institute. *Your Guide to Lowering Your Blood Pressure with DASH. DASH Eating Plan*. 2006. NIH Publication No. 06-4082. http://www.nhlbi.nih.gov/health/public/heart/hbp/dash/new_dash.pdf. Accessed June 23, 2010.

Sacks FM, Svetkey LP, Vollmer WM, Appel LJ, Bray GA, Harsha D, Obaranek E, Conlin PR, Miller ER III, Simons-Morton DG, Karanja N, Lin PH, for the DASH-Sodium Collaborative Research Group. Effects on blood pressure of reduced dietary sodium and the Dietary Approaches to Stop Hypertension (DASH) diet. *N Engl J Med*. 2001;344:3-10.

Savaiano DA et al. Lactose intolerance symptoms assessed by meta-analysis: a grain of truth that leads to exaggeration. *J Nutr*. 2006;136:1107.

LABORATORY
ASSIGNMENTS

LABORATORY ASSIGNMENTS CHART

Laboratory Name	Laboratory Usage: Recommended Chapter(s)
Lifestyle Assessment Inventory	1
Assessing Nutritional Habits	1
Analyzing Your Diet	1 or 2
Setting Goals for a Healthy Diet	1, 2, or 3
Planning a New Diet	1, 2, or 3
What Triggers Your Eating	3
Estimating Daily Caloric Expenditure and the Caloric Deficit Required to Lose 1 Pound of Fat per Week	4
Finding Your Cholesterol Plan	4
Assessing Body Image	5
Weight-Loss Goals and Progress Report	5 and 6 and 11
Wellness Profile	7, 8, 9, 10, or 13
Determining Ideal Body Weight Using Percent Body Fat and the Body Mass Index	11
Warming Up	12
Which Physical Activities Work Best for You?	11, 12, or 13
Using a Pedometer to Count Your Steps	11, 12, or 13
Measuring Cardiorespiratory Fitness: The 1.5-Mile Run Test	11, 12, or 13
Measuring Cardiorespiratory Fitness: The 1-Mile Walk Test	11, 12, or 13
Measuring Cardiorespiratory Fitness: Submaximal Cycle Test	11, 12, or 13
Measuring Cardiorespiratory Fitness: Step Test	11, 12, or 13
Determining Target Heart Rate	11, 12, or 13
Developing Your Personal Exercise Prescription	11, 12, or 13
Determining Rate of Perceived Exertion	11, 12, or 13
Evaluating Fitness Products	13
Managing Time and Establishing Priorities	14
Assessing Your Personality Behavior Pattern	14

NAME _____ DATE _____

Lifestyle Assessment Inventory

The purpose of this lifestyle assessment inventory is to help you identify areas in your life that increase your risk of disease, injury, and possibly premature death. Awareness is the first step in making change.

Put a check by each statement that applies to you. You may select more than one choice per category.

Physical Health

A. Physical Fitness

_____ I exercise for a minimum of 20 to 30 minutes at least 3 days per week.

_____ I walk for 15 to 30 minutes (3 to 7 days per week).

_____ I get lifestyle or occupational physical activity most days of the week.

B. Body Fat

_____ There is no place on my body where I can pinch more than 1 inch of fat.

_____ I am satisfied with the way my body looks.

C. Sleep

_____ I always get 7 to 9 hours of sleep.

_____ I do not have trouble going to sleep.

_____ I generally do not wake up during the night.

D. Diet

_____ I generally eat balanced meals and a variety of food.

_____ I eat fruits and vegetables daily.

_____ I rarely overeat.

_____ I rarely eat large quantities of fatty foods and sweets.

E. Alcohol Use

_____ I consume fewer than two drinks per day.

_____ I never get intoxicated.

_____ I do not binge drink.

F. Tobacco and Drug Use

_____ I never smoke (cigarettes, pipe, cigars, etc.).

_____ I do not use smokeless tobacco.

_____ I use prescription medications only for their intended purpose.

_____ I do not use illegal drugs.

Social Health

_____ I have a happy and satisfying relationship with my spouse or boyfriend/girlfriend.

_____ I have good relationships with my close friends.

_____ I get a great deal of love and support from my family.

_____ I work to have good communication skills.

_____ I am able to express my feelings and emotions to people close to me.

Emotional Health

A. Stress Level

_____ I find it easy to relax.

_____ I rarely feel tense or anxious.

_____ I am able to cope with daily stresses without undue emotional stress.

_____ I have not experienced a major stressful life event in the past year.

B. Mental Health

_____ I do not suffer from depressive or anxiety disorders.

_____ I do not have an eating disorder.

Intellectual Health

_____ I attend class regularly.

_____ I keep informed about current events.

_____ I seek opportunities to learn new things.

_____ I have an open mind about ideas that might be different from mine.

Environmental Health

_____ I am not exposed to second-hand smoke on a regular basis.

_____ I use sunscreen regularly or limit my sun exposure.

_____ I carpool or use physical activity for transportation when possible.

_____ I recycle regularly.

_____ I limit my exposure to harmful environmental contaminants.

Spiritual Health

_____ I have a sense of meaning and purpose in my life.

_____ I am satisfied with my level of spirituality.

_____ I work to develop my spiritual health.

LABORATORY

NAME _____ DATE _____

Evaluating Your Responses

1. What area of health and wellness is your strongest area? What do you do to maintain healthy behaviors for that wellness component?

   _____

   _____

2. What area of health and wellness is your weakest area? What behaviors can you change to improve that area?

   _____

   _____

3. Write a long-term and a short-term goal for improving one health and wellness behavior you seriously want to change this semester.

   _____

   _____

NAME _____ DATE _____

Analyzing Your Diet

The purpose of this exercise is to analyze your eating habits during a 3-day period. For a 3-day period (two weekdays and one weekend day), eat the foods that typically constitute your normal diet. At the end of each day, record on the following chart the foods you ate that day and the amounts of the listed nutrients contained in each. You can use the food labels on your foods to obtain the nutrient values, or refer to the Appendix at the end of this text (you can also use a diet analysis software program, if you have access to one.)

Total the values for each nutrient at the bottom of the chart. Transfer the total to the next chart. At the end of the 3-day period, total the daily values and divide by 3 to get the average dietary intake for each of the nutrients analyzed.

Compare your average intake for each of the nutrients with those recommended at the bottom of the page for your sex and age group. (Remember that this analysis is only as representative of your normal diet as the foods you eat over the 3-day period). Then, answer the following questions:

1. How did you do on calories? Are you taking in more or fewer calories than you should be for your sex, age, and activity level?

   _____

2. Was your fat, sodium, and cholesterol intake higher than it should be?

   _____

3. What nutrients did you eat in inadequate amounts?

   _____

4. What are three substitutions you could have made that would improve the quality of your diet?

   _____

Recommended Dietary Allowances

- Kcal total (total daily energy expenditure) equals body weight multiplied by kcal per pound per day:

  _____ × _____ = _____

  body weight in lb   kcal per lb per day   **kcal total (total daily energy expenditure)**

- Kcal from fat should be no more than 30% of total calories per day:

  _____ × _____ = _____

  30% (0.3)   kcal per day   **recommended MAXIMUM kcal from fat**

- Protein intake should be 12% of total calories per day, or 0.8 to 0.9 gram per kilogram (0.36 g per pound) of body weight. (Pregnant women should add 15 g, and lactating women should add 20 g):

  _____ × _____ = _____

  0.36 g   body weight in lb   **recommended protein intake**

- Carbohydrate intake should be approximately 58% of total calories per day:

  _____ × _____ = _____

  58% (0.58)   kcal per day   **recommended carbohydrate intake**

Fat < 30% of diet; fiber ~30% of diet; saturated fat < 10% of diet; cholesterol < 300 mg.; sodium < 3000 mg

Daily Nutrient Intake

NAME: _____

DATE: _____

Foods	Amount	kcal (total)	kcal from fat	Protein (gm)	Carb. (gm)	Fiber (gm)	Fat (gm)	Fat % (kcal)	Sat. Fat (gm)	Chol. (mg)	Sodium (mg)	Vit. A (I.U.)	Vit. C (mg)	Calcium (mg)	Iron (mg)	Vit. B$_1$ (mg)	Vit. B$_2$ (mg)	Niacin (mg)
Totals																		

NAME _____ DATE _____

Three-Day Nutrient Summary

NAME:

DATE:

Day	kcal (Total)	kcal from Fat	Protein (gm)	Carb. (gm)	Fiber (gm)	Fat (gm)	Fat % (kcal)	Sat. Fat (gm)	Chol. (mg)	Sodium (mg)	Vit. A (IU)	Vit. C (mg)	Calcium (mg)	Iron (mg)	Vit. B$_1$ (mg)	Vit. B$_2$ (mg)	Niacin (mg)
One																	
Two																	
Three																	
Totals																	
Average																	

LABORATORY

NAME _____ DATE _____

Setting Goals for a Healthy Diet

What are your three worst dietary habits?

1. _____
2. _____
3. _____

Check the appropriate boxes in the table below to indicate the changes that you think you need to make to improve your diet.

	Increase	Decrease	Keep the Same
Calories			
Carbohydrates			
Fat			
Protein			
Vitamins			
Minerals			

Based on your selections above, list two short-term and two long-term goals for improving your diet:

Short-term goal 1

_____

Short-term goal 2

_____

Long-term goal 1

_____

Long-term goal 2

_____

NAME _____ DATE _____

Planning a New Diet

The purpose of this exercise is to plan a new diet using the principles outlined in this chapter. After completing the Daily Nutrient Intake lab, you should have a general idea of how your diet may need modification. Follow the example given in the following Sample Diet table to choose foods to build a new diet that meets the recommended dietary goals presented. Fill in the chart on the following page with the requested information obtained from this book's appendix or from package labels. Use the totals for each column and the RDA for each nutrient in the Daily Nutrient Intake lab or the following Recommended Dietary Allowances table to determine your percentage of RDA for each nutrient.

Recommended Dietary Allowances of Micronutrients

Minerals

Life Stage Group	Calcium (mg/d)	Phosphorus (mg/d)	Magnesium (mg/d)	Iron (mg/d)	Zinc (mg/d)	Selenium (mg/d)	Iodine (mg/d)	Copper (mg/d)	Manganese (mg/d)	Fluoride (mg/d)	Chromium (mg/d)	Molybdenum (mg/d)
Infants												
0–6 mo	210*	100*	30*	0.27*	2*	15*	110*	200*	0.003*	0.01*	0.2*	2*
7–12 mo	270*	275*	75*	11	3	20*	130*	220*	0.6*	0.5*	5.5*	3*
Children												
1–3 y	500*	460	80	7	3	20	90	340	1.2*	0.7*	11*	17
4–8 y	800*	500	130	10	5	30	90	440	1.5*	1*	15*	22
Males												
9–13 y	1300*	1250	240	8	8	40	120	700	1.9*	2*	25*	34
14–18 y	1300*	1250	410	11	11	55	150	890	2.2*	3*	35*	43
19–30 y	1000*	700	400	8	11	55	150	900	2.3*	4*	35*	45
31–50 y	1000*	700	420	8	11	55	150	900	2.3*	4*	35*	45
51–70 y	1200*	700	420	8	11	55	150	900	2.3*	4*	30*	45
>70 y	1200*	700	420	8	11	55	150	900	2.3*	4*	30*	45
Females												
9–13 y	1300*	1250	240	8	8	40	120	700	1.6*	2*	21*	34
14–18 y	1300*	1250	360	15	9	55	150	890	1.6*	3*	24*	43
19–30 y	1000*	700	310	18	8	55	150	900	1.8*	3*	25*	45
31–50 y	1000*	700	320	18	8	55	150	900	1.8*	3*	20*	45
51–70 y	1200*	700	320	8	8	55	150	900	1.8*	3*	20*	45
>70 y	1200*	700	320	8	8	55	150	900	1.8*	3*	20*	45
Pregnancy												
≤18 y	1300*	1250	400	27	12	60	220	1000	2.0*	3*	29*	50
19–30 y	1000*	700	350	27	11	60	220	1000	2.0*	3*	30*	50
31–50 y	1000*	700	360	27	11	60	220	1000	2.0*	3*	30*	50
Lactation												
≤18 y	1300*	1250	360	10	13	70	290	1300	2.6*	3*	44*	50
19–30 y	1000*	700	310	9	12	70	290	1300	2.6*	3*	45*	50
31–50 y	1000*	700	320	9	12	70	290	1300	2.6*	3*	45*	50

Vitamins

Life Stage Group	Vitamin A (μg/d)[a]	Vitamin D (μg/d)[b]	Vitamin E (mg/d)[c]	Vitamin K (μg/d)	Thiamin (mg/d)	Riboflavin (mg/d)	Niacin (mg/d)[d]	Pantothenic Acid (mg/d)	Biotin (μg/d)	Vitamin B₆ (mg/d)	Folate (μg/d)[e]	Vitamin B₁₂ (μg/d)	Vitamin C (mg/d)	Choline (mg/d)
Infants														
0–6 mo	400*	5*	4*	2.0*	0.2*	0.3*	2*	1.7*	5*	0.1*	65*	0.4*	40*	125*
7–12 mo	500*	5*	5*	2.5*	0.3*	0.4*	4*	1.8*	6*	0.3*	80*	0.5*	50*	150*
Children														
1–3 y	300	5*	6	30*	0.5	0.5	6	2*	8*	0.5	150	0.9	15	200*
4–8 y	400	5*	7	55*	0.6	0.6	8	3*	12*	0.6	200	1.2	25	250*
Males														
9–13 y	600	5*	11	60*	0.9	0.9	12	4*	20*	1.0	300	1.8	45	375*
14–18 y	900	5*	15	75*	1.2	1.3	16	5*	25*	1.3	400	2.4	75	550*
19–30 y	900	5*	15	120*	1.2	1.3	16	5*	30*	1.3	400	2.4	90	550*
31–50 y	900	5*	15	120*	1.2	1.3	16	5*	30*	1.3	400	2.4	90	550*
51–70 y	900	10*	15	120*	1.2	1.3	16	5*	30*	1.7	400	2.4	90	550*
>70 y	900	15*	15	120*	1.2	1.3	16	5*	30*	1.7	400	2.4	90	550*
Females														
9–13 y	600	5*	11	60*	0.9	0.9	12	4*	20*	1.0	300	1.8	45	375*
14–18 y	700	5*	15	75*	1.0	1.0	14	5*	25*	1.2	400	2.4	65	400*
19–30 y	700	5*	15	90*	1.1	1.1	14	5*	30*	1.3	400	2.4	75	425*
31–50 y	700	5*	15	90*	1.1	1.1	14	5*	30*	1.3	400	2.4	75	425*
51–70 y	700	10*	15	90*	1.1	1.1	14	5*	30*	1.5	400	2.4	75	425*
>70 y	700	15*	15	90*	1.1	1.1	14	5*	30*	1.5	400	2.4	75	425*
Pregnancy														
≤18 y	750	5*	15	75*	1.4	1.4	18	6*	30*	1.9	600	2.6	80	450*
19–30 y	770	5*	15	90*	1.4	1.4	18	6*	30*	1.9	600	2.6	85	450*
31–50 y	770	5*	15	90*	1.4	1.4	18	6*	30*	1.9	600	2.6	85	450*
Lactation														
≤18 y	1200	5*	19	75*	1.4	1.4	17	7*	35*	2.0	500	2.8	115	550*
19–30 y	1300	5*	19	90*	1.4	1.4	17	7*	35*	2.0	500	2.8	120	550*
31–50 y	1300	5*	19	90*	1.4	1.4	17	7*	35*	2.0	500	2.8	120	550*

Source: Reprinted with permission from the National Academies Press. Copyright 1997, 1998, 2000, 2001, 2005 by the National Academy of Sciences. These reports may be accessed via www.nap.edu.

Note: This table is adapted from the DRI reports; see www.nap.edu. It lists Recommended Dietary Allowances (RDAs), with Adequate Intakes (AIs) indicated by an asterisk (*). RDAs and AIs may both be used as goals for individual intake. RDAs are set to meet the needs of almost all (97 percent to 98 percent) individuals in a group. For healthy breastfed infants, the AI is the mean intake. The AI for other life stage and gender groups is believed to cover the needs of all individuals in the group, but lack of data prevents being able to specify with confidence the percentage of individuals covered by this intake.

[a] Given as retinal activity equivalents (RAE).

[b] Also known as calciferol. The DRI values are based on the absence of adequate exposure to sunlight.

[c] Also known as a-tocopherol.

[d] Given as niacin equivalents (NIE), except for infants 0–6 months, which are expressed as preformed niacin.

[e] Given as dietary folate equivalents (DFE).

Sample Diet for a College-Aged Female Weighing 110 Pounds, Assuming Light Daily Activities

	kcal	Fat (g)	Cholesterol (mg)	Sodium (mg)	Carbohydrate (g)	Protein (g)	Vitamin A (RE)*	Vitamin C (mg)	Calcium (mg)
Breakfast									
1/2 grapefruit	38	0.1	0	0	10.7	0.8	2	41.3	14
Whole-grain cereal (1 cup)	127	0	0	244	33	3	0	0	16
Low-fat milk (1 cup)	225	2.6	10	121	42	9	20	1.4	314
1 banana	105	1	0	1	27	1	93	10	7
Snack									
Low-fat yogurt (1 cup)	130	2.6	10	121	44	9	20	1.4	314
Lunch									
Turkey sandwich: whole-wheat bread with mustard	191	3.7	9	784	25	9.4	0	0	78
Baby carrots (10)	36	1	0	35	8	1	1972	8	23
Snack									
1 slice pizza with Parmesan cheese	145	3	8	336	21	8	382	1	117
Dinner									
Broiled salmon (1/2 fillet)	180	5	83	107	0	32	169	0	21
Mushrooms (1/2 cup)	20	0	0	2	4	2	0	3	5
Whole-wheat dinner rolls (2)	150	2	0	272	27	4	0	0	60
Broccoli (3 spears)	26	0	0	25	5	3	1434	87	45
Lima beans (1/2 cup)	90	0	0	15	21	6	332	9	29
Peach (1)	37	0	0	0	10	1	465	6	4
Totals	1500	21	120	2065	247.4	88.2	4907	169.1	883
RDA	1690	<30%	<300	<3000	>58%	40	700	75	1000
% of RDA	89	14	40	68	72	220	953	225	88

*RE = retinol equivalents.

	kcal (g)	Protein (g)	Sat. Fat (g)	Chol. (mg)	Sod. (mg)	Carb. (g)	Vit. A (IU)	Vit. C (mg)	Ca (mg)	Iron (mg)	GI
Breakfast											
Lunch											
Dinner											
Totals											
RDA		<30%*	<10%	<300	3000	>58%	1000	60	1200	12	†
% of RDA											

*Protein intake should be 0.8 g/kg of body weight (0.36 g/lb). Pregnant women should add 15 g, and lactating women should add 20 g.

†For a complete list of the glycemixc index of various foods, visit www.glycemicindex.com

NAME _____ DATE _____

Assessing Nutritional Habits

Read the following scenarios and select which option applies to you. Score your answers according to the instructions at the end.

1. You don't have time to make dinner, so you run out to get "fast food." What do you get?
   a. grilled chicken breast sandwich
   b. supersized burger

2. You go to a movie, find yourself hungry, and cannot resist a snack. Which do you buy?
   a. unbuttered popcorn
   b. candy

3. You're late for work and realize you forgot breakfast. You decide to stop and grab something to eat. What do you pick up?
   a. a banana
   b. a sausage biscuit

4. You decide to go out for a nice dinner at an Italian restaurant. What do you order?
   a. spaghetti with red sauce
   b. five-cheese lasagna

5. It's 3:00 PM, and you didn't have much lunch and need an afternoon snack. What do you reach for?
   a. an apple
   b. M&Ms

6. You stop for ice cream. Which do you pick?
   a. a fruit sorbet
   b. regular ice cream

7. What kind of dessert would you normally choose to eat?
   a. a bowl of mixed berries with a sprinkling of sugar
   b. chocolate cake with frosting

8. What do you use to stir fry vegetables?
   a. olive oil
   b. margarine

9. Which of the following salty snacks would you prefer?
   a. pretzels
   b. potato chips

10. You want cereal for breakfast. Which would you choose?
    a. whole-grain flakes
    b. peanut butter puffs

Interpretation

If you answered "b" to any of the above questions, you chose foods that are high in calories, fat, or sugar. Follow the advice in this chapter and in the MyPyramid food guidance system to improve your food choices.

NAME _____ DATE _____

Determining Ideal Body Weight Using Percent Body Fat and the Body Mass Index

There are several different ways to compute an ideal body weight. Method A of this laboratory enables you to compute and record your ideal body weight using that method. Method B enables you to calculate and record your ideal body weight using the body mass index (BMI) procedure. Choose one of these techniques, and complete the appropriate section.

Method A: Computing Ideal Body Weight Using Percent Body Fat

Step 1: Calculate fat-free weight

100% – your percent body fat estimated from skinfold measurement = _____ % fat-free weight.

Therefore,

_____ % fat-free weight expressed as a decimal $\times$ _____ your body weight in pounds = _____ pounds of fat-free weight.

Step 2: Calculate optimal weight
Remember: Optimal body fat ranges are 10–20% for men and 15–25% for women.

Optimal weight = fat-free weight $\div$ (1.00 – optimal %fat), with optimal %fat expressed as a decimal. Therefore, the low and high optimal weight ranges for your gender are as follows:

For low %fat: Optimal weight _____ pounds
For high %fat: Optimal weight _____ pounds

Method B: Computing Ideal Body Weight Using Body Mass Index (BMI)

The BMI uses the metric system. Therefore, you must express your weight in kilograms (1 kilogram = 2.2 pounds) and your height in meters (1 inch = 0.0254 meter).

Step 1: Compute your BMI

$$BMI = \text{body weight (kg)} \div (\text{height in meters})^2$$
$$\text{Your BMI} = \underline{\hspace{3cm}}$$

Step 2: Calculate your ideal body weight based on BMI*
The ideal BMI is 21.9 to 22.4 for men and 21.3 to 22.1 for women. The formula for computing ideal body weight using BMI is

$$\text{Ideal body weight (kilograms)} = \text{Desired BMI} \times (\text{height in meters})^2$$

Consider the following example as an illustration of the computation of ideal body weight. A man who weighs 60 kilograms and is 1.5 meters tall computes his BMI to be 26.7. His ideal BMI is between 21.9 and 22.4; therefore, his ideal body weight range is as follows:

Low end range: $21.9 \times 2.25 = 49.3$ kilograms
High end of range: $22.4 \times 2.2550.4$ kilograms

Now complete this calculation using your values for BMI.

My ideal body weight range using the BMI method is _____ to _____ kilograms.

*Note: BMI may not be a good method to determine ideal body weight for a highly muscled individual.

LABORATORY

NAME _____ DATE _____

Estimating Daily Caloric Expenditure and the Caloric Deficit Required to Lose 1 Pound of Fat per Week

Part A: Estimating Your Daily Caloric Expenditure

Compute your estimated daily caloric expenditure.

Estimated daily caloric expenditure = _____ calories/day.

Note: For you to maintain current body weight, your caloric intake should equal your daily caloric expenditure.

Part B: Calculating Caloric Intake Required to Promote 1 Pound Per Week of Weight Loss

Recall that 1 pound of fat contains approximately 3500 calories. Therefore, a negative caloric balance of 500 calories per day will result in a weight loss of 1 pound per week. Use the following formula to compute your daily caloric intake to result in a daily caloric deficit of 500 calories.

Estimated daily caloric expenditure − 500 calories (deficit) = Daily caloric intake needed to produce a 500-calorie deficit

In the space provided, compute your daily caloric intake needed to produce 1 pound per week of weight loss.

_____ (estimated caloric expenditure)

− 500 (caloric deficit)

= _____ (target daily caloric intake)

Note: To increase body weight by 1–2 pounds per week, increase daily caloric intake by 90–180 calories per day.

LABORATORY

NAME _____ DATE _____

Weight-Loss Goals and Progress Report

In the spaces provided, record your short-term and long-term weight-loss goals. Then keep a record of your progress on the chart.

Ideal body weight (range): _____

Short-term weight loss goal: _____1–2_____ (pounds/week)

Long-term weight loss goal: _____ pounds

Week No.	Body Weight	Date	Weight Loss
1			
2			
3			
4			
5			
6			
7			
8			
9			
10			
11			
12			
13			
14			
15			

NAME _____ DATE _____

Assessing Body Image

Respond to the questions below to assess your body image.

1. Where do you get your ideas about the "ideal body"? If more than one applies, how do they rank?

    a. TV/movies _____

    b. friends (including boyfriends and girlfriends) _____

    c. parents and family _____

    d. professional athletes _____

2. What other sources contribute to your image of the "ideal body"?

    _____

    _____

    Fill in the blanks to complete the following statements about your body image. Use extra paper if needed.

3. The thing I like most about my body is

    _____

    _____

4. The thing I like least about my body is

    _____

    _____

5. When I eat a big meal, I feel

    _____

    _____

6. When I look in the mirror, I see

    _____

    _____

7. I like/dislike (circle one) shopping for clothes because

    _____

    _____

8. I feel self-conscious when

    _____

    _____

9. Compared to others, I feel my body is

_____

_____

10. In the presence of someone I find attractive, I feel

_____

_____

11. I feel that my appearance is

_____

_____

12. One word to describe my body is

_____

Interpretation

Now review your answers to the previous questions and think about whether they are positive or negative. To improve a negative body image, keep the following strategies in mind:

- Focus on good physical health. Engage in physical activities that you enjoy.
- Remember that your self-worth is not dependent on how you look.
- Avoid chronic, restrained dieting.
- Recognize that there is much more to you than your body. Think about the qualities that you like best about yourself, and be sure to appreciate them.

NAME _____ DATE _____

What Triggers Your Eating?

There are many things that cause us to eat. Usually, just by identifying the triggers that cause you to eat, you can develop a strategy to counter those habits. Use the questions below to determine your motivation for eating. For each statement, check yes or no.

Emotional Triggers

Yes No

___ ___   I cannot lose weight and keep it off.

___ ___   My eating is out of control.

___ ___   Even if I'm not hungry, I eat.

___ ___   I eat when I am stressed or upset.

___ ___   Food gives me great pleasure and I use it as a reward.

___ ___   Eating is usually on my mind.

___ ___   My eating causes problems with weight management.

___ ___   I go on eating "binges" or find myself eating constantly.

___ ___   My eating habits cause me embarrassment.

___ ___   I use food to help me cope with feelings.

Social Triggers

Yes No

___ ___   I eat whenever others around me are eating.

___ ___   If anyone offers food, I take it.

___ ___   Whenever I am in a stressful social situation, I want to eat.

___ ___   Whenever I am in a relaxed social situation, I want to eat.

___ ___   I eat more in a social setting than I do at home.

___ ___   I eat less when others are around to see me.

___ ___   In a social setting, the amount of food I eat depends on the group of people.

___ ___   I eat different foods in a social setting than I do at home.

LABORATORY

Environmental Triggers

Yes No

___ ___   I eat more at restaurants than I do at home.

___ ___   I eat less at restaurants than I do at home.

___ ___   If I smell or see food I can't resist the urge to eat.

___ ___   If I walk by a restaurant or bakery I can't resist the urge to eat.

___ ___   I like to eat while reading or watching TV.

___ ___   I find food comforting in different environmental conditions, such as on a rainy day or in cold weather.

___ ___   I find food comforting when I am in unfamiliar surroundings.

___ ___   If I am outdoors, I feel like I can eat more.

Interpretation

Insignificant influence: If you answered yes to one question within a section or fewer than six questions total, weight management is probably relatively easy for you.

Some influence: If you answered yes to two questions within a section or six to nine questions total, there are issues complicating your weight management. It might help to talk with a health care professional while developing a weight management plan.

Significant influence: If you answered yes to three questions within a section or 10–13 questions total, there are several issues affecting your weight management plan. Speaking with a health care professional or counselor can help you deal with issues that trigger your eating.

Severe influence: If you answered yes to four or more questions within a section or 14 or more questions total, there are many issues that complicate your weight management. Counseling and speaking with a health care professional will help you to develop a weight-management plan.

NAME _____ DATE _____

Finding Your Cholesterol Plan

The following two-step program will guide you through the National Cholesterol Education Program's treatment guidelines. The first step helps you establish your overall coronary risk; the second uses that information to determine your LDL treatment goals and how to reach them. You'll need to know your blood pressure, your total LDL and HDL cholesterol levels, and your triglyceride and fasting glucose levels. If you're not sure of those numbers, ask your doctor and, if necessary, schedule an exam to get them. (Everyone should have a complete lipid profile every 5 years, starting at age 20.)

Step 1: Take the Heart-Attack Risk Test

This test will identify your chance of having a heart attack or dying of coronary disease in the next 10 years. (People with previously diagnosed coronary disease, diabetes, aortic aneurysm, or symptomatic carotid artery disease or peripheral artery disease already face more than a 20 percent risk; they can skip the test and go straight to step 2.) The test uses data from the Framingham Heart Study, the world's longest-running study of cardiovascular risk factors. The test is limited to established, major factors that are easily measured. Circle the point value for each of the risk factors shown.

Age

Years	Women	Men
20–34	−7	−9
35–39	−3	−4
40–44	0	0
45–49	3	3
50–54	6	6
55–59	8	8
60–64	10	10
65–69	12	11
70–74	14	12
75–79	16	13

Total Cholesterol

mg/dL	Age 20–39		Age 40–49		Age 50–59		Age 60–69		Age 70–79	
	Women	Men	Women	Men	Women	Men	Women	Men	Women	Men
<160	0	0	0	0	0	0	0	0	0	0
160–199	4	4	3	3	2	2	1	1	1	0
200–239	8	7	6	5	4	3	2	1	1	0
240–279	11	9	8	6	5	4	3	2	2	1
280+	13	11	10	8	7	5	4	3	2	1

High-Density Lipoprotein (HDL) Cholesterol

mg/dL	Women and Men
60+	−1
50–59	0
40–49	1
<40	2

Systolic Blood Pressure (the Higher Number)

mm/Hg	Treated		Untreated	
	Women	Men	Women	Men
<120	0	0	0	0
120–129	1	0	3	1
130–139	2	1	4	2
140–159	3	1	5	2
>159	4	2	6	3

Smoking

Age 20–39		Age 40–49		Age 50–59		Age 60–69		Age 70–79	
Women	Men	Women	Men	Women	Men	Women	Men	Women	Men
9	8	7	5	4	3	2	1	1	1

Total Your Points _____

Now find your total point score in the men's or women's column to locate your 10-year risk (the far-right column).

Ten-Year Risk for Heart Disease

Women's Score	Men's Score	Your 10-Year Risk
<20	<12	<10%
20–22	12–15	10–20%
>22	>15	>20%

Step 2: Find Your Low-Density Lipoprotein (LDL) Treatment Plan

Consult the table on the next page to learn whether your overall CHD risk indicates that you need to lower your LDL cholesterol level and, if you do, by how much. First, locate your CHD risk in the left column. (That's based on the 10-year heart-attack risk that you just calculated, as well as your CHD risk factors and any heart-threatening diseases you may have.) Then look across that row to see whether you should make lifestyle changes and take cholesterol-lowering medication, based on your current LDL level.

LABORATORY

NAME _____ DATE _____

CHD Risk Group	Start lifestyle changes if your LDL level is . . .*	Add drugs if your LDL level is . . .
Very High 1. Ten-year heart-attack risk of 20% or more *or* 2. History of coronary heart disease, diabetes, peripheral-artery disease, carotid-artery disease, or aortic aneurysm.	100 mg/dl or higher. (Aim for an LDL under 100.) Get retested after 3 months.	130 or higher. (Drugs are optional if your LDL is between 100 and 130.)
High 1. Ten-year heart-attack risk of 10% to 20% *and* 2. Two or more major coronary risk factors.†	130 or higher. (Aim for an LDL under 130.) Get retested after 3 months.	130 or higher and lifestyle changes don't achieve your LDL goal in 3 months.
Moderately High 1. Ten-year heart-attack risk under 10% *and* 2. Two or more major coronary risk factors.†	Same as above.	160 or higher, and lifestyle changes don't achieve your LDL goal in 3 months.‡
Low to Moderate 1. One or no major coronary risk factors.†§	160 or higher. (Aim for an LDL under 160.) Get retested after 3 months.	190 or higher, and lifestyle changes don't achieve your LDL goal in 3 months. (Drugs are optional if your LDL is between 160 and 189.)

*People who have the metabolic syndrome should make lifestyle changes even if their LDL level alone doesn't warrant it. You have the metabolic syndrome if you have three or more of these risk factors: HDL under 40 in men, 50 in women; systolic blood pressure of 130 or more or diastolic pressure of 85 or more; fasting glucose level of 110 to 125; triglycerides level of 150 or more; and waist circumference over 40 inches in men, 35 inches in women. People with the syndrome should limit their carbohydrate intake, get up to 30 to 35 percent of their calories from total fat (more than usually recommended), and make the other lifestyle changes, including restriction of saturated fat.

†The major coronary risk factors are cigarette smoking; coronary disease in a father or brother before age 55 or a mother or sister before age 65; systolic blood pressure of 140 or more, a diastolic pressure of 90 or more, or being on drugs for hypertension; and an HDL level under 40. If your HDL is 60 or more, subtract one risk factor. (High LDL is a major factor, of course, but it's already figured into the table.)

‡Although the goal is to get LDL under 130, the use of drugs in these people usually isn't worthwhile, even if lifestyle steps fail to achieve that goal.

§People in this group usually have a 10-year risk of less than 10%. Those who have higher risk should ask their doctor whether they need more aggressive treatment than shown here.

Source: From Rebecca Donatelle, *Access to Health,* 8th ed. Copyright © 2004. Reprinted by permission of Pearson Education, Inc.

NAME _____ DATE _____

Understanding Your Risk for Cardiovascular Disease

Each of us has a unique level of risk for various diseases. Some of these risks you can take action to change; others are risks that you need to consider as you plan a lifelong strategy for overall risk reduction. Complete each of the following questions, and total your points in each section. If you score between 1 and 5 in any section, consider your risk. The higher the number, the greater your risk. If you answered "Don't know" for any question, talk to your parents or other family members as soon as possible to find out whether you have any unknown risks.

Part I: Assess Your Family Risk for CVD

1. Do any of your primary relatives (mother, father, grandparents, siblings) have a history of heart disease or stroke?

   Yes _____ (1 point)   No _____ (0 points)   Don't know _____

2. Do any of your primary relatives (mother, father, grandparents, siblings) have diabetes?

   Yes _____ (1 point)   No _____ (0 points)   Don't know _____

3. Do any of your primary relatives (mother, father, grandparents, siblings) have high blood pressure?

   Yes _____ (1 point)   No _____ (0 points)   Don't know _____

4. Do any of your primary relatives (mother, father, grandparents, siblings) have a history of high cholesterol?

   Yes _____ (1 point)   No _____ (0 points)   Don't know _____

5. Would you say that your family consumed a high-fat diet (lots of red meat, dairy products, butter or margarine) during your time spent at home?

   Yes _____ (1 point)   No _____ (0 points)   Don't know _____

Total points _____

Part II: Assess Your Lifestyle Risk for CVD

1. Is your total cholesterol level higher than it should be?

   Yes _____ (1 point)   No _____ (0 points)   Don't know _____

2. Do you have high blood pressure?

   Yes _____ (1 point)   No _____ (0 points)   Don't know _____

3. Have you been diagnosed as prediabetic or diabetic?

   Yes _____ (1 point)   No _____ (0 points)   Don't know _____

4. Do you smoke?

   Yes _____ (1 point)   No _____ (0 points)   Don't know _____

5. Would you describe your life as being highly stressful?

   Yes _____ (1 point)   No _____ (0 points)   Don't know _____

Total points _____

LABORATORY

Part III: Assess Your Additional Risks for CVD

1. How would you best describe your current weight?
   a. Lower than what it should be for my height and weight. (0 points)
   b. About what it should be for my height and weight. (0 points)
   c. Higher than it should be for my height and weight. (1 point)

2. How would you describe the level of exercise that you get each day?
   a. Less than what I should be exercising each day. (1 point)
   b. About what I should be exercising each day. (0 points)
   c. More than what I should be each day. (0 points)

3. How would you describe your dietary behaviors?
   a. Eating only the recommended number of calories per day. (0 points)
   b. Eating less than the recommended number of calories each day. (0 points)
   c. Eating more than the recommended number of calories each day. (1 point)

4. Which of the following best describes your typical dietary behavior?
   a. I eat from the major food groups, trying hard to get the recommended fruits and vegetables. (0 points)
   b. I eat too much red meat and consume too much saturated fat from meats and dairy products each day. (1 point)
   c. Whenever possible, I try to substitute olive oil or canola oil for other forms of dietary fat. (0 points)

5. Do you have a history of *Chlamydia* infection?
   a. Yes. (1 point)
   b. No. (0 points)

Total points _____

NAME _____ DATE _____

Assessing Your Genetic Predisposition for Cardiovascular Disease

The following is a family tree that allows you to fill in risk factors and conditions for heart disease in your family members. Remember that heart disease has a genetic component, so examining your relatives' health and lifestyles will provide insight into your future susceptibility to heart disease. Write in risk factors directly related to heart disease. Examples include hypertension, high blood cholesterol, diabetes, stroke, obesity, and heart attack.

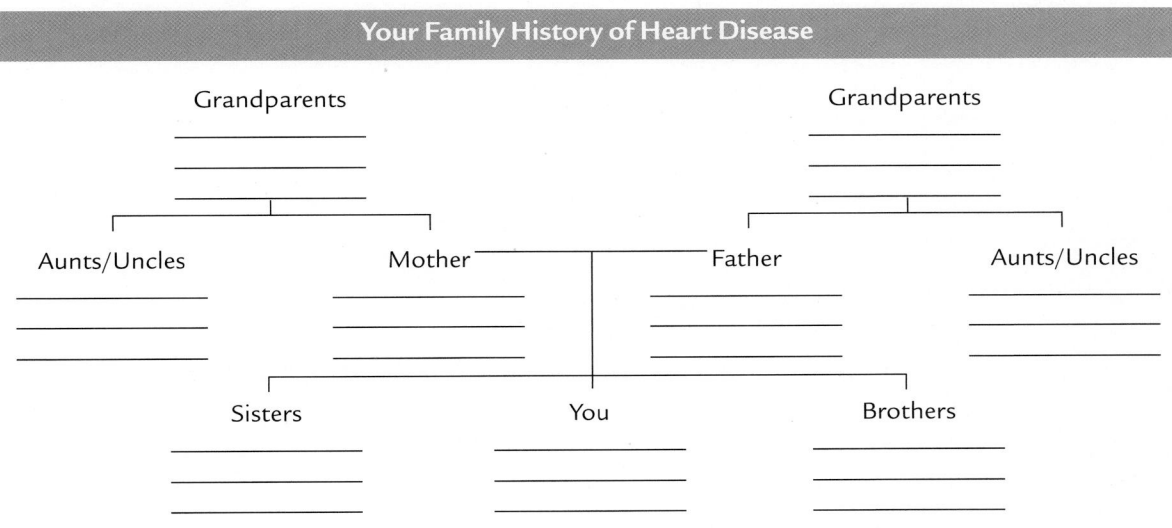

Your Family History of Heart Disease

Grandparents   Grandparents

Aunts/Uncles   Mother   Father   Aunts/Uncles

Sisters   You   Brothers

Note: This family tree can be copied and used for other diseases with an inheritable component, such as cancer.

In the space below, list any diet, behavior, or lifestyle risks in your life that may contribute to heart disease. Examples include high stress level, high-fat diet, physical inactivity, high sodium intake.

_____

_____

_____

Interpretation

Inherited traits can increase your risk of cardiovascular disease. The good news is that you are not destined to develop heart disease or any of the conditions present in your relatives. Lifestyle changes that include moderate exercise and proper diet can reduce your risk of developing cardiovascular diseases. Being aware of health concerns and problems within your family that may be passed on genetically will make you a more informed, health-conscious individual.

LABORATORY

NAME _____ DATE _____

Warming Up

Use the following activities to warm up your body for aerobic activities such as jogging, walking, or cycling. Perform the exercises slowly, holding each stretch for 20 to 30 seconds. Do not bounce or jerk the muscle. Do each stretch at least once and up to three times.

Visit this textbook's companion website to view demonstration videos of these stretches.

Cardiovascular Warm-Up

Walk briskly or jog slowly for 5 minutes.

Stretches

Calf Stretch for Gastrocnemius and Soleus

Stand with your right foot about 1 to 2 feet in front of your left foot, with both feet pointing forward. Keeping your left leg straight, lunge forward by bending your right knee and pushing your left heel backward. Hold this position. Then pull your left foot in slightly and bend your left knee. Shift your weight to your left leg and hold. Repeat this entire sequence with the left leg forward.

Sitting Toe Touch for Hamstrings

Sit on the ground with your right leg straight and your left leg tucked close to your body. Reach toward your out-stretched right foot as far as possible with both hands. Repeat with the left leg.

Step Stretch for Quadriceps and Hip

Step forward and bend your front knee about 90 degrees, keeping your knee directly above your ankle. Stretch the opposite leg back so that it is parallel to the floor. Rotate your hips forward and slightly down to stretch. Your arms can be at your sides or resting on top of your forward thigh. Repeat on the other side.

Leg Hug for the Hip and Back Extensors

Lie flat on your back with both legs straight. Bending your knees, bring your legs up to your torso, and grasp both legs behind the thighs. Pull both legs in to your chest and hold.

Side Stretch for the Torso

Stand with feet shoulder-width apart, knees slightly bent, and pelvis tucked under. Raise one arm over your head, and bend sideways from the waist. Support your torso by placing the hand of your resting arm on your hip or thigh for support. Repeat on the other side.

  You can also repeat these same exercises after a workout to cool down.

1. Did you notice an increase in heart rate during the cardiovascular warm-up? _____

2. In which stretch did you feel the most tightness? _____

3. Do you think the sample warm-up is adequate for the activities you plan to do as part of your exercise program? If not, what exercises would you add?

_____

_____

943

NAME _____ DATE _____

Which Physical Activities Work Best for You?

As you design your personal fitness program, think about the activities you currently enjoy most and least and about new activities you would like to try. Which can you incorporate into your program?

Answer the following questions in the spaces provided.

1. List the fitness/wellness activities in which you have participated or are currently participating. Examples include recreational tennis, high school basketball, or yoga classes.

   _____

2. Which of these activities did you enjoy the most? Why?

   _____

3. What are some new activities you might enjoy? (See the list at the end of the lab for additional options.)

   _____

   _____

4. What components of physical fitness do you think these activities affect? For instance, jogging improves cardiovascular fitness, whereas weight lifting increases muscular strength.

   _____

   _____

5. What areas of physical and mental health would you like to improve? Can you think of any physical activities that would aid in this goal?

   _____

   _____

Examples of Exercise and Physical Activity

- Walking or jogging on a treadmill
- Walking to work instead of driving
- Cycling on an upright or recumbent exercise bike
- Cycling to work instead of driving
- Outdoor walking or jogging
- Outdoor cycling
- Aerobics class
- Kickboxing class
- Weight or resistance training
- Yoga
- Martial arts
- Pilates

- Hiking
- Rock climbing
- Elliptical trainer
- Sport activities (e.g., soccer, basketball, tennis, racquetball)

NAME _____ DATE _____

Using a Pedometer to Count Your Steps

One way to determine your level of daily physical activity is to use a pedometer to measure the number of steps you take in a day. A pedometer is a small portable device that contains a sensor and, often, software applications to estimate the distance walked and the number of calories expended. The accuracy of pedometers can vary from device to device, but many pedometers are reasonably accurate if they are worn in the optimal position (such as on a belt clip). However, carrying a pedometer in a pocket or handbag tends to reduce its accuracy. Moreover, some pedometers record movement other than walking (e.g., bending to tie your shoes), and therefore some "false steps" may show up on your daily step count.

Experts currently recommend 10,000 steps per day to reach a level of physical activity that is considered to be an active lifestyle with positive health benefits. Do you think you meet this goal?

A pedometer worn at the waist.

Directions:

Wear a pedometer for a day and note your number of steps. Write in the total number below. Then, set a goal for the number of steps you want to take per day, and list some strategies for incorporating more steps into your day. Track the number of steps you take every day for the next 2 weeks, and note your progress toward your goal.

Number of steps for day 1: _____   Goal number of steps/day: _____

Number of steps for day 2: _____

Number of steps for day 3: _____

Number of steps for day 4: _____

Number of steps for day 5: _____

Number of steps for day 6: _____

Number of steps for day 7: _____

Number of steps for day 8: _____

Number of steps for day 9: _____

Number of steps for day 10: _____

Number of steps for day 11: _____

Number of steps for day 12: _____

Number of steps for day 13: _____

Number of steps for day 14: _____

Analysis

1. Did you meet your goal for number of daily steps on most days?   Yes/No
2. Are you walking at least the recommended 10,000 steps per day? Yes/No
3. If not, think about how you can incorporate more steps into your daily routine. List below four ways to increase the amount of walking you do daily:

_____

_____

_____

_____

NAME _____ DATE _____

Measuring Cardiorespiratory Fitness: The 1.5-Mile Run Test

The objective of the test is to complete the 1.5-mile distance as quickly as possible. You can complete the run on an oval track or any properly measured course. If the run will take place outside, the test is best conducted in moderate weather conditions; avoid running it on very hot or very cold days. A good strategy is to try to keep a steady pace during the entire distance. Performing a practice test is a good way to get familiar with the distance and determine the ideal pace you can maintain. You should use a stopwatch to get an accurate time. You should attempt this test only if you have met the medical clearance criteria.

Before the test, perform a 5- to 10-minute warm-up. If you become extremely fatigued during the test, slow your pace or walk—do not overstress yourself! If you feel faint or nauseated or experience any unusual pains in your upper body, stop and notify your instructor.

After you complete the test, cool down and record your time and fitness category from Cooper's 1.5-Mile Run Test Table on page 950. Find your age group along the top of the table, and then locate your time range according to your sex. The fitness classifications are along the left of the table.

Test date: _____

Finish time: _____

Fitness category: _____

1. Is your fitness classification what you expected based on your current level of activity? If not, why do you think it was higher or lower than expected?

_____

_____

2. Write fitness goals for maintaining or improving your cardiorespiratory endurance.

_____

_____

Fitness Categories for Cooper's 1.5-Mile Run Test

Fitness Category	Age (years)					
	13–19	20–29	30–39	40–49	50–59	60+
Men						
Very poor	>15:30	>16:00	>16:30	>17:30	>19:00	.20:00
Poor	12:11–15:30	14:01–16:00	14:46–16:30	15:36–17:30	17:01–19:00	19:01–20:00
Average	10:49–12:10	12:01–14:00	12:31–14:45	13:01–15:35	14:31–17:00	16:16–19:00
Good	9:41–10:48	10:46–12:00	11:01–12:30	11:31–13:00	12:31–14:30	14:00–16:15
Excellent	8:37–9:40	9:45–10:45	10:00–11:00	10:30–11:30	11:00–12:30	11:15–13:59
Superior	<8:37	<9:45	<10:00	<10:30	<11:00	<11:15
Women						
Very poor	>18:30	>19:00	>19:30	>20:00	>20:30	>21:00
Poor	16:55–18:30	18:31–19:00	19:01–19:30	19:31–20:00	20:01–20:30	20:31–21:31
Average	14:31–16:54	15:55–18:30	16:31–19:00	17:31–19:30	19:01–20:00	19:31–20:30
Good	12:30–14:30	13:31–15:54	14:31–16:30	15:56–17:30	16:31–19:00	17:31–19:30
Excellent	11:50–12:29	12:30–13:30	13:00–14:30	13:45–15:55	14:30–16:30	16:30–18:00
Superior	<11:50	<12:30	<13:00	<13:45	<14:30	<16:30

Times are given in minutes and seconds. (> = greater than; < = less than)
Source: From Cooper, K. *The Aerobics Program for Total Well-Being.* Bantam Books, New York, 1982. Copyright © 1982 by Kenneth H. Cooper. Used by permission of Bantam Books, a division of Random House, Inc.

NAME _____ DATE _____

Measuring Cardiorespiratory Fitness: The 1-Mile Walk Test

The objective of the test is to walk the 1-mile distance as quickly as possible. You can complete the walk on an oval track or any properly measured course. You should attempt this test only if you have met the medical clearance criteria.

Before the test, perform a 5- to 10-minute warm-up. If you become extremely fatigued during the test, slow your pace—do not overstress yourself! If you feel faint or nauseated or experience any unusual pains in your upper body, stop and notify your instructor.

After you complete the test, cool down and record your time and fitness category from 1-Mile Walk Test Table on page 952. Find your age group along the top of the table, and then locate your time range according to your sex. The fitness classifications are along the left of the table.

Test date: _____

Finish time: _____

Fitness category: _____

1. Is your fitness classification what you expected based on your current level of activity? If not, why do you think it was higher or lower than expected?

   _____

   _____

2. Write fitness goals for maintaining or improving your cardiorespiratory endurance.

   _____

   _____

Fitness Classification for 1-Mile Walk Test

Fitness Category	Age (years)			
	13–19	20–29	30–39	40+
Men				
Very poor	>17:30	>18:00	>19:00	>21:30
Poor	16:01–17:30	16:31–18:00	17:31–19:00	18:31–21:30
Average	14:01–16:00	14:31–16:30	15:31–17:30	16:01–18:30
Good	12:30–14:00	13:00–14:30	13:30–15:30	14:00–16:00
Excellent	<12:30	<13:00	<13:30	<14:00
Women				
Very poor	>18:01	>18:31	>19:31	>20:01
Poor	16:31–18:00	17:01–18:30	18:01–19:30	19:31–20:00
Average	14:31–16:30	15:01–17:00	16:01–18:00	18:01–19:30
Good	13:31–14:30	13:31–15:00	14:01–16:00	14:31–18:00
Excellent	<13:30	<13:30	<14:00	<14:30

Because the 1-mile walk test is designed primarily for older or less conditioned individuals, the fitness categories listed here do not include a "superior" category.

Source: Modified from *Rockport Fitness Walking Test.* Copyright © 1993. The Rockport Company, Inc. All rights reserved. Reprinted by permission of The Rockport Company, Inc.

NAME _____ DATE _____

Measuring Cardiorespiratory Fitness: Submaximal Cycle Test

This lab test is performed with a partner. While you are exercising, your partner will help by setting the workload for the test, checking your pedal rate, and taking your heart rate. The work performed on a cycle ergometer is commonly expressed either in *kilopond meters per minute (KPM)* or in watts. Your instructor will explain how to use the KPM and watts settings to adjust the workload.

Warm up for 3 minutes without using any resistance (unloaded pedaling). Your instructor will tell you how to adjust the workload. Set the appropriate load for your age, sex, and level of conditioning in the table below, and begin pedaling at the rate of 50 revolutions per minute (RPM). Your instructor will set a metronome so you know how fast to pedal. Exercise for a 5-minute period. Your partner will take your heart rate during a 15-second period between minutes 4.5 and 5 of the test.

Cool down for 3 to 5 minutes without resistance. Record your heart rate (15-second count) below, and calculate your relative $\dot{V}O_2$max using the table on the next page. After calculating your relative $\dot{V}O_2$max, locate your fitness category in the table on page 955.

Test date: _____

Heart rate (15-second count) during minute 5 of test: _____

Fitness category: _____

1. Is your fitness classification what you expected based on your current level of activity? If not, why do you think it was higher or lower than expected?

   _____

   _____

2. Write fitness goals for maintaining or improving your cardiorespiratory endurance.

   _____

   _____

Work Rates for Submaximal Cycle Ergometer Fitness Test

Gender	Age (years)	Pedal Speed (RPM)	Load	(watts)
Men				
	Up to 29	50	150	(900 KPM)
	30 and up	50	50	(300 KPM)
Women				
	Up to 29 (or well conditioned)	50	100	(600 KPM)
	30 and up (or poorly conditioned)	50	50	(300 KPM)

Cycle Ergometer Fitness Index for Men and Women

Locate your 15-second heart rate in the left-hand column; then find your estimated $\dot{V}O_2$max in the appropriate column on the right. For example, the second column from the left contains the absolute $\dot{V}O_2$max (expressed in mL/min) for male subjects using the 900-KPM work rate. The third column from the left contains the absolute $\dot{V}O_2$max (expressed in mL/min) for women using the 600-KPM work rate, and so on. After determination of your absolute $\dot{V}O_2$max, calculate your relative $\dot{V}O_2$max (mL/kg/min) by dividing your $\dot{V}O_2$max expressed in mL/min by your body weight in kilograms (1 kilogram = 2.2 pounds). For example, if your body weight is 70 kilograms and your absolute $\dot{V}O_2$max is 2631 mL/min, your relative $\dot{V}O_2$max is approximately 38 mL/kg/min (i.e., 2631 divided by 70 = 37.6). After computing your relative $\dot{V}O_2$max, use Cycle Ergometer to identify your fitness category.

15-Second Heart Rate	Estimated Absolute $\dot{V}O_2$max (mL/min)		
	Men: 900-KPM Work Rate (mL/min)	Women: 600-KPM Work Rate (mL/min)	Men or Women: 300-KPM Work Rate (mL/min)
28	3560	2541	1525
29	3442	2459	1475
30	3333	2376	1425
31	3216	2293	1375
32	3099	2210	1325
33	2982	2127	1275
34	2865	2044	1225
35	2748	1961	1175
36	2631	1878	1125
37	2514	1795	1075
38	2397	1712	1025
39	2280	1629	—
40	2163	1546	—
41	2046	1463	—
42	1929	1380	—
43	1812	1297	—
44	1695	1214	—
45	1578	1131	—

NAME _____ DATE _____

Cardiorespiratory Fitness Norms for Men and Women Based on Estimated $\dot{V}O_2$max Values Determined by the Cycle Ergometer Fitness Test

After determining your relative $\dot{V}O_2$max (mL/kg/min) in the table on the previous page, find your appropriate fitness category.

Age Group (years)	Fitness Categories Based on $\dot{V}O_2$max (mL/kg/min)					
	Very Poor	Poor	Average	Good	Excellent	Superior
Men						
18–25	<30	30–39	40–45	46–60	61–64	>64
26–35	<29	29–38	39–43	44–55	56–59	>59
36–45	<27	27–35	36–40	41–49	50–55	>55
46–45	<25	25–31	32–35	36–45	46–49	>49
56–65	<22	22–28	29–33	34–40	41–43	>43
>65	<20	20–25	26–28	29–34	35–38	>38
Women						
18–25	<30	30–38	39–43	44–54	55–58	>58
26–35	<28	28–33	34–41	42–53	54–58	>58
36–45	<24	24–32	33–36	37–46	47–50	>50
46–55	<22	22–28	29–31	32–41	42–45	>45
56–65	<19	19–25	26–29	30–36	37–40	>40
>65	<17	17–21	22–25	26–30	31–34	>34

Source: Data reprinted from Golding, L., (ed.). *YMCA Fitness Testing and Assessment Manual*, 4th Edition. With permission of the YMCA of the USA, Chicago IL. Copyright © 2000.

LABORATORY

NAME _____ DATE _____

Measuring Cardiorespiratory Fitness: Step Test

To complete this test, you need a step or bench that is approximately 18 inches high, such as a locker room bench or a sturdy chair. The step test lasts for 3 minutes, and then heart rate is assessed in the 3.5 minutes following the test. You will need a metronome to help you maintain the step rate.

   To perform this test, you will step up and down at a rate of 30 complete steps per minute. If you set the metronome to 60 tones per minute, you will step with each tone making a complete step (up, up, down, down) every 2 seconds. Note that it is important that you straighten your knees during the "up" phase of the test. After you complete the test, sit quietly in a chair or on the step bench, and take your heart rate for 30 seconds at the following times:

1 to 1.5 minutes post exercise

2 to 2.5 minutes post exercise

3 to 3.5 minutes post exercise

Visit this textbook's companion website to view a demonstration video of the step test.

Subject steps up onto an 18-inch surface and then down once every
2 seconds. Set metronome to 60 tones per minute.

LABORATORY

Maintaining the 30-step-per-minute cadence and accurately taking your heart rate are very important for getting a good estimate from the step test. To determine your fitness category, add the three 30-second heart rates obtained during the period after exercise.

Record your heart rates below, and use the table on this page to determine your fitness category.

Test date: _____

Recovery heart rate post exercise (bpm)

1–1.5 min: _____

2–2.5 min: _____

3–3.5 min: _____

Total (recovery index): _____

Fitness category: _____

Norms for Cardiorespiratory Fitness Using the Sum of Three Recovery Heart Rates Obtained Following the Step Test

Fitness Category	3-Minute Step Test Recovery Index	
	Women	Men
Superior	95–120	95–117
Excellent	121–135	118–132
Good	136–153	133–147
Average	154–174	148–165
Poor	175–204	166–192
Very Poor	205–233	193–217

Fitness categories are for college-aged men and women (aged 18–25 years) at the University of Florida who performed the test on an 18-inch bench.

LABORATORY

NAME _____ DATE _____

1. Is your fitness classification what you expected based on your current level of activity? If not, why do you think it was higher or lower than expected?

_____

_____

2. Write fitness goals for maintaining or improving your cardiorespiratory endurance.

_____

_____

NAME _____ DATE _____

Assessing Cardiorespiratory Fitness for Individuals with Disabilities

This test uses arm exercise and is for people who cannot perform exercise that requires use of the legs (people in wheelchairs or with leg or foot injuries). To perform this assessment, you will need an arm crank ergometer. Your instructor will adjust the ergometer to the correct height and position for the test.

First, do a warm-up with no resistance. Then your instructor will increase the resistance, and you will perform a 2-minute stage. Rest 5 to 10 minutes. Then, after your instructor increases the workload, perform another 2-minute period of arm exercise. Repeat this cycle until you cannot complete 2 minutes of exercise at a given workload. Your instructor will tell you the workload for the last stage in which you completed the full 2 minutes of exercise. You can use that number, along with the table included in this lab, to determine your $\dot{V}O_2max$. After you find your weight and workload on the table, find the corresponding number and multiple that value by 3.5 to get your $\dot{V}O_2max$. If your weight is not on the table, you can use the following equation to calculate your $\dot{V}O_2max$:

$$\dot{V}O_2max = 3 \times (\text{work rate*})/\text{body weight in kg} \dagger + 3.5$$

The table on page 955 has the fitness classifications that correspond to your $\dot{V}O_2max$. Because this test uses arm exercise, which involves a smaller muscle mass than leg or whole body exercise, your $\dot{V}O_2max$ estimate will be a slight underestimate.

Fitness category: _____

1. Is your fitness classification what you expected based on your current level of activity? If not, why do you think it was higher or lower than expected?

   _____

   _____

2. Write fitness goals for maintaining or improving your cardiorespiratory endurance.

   _____

   _____

* Your instructor will give you this value.

† Weight in kg = weight in lbs ÷ 2.2

LABORATORY

Approximate Energy Requirements in METs* during Arm Ergometry

| Body Weight | | Power Output (kg/g/min and W†) | | | | | |
| kg | lb | 150 | 300 | 450 | 600 | 750 | 900 (kg/m/min) |
		25	50	75	100	125	150 (W)
50	110	3.6	6.1	8.7	11.3	13.9	16.4
60	132	3.1	5.3	7.4	9.6	11.7	13.9
70	154	2.8	4.7	6.5	8.3	10.2	12.0
80	176	2.6	4.2	5.8	7.4	9.0	10.6
90	198	2.4	3.9	5.3	6.7	8.1	9.6
100	220	2.3	3.6	4.9	6.1	7.4	8.7

* 1 MET=3.5 ml/kg/min. This value is your $\dot{V}O_2$ at rest.

† W = watts.

Source: From American College of Sports Medicine. *ACSM's Guideline for Exercise Testing and Prescription,* 7th ed. Philadelphia: Lippincott, Williams, & Wilkins, 2006.

NAME _____ DATE _____

Determining Target Heart Rate

Practice taking your heart rate at both the carotid and radial locations. You can feel the carotid pulse next to the larynx, beneath the lower jaw. The radial pulse is located on the inside of the wrist, directly in line with the base of the thumb. Use a stopwatch to count for 15, 30, and 60 seconds. To determine your heart rate in beats per minute (bpm), multiply your 15-second count by 4, and your 30-second count by 2.

Try locating and taking the heart rate of a classmate at both the radial and carotid locations. Record your resting pulse counts in the spaces provided.

Visit this textbook's companion website to view demonstration videos of locating the radical and carotid pulses.

Carotid Pulse Count (self)	Heart Rate (bpm)	Radial Pulse Count (self)	Heart Rate (bpm)
15 seconds × 4		× 4	
30 seconds × 2		× 2	
60 seconds × 1		× 1	
Carotid Pulse Count (partner)	Heart Rate (bpm)	Radial Pulse Count (partner)	Heart Rate (bpm)
15 seconds × 4		× 4	
30 seconds × 2		× 2	
60 seconds × 1		× 1	

The target heart rate (THR) range is calculated in steps.

Step 1: Calculate your estimated maximal heart rate (HR_{max})

$$HR_{max} = 220 - age \underline{\hspace{2cm}}$$

Step 2: Calculate your heart rate reserve (HRR) by subtracting your resting heart rate from your HR_{max} (use the 60-second count from above).

$$HRR = HR_{max} - resting\ heart\ rate$$
$$HRR = \underline{\hspace{1.5cm}} - \underline{\hspace{1cm}}$$
$$HRR = \underline{\hspace{3cm}}$$

Step 3: Calculate 50% and 85% HRR (use decimal values)

Lower end of THR $= 0.5\,(HRR) = \underline{\hspace{2.5cm}}$
Upper end of THR $= 0.85\,(HRR) = \underline{\hspace{2.5cm}}$

Step 4: Add your resting heart rate back to these values

$$50\% \text{ HRR } + \text{ resting heart rate } = \text{_____}$$
$$85\% \text{ HRR } + \text{ resting heart rate } = \text{_____}$$

THR = _____ bpm to _____ bpm

1. Which of the resting pulses did you find easiest to locate on yourself?

   ____Carotid   ____ Radial

2. Which resting pulse was easiest to locate on your partner?

   ____Carotid   ____ Radial

3. Which of the two locations would you prefer to use when counting exercise heart rate?

   ____Carotid   ____ Radial

   Why? _____

NAME _____ DATE _____

Developing Your Personal Exercise Prescription

Using the following Sample Exercise Programs as models, develop your personal exercise program based on your current fitness level and goals. Record the appropriate information in the spaces provided below.

Sample Exercise Program for Someone with an Initial Low Level of Cardiorespiratory Fitness

General guidelines:

1. Begin each session with a warm-up.

2. Don't progress to the next level until you feel comfortable with your current level of exercise.

3. Monitor your heart rate during each training session.

4. End each session with a cool-down.

5. Be aware of aches and pains. If you are injury prone, choose a low-impact activity mode, and limit your exercise duration to 20 to 30 minutes per day.

Week No.	Phase	Duration (min/day)	Intensity (% of HR_{max})	Frequency (days/wk)
1	Initial conditioning	10	60	3
2	Initial conditioning	10	60	3
3	Initial conditioning	12	60	3
4	Initial conditioning	12	70	3
5	Initial conditioning	15	70	3
6	Initial conditioning	15	70	3
7	Improvement	20	70	3
8	Improvement	20	70	3
9	Improvement	25	70	3
10	Improvement	25	70	3
11	Improvement	30	70	3
12	Improvement	30	70	3
13	Improvement	35	70	3
14	Improvement	35	70	3
15	Improvement	40	70	3
16	Improvement	40	70	3
17	Improvement	40	75	3
18	Improvement	40	75	3
19	Improvement	40	75	3
20	Improvement	40	75	3–4
21	Improvement	40	75	3–4
22	Improvement	40	75	3–4
23	Maintenance	30	75	3–4
24	Maintenance	30	75	3–4
25	Maintenance	30	75	3–4
26	Maintenance	30	75	3–4

LABORATORY

Sample Exercise Program for Someone with an Initial Average Level of Cardiorespiratory Fitness

General guidelines:

1. Begin each session with a warm-up.

2. Don't progress to the next level until you feel comfortable with your current level of exercise.

3. Monitor your heart rate during each training session.

4. End each session with a cool-down.

5. Be aware of aches and pains. If you are injury prone, choose a low-impact activity mode, and limit your exercise duration to 20 to 30 minutes per day.

Week No.	Phase	Duration (min/day)	Intensity (% of HR_{max})	Frequency (days/wk)
1	Initial conditioning	10	70	3
2	Initial conditioning	15	70	3
3	Initial conditioning	15	70	3
4	Initial conditioning	20	70	3
5	Improvement	25	70	3
6	Improvement	25	75	3
7	Improvement	25	75	3
8	Improvement	30	75	3
9	Improvement	30	75	3
10	Improvement	35	75	3
11	Improvement	35	75	3
12	Improvement	40	75	3
13	Improvement	40	75	3
14	Improvement	40	75	3
15	Improvement	40	80	3
16	Improvement	40	80	3–4
17	Improvement	40	80	3–4
18	Improvement	40	80	3–4
19	Maintenance	30	80	3–4
20	Maintenance	30	80	3–4
21	Maintenance	30	80	3–4
22	Maintenance	30	80	3–4

LABORATORY

Sample Exercise Program for Someone with an Initial High Level of Cardiorespiratory Fitness

General guidelines:

1. Begin each session with a warm-up.

2. Don't progress to the next level until you feel comfortable with your current level of exercise.

3. Monitor your heart rate during each training session.

4. End each session with a cool-down.

5. Be aware of aches and pains. If you are injury prone, choose a low-impact activity mode, and limit your exercise duration to 20 to 30 minutes per day.

Week No.	Phase	Duration (min/day)	Intensity (% of HR_{max})	Frequency (days/wk)
1	Initial conditioning	15	75	3
2	Initial conditioning	20	75	3
3	Improvement	25	75	3
4	Improvement	30	75	3
5	Improvement	35	75	3
6	Improvement	40	75	3
7	Improvement	40	75	3–4
8	Improvement	40	75	3–4
9	Improvement	40	80	3–4
10	Improvement	40	80	3–4
11	Improvement	40	80	3–4
12	Improvement	40	80–85	3–4
13	Improvement	40	80–85	3–4
14	Improvement	40	80–85	3–4
15	Maintenance	30	80–85	3–4
16	Maintenance	30	80–85	3–4
17	Maintenance	30	80–85	3–4
18	Maintenance	30	80–85	3–4

LABORATORY

Week No.	Phase	Duration (min/day)	Intensity (% of HHR or RPE)	Frequency (days/week)	Exercise Mode	Comments
1						
2						
3						
4						
5						
6						
7						
8						
9						
10						
11						
12						
13						
14						
15						
16						

NAME _____ DATE _____

Determining Rate of Perceived Exertion

Rate of perceived exertion (RPE) was originally developed to correspond to heart rates. Adding a zero to the numerical rating produces the expected heart rate range for that rating. However, people perceive exertion differently, so ratings do not always match heart rate values. The important thing to learn is the RPE number that corresponds to your threshold of training heart rate and the RPE that represents the upper-limit heart rate of your target heart rate (THR) range. Typically, numerical RPE ratings for exercise in the THR zone will fall between 12 and 16. With practice, you can learn to make accurate ratings.

Use the following RPE scale to rate your exertion.

Scale	Verbal Rating
6	No exertion at all
7	Extremely light
8	
9	Very light
10	
11	Light
12	
13	Somewhat hard
14	
15	Hard (heavy)
16	
17	Very hard
18	
19	Extremely hard
20	Maximal exertion

Perform the following exercises:

1. Walk for 3 minutes at a brisk pace.

2. Jog for 3 minutes at a slow pace.

3. Jog for 3 minutes at a pace that will elevate your heart rate to your threshold level.

After each exercise bout, take your heart rate. Also, rate the intensity of the exercise at the end of minute 3 using the RPE scale above. Record these values on the table that follows.

Next, perform a more intense 3-minute run that elevates your heart rate to the upper one-third of your THR zone. After the run, take your heart rate and give an RPE value.

Activity	Heart Rate (bpm)	Rating of Perceived Exertion
Walk		
Slow jog		
Faster jog (to reach training threshold)		
Intense run		

After you've completed your slow and faster jogs, answer the following questions:

1. Did you reach your heart rate training threshold with the walk or slow jog? ___ Yes ___ No

2. Was your RPE less than 12 for the walk or slow jog? ___ Yes ___ No

3. Was your RPE for the faster jog in the range of 12 to 16? ___ Yes ___ No

4. Did your heart rate reach the upper end of your THR for the run? ___ Yes ___ No

5. Was your RPE in the intense run in the range of 12 to 16? ___ Yes ___ No

6. Was your heart approximately 10 times your RPE? ___ Yes ___ No

7. With practice, do you think you could learn to use the RPE scale to assess your exercise intensity? _____

8. What are the limitations for using heart rate to assess your exercise intensity?

_____

_____

9. What are the limitations for using RPE to assess your exercise intensity?

_____

_____

_____

NAME _____ DATE _____

Managing Time and Establishing Priorities

Often people feel that that there are not enough hours in the day. They feel that at some future point, such as "when I graduate," they will have more time to focus on priorities. Delaying things until the future results in lack of completion. Use the following time management tool to help you budget your time and organize your priorities.

Step 1: Establish Priorities

Rank each priority that applies to you in the list below. Use 1 for the highest priority, 2 for the second highest, and so on. You may add priorities as necessary.

Priority	Rank	Priority	Rank
More time with family	_____	More time for exercise and physical activity	_____
More time with friends	_____	More time to relax	_____
More time for work and professional pursuits	_____	More time to study	_____
More time for leisure and recreaton	_____	More time for myself	_____
More time with boyfriend/girlfriend/spouse	_____	Other: _____	_____

Step 2: Monitor Your Current Time Use

Pick one day of the week, and track what you do each hour of the day.

Time	Activity
5:00 AM	
6:00	
7:00	
8:00	
9:00	
10:00	
11:00	
12:00 PM	
1:00	
2:00	

LABORATORY

Time	Activity
3:00	
4:00	
5:00	
6:00	
7:00	
8:00	
9:00	
10:00	
11:00	
12:00 AM	

Step 3: Analyze Your Current Time Use

1. In what activity can you spend less time? For example, did you watch TV for 3 hours?

   _____

   _____

2. What can you do to spend less time in these activities? How can you replace those activities with ones on your prioritized list?

   _____

   _____

3. During which hours can you spend time doing activities that are important to you?

   _____

   _____

Step 4: Make a Schedule

Write in your planned activities for the next day, and try to stick closely to this schedule.

LABORATORY

NAME _____ DATE _____

Time	Activity
5:00 AM	
6:00	
7:00	
8:00	
9:00	
10:00	
11:00	
12:00 PM	
1:00	
2:00	
3:00	
4:00	
5:00	
6:00	
7:00	
8:00	
9:00	
10:00	
11:00	
12:00 AM	

Were you able to modify your schedule to find time for your priorities? If not, state how you will modify your plan to accommodate your priority activities.

_____

_____

LABORATORY

NAME _____ DATE _____

Assessing Your Personality Behavior Pattern

Circle the position that you feel best reflects your typical behavior in the situations described. Behaviors exhibited by extreme Type A behavior pattern fall to the left, and those exhibited by extreme Type B behavior pattern fall to the right.

Extreme Type A Behavior Pattern						Extreme Type B Behavior Pattern
Fast at doing things	1	2	3	4	5	Slow at doing things (eating, talking, walking)
Unable to wait patiently	1	2	3	4	5	Able to wait patiently
Never late	1	2	3	4	5	Unconcerned about being on time
Very competitive	1	2	3	4	5	Not competitive
Poor listener (I finish other people's sentences for them)	1	2	3	4	5	Good listener
Always in a hurry	1	2	3	4	5	Never in a hurry
Always do two or more things at once	1	2	3	4	5	Take one thing at a time
Speak quickly and forcefully	1	2	3	4	5	Speak slowly and deliberately
Need recognition from others	1	2	3	4	5	Don't worry about what others think
Push myself (and others) hard	1	2	3	4	5	Easygoing
Don't express feelings	1	2	3	4	5	Good at expressing feelings
Few interests outside school or work	1	2	3	4	5	Many hobbies and interests
Very ambitious	1	2	3	4	5	Not ambitious
Eager to get things done	1	2	3	4	5	Deadlines don't bother me

Interpretation

- If the majority of your responses are 1s, then you fall in the **Extreme Type A Behavior Pattern.** This personality behavior pattern is described as extremely competitive, highly committed to work, with an extreme sense of time urgency. Such individuals are extremely goal oriented, and can become hostile if someone gets between them and a goal they have established.

- If the majority of your responses are 2s with a few 1s, then you fall in the **Type A Behavior Pattern**. Type A behavior pattern is characterized by the traits listed for Extreme Type A behavior pattern, but they are moderated somewhat. People who exhibit this behavior pattern are ambitious, competitive, and goal oriented, with a sense of time urgency.

- If your responses are a mixture of the behavior patterns, you are described as a **Balanced Personality**. People with this type of personality get things done, but not at all costs. They can compete but do not feel they have to. They are more laid-back and inclined to give people the benefit of the doubt. They balance leisure time and work time.

- If the majority of your responses are 4s with some 5s, then you fall in the **Type B Behavior Pattern**. People with Type B behavior pattern are easygoing and lack a strong sense of time urgency. They don't like to compete and won't let deadlines interfere with vacation or leisure time. It is not that they are less ambitious than those with Type A behavior pattern; they are just more relaxed.

- If the majority of your responses are 5s, then you fall in the **Extreme Type B Behavior Pattern**. This personality behavior pattern is very relaxed, with no sense of time urgency. In fact, Extreme Type Bs typically don't wear a watch. They try to avoid competition at all costs and never mix leisure time and work time.

Remember: This inventory is only one aspect of your personality. If your responses indicate Type A tendencies, you may want to assess your lifestyle and address some of the more stressful areas.

NAME _____ DATE _____

Assessing Your Risk for Stress-Related Illness

In 1967, Drs. Holmes and Rahe developed a scale of life change events to study the relationship between stress and illness. These events have been updated through the years to better reflect the amount of stress that life changes can bring about. To identify the level of stress in your life, circle each of the following life change events that you have experienced during the past 12 months. Add the assigned life change unit (LCU) values to determine your total LCU score. Refer to the scoring chart below the table to determine your risk of developing a stress-related illness.

Life Event	Life Change Units (LCUs)
Death of spouse, parent, boyfriend/girlfriend	100
Divorce (yourself or your parents)	65
Pregnancy (or causing pregnancy)	65
Marital separation or breakup with boyfriend/girlfriend	60
Jail term or probation	60
Death of other family member (other than spouse, parent, boyfriend/girlfriend)	60
Broken engagement	55
Engagement	50
Serious personal injury or illness	45
Marriage	45
Entering college or beginning next level of school	45
Change in independence or responsibility	45
Any drug or alcohol use	45
Fired at work or expelled from school	45
Change in alcohol or drug use	45
Reconciliation with spouse or significant other	40
Trouble at school	40
Serious health problem of a family member	40
Working while attending school	35

Life Event	Life Change Units (LCUs)
Working more than 40 hours per week	35
Changing course of study	35
Change in frequency of dating	35
Sexual adjustment problems (confusion of sexual identity)	35
Gain new family member (new baby born or parent remarries)	35
Change in work responsibilties	35
Change in financial state	30
Death of a close friend (not family member)	30
Change to a different kind of work	30
Change in number of arguments with spouse, significant other, family, or friends	30
Sleeping fewer than 8 hours per night	25
Trouble with in-laws or family of significant other	25
Outstanding personal achievement (e.g., awards, grades, promotion)	25
Significant other or parents start or stop working	20
Begin or end school	20
Change in living conditions (e.g., visitors in home, change in roommates)	20
Change in personal habits (start or stop a habit, such as smoking or dieting)	20
Chronic allergies	20
Trouble with boss	20
Change in work hours	15
Change in residence	15
Change in religious activity	15
Change to a new school (other than graduation)	10

LABORATORY

NAME _____ DATE _____

Life Event	Life Change Units (LCUs)
Going into debt (you or your family)	10
Change in frequency of family gatherings	10
Vacation	10
Currently in winter holiday season	10
Minor violation of the law	5
Total Life Change Events	

Scoring

- Fewer than 150 LCUs   37% chance of developing a stress-related illness
- 150–299 LCUs   51% chance of developing a stress-related illness
- Over 300 LCUs   80% chance of developing a stress-related illness

Remember: This score indicates your probability or risk of developing a stress-related illness. It does not guarantee that you will develop a stress-related illness. Persons with a low stress tolerance may develop a stress-related illness with fewer than 150 LCUs, and others may remain healthy in spite of high numbers of LCUs. It is your perception of the stressors, as well as your ability to effectively manage them, that influences your chance of developing a stress-related illness. Developing a realistic perception of the stressor(s), plus employing effective coping strategies such as those presented in this chapter, will lessen your chances of becoming ill. If after evaluating the level of stress in your life you would like to learn more about stress management or contact a professional for help in this area, refer to the websites listed at the end of this chapter.

Source: Reprinted from T. H. Holmes and R. H. Rahe, "The Social Readjustment Rating Scale," *Journal of Psychosomatic Research,* Vol. 11, Issue 2, Aug 1967, pp. 213–218, © 1967, with permission from Elsevier Limited.

NAME _____ DATE _____

Determining Your Cancer Risk

The purpose of this laboratory is to increase your awareness of your risk of developing all forms of cancer. Complete the following questions by putting a check under either "Yes" or "No."

    The more times you check "yes," the more risk factors you have for developing cancer. If you check "yes" even once, you should take steps to modify your lifestyle and reduce your risk for cancer. For some specific information about lowering your cancer risks, see the text of this chapter.

	Yes	No
Do you have a family history of cancer?	___	___
Do you have a fair complexion?	___	___
Are you regularly exposed to occupational carcinogens or various types of radiation?	___	___
Is your skin regularly exposed to excessive sunlight?	___	___
Do you consume more than 4 oz of red meat or 1 oz of processed meat per day?	___	___
Do you regularly eat smoked foods?	___	___
Is your diet low in fiber?	___	___
Are you obese?	___	___
Do you consume an excessive amount of alcohol?	___	___
Do you use tobacco products or breathe secondhand tobacco smoke?	___	___

1. How many "yes" responses do you have?

   _____

2. Name any behaviors you can modify or change to reduce your risk for cancer.

   _____

   _____

3. Select one of your modifiable risk factors, and write out steps to change your behavior to reduce your risk. Use the strategies for behavior change to address your risk factor, if applicable.

   _____

   _____

   _____

   _____

LABORATORY

NAME _____ DATE _____

Early Detection

Early detection of cancer is very important in getting prompt and effective treatment. Several screening procedures outlined in this chapter are recommended for early detection of cancer. The purpose of this lab is to assess your behaviors related to early detection of cancer. Check the appropriate box to indicate your current level of participation for each screening.

	Never	Sometimes	As Recommended	N/A
Breast self-exam	____	____	____	____
Clinical breast exam	____	____	____	____
Mammogram	____	____	____	____
Testicular self-exam	____	____	____	____
Clinical testicular exam	____	____	____	____
Colon cancer screening	____	____	____	____
PSA test	____	____	____	____
Pap test	____	____	____	____
Skin exam	____	____	____	____

1. Do you meet the recommendations for cancers screenings based on your age, sex, and risk level?

_____

2. If not, what screenings do you need to start? Make a plan to begin the appropriate screenings recommended for early detection of cancer.

_____

_____

_____

_____

NAME _____ DATE _____

Tobacco Usage Inventory

This laboratory is designed to increase your awareness of your tobacco habits. Habits are sometimes difficult to break because they become unconscious acts. Unrecognized triggers may cause the desire to smoke or use the product. Breaking a habit may be as easy as identifying the trigger and substituting a healthy behavior in place of the unhealthy one.

Over the next 24 hours, take an inventory of the tobacco products you use. Identify the number of tobacco products you use each hour, where you used the product (such as a certain room of the house or in the car), when you used the product (such as after a meal or first thing in the morning), and any other factors, such as being with friends, family, alone, and so on. You must answer each question honestly to provide a valid assessment of your tobacco usage behaviors.

Time of Day	Number of Tobacco Products Used	Location	What Were You Doing Before and During Usage?	Other Factors
12:00 AM				
1:00				
2:00				
3:00				
4:00				
5:00				
6:00				
7:00				
8:00				
9:00				
10:00				
11:00				
12:00 PM				
1:00				
2:00				
3:00				

Time of Day	Number of Tobacco Products Used	Location	What Were You Doing Before and During Usage?	Other Factors
4:00				
5:00				
6:00				
7:00				
8:00				
9:00				
10:00				
11:00				
12:00 AM				

Analyze the above chart, noting any patterns to your use of tobacco. Answer the following questions:

1. Do you smoke or use more than 1 cigarette in any given hour of the day? When?

_____

_____

_____

2. Is there a particular location in your home, at school, or in a favorite restaurant or bar where you prefer to smoke? Where?

_____

_____

_____

3. Do you use tobacco products more often at certain times, such as around meal time, when talking on the phone, or driving in a car?

_____

_____

_____

NAME _____ DATE _____

4. Is there a friend or family member present or do you smoke alone?

_____

_____

_____

Now that you have identified a potential pattern to your tobacco usage, think about ways that you can change that pattern. For example:

- Look at the number of cigarettes that you used during 1 hour, and try cutting the number down by half over the next 2 weeks. Every 2 weeks, cut your usage in half.

- Identify one location from the above chart that you will make off-limits to any tobacco product over the next 2 weeks. Every 2 weeks, add another location to make off-limits. Do not add any new locations to the above list.

- Identify when you use the product and what might be the trigger event. For example, you may find that mealtime, studying, or talking on the telephone triggers your need to smoke. Try substituting a healthy behavior, such as taking a walk after a meal, eating a piece of fruit while studying, or drinking a glass of water when using the telephone.

- Examine the other factors that may influence your tobacco usage. You may find that you smoke only when you are alone or when you are with one particular individual or group of people. Identify a way in which you can continue to socialize with your friends without tobacco. For example, plan on meeting your friends in a smokeless restaurant, bar, or building. If you smoke when alone, try performing other tasks that will keep your hands occupied.

Note that these steps may help you cut down on smoking, but by themselves they may not be enough to kick the habit. Nicotine is a highly addictive substance and may require medical intervention, such as obtaining a prescription for the nicotine patch to help you quit.

NAME _____ DATE _____

Wellness Profile

After reading this book you will be equipped with the knowledge and skills you need to lead a healthy, fit lifestyle. Take the opportunity now to reexamine your strengths in the six areas of wellness. Write your top three strengths for each component of wellness below.

Physical Wellness

Maintaining overall physical health and participating in physical activities. Examples of strengths include cardiorespiratory endurance, balance, and flexibility.

1. _____

2. _____

3. _____

Emotional Wellness

Possessing a positive self-concept and dealing appropriately with your feelings. Strengths may include self-confidence, trust, and optimism.

1. _____

2. _____

3. _____

Intellectual Wellness

Retaining knowledge, thinking critically about issues, making sound decisions, and finding solutions to problems. Examples include inquisitiveness, curiosity, and dedication.

1. _____

2. _____

3. _____

Social Wellness

Developing lasting relationships with family and friends and contributing to the community. Strengths in this area may include compassion and friendliness.

1. _____

2. _____

3. _____

Environmental Wellness

Protecting yourself from environmental hazards and minimizing your negative impact on the environment. Behaviors such as recycling and carpooling are examples of strengths in this aspect of wellness.

1. _____

2. _____

3. _____

Spiritual Wellness

Having a sense of meaning and purpose in life. Behaviors such as prayer, meditation, helping others, and enjoying nature are examples of strengths along this dimension.

1. _____

2. _____

3. _____

Is there an aspect of wellness that you need to develop more fully? If so, which one? What are some specific behaviors you can do now to improve this wellness component in your life?

_____

_____

_____

_____

_____

_____

NAME _____ DATE _____

Evaluating Fitness Products

Complete this activity to evaluate fitness advertisements you see or hear regularly. Find three examples (from magazines, TV or radio ads, or online) of misleading or false claims on fitness or health products. Answer the following questions for each of your products.

1. What are two specific things (images or statements) that are false or misleading in the ad?

   _____

   _____

2. What makes them false? Support your answer with information you learned in class.

   _____

   _____

   _____

3. What are the credentials of the author or person endorsing the project? Is the information provided by an expert in the field of exercise science or physical fitness?

   _____

   _____

   _____

4. Are the benefits of the product realistic?

   _____

   _____

   _____

5. Does the ad contain gimmick words, such as "quick," "spot reduce," or "just minutes a day"?

   _____

   _____

   _____

6. Is the main purpose of the ad to provide useful information or only to sell a product?

   _____

   _____

   _____

LABORATORY

NAME _____ DATE _____

Exercise Training during Pregnancy

Use the following laboratory to design an exercise prescription for a pregnant woman.

Pregnancy and Exercise

Pregnancy places special demands on a woman's body because of the developing fetus's need for calories, protein, vitamins, minerals, and a stable physiological environment. To protect mother and fetus, consult a physician or other health care provider prior to initiating an exercise program.

Design a regular exercise program (at least 3 days per week) for a woman in her second trimester. Keep in mind that she should avoid exercises on her back and should emphasize non-weight-bearing activities. Describe the type of activity and duration of the exercise session. (*Example*: Monday could be lap swimming at a moderate pace for 20 minutes). Don't forget to include specific rest days.

Sunday	Monday	Tuesday	Wednesday	Thursday	Friday	Saturday

LABORATORY

NAME _____ DATE _____

Selecting the Best Health Insurance Plan

The Agency for Healthcare Research and Quality suggests answering the following questions about your health care needs and wants to determine whether a fee-for-service, HMO, or PPO is best for you. This quiz won't answer all of your questions, but it will get you on track to making a sound decision for your health care needs.

For each group, circle the number of the statement (1 or 2) that best describes how you feel:

1. Having complete freedom to choose doctors and hospitals is the most important thing to me in a health plan, even if it costs more.
2. Holding down my costs is the most important thing to me, even if it means limiting some of my choices.

1. I travel a lot or have children that live away from me, and we may need to see doctors in other parts of the country.
2. I do not travel a lot and almost all care for my family will be needed in our local area.

1. I don't mind a health insurance plan that includes filling out forms or keeping receipts and sending them in for payment.
2. I prefer not to fill out forms or keep receipts. I want most of my care covered without a lot of paperwork.

1. In addition to my premiums, I am willing to pay for the cost of routine and preventive care, such as office visits, checkups, and shots. I also like knowing that I can get an appointment for these services when I want one.
2. I want a health plan that includes routine and preventive care. I don't mind if I have to wait for these services to be scheduled or for an available appointment with my doctor.

1. If I need to see a specialist, I probably will ask my doctor for a recommendation, but I want to decide whom to go to and when. I don't want to have to see my primary care doctor each time before I can see a specialist.
2. I don't mind if my primary care doctor must refer me to specialists. If my doctor doesn't think I need special services, that is fine with me.

If your answers are mostly 1's: You want to make your own health care choices, even if it costs you more and takes more paperwork. Fee-for-service may be the best plan for you.

If your answers are mostly 2's: You are willing to give up some choices to hold down your medical costs. You also want help in managing your care. Consider a health maintenance organization.

If your answers are some 1's and some 2's: You might want to look for a plan such as a preferred provider organization that combines some of the features of fee-for-service and those of a health maintenance organization.

LABORATORY

1. According to your responses, what type of plan is best for you? Is this the type of plan you currently have?

   _____

   _____

   _____

2. Are there services with your current plan that do not meet your needs? If so, what are they?

   _____

   _____

   _____

3. What type of plan would better meet your needs?

   _____

   _____

   _____

Source: Agency for Healthcare Research and Quality, Department of Health and Human Services. Checkup on health insurance. www.ahrq.gov/consumer/insuranceqa.

NAME _____ DATE _____

An Exercise Interview with an Older Adult

Interview a friend or family member over age 60 about his or her physical activity and exercise habits. Use the following questions to assess their physical activity habits and to evaluate their activity status.

Interview Questions

1. Do you perform some type of exercise at least 3 times per week? (Be sure to provide the interviewee with some examples of exercise, based on what you've learned in this course.)

   _____

2. If you answered yes to question 1, what types of exercise do you do? How long is each exercise session? What are some benefits you get from your exercise program?

   _____

   _____

   _____

3. If you answered no to question 1, what are some reasons you do not exercise? How do you think an exercise program could affect your health?

   _____

   _____

   _____

4. Do you do things that are not exercise, but that keep you active, such as gardening, other yard work, or heavy housework? If so, what do you do, and how often do you do these activities?

   _____

   _____

   _____

5. How have your exercise and activity habits changed throughout your lifetime? Are you more or less active than you were in the past? How have your choices of activities changed? How has your exercise prescription changed?

   _____

   _____

   _____

LABORATORY

Assessment Questions

1. Does the person you interviewed meet the current physical activity recommendations? If no, what are some changes he or she could make?

_____

_____

_____

2. Does the person you interviewed have an accurate perception of exercise and activity for older adults? If not, what information would you give that person to clarify his or her misperceptions?

_____

_____

_____

3. Does the person you interviewed have a lifetime pattern that is similar to what we see in the general population?

_____

_____

_____

Health Exercise

NAME _____ DATE _____

Stress Index Questionnaire

The purpose of this stress index questionnaire is to increase your awareness of stress in your life. Circle either yes or no to answer each of the following questions.

Yes	No	1. I have frequent arguments.
Yes	No	2. I often get upset at work.
Yes	No	3. I often have neck and/or shoulder pains due to anxiety/stress.
Yes	No	4. I often get upset when I stand in long lines.
Yes	No	5. I often get angry when I listen to the local, national, or world news or read the newspaper.
Yes	No	6. I do not have a sufficient amount of money for my needs.
Yes	No	7. I often get upset when driving.
Yes	No	8. At the end of a workday I often feel stress-related fatigue.
Yes	No	9. I have at least one constant source of stress/anxiety in my life (e.g., conflict with boss, neighbor, mother-in-law).
Yes	No	10. I often have stress-related headaches.
Yes	No	11. I do not practice stress management techniques.
Yes	No	12. I rarely take time for myself.
Yes	No	13. I have difficulty in keeping my feelings of anger and hostility under control.
Yes	No	14. I have difficulty in managing time wisely.
Yes	No	15. I often have difficulty sleeping.
Yes	No	16. I am generally in a hurry.
Yes	No	17. I usually feel that there is not enough time in the day to accomplish what I need to do.
Yes	No	18. I often feel that I am being mistreated by friends or associates.
Yes	No	19. I do not regularly perform physical activity.
Yes	No	20. I rarely get 7 to 9 hours of sleep per night.

Health Exercise

Scoring and Interpretation

Answering yes to any of the questions means that you need to use some form of stress management techniques (see the text for details). Total your yes answers, and use the following scale to evaluate the level of stress in your life.

Number of Yes Answers	Stress Category
6–20	High stress
3–5	Average stress
0–2	Low stress

1. Are you satisfied with your score? If not, name the areas you could target to reduce your level of stress.

_____

_____

_____

2. If you named areas you want to target in the previous question or you are in the high-stress category, what techniques will you employ to help lower your stress level? Write out a specific plan for how you will attempt to use at least of one of the stress management strategies for a specific stressor that you face.

_____

_____

_____

_____

_____

_____

NAME _____ DATE _____

Keeping a Stress Diary

For this exercise, you will need seven copies of this worksheet. Keep a daily stress diary for one week. Indicate the time of day the stressor occurred, your perceived level of stress (10 is the worst stress you have ever felt), any symptoms you experienced, and your response to the symptoms. A response can include, for example, practicing a relaxation technique, getting angry, or doing nothing. At the end of 7 days, analyze your stress diary to determine the greatest sources of stress and the times that they occur. Once you have done this, you will be ready to practice effective stress management techniques.

Time	Level of Perceived Stress (0 to 10)	Cause of Stress	Symptoms of Stress	Your Response
7:00 AM				
8:00				
9:00				
10:00				
11:00				
12:00 PM				
1:00				
2:00				
3:00				
4:00				
5:00				
6:00				
7:00				
8:00				

1. What are the greatest sources of stress in your life, and when do they occur?

_____

_____

2. What are some specific steps you can take to eliminate or minimize these stressors?

_____

_____

APPENDICES

APPENDIX A

Nutrient Values of Foods

The following table of nutrient values is taken from the MyDietAnalysis diet analysis software that is available with this text.* The foods in the table are just a fraction of the foods provided in the software. When using the software, you can quickly find foods shown here by entering the MyDietAnalysis code in the search field. Values are obtained from the USDA Nutrient Database for Standard Reference, Release 19. A "0" indicates that nutrient value is determined to be zero; a blank space indicates that nutrient information is not available.

Ener energy (kilocalories); *Prot* protein; *Carb* carbohydrate; *Fiber* dietary fiber; *Fat* total fat; *Mono* monounsaturated fat; *Poly* polyunsaturated fat; *Sat* saturated fat; *Chol* cholesterol; *Calc* calcium; *Iron* iron; *Mag* magnesium; *Phos* phosphorus; *Sodi* sodium; *Zinc* zinc; *Vit A* vitamin A; *Vit C* vitamin C; *Thia* thiamin; *Ribo* riboflavin; *Niac* niacin; *Vit B$_6$* vitamin B$_6$; *Vit B$_{12}$* vitamin B$_{12}$; *Vit E* vitamin E; *Fol* folate; *Alc* alcohol.

Index to Appendix A

---

*This food composition table has been prepared for Pearson Education, Inc., and is copyrighted by ESHA Research in Salem, Oregon—the developer of the MyDietAnalysis software program.

MDA Code	Food Name	Amt	Wt (g)	Ener (kcal)	Prot (g)	Carb (g)	Fiber (g)	Fat (g)	Mono (g)	Poly (g)
	BEVERAGES									
	Alcoholic									
22831	Beer	12 fl oz	360	157	1	13		0	0	0
34067	Beer, dark	12 fl oz	355.5	150	1	13		0	0	0
34053	Beer, light	12 fl oz	352.9	105	1	5	0	0	0	0
22606	Beer, nonalcoholic	12 fl oz	352.9	73	1	14	0	0	0	0
22849	Beer, pale ale	12 fl oz	360.2	179	2	17		0	0	0
22545	Daiquiri, frozen, from concentrate mix	1 ea	36	101	0	26	0	0	0	0
22514	Gin, 80 proof	1 fl oz	27.8	64	0	0	0	0	0	0
22544	Liqueur, coffee, 63 proof	1 fl oz	34.8	107	0	11	0	0	0	0
34085	Martini, prepared from recipe	1 fl oz	28.2	69	0	1	0	0	0	0
22593	Rum, 80 proof	1 fl oz	27.8	64	0	0	0	0	0	0
22515	Tequila, 80 proof	1 fl oz	27.8	64	0	0	0	0	0	0
22594	Vodka, 80 proof	1 fl oz	27.8	64	0	0	0	0	0	0
22670	Whiskey, 80 proof	1 fl oz	27.8	64	0	0	0	0	0	0
34084	Wine, cooking	1 tsp	4.9	2	0	0	0	0	0	0
22884	Wine, red, Cabernet Sauvignon	1 fl oz	29	24	0	1		0	0	0
22876	Wine, red, Pinot Noir	1 fl oz	29.4	24	0	1		0	0	0
22676	Wine, sake/saki, Japanese	1 fl oz	29.1	39	0	1	0	0	0	0
22861	Wine, white, Sauvignon Blanc	1 fl oz	29.3	24	0	1		0	0	0
	Coffee									
20012	Coffee, brewed w/tap water	1 cup	237	2	0	0	0	0	0	0
20686	Coffee, decaffeinated, brewed w/tap water	1 cup	236.8	0	0	0	0	0	0	0
20439	Coffee, espresso	1 cup	237	5	0	0	0	0	0	0.2
20972	Coffee, espresso, decaffeinated	1 cup	237	0	0	0	0	0	0	0.2
20091	Coffee, decaffeinated, instant	1 cup	179	4	0	1	0	0	0	0
20023	Coffee, instant, prep w/water	1 cup	238.4	5	0	1	0	0	0	0
20402	Coffee, instant, French vanilla cafe, fat & sugar free	1 ea	7	25	0	5	0	0		
	Dairy Mixed Drinks and Mixes									
44	Carob flavor, dry mix, prepared w/whole milk	1 cup	256	192	8	22	1	8	2	0.5
85	Chocolate milk, prepared w/syrup	1 cup	282	254	9	36	1	8	2.1	0.5
46	Hot cocoa, sugar free, w/aspartame, prepared w/water	1 cup	256	74	3	14	1	1	0.2	0
195	Hot cocoa, rich chocolate, w/o add sugar, dry pkt	1 ea	15	50	2	10	1	0		
172	Hot cocoa, rich chocolate, dry pkt	1 ea	28	112	1	21	1	4		
21	Hot cocoa, prep from recipe w/milk	1 cup	250	192	9	27	2	6	1.7	0.1
48	Hot cocoa, prep from dry mix w/water	1 cup	274.7	151	2	32	1	2	0.5	0
166	Hot cocoa, w/marshmallows, dry pkt	1 ea	28	112	1	21	1	4		
39	Drink, chocolate, prepared from dry mix w/whole milk	1 cup	266	226	9	32	1	9	2.2	0.5
34	Chocolate malted milk, prepared from powder w/whole milk	1 cup	265	225	9	30	1	9	2.2	0.6
29	Malted milk, natural, w/o add nutrients, prep from powder w/milk	1 cup	265	233	10	27	0	10	2.4	0.7
41	Drink, strawberry, prep from dry mix w/whole milk	1 cup	266	234	8	33	0	8	2.4	0.3
	Fruit and Vegetable Beverages and Juices									
71080	Apple juice, unsweetened	8.45 fl oz	262	123	0	31	0	0	0	0.1
3010	Apple juice, unsweetened, prepared from frozen concentrate	1 cup	239	112	0	28	0	0	0	0.1
3015	Apricot nectar, w/o add vitamin C, canned	1 cup	251	141	1	36	2	0	0.1	0
72092	Blackberry juice, canned	0.5 cup	120	46	0	9	0	1	0.1	0.4
20277	Capri Sun, fruit punch, pouch	1 ea	210	99	0	26	0	0	0	0
5226	Carrot juice, canned	1 cup	236	94	2	22	2	0	0	0.2
20042	Clam and tomato juice, canned	5.5 oz	166.1	80	1	18	1	0		
3042	Cranberry juice cocktail	1 cup	252.8	137	0	34	0	0	0	0.1

Sat (g)	Chol (mg)	Calc (mg)	Iron (mg)	Mag (mg)	Phos (mg)	Pota (mg)	Sodi (mg)	Zinc (mg)	Vit A (RAE)	Vit C (mg)	Thia (mg)	Ribo (mg)	Niac (mg)	Vit B$_6$ (mg)	Vit B$_{12}$ (µg)	Vit E (mg)	Fol (µg)	Alc (g)
0	0						9								0			14.3
0	0						34											17.06
0	0	11				59	11				0.04	0.04	1.41					14.12
0	0	19				54	10				0.04	0.07	1.41					1.78
0	0						9								0			14.7
0	0	3	0.13	1.1	7	34	123	0.1	0	3.2	0.01	0.01	0	0	0	0	0	0
0	0	0	0.01	0	1	1	0	0	0	0	0	0	0	0	0	0	0	9.29
0	0	0	0.02	1	2	10	3	0	0	0	0	0	0.05	0	0	0	0	9.05
0	0	0	0.01	0.6	1	5	1	0	0	0	0	0	0.01	0	0	0	0	9.56
0	0	0	0.03	0	1	1	0	0	0	0	0	0	0	0	0	0	0	9.29
0	0	0	0.01	0	1	1	0	0	0	0	0	0	0	0	0	0	0	9.29
0	0	0	0	0	1	0	0	0	0	0	0	0	0	0	0	0	0	9.29
0	0	0	0.01	0	1	1	0	0	0	0	0	0	0	0	0	0	0	9.29
0	0	0	0.02	0.5	1	4	31	0	0	0	0	0	0	0	0	0	0	0.16
0																		3.04
0																		3.06
0	0	1	0.03	1.7	2	7	1	0	0	0	0	0	0	0	0	0	0	4.69
0																		3.08
0	0	5	0.02	7.1	7	116	5	0	0	0	0.03	0.18	0.45	0	0	0	4.7	0
0	0	5	0.12	11.8	2	128	5	0	0	0	0	0	0.53	0	0	0	0	0
0.2	0	5	0.31	189.6	17	273	33	0.1	0	0.5	0	0.42	12.34	0	0	0	2.4	0
0.2	0	5	0.31	189.6	17	273	33	0.1	0	0.5	0	0.42	12.34	0	0	0	2.4	0
0	0	5	0.11	9	7	82	4	0	0	0	0	0.03	0.5	0	0	0	0	0
0	0	10	0.1	7.2	7	72	5	0	0	0	0	0	0.56	0	0	0	0	0
0.1	0	4	0.06		16	72	65	0	0									0
4.6	26	251	0.64	25.6	205	335	118	0.9	69	0	0.11	0.45	0.35	0.1	1.08	0.1	12.8	0
4.7	25	251	0.9	50.8	254	409	133	1.2	70	0	0.11	0.47	0.39	0.09	1.07	0.1	14.1	0
0	0	120	1	43.5	179	540	228	0.7	36	0.3	0.05	0.28	0.22	0.06	0.33	0.1	2.6	0
0.1	1	300	0.54	27	135	288	180	0.6		0.3	0.06	0.22	0.18	0.05	0.45	0	5.8	0
2.8	0	28	0.5	27.4	71	0	238	0.4		0	0.03	0.12	0.16	0.03	0.1	0	2	0
3.6	20	262	1.2	57.5	262	492	110	1.6	128	0.5	0.1	0.45	0.33	0.1	1.05	0.1	12.5	0
0.9	3	60	0.47	33	118	269	195	0.6	0	0.5	0.04	0.21	0.22	0.04	0.49	0.2	0	0
4.2	0	22	0.5	16.2	58	142	224	0.2		0	0.03	0.12	0.1	0.03	0.12	0	1.1	0
4.9	24	253	0.8	47.9	234	458	154	1.3	70	0.3	0.11	0.48	0.38	0.09	1.06	0.2	13.3	0
5	26	260	0.56	39.8	241	456	159	1.1	70	0.3	0.14	0.49	0.69	0.12	1.11	0.2	23.8	0
5.4	32	310	0.24	45	281	485	209	1.1	87	0.5	0.21	0.64	1.38	0.17	1.22	0.3	21.2	0
5.1	32	293	0.21	31.9	229	370	128	0.9	69	2.4	0.09	0.42	0.22	0.1	0.88	0.3	13.3	0
0	0	18	0.97	7.9	18	312	8	0.1	0	2.4	0.06	0.04	0.26	0.08	0	0	0	0
0	0	14	0.62	12	17	301	17	0.1	0	1.4	0.01	0.04	0.09	0.08	0	0	0	0
0	0	18	0.95	12.6	23	286	8	0.2	166	1.5	0.02	0.04	0.65	0.06	0	0.8	2.5	0
0	0	14	0.58	25.2	14	162	1	0.5	10	13.6	0.01	0.02	0.54	0.03	0	1.1	12	0
0	0	2	0.06		2	25	21			2.7								0
0.1	0	57	1.09	33	99	689	68	0.4	2256	20.1	0.22	0.13	0.91	0.51	0	2.7	9.4	0
	0	13	0.25	8.3	18	148	601	0.1	12	8.3	0.03	0.02	0.38	0.1	0.05	0.2	13.3	0
0	0	8	0.25	2.5	3	35	5	0.1	1	106.9	0	0	0.1	0	0	0.6	0	0

MDA Code	Food Name	Amt	Wt (g)	Ener (kcal)	Prot (g)	Carb (g)	Fiber (g)	Fat (g)	Mono (g)	Poly (g)
20115	Cranberry juice cocktail, from frozen concentrate	1 cup	249.6	137	0	35	0	0	0	0
3275	Cranberry-grape juice	1 cup	244.8	137	0	34	0	0	0	0.1
20024	Fruit punch, w/added nutrients, canned	1 cup	248	117	0	30	0	0	0	0
20035	Fruit punch, from frozen concentrate	1 cup	247.2	114	0	29	0	0	0	0
20101	Grape drink, canned	1 cup	250.4	153	0	39	0	0	0	0
3165	Grapefruit juice, sweetened, canned	1 cup	250	115	1	28	0	0	0	0.1
3052	Grapefruit juice, unsweetened, canned	1 cup	247	94	1	22	0	0	0	0.1
3053	Grapefruit juice, unsweetened, from frozen concentrate	1 cup	247	101	1	24	0	0	0	0.1
20330	Kool-Aid, cherry, sugar free, w/aspartame & vitamin C	1 ea	9.6	28	1	8	0			
20687	Kool-Aid, tropical punch, sweetened, dry mix, serving	1 ea	17	64	0	16	0	0	0	0
3068	Lemon juice, fresh	1 Tbs	15.2	4	0	1	0	0	0	0
20045	Lemonade, prepared from powder	1 cup	266	112	0	29	0	0	0	0
20047	Lemonade, low cal, w/aspartame, prep from powder	1 cup	236.8	5	0	1	0	0	0	0
20117	Lemonade, pink, from frozen concentrate	1 cup	247.2	99	0	26	0	0	0	0
20000	Lemonade, white, from frozen concentrate	1 cup	248	131	0	34	0	0	0	0
3072	Lime juice, fresh	1 Tbs	15.4	4	0	1	0	0	0	0
20002	Limeade, from frozen concentrate	1 cup	247.2	104	0	26	0	0		
20070	Orange drink, w/added vitamin C, canned	1 cup	248	122	0	31	0	0	0	0
20004	Orange breakfast drink, from powder	1 cup	248	122	0	31	0	0	0	0
71108	Orange juice, unsweetened, box	8.45 fl oz	263	110	2	26	1	0	0.1	0.1
3090	Orange juice, fresh	1 cup	248	112	2	26	0	0	0.1	0.1
3091	Orange juice, unsweetened, from frozen concentrate	1 cup	249	112	2	27	0	0	0	0
3170	Orange-grapefruit juice, unsweetened, canned	1 cup	247	106	1	25	0	0	0	0
3095	Papaya nectar, canned	1 cup	250	142	0	36	2	0	0.1	0.1
3200	Passion fruit juice, purple, fresh	1 cup	247	126	1	34	0	0	0	0.1
3101	Peach nectar, w/o added vitamin C, canned	1 cup	249	134	1	35	1	0	0	0
20059	Pineapple-grapefruit juice, canned	1 cup	250.4	118	1	29	0	0	0	0.1
20025	Pineapple-orange juice, canned	1 cup	250.4	125	3	30	0	0	0	0
3120	Pineapple juice, unsweetened, w/o added vitamin C, canned	1 cup	250	132	1	32	1	0	0	0.1
3128	Prune juice, canned	1 cup	256	182	2	45	3	0	0.1	0
20340	Tang, orange, from dry mix	2 Tbs	25	92	0	25	0	0	0	0
3140	Tangerine juice, sweetened, canned	1 cup	249	124	1	30	0	0	0	0.1
5397	Tomato juice, unsalted, canned	1 cup	243	41	2	10	1	0	0	0.1
20849	Vegetable-fruit juice, mixed	4 oz	113.4	33	0	8	0	0		
20080	Vegetable juice, mixed, canned	1 cup	242	46	2	11	2	0	0	0.1
	Soft Drinks									
20006	Club soda	1 cup	236.8	0	0	0	0	0	0	0
20685	Low-calorie cola, with aspartame, caffeine free	12 fl oz	355.2	4	0	1	0	0	0	0
20843	Cola, w/higher caff	12 fl oz	370	152	0	39	0	0	0	0
20028	Cream soda	1 cup	247.2	126	0	33	0	0	0	0
20008	Ginger ale	1 cup	244	83	0	21	0	0	0	0
20031	Grape soda	1 cup	248	107	0	28	0	0	0	0
20032	Lemon-lime soft drink	1 cup	245.6	98	0	25	0	0		
20027	Pepper-type soft drink	1 cup	245.6	101	0	26	0	0	0	0
20009	Root beer	1 cup	246.4	101	0	26	0	0	0	0
	Tea									
20436	Iced tea, lemon flavor	1 cup	240	86	0	22	0	0	0	0
20040	Instant tea mix w/lemon flavor & saccharin	1 cup	236.8	5	0	1	0	0	0	0
20014	Tea, brewed	1 cup	236.8	2	0	1	0	0	0	0
444	Tea, decaffeinated, brewed	1 cup	236.8	2	0	1	0	0	0	0

Sat (g)	Chol (mg)	Calc (mg)	Iron (mg)	Mag (mg)	Phos (mg)	Pota (mg)	Sodi (mg)	Zinc (mg)	Vit A (RAE)	Vit C (mg)	Thia (mg)	Ribo (mg)	Niac (mg)	Vit B_6 (mg)	Vit B_{12} (µg)	Vit E (mg)	Fol (µg)	Alc (g)
0	0	12	0.22	5	2	35	7	0.1	2	24.7	0.02	0.02	0.03	0.03	0	0	0	0
0.1	0	20	0.02	7.3	10	59	7	0.1	1	78.3	0.02	0.04	0.29	0.07	0	0	2.4	0
0	0	20	0.22	7.4	7	77	94	0	5	73.4	0.01	0.06	0.05	0.03	0	0	2.5	0
0	0	10	0.22	4.9	2	32	10	0	1	108.3	0.02	0.03	0.05	0.01	0	0	2.5	0
0	0	130	0.18	2.5	0	30	40	0.3	0	78.6	0	0.01	0.03	0.01	0	0	0	0
0	0	20	0.9	25	28	405	5	0.1	1	67.2	0.1	0.06	0.8	0.05	0	0.1	25	0
0	0	17	0.49	24.7	27	378	2	0.2	1	72.1	0.1	0.05	0.57	0.05	0	0.1	24.7	0
0	0	20	0.35	27.2	35	336	2	0.1	1	83.2	0.1	0.05	0.54	0.11	0	0.1	9.9	0
		0	0			0	41			53.8					0			0
0	0	28	0.01		13	0	2		0	6								0
0	0	1	0	0.9	1	19	0	0	0	7	0	0	0.02	0.01	0	0	2	0
0	0	29	0.05	2.7	3	3	19	0.1	0	34	0	0	0	0	0	0	0	0
0	0	52	0.09	2.4	24	0	5	0	0	5.9	0	0	0	0	0	0	0	0
0	0	7	0.4	4.9	5	37	7	0.1	0	9.6	0.01	0.05	0.04	0.01	0	0	4.9	0
0	0	10	0.52	5	7	50	7	0.1	0	12.9	0.02	0.07	0.05	0.02	0	0	2.5	0
0	0	2	0.01	1.2	2	18	0	0	0	4.6	0	0	0.02	0.01	0	0	1.5	0
	0	7	0.02	2.5	2	22	5	0	0	5.9	0	0.01	0.02	0.01	0	0	2.5	0
0	0	12	0.1	5	2	45	7	0	2	142.1	0	0	0.03	0	0	0	5	0
0	0	126	0.02	2.5	47	60	10	0	191	73.2	0	0.22	2.54	0.25	0	0	0	0
0	0	21	1.16	28.9	37	460	5	0.2	24	90.5	0.16	0.07	0.83	0.23	0	0.5	47.3	0
0.1	0	27	0.5	27.3	42	496	2	0.1	25	124	0.22	0.07	0.99	0.1	0	0.1	74.4	0
0	0	22	0.25	24.9	40	473	2	0.1	12	96.9	0.2	0.04	0.5	0.11	0	0.5	109.6	0
0	0	20	1.14	24.7	35	390	7	0.2	15	71.9	0.14	0.07	0.83	0.06	0	0.3	34.6	0
0.1	0	25	0.85	7.5	0	78	12	0.4	45	7.5	0.02	0.01	0.38	0.02	0	0.6	5	0
0	0	10	0.59	42	32	687	15	0.1	89	73.6	0	0.32	3.61	0.12	0	0	17.3	0
0	0	12	0.47	10	15	100	17	0.2	32	13.2	0.01	0.03	0.72	0.02	0	0.7	2.5	0
0	0	18	0.78	15	15	153	35	0.2	0	115.2	0.08	0.04	0.67	0.11	0	0	22.5	0
0	0	13	0.68	15	10	115	8	0.2	3	56.3	0.08	0.05	0.52	0.12	0	0.1	22.5	0
0	0	32	0.78	30	20	325	5	0.3	1	25	0.14	0.05	0.5	0.25	0	0	45	0
0	0	31	3.02	35.8	64	707	10	0.5	0	10.5	0.04	0.18	2.01	0.56	0	0.3	0	0
0	0	92	0.02	0	42	48	2	0		60	0	0.17	2	0.2	0	2	0	0
0	0	45	0.5	19.9	35	443	2	0.1	32	54.8	0.15	0.05	0.25	0.08	0	0.4	12.4	0
0	0	24	1.04	26.7	44	556	24	0.4	56	44.5	0.11	0.08	1.64	0.27	0	0.8	48.6	0
	0	3	0.05	1.1	2	22	24	0	118	36.9	0	0	0.02	0.01	0	1.8	0	0
0	0	27	1.02	26.6	41	467	653	0.5	189	67	0.1	0.07	1.76	0.34	0	0.8	50.8	0
0	0	12	0.02	2.4	0	5	50	0.2	0	0	0	0	0	0	0	0	0	0
0	0	11	0.07	0	36	25	14	0	0	0	0.02	0.08	0	0	0	0	0	0
0	0	7	0.07	0	41	11	15	0	0	0	0	0	0	0	0	0	0	0
0	0	12	0.12	2.5	0	2	30	0.2	0	0	0	0	0	0	0	0	0	0
0	0	7	0.44	2.4	0	2	17	0.1	0	0	0	0	0	0	0	0	0	0
0	0	7	0.2	2.5	0	2	37	0.2	0	0	0	0	0	0	0	0	0	0
	0	5	0.27	2.5	0	2	22	0.1	0	0	0	0	0.04	0	0	0	0	0
0.2	0	7	0.1	0	27	2	25	0.1	0	0	0	0	0	0	0	0	0	0
0	0	12	0.12	2.5	0	2	32	0.2	0	0	0	0	0	0	0	0	0	0
0		7	0	2.4	86	46	50	0.1										0
0	0	7	0.12	2.4	2	31	9	0	0	0	0	0	0.05	0	0	0	0	0
0	0	0	0.05	7.1	2	88	7	0	0	0	0	0.03	0	0	0	0	11.8	0
0	0	0	0.05	7.1	2	88	7	0	0	0	0	0.03	0	0	0	0	11.8	0

MDA Code	Food Name	Amt	Wt (g)	Ener (kcal)	Prot (g)	Carb (g)	Fiber (g)	Fat (g)	Mono (g)	Poly (g)
20118	Tea, herbal, chamomile, brewed	1 cup	236.8	2	0	0	0	0	0	0
20036	Tea, herbal, not chamomile, brewed	1 cup	236.8	2	0	0	0	0	0	0
	Other									
20983	Bean beverage	1 cup	230	78	6	13	0	0	0	0
17	Eggnog	1 cup	254	343	10	34	0	19	5.7	0.9
20440	Rice milk, original	1 cup	244.8	120	0	25	0	2	1.3	0.3
20033	Soy milk	1 cup	245	127	11	12	3	5	0.9	1.9
21070	Soy milk, plain, lite	1 cup	245	90	4	15	2	2	0.5	1
21064	Soy milk, vanilla	1 cup	245	190	11	25	5	5	1	3
20041	Water, tap, municipal	1 cup	236.6	0	0	0	0	0	0	0
20076	Wine, nonalcoholic	4 fl oz	116	7	1	1	0	0	0	0
	BREAKFAST CEREALS									
40095	All-Bran/Kellogg's	0.5 cup	30	78	4	22	9	1	0.2	0.6
40295	Apple Cinnamon Cheerios/Gen Mills	0.75 cup	30	120	2	25	1	2	1	0.5
40097	Apple Cinnamon Squares cereal/Kellogg's	0.75 cup	55	182	4	44	5	1	0.3	0.5
40098	Apple Jacks/Kellogg's	1 cup	30	117	1	27	1	1	0.2	0.3
40394	Basic 4/Gen Mills	1 cup	55	210	4	44	3	3	1	0.5
40259	Bran Flakes/Post	0.75 cup	30	96	3	24	5	1		
61211	Bran & malted flour cereal	0.33 cup	29	83	4	23	8	1	0.1	0.3
40032	Cap'n Crunch/Quaker	0.75 cup	27	108	1	23	1	2	0.3	0.2
40297	Cheerios/Gen Mills	1 cup	30	110	3	23	3	2	0.7	0.7
40414	Cinnamon Grahams/Gen Mills	0.75 cup	30	113	2	26	1	1	0.3	0.3
40126	Cinnamon Toast Crunch/Gen Mills	0.75 cup	30	130	1	24	1	4	2.5	0.5
40102	Cocoa Krispies/Kellogg's	0.75 cup	31	118	2	27	1	1	0.1	0.1
40425	Cocoa Puffs/Gen Mills	1 cup	30	120	1	26	2	2	1	0
40325	Corn Chex/Gen Mills	1 cup	30	110	2	26	1	1	0.1	0.2
40195	Corn Flakes/Kellogg's	1 cup	28	101	2	24	1	0	0	0.1
40089	Corn Grits, instant, plain, prepared/Quaker	1 ea	137	93	2	21	1	0	0	0.1
92416	Corn grits, white, quick, enriched, cooked w/water & salt	1 cup	242	143	3	31	1	0	0.1	0.2
40206	Corn Pops/Kellogg's	1 cup	31	117	1	28	0	0	0.1	0.1
40205	Cracklin' Oat Bran/Kellogg's	0.75 cup	55	221	4	39	7	8	2.6	1.6
40179	Cream of Rice, prepared w/salt/Kraft	1 cup	244	127	2	28	0	0	0.1	0.1
40104	Crispix/Kellogg's	1 cup	29	109	2	25	0	0	0.1	0.1
40184	Farina, enriched, prepared w/salt	1 cup	233	112	3	24	1	0	0	0.1
40182	Farina, instant, prepared w/salt	1 cup	241	149	4	32	1	1	0.1	0.3
40130	Fiber One/Gen Mills	0.5 cup	30	60	2	25	14	1	0.1	0.4
40218	Froot Loops/Kellogg's	1 cup	30	118	2	26	1	1	0.1	0.2
40217	Frosted Flakes/Kellogg's	0.75 cup	31	114	1	28	1	0	0	0.1
11916	Frosted Mini Wheats, bite size/Kellogg's	1 cup	55	189	6	45	6	1	0.1	0.6
40048	Granola cereal, prep f/recipe	0.5 cup	61	298	9	32	5	15	5.8	5.6
40277	Grape Nuts/Post	0.5 cup	58	208	6	47	5	1		
40292	Honey Bunches of Oats, Honey Roasted/Post	0.75 cup	30	118	2	25	1	2		
40361	Honey Nut Heaven/Quaker	1 cup	49	192	4	38	3	4	1.7	1
40108	Just Right, Crunchy Blends/Kellogg's	1 cup	55	204	4	46	3	1	0.3	1
40010	Kix/Gen Mills	1.33 cup	30	120	2	25	1	1	0.3	0.4
40011	Life, plain/Quaker	0.75 cup	32	120	3	25	2	1	0.5	0.5
40197	Low-Fat Granola, w/raisins/Kellogg's	0.66 cup	55	201	4	44	3	3	1.3	0.5
40300	Lucky Charms/Gen Mills	1 cup	30	120	2	25	1	1	0.5	0.5
40186	Maltex, prep w/water & salt	1 cup	249	189	6	39	2	1	0.1	0.4
38659	Nutri-Grain Cereal, wheat/Kellogg's	1 oz	28.4	102	2	24	2	0	0	0.1

Sat (g)	Chol (mg)	Calc (mg)	Iron (mg)	Mag (mg)	Phos (mg)	Pota (mg)	Sodi (mg)	Zinc (mg)	Vit A (RAE)	Vit C (mg)	Thia (mg)	Ribo (mg)	Niac (mg)	Vit B_6 (mg)	Vit B_{12} (µg)	Vit E (mg)	Fol (µg)	Alc (g)
0	0	5	0.19	2.4	0	21	2	0.1	2	0	0.02	0.01	0	0	0	0	2.4	0
0	0	5	0.19	2.4	0	21	2	0.1	0	0	0.02	0.01	0	0	0	0	2.4	0
0	0	39	2.88	110.4	212	775	5	0.9	0	0	0.35	0.23	1.43	0.23	0	0.6	138	0
11.3	150	330	0.51	48.3	277	419	137	1.2	116	3.8	0.09	0.48	0.27	0.13	1.14	0.5	2.5	0
0.2	0	20	0.2	9.8	34	69	86	0.2	0	1.2	0.08	0.01	1.91	0.04	0	1.8	90.6	0
0.6	0	93	2.7	61.2	135	304	135	1.1	76	0	0.15	0.12	0.71	0.24	2.99	3.3	39.2	0
0	0	300	1.44	32	150	160	90			0	0.42							0
0.5	0	300	2.7	60	250	370	85			0	0.42							0
0	0	7	0	2.4	0	2	7	0	0	0	0	0	0	0	0	0	0	0
0	0	10	0.46	11.6	17	102	8	0.1	0	0	0	0.01	0.12	0.02	0	0	1.2	0
0.2	0	117	5.28	108.6	345	306	73	3.7	158	6	0.68	0.81	4.44	3.6	5.64	0.4	393	0
0	0	100	4.5	15.9	60	60	120	3.8	149	6	0.38	0.43	5	0.5	1.5	0.2	200.1	0
0.2	0	21	16.23	48.4	154	166	20	1.5	0	0	0.38	0.44	5.01	0.49	1.49	0.3	110	0
0.1	0	8	4.17	16.5	38	36	142	1.5	40	13.8	0.51	0.39	4.62	0.45	1.38	0	93	0
0.5	0	250	4.5	31.9	100	150	320	3.8	150	0	0.37	0.42	5	0.5	1.5	0.6	100.1	0
0.1	0	17	8.1	64.2	152	185	220	1.5		0	0.38	0.43	5	0.5	1.5		99.9	0
0.1	0	22	8.1	80.6	236	275	121	3.7	225	0	0.37	0.43	5	0.5	0	0.7	100	0
0.4	0	4	5.16	15.1	45	54	202	4.3	2	0	0.43	0.48	5.71	0.57	0	0.2	420.1	0
0.4	0	100	8.4	39.9	100	200	210	3.8	150	6	0.38	0.43	5	0.5	1.5	0.2	200.1	0
0.2	0	100	4.5	8.1	20	44	237	3.8	150	6	0.38	0.43	5.01	0.5	1.5	0.1	99.9	0
0.5	0	100	4.5	8.1	40	45	210	3.8	150	6	0.38	0.43	5	0.5	1.5	0.9	99.9	0
0.6	0	5	6.88	11.8	32	61	197	1.5	153	15	0.46	0.7	4.96	1.02	2.15	0.1	197.5	0
0	0	100	4.5	8.1	20	60	160	3.8	0	6	0.38	0.43	5	0.5	1.5	0.2	99.9	0
0.1	0	100	9	15	22	45	280	3.8	136	6	0.38	0.43	5	0.5	1.5	0.1	200.1	0
0.1	0	1	8.12	2.5	10	22	202	0.1	128	6.2	0.6	0.74	6.83	0.96	2.65	0	134.4	0
0	0	8	7.96	9.6	29	38	288	0.2	0	0	0.16	0.19	2.21	0.05	0	0	46.6	0
0.1	0	7	1.45	12.1	27	51	540	0.2	0	0	0.2	0.13	1.75	0.05	0	0	79.9	0
0.1	0	5	1.92	2.2	10	26	120	1.5	143	6	0.37	0.43	4.99	0.5	1.52	0	102	0
3.4	0	33	2.04	67.6	179	248	170	1.7	252	17.6	0.44	0.49	5.67	0.56	1.7	0.5	112.8	0
0	0	7	0.49	7.3	41	49	422	0.4	0	0	0	0	0.98	0.07	0	0	7.3	0
0.1	0	4	9.61	7	28	33	222	2.3	262	8.8	1.27	1.25	8.47	0.98	2.09	0	200.1	0
0	0	9	1.16	4.7	28	30	767	0.2	0	0	0.14	0.1	1.14	0.02	0	0	79.2	0
0.1	0	154	11.95	14.5	43	48	364	0.4	559	0	0.56	0.51	7.45	0.74	0	0	149.4	0
0.1	0	100	4.5	39.9	150	180	105	3.8	1	6	0.38	0.43	5	0.5	1.5	0.3	99.9	0
0.5	0	4	6.12	9.9	34	36	150	5.7	140	14.1	0.68	0.58	7.26	1.1	2.12	0.1	105.6	0
0	0	2	4.5	2.5	11	23	148	0.1	160	6.2	0.37	0.46	5.02	0.5	1.55	0	101.4	0
0.2	0	18	15.4	64.9	162	190	4	1.8	0	0	0.41	0.46	5.39	0.54	1.62	0	107.8	0
2.5	0	48	2.58	106.8	278	329	15	2.5	1	0.7	0.45	0.18	1.31	0.18	0	6.8	50	0
0.2	0	20	16.2	58	139	178	354	1.2		0	0.38	0.42	5	0.5	1.5		99.8	0
0.2	0	6	8.1	16.5	48	52	193	0.3		0	0.38	0.43	5	0.5	1.5		99.9	0
0.5	0	133	6.81	60.3	166	181	216	5.4	216	1.5	0.59	0.67	7.18	0.72	0	1.8	436.6	0
0.1	0	14	16.23	34.1	106	121	338	0.9	376	0	0.38	0.44	5.01	0.49	1.49	1.5	102.3	0
0.1	0	150	8.4	8.1	40	40	220	3.8	138	6	0.38	0.43	5	0.5	1.5	0.1	200.1	0
0.3	0	112	8.95	30.7	133	91	164	4.1	1	0	0.4	0.47	5.5	0.55	0	0.2	416	0
0.6	0	23	1.65	41.2	129	165	135	3.5	206	3.3	0.35	0.38	4.57	1.81	5.5	3.1	369.6	0
0	0	100	4.5	15.9	40	50	200	3.8	150	6	0.38	0.43	5	0.5	1.5	0.1	200.1	0
0.2	0	22	1.79	57.3	177	266	189	1.9	0	0	0.26	0.1	2.37	0.08	0	1.1	29.9	0
0.1	0	8	0.8	22.2	106	77	193	3.7	0	15.1	0.37	0.43	5	0.51	1.51	7.5	100.3	0

MDA Code	Food Name	Amt	Wt (g)	Ener (kcal)	Prot (g)	Carb (g)	Fiber (g)	Fat (g)	Mono (g)	Poly (g)
40434	Oat Bran Cereal/Quaker	1.25 cup	57	212	7	43	6	3	0.9	1.2
40430	Oatmeal Squares/Quaker	1 cup	56	212	6	44	4	2	0.8	1
40073	Oatmeal, apple cinnamon, instant, prep w/water/Quaker	1 ea	149	130	3	26	3	1	0.5	0.4
40018	Puffed Rice/Quaker	1 cup	14	54	1	12	0	0	0	0
40242	Puffed Wheat, fortified	1 cup	12	44	2	10	1	0		0
40209	Raisin Bran/Kellogg's	1 cup	61	195	5	47	7	2	0.3	0.9
40343	Reese's Peanut Butter Puffs/Gen Mills	0.75 cup	30	130	2	23	1	4	1.5	1
40333	Rice Chex/Gen Mills	1.25 cup	31	120	2	26	0	0	0.2	0.2
40210	Rice Krispies/Kellogg's	1.25 cup	33	128	2	28	0	0	0.1	0.1
60887	Shredded Wheat, w/o sugar & salt, round biscuits	2 ea	37.8	127	4	30	5	1	0.1	0.5
60879	Smart Start/Kellogg's	1 cup	50	182	4	43	3	1	0.1	0.4
40211	Special K/Kellogg's	1 cup	31	117	7	22	1	0	0.1	0.2
40066	Sweet Crunch/Quisp/Quaker	1 cup	27	109	1	23	1	2	0.3	0.2
40413	Toasty O's/Malt-O-Meal	1 cup	30	121	4	22	3	2	0.6	0.7
40382	Total, raisin bran/Gen Mills	1 cup	55	170	3	42	5	1	0.1	0.5
40021	Total, wheat/Gen Mills	0.75 cup	30	100	2	23	3	1	0.1	0.2
40306	Trix/Gen Mills	1 cup	30	120	1	26	1	2	0.7	0.5
40335	Wheat Chex/Gen Mills	1 cup	30	108	3	24	3	1	0.1	0.2
40307	Wheaties/Gen Mills	1 cup	30	110	3	24	3	1	0.3	0.4

DAIRY AND CHEESE

See Fats and Oils for butter.

MDA Code	Food Name	Amt	Wt (g)	Ener (kcal)	Prot (g)	Carb (g)	Fiber (g)	Fat (g)	Mono (g)	Poly (g)
7	Buttermilk, low fat, cultured	1 cup	245	98	8	12	0	2	0.6	0.1
500	Cream, half & half	2 Tbs	30	39	1	1	0	3	1	0.1
11953	Kefir, peach	1 cup	225	200	7	23	1	7		
218	Milk, 2%, w/added vitamins A & D	1 cup	245	130	8	13	0	5		
21109	Milk, chocolate, reduced fat w/added calcium	1 cup	250	195	7	30	2	5	1.1	0.2
19	Milk, low fat, chocolate	1 cup	250	158	8	26	1	2	0.8	0.1
11	Milk, condensed, sweetened, canned	2 Tbs	38.2	123	3	21	0	3	0.9	0.1
23	Milk, goat	1 cup	244	168	9	11	0	10	2.7	0.4
22	Milk, human breast	1 cup	246	172	3	17	0	11	4.1	1.2
134	Milk, evaporated, w/added vitamin A, canned	2 Tbs	31.5	42	2	3	0	2	0.7	0.1
10	Milk, evaporated, nonfat/skim, canned	2 Tbs	32	25	2	4	0	0	0	0
68	Milk, nonfat/skim, w/added vitamin A, dry	0.5 cup	60	217	22	31	0	0	0.1	0
6	Milk, nonfat/skim, w/added vitamin A	1 cup	245	83	8	12	0	0	0.1	0
1	Milk, whole, 3.25%	1 cup	244	146	8	11	0	8	2	0.5
20	Milk, whole, chocolate	1 cup	250	208	8	26	2	8	2.5	0.3
2834	Yogurt, blueberry, fruit on the bottom	1 ea	227	220	9	41	1	2		
2315	Yogurt, blueberry, low fat	1 ea	113	110	3	23	0	1		
72636	Yogurt, blueberry, nonfat	1 ea	227	120	7	21	0	0	0	0
72639	Yogurt, creamy vanilla, nonfat	1 ea	227	120	7	21	0	0	0	0
2001	Yogurt, fruit, low fat	1 cup	245	250	11	47	0	3	0.7	0.1
72088	Yogurt, fruit, nonfat	1 cup	245	230	11	47	0	0	0.1	0
2096	Yogurt, lemon, nonfat	1 cup	245	223	13	43	0	0	0.1	0

Cheese

MDA Code	Food Name	Amt	Wt (g)	Ener (kcal)	Prot (g)	Carb (g)	Fiber (g)	Fat (g)	Mono (g)	Poly (g)
1287	American cheese, nonfat slice/Kraft	1 pce	21.3	32	5	2	0	0		
47855	Blue, 1" cube	1 ea	17.3	61	4	0	0	5	1.3	0.1
47859	Brie, 1" cube	1 ea	17	57	4	0	0	5	1.4	0.1
47861	Camembert, 1" cube	1 ea	17	51	3	0	0	4	1.2	0.1
48333	Cheddar, fat free, 1" cube	1 ea	16	24	4	2	0	0	0	0
1440	Cheese, fondue	2 Tbs	26.9	62	4	1	0	4	1	0.1

Sat (g)	Chol (mg)	Calc (mg)	Iron (mg)	Mag (mg)	Phos (mg)	Pota (mg)	Sodi (mg)	Zinc (mg)	Vit A (RAE)	Vit C (mg)	Thia (mg)	Ribo (mg)	Niac (mg)	Vit B_6 (mg)	Vit B_{12} (µg)	Vit E (mg)	Fol (µg)	Alc (g)
0.5	0	109	17.07	95.8	295	250	207	4	165	6.6	0.41	0.47	5.49	0.55	0	1.4	420.1	0
0.5	0	113	17.07	65.5	206	205	269	4.2	167	6.4	0.39	0.48	5.63	0.55	0	1.4	439.6	0
0.2	0	110	3.84	28.3	94	109	165	0.6	322	0.3	0.29	0.35	4.07	0.43	0	0.1	84.9	0
0	0	1	0.4	4.2	17	16	1	0.2	0	0	0.06	0.04	0.49	0	0	0	21.6	0
0	0	3	3.8	17.4	43	42	0	0.3	0	0	0.31	0.22	4.24	0.02	0	0	3.8	0
0.3	0	29	4.64	83	259	372	362	1.5	155	0.4	0.39	0.44	5.18	0.52	1.55	0.5	103.7	0
0.5	0	100	4.5	8.1	60	65	200	3.8	145	6	0.38	0.43	5	0.5	1.5	0.8	99.9	0
0.1	0	100	9	27.6	35	50	270	3.8	150	6	0.38	0.42	5	0.5	1.5	0.2	200	0
0.1	0	3	2	8.2	33	36	314	0.4	170	7.8	0.73	0.74	7.58	1.08	2.01	0	151.1	0
0.2	0	19	1.12	50.3	140	142	2	1.1	0	3.8	0.1	0.05	1.98	0.44	0	0	16.3	0
0.2	0	17	18	24	80	90	275	15.1	376	15	1.55	1.7	20	2	6	13.5	402.5	0
0.1	0	9	8.37	19.2	68	61	224	0.9	230	21	0.53	0.59	7.13	1.98	6.04	4.7	399.9	0
0.4	0	3	4.96	14.8	45	51	200	4.1	11	2.9	0.41	0.47	5.51	0.55	0	0.2	420.1	0
0.4	0	122	9.81	35.7	112	95	269	4.4	65	6.2	0.47	0.6	5.7	0.72	1.84	0.2	156	0
0.2	0	1000	18	31.9	100	310	240	15	149	0	1.5	1.7	20	2	6	13.5	399.8	0
0.1	0	1000	18	24	80	90	190	15	150	60	1.5	1.7	20	2	6	13.5	399.9	0
0.2	0	100	4.5	3.6	20	30	190	3.8	147	6	0.38	0.43	5	0.5	1.5	0.6	99.9	0
0.1	0	60	8.64	24	90	114	252	2.2	90	3.6	0.22	0.26	3	0.3	0.9	0.2	240	0
0.1	0	20	8.4	32.1	100	105	210	7.5	150	6	0.75	0.85	10	1	3	0.4	200.1	0
1.3	10	284	0.12	27	218	370	257	1	17	2.4	0.08	0.38	0.14	0.08	0.54	0.1	12.2	0
2.1	11	32	0.02	3	28	39	12	0.2	29	0.3	0.01	0.04	0.02	0.01	0.1	0.1	0.9	0
6	35	250	0				110			3.6								0
3	20	250	0				125			1.2		0.45						0
2.9	20	485	0.6	35	190	308	165	1	160	0	0.11	1.41	0.41	0.06	0.83	0.1	5	0
1.5	8	288	0.6	32.5	258	425	152	1	145	2.2	0.09	0.41	0.32	0.1	0.85	0	12.5	0
2.1	13	108	0.07	9.9	97	142	49	0.4	28	1	0.03	0.16	0.08	0.02	0.17	0.1	4.2	0
6.5	27	327	0.12	34.2	271	498	122	0.7	139	3.2	0.12	0.34	0.68	0.11	0.17	0.2	2.4	0
4.9	34	79	0.07	7.4	34	125	42	0.4	150	12.3	0.03	0.09	0.44	0.03	0.12	0.2	12.3	0
1.4	9	82	0.06	7.6	64	95	33	0.2	35	0.6	0.01	0.1	0.06	0.02	0.05	0.1	2.5	0
0	1	93	0.09	8.6	62	106	37	0.3	38	0.4	0.01	0.1	0.06	0.02	0.08	0	2.9	0
0.3	12	754	0.19	66	581	1076	321	2.4	392	4.1	0.25	0.93	0.57	0.22	2.42	0	30	0
0.1	5	306	0.07	27	247	382	103	1	149	0	0.11	0.45	0.23	0.09	1.3	0	12.2	0
4.6	24	276	0.07	24.4	222	349	98	1	69	0	0.11	0.45	0.26	0.09	1.07	0.1	12.2	0
5.3	30	280	0.6	32.5	252	418	150	1	66	2.2	0.09	0.41	0.31	0.1	0.83	0.1	12.5	0
1	10	300	0			440	210		0	0								0
0.5	10	100	0				50		0	0								0
0	5	350	0	16	200	320	110		0	0		0.25						0
0	5	350	0	16	200	320	110		0	0		0.25						0
1.7	10	372	0.17	36.8	292	478	142	1.8	25	1.7	0.09	0.44	0.23	0.1	1.15	0	22	0
0.3	5	372	0.17	36.8	292	475	142	1.8	6	1.7	0.1	0.44	0.25	0.1	1.15	0.1	22	0
0.3	4	436	0.21	41.8	343	559	168	2.1	4	1.9	0.11	0.52	0.27	0.12	1.34	0	26.7	0
0.1	3	152	0.01		197	50	276	0.5		0		0.06						0
3.2	13	91	0.05	4	67	44	241	0.5	34	0	0.01	0.07	0.18	0.03	0.21	0	6.2	0
3	17	31	0.08	3.4	32	26	107	0.4	30	0	0.01	0.09	0.06	0.04	0.28	0	11	0
2.6	12	66	0.06	3.4	59	32	143	0.4	41	0	0	0.08	0.11	0.04	0.22	0	10.5	0
0.1	2	110	0.04	5.8	150	46	244	0.5	70	0	0.01	0.08	0.03	0.01	0.18	0	4.3	0
2.3	12	128	0.1	6.2	82	28	36	0.5	29	0	0.01	0.05	0.05	0.01	0.22	0.1	2.2	0.08

MDA Code	Food Name	Amt	Wt (g)	Ener (kcal)	Prot (g)	Carb (g)	Fiber (g)	Fat (g)	Mono (g)	Poly (g)
48288	Cheese substitute	1 oz	28.4	40	6	2	0	0	0.1	0
48313	Cheese spread, cream cheese base	1 Tbs	15	44	1	1	0	4	1.2	0.2
13349	Cheez Whiz/Kraft	2 Tbs	33	91	4	3	0	7		
47940	Colby, low fat, 1" cube	1 ea	17.3	30	4	0	0	1	0.4	0
1013	Cottage cheese, creamed, large curd, not packed	0.5 cup	105	108	13	3	0	5	1.3	0.1
1014	Cottage cheese, 2% fat	0.5 cup	113	102	16	4	0	2	0.6	0.1
47867	Cottage cheese, nonfat, small curd, dry	0.5 cup	113	96	20	2	0	0	0.1	0
1015	Cream cheese	2 Tbs	29	101	2	1	0	10	2.9	0.4
1452	Cream cheese, fat free	2 Tbs	29	28	4	2	0	0	0.1	0
1016	Feta, crumbled	0.25 cup	37.5	99	5	2	0	8	1.7	0.2
47874	Fontina, 1 oz slice	1 ea	28.4	110	7	0	0	9	2.5	0.5
1054	Gouda	1 oz	28.4	101	7	1	0	8	2.2	0.2
1442	Mexican, queso anejo, crumbled	0.25 cup	33	123	7	2	0	10	2.8	0.3
47885	Monterey jack, slice	1 ea	28.4	106	7	0	0	9	2.5	0.3
47887	Mozzarella, whole milk, slice	1 ea	34	102	8	1	0	8	2.2	0.3
47892	Muenster, slice	1 ea	28.4	105	7	0	0	9	2.5	0.2
1075	Parmesan, grated	1 Tbs	5	22	2	0	0	1	0.4	0.1
47900	Provolone, slice	1 ea	28.4	100	7	1	0	8	2.1	0.2
1024	Ricotta, part skim	0.25 cup	62	86	7	3	0	5	1.4	0.2
1064	Ricotta, whole milk	0.25 cup	62	108	7	2	0	8	2.2	0.2
	EGGS AND EGG SUBSTITUTES									
19524	Egg substitute, frozen	0.25 cup	60	96	7	2	0	7	1.5	3.7
19525	Egg substitute, liquid	0.25 cup	62.8	53	8	0	0	2	0.6	1
19526	Egg substitute, powder	1 oz	28.4	126	16	6	0	4	1.5	0.5
19506	Egg whites, raw, large	1 ea	33.4	17	4	0	0	0		
19509	Egg, whole, large, fried	1 ea	46	90	6	0	0	7	2.9	1.2
19515	Egg, whole, hard boiled	1 ea	37	57	5	0	0	4	1.5	0.5
19521	Egg, whole, poached, small	1 ea	37	53	5	0	0	4	1.4	0.5
19516	Egg, whole, scrambled	1 ea	61	102	7	1	0	7	2.9	1.3
19508	Egg yolk, raw, large	1 ea	16.6	53	3	1	0	4	1.9	0.7
	FRUIT									
3512	Apples, Golden Delicious, fresh	1 ea	138	59	0	17	2	0	0	0
71079	Apples, fresh	1 cup	125	65	0	17	3	0	0	0.1
3004	Apples, fresh, peeled, slices	1 cup	110	53	0	14	1	0	0	0
3148	Apples, slices, sweetened, drained, canned	0.5 cup	102	68	0	17	2	0	0	0.1
3331	Applesauce, sweetened, canned, w/salt	0.5 cup	127.5	97	0	25	2	0	0	0.1
3330	Applesauce, unswtnd, w/vitamin C, canned	1 cup	244	105	0	28	3	0	0	0
72101	Apricots, w/heavy syrup, canned, drained	1 cup	182	151	1	39	5	0	0.1	0
3155	Apricots, sweetened, frozen	0.5 cup	121	119	1	30	3	0	0.1	0
3333	Apricots, w/o skin, canned, w/water	0.5 cup	113.5	25	1	6	1	0	0	0
3657	Apricots, raw, sliced	1 cup	165	79	2	18	3	1	0.3	0.1
3210	Avocado, California, fresh	1 ea	173	289	3	15	12	27	17	3.1
71082	Banana, fresh, extra small, 6" or shorter	1 ea	81	72	1	19	2	0	0	0.1
3026	Boysenberries, fresh	0.5 cup	72	31	1	7	4	0	0	0.2
3663	Breadfruit, fresh	1 cup	220	227	2	60	11	1	0.1	0.1
71768	Carambola (starfruit), fresh, small	1 ea	70	22	1	5	2	0	0	0.1
72094	Cherries, maraschino, canned, drained	1 ea	4	7	0	2	0	0	0	0
3403	Cherries, sour, red, canned, w/heavy syrup	0.5 cup	128	116	1	30	1	0	0	0
3159	Cherries, sour, red, frozen, unsweetened	0.5 cup	77.5	36	1	9	1	0	0.1	0.1
3035	Cherries, sour/tart, red, canned in water	0.5 cup	122	44	1	11	1	0	0	0

Sat (g)	Chol (mg)	Calc (mg)	Iron (mg)	Mag (mg)	Phos (mg)	Pota (mg)	Sodi (mg)	Zinc (mg)	Vit A (RAE)	Vit C (mg)	Thia (mg)	Ribo (mg)	Niac (mg)	Vit B$_6$ (mg)	Vit B$_{12}$ (µg)	Vit E (mg)	Fol (µg)	Alc (g)
0.2	2	157	0.26	9.9	142	95	352	0.9	3	0	0.01	0.14	0.04	0.04	0.35	0	2.3	0
2.7	14	11	0.17	0.9	14	17	101	0.1	51	0	0	0.03	0.14	0.01	0.06	0.1	1.8	0
4.3	25	118	0.06		266	79	541	0.5		0.1		0.08						0
0.8	4	72	0.07	2.8	84	11	106	0.3	10	0	0	0.04	0.01	0.01	0.08	0	1.9	0
3	16	63	0.15	5.2	139	88	425	0.4	46	0	0.02	0.17	0.13	0.07	0.65	0	12.6	0
1.4	9	78	0.18	6.8	171	108	459	0.5	24	0	0.03	0.21	0.16	0.09	0.8	0	14.7	0
0.3	8	36	0.26	4.5	118	36	15	0.5	10	0	0.03	0.16	0.18	0.09	0.94	0	17	0
6.4	32	23	0.35	1.7	30	35	86	0.2	106	0	0	0.06	0.03	0.01	0.12	0.1	3.8	0
0.3	2	54	0.05	4.1	126	47	158	0.3	81	0	0.01	0.05	0.05	0.01	0.16	0	10.7	0
5.6	33	185	0.24	7.1	126	23	418	1.1	47	0	0.06	0.32	0.37	0.16	0.63	0.1	12	0
5.5	33	156	0.07	4	98	18	227	1	74	0	0.01	0.06	0.04	0.02	0.48	0.1	1.7	0
5	32	199	0.07	8.2	155	34	233	1.1	47	0	0.01	0.09	0.02	0.02	0.44	0.1	6	0
6.3	35	224	0.16	9.2	147	29	373	1	18	0	0.01	0.07	0.01	0.02	0.46	0.1	0.3	0
5.4	25	212	0.2	7.7	126	23	152	0.9	56	0	0	0.11	0.03	0.02	0.24	0.1	5.1	0
4.5	27	172	0.15	6.8	120	26	213	1	61	0	0.01	0.1	0.04	0.01	0.78	0.1	2.4	0
5.4	27	204	0.12	7.7	133	38	178	0.8	85	0	0	0.09	0.03	0.02	0.42	0.1	3.4	0
0.9	4	55	0.04	1.9	36	6	76	0.2	6	0	0	0.02	0.01	0	0.11	0	0.5	0
4.9	20	215	0.15	8	141	39	249	0.9	67	0	0.01	0.09	0.04	0.02	0.41	0.1	2.8	0
3.1	19	169	0.27	9.3	113	78	78	0.8	66	0	0.01	0.11	0.05	0.01	0.18	0	8.1	0
5.1	32	128	0.24	6.8	98	65	52	0.7	74	0	0.01	0.12	0.06	0.03	0.21	0.1	7.4	0
1.2	1	44	1.19	9	43	128	119	0.6	7	0.3	0.07	0.23	0.08	0.08	0.2	1	9.6	0
0.4	1	33	1.32	5.7	76	207	111	0.8	11	0	0.07	0.19	0.07	0	0.19	0.2	9.4	0
1.1	162	93	0.9	18.5	136	211	227	0.5	105	0.2	0.06	0.5	0.16	0.04	1	0.4	35.5	0
	0	2	0.03	3.7	5	54	55	0	0	0	0	0.15	0.04	0	0.03	0	1.3	0
2	210	27	0.91	6	96	68	94	0.6	91	0	0.03	0.24	0.04	0.07	0.64	0.6	23.5	0
1.2	157	18	0.44	3.7	64	47	46	0.4	63	0	0.02	0.19	0.02	0.04	0.41	0.4	16.3	0
1.1	156	20	0.68	4.4	70	49	109	0.4	51	0	0.03	0.18	0.03	0.05	0.47	0.4	17.4	0
2.2	215	43	0.73	7.3	104	84	171	0.6	87	0.1	0.03	0.27	0.05	0.07	0.47	0.5	18.3	0
1.6	205	21	0.45	0.8	65	18	8	0.4	63	0	0.03	0.09	0	0.06	0.32	0.4	24.2	0
0	0	4	0.28	5.5		104	3	0.1	2	6.9	0.03	0.01	0.14		0			0
0	0	8	0.15	6.2	14	134	1	0	4	5.7	0.02	0.03	0.11	0.05	0	0.2	3.8	0
0	0	6	0.08	4.4	12	99	0	0.1	2	4.4	0.02	0.03	0.1	0.04	0	0.1	0	0
0.1	0	4	0.23	2	5	69	3	0	3	0.4	0.01	0.01	0.07	0.04	0	0.2	0	0
0	0	5	0.45	3.8	9	78	36	0.1	1	2.2	0.02	0.04	0.24	0.03	0	0.1	1.3	0
0	0	7	0.29	7.3	17	183	5	0.1	2	51.7	0.03	0.06	0.46	0.06	0	0.1	2.4	0
0	0	18	0.55	12.7	24	260	7	0.2	266	5.6	0.04	0.04	0.68	0.1	0	1.6	3.6	0
0	0	12	1.09	10.9	23	277	5	0.1	102	10.9	0.02	0.05	0.97	0.07	0	1.1	2.4	0
0	0	9	0.61	10.2	18	175	12	0.1	103	2	0.02	0.03	0.5	0.06	0	1	2.3	0
0	0	21	0.64	16.5	38	427	2	0.3	158	16.5	0.05	0.07	0.99	0.09	0	1.5	14.8	0
3.7	0	22	1.06	50.2	93	877	14	1.2	12	15.2	0.13	0.25	3.31	0.5	0	3.4	154	0
0.1	0	4	0.21	21.9	18	290	1	0.1	2	7	0.03	0.06	0.54	0.3	0	0.1	16.2	0
0	0	21	0.45	14.4	16	117	1	0.4	8	15.1	0.01	0.02	0.47	0.02	0	0.8	18	0
0.1	0	37	1.19	55	66	1078	4	0.3	0	63.8	0.24	0.07	1.98	0.22	0	0.2	30.8	0
0	0	2	0.06	7	8	93	1	0.1	2	24.1	0.01	0.01	0.26	0.01	0	0.1	8.4	0
0	0	2	0.02	0.2	0	1	0	0	0	0	0	0	0	0	0	0	0	0
0	0	13	1.66	7.7	13	119	9	0.1	46	2.6	0.02	0.05	0.22	0.06	0	0.3	10.2	0
0.1	0	10	0.41	7	12	96	1	0.1	34	1.3	0.03	0.03	0.11	0.05	0	0	3.9	0
0	0	13	1.67	7.3	12	120	9	0.1	46	2.6	0.02	0.05	0.22	0.05	0	0.3	9.8	0

MDA Code	Food Name	Amt	Wt (g)	Ener (kcal)	Prot (g)	Carb (g)	Fiber (g)	Fat (g)	Mono (g)	Poly (g)
3038	Cherries, sweet, canned in heavy syrup	1 cup	253	210	2	54	4	0	0.1	0.1
72103	Cherries, sweet, canned, heavy syrup, drained	1 cup	184	153	1	39	5	0	0.1	0.1
3336	Cherries, sweet, canned in juice	0.5 cup	125	68	1	17	2	0	0	0
71731	Chinese gooseberries, fresh, w/o skin	1 ea	91	56	1	13	3	0	0	0.3
72093	Cranberries, dried, sweetened	0.33 cup	40	123	0	33	2	1	0.1	0.3
3673	Cranberries, raw	1 cup	110	51	0	13	5	0	0	0.1
27019	Cranberry-orange relish, canned	0.25 cup	68.8	122	0	32	0	0	0	0
4900	Currants, red or white, raw	0.25 cup	28	16	0	4	1	0	0	0
3192	Currants, Zante, dried	0.25 cup	36	102	1	27	2	0	0	0.1
3044	Dates, Deglet Noor	5 ea	41.5	117	1	31	3	0	0	0
72111	Dates, medjool	1 ea	24	66	0	18	2	0		
3975	Durian, fresh or frozen	1 ea	602	885	9	163	23	32		
5611	Eggplant, pickled	1 cup	136	67	1	13	3	1	0.1	0.4
3677	Figs, raw	1 ea	40	30	0	8	1	0	0	0.1
3045	Fruit cocktail canned in heavy syrup	1 cup	248	181	1	47	2	0	0	0.1
3164	Fruit cocktail canned in juice	1 cup	237	109	1	28	2	0	0	0
3414	Fruit salad canned in heavy syrup	1 cup	255	186	1	49	3	0	0	0.1
44023	Fruit salad canned in juice	0.5 cup	124.5	62	1	16	1	0	0	0
3203	Gooseberries, raw	0.5 cup	75	33	1	8	3	0	0	0.2
3342	Grapefruit, canned in juice	0.5 cup	124.5	46	1	11	0	0	0	0
71976	Grapefruit, fresh	0.5 ea	154	60	1	16	6	0	0	0
3055	Grapes, Thompson seedless, fresh	0.5 cup	80	55	1	14	1	0	0	0
3634	Guava, raw	0.5 cup	82.5	56	2	12	4	1	0.1	0.3
71732	Kiwifruit (Chinese gooseberry) peeled, raw	1 ea	76	46	1	11	2	0	0	0.2
3252	Kumquat, raw	1 ea	19	13	0	3	1	0	0	0
71979	Lemon, fresh	1 ea	58	15	0	5	1	0	0	0
3071	Limes, peeled, fresh	1 ea	67	20	0	7	2	0	0	0
3033	Loganberries, w/heavy syrup, canned	0.5 cup	128	113	1	29	3	0	0	0.1
71743	Lychee (Litchi), shelled, dried	1 ea	2.5	7	0	2	0	0	0	0
71927	Mango, dried	0.33 cup	40	140	0	34	1	0	0	0
3221	Mango, raw	0.5 ea	103.5	67	1	18	2	0	0.1	0.1
3167	Melon balls (cantaloupe & honeydew), frozen	0.5 cup	86.5	29	1	7	1	0	0	0.1
3642	Melon, cantaloupe, fresh, wedge	1 pce	69	23	1	6	1	0	0	0.1
4488	Melon, casaba, raw	1 pce	164	46	2	11	1	0	0	0.1
3644	Melon, honeydew, fresh	1 ea	1280	461	7	116	10	2	0	0.8
3168	Mixed fruit (prune, apricot & pear), dried	1 oz	28.4	69	1	18	2	0	0.1	0
3216	Nectarine, raw	1 cup	138	61	1	15	2	0	0.1	0.2
27011	Olives, black, pitted, canned	1 ea	3.2	4	0	0	0	0	0.3	0
3228	Orange, California navel, fresh	1 ea	140	69	1	18	3	0	0	0
3230	Orange, Florida, fresh	1 ea	151	69	1	17	4	0	0.1	0.1
3085	Orange, fresh	1 ea	184	86	2	22	4	0	0	0
71990	Orange, mandarin, fresh	1 ea	109	50	1	15	3	0		
3721	Papayas, raw	1 ea	152	59	1	15	3	0	0.1	0
3098	Peach, canned in heavy syrup	1 cup	262	194	1	52	3	0	0.1	0.1
57481	Peach, frozen, sweetened	1 cup	250	235	2	60	4	0	0.1	0.2
3726	Peach, peeled, raw	1 ea	79	31	1	8	1	0	0.1	0.1
3106	Pear, d'anjou, fresh	1 ea	209	121	1	32	6	0	0.1	0.1
3106	Pear, raw	1 ea	209	121	1	32	6	0	0.1	0.1
3194	Persimmon, native, raw	1 ea	25	32	0	8	0	0		
72113	Pineapple, fresh, slice	1 pce	84	38	0	10		0		

Sat (g)	Chol (mg)	Calc (mg)	Iron (mg)	Mag (mg)	Phos (mg)	Pota (mg)	Sodi (mg)	Zinc (mg)	Vit A (RAE)	Vit C (mg)	Thia (mg)	Ribo (mg)	Niac (mg)	Vit B6 (mg)	Vit B12 (µg)	Vit E (mg)	Fol (µg)	Alc (g)
0.1	0	23	0.89	22.8	46	367	8	0.3	20	9.1	0.05	0.1	1	0.08	0	0.6	10.1	0
0.1	0	18	0.64	16.6	37	272	6	0.2	22	6.6	0.04	0.08	0.73	0.06	0	0.4	9.2	0
0	0	18	0.72	15	28	164	4	0.1	8	3.1	0.02	0.03	0.51	0.04	0	0.3	5	0
0	7	31	0.28	15.5	31	284	3	0.1	4	84.4	0.02	0.02	0.31	0.06	0	1.3	23	0
0	0	4	0.21	2	3	16	1	0	0	0.1	0	0.01	0.4	0.02	0	0.4	0	0
0	0	9	0.28	6.6	14	94	2	0.1	3	14.6	0.01	0.02	0.11	0.06	0	1.3	1.1	0
0	0	8	0.14	2.8	6	26	22	0.1	3	12.4	0.02	0.01	0.07	0.02	0	0	2.1	0
0	0	9	0.28	3.6	12	77	0	0.1	1	11.5	0.01	0.01	0.03	0.02	0	0	2.2	0
0	0	31	1.17	14.8	45	321	3	0.2	1	1.7	0.06	0.05	0.58	0.11	0	0	3.6	0
0	0	16	0.42	17.8	26	272	1	0.1	0	0.2	0.02	0.03	0.53	0.07	0	0	7.9	0
	0	15	0.22	13	15	167	0	0.1	2	0	0.01	0.01	0.39	0.06			3.6	0
	0	36	2.59	180.6	235	2625	12	1.7	12	119	2.25	1.2	6.47	1.9	0		217	0
0.2	0	34	1.05	8.2	12	16	2277	0.3	4	0	0.07	0.1	0.9	0.19	0	0	27.2	0
0	0	14	0.15	6.8	6	93	0	0.1	3	0.8	0.02	0.02	0.16	0.05	0	0	2.4	0
0	0	15	0.72	12.4	27	218	15	0.2	25	4.7	0.04	0.05	0.93	0.12	0	1	7.4	0
0	0	19	0.5	16.6	33	225	9	0.2	36	6.4	0.03	0.04	0.96	0.12	0	0.9	7.1	0
0	0	15	0.71	12.8	23	204	15	0.2	64	6.1	0.04	0.05	0.88	0.08	0	1	7.6	0
0	0	14	0.31	10	17	144	6	0.2	37	4.1	0.01	0.02	0.44	0.03	0	0.7	3.7	0
0	0	19	0.23	7.5	20	148	1	0.1	11	20.8	0.03	0.02	0.23	0.06	0	0.3	4.5	0
0	0	19	0.26	13.7	15	210	9	0.1	0	42.2	0.04	0.02	0.31	0.02	0	0.1	11.2	0
0		20	0				0		38	66					0			0
0	4	8	0.29	5.6	16	153	2	0.1	2	8.6	0.06	0.06	0.15	0.07	0	0.2	1.6	0
0.2	0	15	0.21	18.2	33	344	2	0.2	26	188.3	0.06	0.03	0.89	0.09	0	0.6	40.4	0
0	0	26	0.24	12.9	26	237	2	0.1	3	70.5	0.02	0.02	0.26	0.05	0	1.1	19	0
0	0	12	0.16	3.8	4	35	2	0	3	8.3	0.01	0.02	0.08	0.01	0	0	3.2	0
0		20	0				5		0	24					0			0
0	3	22	0.4	4	12	68	1	0.1	1	19.5	0.02	0.01	0.13	0.03	0	0.1	5.4	0
0	0	23	0.55	14.1	13	115	4	0.2	3	7.9	0.03	0.04	0.29	0.05	0	0.9	43.5	0
0	0	1	0.04	1	5	28	0	0	0	4.6	0	0.01	0.08	0	0	0	0.3	0
0		80	0.36			10	20	25		1.2					0			0
0.1	0	10	0.13	9.3	11	161	2	0	39	28.7	0.06	0.06	0.6	0.14	0	1.2	14.5	0
0.1	0	9	0.25	12.1	10	242	27	0.1	77	5.4	0.14	0.02	0.55	0.09	0	0.1	22.5	0
0	5	6	0.14	8.3	10	184	11	0.1	117	25.3	0.03	0.01	0.51	0.05	0	0	15	0
0	0	18	0.56	18	8	298	15	0.1	0	35.8	0.02	0.05	0.38	0.27	0	0.1	13.1	0
0.5	77		2.18	128	141	2918	230	1.2	38	230	0.49	0.15	5.35	1.13	0	0.3	243	0
0	0	11	0.77	11.1	22	226	5	0.1	35	1.1	0.01	0.04	0.55	0.05	0	0.2	1.1	0
0	0	8	0.39	12.4	36	277	0	0.2	23	7.5	0.05	0.04	1.55	0.03	0	1.1	6.9	0
0	0	3	0.11	0.1	0	0	28	0	1	0	0	0	0	0	0	0.1	0	0
0	12	60	0.18	15.4	32	232	1	0.1	17	82.7	0.1	0.07	0.6	0.11	0	0.2	48	0
0		65	0.14	15.1	18	255	0	0.1	17	68	0.15	0.06	0.6	0.08	0	0.3	26	0
0		74	0.18	18.4	26	333	0	0.1	20	97.9	0.16	0.07	0.52	0.11	0	0.3	55	0
0		40	0				0		0	30					0			0
0.1	0	36	0.15	15.2	8	391	5	0.1	84	93.9	0.04	0.05	0.51	0.03	0	1.1	57.8	0
0	0	8	0.71	13.1	29	241	16	0.2	45	7.3	0.03	0.06	1.61	0.05	0	1.3	7.9	0
0	0	8	0.93	12.5	28	325	15	0.1	35	235.5	0.03	0.09	1.63	0.04	0	1.6	7.5	0
0	0	5	0.2	7.1	16	150	0	0.1	13	5.2	0.02	0.02	0.64	0.02	0	0.6	3.2	0
0	11	19	0.36	14.6	23	249	2	0.2	2	8.8	0.03	0.05	0.33	0.06	0	0.3	15	0
0	0	19	0.36	14.6	23	249	2	0.2	2	8.8	0.03	0.05	0.33	0.06	0	0.3	14.6	0
0		7	0.62		6	78	0			16.5					0	0.2	2	0
0		11	0.21	10.1	8	105	1	0.1	2	14.2	0.07	0.02	0.39	0.09			9.2	0

MDA Code	Food Name	Amt	Wt (g)	Ener (kcal)	Prot (g)	Carb (g)	Fiber (g)	Fat (g)	Mono (g)	Poly (g)
3748	Plantain, cooked, mashed	1 cup	200	232	2	62	5	0	0	0.1
3121	Plums, fresh	1 ea	66	30	0	8	1	0	0.1	0
3197	Pomegranate, fresh	1 ea	154	105	1	26	1	0	0.1	0.1
3263	Quince, fresh	1 ea	92	52	0	14	2	0	0	0
3766	Raisins, seedless	50 ea	26	78	1	21	1	0	0	0
9758	Raisins, golden, seedless	0.25 cup	40	130	1	31	2	0	0	0
71987	Raspberries, fresh	1 cup	125	50	1	17	8	0	0	0
3133	Rhubarb, frozen, cooked w/sugar	0.5 cup	120	139	0	37	2	0	0	0
3767	Rhubarb, fresh, stalk	1 ea	51	11	0	2	1	0	0	0.1
3761	Shaddock (pomelo or grapefruit), fresh, sections	1 cup	190	72	1	18	2	0		
3354	Strawberries, frozen, sweetened, thawed, whole	0.5 cup	127.5	99	1	27	2	0	0	0.1
3135	Strawberries, fresh, sliced	1 cup	166	53	1	13	3	0	0.1	0.3
3792	Tamarindo, Spanish, fresh, pulp	1 cup	120	287	3	75	6	1	0.2	0.1
3717	Tangerines, fresh, large	1 ea	98	52	1	13	2	0	0.1	0.1
3143	Watermelon, fresh, 1/16 melon	1 pce	286	86	2	22	1	0	0.1	0.1

GRAIN PRODUCTS, GRAINS, AND FLOURS
Breads, Rolls, Bread Crumbs, and Croutons

MDA Code	Food Name	Amt	Wt (g)	Ener (kcal)	Prot (g)	Carb (g)	Fiber (g)	Fat (g)	Mono (g)	Poly (g)
71170	Bagel, cinnamon raisin, mini, 2-1/2"	1 ea	26	71	3	14	1	0	0	0.2
71167	Bagel, egg, mini, 2-1/2"	1 ea	26	72	3	14	1	1	0.1	0.2
42744	Bagel, blueberry, 4", Lender's	1 ea	102	264	11	53	2	2	0.4	0.5
71176	Bagel, oat bran, mini, 2-1/2"	1 ea	26	66	3	14	1	0	0.1	0.1
71152	Bagel, sesame, mini, enriched, w/calcium propionate, 2-1/2"	1 ea	26	67	3	13	1	0	0.1	0.2
42039	Banana bread, homemade w/margarine, slice	1 pce	60	196	3	33	1	6	2.7	1.9
42433	Biscuit	1 ea	82	273	5	28	1	16		
47709	Biscuit, buttermilk, refrigerated dough/Pillsbury	1 ea	64	150	4	29	1	2		
42111	Biscuit, mixed grain, refrigerated dough, 2-1/2"	1 ea	44	116	3	21		2	1.3	0.4
71192	Biscuit, plain, lower fat, refrigerated dough, 2-1/4"	1 ea	21	63	2	12	0	1	0.6	0.2
42004	Bread crumbs, plain, grated, dry	1 Tbs	6.8	27	1	5	0	0	0.1	0.1
42144	Bread crumbs, seasoned, grated, dry	1 Tbs	7.5	29	1	5	0	0	0.1	0.2
42090	Bread, egg, slice	1 pce	40	113	4	19	1	2	0.9	0.4
49144	Bread, garlic, crusty Italian	1 pce	50	186	4	21		10	3.9	1.8
70964	Bread, garlic, frozen, Campione	1 pce	28	101	2	12	1	5		
42119	Bread, Irish soda, homemade	1 pce	28	81	2	16	1	1	0.6	0.4
42069	Bread, oat bran, slice	1 pce	30	71	3	12	1	1	0.5	0.5
42076	Bread, oat bran, reduced calorie, slice	1 pce	23	46	2	9	3	1	0.2	0.4
42136	Bread, wheat bran, slice	1 pce	36	89	3	17	1	1	0.6	0.2
42599	Bread, wheat germ, slice	1 pce	28	73	3	14	1	1	0.4	0.2
42095	Bread, wheat, reduced calorie, slice	1 pce	23	46	2	10	3	1	0.1	0.2
71247	Bread, white, soft, w/o crust, thin slice	1 pce	9	24	1	5	0	0	0.1	0.1
42084	Bread, white, reduced calorie, slice	1 pce	23	48	2	10	2	1	0.2	0.1
71259	Breadsticks, plain, small, 4-1/4" long	1 ea	5	21	1	3	0	0	0.2	0.2
26561	Buns, hamburger/Wonder	1 ea	43	117	3	22	1	2	0.4	0.9
42021	Buns, hot dog/frankfurter	1 ea	43	120	4	21	1	2	0.5	0.8
71364	Buns, hot dog/frankfurter, whole wheat	1 ea	43	114	4	22	3	2	0.5	0.9
42115	Cornbread, prepared from dry mix	1 pce	60	188	4	29	1	6	3.1	0.7
49012	Cornbread, hush puppies, homemade	1 ea	22	74	2	10	1	3	0.7	1.6
42016	Croutons, plain, dry	0.25 cup	7.5	31	1	6	0	0	0.2	0.1
71302	Croutons, seasoned, fast food pkg	1 ea	10	46	1	6	0	2	0.9	0.2
71227	Pita bread, white, enriched, small, 4"	1 ea	28	77	3	16	1	0	0	0.1
71228	Pita bread, whole wheat, small, 4"	1 ea	28	74	3	15	2	1	0.1	0.3

Sat (g)	Chol (mg)	Calc (mg)	Iron (mg)	Mag (mg)	Phos (mg)	Pota (mg)	Sodi (mg)	Zinc (mg)	Vit A (RAE)	Vit C (mg)	Thia (mg)	Ribo (mg)	Niac (mg)	Vit B$_6$ (mg)	Vit B$_{12}$ (µg)	Vit E (mg)	Fol (µg)	Alc (g)
0.1	0	4	1.16	64	56	930	10	0.3	90	21.8	0.09	0.1	1.51	0.48	0	0.3	52	0
0	0	4	0.11	4.6	11	104	0	0.1	11	6.3	0.02	0.02	0.28	0.02	0	0.2	3.3	0
0.1	0	5	0.46	4.6	12	399	5	0.2	8	9.4	0.05	0.05	0.46	0.16	0	0.9	9.2	0
0	0	10	0.64	7.4	16	181	4	0	2	13.8	0.02	0.03	0.18	0.04	0	0.5	2.8	0
0	0	13	0.49	8.3	26	195	3	0.1	0	0.6	0.03	0.03	0.2	0.05	0	0	1.3	0
0	0	20	1.08				10		0	0								0
0	0	20	0.36				0		0	24					0			0
0	0	174	0.25	14.4	10	115	1	0.1	5	4	0.02	0.03	0.24	0.02	0	0.3	6	0
0	0	44	0.11	6.1	7	147	2	0.1	3	4.1	0.01	0.02	0.15	0.01	0	0.2	3.6	0
	0	8	0.21	11.4	32	410	2	0.2	1	115.9	0.06	0.05	0.42	0.07	0	0.2	49.4	0
0	0	14	0.6	7.6	15	125	1	0.1	1	50.4	0.02	0.1	0.37	0.04	0	0.3	5.1	0
0	0	27	0.68	21.6	40	254	2	0.2	2	97.6	0.04	0.04	0.64	0.08	0	0.5	39.8	0
0.3	0	89	3.36	110.4	136	754	34	0.1	2	4.2	0.51	0.18	2.33	0.08	0	0.1	16.8	0
0	0	36	0.15	11.8	20	163	2	0.1	33	26.2	0.06	0.04	0.37	0.08	0	0.2	15.7	0
0	0	20	0.69	28.6	31	320	3	0.3	80	23.2	0.09	0.06	0.51	0.13	0	0.1	8.6	0
0.1	0	5	0.99	7.3	26	38	84	0.3	5	0.2	0.1	0.07	0.8	0.02	0	0.1	28.9	0
0.1	6	3	1.03	6.5	22	18	131	0.2	9	0.2	0.14	0.06	0.9	0.02	0.04	0	22.9	0
0.3	0	57	1.84			158	427	0	0	0	0.27	0.2	4.08	0.06	0		75.5	0
0	0	3	0.8	8.1	29	30	132	0.2	0	0.1	0.09	0.09	0.77	0.01	0	0.1	25.5	0
0.1	0	23	1.57	5.7	23	20	116	0.5	0	0.3	0.16	0.07	1.03	0.02	0	0	37.7	0
1.3	26	13	0.84	8.4	35	80	181	0.2	64	1	0.1	0.12	0.87	0.09	0.06	1.1	19.8	0
3.9	1	30					786			0								0
0.3	0		1.44				570											0
0.6	0	7	1.21	13.2	104	201	295	0.3	0	0	0.17	0.09	1.5	0.03	0	0.4	36.5	0
0.3	0	4	0.65	3.6	98	39	305	0.1	0	0	0.09	0.05	0.72	0.01	0	0	17.4	0
0.1	0	12	0.33	2.9	11	13	50	0.1	0	0	0.07	0.03	0.45	0.01	0.02	0	7.3	0
0.1	0	14	0.37	3.4	13	17	132	0.1	1	0.2	0.07	0.03	0.46	0.01	0	0	8.9	0
0.6	20	37	1.22	7.6	42	46	197	0.3	25	0	0.18	0.17	1.94	0.03	0.04	0.1	42	0
2.4	6		1.18				200											0
0.8			0.3				154											0
0.3	5	23	0.75	6.4	32	74	111	0.2	13	0.2	0.08	0.08	0.67	0.02	0.01	0.3	13.2	0
0.2	0	20	0.94	10.5	42	44	122	0.3	1	0	0.15	0.1	1.45	0.02	0	0.1	24.3	0
0.1	0	13	0.72	12.6	32	23	81	0.2	0	0	0.08	0.05	0.87	0.02	0	0.1	18.6	0
0.3	0	27	1.11	29.2	67	82	175	0.5	0	0	0.14	0.1	1.58	0.06	0	0.1	37.8	0
0.2	0	25	0.97	7.8	34	71	155	0.3	0	0.1	0.1	0.1	1.26	0.02	0.02	0.1	33	0
0.1	0	18	0.68	9	23	28	118	0.3	0	0	0.1	0.07	0.89	0.03	0	0.1	20.9	0
0.1	0	14	0.34	2.1	9	9	61	0.1	0	0	0.04	0.03	0.39	0.01	0	0	10	0
0.1	0	22	0.73	5.3	28	17	104	0.3	0	0.1	0.09	0.07	0.84	0.01	0.06	0	21.8	0
0.1	0	1	0.21	1.6	6	6	33	0	0	0	0.03	0.03	0.26	0	0	0.1	8.1	0
0.4		37	0.95				256											0
0.5	0	59	1.43	9	27	40	206	0.3	0	0	0.17	0.14	1.79	0.03	0.09	0	47.7	0
0.4	0	46	1.04	36.6	96	117	206	0.9	0	0	0.11	0.07	1.58	0.08	0	0.4	12.9	0
1.6	37	44	1.14	12	226	77	467	0.4	26	0.1	0.15	0.16	1.23	0.06	0.1	0.7	33	0
0.5	10	61	0.67	5.3	42	32	147	0.1	9	0	0.08	0.07	0.61	0.02	0.04	0.3	19.6	0
0.1	0	6	0.31	2.3	9	9	52	0.1	0	0	0.05	0.02	0.41	0	0	0	9.9	0
0.5	1	10	0.28	4.2	14	18	124	0.1	1	0	0.05	0.04	0.46	0.01	0.01	0	10.5	0
0	0	24	0.73	7.3	27	34	150	0.2	0	0	0.17	0.09	1.3	0.01	0	0.1	30	0
0.1	0	4	0.86	19.3	50	48	149	0.4	0	0	0.09	0.02	0.8	0.07	0	0.2	9.8	0

MDA Code	Food Name	Amt	Wt (g)	Ener (kcal)	Prot (g)	Carb (g)	Fiber (g)	Fat (g)	Mono (g)	Poly (g)
42159	Rolls, dinner, egg, 2-1/2"	1 ea	35	107	3	18	1	2	1	0.4
71368	Rolls, dinner, homemade w/2% milk, 3-1/2"	1 ea	43	136	4	23	1	3	1.2	0.9
42161	Rolls, French	1 ea	38	105	3	19	1	2	0.7	0.3
71056	Rolls, kaiser, 3-1/2"	1 ea	57	167	6	30	1	2	0.6	1
42297	Tortilla, corn, medium, 6", unsalted	1 ea	26	58	1	12	1	1	0.2	0.3
90645	Taco shells, baked, mini, 3"	1 ea	5	23	0	3	0	1	0.6	0.2
	Crackers									
71277	Cheese crackers, bite size	1 cup	62	312	6	36	1	16	7.5	1.5
43532	Crispbread crackers, rye	1 ea	10	37	1	8	2	0	0	0.1
71451	Goldfish crackers, cheese, low sodium	55 pce	33	166	3	19	1	8	3.9	0.8
43510	Matzoh, whole wheat	1 oz	28.4	100	4	22	3	0	0.1	0.2
71284	Melba toast, plain	1 cup	30	117	4	23	2	1	0.2	0.4
71032	Melba toast, pumpernickel	6 ea	30	117	3	23	2	1	0.3	0.4
43507	Oyster crackers	1 cup	45	193	4	32	1	5	3.2	0.6
43659	Oyster crackers, low sodium	1 cup	45	195	4	32	1	5	2.9	0.8
70963	Ritz crackers, original/Nabisco	5 ea	16	79	1	10	0	4	2.8	0.3
43540	Rusk toast crackers	3 ea	30	122	4	22	1	2	0.8	0.7
43587	Saltine crackers, original/Kraft	5 ea	14	56	1	10	0	1		
43664	Saltines, low sodium, fat free	6 ea	30	118	3	25	1	0	0	0.2
43545	Sandwich crackers, cheese	4 ea	28	134	3	17	1	6	3.2	0.7
43501	Sandwich crackers, cheese, peanut butter	4 ea	28	139	3	16	1	7	3.6	1.4
43546	Sandwich crackers, peanut butter	4 ea	28	138	3	16	1	7	3.9	1.3
44677	Snackwell crackers, wheat/Kraft	1 ea	15	62	1	12	1	2		
43581	Wheat Thins, original/Kraft	16 ea	29	140	3	20	1	6		
43508	Whole wheat crackers	4 ea	32	142	3	22	3	6	1.9	2.1
43570	Whole wheat crackers, low sodium	7 ea	28	124	2	19	3	5	1.6	1.8
	Muffins and Baked Goods									
71035	English muffin, granola	1 ea	66	155	6	31	2	1	0.5	0.4
42723	English muffin, plain/Thomas'	1 ea	57	132	5	26		1	0.2	0.5
42060	English muffin, sourdough, w/calcium proprionate	1 ea	57	129	5	25	2	1	0.2	0.3
42153	English muffin, wheat	1 ea	57	127	5	26	3	1	0.2	0.5
62916	Muffin, blueberry, mini, 1-1/4"	1 ea	11	43	1	5	0	2	0.6	1.1
44521	Muffin, corn, 2-1/4" × 2-1/2"	1 ea	57	174	3	29	2	5	1.2	1.8
44514	Muffin, oat bran, 2-1/4" × 2-1/2"	1 ea	57	154	4	28	3	4	1	2.4
44518	Toaster muffin, blueberry	1 ea	33	103	2	18	1	3	0.7	1.8
44522	Toaster muffin, cornmeal	1 ea	33	114	2	19	1	4	0.9	2.1
	Noodles and Pasta									
66103	Angel hair pasta, semolina, dry	1 ea	56	201	7	41	2	1	0.2	0.8
91313	Bow tie pasta, enriched, dry	1.5 cup	56	204	8	42	2	1		
38048	Chow mein noodles, dry	1 cup	45	237	4	26	2	14	3.5	7.8
38047	Egg pasta, enriched, cooked	0.5 cup	80	110	4	20	1	2	0.5	0.4
38251	Egg pasta, enriched, cooked w/salt	0.5 cup	80	110	4	20	1	2	0.5	0.4
91316	Elbow pasta, enriched, dry	0.5 cup	56	204	8	42	2	1		
38356	Fettuccine pasta, frozen/Kraft	70 g	70	200	8	38	2	2		
91293	Fettuccine pasta, spinach, enriched, dry	1.33 cup	56	202	8	40	2	1	0.1	0.6
38102	Macaroni pasta, enriched, cooked	1 cup	140	221	8	43	3	1	0.2	0.4
38110	Macaroni pasta, whole wheat, cooked	1 cup	140	174	7	37	4	1	0.1	0.3
66121	Pasta shells, small, wheat free, low protein, dry	2 oz	56.7	194	0	48	0	0		
92830	Penne pasta, dry	0.25 ea	57	210	7	41	1	1		
38067	Ramen noodles, cooked	0.5 cup	113.5	77	2	10	1	3	0.6	1.7

Sat (g)	Chol (mg)	Calc (mg)	Iron (mg)	Mag (mg)	Phos (mg)	Pota (mg)	Sodi (mg)	Zinc (mg)	Vit A (RAE)	Vit C (mg)	Thia (mg)	Ribo (mg)	Niac (mg)	Vit B_6 (mg)	Vit B_{12} (µg)	Vit E (mg)	Fol (µg)	Alc (g)
0.6	18	21	1.23	8.8	35	36	191	0.4	2	0	0.18	0.18	1.15	0.02	0.08	0.1	64.4	0
0.8	15	26	1.27	8.2	54	65	178	0.3	37	0.1	0.17	0.18	1.48	0.03	0.06	0.4	38.7	0
0.4	0	35	1.03	7.6	32	43	231	0.3	0	0	0.2	0.11	1.65	0.01	0	0.1	42.9	0
0.3	0	54	1.87	15.4	57	62	310	0.5	0	0	0.27	0.19	2.42	0.02	0	0.2	54.2	0
0.1	0	46	0.36	16.9	82	40	3	0.2	0	0	0.03	0.02	0.39	0.06	0	0	29.6	0
0.2	0	5	0.09	4.2	11	11	19	0.1	0	0	0.01	0	0.09	0.01	0	0	3.4	0
5.8	8	94	2.96	22.3	135	90	617	0.7	18	0	0.35	0.27	2.9	0.34	0.29	0	94.2	0
0	0	3	0.24	7.8	27	32	26	0.2	0	0	0.02	0.01	0.1	0.02	0	0.1	4.7	0
3.2	4	50	1.57	11.9	72	35	151	0.4	6	0	0.19	0.14	1.54	0.18	0.15	0.1	29.4	0
0.1	0	7	1.32	38.1	87	90	1	0.7	0	0	0.1	0.08	1.54	0.05	0		9.9	0
0.1	0	28	1.11	17.7	59	61	249	0.6	0	0	0.12	0.08	1.23	0.03	0	0.1	37.2	0
0.1	0	23	1.1	11.7	55	58	270	0.4	0	0	0.14	0.09	1.42	0.03	0	0.2	25.5	0
0.7	0	31	2.54	9.9	45	69	482	0.4	0	0	0.04	0.2	2.36	0.04	0	0.4	62.6	0
1.3	0	54	2.43	12.2	47	326	286	0.3	0	0	0.25	0.21	2.36	0.02	0	0.1	55.8	0
0.6	0	24	0.65	3.2	48	15	124	0.2	0	0	0.04	0.05	0.61	0.01	0		9.6	0
0.4	23	8	0.82	10.8	46	74	76	0.3	4	0	0.12	0.12	1.39	0.01	0.05	0.2	26.1	0
	0	0	0.67				177		0	0								0
0.1	0	7	2.32	7.8	34	34	191	0.3	0	0	0.16	0.18	1.71	0.03	0	0	37.2	0
1.7	1	72	0.67	10.1	114	120	392	0.2	5	0	0.12	0.19	1.05	0.01	0.03	0.1	28	0
1.2	0	14	0.76	15.7	75	61	199	0.3	0	0	0.15	0.08	1.63	0.04	0.08	0.7	26.3	0
1.4	0	23	0.78	15.4	77	60	201	0.3	0	0	0.14	0.08	1.71	0.04	0	0.6	24.1	0
		22	0.59	6.9	50	28	150	0.3	0	0	0.04	0.06				0		0
0.9	0	19	1.01				262		0	0								0
1.1	0	16	0.99	31.7	94	95	211	0.7	0	0	0.06	0.03	1.45	0.06	0	0.3	9	0
1	0	14	0.86	27.7	83	83	69	0.6	0	0	0.06	0.03	1.27	0.05	0	0.2	7.8	0
0.2	0	129	1.99	27.1	53	103	275	0.9	0	0	0.28	0.21	2.36	0.03	0	0	52.8	0
0.2		103	0.8				197		0	0.1					0.21	1	22.8	0
0.4	0	93	2.28	13.7	52	62	242	0.6	0	1	0.27	0.14	2.32	0.03	0.02	0.2	53.6	0
0.2	0	101	1.64	21.1	61	106	218	0.6	0	0	0.25	0.17	1.91	0.05	0	0.3	36.5	0
0.4	4	4	0.22	1.1	14	11	35	0.1	1	0.1	0.02	0.02	0.15	0	0.01	0.2	5.3	0
0.8	15	42	1.6	18.2	162	39	297	0.3	30	0	0.16	0.19	1.16	0.05	0.05	0.5	45.6	0
0.6	0	36	2.39	89.5	214	289	224	1	0	0	0.15	0.05	0.24	0.09	0.01	0.4	50.7	0
0.5	2	4	0.17	4	19	27	158	0.1	31	0	0.08	0.1	0.67	0.01	0.01	0.3	21.4	0
0.6	4	6	0.49	4.6	50	30	142	0.1	6	0	0.1	0.12	0.76	0.02	0.01	0.5	18.8	0
0.3	0	12	1.61	26.3	90	105	3	0.7	0	0	0.49	0.21	3.34	0.07	0	0.1	111.1	0
0.2	0	10	1.8	30.1	79	81	3	0.6	0	0	0.45	0.25	3				119.8	0
2	0	9	2.13	23.4	72	54	198	0.6	0	0	0.26	0.19	2.68	0.05	0	1.6	40.5	0
0.3	23	10	1.18	16.8	61	30	4	0.5	5	0	0.23	0.11	1.66	0.04	0.07	0.1	67.2	0
0.3	23	10	1.18	16.8	61	30	132	0.5	5	0	0.23	0.11	1.66	0.04	0.07	0.1	67.2	0
0.2	0	10	1.8	30.1	79	81	3	0.6	0	0	0.45	0.25	3				119.8	0
0	0	0	0				140		0	0								0
0.3	1	78	1.8	43.7	117	203	16	0.8	7	0	0.45	0.25	3					0
0.2	0	10	1.79	25.2	81	62	1	0.7	0	0	0.38	0.19	2.36	0.07	0	0.1	102.2	0
0.1	0	21	1.48	42	125	62	4	1.1	0	0	0.15	0.06	0.99	0.11	0	0.4	7	0
0	0	3	0.68			52			0	0.5								0
	0	0	0.72				0		0	0								0
0.8	0	7	0.2	5.2	12	25	401	0.1	1	0	0.01	0.01	0.13	0.01	0	1.2	1.6	0

MDA Code	Food Name	Amt	Wt (g)	Ener (kcal)	Prot (g)	Carb (g)	Fiber (g)	Fat (g)	Mono (g)	Poly (g)
38551	Rice pasta, cooked	0.5 cup	88	96	1	22	1	0	0	0
38094	Soba noodles, cooked	1 cup	114	113	6	24	1	0	0	0
38118	Spaghetti, enriched, cooked	0.5 cup	70	111	4	22	1	1	0.1	0.2
38066	Spaghetti, spinach, cooked	1 cup	140	182	6	37	5	1	0.1	0.4
38274	Spaghetti, unenriched, cooked w/salt	0.5 cup	70	110	4	21	1	1	0.1	0.2
38060	Spaghetti, whole wheat, cooked	1 cup	140	174	7	37	6	1	0.1	0.3
	Flours									
38071	Arrowroot flour	0.25 cup	32	114	0	28	1	0	0	0
38548	Barley flour	0.25 cup	37	128	4	28	4	1	0.1	0.3
38053	Buckwheat flour, whole groat	0.25 cup	30	100	4	21	3	1	0.3	0.3
38005	Corn flour, masa, white, enriched	0.25 cup	28.5	104	3	22	3	1	0.3	0.5
38054	Semolina flour, enriched	0.25 cup	41.8	150	5	30	2	0	0.1	0.2
7565	Soy flour, full fat, stirred, raw	0.25 cup	21	92	7	7	2	4	1	2.4
38087	Triticale flour, whole grain	0.25 cup	32.5	110	4	24	5	1	0.1	0.3
38033	White flour, all purpose, enriched	0.25 cup	31.2	110	3	23	1	0	0	0.1
38277	White bread flour, enriched	0.25 cup	34.2	123	4	25	1	1	0	0.2
38032	Whole wheat flour	0.25 cup	30	102	4	22	4	1	0.1	0.2
	Grains									
38003	Barley, pearled, cooked	0.5 cup	78.5	97	2	22	3	0	0	0.2
38028	Bulgur, wheat, cooked	1 cup	182	151	6	34	8	0	0.1	0.2
38252	Corn, white, dry	0.25 cup	41.5	151	4	31		2	0.5	0.9
38279	Corn, yellow, dry	0.25 cup	41.5	151	4	31	3	2	0.5	0.9
38183	Cornmeal, white, degermed, enriched	0.25 cup	34.5	127	3	27	1	1	0.1	0.3
38004	Cornmeal, yellow, degermed, enriched	0.25 cup	34.5	127	3	27	1	1	0.1	0.3
38076	Couscous, cooked	0.5 cup	78.5	88	3	18	1	0	0	0.1
5470	Hominy, yellow, canned	0.5 cup	80	58	1	11	2	1	0.2	0.3
38052	Millet, cooked	0.5 cup	87	104	3	21	1	1	0.2	0.4
38078	Oat bran, cooked	0.5 cup	109.5	44	4	13	3	1	0.3	0.4
38080	Oats, unprocessed whole grain	0.25 cup	39	152	7	26	4	3	0.8	1
38010	Rice, brown, long grain, cooked	1 cup	195	216	5	45	4	2	0.6	0.6
38082	Rice, brown, med grain, cooked	0.5 cup	97.5	109	2	23	2	1	0.3	0.3
38083	Rice, white, glutinous, cooked	1 cup	174	169	4	37	2	0	0.1	0.1
38256	Rice, white, long grain, enriched, cooked w/salt	1 cup	158	205	4	45	1	0	0.1	0.1
38019	Rice, white, long grain, enriched, instant	1 cup	165	193	4	41	1	1	0.1	0
38097	Rice, white, med grain, cooked	0.5 cup	93	121	2	27	0	0	0.1	0.1
38085	Sorghum, whole grain	0.5 cup	96	325	11	72	6	3	1	1.3
38034	Tapioca, pearl, dry	0.25 cup	38	136	0	34	0	0	0	0
38025	Wheat, germ, crude	0.25 cup	28.8	104	7	15	4	3	0.4	1.7
38068	Wheat, sprouted	0.25 cup	27	53	2	11	0	0	0	0.2
	Pancakes, French Toast, and Waffles									
42155	French toast, frozen	1 pce	59	126	4	19	1	4	1.2	0.7
42156	French toast, homemade w/2% milk	1 pce	65	149	5	16	1	7	2.9	1.7
45192	Pancakes, buttermilk, frozen/Eggo	1 ea	42.5	99	3	16	0	3	1.2	0.9
45118	Pancakes, blueberry, homemade, 6"	1 ea	77	171	5	22	1	7	1.8	3.2
45121	Pancakes, buttermilk, homemade, 6"	1 ea	77	175	5	22	1	7	1.8	3.5
45117	Pancakes, plain, homemade, 6"	1 ea	77	175	5	22	1	7	1.9	3.4
45199	Pancakes, buttermilk, frozen, 4"	1 ea	36	81	2	14	1	2	0.7	0.4
45193	Waffles, homestyle, low fat, frozen/Eggo	1 ea	35	83	2	15	0	1	0.4	0.4
45003	Waffles, plain, homemade, round, 7"	1 ea	75	218	6	25	1	11	2.6	5.1
45197	Waffles, buttermilk, frozen, 4"	1 ea	35	100	2	15	1	3	1.8	0.8

Sat (g)	Chol (mg)	Calc (mg)	Iron (mg)	Mag (mg)	Phos (mg)	Pota (mg)	Sodi (mg)	Zinc (mg)	Vit A (RAE)	Vit C (mg)	Thia (mg)	Ribo (mg)	Niac (mg)	Vit B6 (mg)	Vit B12 (µg)	Vit E (mg)	Fol (µg)	Alc (g)
0	0	4	0.12	2.6	18	4	17	0.2	0	0	0.02	0	0.06	0.01	0		2.6	0
0	0	5	0.55	10.3	28	40	68	0.1	0	0	0.11	0.03	0.58	0.05	0		8	0
0.1	0	5	0.9	12.6	41	31	1	0.4	0	0	0.19	0.1	1.18	0.03	0	0	51.1	0
0.1	0	42	1.46	86.8	151	81	20	1.5	11	0	0.14	0.14	2.14	0.13	0	0	16.8	0
0.1	0	5	0.35	12.6	41	31	92	0.4	0	0	0.01	0.01	0.28	0.03	0	0	4.9	0
0.1	0	21	1.48	42	125	62	4	1.1	0	0	0.15	0.06	0.99	0.11	0	0.4	7	0
0	0	13	0.11	1	2	4	1	0	0	0	0	0	0	0	0		2.2	0
0.1	0	12	0.99	35.5	110	114	1	0.7	0	0	0.14	0.04	2.32	0.15	0	0.2	3	0
0.2	0	12	1.22	75.3	101	173	3	0.9	0	0	0.13	0.06	1.85	0.17	0	0.1	16.2	0
0.2	0	40	2.05	31.4	64	85	1	0.5	0	0	0.41	0.21	2.81	0.11	0	0	66.4	0
0.1	0	7	1.82	19.6	57	78	0	0.4	0	0	0.34	0.24	2.5	0.04	0	0.1	76.5	0
0.6	0	43	1.34	90.1	104	528	3	0.8	1	0	0.12	0.24	0.91	0.1	0	0.4	72.4	0
0.1	0	11	0.84	49.7	104	151	1	0.9	0	0	0.12	0.04	0.93	0.13	0	0.3	24	0
0	0	105	1.46	5.9	186	39	396	0.2	0	0	0.21	0.13	1.82	0.02	0	0	61.2	0
0.1	0	5	1.51	8.6	33	34	1	0.3	0	0	0.28	0.18	2.58	0.01	0	0.1	62.6	0
0.1	0	10	1.16	41.4	104	122	2	0.9	0	0	0.13	0.06	1.91	0.1	0	0.2	13.2	0
0.1	0	9	1.04	17.3	42	73	2	0.6	0	0	0.07	0.05	1.62	0.09	0	0	12.6	0
0.1	0	18	1.75	58.2	73	124	9	1	0	0	0.1	0.05	1.82	0.15	0	0	32.8	0
0.3	0	3	1.12	52.7	87	119	15	0.9	0	0	0.16	0.08	1.51	0.26	0	0.2		0
0.3	0	3	1.12	52.7	87	119	15	0.9	5	0	0.16	0.08	1.51	0.26	0	0.2	7.9	0
0.1	0	1	1.49	12.1	36	52	2	0.2	0	0	0.21	0.14	1.83	0.07	0	0.1	74.2	0
0.1	0	1	1.49	12.1	36	52	2	0.2	4	0	0.21	0.14	1.83	0.07	0	0.1	74.2	0
0	0	6	0.3	6.3	17	46	4	0.2	0	0	0.05	0.02	0.77	0.04	0	0.1	11.8	0
0.1	0	8	0.5	12.8	28	7	168	0.8	5	0	0	0	0.03	0	0	0.1	0.8	0
0.1	0	3	0.55	38.3	87	54	2	0.8	0	0	0.09	0.07	1.16	0.09	0	0	16.5	0
0.2	0	11	0.96	43.8	130	101	1	0.6	0	0	0.18	0.04	0.16	0.03	0	0.1	6.6	0
0.5	0	21	1.84	69	204	167	1	1.5	0	0	0.3	0.05	0.37	0.05	0	0.3	21.8	0
0.4	0	20	0.82	83.8	162	84	10	1.2	0	0	0.19	0.05	2.98	0.28	0	0.1	7.8	0
0.2	0	10	0.52	42.9	75	77	1	0.6	0	0	0.1	0.01	1.3	0.15	0	0.2	3.9	0
0.1	0	3	0.24	8.7	14	17	9	0.7	0	0	0.03	0.02	0.5	0.05	0	0.1	1.7	0
0.1	0	16	1.9	19	68	55	604	0.8	0	0	0.26	0.02	2.33	0.15	0	0.1	91.6	0
0	0	13	2.92	8.2	61	15	7	0.8	0	0	0.12	0.01	2.87	0.08	0	0	115.5	0
0.1	0	3	1.39	12.1	34	27	0	0.4	0	0	0.16	0.01	1.71	0.05	0	0	53.9	0
0.4	0	27	4.22		276	336	6		0	0	0.23	0.14	2.81		0	0.1		0
0	0	8	0.6	0.4	3	4	0	0	0	0	0	0	0	0	0	0	1.5	0
0.5	0	11	1.8	68.8	242	257	3	3.5	0	0	0.54	0.14	1.96	0.37	0	4	80.9	0
0.1	0	8	0.58	22.1	54	46	4	0.4	0	0.7	0.06	0.04	0.83	0.07	0	0	10.3	0
0.9	48	63	1.3	10	82	79	292	0.5	32	0.2	0.16	0.22	1.61	0.29	0.99	0.4	30.7	0
1.8	75	65	1.09	11	76	87	311	0.4	81	0.2	0.13	0.21	1.06	0.05	0.2	0.7	28	0
0.6	5	15	1.32	7.6	145	44	225	0.3		0.6	0.11	0.12	1.47	0.15	0.44	0	22.1	0
1.5	43	159	1.32	12.3	116	106	317	0.4	38	1.7	0.15	0.21	1.17	0.04	0.15		27.7	0
1.4	45	121	1.31	11.6	107	112	402	0.5	23	0.3	0.16	0.22	1.21	0.03	0.14	1.1	29.3	0
1.6	45	169	1.39	12.3	122	102	338	0.4	42	0.2	0.15	0.22	1.21	0.04	0.17	0.7	29.3	0
0.3	6	26	0.79	5	105	45	182	0.1	23	0.1	0.12	0.18	1.05	0.05	0.03	0.1	25.6	0
0.3	9	20	1.95	23.8	28	50	155			0	0.31	0.26	2.59	0.16	0.55		27	0
2.1	52	191	1.73	14.2	142	119	383	0.5	49	0.3	0.2	0.26	1.55	0.04	0.19	1.7	34.5	0
0.5	5	108	1.96	8	126	44	223	0.2	133	0	0.22	0.22	2.65	0.31	1.03	0.4	23.8	0

MDA Code	Food Name	Amt	Wt (g)	Ener (kcal)	Prot (g)	Carb (g)	Fiber (g)	Fat (g)	Mono (g)	Poly (g)
MEAT AND MEAT SUBSTITUTES										
Beef										
10093	Beef, average of all cuts, cooked, 1/4" trim	3 oz	85.1	260	22	0	0	18	7.8	0.7
10705	Beef, average of all cuts, lean, cooked, 1/4" trim	3 oz	85.1	184	25	0	0	8	3.5	0.3
10108	Beef, brisket, whole, braised, 1/4" trim	3 oz	85.1	328	20	0	0	27	11.8	1
10035	Beef, breakfast strips, cured, cooked	3 ea	34	153	11	0	0	12	5.7	0.5
58239	Beef, brisket, flat half, braised, select, 1/8" trim	3 oz	85.1	238	25	0	0	15	6.4	0.5
58051	Beef, chuck clod roast, roasted, 1/4" trim	3 oz	85.1	206	21	0	0	13	6	0.5
58104	Beef, chuck clod steak, braised, 1/4" trim	3 oz	85.1	231	22	0	0	15	6.8	0.6
58099	Beef, chuck tender steak, broiled, 0" trim	3 oz	85.1	136	22	0	0	5	2.3	0.3
58083	Beef, chuck top blade, broiled, choice, 0" trim	3 oz	85.1	193	22	0	0	11	5.3	0.4
10264	Beef, cured, thin sliced	5 pce	21	37	6	1	0	1	0.4	0
10009	Beef, cured, dried, slices	5 pce	21	32	7	1	0	0	0.2	0
10034	Beef, kidney, cooked	3 oz	85.1	134	23	0	0	4	0.6	0.7
10010	Beef, liver, fried	3 oz	85.1	149	23	4	0	4	0.6	0.5
10624	Beef, short ribs, braised, choice, 1/4" trim	3 oz	85.1	401	18	0	0	36	16.1	1.3
10011	Beef, tongue, cooked	3 oz	85.1	242	16	0	0	19	8.6	0.6
10018	Beef, tripe, raw	4 oz	113.4	96	14	0	0	4	1.7	0.2
10133	Beef, whole rib, roasted, 1/4" trim	3 oz	85.1	305	19	0	0	25	10.6	0.9
10008	Corned beef, cured, canned, slices	3 oz	85.1	213	23	0	0	13	5.1	0.5
57710	Corned beef hash, canned/Hormel	1 cup	236	387	21	22	3	24	12.4	0.7
93273	Corned beef hash, canned	3 oz	85.1	140	7	8	1	9	4.5	0.3
58129	Ground beef, hamburger, pan browned, 25% fat	3 oz	85.1	236	22	0	0	15	7.1	0.4
58124	Ground beef, hamburger, pan browned, 20% fat	3 oz	85.1	231	23	0	0	15	6.5	0.4
58119	Ground beef, hamburger, pan browned, 15% fat	3 oz	85.1	218	24	0	0	13	5.6	0.4
58114	Ground beef, hamburger, pan browned, 10% fat	3 oz	85.1	196	24	0	0	10	4.3	0.4
58109	Ground beef, hamburger, pan browned, 5% fat	3 oz	85.1	164	25	0	0	6	2.7	0.3
10791	Porterhouse steak, broiled, 1/4" trim	3 oz	85.1	280	19	0	0	22	9.8	0.9
11487	Porterhouse steak, broiled, 1/8" trim	3 oz	85.1	253	20	0	0	19	8.2	0.7
58257	Rib eye steak, broiled, 0" trim	3 oz	85.1	210	23	0	0	13	5.1	0.5
58324	Rib steak, lean, broiled, choice, 1/8" trim	3 oz	85.1	172	24	0	0	8	3.1	0.3
57709	Roast beef hash, canned/Hormel	1 cup	236	385	21	23	4	24	11.3	0.6
58094	Skirt steak, broiled, 0" trim	3 oz	85.1	187	22	0	0	10	5.2	0.4
58069	Skirt steak, outside, lean, broiled, 0" trim	3 oz	85.1	198	21	0	0	12	6.3	0.5
58328	Strip steak, top loin, lean, broiled, choice, 1/8" trim	3 oz	85.1	171	25	0	0	7	2.9	0.3
10805	T-bone steak, broiled, 1/4" trim	3 oz	85.1	260	20	0	0	19	8.6	0.7
11491	T-bone steak, broiled, 1/8" trim	3 oz	85.1	238	21	0	0	17	7.3	0.6
58299	Top round steak, lean, broiled, select, 1/8" trim	3 oz	85.1	151	27	0	0	4	1.7	0.2
58098	Tri-tip steak, loin, broiled, 0" trim	3 oz	85.1	226	26	0	0	13	6.6	0.5
58258	Tri-tip roast, sirloin, roasted, 0" trim	3 oz	85.1	177	22	0	0	9	4.7	0.3
11550	Veal tongue, braised	3 oz	85.1	172	22	0	0	9	3.9	0.3
11531	Veal, average of all cuts, cooked	3 oz	85.1	197	26	0	0	10	3.7	0.7
11530	Veal, ground, broiled, 8% fat	3 oz	85.1	146	21	0	0	6	2.4	0.5
Chicken										
81185	Chicken, breast, mesquite flavor, fat free, sliced	2 pce	42	34	7	1	0	0	0.1	0
81186	Chicken, breast, oven roasted, fat free, sliced	2 pce	42	33	7	1	0	0	0.1	0
15013	Chicken breast, w/skin, batter fried	3 oz	85.1	221	21	8	0	11	4.6	2.6
15057	Chicken breast, w/o skin, fried	3 oz	85.1	159	28	0	0	4	1.5	0.9
15113	Chicken, dark meat, w/skin, batter fried	3 oz	85.1	254	19	8	0	16	6.5	3.8
15080	Chicken, dark meat, w/skin, roasted	3 oz	85.1	215	22	0	0	13	5.3	3

Sat (g)	Chol (mg)	Calc (mg)	Iron (mg)	Mag (mg)	Phos (mg)	Pota (mg)	Sodi (mg)	Zinc (mg)	Vit A (RAE)	Vit C (mg)	Thia (mg)	Ribo (mg)	Niac (mg)	Vit B_6 (mg)	Vit B_{12} (µg)	Vit E (mg)	Fol (µg)	Alc (g)
7.3	75	9	2.23	18.7	173	266	53	5	0	0	0.07	0.18	3.1	0.28	2.08	0.2	6	0
3.2	73	8	2.54	22.1	198	306	57	5.9	0	0	0.09	0.2	3.51	0.31	2.25	0.1	6.8	0
10.5	80	7	1.91	15.3	159	197	52	4.3	0	0	0.05	0.15	2.55	0.2	1.94	0.2	5.1	0
4.9	40	3	1.07	9.2	80	140	766	2.2	0	0	0.03	0.09	2.2	0.11	1.17	0.1	2.7	0
5.9	60	14	2.04	16.2	153	202	42	5.9	0	0	0.05	0.13	3.55	0.24	1.63	0.4	7.7	0
4.9	64	7	2.39	17	167	287	57	4.9	0	0	0.07	0.19	2.73	0.22	2.41	0.1	7.7	0
5.7	80	8	2.83	16.2	176	220	49	5.8	0	0	0.06	0.19	2.43	0.21	2.33	0.1	6.8	0
1.6	54	7	2.49	19.6	193	249	60	6.7	0	0	0.09	0.2	3.09	0.27	2.88	0.1	6.8	0
3.5	49	6	2.36	20.4	183	255	58	7.5	0	0	0.09	0.19	3.08	0.27	2.88	0.2	6.8	0
0.3	9	2	0.57	4	35	90	302	0.8	0	0	0.02	0.04	1.11	0.07	0.54	0	2.3	0
0.2	17	1	0.61	4.6	41	61	586	0.8	0	0	0.01	0.05	0.69	0.05	0.5	0	1.7	0
0.9	609	16	4.94	10.2	259	115	80	2.4	0	0	0.14	2.53	3.34	0.33	21.19	0.1	70.6	0
1.3	324	5	5.25	18.7	413	299	66	4.5	6590	0.6	0.15	2.91	14.87	0.87	70.74	0.4	221.3	0
15.1	80	10	1.97	12.8	138	191	43	4.2	0	0	0.04	0.13	2.09	0.19	2.23	0.2	4.3	0
6.9	112	4	2.22	12.8	123	157	55	3.5	0	1.1	0.02	0.25	2.97	0.13	2.66	0.3	6	0
1.5	138	78	0.67	14.7	73	76	110	1.6	0	0	0	0.07	1	0.02	1.58	0.1	5.7	0
10	71	9	1.99	17	149	256	54	4.6	0	0	0.06	0.14	2.9	0.2	2.16	0.2	6	0
5.3	73	10	1.77	11.9	94	116	856	3	0	0	0.02	0.13	2.07	0.11	1.38	0.1	7.7	0
10.2	76	45	2.36	30.7		406	1003	3.3	0	2.1								0
3.7	27	16	0.85	11.1	48	146	362	1.2	0	0.8	0.06	0.04	1.34	0.2	0.35	0	6	0
6	76	29	2.24	18.7	182	301	79	5.3	0	0	0.04	0.16	4.55	0.37	2.5	0.4	10.2	0
5.6	76	24	2.37	19.6	192	323	77	5.4	0	0	0.04	0.16	4.96	0.36	2.43	0.4	9.4	0
5	77	19	2.49	21.3	203	346	76	5.6	0	0	0.04	0.16	5.38	0.36	2.37	0.4	8.5	0
4	76	14	2.62	23	213	368	74	5.8	0	0	0.04	0.16	5.79	0.36	2.31	0.4	6.8	0
2.9	76	8	2.75	23.8	224	391	72	6	0	0	0.04	0.17	6.2	0.36	2.25	0.3	6	0
8.7	61	7	2.28	17	151	217	53	3.5	0	0	0.08	0.18	3.28	0.28	1.8	0.2	6	0
7.2	60	7	2.33	19.6	159	273	54	3.9	0	0	0.09	0.19	3.46	0.3	1.83	0.2	6	0
4.9	94	17	1.49	19.6	180	289	48	4.2	0	0	0.06	0.11	6.18	0.49	1.36	0.4	6.8	0
2.9	72	14	1.63	20.4	186	300	49	4.5	0	0	0.06	0.12	7.1	0.5	1.51	0.4	7.7	0
9.9	73	42	2.36	33		432	793	3.3	0	1.9								0
4	51	9	2.36	20.4	196	246	64	6.2	0	0	0.08	0.16	3.19	0.27	3.17	0.1	6	0
5.1	49	9	2.26	21.3	188	334	80	4.9	0	0	0.1	0.17	3.69	0.42	3.66	0.1	6.8	0
2.7	67	14	1.68	21.3	192	308	51	4.7	0	0	0.07	0.13	7.32	0.52	1.55	0.3	8.5	0
7.6	55	6	2.63	18.7	157	240	57	3.7	0	0	0.08	0.18	3.37	0.29	1.81	0.2	6	0
6.4	53	7	2.41	20.4	164	286	56	4	0	0	0.09	0.19	3.52	0.3	1.85	0.2	6	0
1.4	52	6	2.26	18.7	176	230	37	4.7	0	0	0.06	0.15	4.63	0.35	1.38	0.3	9.4	0
4.9	58	10	3.1	22.1	226	372	61	6	0	0	0.11	0.24	3.6	0.38	2.41	0.1	8.5	0
3.5	71	16	1.41	18.7	171	275	45	4	0	0	0.06	0.11	5.9	0.46	1.3	0.3	6.8	0
3.7	203	8	1.78	15.3	141	138	54	3.8	0	5.1	0.06	0.3	1.25	0.13	4.51	2.1	7.7	0
3.6	97	19	0.98	22.1	203	277	74	4.1	0	0	0.05	0.27	6.78	0.26	1.34	0.3	12.8	0
2.6	88	14	0.84	20.4	185	287	71	3.3	0	0	0.06	0.23	6.83	0.33	1.08	0.1	9.4	0
0.1	15	2	0.13	15.1	108	133	437	0.3	0	0	0.01	0.01	1.15	0.05	0.03	0	0.4	0
0.1	15	3	0.13	3.8	25	28	457	0.1	0	0	0.01	0.01	1.44	0.06	0.04	0	0.4	0
3	72	17	1.06	20.4	157	171	234	0.8	17	0	0.1	0.12	8.96	0.37	0.26	0.9	12.8	0
1.1	77	14	0.97	26.4	209	235	67	0.9	6	0	0.07	0.11	12.58	0.54	0.31	0.4	3.4	0
4.2	76	18	1.23	17	123	157	251	1.8	26	0	0.1	0.19	4.77	0.21	0.23	1	15.3	0
3.7	77	13	1.16	18.7	143	187	74	2.1	51	0	0.06	0.18	5.41	0.26	0.25	0.5	6	0

MDA Code	Food Name	Amt	Wt (g)	Ener (kcal)	Prot (g)	Carb (g)	Fiber (g)	Fat (g)	Mono (g)	Poly (g)
15026	Chicken, dark meat, w/o skin, fried	3 oz	85.1	203	25	2	0	10	3.7	2.4
15030	Chicken drumstick, w/skin, batter fried	3 oz	85.1	228	19	7	0	13	5.5	3.2
15042	Chicken drumstick, w/o skin, fried	3 oz	85.1	166	24	0	0	7	2.5	1.7
58216	Chicken feet, cooked	1 oz	28.4	61	6	0	0	4	1.6	0.8
15105	Chicken giblets, chopped, fried	1 cup	145	402	47	6	0	20	6.4	4.9
15106	Chicken giblets, chopped, simmered	1 cup	145	229	39	1	0	7	1.4	1.2
15025	Chicken gizzard, average, chopped, simmered	3 oz	85.1	124	26	0	0	2	0.4	0.3
15151	Chicken leg, w/skin, batter fried	3 oz	85.1	232	19	7	0	14	5.6	3.3
81432	Chicken leg, skinless, fried	1 ea	94	196	27	1	0	9	3.2	2.1
15111	Chicken, light meat, w/skin, batter fried	3 oz	85.1	236	20	8	0	13	5.4	3.1
15077	Chicken, light meat, w/skin, roasted	3 oz	85.1	189	25	0	0	9	3.6	2
15031	Chicken, light meat, w/o skin, fried	3 oz	85.1	163	28	0	0	5	1.7	1.1
15072	Chicken, whole, w/skin, batter fried	3 oz	85.1	246	19	8	0	15	6	3.5
15214	Chicken, whole, w/o skin, fried	3 oz	85.1	186	26	1	0	8	2.9	1.8
15000	Chicken, whole, w/o skin, roasted	3 oz	85.1	162	25	0	0	6	2.3	1.4
15036	Chicken thigh, w/skin, batter fried	3 oz	85.1	236	18	8	0	14	5.7	3.3
15011	Chicken thigh, w/o skin, fried	3 oz	85.1	186	24	1	0	9	3.3	2.1
15095	Chicken, whole, w/giblet & neck, batter fried	3 oz	85.1	248	19	8	0	15	6.1	3.5
15094	Chicken, whole, w/giblet & neck, raw	4 oz	113.4	242	21	0	0	17	6.9	3.6
15097	Chicken, whole, w/giblet & neck, roasted	3 oz	85.1	199	23	0	0	11	4.4	2.5
15034	Chicken wing, w/skin, batter fried	3 oz	85.1	276	17	9	0	19	7.6	4.3
15048	Chicken wing, w/o skin, fried	3 oz	85.1	180	26	0	0	8	2.6	1.8
15059	Chicken wing, w/o skin, roasted	3 oz	85.1	173	26	0	0	7	2.2	1.5
	Turkey									
13125	Turkey bacon	1 oz	28.4	71	4	0	0	6	2.1	1.3
51151	Turkey bacon, cooked	1 oz	28.4	108	8	1	0	8	3.1	1.9
16073	Turkey giblets, simmered	1 cup	145	289	30	1	0	17	7.2	1.8
51098	Turkey, thick slice, breaded & batter fried, 3" × 2" × 3/8"	1 ea	42	119	6	7	0	8	3.1	2
16308	Turkey, roast, light & dark meat, seasoned, from frozen	1 cup	135	209	29	4	0	8	1.6	2.2
16110	Turkey breast, w/skin, roasted	3 oz	85.1	130	25	0	0	3	1	0.6
16038	Turkey breast, w/o skin, roasted	3 oz	85.1	115	26	0	0	1	0.1	0.2
16101	Turkey, dark meat, w/skin, roasted	3 oz	85.1	155	24	0	0	6	1.9	1.6
16099	Turkey, light meat, w/skin, roasted	3 oz	85.1	140	24	0	0	4	1.4	0.9
16003	Turkey, ground patty, 13% fat, cooked, 4 oz raw	1 ea	82	193	22	0	0	11	4	2.6
	Lamb									
40422	Lamb, Australian, loin, lean, broiled, 1/8" trim	3 oz	85.1	163	23	0	0	7	3	0.3
13604	Lamb, average of all cuts, cooked, choice, 1/4" trim	3 oz	85.1	250	21	0	0	18	7.5	1.3
13616	Lamb, average of all cuts, lean, cooked, choice, 1/4" trim	3 oz	85.1	175	24	0	0	8	3.5	0.5
13669	Lamb, ground, cooked	3 oz	85.1	241	21	0	0	17	7.1	1.2
13522	Lamb, kabob meat, lean, broiled, 1/4" trim	3 oz	85.1	158	24	0	0	6	2.5	0.6
	Pork									
12000	Bacon, broiled/pan fried/roasted, medium slice	3 pce	19	103	7	0	0	8	3.5	0.9
28143	Canadian bacon/Hormel	1 ea	56	68	9	1		3	1.4	0.3
12212	Ham, cured, extra lean, 5% fat, roasted	1 cup	140	203	29	2	0	8	3.7	0.8
12211	Ham, cured, 11% fat, roasted	1 cup	140	249	32	0	0	13	6.2	2
12309	Pork, average of retail cuts, cooked	3 oz	85.1	232	23	0	0	15	6.5	1.2
12097	Pork, ribs, backribs, roasted	3 oz	85.1	315	21	0	0	25	11.5	2
58237	Pork, stomach, cooked	3 oz	85.1	134	18	0	0	6	1.8	0.6
12099	Pork, ground, cooked	3 oz	85.1	253	22	0	0	18	7.9	1.6
12178	Pork, pigs feet, simmered	3 oz	85.1	197	19	0	0	14	6.8	1.3

Sat (g)	Chol (mg)	Calc (mg)	Iron (mg)	Mag (mg)	Phos (mg)	Pota (mg)	Sodi (mg)	Zinc (mg)	Vit A (RAE)	Vit C (mg)	Thia (mg)	Ribo (mg)	Niac (mg)	Vit B_6 (mg)	Vit B_{12} (µg)	Vit E (mg)	Fol (µg)	Alc (g)
2.7	82	15	1.27	21.3	159	215	83	2.5	20	0	0.08	0.21	6.02	0.31	0.28	0.5	7.7	0
3.5	73	14	1.15	17	125	158	229	2	22	0	0.1	0.18	4.34	0.23	0.24	1	15.3	0
1.8	80	10	1.12	20.4	158	212	82	2.7	15	0	0.07	0.2	5.23	0.33	0.3	0.4	7.7	0
1.1	24	25	0.26	1.4	24	9	19	0.2	9	0	0.02	0.06	0.11	0	0.13	0.1	24.4	0
5.5	647	26	14.96	36.2	415	478	164	9.1	5194	12.6	0.14	2.21	15.93	0.88	19.3	3.6	549.6	0
1.9	641	20	10.21	20.3	419	325	97	6.1	2542	18.1	0.21	1.53	9.61	0.58	13.69	0.7	372.6	0
0.6	315	14	2.71	2.6	161	152	48	3.8	0	0	0.02	0.18	2.66	0.06	0.89	0.2	4.3	0
3.6	77	15	1.19	17	129	161	237	1.8	23	0	0.1	0.19	4.62	0.23	0.24	1	15.3	0
2.3	93	12	1.32	23.5	181	239	90	2.8	19	0	0.08	0.23	6.29	0.37	0.32		8.5	0
3.5	71	17	1.07	18.7	143	157	244	0.9	20	0	0.1	0.13	7.79	0.33	0.24	0.9	13.6	0
2.6	71	13	0.97	21.3	170	193	64	1	28	0	0.05	0.1	9.48	0.44	0.27	0.3	2.6	0
1.3	77	14	0.97	24.7	197	224	69	1.1	8	0	0.06	0.11	11.37	0.54	0.31	0.3	3.4	0
3.9	74	18	1.17	17.9	132	157	248	1.4	24	0	0.1	0.16	5.99	0.26	0.24	1.1	15.3	0
2.1	80	14	1.15	23	174	219	77	1.9	15	0	0.07	0.17	8.22	0.41	0.29	0.4	6	0
1.7	76	13	1.03	21.3	166	207	73	1.8	14	0	0.06	0.15	7.81	0.4	0.28	0.2	5.1	0
3.8	79	15	1.23	17.9	132	163	245	1.7	25	0	0.1	0.19	4.86	0.22	0.24	1	16.2	0
2.4	87	11	1.24	22.1	169	220	81	2.4	18	0	0.07	0.22	6.06	0.32	0.28	0.5	7.7	0
4	88	18	1.52	17.9	134	162	242	1.6	154	0.3	0.1	0.21	6.03	0.27	0.71	1.1	27.2	0
4.8	102	12	1.49	22.7	169	214	79	1.7	263	2.9	0.07	0.21	7.53	0.39	1.26	0.4	34	0
3.1	91	13	1.41	19.6	155	180	67	1.8	163	0.4	0.05	0.19	6.73	0.32	0.8	0.3	24.7	0
5	67	17	1.1	13.6	103	117	272	1.2	29	0	0.09	0.13	4.48	0.26	0.21	0.9	15.3	0
2.1	71	13	0.97	17.9	140	177	77	1.8	15	0	0.04	0.11	6.16	0.5	0.29	0.3	3.4	0
1.9	72	14	0.99	17.9	141	179	78	1.8	15	0	0.04	0.11	6.22	0.5	0.29	0.2	3.4	0
1.5	26	11	0.41	5.4	57	59	344	0.7	0	0							2.3	0
2.4	28	3	0.6	8.2	131	112	649	0.9	0	0	0.02	0.07	1	0.09	0.1	0.3	2.6	0
5.7	419	9	11.18	26.1	335	392	93	4.5	15569	19.9	0.04	2.18	10.15	0.84	48.21	0.1	485.8	0
2	32	6	0.92	6.3	113	116	336	0.6	4	0	0.04	0.08	0.97	0.08	0.1	0.4	17.2	0
2.6	72	7	2.2	29.7	329	402	918	3.4	0	0	0.06	0.22	8.47	0.36	2.05	0.5	6.8	0
0.7	77	13	1.34	23.8	184	237	45	1.5	0	0	0.03	0.11	5.92	0.43	0.31	0.2	5.1	0
0.2	71	10	1.3	24.7	191	248	44	1.5	0	0	0.04	0.11	6.38	0.48	0.33	0.1	5.1	0
1.8	100	23	1.98	19.6	162	202	65	3.3	0	0	0.04	0.2	2.85	0.28	0.31	0.7	7.7	0
1.1	81	15	1.37	22.1	174	223	49	1.8	0	0	0.03	0.12	5.34	0.42	0.31	0.1	5.1	0
2.8	84	20	1.58	19.7	161	221	88	2.3	0	0	0.04	0.14	3.95	0.32	0.27	0.3	5.7	0
3.1	69	18	1.86	22.1	187	289	68	3			0.15	0.28	6.94	0.44	1.71			0
7.5	83	14	1.6	19.6	160	264	61	3.8	0	0	0.09	0.21	5.67	0.11	2.17	0.1	15.3	0
2.9	78	13	1.74	22.1	179	293	65	4.5	0	0	0.09	0.24	5.38	0.14	2.22	0.2	19.6	0
6.9	83	19	1.52	20.4	171	288	69	4	0	0	0.09	0.21	5.7	0.12	2.22	0.2	16.2	0
2.2	77	11	1.99	26.4	191	285	65	4.9	0	0	0.09	0.26	5.63	0.12	2.58	0.2	19.6	0
2.6	21	2	0.27	6.3	101	107	439	0.7	2	0	0.08	0.05	2.11	0.07	0.23	0.1	0.4	0
1	27	3	0.5	10.6		156	569	1	0	0.8								0
2.5	74	11	2.07	19.6	274	402	1684	4	0	0	1.06	0.28	5.63	0.56	0.91	0.4	4.2	0
4.4	83	11	1.88	30.8	393	573	2100	3.5	0	0	1.02	0.46	8.61	0.43	0.98	0.4	4.2	0
5.3	77	21	0.94	20.4	197	301	53	2.5	2	0.3	0.66	0.28	4.19	0.34	0.66	0.2	5.1	0
9.4	100	38	1.17	17.9	166	268	86	2.9	3	0.3	0.36	0.17	3.02	0.26	0.54	0.4	2.6	0
2.5	269	13	1.05	12.8	110	72	34	2.5	0	0	0.03	0.16	1.17	0.02	0.41	0.1	2.6	0
6.6	80	19	1.1	20.4	192	308	62	2.7	2	0.6	0.6	0.19	3.58	0.33	0.46	0.2	5.1	0
3.7	91	0	0.83	4.3	70	28	62	0.9	0	0	0.01	0.05	0.5	0.03	0.35	0.1	1.7	0

MDA Code	Food Name	Amt	Wt (g)	Ener (kcal)	Prot (g)	Carb (g)	Fiber (g)	Fat (g)	Mono (g)	Poly (g)
	Game Meats									
51147	Dove, whole, cooked	3 oz	85.1	186	20	0	0	11	4.6	2.3
16063	Duck, liver, raw, domesticated	1 ea	44	60	8	2	0	2	0.3	0.3
40567	Deer loin, lean, 1" thick steak, broiled	3 oz	85.1	128	26	0	0	2	0.3	0.1
14009	Bison, roasted	3 oz	85.1	122	24	0	0	2	0.8	0.2
15240	Cornish game hen, whole, w/skin, roasted	3 oz	85.1	221	19	0	0	15	6.8	3.1
15242	Cornish game hen, whole, w/o skin, roasted	3 oz	85.1	114	20	0	0	3	1.1	0.8
16020	Duck breast, w/o skin, raw, wild	4 oz	113.4	139	23	0	0	5	1.4	0.7
16019	Duck, whole, w/skin, raw, wild	4 oz	113.4	239	20	0	0	17	7.7	2.3
51149	Quail, whole, cooked	3 oz	85.1	199	21	0	0	12	4.2	3
16013	Quail, whole, w/skin, raw	4 oz	113.4	218	22	0	0	14	4.7	3.4
14004	Rabbit, domestic, roasted	3 oz	85.1	168	25	0	0	7	1.8	1.3
51111	Pigeon, whole, w/skin, raw	4 oz	113.4	333	21	0	0	27	11	3.5
	Lunch Meats									
13103	Beef, chopped, smoked & cured, 1 oz slice	1 pce	28.4	38	6	1	0	1	0.5	0.1
13335	Beef, smoked, sliced/Carl Buddig	1 pce	71	99	14	0	0	5		0.2
13000	Beef, thin slice	1 oz	28.4	42	5	0	0	2	0.9	0.1
57871	Beerwurst, pork & beef salami, 2-3/4" × 1/16" slice	1 pce	6	17	1	0	0	1	0.6	0.1
58275	Bologna, beef & pork, low fat, 1" cube	1 ea	14	32	2	0	0	3	1.3	0.2
58280	Bologna, beef, low fat, medium slice	1 ea	28	57	3	1	0	4	1.8	0.1
58212	Bologna, beef, reduced sodium, thin slice	1 pce	14	44	2	0	0	4	1.9	0.1
13157	Chicken breast, oven roasted, deluxe/Louis Rich	1 oz	28.4	29	5	1	0	1	0.2	0.1
90737	Chicken salad, lunchmeat spread, canned/Spreadables	1 ea	118	171	6	12		11	3.5	4.2
13306	Corned beef/Carl Buddig	1 ea	71	101	14	1	0	5		0.2
13264	Ham, slices, regular, 11% fat	1 cup	135	220	22	5	2	12	5.9	1.1
13206	Lunchmeat loaf, old fashioned/Oscar Mayer	1 pce	28	65	4	2	0	5	2.2	0.7
13049	Lunchmeat loaf, olive, w/pork, 4" × 4" × 3/32" slice	1 pce	28.4	67	3	3	0	5	2.2	0.5
13337	Pastrami, beef, smoked/Carl Buddig	1 oz	28.4	40	6	0	0	2		0.1
13101	Pastrami, beef, cured, 1 oz slice	1 oz	28.4	41	6	0	0	2	0.6	0.1
13020	Pastrami, turkey, slices	2 pce	56.7	70	9	2	0	2	0.8	0.6
13215	Salami, cotto, beef, slice/Oscar Mayer	1 oz	28.4	59	4	1	0	4	2	0.2
11913	Spam, pork & ham, canned/Spam	1 ea	56.7	176	8	2	0	15	7.8	1.7
13123	Turkey bologna/Louis Rich	1 oz	28.4	52	3	1	0	4	1.5	1
16160	Turkey breast slice, 3-1/2" slice	1 pce	21	22	4	1	0	0	0.1	0.1
57889	Turkey ham, cured thigh meat, 8 oz package	1 ea	227	286	40	5	0	11	4.3	3
58279	Turkey ham, extra lean, package	1 cup	138	163	27	2	0	5	1.2	1.6
13144	Turkey salami/Louis Rich	1 ea	28	41	4	0	0	3	0.9	0.7
	Sausage									
58009	Bacon & beef sticks	2 oz	56.7	293	16	0	0	25	12.4	2.4
58230	Beef sausage, cooked from fresh	2 oz	56.7	188	10	0	0	16	7.2	0.5
58228	Beef sausage, precooked	2 oz	56.7	230	9	0	0	21	9.3	0.6
13077	Blood sausage, 5" × 4-5/8" × 1/16" slice	1 pce	25	95	4	0	0	9	4	0.9
13079	Bratwurst, pork, cooked	1 ea	85	283	12	2	0	25	12.5	2.2
58012	Bratwurst, pork, beef & turkey, light, smoked	3 oz	85.1	158	12	1	0	12	6.1	0.7
13180	Braunschweiger liver sausage, sliced/Oscar Mayer	1 pce	28	93	4	1	0	8	4.2	1
13070	Chorizo, pork & beef sausage, 4" link	1 ea	60	273	14	1	0	23	11	2.1
13190	Frank, beef, bun length/Oscar Mayer	1 ea	57	185	6	2	0	17	8.3	0.5
13250	Frank, beef, fat free/Oscar Mayer	1 ea	50	39	7	3	0	0	0.1	0
13191	Frank, beef/Oscar Mayer	1 ea	45	147	5	1	0	14	6.6	0.6
13129	Frank, turkey & chicken/Louis Rich	1 ea	45	85	5	2	0	6	2.5	1.4

Sat (g)	Chol (mg)	Calc (mg)	Iron (mg)	Mag (mg)	Phos (mg)	Pota (mg)	Sodi (mg)	Zinc (mg)	Vit A (RAE)	Vit C (mg)	Thia (mg)	Ribo (mg)	Niac (mg)	Vit B$_6$ (mg)	Vit B$_{12}$ (µg)	Vit E (mg)	Fol (µg)	Alc (g)
3.2	99	14	5.03	22.1	283	218	49	3.3	24	2.5	0.24	0.3	6.47	0.49	0.35	0.1	5.1	0
0.6	227	5	13.43	10.6	118	101	62	1.4	5273	2	0.25	0.39	2.86	0.33	23.76	0.6	324.7	0
0.7	67	5	3.48	25.5	236	339	49	3.1	0	0	0.24	0.44	9.15	0.64	1.56	0.5	7.7	0
0.8	70	7	2.91	22.1	178	307	49	3.1	0	0	0.09	0.23	3.16	0.34	2.43	0.3	6.8	0
4.3	111	11	0.77	15.3	124	208	54	1.3	27	0.4	0.06	0.17	5.02	0.26	0.24	0.3	1.7	0
0.8	90	11	0.66	16.2	127	213	54	1.3	17	0.5	0.06	0.19	5.34	0.3	0.26	0.2	1.7	0
1.5	87	3	5.11	24.9	211	304	65	0.8	18	7	0.47	0.35	3.91	0.71	0.86	0.3	28.4	0
5.7	91	6	4.72	22.7	191	282	64	0.9	29	5.9	0.4	0.31	3.76	0.6	0.74	0.8		0
3.4	73	13	3.77	18.7	237	184	44	2.6	60	2	0.19	0.26	6.74	0.53	0.31	0.6	5.1	0
3.8	86	15	4.5	26.1	312	245	60	2.7	83	6.9	0.28	0.29	8.55	0.68	0.49	0.8	9.1	0
2	70	16	1.93	17.9	224	326	40	1.9	0	0	0.08	0.18	7.17	0.4	7.06	0.7	9.4	0
9.6	108	14	4.01	24.9	281	226	61	2.5	83	5.9	0.24	0.25	6.86	0.46	0.45	0.1	6.8	0
0.5	13	2	0.81	6	51	107	357	1.1	0	0	0.02	0.05	1.3	0.1	0.49		2.3	0
1.8	48	10	1.6			239	1016				0.06	0.17	2.74					0
0.8	20	3	0.59	5.4	48	122	401	1.1	0	0	0.02	0.05	1.21	0.1	0.73	0.1	3.1	0
0.5	4	2	0.1	1.1	8	15	44	0.1	0	0	0.01	0.01	0.18	0.01	0.07	0	0.3	0
1	5	2	0.09	1.7	25	22	155	0.2	0	0	0.02	0.02	0.36	0.03	0.18	0	0.7	0
1.5	12	3	0.28	3.4	50	41	330	0.5	0	0.3	0.01	0.03	0.7	0.04	0.39	0.1	1.4	0
1.6	8	2	0.2	1.4	11	22	95	0.3	0	0	0.01	0.02	0.37	0.03	0.2	0	0.7	0
0.2	14	2	0.33	6.8	76	75	337	0.2	0	0								0
2.3	31						552		0									0
2	46	12	1.7			250	953				0.06	0.17	2.98					0
4	77	32	1.38	29.7	207	387	1760	1.8	0	5.4	0.85	0.24	3.92	0.44	0.57	0.1	9.4	0
1.6	17	32	0.37	6.4	58	82	332	0.5	0	0								0
1.7	11	31	0.15	5.4	36	84	421	0.4	17	0	0.08	0.07	0.52	0.07	0.36	0.1	0.6	0
0.9	18	5	0.7			104	300				0.03	0.07	1.16					0
0.8	19	3	0.63	5.4	50	67	251	1.4	9	0.4	0.02	0.05	1.21	0.08	0.52	0.1	2	0
0.7	39	6	2.38	7.9	113	196	556	1.2	2	9.1	0.03	0.14	2	0.15	0.14	0.1	2.8	0
1.9	24	2	0.77	4.8	64	59	372	0.6		0								0
5.6	40	8	0.51	7.9		130	776	1	0	0.5							1.7	0
1.1	19	35	0.47	6.2	56	43	306	0.5	0	0							1.7	0
0.1	9	2	0.3	4.4	34	63	213	0.3	2	1.2	0.03	0.07	0.02	0.03	0.02	0	0.8	0
3.5	163	18	5.31	49.9	667	651	2529	5.9	16	0	0.07	0.34	4.81	0.47	0.52	1.5	15.9	0
1.8	92	7	1.86	27.6	420	413	1432	3.3	0	0	0.07	0.34	4.87	0.32	0.36	0.5	8.3	0
0.8	21	11	0.35	6.2	74	60	281	0.6	0	0								0
9.1	58	8	1.05	9.6	81	218	805	1.8	0	0	0.34	0.16	2.76	0.28	1.08	0.2	1.1	0
6.2	46	6	0.89	7.9	80	146	370	2.5	7	0	0.03	0.09	2.04	0.18	1.14	0.1	1.7	0
8.6	47	9	0.87	7.4	105	133	516	1.7	14	0.4	0.02	0.07	1.82	0.11	1.15	0.3	2.8	0
3.3	30	2	1.6	2	6	10	170	0.3	0	0	0.02	0.03	0.3	0.01	0.25	0	1.2	0
8.6	63	24	0.45	17.8	191	220	719	2.1	0	0	0.53	0.22	3.94	0.35	0.68	0	2.6	0
	48	12	0.8	11.9	112	209	836	2.3	0	0	0.08	0.14	1.57	0.18	1.36	0	4.3	0
3	50	3	2.94	3.9	56	57	325	1	1322	2.5	0.06	0.45	2.57	0.09	5.26	0	13.2	0
8.6	53	5	0.95	10.8	90	239	741	2	0	0	0.38	0.18	3.08	0.32	1.2	0.1	1.2	0
7.1	34	7	0.89	8.6	60	90	584	1.3	0	0							6.3	0
0.1	15	10	0.98	9.5	64	234	464	1.2	0	0								0
5.6	25	4	0.6	5.8	63	58	461	1	0	0	0.02	0.05	1.03	0.03	0.73		2.7	0
1.7	41	59	0.98	10.4	66	72	511	0.8	0	0								0

MDA Code	Food Name	Amt	Wt (g)	Ener (kcal)	Prot (g)	Carb (g)	Fiber (g)	Fat (g)	Mono (g)	Poly (g)
57877	Frankfurter, beef, 5" × 3/4"	1 ea	45	148	5	2	0	13	6.4	0.5
58027	Frankfurter, beef, cooked	1 ea	52	170	6	2	0	15	7.4	0.6
13260	Frankfurter, chicken	1 ea	45	116	6	3	0	9	3.8	1.8
13012	Frankfurter, turkey	1 ea	45	102	6	1	0	8	2.5	2.2
57890	Italian sausage, pork, cooked, 1/4 lb	1 ea	83	286	16	4	0	23	9.9	2.7
13043	Kielbasa, beef, pork & nonfat dry milk, slice	1 pce	26	81	3	1	0	7	3.4	0.8
58020	Kielbasa, Polish, turkey & beef, smoked	3 oz	85.1	192	11	3	0	15	7	2
13044	Knockwurst, beef & pork, link, 4" long	1 ea	68	209	8	2	0	19	8.7	2
13019	Liverwurst, pork, 2-1/2" × 1/4" slice	1 pce	18	59	3	0	0	5	2.4	0.5
13021	Pepperoni, beef & pork, slice	1 pce	5.5	26	1	0	0	2	1	0.1
13022	Polish sausage, pork, 10" × 1-1/4"	1 ea	227	740	32	4	0	65	30.7	7
13185	Pork sausage, cooked/Oscar Mayer	2 ea	48	165	8	0	0	15	7.1	1.8
58227	Pork sausage, precooked	3 oz	85	321	12	0	0	30	12.9	4.1
13184	Smokie sausage links/Oscar Mayer	1 ea	43	130	5	1	0	12	5.7	1.2
13200	Summer sausage, Thuringer Cervelat, slice/Oscar Mayer	2 ea	46	140	7	0	0	12	5.6	1
58007	Turkey sausage, breakfast link, mild	2 ea	56	132	9	1	0	10	2.8	1.8
58219	Turkey, pork, and beef sausage, low fat, smoked	2 oz	56	57	4	6	0	1	0.6	0.2
	Meat Substitutes									
27044	Bacon bits, meatless	1 Tbs	7	33	2	2	1	2	0.4	0.9
7509	Bacon strips, meatless	3 ea	15	46	2	1	0	4	1.1	2.3
7558	Beef substitute, fillet	1 ea	85	246	20	8	5	15	3.7	7.9
7561	Beef substitute, patty	1 ea	56	110	12	4	3	5	1.2	2.6
62359	Breakfast patty, vegetarian/Morningstar Farms	1 ea	38	81	10	3	2	3	0.7	1.8
91055	Burger, vegetarian, Grillers Vegan/Morningstar Farms	1 ea	85	114	14	8	5	3	1	1.4
7725	Burger crumbles, vegetarian, Grillers Recipe Crumbles/Morningstar Farms	0.5 cup	55	82	11	5	2	2	0.5	1.4
7547	Chicken, vegetarian	1 cup	168	376	40	6	6	21	4.6	12.2
7722	Garden Veggie Patties, frozen/Morningstar Farms	1 ea	67	111	12	10	3	3	0.7	1.6
7674	Harvest Burger, vegetarian, original, frozen/Gardetto's	1 ea	90	138	18	7	6	4	2.1	0.3
90626	Sausage, vegetarian, slices	1 ea	28	72	5	3	1	5	1.3	2.6
7554	Soy burger	1 ea	70	136	15	5	3	6	1.2	2.5
7726	Spicy Black Bean Burger/Morningstar Farms	1 ea	78	150	12	15	3	5	1.2	2.4
	NUTS AND SEEDS									
4642	Beechnuts, dried	2 oz	56.7	327	4	19	2	28	12.4	11.4
4757	Butternuts, dried	1 ea	3	18	1	0	0	2	0.3	1.3
63195	Cashews, raw	2 oz	56.7	314	10	17	2	25	13.5	4.4
4519	Cashews, dry roasted, salted	0.25 cup	34.2	196	5	11	1	16	9.3	2.7
4645	Chinese chestnuts, dried	1 oz	28.4	103	2	23	1	1	0.3	0.1
63429	Filberts, dry roasted, unsalted	1 oz	28	181	4	5	3	17	13.1	2.4
63081	Flax seeds, whole	1 Tbs	11.2	60	2	3	3	5	0.8	3.2
4728	Macadamia nuts, dry roasted, unsalted	1 cup	134	962	10	18	11	102	79.4	2
4592	Mixed nuts, w/peanuts, dry roasted, salted	0.25 cup	34.2	203	6	9	3	18	10.7	3.7
4626	Peanut butter, chunky	2 Tbs	32	188	8	7	3	16	7.9	4.7
4756	Peanuts, dry roasted, unsalted	30 ea	30	176	7	6	2	15	7.4	4.7
4696	Peanuts, raw	0.25 cup	36.5	207	9	6	3	18	8.9	5.7
4540	Pistachios, dry roasted, salted	0.25 cup	32	182	7	9	3	15	7.7	4.4
4565	Pumpkin seeds/squash kernels, roasted, unsalted	0.25 cup	56.8	296	19	8	2	24	7.4	10.9
4523	Sesame seeds, whole, dried	0.25 cup	36	206	6	8	4	18	6.8	7.8
4551	Sunflower seeds, dry roasted, unsalted	0.25 cup	32	186	6	8	4	16	3	10.5
	SEAFOOD									
19041	Abalone, fried, mixed species	3 oz	85.1	161	17	9	0	6	2.3	1.4

Sat (g)	Chol (mg)	Calc (mg)	Iron (mg)	Mag (mg)	Phos (mg)	Pota (mg)	Sodi (mg)	Zinc (mg)	Vit A (RAE)	Vit C (mg)	Thia (mg)	Ribo (mg)	Niac (mg)	Vit B_6 (mg)	Vit B_{12} (µg)	Vit E (mg)	Fol (µg)	Alc (g)
5.3	24	6	0.68	6.3	72	70	513	1.1	0	0	0.02	0.07	1.07	0.04	0.77	0.1	2.2	0
5.9	29	6	0.81	7.3	89	76	600	1.2	0		0.02	0.07	1.22	0.05	0.86	0.1	3.6	0
2.5	45	43	0.9	4.5	48	38	616	0.5	18	0	0.03	0.05	1.39	0.14	0.11	0.1	1.8	0
2.7	48	48	0.83	6.3	60	81	642	1.4	0	0	0.02	0.08	1.86	0.1	0.13	0.3	3.6	0
7.9	47	17	1.19	14.9	141	252	1002	2	8	0.1	0.52	0.19	3.46	0.27	1.08	0.2	4.2	0
2.6	17	11	0.38	4.2	38	70	280	0.5	0	0	0.06	0.06	0.75	0.05	0.42	0.1	1.3	0
5.3	60		1.06				1021		0	12.6								0
6.9	41	7	0.45	7.5	67	135	632	1.1	0	0	0.23	0.1	1.86	0.12	0.8	0.4	1.4	0
1.9	28	5	1.15	2.2	41	31	155	0.4	1495	0	0.05	0.19	0.77	0.03	2.42	0.1	5.4	0
0.9	6	1	0.08	1	10	17	98	0.2	0	0	0.03	0.01	0.3	0.02	0.09	0	0.3	0
23.4	159	27	3.27	31.8	309	538	1989	4.4	0	2.3	1.14	0.34	7.82	0.43	2.22	0.5	4.5	0
5.1	37	8	0.83	8.6	76	114	401	1.2	0	0								0
9.9	63	116	0.78	11	234	261	639	1.3	16	0.6	0.18	0.13	3.44	0.13	0.6	0.5	0.8	0
4	27	4	0.5	7.3	103	77	433	0.9	0	0								0
4.9	39	4	1.03	6.9	60	105	658	1		0	0.11	0.13	2.02	0.14	1.73		2.3	0
4.4	34	18	0.6	14	104	110	328	1.2	0	17	0.04	0.1	2.06	0.21	0.24	0.2	4.5	0
0.5	12	6	1.23	9	41	136	446	0.7	0	1.1	0.07	0.04	0.87	0.06	0.16	0.1	3.4	0
0.3	0	7	0.05	6.6	15	10	124	0.1	0	0.1	0.04	0	0.11	0.01	0.08	0.5	8.9	0
0.7	0	3	0.36	2.8	10	26	220	0.1	1	0	0.66	0.07	1.13	0.07	0	1	6.3	0
2.4	0	81	1.7	19.6	382	510	416	1.2	0	0	0.94	0.76	10.2	1.27	3.57	2.9	86.7	0
0.8	0	16	1.18	10.1	193	101	308	1	0	0	0.5	0.34	5.6	0.67	1.34	1	43.7	0
0.4	1	17	2.04	1.1	116	125	255	0.5	0	0	5.53	0.21	3.83	0.31	2.39		0.3	0
0.4	0	31	2.51	16.2	188	423	336	0.7	0	0	0.26	0.55	4.11	0.2	0	0	245.6	0
0.3	0	31	3.05	25.8	111	117	236	0.9	0	0	0.69	0.19	7.83	0.79	4.97	0.3		0
3.1	0	59	5.49	28.6	563	91	1191	1.2	0	0	1.15	0.41	2.44	1.18	3.66	4.5	127.7	0
0.4	1	40	1.47	29.5	110	142	349	0.7	21	0	7.5	0.17	0	0	0	0.5	59	0
1	0	102	3.85	70.2	225	432	411	8.1	0	0	0.31	0.2	6.3	0.39	0	1.6	21.6	0
0.8	0	18	1.04	10.1	63	65	249	0.4	0	0	0.66	0.11	3.13	0.23	0	0.6	7.3	0
0.8	0	20	1.47	12.6	241	126	385	1.3	0	0	0.63	0.42	7	0.84	1.68	1.2	54.6	0
0.6	2	44	3.37	43.7	162	314	458	0.8		0	7.36	0.3	0	0.21	0.07	0.4		0
3.2	0	1	1.39	0	0	577	22	0.2	0	8.8	0.17	0.21	0.5	0.39	0		64.1	0
0	0	2	0.12	7.1	13	13	0	0.1	0	0.1	0.01	0	0.03	0.02	0	0.1	2	0
4.4	0	21	3.79	165.6	336	374	7	3.3	0	0.3	0.24	0.03	0.6	0.24	0	0.5	14.2	0
3.1	0	15	2.05	88.9	168	193	219	1.9	0	0	0.07	0.07	0.48	0.09	0	0.3	23.6	0
0.1	0	8	0.65	38.9	44	206	1	0.4	5	16.6	0.07	0.08	0.37	0.19	0	0.3	31.2	0
1.3	0	34	1.23	48.4	87	211	0	0.7	1	1.1	0.09	0.03	0.57	0.17	0	4.3	24.6	0
0.4	0	29	0.64	43.9	72	91	3	0.5	0	0.1	0.18	0.02	0.34	0.05	0	0	9.7	0
16	0	94	3.55	158.1	265	486	5	1.7	0	0.9	0.95	0.12	3.05	0.48	0	0.8	13.4	0
2.4	0	24	1.27	77	149	204	229	1.3	0	0.1	0.07	0.07	1.61	0.1	0	3.7	17.1	0
2.6	0	14	0.61	51.2	102	238	156	0.9	0	0	0.03	0.04	4.38	0.13	0	2	29.4	0
2.1	0	16	0.68	52.8	107	197	2	1	0	0	0.13	0.03	4.06	0.08	0	2.1	43.5	0
2.5	0	34	1.67	61.3	137	257	7	1.2	0	0	0.23	0.05	4.4	0.13	0	3	87.6	0
1.8	0	35	1.34	38.4	155	333	130	0.7	4	0.7	0.27	0.05	0.46	0.41	0	0.6	16	0
4.5	0	24	8.49	303.3	666	458	10	4.2	11	1	0.12	0.18	0.99	0.05	0	0	32.4	0
2.5	0	351	5.24	126.4	226	168	4	2.8	0	0	0.28	0.09	1.63	0.28	0	0.1	34.9	0
1.7	0	22	1.22	41.3	370	272	1	1.7	0	0.4	0.03	0.08	2.25	0.26	0	8.4	75.8	0
1.4	80	31	3.23	47.7	185	242	503	0.8	2	1.5	0.19	0.11	1.62	0.13	0.59	5.1	11.9	0

MDA Code	Food Name	Amt	Wt (g)	Ener (kcal)	Prot (g)	Carb (g)	Fiber (g)	Fat (g)	Mono (g)	Poly (g)
17029	Bass, freshwater, mixed species, fillet, baked/broiled	3 oz	85.1	124	21	0	0	4	1.6	1.2
17104	Bass, striped, fillet, baked/broiled	3 oz	85.1	106	19	0	0	3	0.7	0.9
50710	Bouillon/fish broth	1 cup	244	39	5	1	0	1	0.3	0.4
71707	Calamari, mixed species, fried	3 oz	85.1	149	15	7	0	6	2.3	1.8
17032	Carp, fillet, raw	4 oz	113.4	144	20	0	0	6	2.6	1.6
17088	Catfish, channel, fillet, breaded, fried	3 oz	85.1	195	15	7	1	11	4.8	2.8
17179	Catfish, channel, farmed, fillet, baked/broiled	3 oz	85.1	129	16	0	0	7	3.5	1.2
19002	Clams, mixed species, canned, drained	3 oz	85.1	126	22	4	0	2	0.1	0.5
71140	Clams, mixed species, raw	4 oz	113.4	84	14	3	0	1	0.1	0.3
17037	Cod, Atlantic, fillet, baked/broiled	3 oz	85.1	89	19	0	0	1	0.1	0.2
17107	Cod, Pacific, fillet, baked/broiled	3 oz	85.1	89	20	0	0	1	0.1	0.3
72116	Conch, baked/broiled	3 oz	85.1	111	22	1	0	1	0.3	0.2
19036	Crab, Alaska king, leg, steamed	3 oz	85.1	83	16	0	0	1	0.2	0.5
19037	Crab, Alaska king, imitation	3 oz	85.1	81	6	13	0	0	0.1	0.1
71722	Crawdads, farmed, mixed species, steamed	3 oz	85.1	74	15	0	0	1	0.2	0.4
17289	Eel, mixed species, fillet, w/o bone, baked/broiled	3 oz	85.1	201	20	0	0	13	7.8	1
7549	Fish sticks, vegetarian	1 ea	28	81	6	3	2	5	1.2	2.6
17090	Haddock, fillet, baked/broiled	3 oz	85.1	95	21	0	0	1	0.1	0.3
17291	Halibut, Atlantic/Pacific, fillet, baked/broiled	3 oz	85.1	119	23	0	0	3	0.8	0.8
17111	Halibut, Greenland, fillet, baked/broiled	3 oz	85.1	203	16	0	0	15	9.1	1.5
17047	Herring, Atlantic, fillet, baked/broiled	3 oz	85.1	173	20	0	0	10	4.1	2.3
17112	Herring, Pacific, fillet, baked/broiled	3 oz	85.1	213	18	0	0	15	7.5	2.6
17049	Mackerel, Atlantic, fillet, baked/broiled	3 oz	85.1	223	20	0	0	15	6	3.7
17115	Mackerel, king, fillet, baked/broiled	3 oz	85.1	114	22	0	0	2	0.8	0.5
19044	Mussels, blue, steamed	3 oz	85.1	146	20	6	0	4	0.9	1
19048	Octopus, steamed	3 oz	85.1	140	25	4	0	2	0.3	0.4
19089	Oysters, eastern, farmed, raw	4 oz	113.4	67	6	6	0	2	0.2	0.7
17094	Perch, mixed species, fillet, baked/broiled	3 oz	85.1	100	21	0	0	1	0.2	0.4
17093	Perch, ocean, Atlantic, fillet, baked/broiled	3 oz	85.1	103	20	0	0	2	0.7	0.5
17095	Pike, northern, fillet, baked/broiled	3 oz	85.1	96	21	0	0	1	0.2	0.2
17118	Pike, walleye, fillet, baked/broiled	3 oz	85.1	101	21	0	0	1	0.3	0.5
17096	Pollock, walleye, fillet, baked/broiled	3 oz	85.1	96	20	0	0	1	0.1	0.4
17073	Pompano, Florida, fillet, baked/broiled	3 oz	85.1	180	20	0	0	10	2.8	1.2
17074	Rockfish, Pacific, mixed species, fillet, baked/broiled	3 oz	85.1	103	20	0	0	2	0.4	0.5
17035	Roe, black/red, granular	1 Tbs	16	40	4	1	0	3	0.7	1.2
17120	Roe, mixed species, baked/broiled	3 oz	85.1	174	24	2	0	7	1.8	2.9
17121	Orange roughy, fillet, baked/broiled	3 oz	85.1	89	19	0	0	1	0.4	0.2
17181	Salmon, Atlantic, farmed, fillet, baked/broiled	3 oz	85.1	175	19	0	0	11	3.8	3.8
17123	Salmon, Atlantic, fillet, baked/broiled, wild	3 oz	85.1	155	22	0	0	7	2.3	2.8
17099	Salmon, sockeye, fillet, baked/broiled	3 oz	85.1	184	23	0	0	9	4.5	2.1
17086	Sea bass, mixed species, fillet, baked/broiled	3 oz	85.1	106	20	0	0	2	0.5	0.8
17023	Sea trout, mixed species, fillet, baked/broiled	3 oz	85.1	113	18	0	0	4	1	0.8
17076	Shark, mixed species, batter dipped, fried	3 oz	85.1	194	16	5	0	12	5.1	3.1
17100	Smelt, rainbow, baked/broiled	3 oz	85.1	106	19	0	0	3	0.7	1
17022	Snapper, mixed species, fillet, baked/broiled	3 oz	85.1	109	22	0	0	1	0.3	0.5
71139	Sturgeon, mixed species, baked/broiled, 4.5 × 2-1/8 × 7/8	3 oz	85.1	115	18	0	0	4	2.1	0.8
17079	Sturgeon, mixed species, smoked	3 oz	85.1	147	27	0	0	4	2	0.4
17066	Swordfish, fillet, baked/broiled	3 oz	85.1	132	22	0	0	4	1.7	1
17185	Trout, rainbow, farmed, fillet, baked/broiled	3 oz	85.1	144	21	0	0	6	1.8	2
17082	Trout, rainbow, wild, fillet, baked/broiled	3 oz	85.1	128	20	0	0	5	1.5	1.6

Sat (g)	Chol (mg)	Calc (mg)	Iron (mg)	Mag (mg)	Phos (mg)	Pota (mg)	Sodi (mg)	Zinc (mg)	Vit A (RAE)	Vit C (mg)	Thia (mg)	Ribo (mg)	Niac (mg)	Vit B$_6$ (mg)	Vit B$_{12}$ (µg)	Vit E (mg)	Fol (µg)	Alc (g)
0.9	74	88	1.63	32.3	218	388	77	0.7	30	1.8	0.07	0.08	1.3	0.12	1.97	0.6	14.5	0
0.6	88	16	0.92	43.4	216	279	75	0.4	26	0	0.1	0.03	2.18	0.29	3.75	0.5	8.5	0
0.3	0	73	0.51	2.4	73	210	776	0.2	2	0	0	0.07	3.34	0.02	0.24	0.4	9.8	0
1.6	221	33	0.86	32.3	214	237	260	1.5	9	3.6	0.05	0.39	2.21	0.05	1.05	1.6	11.9	0
1.2	75	46	1.41	32.9	471	378	56	1.7	10	1.8	0.13	0.06	1.86	0.22	1.74	0.7	17	0
2.8	69	37	1.22	23	184	289	238	0.7	7	0	0.06	0.11	1.94	0.16	1.62	1.1	25.5	0
1.5	54	8	0.7	22.1	208	273	68	0.9	13	0.7	0.36	0.06	2.14	0.14	2.38	1.1	6	0
0.2	57	78	23.79	15.3	288	534	95	2.3	154	18.8	0.13	0.36	2.85	0.09	84.16	0.5	24.7	0
0.1	39	52	15.85	10.2	192	356	64	1.6	102	14.7	0.09	0.24	2	0.07	56.06	0.4	18.1	0
0.1	47	12	0.42	35.7	117	208	66	0.5	12	0.9	0.07	0.07	2.14	0.24	0.89	0.7	6.8	0
0.1	40	8	0.28	26.4	190	440	77	0.4	9	2.6	0.02	0.04	2.11	0.39	0.89	0.3	6.8	0
0.3	55	83	1.2	202.5	185	139	130	1.5	6	0	0.05	0.07	0.89	0.05	4.47	5.4	152.3	0
0.1	45	50	0.65	53.6	238	223	912	6.5	8	6.5	0.05	0.05	1.14	0.15	9.79	0.8	43.4	0
0.1	17	11	0.33	36.6	240	77	716	0.3	0	0	0.03	0.07	0.53	0.11	0.49	0.1	0	0
0.2	117	43	0.94	28.1	205	203	83	1.3	13	0.4	0.04	0.07	1.42	0.11	2.64	0.8	9.4	0
2.6	137	22	0.54	22.1	236	297	55	1.8	968	1.5	0.16	0.04	3.82	0.07	2.46	4.3	14.5	0
0.8	0	27	0.56	6.4	126	168	137	0.4	0	0	0.31	0.25	3.36	0.42	1.18	1.1	28.6	0
0.1	63	36	1.15	42.6	205	340	74	0.4	16	0	0.03	0.04	3.94	0.29	1.18	0.4	11.1	0
0.4	35	51	0.91	91.1	243	490	59	0.5	46	0	0.06	0.08	6.06	0.34	1.17	0.9	11.9	0
2.6	50	3	0.72	28.1	179	293	88	0.4	15	0	0.06	0.09	1.64	0.41	0.82	1.1	0.9	0
2.2	66	63	1.2	34.9	258	357	98	1.1	31	0.6	0.1	0.25	3.51	0.3	11.18	1.2	10.2	0
3.6	84	90	1.23	34.9	248	461	81	0.6	30	0	0.06	0.22	2.4	0.44	8.19	1.1	5.1	0
3.6	64	13	1.34	82.5	237	341	71	0.8	46	0.3	0.14	0.35	5.83	0.39	16.17	1.6	1.7	0
0.4	58	34	1.94	34.9	271	475	173	0.6	214	1.4	0.1	0.49	8.9	0.43	15.32	1.5	7.7	0
0.7	48	28	5.72	31.5	243	228	314	2.3	77	11.6	0.26	0.36	2.55	0.09	20.42	1.2	64.7	0
0.4	82	90	8.12	51.1	237	536	391	2.9	77	6.8	0.05	0.06	3.22	0.55	30.64	1	20.4	0
0.5	28	50	6.55	37.4	105	141	202	43	9	5.3	0.12	0.07	1.44	0.07	18.37	0.8	20.4	0
0.2	98	87	0.99	32.3	219	293	67	1.2	9	1.4	0.07	0.1	1.62	0.12	1.87	1.3	5.1	0
0.3	46	117	1	33.2	236	298	82	0.5	12	0.7	0.11	0.11	2.07	0.23	0.98	1.4	8.5	0
0.1	43	62	0.6	34	240	282	42	0.7	20	3.2	0.06	0.07	2.38	0.11	1.96	0.2	14.5	0
0.3	94	120	1.42	32.3	229	425	55	0.7	20	0	0.27	0.17	2.38	0.12	1.97	0.2	14.5	0
0.2	82	5	0.24	62.1	410	329	99	0.5	21	0	0.06	0.06	1.4	0.06	3.57	0.7	3.4	0
3.8	54	37	0.57	26.4	290	541	65	0.6	31	0	0.58	0.13	3.23	0.2	1.02	1.2	14.5	0
0.4	37	10	0.45	28.9	194	443	66	0.5	60	0	0.04	0.07	3.34	0.23	1.02	1.3	8.5	0
0.6	94	44	1.9	48	57	29	240	0.2	90	0	0.03	0.1	0.02	0.05	3.2	1.1	8	0
1.6	408	24	0.66	22.1	438	241	100	1.1	77	14	0.24	0.81	1.87	0.16	9.82	7.2	78.3	0
0	68	9	0.96	15.3	87	154	59	0.3	20	0	0.04	0.05	1.55	0.06	0.4	1.6	4.3	0
2.1	54	13	0.29	25.5	214	327	52	0.4	13	3.1	0.29	0.11	6.85	0.55	2.38	0.8	28.9	0
1.1	60	13	0.88	31.5	218	534	48	0.7	11	0	0.23	0.41	8.58	0.8	2.6	1.1	24.7	0
1.6	74	6	0.47	26.4	235	319	56	0.4	54	0	0.18	0.15	5.68	0.19	4.94	1.1	4.3	0
0.6	45	11	0.31	45.1	211	279	74	0.4	54	0	0.11	0.13	1.62	0.39	0.26	0.5	5.1	0
1.1	90	19	0.3	34	273	372	63	0.5	30	0	0.06	0.18	2.49	0.39	2.94	0.2	5.1	0
2.7	50	43	0.94	36.6	165	132	104	0.4	46	0	0.06	0.08	2.37	0.26	1.03	0.9	12.8	0
0.5	77	66	0.98	32.3	251	317	66	1.8	14	0	0.01	0.12	1.5	0.14	3.38	0.5	4.3	0
0.3	40	34	0.2	31.5	171	444	49	0.4	30	1.4	0.05	0	0.29	0.39	2.98	0.5	5.1	0
1	66	14	0.77	38.3	231	310	59	0.5	224	0	0.07	0.08	8.6	0.2	2.13	0.5	14.5	0
0.9	68	14	0.79	40	239	323	629	0.5	238	0	0.08	0.08	9.45	0.23	2.47	0.4	17	0
1.2	43	5	0.89	28.9	287	314	98	1.3	35	0.9	0.04	0.1	10.03	0.32	1.72	0.5	1.7	0
1.8	58	73	0.28	27.2	226	375	36	0.4	73	2.8	0.2	0.07	7.48	0.34	4.23	0	20.4	0
1.4	59	73	0.32	26.4	229	381	48	0.4	13	1.7	0.13	0.08	4.91	0.29	5.36	0.4	16.2	0

MDA Code	Food Name	Amt	Wt (g)	Ener (kcal)	Prot (g)	Carb (g)	Fiber (g)	Fat (g)	Mono (g)	Poly (g)
56007	Tuna salad, lunchmeat spread	2 Tbs	25.6	48	4	2	0	2	0.7	1.1
17101	Tuna, bluefin, fillet, baked/broiled	3 oz	85.1	157	25	0	0	5	1.7	1.6
17177	Tuna, yellowfin, fillet, baked/broiled	3 oz	85.1	118	26	0	0	1	0.2	0.3
17151	Tuna, white, w/water, drained, can	3 oz	85.1	109	20	0	0	3	0.7	0.9
17083	Tuna, white, canned, w/oil, drained	3 oz	85.1	158	23	0	0	7	2.8	2.5
17162	Whitefish, mixed species, fillet, baked/broiled	3 oz	85.1	146	21	0	0	6	2.2	2.3
17164	Yellowtail, mixed species, fillet, baked/broiled	3 oz	85.1	159	25	0	0	6		

VEGETABLES AND LEGUMES
Beans

MDA Code	Food Name	Amt	Wt (g)	Ener (kcal)	Prot (g)	Carb (g)	Fiber (g)	Fat (g)	Mono (g)	Poly (g)
92132	Baked beans, unsalted, canned	1 cup	253	266	12	52	14	1	0.1	0.4
7038	Baked beans, plain/vegetarian, canned	1 cup	254	239	12	54	10	1	0.2	0.3
56101	Baked beans, w/franks, canned	0.5 cup	129.5	184	9	20	9	9	3.7	1.1
5197	Bean sprouts, mung, mature, canned, drained	1 cup	125	15	2	3	1	0	0	0
7012	Black beans, mature, cooked	1 cup	172	227	15	41	15	1	0.1	0.4
92152	Chili beans, ranch style bbq, cooked	1 cup	253	245	13	43	11	3	0.2	1.4
9574	Black eyed peas, immature, cooked w/salt	1 cup	165	155	5	33	8	1	0.1	0.3
90018	Cowpeas, mature, cooked w/salt	1 cup	171	198	13	35	11	1	0.1	0.4
7057	Cowpeas, mature, w/pork, canned	0.5 cup	120	100	3	20	4	2	0.8	0.3
9583	Fava beans (broadbeans), mature, cooked w/salt	1 cup	170	187	13	33	9	1	0.1	0.3
7913	Fava beans, immature, in pod	1 cup	126	111	10	22		1	0.1	0.4
7219	Golden gram beans, mature, cooked	1 cup	202	212	14	39	15	1	0.1	0.3
7217	Golden gram beans, mature	1 cup	207	718	49	130	34	2	0.3	0.8
7081	Hummus, garbanzo or chick pea spread, homemade	1 Tbs	15.4	27	1	3	1	1	0.8	0.3
7087	Kidney beans, all types, mature, canned	1 cup	256	215	13	37	11	2	0.7	0.5
7047	Kidney beans, red, mature, cooked	1 cup	177	225	15	40	13	1	0.1	0.5
7006	Lentils, mature, cooked	1 cup	198	230	18	40	16	1	0.1	0.3
90021	Lima beans, baby, cooked w/salt	1 cup	182	229	15	42	14	1	0.1	0.3
7010	Lima beans, large, mature, cooked	1 cup	188	216	15	39	13	1	0.1	0.3
7011	Lima beans, large, mature, canned	1 cup	241	190	12	36	12	0	0	0.2
5850	Lima beans, baby, immature, cooked from frozen w/salt	0.5 cup	90	94	6	18	5	0	0	0.1
7022	Navy beans, mature, cooked	1 cup	182	255	15	47	19	1	0.2	0.8
7122	Navy beans, mature, canned	1 cup	262	296	20	54	13	1	0.1	0.5
7051	Pinto beans, mature, canned	1 cup	240	206	12	37	11	2	0.4	0.7
5854	Pinto beans, immature, cooked from frozen w/salt	3 oz	85.1	138	8	26	7	0	0	0.2
5856	Snap beans, green, cooked w/salt	1 cup	125	44	2	10	4	0	0	0.2
6748	Snap beans, green, fresh, 4" long	10 ea	55	17	1	4	2	0	0	0
5857	Snap beans, yellow, cooked w/salt	1 cup	125	44	2	10	4	0	0	0.2
5320	Snap beans, yellow, fresh	0.5 cup	55	17	1	4	2	0	0	0
90026	Peas, green, split, mature, cooked w/salt	0.5 cup	98	114	8	20	8	0	0.1	0.2
7053	White beans, mature, cooked	1 cup	179	249	17	45	11	1	0.1	0.3
7054	White beans, mature, canned	1 cup	262	299	19	56	13	1	0.1	0.3
7052	Yellow beans, mature, cooked	1 cup	177	255	16	45	18	2	0.2	0.8

Fresh Vegetables

MDA Code	Food Name	Amt	Wt (g)	Ener (kcal)	Prot (g)	Carb (g)	Fiber (g)	Fat (g)	Mono (g)	Poly (g)
90542	Arrowroot, fresh	1 ea	33	21	1	4	0	0	0	0
9577	Artichokes, French, cooked w/salt, medium	1 ea	20	10	1	2	1	0	0	0
5723	Artichokes, globe, frozen	3 oz	85.1	32	2	7	3	0	0	0.2
6033	Arugula greens, chopped, fresh	1 cup	20	5	1	1	0	0	0	0.1
5841	Asparagus, cooked w/salt	0.5 cup	90	20	2	4	2	0	0	0.1
90406	Asparagus spears, tips, fresh, 2" long or less	10 ea	35	9	1	1	1	0	0	0
5863	Beet greens, cooked w/salt, drained, 1" pieces	1 cup	144	39	4	8	4	0	0.1	0.1

Sat (g)	Chol (mg)	Calc (mg)	Iron (mg)	Mag (mg)	Phos (mg)	Pota (mg)	Sodi (mg)	Zinc (mg)	Vit A (RAE)	Vit C (mg)	Thia (mg)	Ribo (mg)	Niac (mg)	Vit B_6 (mg)	Vit B_{12} (µg)	Vit E (mg)	Fol (µg)	Alc (g)
0.4	3	4	0.26	4.9	46	46	103	0.1	6	0.6	0.01	0.02	1.72	0.02	0.31	0.2	2	0
1.4	42	9	1.11	54.5	277	275	43	0.7	644	0	0.24	0.26	8.97	0.45	9.26	1.1	1.7	0
0.3	49	18	0.8	54.5	208	484	40	0.6	17	0.9	0.43	0.05	10.16	0.88	0.51	0.5	1.7	0
0.7	36	12	0.83	28.1	185	202	321	0.4	5	0	0.01	0.04	4.93	0.18	1	0.7	1.7	0
1.1	26	3	0.55	28.9	227	283	337	0.4	4	0	0.01	0.07	9.95	0.37	1.87	2	4.3	0
1	66	28	0.4	35.7	294	346	55	1.1	33	0	0.15	0.13	3.27	0.29	0.82	0.2	14.5	0
	60	25	0.54	32.3	171	458	43	0.6	26	2.5	0.15	0.04	7.42	0.16	1.06	0.2	3.4	0
0.3	0	126	0.73	81	263	749	3	3.5	13	7.8	0.38	0.15	1.09	0.33	0	1.3	60.7	0
0.2	0	86	3.02	68.6	188	569	871	5.8	13	0	0.24	0.1	1.09	0.21	0	0.4	30.5	0
3	8	62	2.24	36.3	135	304	557	2.4	5	3	0.08	0.07	1.17	0.06	0.44	0.6	38.8	0
0	0	18	0.54	11.2	40	34	175	0.4	1	0.4	0.04	0.09	0.27	0.04	0	0	12.5	0
0.2	0	46	3.61	120.4	241	611	2	1.9	0	0	0.42	0.1	0.87	0.12	0	0.1	256.3	0
0.4	0	78	4.71	113.8	390	1138	1834	5.1	3	4.3	0.1	0.38	0.91	0.68	0.03	0.5	65.8	0
0.2	0	211	1.85	85.8	84	690	396	1.7	66	3.6	0.17	0.24	2.31	0.11	0	0.4	209.6	0
0.2	0	41	4.29	90.6	267	475	410	2.2	2	0.7	0.35	0.09	0.85	0.17	0	0.5	355.7	0
0.7	8	20	1.7	51.6	115	214	420	1.2	0	0.2	0.08	0.06	0.52	0.05	0	0.6	61.2	0
0.1	0	61	2.55	73.1	212	456	410	1.7	2	0.5	0.16	0.15	1.21	0.12	0	0	176.8	0
0.1	0	47	1.95	41.6	163	418	32	1.3	21	4.7	0.17	0.37	2.83	0.13	0		186.5	0
0.2	0	55	2.83	97	200	537	4	1.7	2	2	0.33	0.12	1.17	0.14	0	0.3	321.2	0
0.7	0	273	13.95	391.2	760	2579	31	5.5	12	9.9	1.29	0.48	4.66	0.79	0	1.1	1293.8	0
0.2	0	8	0.24	4.5	17	27	37	0.2	0	1.2	0.01	0.01	0.06	0.06	0	0.1	9.1	0
0.3	0	87	3	69.1	230	607	758	1.2	0	3.1	0.3	0.13	1.05	0.19	0	0.1	92.2	0
0.1	0	50	5.2	79.6	251	713	4	1.9	0	2.1	0.28	0.1	1.02	0.21	0	1.5	230.1	0
0.1	0	38	6.59	71.3	356	731	4	2.5	1	3	0.33	0.14	2.1	0.35	0	0.2	358.4	0
0.2	0	53	4.37	96.5	231	730	435	1.9	0	0	0.29	0.1	1.2	0.14	0	0.3	273	0
0.2	0	32	4.49	80.8	209	955	4	1.8	0	0	0.3	0.1	0.79	0.3	0	0.3	156	0
0.1	0	51	4.36	94	178	530	810	1.6	0	0	0.13	0.08	0.63	0.22	0	0.2	120.5	0
0.1	0	25	1.76	50.4	101	370	238	0.5	7	5.2	0.06	0.05	0.69	0.1	0	0.6	14.4	0
0.2	0	126	4.3	96.5	262	708	0	1.9	0	1.6	0.43	0.12	1.18	0.25	0	0	254.8	0
0.3	0	123	4.85	123.1	351	755	1174	2	0	1.8	0.37	0.14	1.28	0.27	0	2	162.4	0
0.4	0	103	3.5	64.8	221	583	706	1.7	0	2.2	0.24	0.15	0.7	0.18	0	1.4	144	0
0	0	44	2.31	46	85	550	271	0.6	0	0.6	0.23	0.09	0.54	0.17	0	0.3	28.9	0
0.1	0	55	0.81	22.5	36	182	299	0.3	44	12.1	0.09	0.12	0.77	0.07	0	0.6	41.2	0
0	0	20	0.57	13.8	21	115	3	0.1	19	9	0.05	0.06	0.41	0.04	0	0.2	20.4	0
0.1	0	58	1.6	31.2	49	374	299	0.5	5	12.1	0.09	0.12	0.77	0.07	0	0.6	41.2	0
0	0	20	0.57	13.8	21	115	3	0.1	3	9	0.05	0.06	0.41	0.04	0	0.1	20.4	0
0.1	0	14	1.26	35.3	97	355	233	1	0	0.4	0.19	0.05	0.87	0.05	0	0	63.7	0
0.2	0	161	6.62	112.8	202	1004	11	2.5	0	0	0.21	0.08	0.25	0.17	0	1.7	145	0
0.2	0	191	7.83	133.6	238	1189	13	2.9	0	0	0.25	0.1	0.3	0.2	0	2.1	170.3	0
0.5	0	110	4.39	131	324	575	9	1.9	0	3.2	0.33	0.18	1.25	0.23	0	0.9	143.4	0
0	0	2	0.73	8.2	32	150	9	0.2	0	0.6	0.05	0.02	0.56	0.09	0		111.5	0
0	0	9	0.26	12	17	71	66	0.1	2	2	0.01	0.01	0.2	0.02	0	0	10.2	0
0.1	0	16	0.43	23	49	211	40	0.3	7	4.5	0.05	0.12	0.73	0.07	0	0.1	107.2	0
0	0	32	0.29	9.4	10	74	5	0.1	24	3	0.01	0.02	0.06	0.01	0	0.1	19.4	0
0	0	21	0.82	12.6	49	202	216	0.5	45	6.9	0.15	0.13	0.98	0.07	0	1.4	134.1	0
0	0	8	0.75	4.9	18	71	1	0.2	13	2	0.05	0.05	0.34	0.03	0	0.4	18.2	0
0	0	164	2.74	97.9	59	1309	687	0.7	552	35.9	0.17	0.42	0.72	0.19	0	2.6	20.2	0

MDA Code	Food Name	Amt	Wt (g)	Ener (kcal)	Prot (g)	Carb (g)	Fiber (g)	Fat (g)	Mono (g)	Poly (g)
5312	Beet greens, fresh	0.5 cup	19	4	0	1	1	0	0	0
5862	Beets, cooked w/salt, drained, slices	0.5 cup	85	37	1	8	2	0	0	0.1
6755	Beets, canned, drained, slices	1 cup	170	53	2	12	3	0	0	0.1
5573	Beets, fresh, slices	0.5 cup	68	29	1	7	2	0	0	0
9160	Belgian endive, fresh, head	0.5 cup	45	8	0	2	1	0	0	0
5558	Broccoli, stalk, fresh	1 ea	114	32	3	6	4	0	0	0.2
6091	Broccoli, cooked w/salt, drained, chopped	0.5 cup	78	22	2	4	3	0	0	0.1
7909	Broccoli, Chinese, cooked	1 cup	88	19	1	3	2	1	0	0.3
9542	Broccoli raab, cooked	3 oz	85.1	28	3	3	2	0	0	0.1
9541	Broccoli raab, fresh, stalk	3 oz	85.1	19	3	2	2	0	0	0.1
5870	Brussels sprouts, cooked w/salt, drained	0.5 cup	78	32	2	7	2	0	0	0.2
5036	Cabbage, fresh, shredded	1 cup	70	18	1	4	2	0	0	0
5878	Cabbage, cooked w/salt, drained, shredded	0.5 cup	75	17	1	4	1	0	0	0
5608	Cabbage, pickled, Japanese style	0.5 cup	75	22	1	4	2	0	0	0
5609	Cabbage, mustard, salted	1 cup	128	36	1	7	4	0	0	0.1
9591	Cabbage, pak choi, shredded, cooked w/salt, drained	0.5 cup	85	10	1	2	1	0	0	0.1
5040	Cabbage, petsai, fresh, chopped	1 cup	76	12	1	2	1	0	0	0.1
5880	Cabbage, red, cooked w/salt, drained, shredded	0.5 cup	75	22	1	5	2	0	0	0
5042	Cabbage, red, fresh, shredded	0.5 cup	35	11	1	3	1	0	0	0
9550	Carrots, dehydrated	1 Tbs	4.6	16	0	4	1	0	0	0
90605	Carrots, fresh, baby, large	1 ea	15	5	0	1	0	0	0	0
5887	Carrots, cooked w/salt, slices	0.5 cup	78	27	1	6	2	0	0	0.1
5199	Carrots, canned, drained, slices	0.5 cup	73	18	0	4	1	0	0	0.1
5045	Carrots, fresh, whole, 7-1/2" long	1 ea	72	30	1	7	2	0	0	0.1
5049	Cauliflower, fresh	0.5 cup	50	12	1	3	1	0	0	0
5891	Cauliflower, cooked w/salt, drained, 1" pces	0.5 cup	62	14	1	3	1	0	0	0.1
5894	Celery, cooked w/salt, drained, diced	0.5 cup	75	14	1	3	1	0	0	0.1
90436	Celery, stalk, small, 5" long, fresh	1 ea	17	3	0	1	0	0	0	0
9203	Chicory, red leafed, fresh, shredded	1 cup	40	9	1	2	0	0	0	0
6093	Collard greens, chopped, cooked w/salt, drained	1 cup	190	49	4	9	5	1	0	0.3
5060	Collard greens, chopped, fresh	1 cup	36	11	1	2	1	0	0	0.1
6801	Corn, yellow, sweet, ear, fresh, small, 5.5"-6.5" long	1 ea	73	63	2	14	2	1	0.3	0.4
7202	Corn, white, sweet, kernels from small ear, fresh	1 ea	73	63	2	14	2	1	0.3	0.4
5900	Corn, yellow, sweet, kernels, cooked w/salt, drained	0.5 cup	82	89	3	21	2	1	0.3	0.5
5241	Dandelion greens, fresh	1 cup	55	25	1	5	2	0	0	0.2
9221	Dasheen, cooked w/salt, slices	0.5 cup	66	94	0	23	3	0	0	0
5908	Eggplant, cooked w/salt, drained, 1" cubes	1 cup	99	35	1	9	2	0	0	0.1
5202	Endive greens, fresh, chopped	0.5 cup	25	4	0	1	1	0	0	0
5450	Fennel, bulb, fresh, slices	0.5 cup	43.5	13	1	3	1	0		
5373	Garden cress greens, fresh, sprigs	20 ea	20	6	1	1	0	0	0	0
7270	Hearts of palm, canned	0.5 cup	73	20	2	3	2	0	0.1	0.1
9182	Jicama, fresh, slices	1 cup	120	46	1	11	6	0	0	0.1
5915	Kale, cooked w/salt, drained, chopped	0.5 cup	65	18	1	4	1	0	0	0.1
9191	Kale, borecole, fresh, chopped	1 cup	67	34	2	7	1	0	0	0.2
5918	Kohlrabi, cooked w/salt, drained, slices	1 cup	165	48	3	11	2	0	0	0.1
5078	Kohlrabi, fresh	0.5 cup	67.5	18	1	4	2	0	0	0
90182	Ladies fingers, fresh, pods, 3" long	8 ea	95	29	2	7	3	0	0	0
5205	Leeks, bulb & lower leaf, fresh, chopped	0.5 cup	44.5	27	1	6	1	0	0	0.1
5920	Leeks, bulb & lower leaf, cooked w/salt, chopped	1 ea	124	38	1	9	1	0	0	0.1
90445	Lettuce, butterhead, fresh, leaf, small	1 pce	5	1	0	0	0	0	0	0

Sat (g)	Chol (mg)	Calc (mg)	Iron (mg)	Mag (mg)	Phos (mg)	Pota (mg)	Sodi (mg)	Zinc (mg)	Vit A (RAE)	Vit C (mg)	Thia (mg)	Ribo (mg)	Niac (mg)	Vit B$_6$ (mg)	Vit B$_{12}$ (µg)	Vit E (mg)	Fol (µg)	Alc (g)
0	0	22	0.49	13.3	8	145	43	0.1	60	5.7	0.02	0.04	0.08	0.02	0	0.3	2.8	0
0	0	14	0.67	19.6	32	259	242	0.3	2	3.1	0.02	0.03	0.28	0.06	0	0	68	0
0	0	26	3.09	28.9	29	252	330	0.4	2	7	0.02	0.07	0.27	0.1	0	0.1	51	0
0	0	11	0.54	15.6	27	221	53	0.2	1	3.3	0.02	0.03	0.23	0.05	0	0	74.1	0
0	0	9	0.11	4.5	12	95	1	0.1	0	1.3	0.03	0.01	0.07	0.02	0		16.6	0
0.1	0	55	1	28.5	75	370	31	0.5	23	106.2	0.07	0.14	0.73	0.18	0	0.5	80.9	0
0	0	31	0.52	16.4	52	229	204	0.4	76	32.8	0.05	0.1	0.43	0.16	0	1.1	84.2	0
0.1	0	88	0.49	15.8	36	230	6	0.3	72	24.8	0.08	0.13	0.38	0.06	0	0.4	87.1	0
0	0	100	1.08	23	70	292	48	0.5	193	31.5	0.14	0.12	1.71	0.19		2.2	60.4	0
0	0	92	1.82	18.7	62	167	28	0.7	112	17.2	0.14	0.11	1.04	0.15		1.4	70.6	0
0.1	0	28	0.94	15.6	44	247	200	0.3	30	48.4	0.08	0.06	0.47	0.14	0	0.3	46.8	0
0	0	28	0.33	8.4	18	119	13	0.1	4	25.6	0.04	0.03	0.16	0.09	0	0.1	30.1	0
0	0	36	0.13	11.2	25	147	191	0.2	3	28.1	0.05	0.03	0.19	0.08	0	0.1	22.5	0
0	0	36	0.37	9	32	640	208	0.2	7	0.5	0	0.03	0.14	0.08	0	0.1	31.5	0
0	0	86	0.9	19.2	35	315	918	0.4	63	0	0.05	0.12	0.92	0.38	0	0	92.2	0
0	0	79	0.88	9.4	25	315	230	0.1	180	22.1	0.03	0.05	0.36	0.14	0	0.1	34.8	0
0	0	59	0.24	9.9	22	181	7	0.2	12	20.5	0.03	0.04	0.3	0.18	0	0.1	60	0
0	0	32	0.5	12.8	25	196	183	0.2	2	8.1	0.05	0.04	0.29	0.17	0	0.1	18	0
0	0	16	0.28	5.6	10	85	9	0.1	20	20	0.02	0.02	0.15	0.07	0	0	6.3	0
0	0	10	0.18	5.4	16	117	13	0.1	249	0.7	0.02	0.02	0.3	0.05	0	0.3	2.5	0
0	0	5	0.13	1.5	4	36	12	0	104	0.4	0	0.01	0.08	0.02	0	0.1	4	0
0	0	23	0.27	7.8	23	183	236	0.2	671	2.8	0.05	0.03	0.5	0.12	0	0.8	1.6	0
0	0	18	0.47	5.8	18	131	177	0.2	407	2	0.01	0.02	0.4	0.08	0	0.5	6.6	0
0	0	24	0.22	8.6	25	230	50	0.2	606	4.2	0.05	0.04	0.71	0.1	0	0.5	13.7	0
0	0	11	0.22	7.5	22	152	15	0.1	0	23.2	0.03	0.03	0.26	0.11	0	0	28.5	0
0	0	10	0.2	5.6	20	88	150	0.1	1	27.5	0.03	0.03	0.25	0.11	0	0	27.3	0
0	0	32	0.31	9	19	213	245	0.1	22	4.6	0.03	0.04	0.24	0.06	0	0.3	16.5	0
0	0	7	0.03	1.9	4	44	14	0	4	0.5	0	0.01	0.05	0.01	0	0	6.1	0
0	0	8	0.23	5.2	16	121	9	0.2	0	3.2	0.01	0.01	0.1	0.02	0	0.9	24	0
0.1	0	266	2.2	38	57	220	479	0.4	771	34.6	0.08	0.2	1.09	0.24	0	1.7	176.7	0
0	0	52	0.07	3.2	4	61	7	0	120	12.7	0.02	0.05	0.27	0.06	0	0.8	59.8	0
0.1	0	1	0.38	27	65	197	11	0.3	7	5	0.15	0.04	1.24	0.04	0	0.1	33.6	0
0.1	0	1	0.38	27	65	197	11	0.3	0	5	0.15	0.04	1.24	0.04	0	0.1	33.6	0
0.2	0	2	0.5	26.2	84	204	207	0.4	11	5.1	0.18	0.06	1.32	0.05	0	0.1	37.7	0
0.1	0	103	1.7	19.8	36	218	42	0.2	136	19.2	0.1	0.14	0.44	0.14	0	2.6	14.8	0
0	0	12	0.48	19.8	50	319	166	0.2	3	3.3	0.07	0.02	0.34	0.22	0	1.9	12.5	0
0	0	6	0.25	10.9	15	122	237	0.1	2	1.3	0.08	0.02	0.59	0.09	0	0.4	13.9	0
0	0	13	0.21	3.8	7	78	6	0.2	27	1.6	0.02	0.02	0.1	0	0	0.1	35.5	0
0		21	0.32	7.4	22	180	23	0.1	3	5.2	0	0.01	0.28	0.02	0		11.7	0
0	0	16	0.26	7.6	15	121	3	0	69	13.8	0.02	0.05	0.2	0.05	0	0.1	16	0
0.1	0	42	2.28	27.7	47	129	311	0.8	0	5.8	0.01	0.04	0.32	0.02	0		28.5	0
0	0	14	0.72	14.4	22	180	5	0.2	1	24.2	0.02	0.03	0.24	0.05	0	0.6	14.4	0
0	0	47	0.58	11.7	18	148	168	0.2	443	26.6	0.03	0.05	0.32	0.09	0	0.6	8.4	0
0.1	0	90	1.14	22.8	38	299	29	0.3	515	80.4	0.07	0.09	0.67	0.18	0	0.5	19.4	0
0	0	41	0.66	31.4	74	561	424	0.5	3	89.1	0.07	0.03	0.64	0.25	0	0.9	19.8	0
0	0	16	0.27	12.8	31	236	14	0	1	41.8	0.03	0.01	0.27	0.1	0	0.3	10.8	0
0	0	77	0.76	54.2	60	288	8	0.6	18	20	0.19	0.06	0.95	0.2	0	0.3	83.6	0
0	0	26	0.93	12.5	16	80	9	0.1	37	5.3	0.03	0.01	0.18	0.1	0	0.4	28.5	0
0	0	37	1.36	17.4	21	108	305	0.1	2	5.2	0.03	0.02	0.25	0.14	0	0.8	29.8	0
0	0	2	0.06	0.6	2	12	0	0	8	0.2	0	0	0.02	0	0	0	3.6	0

MDA Code	Food Name	Amt	Wt (g)	Ener (kcal)	Prot (g)	Carb (g)	Fiber (g)	Fat (g)	Mono (g)	Poly (g)
5089	Lettuce, romaine, fresh, inner leaf	2 pce	20	3	0	1	0	0	0	0
5087	Lettuce, green leaf, fresh, leaf	2 pce	20	3	0	1	0	0	0	0
9545	Lettuce, red leaf, fresh, shredded	1 cup	28	4	0	1	0	0		
7949	Mushrooms, oyster, fresh, small	1 ea	15	5	0	1	0	0	0	0
5926	Mushrooms, shiitake, cooked w/salt, pieces	1 cup	145	78	2	20	3	0	0.1	0
51069	Mushrooms, crimini, fresh	2 ea	28	8	1	1	0	0	0	0
90457	Mushrooms, canned, drained, caps	8 ea	47	12	1	2	1	0	0	0.1
51067	Mushrooms, portabella, fresh, small	1 oz	28	7	1	1	0	0	0	0
5927	Mustard greens, cooked w/salt, drained, chopped	0.5 cup	70	10	2	1	1	0	0.1	0
5207	Mustard greens, fresh, chopped	1 cup	56	15	2	3	2	0	0.1	0
6971	Okra, cooked w/salt, drained, slices	0.5 cup	80	18	1	4	2	0	0	0
6074	Onion, cooked w/salt, drained	0.5 cup	105	44	1	10	1	0	0	0.1
90472	Onion, yellow, fresh, small, whole	1 ea	70	28	1	7	1	0	0	0
90487	Onion, spring, tops & bulb, fresh, small, 3" long	1 ea	5	2	0	0	0	0	0	0
9548	Onion, sweet, fresh	1 oz	28	9	0	2	0	0		
9547	Onion, green, tops only, fresh, stalk	1 Tbs	6	2	0	0	0	0	0	0
5936	Parsnips, cooked w/salt, drained, slices	0.5 cup	78	55	1	13	3	0	0.1	0
5211	Parsnips, fresh, slices	0.5 cup	66.5	50	1	12	3	0	0.1	0
5281	Peas & carrots, canned, w/liquid	0.5 cup	127.5	48	3	11	3	0	0	0.2
6096	Pea pods, cooked w/salt, drained	1 cup	160	64	5	10	4	0	0	0.2
6836	Pea pods, fresh, chopped	1 cup	98	41	3	7	3	0	0	0.1
5938	Peas, green, cooked w/salt, drained	0.5 cup	80	67	4	13	4	0	0	0.1
5116	Peas, green, fresh	1 cup	145	117	8	21	7	1	0.1	0.3
9611	Peppers, green chili, canned	0.5 cup	69.5	15	1	3	1	0	0	0.1
7932	Peppers, jalapeno, fresh, sliced	1 cup	90	27	1	5	2	1	0	0.3
9632	Peppers, serrano, fresh	1 cup	105	34	2	7	3	0	0	0.2
90493	Peppers, bell, green, sweet, fresh, strips	10 pce	27	5	0	1	0	0	0	0
9549	Peppers, bell, green, sweet, sauteed	1 oz	28	36	0	1	1	3	0.7	1.7
6990	Peppers, bell, red, sweet, fresh, ring, 3" × 1/4" thick	1 ea	10	3	0	1	0	0	0	0
9551	Peppers, bell, red, sweet, sauteed	1 oz	28	37	0	2	1	4	0.6	1.6
9300	Peppers, bell, yellow, sweet, fresh, med	1 ea	119	32	1	8	1	0		
90589	Pickles, sweet, spear	1 ea	20	16	0	4	0	0	0	0
92209	Pickles, bread & butter	1 ea	8	6	0	2	0	0	0	0
5228	Pimentos, canned, slices	20 pce	20	5	0	1	0	0	0	0
9251	Potatoes, red, w/skin, baked, small, 1-3/4" to 2-1/2"	1 ea	138	123	3	27	2	0	0	0.1
9245	Potatoes, russet, w/skin, baked, small, 1-3/4"-2-1/2"	1 ea	138	134	4	30	3	0	0	0.1
90564	Potatoes, peeled, cooked w/salt, large, 3" to 4-1/4"	1 ea	299.6	258	5	60	6	0	0	0.1
5950	Potatoes, skin, baked w/salt	1 ea	58	115	2	27	5	0	0	0
5964	Pumpkin, canned, w/salt	0.5 cup	122.5	42	1	10	4	0	0	0
90505	Radishes, fresh, small	10 ea	20	3	0	1	0	0	0	0
5969	Rutabaga, cooked w/salt, drained, mashed	0.5 cup	120	47	2	10	2	0	0	0.1
6859	Seaweed, oarweed, fresh, Laminaria spp.	0.5 cup	40	17	1	4	1	0	0	0
5260	Seaweed, spirulina, dried	0.5 cup	59.5	173	34	14	2	5	0.4	1.2
5427	Shallots, chopped, fresh	1 Tbs	10	7	0	2	0	0	0	0
9212	Silverbeet greens, cooked w/salt, drained, chopped	0.5 cup	87.5	18	2	4	2	0		
5972	Spinach, cooked w/salt, drained	0.5 cup	90	21	3	3	2	0	0	0.1
5149	Spinach, canned, drained	0.5 cup	107	25	3	4	3	1	0	0.2
5146	Spinach, fresh, chopped	1 cup	30	7	1	1	1	0	0	0
5982	Squash, acorn, baked w/salt, cubes	0.5 cup	102.5	57	1	15	5	0	0	0.1
5984	Squash, butternut, baked w/salt, cubes	0.5 cup	102.5	41	1	11	3	0	0	0

Sat (g)	Chol (mg)	Calc (mg)	Iron (mg)	Mag (mg)	Phos (mg)	Pota (mg)	Sodi (mg)	Zinc (mg)	Vit A (RAE)	Vit C (mg)	Thia (mg)	Ribo (mg)	Niac (mg)	Vit B$_6$ (mg)	Vit B$_{12}$ (µg)	Vit E (mg)	Fol (µg)	Alc (g)
0	0	7	0.19	2.8	6	49	2	0	58	4.8	0.01	0.01	0.06	0.01	0	0	27.2	0
0	0	7	0.17	2.6	6	39	6	0	74	3.6	0.01	0.02	0.08	0.02	0	0.1	7.6	0
		9	0.34	3.4	8	52	7	0.1	105	1	0.02	0.02	0.09	0.03		0	10.1	0
0	0	0	0.2	2.7	18	63	3	0.1	0	0	0.02	0.05	0.74	0.02	0	0	4	0
0.1	0	4	0.64	20.3	42	170	348	1.9	0	0.4	0.05	0.25	2.17	0.23	0	0	30.4	0
0	0	5	0.11	2.5	34	125	2	0.3	0	0	0.03	0.14	1.06	0.03	0.03	0	3.9	0
0	0	5	0.37	7	31	61	200	0.3	0	0	0.04	0.01	0.75	0.03	0	0	5.6	0
0	0	2	0.17	3.1	36	136	2	0.2	0	0	0.02	0.13	1.26	0.03	0.01	0	6.2	0
0	0	52	0.49	10.5	29	141	176	0.1	221	17.7	0.03	0.04	0.3	0.07	0	0.8	51.1	0
0	0	58	0.82	17.9	24	198	14	0.1	294	39.2	0.04	0.06	0.45	0.1	0	1.1	104.7	0
0	0	62	0.22	28.8	26	108	193	0.3	11	13	0.11	0.04	0.7	0.15	0	0.2	36.8	0
0	0	23	0.25	11.6	37	174	251	0.2	0	5.5	0.04	0.02	0.17	0.14	0	0	15.8	0
0	0	16	0.15	7	20	102	3	0.1	0	5.2	0.03	0.02	0.08	0.08	0	0	13.3	0
0	0	4	0.07	1	2	14	1	0	2	0.9	0	0	0.03	0	0	0	3.2	0
	0	6	0.07	2.5	8	33	2	0	0	1.3	0.01	0.01	0.04	0.04		0	6.4	0
0	0	4	0.12	1.2	2	16	0	0	12	2.7	0	0.01	0.01	0	0	0	0.8	0
0	0	29	0.45	22.6	54	286	192	0.2	0	10.1	0.06	0.04	0.56	0.07	0	0.8	45.2	0
0	0	24	0.39	19.3	47	249	7	0.4	0	11.3	0.06	0.03	0.47	0.06	0	1	44.6	0
0.1	0	29	0.96	17.8	59	128	332	0.7	368	8.4	0.09	0.07	0.74	0.11	0	0.2	23	0
0.1	0	67	3.15	41.6	88	384	384	0.6	83	76.6	0.2	0.12	0.86	0.23	0	0.6	46.4	0
0	0	42	2.04	23.5	52	196	4	0.3	53	58.8	0.15	0.08	0.59	0.16	0	0.4	41.2	0
0	0	22	1.23	31.2	94	217	191	1	32	11.4	0.21	0.12	1.62	0.17	0	0.1	50.4	0
0.1	0	36	2.13	47.8	157	354	7	1.8	55	58	0.39	0.19	3.03	0.25	0	0.2	94.2	0
0	0	25	0.92	2.8	8	79	276	0.1	4	23.8	0.01	0.02	0.44	0.08	0		37.5	0
0.1	0	9	0.63	17.1	28	194	1	0.2	36	39.9	0.13	0.05	1.01	0.46	0	0.4	42.3	0
0.1	0	12	0.9	23.1	42	320	10	0.3	49	47.1	0.06	0.09	1.61	0.53	0	0.7	24.2	0
0	0	3	0.09	2.7	5	47	1	0	5	21.7	0.02	0.01	0.13	0.06	0	0.1	2.7	0
0.4	0	2	0.08	2.2	4	38	5	0	4	49.6	0.01	0.01	0.16	0.05	0	0.4	0.6	0
0	0	1	0.04	1.2	3	21	0	0	16	12.8	0.01	0.01	0.1	0.03	0	0.2	4.6	0
0.4	0	2	0.13	3.4	6	54	6	0	39	45.6	0.02	0.03	0.27	0.1	0	0.9	0.6	0
0	0	13	0.55	14.3	29	252	2	0.2	12	218.4	0.03	0.03	1.06	0.2	0	0.8	30.9	0
0	0	12	0.05	1.4	4	20	91	0	8	0.1	0.01	0.01	0.02	0	0	0.1	0.2	0
0	0	3	0.03	0.2	2	16	54	0	1	0.7	0	0	0	0	0	0	0.3	0
0	0	1	0.34	1.2	3	32	3	0	27	17	0	0.01	0.12	0.04	0	0.1	1.2	0
0	0	12	0.97	38.6	99	752	17	0.6	1	17.4	0.1	0.07	2.2	0.29	0	0.1	37.3	0
0	0	25	1.48	41.4	98	759	19	0.5	1	17.8	0.09	0.07	1.86	0.49	0	0.1	35.9	0
0.1	0	24	0.93	59.9	120	983	722	0.8	0	22.2	0.29	0.06	3.93	0.81	0	0	27	0
0	0	20	4.08	24.9	59	332	149	0.3	1	7.8	0.07	0.06	1.78	0.36	0	0	12.8	0
0.2	0	32	1.7	28.2	43	252	295	0.2	953	5.1	0.03	0.07	0.45	0.07	0	1.3	14.7	0
0	0	5	0.07	2	4	47	8	0.1	0	3	0	0.01	0.05	0.01	0	0	5	0
0	0	58	0.64	27.6	67	391	305	0.4	0	22.6	0.1	0.05	0.86	0.12	0	0.4	18	0
0.1	0	67	1.14	48.4	17	36	93	0.5	2	1.2	0.02	0.06	0.19	0	0	0.3	72	0
1.6	0	71	16.96	116	70	811	624	1.2	17	6	1.42	2.18	7.63	0.22	0	3	55.9	0
0	0	4	0.12	2.1	6	33	1	0	6	0.8	0.01	0	0.02	0.03	0	0	3.4	0
	0	51	1.98	75.2	29	480	363	0.3	268	15.8	0.03	0.08	0.32	0.07	0	1.7	7.9	0
0	0	122	3.21	78.3	50	419	275	0.7	472	8.8	0.09	0.21	0.44	0.22	0	1.9	131.4	0
0.1	0	136	2.46	81.3	47	370	29	0.5	524	15.3	0.02	0.15	0.42	0.11	0	2.1	104.9	0
0	0	30	0.81	23.7	15	167	24	0.2	141	8.4	0.02	0.06	0.22	0.06	0	0.6	58.2	0
0	0	45	0.95	44.1	46	448	246	0.2	22	11.1	0.17	0.01	0.9	0.2	0	0.1	19.5	0
0	0	42	0.62	29.7	28	291	246	0.1	572	15.5	0.07	0.02	0.99	0.13	0	1.3	19.5	0

MDA Code	Food Name	Amt	Wt (g)	Ener (kcal)	Prot (g)	Carb (g)	Fiber (g)	Fat (g)	Mono (g)	Poly (g)
6922	Squash, spaghetti, cooked w/salt, drained	0.5 cup	77.5	21	1	5	1	0	0	0.1
5975	Squash, summer, all types, cooked w/salt, drained	0.5 cup	90	18	1	4	1	0	0	0.1
5981	Squash, winter, all types, baked w/salt, cubes	0.5 cup	102.5	40	1	9	3	1	0	0.3
5989	Succotash, cooked w/salt, drained	0.5 cup	96	107	5	23	5	1	0.1	0.4
6924	Sweet potatoes, dark orange, baked in skin w/salt	0.5 cup	100	90	2	21	3	0	0	0.1
5555	Sweet potatoes, dark orange, canned, w/syrup, drained	1 cup	196	212	3	50	6	1	0	0.3
5445	Tomatillo, fresh, medium	1 ea	34	11	0	2	1	0	0.1	0.1
5476	Tomato puree, canned	0.5 cup	125	48	2	11	2	0	0	0.1
5180	Tomato sauce, canned	0.5 cup	122.5	29	2	7	2	0	0	0.1
5474	Tomatoes, red, stewed, canned	0.5 cup	127.5	33	1	8	1	0	0	0.1
6887	Tomato, red, whole, w/tomato juice, canned	1 ea	190	32	1	8	2	0	0	0.1
90532	Tomato, red, fresh, year round avg, small/thin slices	1 pce	15	3	0	1	0	0	0	0
5447	Tomatoes, sun dried	10 pce	20	52	3	11	2	1	0.1	0.2
9299	Tomato, yellow, cherry, fresh	1 ea	17	3	0	1	0	0	0	0
6949	Tung sun, slices, cooked w/salt, drained, 1/2" slices	1 cup	120	13	2	2	1	0	0	0.1
6737	Tung sun, slices, fresh	1 cup	151	41	4	8	3	0	0	0.2
6004	Turnip greens, cooked w/salt, drained, chopped	0.5 cup	72	14	1	3	3	0	0	0.1
6002	Turnips, cooked w/salt, drained, mashed	0.5 cup	115	25	1	6	2	0	0	0
7955	Wasabi, root, fresh	1 ea	169	184	8	40	13	1		
5388	Water chestnuts, Chinese, canned, w/liquid	4 ea	28	14	0	3	1	0	0	0
5223	Watercress greens, fresh, sprig	10 ea	25	3	1	0	0	0	0	0
6010	Yams, tropical, cooked/baked w/salt, drained, cubes	0.5 cup	68	78	1	18	3	0	0	0
5306	Yams, tropical, fresh, cubes	0.5 cup	75	88	1	21	3	0	0	0.1
9197	Yuca, fresh	1 cup	206	330	3	78	4	1	0.2	0.1
90525	Zucchini, w/skin, fresh, small	1 ea	118	19	1	4	1	0	0	0.1
6921	Zucchini, w/skin, cooked w/salt, drained, mashed	0.5 cup	120	19	1	5	2	0	0	0
	Soy and Soy Products									
7503	Miso	1 Tbs	17.2	34	2	5	1	1	0.2	0.6
7508	Natto, fermented soybeans	1 cup	175	371	31	25	9	19	4.3	10.9
7564	Tempeh	0.5 cup	83	160	15	8		9	2.5	3.2
7015	Soybeans, mature, cooked	1 cup	172	298	29	17	10	15	3.4	8.7
7014	Soybeans, mature, dry	0.25 cup	46.5	193	17	14	4	9	2	5.2
4707	Soybeans, mature, roasted, salted	0.25 cup	43	203	15	14	8	11	2.4	6.2
7585	Soymeal, defatted, raw	0.5 cup	61	207	27	24		1	0.2	0.6
71584	Soy yogurt, peach/Silk	1 ea	170.1	170	4	32	1	2		
7542	Tofu, firm, silken, 1" slice/Mori-Nu	3 oz	85.1	53	6	2	0	2	0.5	1.3
7799	Tofu, firm, silken, light, 1" slice/Mori-Nu	3 oz	85.1	31	5	1	0	1	0.1	0.4
7541	Tofu, soft, silken, 1" slice/Mori-Nu	3 oz	85.1	47	4	2	0	2	0.4	1.3
7546	Tofu yogurt, tofu	1 cup	262	246	9	42	1	5	1	2.7
	MEALS AND DISHES									
	Homemade									
57482	Coleslaw	0.5 cup	60	47	1	7	1	2	0.4	0.8
56102	Falafel patty, 2-1/4"	1 ea	17	57	2	5		3	1.7	0.7
53125	Mole poblano	2 Tbs	30.3	50	1	4	1	3		
56005	Potato salad	0.5 cup	125	179	3	14	2	10	3.1	4.7
5786	Potatoes au gratin, w/butter	1 cup	245	323	12	28	4	19	5.3	0.7
56076	Spinach souffle	1 cup	136	233	11	8	1	18	4.1	0.8
92216	Tortellini pasta, cheese filled	1 cup	108	332	15	51	2	8	2.2	0.5
	Packaged or Canned Meals or Dishes									
57705	Egg noodles, w/creamy alfredo sauce, dry mix/Lipton	1 ea	124	518	19	77		15	4.8	1.5

Sat (g)	Chol (mg)	Calc (mg)	Iron (mg)	Mag (mg)	Phos (mg)	Pota (mg)	Sodi (mg)	Zinc (mg)	Vit A (RAE)	Vit C (mg)	Thia (mg)	Ribo (mg)	Niac (mg)	Vit B$_6$ (mg)	Vit B$_{12}$ (µg)	Vit E (mg)	Fol (µg)	Alc (g)
0	0	16	0.26	8.5	11	91	197	0.2	5	2.7	0.03	0.02	0.63	0.08	0	0.1	6.2	0
0.1	0	24	0.32	21.6	35	173	213	0.4	10	5	0.04	0.04	0.46	0.06	0	0.1	18	0
0.1	0	14	0.34	8.2	20	448	243	0.3	268	9.8	0.09	0.02	0.72	0.07	0	0.1	28.7	0
0.1	0	16	1.46	50.9	112	394	243	0.6	14	7.9	0.16	0.09	1.27	0.11	0	0.3	31.7	0
0.1	0	38	0.69	27	54	475	246	0.3	961	19.6	0.11	0.11	1.49	0.29	0	0.7	6	0
0.1	0	33	1.86	23.5	49	378	76	0.3	898	21.2	0.05	0.07	0.67	0.12	0	2.3	15.7	0
0	0	2	0.21	6.8	13	91	0	0.1	2	4	0.01	0.01	0.63	0.02	0	0.1	2.4	0
0	0	22	2.22	28.8	50	549	499	0.5	32	13.3	0.03	0.1	1.83	0.16	0	2.5	13.8	0
0	0	16	1.25	19.6	32	405	642	0.2	21	8.6	0.03	0.08	1.19	0.12	0	1.7	13.5	0
0	0	43	1.7	15.3	26	264	282	0.2	11	10.1	0.06	0.04	0.91	0.02	0	1.1	6.4	0
0	0	59	1.84	20.9	36	357	272	0.3	11	17.7	0.09	0.1	1.35	0.21	0	1.3	15.2	0
0	0	2	0.04	1.6	4	36	1	0	6	1.9	0.01	0	0.09	0.01	0	0.1	2.2	0
0.1	0	22	1.82	38.8	71	685	419	0.4	9	7.8	0.11	0.1	1.81	0.07	0	0	13.6	0
0	0	2	0.08	2	6	44	4	0	0	1.5	0.01	0.01	0.2	0.01	0		5.1	0
0.1	0	14	0.29	3.6	24	640	288	0.6	0	0	0.02	0.06	0.36	0.12	0	0.8	2.4	0
0.1	0	20	0.76	4.5	89	805	6	1.7	2	6	0.23	0.11	0.91	0.36	0	1.5	10.6	0
0	0	99	0.58	15.8	21	146	191	0.1	274	19.7	0.03	0.05	0.3	0.13	0	1.4	85	0
0	0	25	0.25	9.2	22	155	329	0.2	0	13.3	0.03	0.03	0.34	0.08	0	0	10.4	0
	0	216	1.74	116.6	135	960	29	2.7	3	70.8	0.22	0.19	1.26	0.46	0		30.4	0
0	0	1	0.24	1.4	5	33	2	0.1	0	0.4	0	0.01	0.1	0.04	0	0.1	1.7	0
0	0	30	0.05	5.2	15	82	10	0	59	10.8	0.02	0.03	0.05	0.03	0	0.2	2.2	0
0	0	10	0.35	12.2	33	456	166	0.1	4	8.2	0.06	0.02	0.38	0.16	0	0.3	10.9	0
0	0	13	0.41	15.8	41	612	7	0.2	5	12.8	0.08	0.02	0.41	0.22	0	0.3	17.2	0
0.2	0	33	0.56	43.3	56	558	29	0.7	2	42.4	0.18	0.1	1.76	0.18	0	0.4	55.6	0
0	0	18	0.41	20.1	45	309	12	0.3	12	20.1	0.06	0.17	0.57	0.26	0	0.1	34.2	0
0	0	16	0.42	26.4	48	304	287	0.2	67	5.5	0.05	0.05	0.51	0.09	0	0.1	20.4	0
0.2	0	10	0.43	8.3	27	36	641	0.4	1	0	0.02	0.04	0.16	0.03	0.01	0	3.3	0
2.8	0	380	15.05	201.2	304	1276	12	5.3	0	22.8	0.28	0.33	0	0.23	0	0	14	0
1.8	0	92	2.24	67.2	221	342	7	0.9	0	0	0.06	0.3	2.19	0.18	0.07	0	19.9	0
2.2	0	175	8.84	147.9	421	886	2	2	4	2.9	0.27	0.49	0.69	0.4	0	0.6	92.9	0
1.3	0	129	7.3	130.2	327	836	1	2.3	0	2.8	0.41	0.4	0.75	0.18	0	0.4	174.4	0
1.6	0	59	1.68	62.4	156	632	70	1.4	4	0.9	0.04	0.06	0.61	0.09	0	0.4	90.7	0
0.2	0	149	8.36	186.7	428	1519	2	3.1	1	0	0.42	0.15	1.58	0.35	0		184.8	0
0	0	500	0				20			0								0
0.3	0	27	0.88	23	77	165	31	0.5	0	0	0.09	0.03	0.21	0.01	0	0.2		0
0.1	0	31	0.64	8.5	69	54	72	0.3	0	0	0.03	0.02	0.09	0	0	0.1		0
0.3	0	26	0.7	24.7	53	153	4	0.4	0	0	0.09	0.03	0.26	0.01	0	0.2		0
0.7	0	309	2.78	104.8	100	123	92	0.8	5	6.6	0.16	0.05	0.63	0.05	0	0.8	15.7	0
0.2	5	27	0.35	6	19	109	14	0.1	32	19.6	0.04	0.04	0.16	0.08	0	0.1	16.2	0
0.4	0	9	0.58	13.9	33	99	50	0.3	0	0.3	0.02	0.03	0.18	0.02	0	0.2	15.8	0
	0	7	0.56	9.7	25	99	41	0.1	45	0	0.01	0	0.5	0.08	0.01	0.4	8.5	0
1.8	85	24	0.81	18.8	65	318	661	0.4	40	12.5	0.1	0.07	1.11	0.18	0	2.3	8.8	0
11.6	56	292	1.57	49	277	970	1061	1.7	157	24.3	0.16	0.28	2.43	0.43	0	0.5	27	0
8.3	160	224	1.62	40.8	192	318	770	1.2	325	9.9	0.11	0.36	0.66	0.13	0.53	1.3	99.3	0
3.9	45	164	1.62	22.7	229	96	372	1.1	41	0	0.34	0.33	2.91	0.05	0.17	0.2	79.9	0
5.7	139	157	3.74			2195												0

MDA Code	Food Name	Amt	Wt (g)	Ener (kcal)	Prot (g)	Carb (g)	Fiber (g)	Fat (g)	Mono (g)	Poly (g)
90098	Beef ravioli, w/tomato & meat sauce, canned, svg/Chef Boyardee	1 ea	244	224	8	33	1	7	2.7	0.3
25279	Beefaroni, w/tomato sauce, canned, svg/Chef Boyardee	1 ea	212.6	196	7	29	1	6	2.4	0.3
56976	Sweet Sue chicken & dumplings, canned/Bryan Foods	1 cup	240	218	15	23	3	7	3	1.6
57658	Chili con carne, w/beans, canned	1 cup	222	269	16	25	9	12	4.8	0.9
56001	Chili w/beans, canned	1 cup	256	287	15	30	11	14	6	0.9
57700	Chili w/o beans, canned/Hormel	1 cup	236	194	17	18	3	7	2.2	0.8
57703	Chili, vegetarian, w/beans, canned/Hormel	1 cup	247	205	12	38	10	1	0.1	0.4
50317	Chili w/beans, canned/Chef-Mate	1 cup	253	420	18	34	8	24	10.7	1.4
90738	Cheeseburger macaroni pasta/Hamburger Helper	1.5 oz	42.5	168	5	27		4		
57068	Macaroni & cheese, original, dry mix, svg/Kraft	1 ea	70	259	11	48	1	3		
90103	Mini beef ravioli, w/tomato sauce, canned, svg/Chef Boyardee	1 ea	252	232	8	31	3	8	3.4	0.4
90508	Sauerkraut, canned, drained	0.5 cup	71	13	1	3	2	0	0	0
47708	Spaghetti, w/meatballs & tomato sauce, canned/Chef Boyardee	1 ea	240	240	10	29	3	9	3.9	0.8
57484	Scalloped potatoes, from dry w/whole milk & butter	1 ea	822	764	17	105	9	35	10	1.6
42147	Stuffing, cornbread, from dry mix	0.5 cup	100	179	3	22	3	9	3.9	2.7
42037	Stuffing, plain, from dry mix	0.5 cup	100	177	3	22	3	9	3.8	2.6
57701	Turkey chili w/beans, canned/Hormel	1 cup	247	203	19	26	6	3	0.4	1.2
90739	Macaroni & cheese, whole wheat, dry mix, svg/Hodgson Mill	1 ea	70	263	10	48	5	3		
	Frozen Meals or Dishes									
50	Beef, sliced, w/gravy & vegetables/Freezer Queen	1 ea	255	207	15	26	4	5	1.2	1.7
70943	Beef & bean burrito, svg/Las Campanas	1 ea	114	296	9	38	1	12	5.5	0.8
70961	Beef & bean chimichanga/Fiesta Café	1 ea	227	422	24	56	6	12	3.9	3.5
70948	Beef enchilada & tamale, w/beans & rice/Patio	1 ea	376	508	14	68	8	20	7.7	2.7
11112	Beef macaroni, svg	1 ea	226.8	200	13	32	4	2	1.1	0.3
70893	Beef pot pie	1 ea	198	449	13	44	2	24	9.7	2.7
83051	Beef pot roast w/whipped potatoes, homestyle/Stouffer's	1 ea	255	184	13	21	3	5	2.6	1
83027	Beef stir fry w/rice, vegetables & sauce, svg/Tyson	1 ea	405	433	26	71		5		
57474	Beef stroganoff, w/peas & carrots/Marie Callender's	1 ea	368	420	25	40	7	18	5.5	4.1
56915	Broccoli w/cheese flavored sauce/Gardetto's	0.5 cup	84	56	2	7		2	0.8	0.2
56738	Cabbage, stuffed, w/whipped potato/Lean Cuisine	1 ea	269	196	11	24	4	6	3	0.9
16310	Chicken, French recipe, w/potato, vegetables, sauce/Budget Gourmet	1 ea	255	178	23	9	6	6	2.7	0.5
70949	Chicken, roasted, w/garlic sauce, pasta, vegetables/Tyson	1 ea	255	214	17	22	4	7	2.3	2.1
1746	Chicken, thigh, fried, w/mashed potatoes & corn/Banquet	1 ea	228	388	22	30	4	20	8.1	5.3
15974	Chicken & noodles, escalloped/Stouffer's	1 ea	283	419	17	31		25	7	12.3
16195	Chicken & vegetables w/vermicelli/Lean Cuisine	1 ea	297	232	20	26	4	5	1.8	1.1
15965	Chicken a l'orange w/broccoli & rice/Lean Cuisine	1 ea	255	268	24	39		2	0.5	0.4
83052	Chicken alfredo, fettuccine/Stouffer's Lunch Express	1 ea	272	373	19	33	4	18	6.3	2.4
16220	Chicken, BBQ glazed, w/sauce & vegetables/Weight Watchers	1 ea	209	217	19	26		4	1.6	1.1
83053	Chicken cacciatore, w/pasta & vegetables/Healthy Choice	1 ea	354	266	22	36	5	4	2.4	0.6
70945	Chicken cordon bleu, svg/Barber Food	1 ea	168	344	26	15		20	8.2	3.2
16198	Chicken enchilada w/rice & cheese sauce/Stouffer's	1 ea	283	424	15	61	4	13	2.7	0.9
83028	Chicken fajita kit, svg/Tyson	1 ea	107	128	7	17	2	4	1.1	1.6
70931	Chicken mesquite BBQ, w/corn & potato/Tyson	1 ea	255	321	18	45	4	8	2.7	0.5
70582	Chicken nuggets w/mac & cheese, corn, pudding	1 ea	257	457	19	51	7	20	7.9	4.9
70899	Chicken pot pie	1 ea	217	484	13	43	2	29	12.5	4.5
16266	Chicken teriyaki w/rice medley & broccoli/Healthy Choice	1 ea	312	250	16	36	9	5	1.7	1.4
6247	Creamed spinach/Stouffer's	0.5 cup	125	169	3	9	2	13	2.8	4.5
70918	Croissant Pockets chicken broccoli cheddar sandwich	1 ea	128	301	11	39	1	11	4.4	1.7
70895	Egg, scrambled, & sausage, w/hashbrowns	1 ea	177	361	13	17	1	27	12.7	3.6
90565	French fries, heated w/salt	10 ea	50	100	2	16	2	4	2.4	0.4

Sat (g)	Chol (mg)	Calc (mg)	Iron (mg)	Mag (mg)	Phos (mg)	Pota (mg)	Sodi (mg)	Zinc (mg)	Vit A (RAE)	Vit C (mg)	Thia (mg)	Ribo (mg)	Niac (mg)	Vit B_6 (mg)	Vit B_{12} (µg)	Vit E (mg)	Fol (µg)	Alc (g)
2.8	7	27	1.63			354	910			0								0
2.5	6	23	1.42				793			0								0
1.8	36		2.57				946		0									0
3.9	29	84	5.79	64.4	215	608	941	2.3		3.1	0.12	0.22	2.16	0.28	1.44	0.3	57.7	0
6	44	120	8.78	115.2	394	934	1336	5.1	44	4.4	0.12	0.27	0.92	0.34	0	1.5	58.9	0
2.2	35	50	2.6	37.8		349	970	2.6		0								0
0.1	0	96	3.46	81.5		803	778	1.7		1.2								0
10.1	40	71	3.8	45.5	167	511	1280	3.9		0	0.11	0.2	3.48	0.23	1.44	1.2		0
1.2	4						863											0
1.3	10	92	2.56	40	265	296	561			0.4	0.67	0.41	4.54				65.1	0
3.5	8	30	2.57				935		50	0								0
0	0	21	1.04	9.2	14	121	469	0.1	1	10.4	0.01	0.02	0.1	0.09	0	0.1	17	0
3.8	17	26	1.97				864		0	1.4								0
21.6	90	296	3.12	115.1	460	1669	2803	2.1	288	27.1	0.16	0.46	8.46	0.35	0	1.2	82.2	0
1.8	0	26	0.94	13	34	62	455	0.2	78	0.8	0.12	0.09	1.25	0.04	0.01	0.9	97	0
1.7	0	32	1.09	12	42	74	543	0.3	118	0	0.14	0.11	1.48	0.04	0.01	1.4	39	0
0.7	35	116	3.46	69.2		682	1198	2.7		1.5								0
1	6	80	1.83				428											0
																		0
1.3	31						648		529									0
4.2	13		3.11				579		0									0
2.2	36		6.81				804		0	5.9								0
6.8	26	241	2.86				1812		30	4.9								0
0.6	14	43	2.56	34	127	345	420	1.2	52	54.9	0.26	0.15	2.94	0.18	0.11	1.6	99.8	0
8.5	38						737		51									0
1.4	20	71	1.58			895	768			3.3	0.18	0.15	3.03					0
							1584			25.1								0
7.2	63	77	2.06				1343			0								0
0.4		45	0.54			403		29.7										0
1.7	13	89	1.51		732	710		0.5	0.22	1		2.58						0
1.4	26					864		115										0
1.3	28		1.56			467												0
4.4	68	135	1.62			604			2.7									0
6	76	116	1.13		329		1211	0	0									0
1.9	30	163	1.43		692	633				2.7	0.27	0.24	6.62					0
0.4	46	20	0.36		430	360	1		18.1									0
7	57	147				588			24.2									0
1	48		1.09			405		0	21.5									0
1	32	53	2.23	255		750	552											0
5.7	81	144					754											0
7.4	51	300	2.18			243	855			4								0
0.9	12	21	1.13				368			20								0
2.6	26						793			0								0
5.6	57	85	2.78				843			0								0
9.7	41	33	2.06	23.9	119	256	857	1	256	1.5	0.25	0.36	4.13	0.2	0.15	3.8	41.2	0
1.6	22	31	0.59		225	424	596			43.7								0
3.7	16	141	1.06			245	335			5.9					0			0
3.4	37		3.8				652			6.3								0
7.3	283		1.66				772		0									0
0.6	0	4	0.62	11	41	209	133	0.2	0	5.1	0.06	0.01	1.04	0.15	0	0.1	6	0

MDA Code	Food Name	Amt	Wt (g)	Ener (kcal)	Prot (g)	Carb (g)	Fiber (g)	Fat (g)	Mono (g)	Poly (g)
56762	Green peppers, stuffed w/beef, w/tomato sauce/Stouffer's	0.5 ea	219.5	160	8	19	3	6	2.2	0.4
70917	Hot Pockets beef cheddar pocket sandwich	1 ea	142	403	16	39		20	6.7	1.2
70434	Italian sausage lasagne/The Budget Gourmet	1 ea	298	456	21	40	3	24	9.8	2
56757	Lasagna w/meat sauce, fzn, svg	1 ea	215	249	17	27	2	8	2.8	0.5
70921	Lean Pockets, chicken supreme	1 ea	128	233	10	34		6	2.5	1
11029	Macaroni, w/beef & tomato sauce/Lean Cuisine	1 ea	283	258	17	37	5	4	1.7	0.6
5587	Mashed potatoes, granules w/milk, prep w/water & margarine	0.5 cup	105	122	2	17	1	5	2.1	1.4
11107	Meatloaf w/sauce, potato, carrot/Banquet	1 ea	453	612	29	34	6	40	17.3	7.2
90491	Onion rings, breaded, pan-fried	1 cup	48	195	3	18	1	13	5.2	2.5
70898	Pizza, pepperoni, cooked, svg	1 ea	146	432	16	42	3	22	10	3.4
81146	Sausage w/biscuit sandwich/Jimmy Dean	1 ea	48	192	5	12	1	14		
70935	Salisbury steak w/red potato & vegetables/Budget Gourmet	1 ea	311	261	18	34	7	6	1.8	0.9
56703	Spaghetti, w/meat sauce/Lean Cuisine	1 ea	326	284	14	49	5	4	1.3	0.9
70960	Spaghetti w/meatballs & pomodoro sauce, low fat/Michelina's	1 ea	284	312	14	49	6	7	2.6	1.1
70959	Spinach, au gratin, frozen/The Budget Gourmet	1 ea	155	222	7	11	2	17		
70958	Stir fry rice & vegetables w/soy sauce/Hanover	1 cup	137	130	5	27	2	0		
11099	Swedish meatballs w/pasta/Lean Cuisine	1 ea	258	273	22	31	3	7	2.6	0.9
16930	Turkey, country roast, w/gravy mushroom & rice/Healthy Choice	1 ea	240	223	19	28	3	4	1.8	0.9
70892	Turkey pot pie	1 ea	397	699	26	70	4	35	13.7	5.5
16306	Turkey w/gravy, 5 oz pkg	1 ea	141.8	95	8	7	0	4	1.4	0.7
70936	Turkey w/gravy dressing & broccoli/Marie Callender's	1 ea	397	504	31	52		19	8.2	1.7
6999	Vegetables, mixed, from frozen w/salt, drained, 10 oz pkg	1 ea	275	165	8	36	12	0	0	0.2

SNACK FOODS AND GRANOLA BARS

MDA Code	Food Name	Amt	Wt (g)	Ener (kcal)	Prot (g)	Carb (g)	Fiber (g)	Fat (g)	Mono (g)	Poly (g)
3307	Banana chips	1 oz	28.4	147	1	17	2	10	0.6	0.2
10051	Beef jerky, large piece	1 ea	19.8	81	7	2	0	5	2.2	0.2
10052	Beef meat stick, smoked	1 ea	19.8	109	4	1		10	4.1	0.9
63331	Breakfast bar w/oats, raisins & coconut	1 ea	43	200	4	29	1	8	0.8	0.7
53227	Cereal bar, mixed berry/Kellogg's	1 ea	37	137	2	27	1	3	1.8	0.4
61251	Cheese puffs & twists, corn based, low fat	1 oz	28.4	123	2	21	3	3	1	1.6
44032	Chex snack mix, traditional	1 cup	42.5	181	5	28	2	7		
44034	Corn Nuts, BBQ	1 oz	28.4	124	3	20	2	4	2.1	0.9
44031	Corn Nuts, original	1 oz	28.4	127	2	20	2	4	2.7	0.9
44212	Fruit leather, bar	1 ea	23	81	0	18	1	1	0.1	0
11594	Fruit leather, berry, w/vitamin C/Fruit Roll-Ups	2 ea	28	104	0	24		1	0.5	0
44214	Fruit leather pieces, 0.75 oz package	1 ea	21.3	76	0	18	0	1	0.3	0.1
23404	Fruit leather, roll, large	1 ea	21	78	0	18	0	1	0.3	0.1
23103	Granola bar, peanut butter, hard	1 ea	23.6	114	2	15	1	6	1.7	2.9
23059	Granola bar, plain, hard	1 ea	24.5	115	2	16	1	5	1.1	3
23101	Granola bar, chocolate chip, hard	1 ea	23.6	103	2	17	1	4	0.6	0.3
23096	Granola bar, chocolate chip, chocolate coated, soft, 1.25 oz	1 ea	35.4	165	2	23	1	9	2.8	0.6
23107	Granola bar, nut & raisin, uncoated, soft	1 oz	28.4	129	2	18	2	6	1.2	1.6
23104	Granola bar, plain, uncoated, soft	1 ea	28.4	126	2	19	1	5	1.1	1.5
44036	Oriental mix, rice based	1 oz	28.4	144	5	15	4	7	2.8	3
44022	Popcorn cake	1 ea	10	38	1	8	0	0	0.1	0.1
44012	Popcorn, air popped	1 cup	8	31	1	6	1	0	0.1	0.2
44014	Popcorn, caramel coated, w/o peanuts	1 oz	28.4	122	1	22	1	4	0.8	1.3
44038	Popcorn, cheese flavored	1 cup	11	58	1	6	1	4	1.1	1.7
44066	Popcorn, low fat, low sodium, microwave	1 cup	8	34	1	6	1	1	0.3	0.3
44013	Popcorn, oil popped, microwaved	1 cup	11	64	1	5	1	5	1.1	2.6
61252	Popcorn, sugar syrup/caramel, fat free	1 cup	37.3	142	1	34	1	1	0.1	0.2

Sat (g)	Chol (mg)	Calc (mg)	Iron (mg)	Mag (mg)	Phos (mg)	Pota (mg)	Sodi (mg)	Zinc (mg)	Vit A (RAE)	Vit C (mg)	Thia (mg)	Ribo (mg)	Niac (mg)	Vit B$_6$ (mg)	Vit B$_{12}$ (µg)	Vit E (mg)	Fol (µg)	Alc (g)
2.2	18	37	1.49			347	623			25.7	0.13	0.11	1.4					0
8.8	53	337	2.93				906		0									0
8.2	48	316	2.68				903											0
4.1	28	148	1.31			340	671			1.3	0.13	0.11	1.38					0
1.9	23	122					562		38									0
1.7	17	85	1.78			773	569			2.3	0.2	0.08	3.28					0
1.3	2	36	0.21	21	67	165	180	0.3	49	6.8	0.09	0.09	0.91	0.17	0.11	0.5	8.4	0
15.5	113	77	3.94				1943			7.7								0
4.1	0	15	0.81	9.1	39	62	180	0.2	5	0.7	0.13	0.07	1.73	0.04	0	0.3	31.7	0
7.1	22	220	3.52	35	302	289	902	2.2	0	2.8	0.33	0.34	3.61	0.14	0.83	1.6	68.6	0
4.3	16	38	0.79				441											0
2	44		3.05				494		72	51								0
1.1	13	101	2.38			574	548			2.9	0.33	0.2	3.88					0
2.2	14		2.93				1011		26	8.8								0
7.6	42	243	1.95				654			27.1								0
							636			16.3								0
2.8	49	114	2.58	43.9	206	560	614	3.7	0	0	0.23	0.28	4.21	0.31	1.01	0.3	31.9	0
1.2	26	22	1.03				437											0
11.4	64		3.97				1390		351									0
1.2	26	20	1.32	11.3	115	86	786	1	18	0	0.03	0.18	2.55	0.14	0.34	0.5	5.7	0
9.1	79	131	4.37				2037			23.8								0
0.1	0	69	2.25	60.5	140	465	745	1.3	588	8.8	0.2	0.33	2.34	0.2	0	1.2	52.2	0
8.2	0	5	0.36	21.6	16	152	2	0.2	1	1.8	0.02	0	0.2	0.07	0	0.1	4	0
2.1	10	4	1.07	10.1	81	118	438	1.6	0	0	0.03	0.03	0.34	0.04	0.2	0.1	26.5	0
4.1	26	13	0.67	4.2	36	51	293	0.5	3	1.3	0.03	0.09	0.9	0.04	0.2	0.1	0	0
5.5	0	26	1.37	43.4	119	140	120	0.7	3	0.4	0.12	0.05	0.75	0.15	0	0.4	34.8	0
0.6	0	14	1.81	9.6	36	70	110	1.5		0	0.37	0.41	5	0.52	0	0	40	0
0.6	0	101	0.36	11.6	101	81	365	0.6	12	6.1	0.15	0.17	2.03	0.2	0.61	1.2	27.5	0
2.4	0	15	10.5	26.8	79	114	432	0.9	3	20.2	0.66	0.21	7.16	0.66	5.27	0.1	21.2	0
0.7	0	5	0.48	31	80	81	277	0.5	5	0.1	0.1	0.04	0.43	0.05	0	0.3	0	0
0.7	0	3	0.47	32.1	78	79	156	0.5	0	0	0.01	0.04	0.48	0.07	0	0.6	0	0
0.9	0	7	0.18	5.1	13	32	18	0	1	16.1	0.01	0.01	0.02	0.07	0	0.1	0.9	0
0.3	0						89			33.6								0
0.1	0	4	0.16	3	5	35	86	0	1	11.9	0.01	0.02	0.02	0.06	0	0.1	0.9	0
0.1	0	7	0.21	4.2	7	62	67	0	1	25.2	0.02	0	0.02	0.06	0	0.1	0.4	0
0.8	0	10	0.57	13	33	69	67	0.3	0	0	0.05	0.02	0.46	0.02	0	0.3	4.2	0
0.6	0	15	0.72	23.8	68	82	72	0.5	2	0.2	0.06	0.03	0.39	0.02	0	0.3	5.6	0
2.7	0	18	0.72	17	48	59	81	0.5	0	0	0.04	0.02	0.13	0.01	0	0.2	3.1	0
5	2	36	0.82	23.4	70	111	71	0.5	2	0	0.03	0.09	0.25	0.04	0.2	0.4	9.2	0
2.7	0	24	0.62	25.8	68	111	72	0.5	1	0	0.05	0.05	0.74	0.03	0.07	0.3	8.5	0
2.1	0	30	0.73	21	65	92	79	0.4	0	0	0.08	0.05	0.15	0.03	0.11	0.3	6.8	0
1.1	0	15	0.69	33.5	74	93	117	0.8	0	0.1	0.09	0.04	0.88	0.02	0	1.6	10.8	0
0	0	1	0.19	15.9	28	33	29	0.4	0	0	0.01	0.02	0.6	0.02	0	0	1.8	0
0	0	1	0.26	11.5	29	26	1	0.2	1	0	0.01	0.01	0.18	0.01	0	0	2.5	0
1	1	12	0.49	9.9	24	31	59	0.2	1	0	0.02	0.02	0.62	0.01	0	0.3	1.4	0
0.7	1	12	0.25	10	40	29	98	0.2	4	0.1	0.01	0.03	0.16	0.03	0.06	0	1.2	0
0.1	0	1	0.18	12.1	21	19	39	0.3	1	0	0.03	0.01	0.17	0.01	0	0.4	1.4	0
0.8	0	0	0.22	8.7	22	20	116	0.3	1	0	0.01	0.01	0.13	0.01	0	0.3	2.8	0
0.1	0	7	0.3	10.1	21	41	107	0.2	1	0	0.01	0.02	0.13	0.02	0	0	1.5	0

MDA Code	Food Name	Amt	Wt (g)	Ener (kcal)	Prot (g)	Carb (g)	Fiber (g)	Fat (g)	Mono (g)	Poly (g)
12080	Pork skins, plain	1 oz	28	153	17	0	0	9	4.1	1
61249	Potato chips, fat free, w/olestra	1 oz	28	77	2	17	2	0	0	0.1
44043	Potato chips, reduced fat	1 oz	28.4	134	2	19	2	6	1.4	3.1
44076	Potato chips, unsalted, plain	1 oz	28.4	152	2	15	1	10	2.8	3.5
5437	Potato chips, sour cream & onion	1 oz	28.4	151	2	15	1	10	1.7	4.9
61257	Potato chips, reduced fat, unsalted	1 oz	28.4	138	2	19	2	6	1.4	3.1
44015	Pretzels, hard	5 pce	30	114	3	24	1	1	0.4	0.2
44079	Pretzels, hard, unsalted, w/enriched flour	10 ea	60	229	5	48	2	2	0.8	0.7
61182	Pretzels, soft, medium	1 ea	115	389	9	80	2	4	1.2	1.1
44053	Rice cake, brown rice & sesame seed	2 ea	18	71	1	15	1	1	0.2	0.2
44021	Rice cake, brown rice, plain	1 ea	9	35	1	7	0	0	0.1	0.1
44020	Taro chips	1 oz	28.4	141	1	19	2	7	1.3	3.7
44058	Trail mix, regular	0.25 cup	37.5	173	5	17	2	11	4.7	3.6
44059	Trail mix, w/chocolate chips, salted nuts & seeds	0.25 cup	36.2	175	5	16	2	12	4.9	4.1

SOUPS

MDA Code	Food Name	Amt	Wt (g)	Ener (kcal)	Prot (g)	Carb (g)	Fiber (g)	Fat (g)	Mono (g)	Poly (g)
92160	Bean & ham, canned, reduced sodium, prepared w/water	0.5 cup	128	95	5	17	5	1	0.5	0.3
50151	Bean & bacon, dehydrated, prepared w/water	1 cup	265	106	5	16	9	2	0.9	0.2
92192	Beef & mushroom, canned, chunky, low sodium	1 cup	251	173	11	24	1	6	1	0.2
50398	Beef barley, canned, ready-to-serve/Progresso	1 cup	241	142	11	20	3	2	0.7	0.3
50198	Beef mushroom, canned, prepared w/water	1 cup	244	73	6	6	0	3	1.2	0.1
57659	Beef stew, canned, serving	1 ea	232	220	11	16	3	12	5.5	0.5
50155	Cauliflower, dehydrated, prepared w/water	1 cup	256.1	69	3	11		2	0.7	0.6
50077	Chicken gumbo, canned, prepared w/water	1 cup	244	56	3	8	2	1	0.7	0.3
50080	Chicken mushroom, canned, prepared w/water	1 cup	244	132	4	9	0	9	4	2.3
50081	Chicken noodle, canned, chunky, ready-to-serve	1 cup	240	175	13	17	4	6	2.7	1.5
50085	Chicken rice, canned, chunky, ready-to-serve	1 cup	240	127	12	13	1	3	1.4	0.7
50088	Chicken vegetable, canned, chunky, ready-to-serve	1 cup	240	166	12	19	0	5	2.2	1
90238	Chicken, canned, chunky	1 cup	240	170	12	17	1	6	2.8	1.3
50021	Clam chowder, Manhattan style, canned, prepared w/water	1 cup	244	78	2	12	1	2	0.4	1.3
50402	Cream of broccoli, canned/Progresso Healthy Classics	1 cup	244	88	2	13	2	3	0.9	0.6
50016	Cream of celery, canned, prepared w/water	1 cup	244	90	2	9	1	6	1.3	2.5
50049	Cream of mushroom, canned, prepared w/water	1 cup	244	129	2	9	0	9	1.7	4.2
50197	Cream of potato, canned, prepared w/water	1 cup	244	73	2	11	0	2	0.6	0.4
50697	Cup of Noodles, ramen noodle soup, chicken flavor, dry	1 ea	64	296	6	37		14		
50050	Green pea, canned, prepared w/water	1 cup	250	165	9	27	5	3	1	0.4
50009	Minestrone, canned, prepared w/water	1 cup	241	82	4	11	1	3	0.7	1.1
92163	Ramen noodle soup, any flavor, dry	0.5 cup	38	172	4	25	1	6	2.4	1
50690	Shark fin soup, restaurant prepared	1 cup	216	99	7	8	0	4	1.3	0.7
50025	Split pea soup, w/ham, canned, prepared w/water	1 cup	253	190	10	28	2	4	1.8	0.6
50689	Stock, fish, homemade	1 cup	233	40	5	0	0	2	0.5	0.3
50043	Tomato vegetable, from dry mix, w/water	1 cup	253	56	2	10	1	1	0.3	0.1
50028	Tomato, canned, prepared w/water	1 cup	244	85	2	17	0	2	0.4	1
50014	Vegetable beef, canned, prepared w/water	1 cup	244	78	6	10	0	2	0.8	0.1
92189	Vegetable chicken, low sodium	1 cup	241	166	12	21	1	5	2.2	1
7559	Vegetarian stew	1 cup	247	304	42	17	3	7	1.8	3.8
50013	Vegetable, vegetarian, canned, prepared w/water	1 cup	241	72	2	12	0	2	0.8	0.7

BABY FOODS

MDA Code	Food Name	Amt	Wt (g)	Ener (kcal)	Prot (g)	Carb (g)	Fiber (g)	Fat (g)	Mono (g)	Poly (g)
61234	Infant cereal, brown rice, instant	1 Tbs	3.7	15	0	3	0	0	0	0
60619	Infant cereal, rice, dry	1 Tbs	2.5	10	0	2	0	0	0	0.1
60844	Infant cookie, banana/Gerber	1 ea	8	34	1	6	0	1		

Sat (g)	Chol (mg)	Calc (mg)	Iron (mg)	Mag (mg)	Phos (mg)	Pota (mg)	Sodi (mg)	Zinc (mg)	Vit A (RAE)	Vit C (mg)	Thia (mg)	Ribo (mg)	Niac (mg)	Vit B$_6$ (mg)	Vit B$_{12}$ (µg)	Vit E (mg)	Fol (µg)	Alc (g)
3.2	27	8	0.25	3.1	24	36	515	0.2	3	0.1	0.03	0.08	0.43	0.01	0.18	0.1	0	0
0.1	0	10	0.67	19.3	49	325	155	1	0	7.9	0.09	0.01	1.22	0.04	0	0	23.2	0
1.2	0	6	0.38	25.3	55	495	140	0	0	7.3	0.06	0.08	1.99	0.19	0	1.6	7.7	0
3.1	0	7	0.46	19	47	362	2	0.3	0	8.8	0.05	0.06	1.09	0.19	0	2.6	12.8	0
2.5	2	20	0.45	21	50	378	178	0.3	4	10.6	0.05	0.06	1.14	0.19	0.28	1.4	17.6	0
1.2	0	6	0.38	25.3	55	495	2	0.3	0	7.3	0.06	0.08	1.99	0.19	0	1.6	2.8	0
0.1	0	5	1.56	8.7	34	41	407	0.4	0	0	0.15	0.1	1.54	0.01	0	0.1	55.8	0
0.4	0	22	2.59	21	68	88	173	0.5	0	0	0.28	0.37	3.15	0.07	0	0.2	102.6	0
0.8	3	26	4.51	24.2	91	101	1615	1.1	0	0	0.47	0.33	4.91	0.02	0	0.6	27.6	0
0.1	0	2	0.28	24.5	68	52	41	0.5	0	0.5	0.01	0.02	1.3	0.03	0	0	3.2	0
0.1	0	1	0.13	11.8	32	26	29	0.3	0	0	0.01	0.01	0.7	0.01	0	0.1	1.9	0
1.8	0	17	0.34	23.9	37	214	97	0.1	2	1.4	0.05	0.01	0.15	0.12	0	3.2	5.7	0
2.1	0	29	1.14	59.2	129	257	86	1.2	0	0.5	0.17	0.07	1.77	0.11	0	1.3	26.6	0
2.2	1	39	1.23	58.3	140	235	44	1.1	1	0.5	0.15	0.08	1.59	0.09	0	3.9	23.5	0
0.3	3	49	1.31	24.3	17	202	239	0.7	45	1.4	0.07	0.04	0.41	0.06	0.04	0.5	37.1	0
1	3	56	1.32	29.2	90	326	928	0.7	3	1.1	0.05	0.27	0.4	0.03	0.03	0.6	8	0
4.1	15	33	2.43	5	126	351	63	2.8	246	7.5	0.1	0.28	2.84	0.15	0.65	0.6	12.6	0
0.7	19	29	1.86	31.3	118	366	470	1.5		3.6	0.13	0.13	2.92	0.19	0.36	0.3	24.1	0
1.5	7	5	0.88	9.8	34	154	942	1.5	0	4.6	0.04	0.06	0.95	0.05	0.2		9.8	0
5.2	37	28	1.65	32.5	128	404	947	1.9	204	10.2	0.17	0.14	2.86	0.3	0.86	0.3	25.5	0
0.3	0	10	0.51	2.6	51	105	843	0.3	0	2.6	0.08	0.08	0.51	0.03	0.18		2.6	0
0.3	5	24	0.9	4.9	24	76	954	0.4	7	4.9	0.02	0.05	0.66	0.06	0.02	0.4	4.9	0
2.4	10	29	0.88	9.8	27	154	942	1	56	0	0.02	0.11	1.63	0.05	0.05	1.2	0	0
1.4	19	24	1.44	9.6	72	108	850	1	67	0	0.07	0.17	4.32	0.05	0.31	0.3	38.4	0
1	12	34	1.87	9.6	72	108	888	1	293	3.8	0.02	0.1	4.1	0.05	0.31	0.6	4.8	0
1.4	17	26	1.46	9.6	106	367	1068	2.2	300	5.5	0.04	0.17	3.29	0.1	0.24	0.1	12	0
1.9	29	24	1.66	7.2	108	168	850	1	65	1.2	0.08	0.17	4.22	0.05	0.24	0.3	4.8	0
0.4	2	27	1.63	12.2	41	188	578	1	56	3.9	0.03	0.04	0.82	0.1	4.05	0.3	9.8	0
0.7	5	41	1.22	14.6	39	161	578	0.3		5.9	0.03	0.06	0.32	0.07	0	0.4	29.3	0
1.4	15	39	0.63	7.3	37	122	949	0.1	56	0.2	0.03	0.05	0.33	0.01	0.24	0.9	2.4	0
2.4	2	46	0.51	4.9	49	100	881	0.6	15	1	0.05	0.09	0.72	0.01	0.05	1	4.9	0
1.2	5	20	0.49	2.4	46	137	1000	0.6	71	0	0.03	0.04	0.54	0.04	0.05	0	2.4	0
6.3			2.18				1434		20									0
1.4	0	28	1.95	40	125	190	918	1.7	10	1.7	0.11	0.07	1.24	0.05	0	0.4	2.5	0
0.6	2	34	0.92	7.2	55	313	911	0.7	118	1.2	0.05	0.04	0.94	0.1	0	0.1	36.2	0
2.9	0	6	1.62	9.1	41	46	441	0.2	0	0	0.25	0.17	2.05	0.02	0	0.8	55.9	0
1.1	4	22	2.03	15.1	45	114	1082	1.8	0	0.2	0.06	0.08	1.06	0.06	0.41	6.9	19.4	0
1.8	8	23	2.28	48.1	213	400	1007	1.3	23	1.5	0.15	0.08	1.47	0.07	0.25	0.2	2.5	0
0.5	2	7	0.02	16.3	130	336	363	0.1	5	0.2	0.08	0.18	2.76	0.09	1.61	0.4	4.7	0
0.4	0	8	0.63	20.2	30	104	1146	0.2	10	6.1	0.06	0.05	0.79	0.05	0	0.4	10.1	0
0.4	0	12	1.76	7.3	34	264	695	0.2	24	66.4	0.09	0.05	1.42	0.11	0	2.3	14.6	0
0.9	5	17	1.12	4.9	41	173	791	1.5	95	2.4	0.04	0.05	1.03	0.08	0.32	0.4	9.8	0
1.4	17	27	1.47	9.6	106	369	84	2.2	333	5.5	0.05	0.17	3.3	0.1	0.24	0.7	43.4	0
1.2	0	77	3.21	313.7	543	296	988	2.7	116	0	1.73	1.48	29.64	2.72	5.43	1.2	254.4	0
0.3	0	22	1.08	7.2	34	210	822	0.5	116	1.4	0.05	0.05	0.92	0.06	0	0.4	9.6	0
0	0	2	1.76	1	10	14	0	0	0	0	0.03	0.01	0.59	0.04	0	0	0.6	0
0	0	21	1.19	5.2	15	10	1	0	0	0.1	0.07	0.06	0.78	0.01	0	0.1	0.6	0
0.2		120	3	2.8	14	33	1	2.4	122	0.1	0.03	0.03	1.35	0.02		2		0

MDA Code	Food Name	Amt	Wt (g)	Ener (kcal)	Prot (g)	Carb (g)	Fiber (g)	Fat (g)	Mono (g)	Poly (g)
60419	Infant dessert, apricot tapioca—Nature's Goodness	6.25 Tbs	100	66	0	16	0	0		
60192	Infant dessert, vanilla custard pudding/3rd Foods	1 ea	170	163	4	31		3		
60778	Infant dinner, beef & carrots, strained/Heinz	1 ea	113.4	64	4	4	2	4		
60871	Infant dinner, broccoli chicken, strained	1 ea	113.4	48	4	4	2	2	0.6	0.4
60793	Infant vegetable, peas, strained/Nature's Goodness	1 ea	113.4	65	5	11	4	0		
62354	Infant formula, Lactofree, w/iron/Mead Johnson	0.125 cup	30.5	19	0	2	0	1	0.4	0.2
60135	Infant formula, low iron/Similac	1 fl-oz	31	20	0	2	0	1	0.4	0.2
60299	Infant formula, soy, w/iron/Isomil	1 fl-oz	30.5	20	0	2	0	1	0.4	0.3
62586	Child formula, soy, preppowder/Enfamil	1 fl-oz	30.5	20	1	2	0	1	0.3	0.2

DESSERTS, CANDIES, AND PASTRIES

Brownies and Fudge

MDA Code	Food Name	Amt	Wt (g)	Ener (kcal)	Prot (g)	Carb (g)	Fiber (g)	Fat (g)	Mono (g)	Poly (g)
62904	Brownie, square, large, 2-3/4" × 7/8"	1 ea	56	227	3	36	1	9	5	1.3
47019	Brownie, homemade, 2" square	1 ea	24	112	1	12	1	7	2.6	2.3
23127	Fudge, chocolate marshmallow, w/nuts, homemade	1 pce	22	104	1	15	0	5	1.2	0.9
23026	Fudge, chocolate, w/nuts, homemade	1 pce	19	88	1	13	0	4	0.7	1.4
23025	Fudge, chocolate, homemade	1 pce	17	70	0	13	0	2	0.5	0

Cakes, Pies, and Donuts

MDA Code	Food Name	Amt	Wt (g)	Ener (kcal)	Prot (g)	Carb (g)	Fiber (g)	Fat (g)	Mono (g)	Poly (g)
46062	Cake, chocolate, homemade, w/o frosting, 9"	1 pce	95	340	5	51	2	14	5.7	2.6
46092	Coffee cake, w/cheese, 1/6 of 16 oz	1 pce	76	258	5	34	1	12	5.4	1.3
46096	Coffee cake, creme filled, w/chocolate frosting, 1/6 of 19 oz	1 pce	90	298	4	48	2	10	5.1	1.3
46003	Cake, white, w/coconut frosting, homemade, 1/12 of 9"	1 pce	112	399	5	71	1	12	4.1	2.4
46085	Cake, white, w/o frosting, homemade, 9"	1 pce	74	264	4	42	1	9	3.9	2.3
46091	Cake, yellow, w/o frosting, homemade, 8"	1 pce	68	245	4	36	0	10	4.2	2.4
49001	Cheesecake, no bake, from dry mix, 1/12 of 9"	1 pce	99	271	5	35	2	13	4.5	0.8
46426	Cupcake, chocolate, w/frosting, low fat	1 ea	43	131	2	29	2	2	0.8	0.2
46011	Cupcake, snack, chocolate, w/frosting & cream filling	1 ea	50	200	2	30	2	8	4.3	0.9
42721	Ding Dongs, w/cream filling/Hostess	1 ea	80	368	3	45	2	19	4	1.2
71338	Doughnut, chocolate, glazed/sugared, 3-3/4"	1 ea	60	250	3	34	1	12	6.8	1.5
71337	Doughnut, w/chocolate icing, large, 3-1/2"	1 ea	57	258	3	29	1	14	4.9	1.1
45525	Doughnut, glazed/sugared, medium, 3"	1 ea	45	192	2	23	1	10	5.7	1.3
71335	Doughnut holes	1 ea	14	59	1	6	0	3	1.8	0.4
45527	Doughnut, French crullers, glazed, 3"	1 ea	41	169	1	24	0	8	4.3	0.9
45563	Doughnut, creme filled, 3-1/2" oval	1 ea	85	307	5	26	1	21	10.3	2.6
46000	Gingerbread, homemade, 1/9 of 8" square	1 pce	74	263	3	36	1	12	5.3	3.1
46001	Sponge cake, 1/12 of 16 oz	1 pce	38	110	2	23	0	1	0.4	0.2
48044	Pie filling, pumpkin, canned	0.5 cup	135	140	1	36	11	0	0	0

Candy

MDA Code	Food Name	Amt	Wt (g)	Ener (kcal)	Prot (g)	Carb (g)	Fiber (g)	Fat (g)	Mono (g)	Poly (g)
51150	Candied fruit	1 oz	28.4	91	0	23	0	0	0	0
23074	Candy, hard, dietetic/low calorie	1 pce	3	11	0	3	0	0	0	0
4148	Candy, Bit O Honey/Nestle	6 pce	40	150	1	32	0	3	0.4	0.1
23115	Candy, butterscotch	5 pce	30	117	0	27	0	1	0.3	0
23015	Candy, caramels	1 pce	10.1	39	0	8	0	1	0.2	0.4
92202	Candy, caramel, w/nuts, chocolate covered	1 ea	14	66	1	8	1	3	1.3	0.8
90671	Candy, jellybeans, large	10 ea	28.4	106	0	27	0	0		
90690	Candy, M & M's milk chocolate peanut, 1.67 oz pkg	1 ea	47.3	244	5	29	2	12	3.8	1.6
90691	Candy, M & M's milk chocolate, 1.48 oz box	1 ea	42	207	2	30	1	9	1.4	0.2
92212	Candy, milk chocolate covered coffee beans	1 oz	28.4	146	2	18	2	7	1.7	0.2
23419	Candy, milk chocolate covered peanuts	10 pce	40	208	5	20	2	13	5.2	1.7
23022	Candy, milk chocolate covered raisins	1.5 oz	42.5	166	2	29	2	6	2	0.2
90682	Candy, milk chocolate w/almonds, 1.55 oz bar	1 ea	43.9	231	4	23	3	15	5.9	1

Sat (g)	Chol (mg)	Calc (mg)	Iron (mg)	Mag (mg)	Phos (mg)	Pota (mg)	Sodi (mg)	Zinc (mg)	Vit A (RAE)	Vit C (mg)	Thia (mg)	Ribo (mg)	Niac (mg)	Vit B$_6$ (mg)	Vit B$_{12}$ (µg)	Vit E (mg)	Fol (µg)	Alc (g)
0		9	0.25		6	63	9	0		61.6	0.02	0.01	0.14	0.01				0
		95	0.51	9.9	114	112	42	0.7			0.03	0.15	0.12	0.05				0
		27	0.54		39	164	16			0.3	0.02	0.05	0.83	0.08				0
0.5	7	46	0.65	13.6	67	192	22	0.7	26	21.5	0.02	0.1	0.88	0.1	0.01	1	51	0
0.1		22	1		78	136	2		23	0	0.11	0.09	1.35					0
0.5	0	16	0.36	1.5	11	22	6	0.2	18	2.4	0.02	0.03	0.2	0.01	0.06	0.3	3.4	0
0.4	1	16	0.04	1.2	9	21	5	0.2	18	1.8	0.02	0.03	0.21	0.01	0.05	0.4	3.1	0
0.4	0	21	0.36	1.5	15	22	9	0.1	18	1.8	0.01	0.02	0.27	0.01	0.09	0.4	3	0
0.4	0	39	0.4	2.1	26	24	7	0.2	18	2.4	0.02	0.02	0.2	0.01	0.06	0.3	3.4	0
2.4	10	16	1.26	17.4	57	83	175	0.4	11	0	0.14	0.12	0.96	0.02	0.04	0.1	26.3	0
1.8	18	14	0.44	12.7	32	42	82	0.2	42	0.1	0.03	0.05	0.24	0.02	0.04	0.7	7	0
2.3	5	11	0.24	10.1	19	37	17	0.2	15	0.1	0.01	0.02	0.05	0.01	0.01	0.2	2.4	0
1.1	2	10	0.37	10.4	21	34	8	0.3	7	0	0.01	0.02	0.06	0.02	0.01	0	3	0
1	2	8	0.3	6.1	12	22	8	0.2	7	0	0	0.01	0.03	0	0.02	0	0.7	0
5.2	55	57	1.53	30.4	101	133	299	0.7	38	0.2	0.13	0.2	1.08	0.04	0.15	1.5	25.6	0
4.1	65	45	0.49	11.4	77	220	258	0.4	65	0.1	0.08	0.1	0.52	0.04	0.26	1.2	29.6	0
2.5	62	34	0.46	13.5	68	70	291	0.4	33	0.1	0.07	0.07	0.76	0.04	0.18	1.6	36.9	0
4.4	1	101	1.3	13.4	78	111	318	0.4	14	0.1	0.14	0.21	1.19	0.03	0.07	0.1	34.7	0
2.4	1	96	1.12	8.9	69	70	242	0.2	11	0.1	0.14	0.18	1.13	0.02	0.06	0.1	28.1	0
2.7	37	99	1.12	8.2	80	62	233	0.3	27	0.1	0.12	0.16	0.99	0.02	0.11	0.8	23.1	0
6.6	29	170	0.47	18.8	232	209	376	0.5	95	0.5	0.12	0.26	0.49	0.05	0.31	1.1	29.7	0
0.5	0	15	0.66	10.8	79	96	178	0.2	0	0	0.02	0.06	0.31	0	0	0.8	6.4	0
2.4	0	58	1.8	18	44	88	194	0.5	0	0.9	0.02	0.04	0.46	0.07	0.03	0.5	13	0
11	14	3	1.84				241											0
3.1	34	128	1.36	20.4	97	64	204	0.3	7	0.1	0.03	0.04	0.28	0.02	0.06	0.1	27	0
7.7	11	14	2.28	17.1	120	115	235	0.6	2	0.7	0.09	0.07	0.91	0.01	0.06	1.2	37	0
2.7	14	27	0.48	7.6	53	46	181	0.2	1	0	0.1	0.09	0.68	0.01	0.11	0.4	20.7	0
1	1	4	0.42	2.2	37	16	78	0.1	0	0.2	0.03	0.02	0.28	0	0.01	0.3	11.2	0
1.9	5	11	0.99	4.9	50	32	141	0.1	1	0	0.07	0.09	0.87	0.01	0.02	0.1	17.2	0
4.6	20	21	1.56	17	65	68	263	0.7	10	0	0.29	0.13	1.91	0.06	0.12	0.2	59.5	0
3.1	24	53	2.13	51.8	40	325	242	0.3	10	0.1	0.14	0.12	1.29	0.14	0.04	1.8	24.4	0
0.3	39	27	1.03	4.2	52	38	93	0.2	17	0	0.09	0.1	0.73	0.02	0.09	0.1	17.9	0
0.1	0	50	1.43	21.6	61	186	281	0.4	560	4.7	0.02	0.16	0.5	0.21	0	1.1	47.2	0
0	0	5	0.05	1.1	1	16	28	0	0	0	0	0	0	0	0	0	0	0
0	0	0	0	0	0	0	0	0	0	0	0	0	0	0	0	0	0	0
2.2	0	14	0.08	2.8	11	18	118	0.2	0	0.3	0.02	0.02	0.03	0	0.02	0.1	0.8	0
0.6	3	1	0	0	0	1	117	0	8	0	0	0	0	0	0	0	0	0
0.3	1	14	0.01	1.7	12	22	25	0	1	0	0.01	0.03	0.01	0.01	0.03	0	0.4	0
0.7	0	11	0.24	11.3	23	62	3	0.3	6	0.2	0.01	0.02	0.67	0.02	0	0.2	12.9	0
	0	1	0.04	0.6	1	11	14	0	0	0	0	0	0	0	0	0	0	0
4.8	4	48	0.55	32.6	90	164	24	0.8	10	0	0.03	0.05	1.59	0.04	0.15	1.3	26	0
5.5	6	44	0.47	18.9	62	112	26	0.6	24	0.2	0.03	0.09	0.12	0.01	0.18	0.6	3.4	0
3.5	6	48	0.65	18.2	53	117	20	0.5	12	0	0.03	0.09	0.09	0.01	0.15	0.5	2.8	0
5.8	4	42	0.52	38.4	85	201	16	1	14	0	0.05	0.07	1.7	0.08	0.18	1.4	3.2	0
3.7	1	37	0.73	19.1	61	218	15	0.3	10	0.1	0.04	0.07	0.17	0.03	0.08	0.4	3	0
7.5	8	98	0.72	39.5	116	195	32	0.6	19	0.1	0.03	0.19	0.33	0.02	0.14	2	6.1	0

MDA Code	Food Name	Amt	Wt (g)	Ener (kcal)	Prot (g)	Carb (g)	Fiber (g)	Fat (g)	Mono (g)	Poly (g)
91509	Candy, milk chocolate, w/almonds, bites/Hershey's Bites	17 pce	39	214	4	20	1	14	5.6	0.9
92201	Candy, nougat w/almonds	1 ea	14	56	0	13	0	0	0	0
23081	Candy, peanut brittle, homemade	1.5 oz	42.5	207	3	30	1	8	3.4	1.9
90698	Candy, Rolo, caramels in milk chocolate, 1.74 oz roll	1 ea	49.3	234	3	33	0	10	1	0.1
23142	Candy, sesame crunch	20 pce	35	181	4	18	3	12	4.4	5.1
90702	Candy, Starburst, fruit chews, original	1 oz	28.4	116	0	23	0	2	0	0
92198	Candy, Twizzlers strawberry twists	4 pce	45	158	1	36	0	1		
90661	Candy, York peppermint patty, small, .6 oz	1 ea	17	65	0	14	0	1	0.1	0
90681	Candy bar, milk chocolate, mini	1 ea	7	37	1	4	0	2	0.9	0.1
90685	Candy bar, milk chocolate, w/crisped rice, mini	1 ea	10	50	1	6	0	3	0.9	0.1
23145	Candy bar, sweet chocolate, 1.45 oz bar	1 ea	41.1	208	2	24	2	14	4.6	0.4
90704	Candy bar, 3 Musketeers, 0.8 oz bar	1 ea	22.7	97	1	18	0	3	0.5	0.1
23405	Candy bar, Almond Joy, fun size, .7 oz	1 ea	19.8	95	1	12	1	5	1	0.2
90679	Candy bar, Baby Ruth, 2.28 oz bar	1 ea	64.6	297	3	42	1	14	3.6	1.7
90653	Candy bar, Butterfinger, 1.6 oz bar	1 ea	45.4	208	2	33	1	9	2.3	1.4
23116	Candy bar, Caramello, 1.6 oz bar	1 ea	45.4	210	3	29	1	10	2.4	0.3
23060	Candy bar, Kit Kat, 1.5 oz bar	1 ea	42.5	220	3	27	0	11	2.5	0.4
23061	Candy bar, Krackel, 1.5 oz bar	1 ea	42.5	218	3	27	1	11	2.7	0.2
23037	Candy bar, Mars almond, 1.76 oz bar	1 ea	50	234	4	31	1	12	5.3	2
90688	Candy bar, Milky Way, 2.05 oz bar	1 ea	58.1	263	2	41	1	10	1.3	0.2
23062	Candy bar, Mr. Goodbar, 1.75 oz bar	1 ea	49.6	267	5	27	2	16	4.1	2.2
23135	Candy bar, Oh Henry!, 2 oz bar	1 ea	56.7	262	4	37	1	13	3.1	1.5
23036	Candy bar, Skor, toffee bar, 1.4 oz bar	1 ea	39.7	212	1	25	1	13	3.7	0.5
23057	Candy bar, Special Dark, sweet chocolate, 1.45 oz bar	1 ea	41.1	218	2	24	3	13	2.1	0.2
23149	Candy bar, Twix, caramel, 2 oz pkg	1 ea	56.7	285	3	37	1	14	1.2	0.2
90712	Chewing gum, small pieces	10 pce	16	40	0	11	0	0	0	0

Cookies

MDA Code	Food Name	Amt	Wt (g)	Ener (kcal)	Prot (g)	Carb (g)	Fiber (g)	Fat (g)	Mono (g)	Poly (g)
47026	Animal crackers	10 ea	12.5	56	1	9	0	2	1	0.2
90636	Chocolate chip cookie, enriched, higher fat, large 3.5"-4"	1 ea	40	196	2	26	1	10	5.3	0.6
47037	Chocolate chip cookie, homemade w/butter, 2-1/4"	2 ea	32	156	2	19	1	9	2.6	1.5
47032	Chocolate chip cookie, lower fat	3 ea	30	136	2	22	1	5	1.8	1.4
47001	Chocolate chip cookie, soft	2 ea	30	137	1	18	1	7	3.9	1
43527	Chocolate coated graham crackers, 2-1/2" square	2 ea	28	136	2	19	1	6	2.2	0.3
47006	Chocolate sandwich cookie, creme filled	3 ea	30	140	2	21	1	6	3.2	0.7
47042	Coconut macaroon, homemade, 2"	1 ea	24	97	1	17	0	3	0.1	0
62905	Fig bar	1 ea	56.7	197	2	40	3	4	1.7	1.6
47043	Fortune cookie	3 ea	24	91	1	20	0	1	0.3	0.1
90638	Gingersnap, large, 3-1/2" to 4"	1 ea	32	133	2	25	1	3	1.7	0.4
71272	Graham crackers, cinnamon, small rectangle pieces	4 ea	14	59	1	11	0	1	0.6	0.5
45787	Little Debbie Nutty Bars wafer, w/peanut butter, chocolate covered	1 ea	57	312	5	31		19		
90639	Molasses cookie, large, 3-1/2" to 4"	1 ea	32	138	2	24	0	4	2.3	0.6
47706	Molasses cookie, home style/Archway	1 ea	26	105	1	18	0	3	1.3	0.3
90640	Oatmeal cookie, big, 3-1/2" to 4"	1 ea	25	112	2	17	1	5	2.5	0.6
47003	Oatmeal raisin cookie, homemade, 2-5/8"	1 ea	15	65	1	10	0	2	1	0.8
47010	Peanut butter cookie, homemade, 3"	1 ea	20	95	2	12	0	5	2.2	1.4
47549	Peanut butter cookie, home style/Archway	1 ea	21	101	2	12	1	5	2.1	0.9
47059	Peanut butter sandwich cookie	2 ea	28	134	2	18	1	6	3.1	1.1
47062	Shortbread pecan cookie, 2"	2 ea	28	152	1	16	1	9	5.2	1.2
47007	Shortbread cookie, plain, 1-5/8" square	4 ea	32	161	2	21	1	8	4.3	1
47559	Sugar cookie, home style/Archway	1 ea	24	99	1	17	0	3	1.2	0.3

Sat (g)	Chol (mg)	Calc (mg)	Iron (mg)	Mag (mg)	Phos (mg)	Pota (mg)	Sodi (mg)	Zinc (mg)	Vit A (RAE)	Vit C (mg)	Thia (mg)	Ribo (mg)	Niac (mg)	Vit B$_6$ (mg)	Vit B$_{12}$ (µg)	Vit E (mg)	Fol (µg)	Alc (g)
6.8	7	86	0.58	23	89	184	29	0.5		0.7	0.03	0.15	0.24	0.03		0.2	6.2	0
0.2	0	4	0.08	4.5	8	15	5	0.1	0	0	0	0.02	0.07	0		0.4	0.7	0
1.8	5	11	0.52	17.8	45	71	189	0.4	17	0	0.06	0.02	1.12	0.03	0	1.1	19.6	0
7.2	6	71	0.21	0	35	93	93	0	17	0.4	0.01	0.06	0.02	0	0.16	0.5	0	0
1.6	0	229	1.49	87.8	148	113	58	1.3	0	0	0.19	0.06	1.3	0.19	0	0.1	18.2	0
2.2	0	0	0	0.3	1	1	1	0		16.7	0	0	0	0	0	0.1	0.3	0
0	0	0	0.23				129		0	0								0
0.7	0	2	0.16	10.7	0	19	5	0.1		0	0.01	0.02	0.14			0	0	0
1	2	13	0.16	4.4	15	26	6	0.1	3	0	0.01	0.02	0.03	0	0.04	0.1	0.8	0
1.6	2	17	0.08	4.9	19	34	14	0.1	6	0	0.01	0.03	0.05	0.01	0.06	0.2	1.5	0
8.3	0	10	1.13	46.4	60	119	7	0.6	0	0	0.01	0.1	0.28	0.02	0	0.1	1.2	0
2	1	12	0.15	6.6	16	30	44	0.1	5	0	0.01	0.01	0.05	0	0.04	0.2	0.9	0
3.5	1	13	0.25	13.1	22	50	28	0.2		0.1	0.01	0.03	0.09	0.01	0.02	0		0
7.8	0	30	0.41	27.8	61	161	149	0.5	0	0	0.04	0.08	0.81	0.03	0.04	0.6	7.8	0
4.3	0	16	0.36	21.8	44	100	104	0.5	0	0	0.05	0.03	1.2	0.03	0.02	0.8	12.7	0
5.8	12	97	0.49	19.1	68	155	55	0.4		0.8	0.02	0.18	0.52	0.02	0.29	0.1		0
7.6	5	53	0.42	15.7	57	98	23	0	10	0	0.05	0.09	0.21	0.01	0.24	0.1	6	0
6.8	5	67	0.45	5.5	52	138	83	0.2		0.3	0.02	0.08	0.11	0.02	0.25	0	2.6	0
3.6	8	84	0.55	36	117	162	85	0.6	8	0.3	0.02	0.16	0.47	0.03	0.18	3.9	4.5	0
7	5	67	0.28	11.6	39	72	97	0.4	19	0.4	0.03	0.08	0.09	0.01	0.1	0.5	2.3	0
7	5	55	0.69	23.3	81	195	20	0.5	17	0.4	0.07	0.07	1.71	0.03	0.16	1.6	18.8	0
5.4	4	39	0.28	28.9	79	147	109	0.7	0	0	0.08	0.07	1.44	0.05	0.11	1.3	24.9	0
7.5	21	52	0.23	4	24	61	126	0.1		0.2	0.01	0.04	0.05	0.01	0.11	0	1.2	0
	2	12	0.88	12.7	21	206	2	0	0	0	0	0	0	0	0	0.1	0	0
10.8	4	60	0.46	15.3	60	105	112	0.5	12	0.3	0.09	0.12	0.63	0.01	0.16	0.7	14.7	0
0	0	0	0	0	0	0	0	0	0	0	0	0	0	0	0	0	0	0
0.4	0	5	0.34	2.2	14	12	49	0.1	0	0	0.04	0.04	0.43	0	0.01	0	12.9	0
3.1	0	14	1.43	19.2	46	59	119	0.3	0	0	0.1	0.09	0.96	0.02	0	0.6	25.2	0
4.5	22	12	0.79	17.6	32	71	109	0.3	44	0.1	0.06	0.06	0.44	0.03	0.03	0.3	10.6	0
1.1	0	6	0.92	8.4	25	37	113	0.2	0	0	0.09	0.08	0.83	0.08	0	0.5	21	0
2.2	0	4	0.72	10.5	15	28	98	0.1	0	0	0.03	0.06	0.49	0.05	0	0.9	11.7	0
3.7	0	16	1	16.2	38	59	81	0.3	1	0	0.04	0.06	0.61	0.02	0	0.1	5.6	0
1.1	0	6	1.18	14.4	28	56	145	0.3	0	0	0.05	0.04	0.8	0	0.01	0.5	15.9	0
2.7	0	2	0.18	5	10	37	59	0.2	0	0	0	0.03	0.03	0.02	0.01	0	1	0
0.6	0	36	1.64	15.3	35	117	198	0.2	5	0.2	0.09	0.12	1.06	0.04	0.05	0.4	19.8	0
0.2	0	3	0.35	1.7	8	10	66	0	0	0	0.04	0.03	0.44	0	0	0	15.8	0
0.8	0	25	2.05	15.7	27	111	209	0.2	0	0	0.06	0.09	1.04	0.03	0	0.3	27.8	0
0.2	0	3	0.52	4.2	15	19	85	0.1	0	0	0.03	0.04	0.58	0.01	0	0	6.4	0
3.6							127			1.1								0
1	0	24	2.06	16.6	30	111	147	0.1	0	0	0.11	0.08	0.97	0.03	0	0	28.5	0
0.7	6	8	1.22			30	150				0	0.08	0.06	0.7				17.9	0
1.1	0	9	0.64	8.2	34	36	96	0.2	1	0.1	0.07	0.06	0.56	0.02	0	0.1	14.8	0
0.5	5	15	0.4	6.3	24	36	81	0.1	21	0.1	0.04	0.02	0.19	0.01	0.01	0.4	4.5	0
0.9	6	8	0.45	7.8	23	46	104	0.2	27	0	0.04	0.04	0.7	0.02	0.02	0.8	11	0
1.1	8	7	0.57			44	85			0	0.05	0.04	0.92					0
1.4	0	15	0.73	13.7	53	54	103	0.3	0	0	0.09	0.07	1.05	0.04	0.06	0.5	17.1	0
2.3	9	8	0.68	5	24	20	79	0.2	0	0	0.08	0.06	0.69	0.01	0	1.1	17.6	0
2	6	11	0.88	5.4	35	32	146	0.2	6	0	0.11	0.11	1.07	0.03	0.03	0.1	22.4	0
0.7	4	6	0.59			21	154			0	0.08	0.06	0.62				18.7	0

MDA Code	Food Name	Amt	Wt (g)	Ener (kcal)	Prot (g)	Carb (g)	Fiber (g)	Fat (g)	Mono (g)	Poly (g)
47690	Sugar cookie, fat free, home style/Archway	1 ea	20	71	1	17	0	0	0	0.1
62907	Sugar cookie, from refrigerated dough, pre-sliced	1 ea	23	111	1	15	0	5	3	0.7
90642	Sugar wafer cookie, creme filled, small, 2-1/2" × 3/4" × 1/4"	1 ea	3.5	18	0	2	0	1	0.4	0.3
90643	Vanilla sandwich cookie, creme filled, oval 3-1/8" × 1-1/4"	2 ea	30	145	1	22	0	6	2.5	2.3
47072	Vanilla wafer, higher fat	4 ea	24	114	1	17	0	5	2.7	0.6
	Custards, Gelatin, and Puddings									
2622	Custard, egg, from dry mix w/2% milk	0.5 cup	133	148	5	23	0	4	1.1	0.3
2613	Custard, egg, from dry mix w/whole milk	0.5 cup	133	161	5	23	0	5	1.6	0.3
57896	Custard, flan, dry mix, serving	1 ea	21	73	0	19	0	0	0	0
23052	Gelatin dessert, from dry mix w/water	0.5 cup	135	84	2	19	0	0	0	0
23360	Gelatin dessert, Jell-O, strawberry, sugar free, low calorie w/aspartame, dry mix serving	1 ea	2.5	8	1	0	0	0		
2632	Pudding, banana, ready-to-eat, 5 oz can	1 ea	141.8	180	3	30	0	5	2.2	1.9
57894	Pudding, chocolate, ready-to-eat, snack can	1 ea	113.4	158	3	26	1	5	1.9	1.6
2612	Pudding, vanilla, ready-to-eat, snack can	1 ea	113.4	147	3	25	0	4	1.7	0.5
2764	Pudding, Jell-O, vanilla, fat free, snack cup	1 ea	113	104	2	23	0	0		
2757	Pudding, Jell-O, vanilla, sugar free, reduced calorie, instant, serving	1 ea	8	26	0	6	0	0		
2651	Pudding, rice, ready-to-eat, 5 oz can	1 ea	141.8	231	3	31	0	11	4.6	4
57902	Pudding, tapioca, ready-to-eat, snack can	1 ea	113.4	135	2	22	0	4	2.6	0.4
	Ice Cream and Frozen Desserts									
71819	Frozen yogurt, chocolate, nonfat, w/artificial sweetener	1 cup	186	199	8	37	2	1	0.4	0.1
72124	Frozen yogurt, all flavors, not chocolate	1 cup	174	221	5	38	0	6	1.7	0.2
49111	Ice cream cone, wafer/cake type, large	1 ea	29	121	2	23	1	2	0.5	0.9
49014	Ice cream cone, sugar, rolled type	1 ea	10	40	1	8	0	0	0.1	0.1
52152	Ice cream bar, Eskimo Pie, vanilla, dark chocolate coated	1 ea	50	166	2	12		12		
2010	Ice cream, vanilla, light, soft serve	0.5 cup	88	111	4	19	0	2	0.7	0.1
90723	Popsicle, 2 fl oz bar	1 ea	59	47	0	11	0	0	0	0
	Pastries									
45788	Apple turnover, frozen/Pepperidge Farm	1 ea	89	284	4	31	2	16		
42264	Cinnamon rolls, w/icing, refrigerated dough/Pillsbury	1 ea	44	145	2	23	0	5		
45675	Éclair shell, homemade, 5" × 2" × 1-3/4"	1 ea	48	174	4	11	0	12	5.3	3.5
71299	Croissant, butter, large	1 ea	67	272	5	31	2	14	3.7	0.7
71301	Croissant, cheese, large	1 ea	67	277	6	31	2	14	4.4	1.6
45572	Danish, cheese	1 ea	71	266	6	26	1	16	8	1.8
71330	Danish, cinnamon nut, 15 oz ring	1 pce	53.2	229	4	24	1	13	7.3	2.3
70913	Crust, pie, Nilla, ready to use/Nabisco	1 ea	28	144	1	18	0	8	5.2	0.4
49015	Strudel, apple	1 pce	71	195	2	29	2	8	2.3	3.8
42164	Sweet roll, cheese	1 ea	66	238	5	29	1	12	6	1.3
42166	Sweet roll, cinnamon, frosted, from refrigerated dough	1 ea	30	109	2	17	1	4	2.2	0.5
71367	Sweet roll, cinnamon raisin, large	1 ea	83	309	5	42	2	14	4	6.2
45683	Toaster pastry, brown sugar & cinnamon	1 ea	50	206	3	34	0	7	4	0.9
45593	Toaster pastry, Pop Tarts, apple cinnamon	1 ea	52	205	2	37	1	5	3.1	1.4
45763	Toaster pastry, Pop Tarts, apple cinnamon, frosted, low fat	1 ea	52	191	2	40	1	3	1.5	0.8
45768	Toaster pastry, Pop Tarts, chocolate fudge, frosted, low fat	1 ea	52	190	3	40	1	3	1.2	0.9
45601	Toaster pastry, Pop Tarts, chocolate fudge, frosted	1 ea	52	201	3	37	1	5	2.7	1.1
	Toppings and Frostings									
23000	Apple butter	1 Tbs	18	31	0	8	0	0	0	0
23070	Caramel topping	2 Tbs	41	103	1	27	0	0	0	0
23014	Chocolate fudge topping	2 Tbs	38	133	2	24	1	3	1.5	0.1
46039	Cream cheese frosting, 16 oz can	1 oz	28.4	118	0	19	0	5	1.1	1.7

Sat (g)	Chol (mg)	Calc (mg)	Iron (mg)	Mag (mg)	Phos (mg)	Pota (mg)	Sodi (mg)	Zinc (mg)	Vit A (RAE)	Vit C (mg)	Thia (mg)	Ribo (mg)	Niac (mg)	Vit B_6 (mg)	Vit B_{12} (µg)	Vit E (mg)	Fol (µg)	Alc (g)
0.1	0	3	0.44			12	80		0	0	0.06	0.04	0.5				15.2	0
1.4	7	21	0.42	1.8	43	37	108	0.1	3	0	0.04	0.03	0.55	0.01	0.02	0	16.1	0
0.1	0	1	0.07	0.4	2	2	5	0	0	0	0	0.01	0.09	0	0	0.1	1.8	0
0.9	0	8	0.66	4.2	22	27	105	0.1	0	0	0.08	0.07	0.81	0.01	0	0.5	15	0
1.2	0	6	0.53	2.9	15	26	73	0.1	0	0	0.09	0.05	0.71	0.01	0.01	0.3	10.3	0
1.8	64	193	0.47	25.3	184	298	118	0.7	81	1.1	0.07	0.28	0.17	0.09	0.6	0.3	12	0
2.8	70	190	0.47	25.3	181	294	117	0.7	49	1.1	0.07	0.28	0.17	0.09	0.59	0.1	12	0
0	0	5	0.02	0	0	32	91	0	0	0	0	0	0	0	0	0	0	0
0	0	4	0.03	1.4	30	1	101	0	0	0	0	0.01	0	0	0	0	1.4	0
0	0	1	0.03		34	0	57		0	0								0
0.8	0	121	0.18	11.3	98	156	278	0.4	9	0.7	0.03	0.21	0.23	0.03	0.26	0	2.8	0
0.8	3	102	0.58	23.8	91	204	146	0.5	12	2	0.03	0.18	0.39	0.03	0	0.3	3.4	0
1.7	8	100	0.15	9.1	77	128	153	0.3	7	0	0.02	0.16	0.29	0.01	0.11	0	3.4	0
0.2	2	86	0.05		115	123	241			0.3								0
0	0	12	0.01		189	2	332		0	0								0
1.7	1	74	0.43	11.3	96	85	121	0.7	35	0.7	0.03	0.1	0.23	0.04	0.3	2	4.3	0
1.1	1	95	0.26	9.1	90	109	180	0.3	0	0.8	0.02	0.11	0.35	0.02	0.24	0.3	3.4	0
0.9	7	296	0.07	74.4	240	631	151	0.9	4	1.3	0.07	0.33	0.37	0.07	0.91	0.1	22.3	0
4	23	174	0.8	17.4	155	271	110	0.5	85	1.2	0.07	0.31	0.12	0.07	0.12	0.2	7	0
0.4	0	7	1.04	7.5	28	32	41	0.2	0	0	0.07	0.1	1.28	0.01	0	0.2	50.2	0
0.1	0	4	0.44	3.1	10	14	32	0.1	0	0	0.05	0.04	0.51	0.01	0	0	14	0
7.2	14	60					34											0
1.4	11	138	0.05	12.3	106	194	62	0.5	26	0.8	0.05	0.17	0.1	0.04	0.44	0.1	4.4	0
0	0	0	0.32	0.6	0	9	4	0.1	0	0.4	0	0	0	0	0	0	0	0
4			1.22				176			0								0
1.5	0		0.72				340											0
2.7	94	17	0.97	5.8	57	47	267	0.4	133	0	0.1	0.17	0.75	0.04	0.19	1.3	25.4	0
7.8	45	25	1.36	10.7	70	79	498	0.5	138	0.1	0.26	0.16	1.47	0.04	0.11	0.6	59	0
7.1	38	36	1.44	16.1	87	88	372	0.6	137	0.1	0.35	0.22	1.45	0.05	0.21	1	49.6	0
4.8	11	25	1.14	10.6	77	70	320	0.5	25	0.1	0.13	0.18	1.42	0.03	0.12	0.2	42.6	0
3.1	24	50	0.96	17	59	51	193	0.5	5	0.9	0.12	0.13	1.22	0.06	0.11	0.4	44.2	0
1.4	3	11	0.5	2.2	23	19	63	0.1			0.05	0.05	0.7	0.01	0.03		8.4	0
1.5	4	11	0.3	6.4	23	106	191	0.1	5	1.2	0.03	0.02	0.23	0.03	0.16	1	19.9	0
4	50	78	0.5	12.5	65	90	236	0.4		0.1	0.1	0.09	0.55	0.05	0.2	1.3	28.4	0
1	0	10	0.8	3.6	104	19	250	0.1	0	0.1	0.12	0.07	1.09	0.01	0.02	0.5	16.5	0
2.6	55	60	1.33	14.1	63	92	318	0.5	51	1.7	0.27	0.22	1.98	0.09	0.12	1.7	59.8	0
1.8	0	17	2.02	12	66	57	212	0.3	148	0.1	0.19	0.29	2.29	0.21	0.11	0.9	14.5	0
0.9	0	12	1.82	5.7	28	47	174	0.3		0	0.15	0.17	1.98	0.2	0	0	41.6	0
0.6	0	6	1.82	4.7	21	28	206	0.2		0	0.16	0.16	1.98	0.21	0	0	52	0
0.5	0	14	1.82	14.6	40	62	249	0.3		0	0.16	0.16	1.98	0.21	0	0	52	0
1	0	20	1.82	15.1	44	82	203	0.3		0	0.16	0.16	1.98	0.21	0	0	52	0
0	0	3	0.06	0.9	1	16	3	0	0	0.2	0	0	0.01	0.01	0	0	0.2	0
0	0	22	0.08	2.9	19	34	143	0.1	11	0.1	0	0.04	0.02	0.01	0.04	0	0.8	0
1.5	1	38	0.6	24.3	64	171	131	0.3	2	0	0.03	0.11	0.14	0.03	0.11	0.9	1.9	0
1.3	0	1	0.05	0.6	1	10	54	0	0	0	0	0	0	0	0	1.2	0	0

MDA Code	Food Name	Amt	Wt (g)	Ener (kcal)	Prot (g)	Carb (g)	Fiber (g)	Fat (g)	Mono (g)	Poly (g)
54334	Hazelnut spread, chocolate flavored	1 oz	28	151	2	17	2	8	4.6	1.9
23164	Strawberry topping	2 Tbs	42.5	108	0	28	0	0	0	0
510	Whipped cream, pressurized	2 Tbs	7.5	19	0	1	0	2	0.5	0.1
514	Whipped topping, pressurized	2 Tbs	8.8	23	0	1	0	2	0.2	0
508	Whipped topping, semi-solid, frozen	2 Tbs	9.4	30	0	2	0	2	0.2	0
54387	Whipped topping, low fat, frozen	2 Tbs	9.4	21	0	2	0	1	0.1	0
	FATS AND OILS									
44469	Butter, light, salted	1 Tbs	13	65	0	0	0	7	2.1	0.3
44470	Butter, light, unsalted	1 Tbs	13	65	0	0	0	7	2.1	0.3
44952	Butter, salted, organic	1 Tbs	14	100	0	0	0	11		
90210	Butter, unsalted, stick	1 Tbs	14	100	0	0	0	11	2.9	0.4
90209	Butter, salted, whipped, stick	1 Tbs	9.4	67	0	0	0	8	2.2	0.3
8003	Fat, bacon grease	1 tsp	4.3	39	0	0	0	4	1.9	0.5
8005	Fat, chicken	1 Tbs	12.8	115	0	0	0	13	5.7	2.7
8107	Fat, lard	1 Tbs	12.8	115	0	0	0	13	5.8	1.4
8135	Margarine & butter, blend, w/soybean oil	1 Tbs	14.2	101	0	0	0	11	4.3	3.4
44476	Margarine, 80% fat, tub	1 Tbs	14.2	102	0	0	0	11	5.1	4
8067	Oil, fish, cod liver	1 Tbs	13.6	123	0	0	0	14	6.4	3.1
8084	Oil, canola	1 Tbs	14	124	0	0	0	14	8.2	4.1
8008	Oil, olive, salad or cooking	1 Tbs	13.5	119	0	0	0	14	9.8	1.4
8111	Oil, safflower, salad or cooking, greater than 70% oleic	1 Tbs	13.6	120	0	0	0	14	10.2	2
8027	Oil, sesame, salad or cooking	1 Tbs	13.6	120	0	0	0	14	5.4	5.7
44483	Shortening, household, vegetable	1 Tbs	12.8	113	0	0	0	13	5.3	3.6
8007	Shortening, household, hydrogenated soybean & cottonseed oil	1 Tbs	12.8	113	0	0	0	13	5.7	3.3
	CONDIMENTS, SAUCES, AND SYRUPS									
53382	Sauce, barbecue, hickory smoke/Kraft	2 Tbs	34	39	0	9	0	0		
1708	Sauce, barbecue, original/Bull's Eye	2 Tbs	36	63	0	15		0		
27001	Catsup	1 ea	6	6	0	2	0	0	0	0
53523	Cheese sauce, ready-to-serve	0.25 cup	63	110	4	4	0	8	2.4	1.6
54388	Cream substitute, light, powder	1 Tbs	5.9	25	0	4	0	1	0.7	0
63334	Dietetic syrup	1 Tbs	15	6	0	7	0	0	0	0
53636	Enchilada sauce/La Victoria	0.25 cup	60.3	20	0	3	0	1		
53474	Fish sauce	2 Tbs	36	13	2	1	0	0	0	0
50939	Gravy, brown, homestyle, savory, canned/Heinz	0.25 cup	60	25	1	3		1	0.3	0
53472	Hoisin sauce	2 Tbs	32	70	1	14	1	1	0.3	0.5
9533	Hollandaise sauce, w/butter fat, from dehydrated w/water, packet	1 ea	204	188	4	11	1	16	4.7	0.7
27004	Horseradish	1 tsp	5	2	0	1	0	0	0	0
92174	Hot sauce, chili, from immature green peppers	1 Tbs	15	3	0	1	0	0	0	0
92173	Hot sauce, chili, from mature red peppers	1 Tbs	15	3	0	1	0	0	0.1	0
23003	Jelly	1 Tbs	19	51	0	13	0	0	0	0
25002	Maple syrup	1 Tbs	20	52	0	13	0	0	0	0
23005	Marmalade, orange	1 Tbs	20	49	0	13	0	0	0	0
44697	Mayonnaise, light	1 Tbs	15	49	0	1	0	5	1.2	2.7
8145	Mayonnaise, soybean & safflower oil	1 Tbs	13.8	99	0	0	0	11	1.8	7.6
8502	Miracle Whip, light	1 Tbs	16	37	0	2	0	3		
435	Mustard, yellow	1 tsp	5	3	0	0	0	0	0.1	0
53656	Nacho cheese sauce w/jalapenos, medium/La Victoria	0.25 cup	71.6	122	1	7	0	10	4.5	1.8
53473	Oyster sauce	2 Tbs	8	4	0	1	0	0	0	0
23042	Pancake syrup	1 Tbs	20	47	0	12	0	0	0	0
23172	Pancake syrup, reduced calorie	1 Tbs	15	25	0	7	0	0	0	0

Sat (g)	Chol (mg)	Calc (mg)	Iron (mg)	Mag (mg)	Phos (mg)	Pota (mg)	Sodi (mg)	Zinc (mg)	Vit A (RAE)	Vit C (mg)	Thia (mg)	Ribo (mg)	Niac (mg)	Vit B$_6$ (mg)	Vit B$_{12}$ (µg)	Vit E (mg)	Fol (µg)	Alc (g)
1.5	0	30	1.23	17.9	43	114	11	0.3	0	0	0.03	0.05	0.12	0.02	0.08	1.4	3.9	0
0	0	3	0.12	1.7	2	22	9	0	0	5.8	0	0.01	0.07	0.01	0	0	2.6	0
1	6	8	0	0.8	7	11	10	0	14	0	0	0	0.01	0	0.02	0	0.2	0
1.7	0	0	0	0.1	2	2	5	0	0	0	0	0	0	0	0	0.1	0	0
2	0	1	0.01	0.2	1	2	2	0	1	0	0	0	0	0	0	0.1	0	0
1.1	0	7	0.01	0.7	7	9	7	0	0	0	0	0.01	0.01	0	0.02	0	0.3	0
4.5	14	6	0.14	0.6	4	9	58	0	60	0	0	0.01	0	0	0.02	0.2	0.1	0
4.5	14	6	0.14	0.6	4	9	5	0	60	0	0	0.01	0	0	0.02	0.2	0.1	0
7	30	0	0				75			0								0
7.2	30	3	0	0.3	3	3	2	0	96	0	0	0	0.01	0	0.02	0.3	0.4	0
4.7	21	2	0.02	0.2	2	2	78	0	64	0	0	0	0	0	0.01	0.2	0.3	0
1.7	4	0	0	0	0	0	6	0	0	0	0	0	0	0	0	0	0	0
3.8	11	0	0	0	0	0	0	0	0	0	0	0	0	0	0	0.3	0	0
5	12	0	0	0	0	0	0	0	0	0	0	0	0	0	0	0.1	0	0
2	2	1	0.01	0.1	1	3	90	0	116	0	0	0	0	0	0	0.6	0.3	0
1.8	0	4	0	0.3	3	5	153	0	116	0	0	0	0	0	0.01	0.7	0.1	0
3.1	78	0	0	0	0	0	0	0	4080	0	0	0	0	0	0	0.4	0	0
1	0	0	0	0	0	0	0	0	0	0	0	0	0	0	0	2.4	0	0
1.9	0	0	0.08	0	0	0	0	0	0	0	0	0	0	0	0	1.9	0	0
0.8	0	0	0	0	0	0	0	0	0	0	0	0	0	0	0	4.6	0	0
1.9	0	0	0	0	0	0	0	0	0	0	0	0	0	0	0	0.2	0	0
3.2	0	0	0.01	0	0	0	1	0	0	0	0	0	0	0	0	0.1	0	0
3.2	0	0	0	0	0	0	0	0	0	0	0	0	0	0	0	0.1	0	0
0	0	5	0.21		3	28	418			0.1								0
							302											0
0	0	1	0.03	1.1	2	23	67	0	3	0.9	0	0.01	0.09	0.01	0	0.1	0.6	0
3.8	18	116	0.13	5.7	99	19	522	0.6	50	0.3	0	0.07	0.02	0.01	0.09	0.2	2.5	0
0.2	0	0	0	0	8	53	14	0	0	0	0	0	0	0	0	0	0.1	0
0	0	0	0	0	0	0	3	0	0	0	0	0	0	0	0	0	0	0
	0	7	0.07				397		70	2.7								0
0	0	15	0.28	63	3	104	2779	0.1	1	0.2	0	0.02	0.83	0.14	0.17	0	18.4	0
0.3	2						352											0
0.2	1	10	0.32	7.7	12	38	517	0.1	0	0.1	0	0.07	0.37	0.02	0	0.1	7.4	0
9.1	41	98	0.71	6.1	100	98	1232	0.6	120	0.2	0.04	0.14	0.04	0.41	0.61	0.6	10.2	0
0	0	3	0.02	1.4	2	12	16	0	0	1.2	0	0	0.02	0	0	0	2.8	0
0	0	1	0.06	1.8	2	85	4	0	4	10.2	0	0	0.1	0.02	0	0.1	1.8	0
0	0	1	0.08	1.8	2	85	4	0	3	4.5	0	0.01	0.09	0.02	0	0.1	1.6	0
0	0	1	0.04	1.1	1	10	6	0	0	0.2	0	0	0.01	0	0	0	0.4	0
0	0	13	0.24	2.8	0	41	2	0.8	0	0	0	0	0.01	0	0	0	0	0
0	0	8	0.03	0.4	1	7	11	0	1	1	0	0.01	0.01	0	0	0	1.8	0
0.8	5	1	0.05	0.3	5	6	101	0	3	0	0	0	0	0	0	0.5	0.6	0
1.2	8	2	0.07	0.1	4	5	78	0	12	0	0	0	0	0.08	0.04	3	1.1	0
0.5	4	1	0.03		2	4	131			0						0.1		0
0	0	3	0.08	2.4	5	7	57	0	0	0.1	0.02	0	0.03	0	0	0	0.4	0
2.7	4	64	0.86				548			1.1								0
0	0	3	0.01	0.3	2	4	219	0	0	0	0	0.01	0.12	0	0.03	0	1.2	0
0	0	1	0.01	0.4	2	3	16	0	0	0	0	0	0	0	0	0	0	0
0	0	0	0	0	6	0	30	0	0	0	0	0	0	0	0	0	0	0

MDA Code	Food Name	Amt	Wt (g)	Ener (kcal)	Prot (g)	Carb (g)	Fiber (g)	Fat (g)	Mono (g)	Poly (g)
23090	Pancake syrup, w/butter	1 Tbs	19.7	58	0	15	0	0	0.1	0
53650	Pasta sauce, smooth, jar, Old World Style/Ragu	0.5 cup	125	80	2	12	3	3	0.5	1.3
53524	Pasta sauce, spaghetti/marinara, ready-to-serve	0.5 cup	125	92	2	14	1	3	1	1.3
53470	Pepper/hot sauce, ready-to-serve	1 tsp	4.7	1	0	0	0	0	0	0
53461	Plum sauce, ready-to-serve	2 Tbs	38.1	70	0	16	0	0	0.1	0.2
92229	Preserves	1 Tbs	20	56	0	14	0	0	0	0
90594	Relish, pickle, sweet, packet	1 ea	10	13	0	4	0	0	0	0
53651	Salsa, chili, chunky, canned/La Victoria	2 Tbs	30	9	0	2	0	0		
53642	Salsa, green chili, mild/La Victoria	2 Tbs	30.5	8	0	1	0	0		
53638	Salsa, green, Jalapena/La Victoria	2 Tbs	30.2	10	0	1	0	0		
53637	Salsa, red, Jalapeno/La Victoria	2 Tbs	30.5	12	0	2	0	0		
90280	Salsa, ready-to-serve, packet	1 ea	8.9	2	0	1	0	0	0	0
53646	Salsa, picante, mild/La Victoria	2 Tbs	30.5	8	0	1	0	0		
504	Sour cream, cultured	2 Tbs	28.8	62	1	1	0	6	1.7	0.2
54383	Sour cream, fat free	1 oz	28	21	1	4	0	0	0	0
505	Sour cream, imitation, cultured	2 Tbs	28.8	60	1	2	0	6	0.2	0
54381	Sour cream, light	1 oz	28	38	1	2	0	3	0.9	0.1
515	Sour cream, reduced fat, cultured	2 Tbs	30	40	1	1	0	4	1	0.1
516	Sour dressing, non-butterfat, cultured, filled cream-type	1 Tbs	14.7	26	0	1	0	2	0.3	0.1
53063	Soy sauce, tamari	1 Tbs	18	11	2	1	0	0	0	0
90035	Soy sauce, low sodium	1 Tbs	18	10	1	2	0	0	0	0
53357	Sweet & sour sauce/Nestle	2 Tbs	33	40	0	8	0	1	0.2	0.4
91056	Taco sauce, green, medium/La Victoria	1 Tbs	15.1	5	0	1	0	0		
53652	Taco sauce, red, mild/La Victoria	1 Tbs	15.7	7	0	1	0	0		
4655	Tahini, from roasted & toasted kernels	1 Tbs	15	89	3	3	1	8	3	3.5
53004	Teriyaki sauce	1 Tbs	18	15	1	3	0	0	0	0
53468	White sauce, medium, homemade	1 cup	250	368	10	23	1	27	11.1	7.2
53099	Worcestershire sauce	1 Tbs	17	11	0	3	0	0	0	0
27175	Yeast extract spread	1 tsp	6	9	2	1	0	0	0	0
	Salad Dressing									
44497	Thousand island, fat free	1 Tbs	16	21	0	5	1	0	0.1	0.1
8024	Thousand island	1 Tbs	15.6	58	0	2	0	5	1.2	2.8
8013	Blue cheese	2 Tbs	30.6	154	1	2	0	16	3.8	8.5
92511	Caesar	2 Tbs	30	150	1	1	0	16		
90232	French, packet	1 ea	12.3	56	0	2	0	6	1	2.6
44467	French, fat free	1 Tbs	16	21	0	5	0	0	0	0
8255	French, reduced fat, unsalted	1 Tbs	16.3	38	0	5	0	2	1	0.8
92510	Italian	2 Tbs	30	140	0	2	0	15		
44498	Italian, fat free	1 Tbs	14	7	0	1	0	0	0	0
44499	Ranch, fat free	1 oz	28.4	34	0	8	0	1		
44696	Ranch, reduced fat	1 Tbs	15	33	0	2	0	3	0.8	0.7
8022	Russian	1 Tbs	15.3	54	0	5	0	4	0.9	2.3
8144	Sesame seed	2 Tbs	30.6	136	1	3	0	14	3.6	7.7
8035	Vinegar & oil, homemade	2 Tbs	31.2	140	0	1	0	16	4.6	7.5
	SPICES, FLAVORS, AND SEASONINGS									
26000	Allspice, ground	1 tsp	1.9	5	0	1	0	0	0	0
26106	Anise seed	1 tsp	2.1	7	0	1	0	0	0.2	0.1
26001	Basil, dried	1 tsp	1.4	4	0	1	1	0	0	0
26107	Bay leaf, crumbled	1 tsp	0.6	2	0	0	0	0	0	0
9518	Celery flakes, dried	0.5 oz	14.2	45	2	9	4	0	0.1	0.1

Sat (g)	Chol (mg)	Calc (mg)	Iron (mg)	Mag (mg)	Phos (mg)	Pota (mg)	Sodi (mg)	Zinc (mg)	Vit A (RAE)	Vit C (mg)	Thia (mg)	Ribo (mg)	Niac (mg)	Vit B$_6$ (mg)	Vit B$_{12}$ (µg)	Vit E (mg)	Fol (µg)	Alc (g)
0.2	1	0	0.02	0.4	2	1	19	0	3	0	0	0	0	0	0	0	0	0
0.4	0		1.02				756		32									0
0.5	0	34	1.06	26.2	45	470	601	0.7	34	3.9	0.03	0.08	4.9	0.22	0	2.5	13.8	0
0	0	0	0.02	0.2	1	7	124	0	0	3.5	0	0	0.01	0.01	0	0	0.3	0
0.1	0	5	0.54	4.6	8	99	205	0.1	1	0.2	0.01	0.03	0.39	0.03	0	0.1	2.3	0
0	0	4	0.1	0.8	4	15	6	0	0	1.8	0	0.02	0.01	0	0	0	2.2	0
0	0	0	0.09	0.5	1	2	81	0	4	0.1	0	0	0.02	0	0	0	0.1	0
		4	0.01				148		3	3.2								0
		5	0.28				175		7	4.1								0
	0	5	0.12				181		4	3.6								0
	0	6	0.05				149		43	9.8								0
0	0	2	0.04	1.3	3	26	53	0	1	0.2	0	0	0.01	0.02	0	0.1	0.4	0
	0	5	0.03				182		6	1.9								0
3.8	13	33	0.02	3.2	24	41	15	0.1	51	0.3	0.01	0.04	0.02	0	0.09	0.2	3.2	0
0	3	35	0	2.8	27	36	39	0.1	20	0	0.01	0.04	0.02	0.01	0.08	0	3.1	0
5.1	0	1	0.11	1.7	13	46	29	0.3	0	0	0	0	0	0	0	0.2	0	0
1.8	10	39	0.02	2.8	20	59	20	0.1	25	0.3	0.01	0.03	0.02	0.01	0.12	0.1	3.1	0
2.2	12	31	0.02	3	28	39	12	0.2	31	0.3	0.01	0.04	0.02	0	0.09	0.1	3.3	0
2	1	17	0	1.5	13	24	7	0.1	0	0.1	0.01	0.02	0.01	0	0.05	0.2	1.8	0
0	0	4	0.43	7.2	23	38	1005	0.1	0	0	0.01	0.03	0.71	0.04	0	0	3.2	0
0	0	3	0.36	6.1	20	32	600	0.1	0	0	0.01	0.02	0.6	0.03	0	0	2.9	0
0.1	0	6	0.28	2.3	3	22	116	0	0	0	0.01	0	0.07	0.01	0	0.1	0.7	0
		1	0.01				96		1	0.7								0
		3	0.03				103		13	2.8								0
1.1	0	64	1.34	14.2	110	62	17	0.7	0	0	0.18	0.07	0.82	0.02	0	0	14.7	0
0	0	4	0.31	11	28	40	690	0	0	0	0.01	0.01	0.23	0.02	0	0	3.6	0
7.1	18	295	0.83	35	245	390	885	1	225	2	0.17	0.46	1.01	0.1	0.7	0.7	20	0
0	0	18	0.9	2.2	10	136	167	0	1	2.2	0.01	0.02	0.12	0	0	0	1.4	0
0	0	5	0.22	10.8	6	156	216	0.1	0	0	0.58	0.86	5.82	0.08	0.03	0	60.6	0
0	1	2	0.04	0.6	0	20	117	0	0	0	0.04	0.01	0.04	0	0	0.1	1.9	0
0.8	4	3	0.18	1.2	4	17	135	0	2	0	0.23	0.01	0.07	0	0	0.6	0	0
3	5	25	0.06	0	23	11	335	0.1	21	0.6	0	0.03	0.03	0.01	0.08	1.8	8.6	0
3	5	0	0.36				280		0	0								0
0.7	0	3	0.1	0.6	2	8	103	0	3	0	0	0.01	0.02	0	0.02	0.6	0	0
0	0	1	0.09	0.5	0	13	128	0	1	0	0	0	0.02	0	0	0	2.2	0
0.2	0	2	0.14	1.3	3	17	5	0	4	0	0	0.01	0.08	0.01	0	0.5	0.3	0
2.5	0	0	0				360		0	0								0
0	0	4	0.06	0.7	15	14	158	0.1	1	0.1	0	0.01	0.02	0	0.04	0.1	1.7	0
	2	14	0.3	2.3	32	32	214	0.1	0	0	0.01	0.01	0	0.01	0	0.1	1.7	0
0.2	3	19	0.13	0.9	29	20	140	0.1	3	0.1	0	0	0	0	0	0.2	0.6	0
0.6		3	0.11	1.5	3	26	144	0	7	0.7	0	0.01	0.09	0.01	0	0.5	0.8	0
1.9	0	6	0.18	0	11	48	306	0	1	0	0	0	0	0	0	1.5	0	0
2.8	0	0	0	0	0	2	0	0	0	0	0	0	0	0	0	1.4	0	0
0	0	13	0.13	2.6	2	20	1	0	1	0.7	0	0	0.05	0	0	0	0.7	0
0	0	14	0.78	3.6	9	30	0	0.1	0	0.4	0.01	0.01	0.06	0.01	0	0	0.2	0
0	0	30	0.59	5.9	7	48	0	0.1	7	0.9	0	0	0.1	0.03	0	0.1	3.8	0
0	0	5	0.26	0.7	1	3	0	0	2	0.3	0	0	0.01	0.01	0	0	1.1	0
0.1	0	83	1.11	27.8	57	623	204	0.4	14	12.3	0.06	0.07	0.66	0.07	0	0.8	15.2	0

MDA Code	Food Name	Amt	Wt (g)	Ener (kcal)	Prot (g)	Carb (g)	Fiber (g)	Fat (g)	Mono (g)	Poly (g)
26040	Celery seeds	1 tsp	2	8	0	1	0	1	0.3	0.1
26002	Chili pepper, powdered	1 tsp	2.6	8	0	1	1	0	0.1	0.2
26003	Cinnamon, ground	1 tsp	2.3	6	0	2	1	0	0	0
26019	Clove, ground	1 tsp	2.1	7	0	1	1	0	0	0.1
26041	Coriander seeds	1 tsp	1.8	5	0	1	1	0	0.2	0
26036	Cumin seeds	1 tsp	2.1	8	0	1	0	0	0.3	0.1
26004	Curry blend, powder	1 tsp	2	6	0	1	1	0	0.1	0.1
26109	Dill seed	1 tsp	2.1	6	0	1	0	0	0.2	0
26105	Fennel seed	1 tsp	2	7	0	1	1	0	0.2	0
26007	Garlic powder	1 tsp	2.8	9	0	2	0	0	0	0
26023	Ginger, ground	1 tsp	1.8	6	0	1	0	0	0	0
90442	Ginger root, fresh	1 tsp	2	2	0	0	0	0	0	0
3067	Lemon peel, fresh	1 Tbs	6	3	0	1	1	0	0	0
26110	Mustard seed, yellow	1 tsp	3.3	15	1	1	0	1	0.7	0.2
26026	Nutmeg, ground	1 tsp	2.2	12	0	1	0	1	0.1	0
26008	Onion powder	1 tsp	2.1	7	0	2	0	0	0	0
26010	Paprika	1 tsp	2.1	6	0	1	1	0	0	0.2
26035	Parsley, dried	1 tsp	0.3	1	0	0	0	0	0	0
90212	Pepper, black, dash	1 ea	0.1	0	0	0	0	0	0	0
26015	Poppy seed	1 tsp	2.8	15	1	1	0	1	0.2	0.9
26030	Rosemary, dried	1 tsp	1.2	4	0	1	1	0	0	0
26111	Saffron	1 tsp	0.7	2	0	0	0	0	0	0
26014	Salt, table	0.25 tsp	1.5	0	0	0	0	0	0	0
26033	Thyme, ground	1 tsp	1.4	4	0	1	1	0	0	0
26034	Turmeric, ground	1 tsp	2.2	8	0	1	0	0	0	0
26624	Vanilla extract	1 tsp	4.3	12	0	1	0	0	0	0

BAKING INGREDIENTS

MDA Code	Food Name	Amt	Wt (g)	Ener (kcal)	Prot (g)	Carb (g)	Fiber (g)	Fat (g)	Mono (g)	Poly (g)
28001	Baker's yeast, dry active, package	1 ea	7	21	3	3	1	0	0.2	0
28003	Baking soda	1 tsp	4.6	0	0	0	0	0	0	0
25005	Brown sugar, packed	1 tsp	4.6	17	0	4	0	0	0	0
23010	Baking chocolate, unsweetened, square	1 ea	28.4	142	4	8	5	15	4.6	0.4
23418	Baking chocolate, Mexican, square	1 ea	20	85	1	15	1	3	1	0.2
90657	Chocolate chips, semi sweet, mini	0.25 cup	43.2	207	2	27	3	13	4.3	0.4
4649	Coconut cream, canned	1 Tbs	18.5	36	0	2	0	3	0.1	0
4527	Coconut water, fresh	1 cup	240	46	2	9	3	0	0	0
4574	Coconut, dried, flaked, sweetened, package	2 Tbs	9.2	42	0	5	1	3	0.1	0
4510	Coconut, dried, unsweetened	2 Tbs	9.2	61	1	2	1	6	0.3	0.1
25203	Corn syrup, high fructose	1 Tbs	19.4	55	0	15	0	0	0	0
25000	Corn syrup, light	1 Tbs	20.5	58	0	16	0	0		
26017	Cream of tartar	1 tsp	3	8	0	2	0	0		0
25006	Granulated white sugar	1 tsp	4.2	16	0	4	0	0	0	0
25001	Honey, strained/extracted	1 Tbs	21.2	64	0	17	0	0	0	0
25202	Maple sugar	1 tsp	3	11	0	3	0	0	0	0
25003	Molasses	1 Tbs	20.5	59	0	15	0	0	0	0
25111	Sorghum syrup	1 Tbs	21	61	0	16	0	0	0	0
27007	Vinegar, cider	1 Tbs	15	3	0	0	0	0	0	0
92153	Vinegar, distilled	1 Tbs	17	3	0	0	0	0	0	0
92129	Wheat gluten, vital	1 oz	28.4	105	21	4	0	1	0	0.2

Sat (g)	Chol (mg)	Calc (mg)	Iron (mg)	Mag (mg)	Phos (mg)	Pota (mg)	Sodi (mg)	Zinc (mg)	Vit A (RAE)	Vit C (mg)	Thia (mg)	Ribo (mg)	Niac (mg)	Vit B$_6$ (mg)	Vit B$_{12}$ (µg)	Vit E (mg)	Fol (µg)	Alc (g)
0	0	35	0.9	8.8	11	28	3	0.1	0	0.3	0.01	0.01	0.06	0.02	0	0	0.2	0
0.1	0	7	0.37	4.4	8	50	26	0.1	39	1.7	0.01	0.02	0.21	0.1	0	0.8	2.6	0
0	0	28	0.88	1.3	1	12	1	0	0	0.7	0	0	0.03	0.01	0	0	0.7	0
0.1	0	14	0.18	5.5	2	23	5	0	1	1.7	0	0.01	0.03	0.01	0	0.2	2	0
0	0	13	0.29	5.9	7	23	1	0.1	0	0.4	0	0.01	0.04		0		0	0
0	0	20	1.39	7.7	10	38	4	0.1	1	0.2	0.01	0.01	0.1	0.01	0	0.1	0.2	0
0	0	10	0.59	5.1	7	31	1	0.1	1	0.2	0.01	0.01	0.07	0.02	0	0.4	3.1	0
0	0	32	0.34	5.4	6	25	0	0.1	0	0.4	0.01	0.01	0.06	0.01	0	0	0.2	0
0	0	24	0.37	7.7	10	34	2	0.1	0	0.4	0.01	0.01	0.12	0.01	0			0
0	0	2	0.08	1.6	12	31	1	0.1	0	0.5	0.01	0	0.02	0.08	0	0	0.1	0
0	0	2	0.21	3.3	3	24	1	0.1	0	0.1	0	0	0.09	0.02	0	0.3	0.7	0
0	0	0	0.01	0.9	1	8	0	0	0	0.1	0	0	0.02	0	0	0	0.2	0
0	0	8	0.05	0.9	1	10	0	0	0	7.7	0	0	0.02	0.01	0	0	0.8	0
0	0	17	0.33	9.8	28	23	0	0.2	0	0.1	0.02	0.01	0.26	0.01	0	0.1	2.5	0
0.6	0	4	0.07	4	5	8	0	0	0	0.1	0.01	0	0.03	0	0	0	1.7	0
0	0	8	0.05	2.6	7	20	1	0	0	0.3	0.01	0	0.01	0.03	0	0	3.5	0
0	0	4	0.5	3.9	7	49	1	0.1	55	1.5	0.01	0.04	0.32	0.08	0	0.6	2.2	0
0	0	4	0.29	0.7	1	11	1	0	2	0.4	0	0	0.02	0	0	0	0.5	0
0	0	0	0.03	0.2	0	1	0	0	0	0	0	0	0	0	0	0	0	0
0.1	0	41	0.26	9.3	24	20	1	0.3	0	0.1	0.02	0	0.03	0.01	0	0	1.6	0
0.1	0	15	0.35	2.6	1	11	1	0	2	0.7	0.01	0.01	0.01	0.02	0	0	3.7	0
0	0	1	0.08	1.8	2	12	1	0	0	0.6	0	0	0.01	0.01	0	0	0.7	0
0	0	0	0	0	0	0	581	0	0	0	0	0	0	0	0	0	0	0
0	0	26	1.73	3.1	3	11	1	0.1	3	0.7	0.01	0.01	0.07	0.01	0	0.1	3.8	0
0.1	0	4	0.91	4.2	6	56	1	0.1	0	0.6	0	0.01	0.11	0.04	0	0.1	0.9	0
0	0	0	0.01	0.5	0	6	0	0	0	0	0	0	0.02	0	0	0	0	1.48
0	0	4	1.16	6.9	90	140	4	0.4	0	0	0.17	0.38	2.78	0.11	0	0	163.8	0
0	0	0	0	0	0	0	1259	0	0	0	0	0	0	0	0	0	0	0
0	0	4	0.09	1.3	1	16	2	0	0	0	0	0	0	0	0	0	0	0
9.2	0	29	4.94	92.9	114	236	7	2.7	0	0	0.04	0.03	0.38	0.01	0	0.1	8	0
1.7	0	7	0.44	19	28	79	1	0.3	0	0	0.01	0.02	0.37	0.01	0	0.1	1	0
7.7	0	14	1.35	49.7	57	158	5	0.7	0	0	0.02	0.04	0.18	0.02	0	0.1	5.6	0
2.9	0	0	0.09	3.1	4	19	9	0.1	0	0.3	0	0.01	0.01	0.01	0	0	2.6	0
0.4	0	58	0.7	60	48	600	252	0.2	0	5.8	0.07	0.14	0.19	0.08	0	0	7.2	0
2.4	0	1	0.14	4.7	9	33	26	0.1	0	0	0	0	0.06	0	0	0	0.3	0
5.3	0	2	0.31	8.3	19	50	3	0.2	0	0.1	0.01	0.01	0.06	0.03	0	0	0.8	0
0	0	0	0.01	0	0	0	0	0	0	0	0	0	0	0	0	0	0	0
	0	3	0	0.2	0	0	13	0.1	0	0	0.01	0	0	0	0	0	0	0
0	0	0	0.11	0.1	0	495	2	0	0	0	0	0	0	0	0	0	0	0
0	0	0	0	0	0	0	0	0	0	0	0	0	0	0	0	0	0	0
0	0	1	0.09	0.4	1	11	1	0	0	0.1	0	0.01	0.03	0.01	0	0	0.4	0
0	0	3	0.05	0.6	0	8	0	0.2	0	0	0	0	0	0	0	0	0	0
0	0	42	0.97	49.6	6	300	8	0.1	0	0	0.01	0	0.19	0.14	0	0	0	0
0	0	32	0.8	21	12	210	2	0.1	0	0	0.02	0.03	0.02	0.14	0	0	0	0
0	0	1	0.03	0.8	1	11	1	0	0	0	0	0	0	0	0	0	0	0
0	0	1	0.01	0.2	1	0	0	0	0	0	0	0	0	0	0	0	0	0
0.1	0	40	1.48	7.1	74	28	8	0.2	0	0	0	0	0	0	0	0	0	0

MDA Code	Food Name	Amt	Wt (g)	Ener (kcal)	Prot (g)	Carb (g)	Fiber (g)	Fat (g)	Mono (g)	Poly (g)
	FAST FOOD									
	Generic Fast Food									
6178	Baked potatoes w/cheese sauce & bacon	1 ea	299	451	18	44		26	9.7	4.8
6177	Baked potatoes w/cheese sauce	1 ea	296	474	15	47		29	10.7	6
6181	Baked potatoes w/sour cream & chives	1 ea	302	393	7	50		22	7.9	3.3
66025	Burrito, bean	1 ea	108.5	224	7	36	4	7	2.4	0.6
56629	Burrito, bean & cheese	1 ea	93	189	8	27		6	1.2	0.9
66024	Burrito, beef	1 ea	110	262	13	29	1	10	3.7	0.4
66023	Burrito, beef, bean & cheese	1 ea	101.5	165	7	20	2	7	2.2	0.5
56600	Breakfast biscuit w/egg sandwich	1 ea	136	373	12	32	1	22	9.1	6.4
56601	Breakfast biscuit w/egg & bacon	1 ea	150	458	17	29	1	31	13.4	7.5
56602	Breakfast biscuit w/egg & ham	1 ea	192	461	20	35	1	27	11	7.7
66028	Breakfast biscuit w/egg & sausage	1 ea	180	581	19	41	1	39	16.4	4.4
66029	Breakfast biscuit w/egg, cheese & bacon	1 ea	144	461	18	33	1	29	14.1	3.5
56604	Biscuit w/ham sandwich	1 ea	113	386	13	44	1	18	4.8	1
66030	Biscuit w/sausage sandwich	1 ea	124	485	12	40	1	32	12.8	3
66013	Cheeseburger, double, w/condiments & vegetables	1 ea	166	417	21	35		21	7.8	2.7
66016	Cheeseburger, double	1 ea	155	477	27	32	1	27	9	0.9
56651	Cheeseburger w/bacon & condiments	1 ea	195	550	31	37	3	31	10.6	1.3
56649	Cheeseburger w/condiments & vegetables	1 ea	219	453	25	37	3	23	7.7	0.7
15063	Chicken drumstick & thigh, dark meat, breaded & fried	3 oz	85.1	248	17	9	1	15	6.3	3.6
15064	Chicken breast & wing, white meat, breaded & fried	3 oz	85.1	258	19	10	1	15	6.4	3.5
56656	Chicken fillet sandwich w/cheese	1 ea	228	632	29	42		39	13.7	9.9
56000	Chicken fillet sandwich, plain	1 ea	182	515	24	39		29	10.4	8.4
50312	Chili con carne	1 cup	253	256	25	22		8	3.4	0.5
56635	Chimichanga, beef & cheese	1 ea	183	443	20	39		23	9.4	0.7
19110	Clams, breaded & fried	3 oz	85.1	334	9	29		20	8.5	5
5461	Cole slaw	0.75 cup	99	147	1	13		11	2.4	6.4
6175	Corn cob w/butter	1 ea	146	155	4	32		3	1	0.6
56668	Corn dog	1 ea	175	460	17	56		19	9.1	3.5
56606	Croissant sandwich w/egg & cheese	1 ea	127	368	13	24		25	7.5	1.4
56607	Croissant sandwich w/egg, cheese & bacon	1 ea	129	413	16	24		28	9.2	1.8
56608	Croissant sandwich w/egg, cheese & ham	1 ea	152	474	19	24		34	11.4	2.4
45588	Danish, cheese	1 ea	91	353	6	29		25	15.6	2.4
45513	Danish, fruit	1 ea	94	335	5	45		16	10.1	1.6
66021	Enchilada, cheese	1 ea	163	319	10	29		19	6.3	0.8
66022	Enchilada, beef & cheese	1 ea	192	323	12	30		18	6.1	1.4
66020	Enchirito, beef, bean & cheese	1 ea	193	344	18	34		16	6.5	0.3
42064	English muffin w/butter	1 ea	63	189	5	30	2	6	1.5	1.3
66031	English muffin sandwich, w/cheese & sausage	1 ea	115	393	15	29	1	24	10.1	2.7
66032	English muffin sandwich, w/egg, cheese & bacon	1 ea	146	308	18	28	2	13	5	1.7
66010	Fish sandwich, w/tartar sauce	1 ea	158	431	17	41	0	23	7.7	8.2
66011	Fish sandwich, w/cheese & tartar sauce	1 ea	183	523	21	48	0	29	8.9	9.4
90736	French fries, fried in vegetable oil, medium	1 ea	134	427	5	50	5	23	13.3	4
42354	French toast sticks	5 pce	141	513	8	58	3	29	12.6	9.9
42353	French toast w/butter	2 pce	135	356	10	36	0	19	7.1	2.4
56638	Frijoles (beans) w/cheese	0.5 cup	83.5	113	6	14		4	1.3	0.3
56664	Ham & cheese sandwich	1 ea	146	352	21	33		15	6.7	1.4
56665	Ham, egg & cheese sandwich	1 ea	143	347	19	31		16	5.7	1.7
69150	Hamburger w/condiments	1 ea	171.5	439	27	38	2	20	9	2.1

Sat (g)	Chol (mg)	Calc (mg)	Iron (mg)	Mag (mg)	Phos (mg)	Pota (mg)	Sodi (mg)	Zinc (mg)	Vit A (RAE)	Vit C (mg)	Thia (mg)	Ribo (mg)	Niac (mg)	Vit B$_6$ (mg)	Vit B$_{12}$ (µg)	Vit E (mg)	Fol (µg)	Alc (g)
10.1	30	308	3.14	68.8	347	1178	972	2.2	188	28.7	0.27	0.24	3.98	0.75	0.33		29.9	0
10.6	18	311	3.02	65.1	320	1166	382	1.9	252	26	0.24	0.21	3.34	0.71	0.18		26.6	0
10	24	106	3.11	69.5	184	1383	181	0.9	266	33.8	0.27	0.18	3.71	0.79	0.21		33.2	0
3.4	2	56	2.26	43.4	49	327	493	0.8	8	1	0.31	0.3	2.03	0.15	0.54	0.9	43.4	0
3.4	14	107	1.13	40	90	248	583	0.8	49	0.8	0.11	0.35	1.79	0.12	0.45		37.2	0
5.2	32	42	3.05	40.7	87	370	746	2.4	7	0.6	0.12	0.46	3.22	0.15	0.98	0.6	64.9	0
3.6	62	65	1.87	25.4	70	205	495	1.2	75	2.5	0.15	0.36	1.93	0.11	0.55	0.4	37.6	0
4.7	245	82	2.9	19	388	238	891	1	180	0.1	0.3	0.49	2.15	0.11	0.63	3.3	57.1	0
8	352	189	3.74	24	238	250	999	1.6	108	2.7	0.14	0.23	2.4	0.14	1.03	2	60	0
5.9	300	221	4.55	30.7	317	319	1382	2.2	236	0	0.67	0.6	2	0.27	1.19	2.3	65.3	0
15	302	155	3.96	25.2	490	320	1141	2.2	160	0	0.5	0.45	3.6	0.2	1.37	2.8	64.8	0
11.1	252	157	2.94	20.2	459	230	1250	1.5		2.3	0.34	0.52	2.57	0.1	1.05	1.4	105.1	0
11.4	25	160	2.72	22.6	554	197	1433	1.6	31	0.1	0.51	0.32	3.48	0.14	0.03	1.7	38.4	0
14.2	35	128	2.58	19.8	446	198	1071	1.6	13	0.1	0.4	0.29	3.27	0.11	0.51	1.4	45.9	0
8.7	60	171	3.42	29.9	242	335	1051	3.5	71	1.7	0.35	0.28	8.05	0.18	1.93		61.4	0
11	85	279	3.67	32.6	284	335	963	4.3	99	0	0.29	0.44	6.79	0.29	2.14	1.2	77.5	0
11.9	98	267	4.04	44.8	353	464	1314	5.2	82	1.4	0.34	0.68	8.25	0.47	2.44		95.6	0
8.5	74	208	4.07	41.6	261	460	843	4.8		4.2	0.32	0.62	7.29		2.21		102.9	0
4.1	95	20	0.92	21.3	138	256	434	1.9	38	0	0.08	0.25	4.14	0.19	0.48	0.8	14.5	0
4.1	77	31	0.77	19.6	160	295	509	0.8	30	0	0.08	0.15	6.25	0.3	0.35	0.8	15.3	0
12.4	78	258	3.63	43.3	406	333	1238	2.9	164	3	0.41	0.46	9.07	0.41	0.46		109.4	0
8.5	60	60	4.68	34.6	233	353	957	1.9	31	8.9	0.33	0.24	6.81	0.2	0.38		100.1	0
3.4	134	68	5.19	45.5	197	691	1007	3.6	83	1.5	0.13	1.14	2.48	0.33	1.14	1.6	45.5	0
11.2	51	238	3.84	60.4	187	203	957	3.4	132	2.7	0.38	0.86	4.67	0.22	1.3		91.5	0
4.9	65	15	2.26	23	176	197	617	1.2	27	0	0.15	0.2	2.12	0.03	0.82		31.5	0
1.6	5	34	0.72	8.9	36	177	267	0.2	36	8.3	0.04	0.03	0.08	0.11	0.18	4	38.6	0
1.6	6	4	0.88	40.9	108	359	29	0.9	34	6.9	0.25	0.1	2.18	0.32	0		43.8	0
5.2	79	102	6.18	17.5	166	262	973	1.3	60	0	0.28	0.7	4.17	0.09	0.44	0.7	103.2	0
14.1	216	244	2.2	21.6	348	174	551	1.8	277	0.1	0.19	0.38	1.51	0.1	0.77		47	0
15.4	215	151	2.19	23.2	276	201	889	1.9	142	2.2	0.35	0.34	2.19	0.12	0.86		45.2	0
17.5	213	144	2.13	25.8	336	272	1081	2.2	131	11.4	0.52	0.3	3.19	0.23	1		45.6	0
5.1	20	70	1.85	15.5	80	116	319	0.6	45	2.6	0.26	0.21	2.55	0.05	0.23		54.6	0
3.3	19	22	1.4	14.1	69	110	333	0.5	25	1.6	0.29	0.21	1.8	0.06	0.24	0.8	31	0
10.6	44	324	1.32	50.5	134	240	784	2.5	99	1	0.08	0.42	1.91	0.39	0.75	1.5	65.2	0
9	40	228	3.07	82.6	167	574	1319	2.7	98	1.3	0.1	0.4	2.52	0.27	1.02	1.5	67.2	0
7.9	50	218	2.39	71.4	224	560	1251	2.8	89	4.6	0.17	0.69	2.99	0.21	1.62	1.5	94.6	0
2.4	13	103	1.59	13.2	85	69	386	0.4	32	0.8	0.25	0.32	2.61	0.04	0.02	0.1	56.7	0
9.9	59	168	2.25	24.2	186	215	1036	1.7	101	1.3	0.7	0.25	4.14	0.15	0.68	1.3	66.7	0
5	250	161	2.6	24.8	288	212	777	1.7	188	1.9	0.53	0.48	3.55	0.16	0.72	0.6	73	0
5.2	55	84	2.61	33.2	212	340	615	1	33	2.8	0.33	0.22	3.4	0.11	1.07	0.9	85.3	0
8.1	68	185	3.5	36.6	311	353	939	1.2	130	2.7	0.46	0.42	4.23	0.11	1.08	1.8	91.5	0
5.3	0	17	1.84	45.6	185	737	260	1	0	3.6	0.23	0.09	3.35	0.51	0	1	40.2	0
4.7	75	78	2.96	26.8	123	127	499	0.9	0	0	0.23	0.25	2.96	0.25	0.07	2.3	197.4	0
7.7	116	73	1.89	16.2	146	177	513	0.6	136	0.1	0.58	0.5	3.92	0.05	0.36		72.9	0
2	18	94	1.12	42.6	88	302	441	0.9	18	0.8	0.07	0.17	0.74	0.1	0.34		55.9	0
6.4	58	130	3.24	16.1	152	291	771	1.4	96	2.8	0.31	0.48	2.69	0.2	0.54	0.3	75.9	0
7.4	246	212	3.1	25.7	346	210	1005	2	166	2.7	0.43	0.56	4.2	0.16	1.23	0.6	75.8	0
8.6	69	149	2.97	41.2	208	386	641	5.2		0.5	0.27	0.34	7.97	0.25	2.85	0.1	37.7	0

MDA Code	Food Name	Amt	Wt (g)	Ener (kcal)	Prot (g)	Carb (g)	Fiber (g)	Fat (g)	Mono (g)	Poly (g)
56662	Hamburger, double, w/condiments & vegetables	1 ea	226	540	34	40		27	10.3	2.8
56661	Hamburger, w/condiments & vegetables	1 ea	218	429	25	38	3	20	7.2	0.5
56659	Hamburger, w/condiments & vegetables	1 ea	110	279	13	27		13	5.3	2.6
66007	Hamburger, plain	1 ea	90	266	13	30	1	10	3.5	0.2
5463	Hash browns	0.5 cup	72	235	2	23	2	16		
56667	Hot dog w/chili & bun	1 ea	114	296	14	31		13	6.6	1.2
66004	Hot dog, plain	1 ea	98	242	10	18		15	6.9	1.7
56666	Hush puppies, cornbread	5 pce	78	257	5	35	3	12	7.8	0.4
2032	Hot fudge sundae	1 ea	158	284	6	48	0	9	2.3	0.8
6185	Mashed potatoes	0.5 cup	121	100	3	20		1	0.4	0.4
90214	Mayonnaise, soybean oil, packet	1 ea	10	72	0	0	0	8	2	4.3
71129	Milk shake, chocolate, small, 12 fl oz	1 ea	249.6	317	8	51	5	9	2.7	0.3
71132	Milk shake, vanilla, small, 12 fl oz	1 ea	249.6	369	8	49	2	16	4.5	0.8
56639	Nachos, w/cheese	7 pce	113	346	9	36		19	8	2.2
56641	Nachos w/cheese, beans, beef & peppers	7 pce	225	502	17	49		27	9.7	5
6176	Onion rings	8 pce	78.1	259	3	29		15	6.3	0.6
19109	Oysters, breaded & battered, fried	3 oz	85.1	226	8	24	0	11	4.2	2.8
45122	Pancakes, w/butter & syrup	1 ea	116	260	4	45	1	7	2.6	1
6173	Potato salad	0.333 cup	95	108	1	13		6	1.6	2.9
56619	Pizza, pepperoni, frozen, 12" or 1/8 pce	1 pce	108	275	15	30		11	4.8	1.8
56669	Roast beef sandwich, w/cheese	1 ea	176	473	32	45		18	3.7	3.5
66003	Roast beef sandwich, plain	1 ea	139	346	22	33		14	6.8	1.7
56643	Taco salad	1.5 cup	198	279	13	24		15	5.2	1.7
56644	Taco salad, w/chili con carne	1.5 cup	261	290	17	27		13	4.5	1.5
19115	Shrimp, breaded & fried	4 ea	93.7	260	11	23		14	9.9	0.4
56670	Steak sandwich	1 ea	204	459	30	52		14	5.3	3.3
56671	Submarine sandwich, w/cold cuts	1 ea	228	456	22	51	2	19	8.2	2.3
56673	Submarine sandwich, w/tuna salad	1 ea	256	584	30	55		28	13.4	7.3
57531	Taco, small	1 ea	171	371	21	27		21	6.6	1
66017	Tostada, bean & cheese	1 ea	144	223	10	27		10	3.1	0.7
56645	Tostada, beef & cheese	1 ea	163	315	19	23		16	3.3	1
	Arby's									
6429	Baked potato w/broccoli & cheese	1 ea	384	517	12	69	8	21		
8988	Beef melt sandwich, w/cheddar	1 ea	150	320	16	36	2	14		
9014	Breakfast sandwich, bacon, egg & cheese, w/biscuit	1 ea	144	420	15	27	1	25		
9008	Cheese sticks, mozzarella, breaded & fried	1 ea	137	426	18	38	2	28		
9011	Chicken tenders, 5 piece serving	1 ea	192	555	37	41	3	27		
69043	French dip submarine sandwich, w/au jus	1 ea	285	453	29	49	3	18		
8987	French fries, curly, large	1 ea	198	631	8	73	7	37		
9006	French fries, homestyle, large	1 ea	212.6	565	6	82	6	37		
8998	Grilled chicken caesar salad	1 ea	338	230	33	8	3	8		
69046	Grilled chicken sandwich, deluxe	1 ea	252	450	29	37	2	22		
9001	Grilled chicken sandwich, grilled	1 ea	174	280	29	30	3	5		
8991	Ham & swiss submarine sandwich, hot	1 ea	278	501	28	46	2	18		
69055	Philly beef & swiss submarine sandwich	1 ea	311	678	35	47	4	36		
56336	Roast beef sandwich, regular	1 ea	157	326	20	35	1	14		
53256	Sauce, Arby's, packet	1 ea	14	15	0	4	0	0		
9018	Sauce, barbecue, dipping, svg	1 serving	28.4	45	0	11	0	0		

Source: Arby's

Sat (g)	Chol (mg)	Calc (mg)	Iron (mg)	Mag (mg)	Phos (mg)	Pota (mg)	Sodi (mg)	Zinc (mg)	Vit A (RAE)	Vit C (mg)	Thia (mg)	Ribo (mg)	Niac (mg)	Vit B$_6$ (mg)	Vit B$_{12}$ (µg)	Vit E (mg)	Fol (µg)	Alc (g)
10.5	122	102	5.85	49.7	314	570	791	5.7	5	1.1	0.36	0.38	7.57	0.54	4.07		76.8	0
6.9	68	150	4.29	41.4	222	462	676	4.8		4.4	0.33	0.6	7.72		2.2		106.8	0
4.1	26	63	2.63	22	124	227	504	2.1	4	1.6	0.23	0.2	3.68	0.12	0.88	0.8	51.7	0
3.2	30	124	2.74	18.9	110	174	396	2	0	0	0.26	0.25	4.81	0.13	0.9	0.5	66.6	0
	0	12	0.48	13.7	79	256	373	0.2	0	2.1	0.1	0.06	1.21	0.16	0	0.7	14.4	0
4.9	51	19	3.28	10.3	192	166	480	0.8	3	2.7	0.22	0.4	3.74	0.05	0.3		73	0
5.1	44	24	2.31	12.7	97	143	670	2	0	0.1	0.24	0.27	3.65	0.05	0.51	0.3	48	0
2.7	135	69	1.43	16.4	190	188	965	0.4	9	0	0	0.02	2.03	0.1	0.17		57.7	0
5	21	207	0.58	33.2	228	395	182	0.9	58	2.4	0.06	0.3	1.07	0.13	0.65	0.7	9.5	0
0.6	2	25	0.57	21.8	67	356	275	0.4	13	0.5	0.11	0.06	1.45	0.28	0.06		9.7	0
1.2	4	2	0.05	0.1	3	3	57	0	8	0	0	0	0	0.06	0.03	0.5	0.8	0
5.8	32	282	0.77	42.4	255	499	242	1	65	1	0.14	0.61	0.4	0.12	0.85	0.3	12.5	0
9.9	57	287	1.15	32.4	245	414	202	1.4	227	0	0.06	1.65	0.53	0.15	0.55	0.6	0	0
7.8	18	272	1.28	55.4	276	172	816	1.8	149	1.2	0.19	0.37	1.54	0.2	0.82		10.2	0
11	18	340	2.45	85.5	342	398	1588	3.2	385	4.3	0.2	0.61	2.95	0.36	0.9		33.8	0
6.5	13	69	0.8	14.8	81	122	405	0.3	1	0.5	0.08	0.09	0.87	0.05	0.12	0.3	51.5	0
2.8	66	17	2.73	14.5	120	111	414	9.6	66	2.6	0.19	0.21	2.71	0.02	0.62		18.7	0
2.9	29	64	1.31	24.4	238	125	552	0.5	41	1.7	0.2	0.28	1.69	0.06	0.12	0.7	25.5	0
1	57	13	0.69	7.6	53	256	312	0.2	28	1	0.07	0.1	0.26	0.14	0.11		23.8	0
3.4	22	98	1.43	13	114	232	406	0.8	80	2.5	0.21	0.36	4.63	0.09	0.28		56.2	0
9	77	183	5.05	40.5	401	345	1633	5.4	58	0	0.39	0.46	5.9	0.33	2.06		63.4	0
3.6	51	54	4.23	30.6	239	316	792	3.4	11	2.1	0.38	0.31	5.87	0.26	1.22	0.2	57	0
6.8	44	192	2.28	51.5	143	416	762	2.7	71	3.6	0.1	0.36	2.46	0.22	0.63		83.2	0
6	5	245	2.66	52.2	154	392	885	3.3	258	3.4	0.16	0.5	2.53	0.52	0.73		91.4	0
3.1	114	48	1.69	22.5	197	105	826	0.7	21	0	0.12	0.52	0	0.04	0.08		57.2	0
3.8	73	92	5.16	49	298	524	798	4.5	20	5.5	0.41	0.37	7.3	0.37	1.57		89.8	0
6.8	36	189	2.51	68.4	287	394	1651	2.6	71	12.3	1	0.8	5.49	0.14	1.09		86.6	0
5.3	49	74	2.64	79.4	220	335	1293	1.9	46	3.6	0.46	0.33	11.34	0.23	1.61		102.4	0
11.4	56	221	2.41	70.1	203	474	802	3.9	108	2.2	0.15	0.44	3.21	0.24	1.04	1.9	68.4	0
5.4	30	210	1.89	59	117	403	543	1.9	45	1.3	0.1	0.33	1.32	0.16	0.69	1.2	43.2	0
10.4	41	217	2.87	63.6	179	572	896	3.7	51	2.6	0.1	0.55	3.15	0.23	1.17		75	0
10.9	46	174	3.82				756			82.2								0
	645	80	2.7				850			0								0
7.3	153	137	0.82				1318			0								0
12.9	45	380	0.99				1370			0.6								0
4.8	61	330	2.63				1742			0.9								0
7.2	59	61	4.38				2843	0		0.6								0
6.8	0	80	3.24				1476			9.6								0
6.7	0	50	1.62				1027			12.6								0
3.5	80	200	1.8				920			42								0
4	110	60	2.7			722	1050			1.2	0.34	0.32	14.9					0
1.5	55	80	1.8				1170			0								0
4.2	55	282	3.26				1840			10.3								0
10.9	91	314	4.56				1968			9.1								0
5.5	45	61	3.67				972	0		0								0
0	0	0	0				177	0		1.2								0
0	0	10	0.18				348			0.6								0

MDA Code	Food Name	Amt	Wt (g)	Ener (kcal)	Prot (g)	Carb (g)	Fiber (g)	Fat (g)	Mono (g)	Poly (g)
	Burger King									
56352	Cheeseburger	1 ea	133	380	19	32	4	20	7.6	2
56355	Cheeseburger, Whopper	1 ea	316	790	35	53	3	48	16	12
56357	Cheeseburger, Whopper, double	1 ea	399	1061	58	54	6	68	25.1	11.9
9087	Chicken tenders, 4 piece serving	1 ea	62	179	11	11	1	10	5.9	1.3
9065	French fries, large	1 ea	160	530	6	64	5	28	17.7	1.8
56351	Hamburger	1 ea	121	333	17	33	2	15	6.4	1.5
56354	Hamburger, Whopper	1 ea	291	678	31	54	5	37	13.6	9.9
9071	Hash browns, rounds, medium	1 ea	128	472	4	44	4	31	17.6	4.1
2127	Milk shake, chocolate, medium	1 ea	397	440	13	80	4	8		
2129	Milk shake, vanilla, medium	1 ea	397	667	13	76	0	35	9.8	1.7
9041	Onion rings, large	1 ea	137	480	7	60	5	23		
69071	Sandwich, breakfast, bacon, egg & cheese, w/biscuit	1 ea	189	692	27	51	1	61		
57002	Sandwich, Chicken Broiler	1 ea	258	550	30	52	3	25		
9084	Sandwich, croissant w/sausage & cheese	1 ea	107	402	15	25	1	27	12.9	3.3
	Source: Burger King Corporation									
	Chik-Fil-A									
69185	Chicken breast fillet, chargrilled	1 ea	79	100	20	1	0	2		
15263	Chicken nuggets, 8 piece serving	1 ea	113	260	26	12	1	12		
15262	Chick-N-Strips, 4 piece serving	1 ea	108	250	25	12	0	11		
52138	Cole slaw, small	1 ea	105	210	1	14	2	17		
48214	Pie, lemon, slice	1 pce	113	320	7	51	3	10		
52134	Salad, garden, chicken, chargrilled	1 ea	278	180	23	8	3	6		
52137	Salad, side	1 ea	164	80	5	6	2	5		
69155	Sandwich, chicken salad, w/whole wheat	1 ea	153	350	20	32	5	15		
69189	Sandwich, chicken deluxe	1 ea	208	420	28	39	2	16		
69176	Sauce, honey mustard, dipping, packet	1 ea	28	45	0	10	0	0	0	0
69182	Wrap, chicken, spicy	1 ea	225	390	31	51	3	7		
	Source: Chik-Fil-A									
	Dairy Queen									
56372	Cheeseburger, double, homestyle	1 ea	219	540	35	30	2	31		
72142	Frozen dessert, banana split, large	1 ea	527	810	17	134	2	23		
71693	Frozen dessert, Brownie Earthquake	1 ea	304	740	10	112	0	27		
72139	Frozen dessert, chocolate cookie dough, large	1 ea	560	1320	21	193	0	52		
72134	Frozen dessert, sundae, chocolate, large	1 ea	333	580	11	100	1	15		
72138	Frozen dessert, Oreo, large	1 ea	500	1010	19	148	2	37		
72135	Frozen dessert, sundae, strawberry, large	1 ea	333	500	10	83	1	15		
72137	Frozen dessert, Triple Chocolate Utopia	1 ea	284	770	12	96	5	39		
2222	Ice cream cone, chocolate, medium	1 ea	198	340	8	53	0	11		
2136	Ice cream cone, dipped, medium	1 ea	220	490	8	59	1	24		
2143	Ice cream cone, vanilla, medium	1 ea	213	355	9	57	0	10		
2134	Ice cream sandwich	1 ea	85	200	4	31	1	6		
72129	Milk shake, chocolate malt, large	1 ea	836	1320	29	222	2	35		
	Source: International Dairy Queen, Inc.									
	Domino's Pizza									
91365	Breadsticks	1 ea	37.2	116	3	18	1	4		
91369	Chicken, buffalo wings	1 ea	24.9	50	6	2	0	2		
56386	Pizza, cheese, hand tossed, 12"	2 pce	159	375	15	55	3	11		
91356	Pizza, Deluxe Feast, hand tossed, 12"	2 pce	200.8	465	19	57	3	18		
91358	Pizza, MeatZZa Feast, hand tossed, 12"	2 pce	216.2	560	26	57	3	26		

Sat (g)	Chol (mg)	Calc (mg)	Iron (mg)	Mag (mg)	Phos (mg)	Pota (mg)	Sodi (mg)	Zinc (mg)	Vit A (RAE)	Vit C (mg)	Thia (mg)	Ribo (mg)	Niac (mg)	Vit B$_6$ (mg)	Vit B$_{12}$ (µg)	Vit E (mg)	Fol (µg)	Alc (g)
9.1	60	124	3.32	31.9	190	237	801	3.2		0.3	0.4	0.32	4.52	0.12		0.1		0
18.3	114	259	6.32	56.9	357	534	1431	5.1		0.6	0.67	0.63	8.09	0.23		0.3	161.2	0
27.9	188	311	21.15	75.8	511	754	1544	14		0.8	1.07	0.84	11.97	0.45		0.2	107.7	0
2.6	32	9	0.38	15.5	141	163	447	0.4		0.4	0.08	0.07	4.64	0.22		0.5	4.3	0
7		14	2.06	48	229	757	728	1.8		1.1	0.28	0.05	3.75	0.28		1.2		0
6.1	42	62	3.05	29	144	220	551	2.6		0.2	0.4	0.27	4.78	0.12		0	77.4	0
12.4	87	113	12.72	52.4	262	492	911	8.2		0.6	0.63	0.51	8.36	0.26		0.4	136.8	0
7.6	0	20	0.88	24.3	141	467	654	0.4	0	2	0.2	0.11	2.31	0.29	0	1.4		0
5	35	350	1.8				270			0								0
21.2	123	413	1.67	47.6	385	607	397	2.7		0	0	0.71	0.36	0.12	1.43	1.3		0
6	0	150	0				690	0		0								0
18.6	253	200	3.59				2130			0								0
5	105	60	3.6				1110			6								0
9.2	46	114	2	20.3	169	219	837	1.5		0	0.35	0.34	4.38	0.19	0.59	1		0
0	60	0	0.36				690	0		0								0
2.5	70	40	1.08				1090	0		0								0
2.5	70	40	1.08				570	0		0								0
2.5	20	40	0.36				180			27								0
3.5	110	150	0				220			4.8								0
3	70	150	0.36				730			6								0
2.5	15	150	0				110			4.8								0
3	65	150	1.8				880	0		0								0
3.5	60	100	2.7				1300			2.4								0
0	0	0	0				150	0		0								0
3.5	70	200	3.6				1150			4.8								0
16	115	250	4.5				1130			3.6								0
15	70	600	2.7				360			12								0
16	50	250	1.8				350			0								0
26	90	600	4.5				670			2.4								0
10	45	350	1.8				260			1.2								0
18	70	600	4.5				770			2.4								0
9	45	400	1.8				230			18								0
17	55	300	1.8				390			1.2								0
7	30	250	1.8				160			1.2								0
13	30	250	1.8				190			2.4								0
6.5	32	269	1.94				172			2.6								0
3	10	80	1.08				140			0								0
22	110	900	3.6				670			4.8								0
0.8	0	6	0.87				152			0.1								0
0.6	26	6	0.32				175			0.1								0
4.8	23	187	2.99				776			0								0
7.7	40	199	3.56				1063			1.4								0
11.4	64	282	3.72				1463			0.1								0

MDA Code	Food Name	Amt	Wt (g)	Ener (kcal)	Prot (g)	Carb (g)	Fiber (g)	Fat (g)	Mono (g)	Poly (g)
91361	Pizza, Pepperoni Feast, hand tossed, 12"	2 pce	196.1	534	24	56	3	25		
91357	Pizza, Veggie Feast, hand tossed, 12"	2 pce	203.2	439	19	57	4	16		
	Source: Domino's Pizza Incorporated									
	Hardee's									
9295	Apple turnover	1 ea	91	270	4	38		12		
42330	Biscuit, cinnamon 'n raisin	1 ea	75	250	2	42		8		
15201	Chicken wing, serving	1 ea	66	200	10	23	0	8		
9278	Hot dog, w/chili	1 ea	160	451	15	24	2	32		
9284	Chicken strips, breaded & fried, 5 piece serving	1 ea	92	201	18	13	0	8		
9277	Hamburger, Monster	1 ea	278	949	53	35	2	67		
9275	Hamburger, Six Dollar	1 ea	353	911	41	50	2	61		
2247	Ice cream cone, twist	1 ea	118	180	4	34		2		
6147	French fries, large	1 ea	150	440	5	59	0	21		
9281	Sandwich, chicken, bbq, grilled	1 ea	171	268	24	34	2	3		
56423	Sandwich, fish, Fisherman's Fillet	1 ea	221	530	25	45		28		
	Source: Hardee's Food Systems, Inc.									
	Jack in the Box									
56437	Cheeseburger, Jumbo Jack	1 ea	296	714	26	56	3	43		
62547	Cheeseburger, bacon ultimate	1 ea	302	974	41	47	2	69		
57014	Chicken teriyaki bowl	1 ea	502	670	26	128	3	4		
56445	Egg roll, 3 piece serving	1 ea	170	400	14	44	6	19		
6425	French fries, curly, medium	1 ea	125	404	6	44	4	23		
6150	French fries, natural cut, small	1 ea	113	306	5	40	3	14		
62558	French toast, original, sticks, serving	1 ea	120	466	7	58	4	23		
56433	Hamburger	1 ea	104	273	14	26	1	12		
62560	Milk shake, cappuccino, medium	1 ea	419	630	11	80	0	29		
2964	Milk shake, Oreo cookie, medium	1 ea	419	941	15	112	1	46		
2165	Milk shake, vanilla, medium	1 ea	332	664	13	75	1	34		
56446	Onion rings, serving	1 ea	120	504	6	51	3	30		
62551	Potato wedges, bacon cheddar, serving	1 ea	268	692	21	53	6	44		
8368	Salad dressing, blue cheese, packet	1 ea	57	210	1	11	0	15		
8449	Salad dressing, Italian, low cal, serving	1 ea	57	25	0	2	0	2		
52088	Salad, garden chicken	1 ea	253	200	23	8	3	9		
56441	Sandwich, chicken fajita pita	1 ea	230	317	24	33	3	11		
56431	Sandwich, breakfast, sausage w/croissant	1 ea	181	603	22	38	2	41		
56377	Taco, beef, regular	1 ea	90	189	6	18	2	9		
	Source: Jack in the Box									
	KFC									
42331	Biscuit, buttermilk	1 ea	57	190	2	23	0	10		
15169	Chicken breast, extra crispy	1 ea	162	460	34	19	0	28		
15185	Chicken breast, hot & spicy	1 ea	179	460	33	20	0	27		
15163	Chicken breast, original recipe	1 ea	161	380	40	11	0	19		
81292	Chicken breast, original recipe, w/o skin or breading	1 ea	108	140	29	0	0	3		
81293	Chicken, drumstick, original recipe	1 ea	59	140	14	4	0	8		
15166	Chicken thigh, original recipe	1 ea	126	360	22	12	0	25		
416	Chicken wing, pieces, honey bbq	6 ea	157	540	25	36	1	33		
56451	Cole slaw, serving	1 ea	130	190	1	22	3	11		
9535	Corn, cob, small	1 ea	82	76	3	13	4	2		
2897	Dessert, strawberry shortcake, Lil Bucket	1 ea	99	200	2	34	0	6		
56681	Macaroni & cheese	1 ea	287	130	5	15	1	6		

Sat (g)	Chol (mg)	Calc (mg)	Iron (mg)	Mag (mg)	Phos (mg)	Pota (mg)	Sodi (mg)	Zinc (mg)	Vit A (RAE)	Vit C (mg)	Thia (mg)	Ribo (mg)	Niac (mg)	Vit B$_6$ (mg)	Vit B$_{12}$ (µg)	Vit E (mg)	Fol (µg)	Alc (g)
10.9	57	279	3.4				1349			0.1								0
7.1	34	279	3.44				987			1.3								0
4	0						250											0
2	0						350											0
2	30						740											0
12	55						1238											0
1.7	25						736											0
25	185						1573											0
27	137						1584											0
1	10						120											0
3	0						520											0
1	60						697											0
7	75						1280											0
16.6	72					424	1356											0
26.8	125					482	1823											0
1	15	100	4.5			620	1730			24								0
6	15					430	920											0
4.4	0					581	882											0
3.5	0					715	502											0
5	25					119	446											0
5.3	35					220	529											0
17	90	350	0			710	320			0								0
25.8	157					913	488											0
21	134					734	256											0
6.1	0					141	424											0
14.8	49					951	1581											0
2.5	25	20	0			40	750	0		0								0
0	0	10	0			40	670	0		0								0
4	65	200	0.72			560	420			12								0
4.7	69					475	928											0
13.5	265					270	801											0
3.6	18					225	320											0
2	0	0	0.72				580	0		0								0
8	135	0	1.44				1230	0		0								0
8	130	0	1.14				1450	0		0								0
6	145	0	1.8				1150	0		0								0
1	95	0	0.72				410	0		0								0
2	75	0	0.72				440	0		0								0
7	165	0	1.14				1060	0		0								0
7	150	60	2.7				1130			4.8								0
2	5	40	0				300			24								0
0.5	0	30	0.55				5	0		3								0
4	20	20	0				110	0		0								0
2	5	100	0.72				610			24								0

MDA Code	Food Name	Amt	Wt (g)	Ener (kcal)	Prot (g)	Carb (g)	Fiber (g)	Fat (g)	Mono (g)	Poly (g)
56453	Mashed potatoes w/gravy, serving	1 ea	136	130	2	18	1	4		
45166	Pecan pie, Colonel's Pies, slice	1 pce	95	370	4	55	2	15		
81090	Pot pie, chicken, chunky	1 ea	423	770	29	70	5	40		
56454	Potato salad, serving	1 ea	128	180	2	22	1	9		
49148	Sandwich, chicken, honey bbq flavor, w/sauce	1 ea	147	300	21	41	4	6		
81301	Sandwich, chicken, tender roasted, w/o sauce	1 ea	177	260	31	23	1	5		
81093	Sandwich, chicken, tender roasted, w/sauce	1 ea	196	390	31	24	1	19		
81302	Sandwich, chicken, Twister	1 ea	252	670	27	55	3	38		

Source: Yum! Brands, Inc.

Long John Silver's

MDA Code	Food Name	Amt	Wt (g)	Ener (kcal)	Prot (g)	Carb (g)	Fiber (g)	Fat (g)	Mono (g)	Poly (g)
91388	Cheese sticks, breaded, fried	3 ea	45	140	4	12	1	8		
91390	Clam chowder, serving	1 ea	227	220	9	23	1	10		
56477	Cornbread, hush puppies, serving	1 ea	23	60	1	9	1	2		
56461	Fish, batter dipped, regular	1 pce	92	230	11	16	0	13		
92415	Fish, cod, baked, serving	1 ea	100.7	120	21	0	0	5		
91392	Sandwich, fish, batter dipped, ultimate	1 ea	199	500	20	48	3	25		
92290	Shrimp, battered, 4 piece serving	1 ea	65.8	197	7	14	0	13		
92292	Shrimp, crunchy, breaded, fried, basket	1 ea	114	340	12	32	2	19		

Source: Yum! Brands, Inc.

McDonald's

MDA Code	Food Name	Amt	Wt (g)	Ener (kcal)	Prot (g)	Carb (g)	Fiber (g)	Fat (g)	Mono (g)	Poly (g)
81465	Breakfast, big, w/eggs, sausage, hashbrowns, biscuit	1 ea	266	742	27	46	3	52	22.9	7.5
56675	Burrito, sausage, breakfast	1 ea	113	296	13	24	1	17	6.5	2.4
69010	Cheeseburger, Big Mac	1 ea	219	563	26	44	4	33	7.6	0.7
81458	Cheeseburger, double	1 ea	173	458	26	34	1	26	8.6	0.8
69012	Cheeseburger, Quarter Pounder	1 ea	199	513	29	40	3	28	9.2	0.9
49152	Chicken McNuggets, 6 piece serving	6 pce	100	264	16	16	0	15	6.2	5
42334	Croutons, serving	1 ea	12	50	1	9	1	1		
42335	Danish, apple	1 ea	105	340	5	47	2	15		
72902	Dessert, apple dipper, w/low fat caramel sauce	1 ea	89	99	0	23		1	0.2	0
81440	French fries, large	1 ea	171	576	6	70	7	31	13.8	8
2171	Hot fudge sundae	1 ea	179	333	7	54	1	11	1.9	0.4
69008	Hamburger	1 ea	105	265	13	32	1	10	3.3	0.2
69011	Hamburger, Quarter Pounder	1 ea	171	417	24	38	3	20	7.2	0.5
6155	Hash browns	1 ea	53	136	1	13	2	9	3.9	2.2
1747	McFlurry, frozen dessert, Butterfinger	1 ea	348	620	16	90	1	22		
72913	Milk shake, chocolate, triple thick, large	1 ea	713	1162	26	199	1	32	8	1.5
81453	Pancakes, hotcake, w/2 pats margarine & syrup	1 ea	221	601	9	102	2	18	1.9	4.6
81154	Parfait, fruit n' yogurt, w/o granola	1 ea	142	128	4	25	1	2	0	0
48136	Pie, apple	1 ea	77	249	2	34	2	12	7.1	0.8
69218	Salad, bacon ranch, w/crispy chicken	1 ea	316	335	27	21	3	18	6.2	4
608	Salad, caesar, w/chicken, shaker	1 ea	163	100	17	3	2	2		
61674	Salad, California cobb, w/grilled chicken	1 ea	325	273	34	11	3	11	3.8	1.4
57764	Salad, chef, shaker	1 ea	206	150	17	5	2	8		
61667	Salad, fruit & walnut	1 ea	264	312	5	44		13	2.1	8.5
81466	Sandwich, breakfast, McGriddle w/bacon, egg & cheese	1 ea	168	457	20	44	1	22	7.9	3
69013	Sandwich, Filet-O-Fish	1 ea	141	400	15	40	1	20	4.3	7
81456	Sandwich, Filet-O-Fish, w/o tartar sauce	1 ea	123	289	15	40	1	11	2.2	1.8
53176	Sauce, barbecue, packet	1 ea	28	46	0	10	0	0	0.1	0.1
53177	Sauce, sweet & sour, packet	1 ea	28	48	0	11	0	0	0.1	0.1
12230	Sausage, pork, serving	1 ea	43	170	6	0	0	16		
42747	Sweet roll, cinnamon	1 ea	105	418	8	56	2	19	9.5	3

Source: McDonald's Nutrition Information Center

Sat (g)	Chol (mg)	Calc (mg)	Iron (mg)	Mag (mg)	Phos (mg)	Pota (mg)	Sodi (mg)	Zinc (mg)	Vit A (RAE)	Vit C (mg)	Thia (mg)	Ribo (mg)	Niac (mg)	Vit B6 (mg)	Vit B12 (µg)	Vit E (mg)	Fol (µg)	Alc (g)
1	0	0	0.36				380			2.4								0
2.5	40	0	1.44				190			0								0
15	115	0	3.6				1680			0								0
1.5	5	0	0.36				470		0	6								0
1.5	50	60	2.7				640			2.4								0
1.5	65	40	1.8				690	0		0								0
4	70	40	1.8				810	0		0								0
7	60	150	2.7				1650			4.8								0
2	10	100	0.72				320			0								0
4	25	150	0.72				810			0								0
0.5	0	20	0.36				200	0		0								0
4	30	20	1.8				700	0		4.8								0
1	90	20	0.72				240			0								0
8	50	150	3.6				1310			9								0
4.1	64	23	0.83				579	0		2.8								0
5	105	500	1.8				720	0		0								0
13.6	466	130	5	37.2	684	545	1463	2.6	189	1.6	0.61	0.94	6.04	0.46	1.54	3.3	196.8	0
6.1	173	203	1.84	19.2	247	155	763	1.3	97	0.9	0.18	0.33	1.92	0.41	0.61	0.2	70.1	0
8.3	79	254	4.38	43.8	267	396	1007	4.2		0.9	0.39	0.46	7.41	0.37	1.93	0.1	100.7	0
10.5	83	277	3.68	34.6	280	375	1137	4.2		0.7	0.28	0.43	6.68		2.04		77.8	0
11.2	94	287	4.18	43.8	320	436	1152	5.2		1.6	0.33	0.7	7.66	0.19	2.51	0.4	101.5	0
3.3	39	14	0.78	22	332	251	699	0.6		1	0.16	0.11	7.4	0.4	0.33		28	0
0	0	20	0.36	3.9	18	26	105	0.1	0	0.2	0.08	0.05	0.57	0.02	0.02		5.1	0
3	20	60	1.44		0	113	340			15	0.3	0.17	2					0
0.4	3	57	0.1				36	0.1	11	188.3	0.02	0.03	0	0.01	0	0.1	0	0
6.1	0	27	1.76	54.7	226	958	332	0.8	0	8.4	0.56	0.06	4.72	0.89		3.5	102.6	0
6.4	23	249	1.49	34	229	440	168	1	145		0.08	0.4	0.27	0.09	0.98	0.3	0	0
3.1	28	127	2.77	21	112	213	532	2		0.6	0.26	0.25	4.77	0.1	0.87	0.1	67.2	0
6.9	67	144	4.12	37.6	212	388	730	4.6		1.5	0.31	0.59	7.61	0.25	2.19	0.1	95.8	0
1.6	0	10	0.4	11.1	57	207	289	0.2	0	1.6	0.06	0.01	1.19	0.13		1	20.1	0
14	70	450	0.36				260			2.4								0
16.4	100	870	3.85	114.1	749	1611	506	3.6	649		0.28	1.53	0.94	0.36	3.85	0	7.1	0
1.8	20	126	2.83	28.7	391	276	625	0.6		0	0.45	0.4	3.24	0.11	0.02		143.6	0
0	7	124	0.51	17	101	234	54	0.4		20.6	0.05	0.17	0.27		0.28		15.6	0
3.1		15	1.53	5.4	28	49	153	0.2		24.9	0.23	0.16	2.03	0.04		1.5	87	0
5	70	149	2.05				1112			31.6	0.19	0.22	9.56		0.41		154.8	0
1.5	40	100	1.08				240			12								0
4.8	143	143	2.21				1079			31.9	0.18	0.33	11.67				149.5	0
3.5	95	150	1.44				740			15								0
1.8	5	172	0.9	34.3	129		84	0.7		383.6	0.1	0.15	0.27	0.25	0.16		13.2	0
7.1	247	183	2.77				1263	3		0.21	0.5	2.22					89	0
3.7	39	164	2.07	28.2	166	247	633	0.7		0	0.36	0.26	3.4	0.06	1.03	1.6	70.5	0
2.1	31	159	2	28.3	161	237	520	0.7		0	0.35	0.25	3.41		0.98		70.1	0
0		3	0.11	3.6	8	55	255	0		3	0	0.01	0.01	0.19	0.02	0.3	2.2	0
0		2	0.18	1.7	4	28	156	0		2	0.3	0.05	0.01	0.11	0.01	0.2	0	0
5	35	7	0.36	6.6	59	102	290	0.8	0	0	0.18	0.06	1.7	0.09	0.35	0.3		0
4.7	61	60	1.81	20	109	147	397	0.9	132	0	0.32	0.28	2.53	0.11		1.9	108.2	0

MDA Code	Food Name	Amt	Wt (g)	Ener (kcal)	Prot (g)	Carb (g)	Fiber (g)	Fat (g)	Mono (g)	Poly (g)
	Pizza Hut									
92497	Breadsticks, cheese	1 ea	67	200	7	21	1	10		
92526	Dessert pizza, cherry, slice	1 pce	102	240	4	47	1	4		
92519	Pasta Bakes, primavera w/chicken, serving	1 ea	540	1050	52	97	6	50		
57394	Pizza, beef, med, 12"	1 pce	91	230	11	21	2	11		
56489	Pizza, cheese, med, 12"	1 pce	96	260	11	30	2	10	2.8	1.8
56481	Pizza, cheese, pan, med, 12"	1 pce	100	280	12	30	2	13	3.2	2.8
57781	Pizza, chicken supreme, med, 12"	1 pce	120	230	14	30	2	6		
830	Pizza, super supreme, med, 12"	1 pce	127	309	14	33	3	14	5	2.2
92483	Pizza, green pepper onion & tomato, med, 12"	1 pce	104	150	6	24	2	4		
92482	Pizza, ham pine & tomato, med, 12"	1 pce	99	160	8	24	2	4		
57810	Pizza, Meat Lover's, med, 12"	1 pce	169	450	21	43	3	21		
56486	Pizza, pepperoni, med, 12"	1 pce	77	210	10	21	1	10		
57811	Pizza, Veggie Lover's, med, 12"	1 pce	172	360	16	45	3	14		

Source: Yum! Brands, Inc.

MDA Code	Food Name	Amt	Wt (g)	Ener (kcal)	Prot (g)	Carb (g)	Fiber (g)	Fat (g)	Mono (g)	Poly (g)
	Subway									
47658	Cookie, chocolate chip, M & M's	1 ea	45	220	2	30	1	10		
52119	Salad, chicken breast, roasted	1 ea	303	140	16	12	3	3		
52115	Salad, club	1 ea	322	150	17	12	3	4		
52118	Salad, tuna, w/light mayonnaise	1 ea	314	240	13	10	3	16		
52113	Salad, veggie delite	1 ea	233	50	2	9	3	1		
91761	Sandwich, chicken teriyaki, w/sweet onion, on white bread, 6"	1 ea	269	380	26	59	4	5		
69117	Sandwich, club, on white bread, 6"	1 ea	255	320	24	46	4	6		
69113	Sandwich, cold cut trio, on white bread, 6"	1 ea	257	440	21	47	4	21		
91763	Sandwich, ham w/honey mustard, on white bread, 6"	1 ea	232	310	18	52	4	5		
69139	Sandwich, Italian BMT, on white bread, 6"	1 ea	248	480	23	46	4	24		
69129	Sandwich, meatball, on white bread, 6"	1 ea	287	530	24	53	6	26		
69103	Sandwich, roast beef, deli style	1 ea	151	220	13	35	3	4		
69143	Sandwich, tuna, w/light mayonnaise, on white bread, 6"	1 ea	255	450	20	46	4	22		
69101	Sandwich, turkey, deli style	1 ea	151	220	13	36	3	4		
69109	Sandwich, veggie delite, on white bread, 6"	1 ea	166	230	9	44	4	3		
91778	Soup, chicken noodle, roasted	1 cup	240	90	7	7	1	4		
91791	Soup, cream of broccoli	1 cup	240	130	5	15	2	6		
91783	Soup, minestrone	1 cup	240	70	3	11	2	1		
91788	Soup, rice, brown & wild, w/chicken	1 cup	240	190	6	17	2	11		

Source: Subway International

MDA Code	Food Name	Amt	Wt (g)	Ener (kcal)	Prot (g)	Carb (g)	Fiber (g)	Fat (g)	Mono (g)	Poly (g)
	Taco Bell									
92107	Border Bowl, chicken, zesty	1 ea	417	730	23	65	12	42		
56519	Burrito, bean	1 ea	198	404	16	55	8	14	5.9	1.7
56522	Burrito, beef, supreme	1 ea	248	469	20	52	8	20	8.1	2
57668	Burrito, chicken, fiesta	1 ea	184	370	18	48	3	12		
56691	Burrito, seven layer	1 ea	283	530	18	67	10	22		
92113	Burrito, steak, grilled, Stuft	1 ea	325	680	31	76	8	28		
92118	Chalupa, beef, nacho cheese	1 ea	153	380	12	33	3	22		
92120	Chalupa, chicken, Baja	1 ea	153	400	17	30	2	24		
92122	Chalupa, steak, supreme	1 ea	153	370	15	29	2	22		
45585	Cinnamon twists, serving	1 ea	35	160	1	28	0	5		
57666	Gordita, beef, Baja	1 ea	153	350	14	31	4	19		
57669	Gordita, chicken, Baja	1 ea	153	320	17	29	2	15		
57662	Gordita, steak, Baja	1 ea	153	320	15	29	2	16		

Sat (g)	Chol (mg)	Calc (mg)	Iron (mg)	Mag (mg)	Phos (mg)	Pota (mg)	Sodi (mg)	Zinc (mg)	Vit A (RAE)	Vit C (mg)	Thia (mg)	Ribo (mg)	Niac (mg)	Vit B$_6$ (mg)	Vit B$_{12}$ (µg)	Vit E (mg)	Fol (µg)	Alc (g)
3.5	15	100	3.6				340			0								0
0.5	0	20	1.08				250			6								0
12	75	800	5.4				2760			6								0
5	25	150	1.8				710			3.6								0
4.8	23	201	1.87	21.1	239	166	658	1.6	71	0	0.25	0.25	3.16	0.11	0.67	0.7		0
5.2	21	208	1.86	21	241	168	624	1.6	74	0	0.24	0.25	3.91	0.11	0.64	1.1		0
3	25	150	1.8				550			6								0
5.8	25	164	2.54	29.2	254	296	875	1.8	46	0	0.34	0.31	4.55	0.19	0.79	1		0
1.5	10	80	1.44				360			21								0
2	15	80	1.44				470			12								0
10	55	250	2.7				1250			9								0
4.5	25	150	1.44				550			2.4								0
7	35	250	2.7				980			9								0
4	15	0	1.08				105	0		0								0
1	45	40	1.08				800			30								0
1.5	35	40	18				1110			30								0
4	40	100	1.08				880			30								0
0	0	40	1.08				310			30								0
1.5	50	80	3.6				1100			27								0
2	35	60	5.4				1300			21								0
7	55	150	5.4				1680			24								0
1.5	25	60	3.6				1260			24								0
9	55	150	3.6				1900			24								0
10	55	150	5.4				1360			27								0
2	15	60	5.4				660			12								0
6	40	15	3.6				1190			24								0
1.5	15	60	3.6				730			12								0
1	0	60	3.6				510			21								0
1	20	20	0				1180			3.6								0
0	10	150	0				860			12								0
0	10	40	0				1030			6								0
4.5	20	300	0				990			24								0
9	45	150	3.6				1640			9								0
4.8	18	232	4.57	61.4	337	533	1216	1.7	6		0.4	0.3	3.39	0.24	0	1	99	0
7.6	40	231	5.6	62	337	608	1424	2.6	10		0.38	0.37	4.33	0.26	1.24	1.1	111.6	0
3.5	30	200	2.7				1090			3.6								0
8	25	300	3.6				1360			4.8								0
8	55	300	4.5				1940			3.6								0
7	20	100	1.44				740			6								0
6	40	100	1.08				690			3.6								0
8	35	100	1.44				520			3.6								0
1	0	0	0.36				150	0		0								0
5	30	150	2.7				750			4.8								0
3.5	40	100	1.8				690			3.6								0
4	30	100	1.8				680			3.6								0

MDA Code	Food Name	Amt	Wt (g)	Ener (kcal)	Prot (g)	Carb (g)	Fiber (g)	Fat (g)	Mono (g)	Poly (g)
56530	Guacamole, serving	1 ea	21	35	0	2	1	3		
38561	Mexican rice, serving	1 ea	131	210	6	23	3	10		
56534	Nachos, BellGrande, svg	1 ea	308	780	20	80	12	43		
56536	Pintos & cheese, serving	1 ea	128	180	10	20	6	7		
56531	Pizza, Mexican	1 ea	216	550	21	46	7	31		
57689	Quesadilla, chicken	1 ea	184	540	28	40	3	30		
92098	Salsa, fiesta	1 ea	21	5	0	1		0	0	0
53186	Sauce, border, hot, packet	1 ea	11	4	0	0	0	0	0	0
92105	Southwest steak bowl	1 ea	443	700	30	73	13	32		
56524	Taco, beef	1 ea	78	184	8	14	3	11	4.2	1.6
57671	Taco, Double Decker, supreme	1 ea	191	380	15	40	6	18		
56693	Taco, soft, steak	1 ea	127	286	15	22	2	15	5	4.4
56537	Salad, taco, w/salsa & shell	1 ea	533	906	36	80	16	49	21.2	4
56528	Tostada	1 ea	170	250	11	29	7	10		

Source: Taco Bell/Yum! Brands, Inc.

Wendy's

MDA Code	Food Name	Amt	Wt (g)	Ener (kcal)	Prot (g)	Carb (g)	Fiber (g)	Fat (g)	Mono (g)	Poly (g)
56579	Baked potato bacon cheese	1 ea	380	580	18	79	7	22		
56582	Baked potato, w/sour cream & chives	1 ea	312	370	7	73	7	6		
81445	Cheeseburger, classic single	1 ea	236	522	35	34	3	27	10.4	3.3
56571	Cheeseburger, w/bacon, jr	1 ea	165	380	20	34	2	19		
15176	Chicken nuggets, 5 piece serving	1 ea	75	250	12	12	0	17	8.5	4.3
50311	Chili, small	1 ea	227	200	17	21	5	6		
6169	French fries, Biggie	1 ea	159	507	6	63	6	26	13.5	5.9
2177	Frozen dessert, dairy, medium	1 ea	298	393	10	70	10	8	2.1	0.3
56574	Hamburger, Big Bacon Classic	1 ea	282	570	34	46	3	29		
56566	Hamburger, classic single	1 ea	218	464	28	37	3	23	8.9	3.4
8457	Salad dressing, blue cheese, packet	1 ea	71	290	2	3	0	30		
8461	Salad dressing, French, fat free, packet	1 ea	71	90	0	21	1	0	0	0
71595	Salad dressing, Oriental sesame, packet	1 ea	71	280	2	21	0	21		
81444	Sandwich, chicken fillet, homestyle	1 ea	230	492	32	50	3	19	6.7	7.1
81443	Sandwich, chicken, Ultimate Grill	1 ea	225	403	33	42	2	11	3.3	4.1
52080	Salad, caesar, w/o dressing, side	1 ea	99	70	7	2	1	4		
71592	Salad, chicken, mandarin, w/o dressing	1 ea	348	150	20	17	3	2		
52083	Salad, garden, w/o dressing, side	1 ea	167	35	2	7	3	0	0	0

Source: Wendy's Foods International

Sat (g)	Chol (mg)	Calc (mg)	Iron (mg)	Mag (mg)	Phos (mg)	Pota (mg)	Sodi (mg)	Zinc (mg)	Vit A (RAE)	Vit C (mg)	Thia (mg)	Ribo (mg)	Niac (mg)	Vit B_6 (mg)	Vit B_{12} (µg)	Vit E (mg)	Fol (µg)	Alc (g)
0	0	0	0				100		0	0								0
4	15	100	1.8				740			4.8								0
13	35	200	2.7				1300			6								0
3.5	15	150	1.08				700			3.6								0
11	45	350	3.6				1030			6								0
13	80	500	1.8				1380			2.4								0
0	0	0	0				60	5		2.4								0
0	0	0	0				102			0								0
8	55	200	6.3				2050			9								0
3.6	24	62	1.47	25.7	139	168	349	1.7	3		0.07	0.15	1.5	0.11	0.75	0.5	14.8	0
8	40	150	2.7				820			4.8								0
4.3	39	149	2.82	26.7	197	232	700	2.7	1		0.39	0.25	3.78	0.11	1.22	0.5	47	0
15.9	101	506	9.43	143.9	549	1221	1935	6.2	16		0.8	0.56	8.02	0.55	2.13	2.9	229.2	0
4	15	150	1.44				710			4.8								0
6	40	200	3.6			1410	950			42								0
4	15	60	3.6			1230	40			36								0
12.3	90	177	5.52	44.8	297	441	1123	6.1		1.2	0.61	0.6	7.53	0.25	3.63			0
7	55	150	3.6			320	890			9								0
3.7	38	18	0.56	18	215	177	509	0.5		1	0.06	0.09	4.53	0.19	0.25			0
2.5	35	80	1.8			470	870			2.4								0
5.1		24	3.07	54.1	218	914	273	0.8		8.1	0.28	0.1	3.95	0.62			27	0
4.9	48	381	3.1	59.6	334	551	292	1.3		0	0.18	2.15	1.04	0	1.76			0
12	100	200	5.4			580	1460			15								0
8	76	74	5.95	39.2	225	425	861	5.4		1.1	0.6	0.45	7.03	0.25	3.16			0
6	45	60	1.08			25	870			0								0
0	0	0	0.72			10	240	0		0								0
3	0	20	0.72			40	620	0		0								0
3.7	71	53	3.45	55.2	370	524	922	1.4		0.7	0.68	0.3	7.59	0.43	0.76			0
2.3	90	56	3.49	54	378	497	961	1.3		2.5	0.88	0.58	9.36	0.32	0.74			0
2	15	150	1.08			280	250			21								0
0	10	60	1.8			420	650			30								0
0	0	40	0.72			350	20		350	18								0

APPENDIX B Calculations and Conversions

Calculation and Conversion Aids

Commonly Used Metric Units

millimeter (mm): one-thousandth of a meter (0.001)
centimeter (cm): one-hundredth of a meter (0.01)
kilometer (km): one thousand times a meter (1000)
kilogram (kg): one thousand times a gram (1000)
milligram (mg): one-thousandth of a gram (0.001)
microgram (µg): one-millionth of a gram (0.000001)
milliliter (ml): one-thousandth of a liter (0.001)

International Units

Some vitamin supplements may report vitamin content as International Units (IU).

To convert IU to:

- Micrograms of vitamin D (cholecalciferol), divide the IU value by 40 or multiply by 0.025.
- Milligrams of vitamin E (alpha-tocopherol), divide the IU value by 1.5 if vitamin E is from natural sources. Divide the IU value by 2.22 if vitamin E is from synthetic sources.
- Vitamin A: 1 IU = 0.3 µg retinol or 3.6 µg beta-carotene

Retinol Activity Equivalents

Retinol Activity Equivalents (RAE) are a standardized unit of measure for vitamin A. RAE account for the various differences in bioavailability from sources of vitamin A. Many supplements will report vitamin A content in IU, as shown above, or Retinol Equivalents (RE).

1 RAE = 1 µg retinol
12 µg beta-carotene
24 µg other vitamin A carotenoids

To calculate RAE from the RE value of vitamin carotenoids in foods, divide RE by 2.

For vitamin A supplements and foods fortified with vitamin A, 1 RE = 1 RAE.

Folate

Folate is measured as Dietary Folate Equivalents (DFE). DFE account for the different factors affecting bioavailability of folate sources.

1 DFE = 1 µg food folate
0.6 µg folate from fortified foods
0.5 µg folate supplement taken on an empty stomach
0.6 µg folate as a supplement consumed with a meal

To convert micrograms of synthetic folate, such as that found in supplements or fortified foods, to DFE:

µg synthetic folate × 1.7 = µg DFE

For naturally occurring food folate, such as spinach, each microgram of folate equals 1 microgram DFE:

µg folate = µg DFE

Conversion Factors

Use the following table to convert U.S. measurements to metric equivalents:

Original Unit	Multiply by	To Get
ounces avdp	28.3495	grams
ounces	0.0625	pounds
pounds	0.4536	kilograms
pounds	16	ounces
grams	0.0353	ounces
grams	0.002205	pounds
kilograms	2.2046	pounds
liters	1.8162	pints (dry)
liters	2.1134	pints (liquid)
liters	0.9081	quarts (dry)
liters	1.0567	quarts (liquid)
liters	0.2642	gallons (U.S.)
pints (dry)	0.5506	liters
pints (liquid)	0.4732	liters
quarts (dry)	1.1012	liters
quarts (liquid)	0.9463	liters
gallons (U.S.)	3.7853	liters
millimeters	0.0394	inches
centimeters	0.3937	inches
centimeters	0.03281	feet
inches	25.4000	millimeters
inches	2.5400	centimeters
inches	0.0254	meters
feet	0.3048	meters
meters	3.2808	feet
meters	1.0936	yards
cubic feet	0.0283	cubic meters
cubic meters	35.3145	cubic feet
cubic meters	1.3079	cubic yards
cubic yards	0.7646	cubic meters

Length: U.S. and Metric Equivalents

¼ inch = 0.6 centimeters
1 inch = 2.5 centimeters
1 foot = 0.3048 meter
         30.48 centimeters
1 yard = 0.91144 meter
1 millimeter = 0.03937 inch
1 centimeter = 0.3937 inch
1 decimeter = 3.937 inches
1 meter = 39.37 inches
          1.094 yards
1 micrometer = 0.00003937 inch

Weights and Measures

Food Measurement Equivalencies from U.S. to Metric

Capacity

⅛ teaspoon = 1 milliliter
¼ teaspoon = 1.25 milliliters
½ teaspoon = 2.5 milliliters
1 teaspoon = 5 milliliters
1 tablespoon = 15 milliliters
1 fluid ounce = 28.4 milliliters
¼ cup = 60 milliliters
⅓ cup = 80 milliliters
½ cup = 120 milliliters
1 cup = 225 milliliters
1 pint (2 cups) = 473 milliliters
1 quart (4 cups) = 0.95 liter
1 liter (1.06 quarts) = 1,000 milliliters
1 gallon (4 quarts) = 3.84 liters

Weight

0.035 ounce = 1 gram
1 ounce = 28 grams
¼ pound (4 ounces) = 114 grams
1 pound (16 ounces) = 454 grams
2.2 pounds (35 ounces) = 1 kilogram

U.S. Food Measurement Equivalents

3 teaspoons = 1 tablespoon
½ tablespoon = 1½ teaspoons
2 tablespoons = ⅛ cup
4 tablespoons = ¼ cup
5 tablespoons + 1 teaspoon = ⅓ cup
8 tablespoons = ½ cup
10 tablespoons + 2 teaspoons = ⅔ cup
12 tablespoons = ¾ cup
16 tablespoons = 1 cup
2 cups = 1 pint
4 cups = 1 quart
2 pints = 1 quart
4 quarts = 1 gallon

Volumes and Capacities

1 cup = 8 fluid ounces
½ liquid pint
1 milliliter = 0.061 cubic inches
1 liter = 1.057 liquid quarts
0.908 dry quart
61.024 cubic inches
1 U.S. gallon = 231 cubic inches
3.785 liters
0.833 British gallon
128 U.S. fluid ounces

1 British Imperial gallon = 277.42 cubic inches
1.201 U.S. gallons
4.546 liters
160 British fluid ounces
1 U.S. ounce, liquid or fluid = 1.805 cubic inches
29.574 milliliters
1.041 British fluid ounces
1 pint, dry = 33.600 cubic inches
0.551 liter
1 pint, liquid = 28.875 cubic inches
0.473 liter
1 U.S. quart, dry = 67.201 cubic inches
1.101 liters
1 U.S. quart, liquid = 57.75 cubic inches
0.946 liter
1 British quart = 69.354 cubic inches
1.032 U.S. quarts, dry
1.201 U.S. quarts, liquid

Energy Units

Commonly Used Energy Units

1 kilocalorie (kcal) = 4.2 kilojoules
1 millijoule (MJ) = 240 kilocalories
1 kilojoule (kJ) = 0.24 kcal
1 gram carbohydrate = 4 kcal
1 gram fat = 9 kcal
1 gram protein = 4 kcal

Temperature Standards

	°Fahrenheit	°Celsius
Body temperature	98.6°	37°
Comfortable room temperature	65–75°	18–24°
Boiling point of water	212°	100°
Freezing point of water	32°	0°

Temperature Scales
To Convert Fahrenheit to Celsius:
$[(°F - 32) \times 5]/9$

1. Subtract 32 from °F
2. Multiply (°F − 32) by 5, then divide by 9

To Convert Celsius to Fahrenheit:
$[(°C \times 9)/5] + 32$

1. Multiply °C by 9, then divide by 5
2. Add 32 to (°C × 9/5)

APPENDIX C Foods Containing Caffeine

Source: Values are obtained from the USDA Nutrient Database for Standard Reference, Release 18.

Beverages

Food Name	Serving	Caffeine/serving (mg)
Beverage mix, chocolate flavor, dry mix, prep w/milk	1 cup (8 fl.oz)	7.98
Beverage mix, chocolate malt powder, fortified, prepared w/milk	1 cup (8 fl. oz)	5.3
Beverage mix, chocolate malted milk powder, no added nutrients, prepared w/milk	1 cup (8 fl. oz)	7.95
Beverage, chocolate syrup w/o added nutrients, prepared w/milk	1 cup (8 fl. oz)	5.64
Beverage, chocolate syrup, fortified, mixed w/milk	1 cup milk and 1 tbsp syrup	2.63
Cocoa mix w/aspartame and calcium and phosphorus, no sodium or vitamin A, low kcal, dry, prepared	6 fl. oz water and 0.53 oz packet	5
Cocoa mix w/aspartame, dry, low kcal, prepared w/water	1 packet dry mix with 6 fl. oz water	1.92
Cocoa mix, dry mix	1 serving (3 heaping tsp or 1 envelope)	5.04
Cocoa mix, dry, w/o added nutrients, prepared w/water	1 oz packet with 6 fl. oz water	4.12
Cocoa mix, fortified, dry, prepared w/water	6 fl. oz H_2O and 1 packet	6.27
Cocoa, dry powder, hi-fat or breakfast, plain	1 piece	6.895
Cocoa, hot, homemade w/whole milk	1 cup	5
Coffee liqueur 53 proof	1 fl. oz	9.048
Coffee liqueur 63 proof	1 fl. oz	9.048
Coffee w/cream liqueur, 34 proof	1 fl. oz	2.488
Coffee mix w/sugar (cappuccino), dry, prepared w/water	6 fl. oz H_2O and 2 rounded tsp mix	74.88
Coffee mix w/sugar (French), dry, prepared w/water	6 fl. oz H_2O and 2 rounded tsp mix	51.03
Coffee mix w/sugar (mocha), dry, prepared w/water	6 fl. oz H_2O and 2 rounded tsp mix	33.84
Coffee, brewed	1 cup (8 fl. oz)	85.32
Coffee, brewed, prepared with tap water, decaffeinated	1 cup (8 fl. oz)	2.37
Coffee, instant, prepared	1 fl. oz	7.748
Coffee, instant, regular, powder, half the caffeine	1 cup (8 fl. oz)	3723.27
Coffee, instant powder, decaffeinated, prepared	6 fl. oz	1.79
Coffee and cocoa (mocha) powder, with whitener and low-calorie sweetener	1 cup	405.48
Coffee, brewed, espresso, restaurant-prepared	1 fl. oz	60.081
Coffee, brewed, espresso, restaurant-prepared, decaffeinated	1 cup (8 fl.oz)	2.37
Energy drink, with caffeine, niacin, pantothenic acid, vitamin B_6	1 fl. oz	9.517
Milk beverage mix, dairy drink w/aspartame, low kcal, dry, prep	6 fl. oz	4.08
Milk, lowfat, 1% fat, chocolate	1 cup	5
Milk, whole, chocolate	1 cup	5
Soft drink, cola w/caffeine	1 fl. oz	2
Soft drink, cola, w/higher caffeine	1 fl. oz	8.37
Soft drink, cola or pepper type, low kcal w/saccharin and caffeine	1 fl. oz	3.256
Soft drink, cola, low kcal w/saccharin and aspartame, w/caffeine	1 fl. oz	4.144
Soft drink, lemon-lime soda, w/caffeine	1 fl. oz	4.605
Soft drink, low kcal, not cola or pepper, with aspartame and caffeine	1 fl. oz	4.44
Soft drink, pepper type	1 fl. oz	3.07
Tea mix, instant w/lemon flavor, w/saccharin, dry, prepared	1 cup (8 fl. oz)	16.59
Tea mix, instant w/lemon, unsweetened, dry, prepared	1 cup (8 fl. oz)	26.18
Tea mix, instant w/sugar and lemon, dry, no added vitamin C, prepared	1 cup (8 fl. oz)	28.49
Tea mix, instant, unsweetened, dry, prepared	1 cup (8 fl. oz)	30.81
Tea, brewed	1 cup (8 fl. oz)	47.4
Tea, brewed, prepared with tap water, decaffeinated	1 cup (8 fl. oz)	2.37
Tea, instant, unsweetened, powder, decaffeinated	1 tsp	1.183
Tea, instant, w/sugar, lemon-flavored, w/added vitamin C, dry prepared	1 cup (8 fl. oz)	28.49
Tea, instant, with sugar, lemon-flavored, decaffeinated, no added vitamin	1 cup	9.1

Cake, Cookies, and Desserts

Food Name	Serving	Caffeine/serving (mg)
Brownies, commercially prepared, Little Debbie	1 oz	0.567
Cake, chocolate pudding, dry mix	1 oz	1.701
Cake, chocolate, dry mix, regular	1 oz	3.118
Cake, German chocolate pudding, dry mix	1 oz	1.985
Cake, marble pudding, dry mix	1 oz	1.985
Candies, chocolate covered, caramel with nuts	1 cup	3.534
Candies, chocolate covered, dietetic or low calorie	1 cup	16.74
Candy, milk chocolate w/almonds	1 bar (1.45 oz)	9.02
Candy, milk chocolate w/rice cereal	1 bar (1.4 oz)	9.2
Candy, raisins, milk chocolate coated	1 cup	45
Chocolate chips, semisweet	1 cup chips (6 oz package)	104.16
Chocolate, baking, unsweetened, square	1 cup, grated	105.6
Chocolate, baking, Mexican, squares	1 tablet	2.8
Chocolate, sweet	1 oz	18.711
Cookie cake, Snackwell's Fat Free Devil's Food, Nabisco	1 serving	1.28
Cookie, Snackwell's Caramel Delights, Nabisco	1 serving	1.44
Cookie, chocolate chip, enriched, commercially prepared	1 oz	3.118
Cookie, chocolate chip, homemade w/margarine	1 oz	4.536
Cookie, chocolate chip, lower fat, commercially prepared	1 oz	1.985
Cookie, chocolate chip, refrigerated dough	1 portion, dough spoon from roll	2.61
Cookie, chocolate chip, soft, commercially prepared	1 oz	1.985
Cookie, chocolate wafers	1 cup, crumbs	7.84
Cookie, graham crackers, chocolate coated	1 oz	13.041
Cookie, sandwich, chocolate, cream filled	1 oz	3.686
Cookie, sandwich, chocolate, cream filled, special dietary	1 oz	0.85
Cupcakes, chocolate w/frosting, low-fat	1 oz	0.567
Donut, cake, chocolate w/sugar or glaze	1 oz	0.284
Donut, cake, plain w/chocolate icing	1 oz	0.567
Fast food, ice cream sundae, hot fudge	1 sundae	1.58
Fast food, milk beverage, chocolate shake	1 cup (8 fl. oz)	1.66
Frosting, chocolate, creamy, ready to eat	2 tbsp creamy	0.82
Frozen yogurts, chocolate	1 cup	5.58
Fudge, chocolate w/nuts, homemade	1 oz	1.984
Granola bar, soft, milk chocolate coated, peanut butter	1 oz	0.85
Granola bar, with coconut, chocolate coated	1 cup	5.58
Ice cream, chocolate	1 individual (3.5 fl. oz)	1.74
Ice cream, chocolate, light	1 oz	0.85
Ice cream, chocolate, rich	1 cup	5.92
M&M's Peanut Chocolate	1 cup	18.7
M&M's Plain Chocolate	1 cup	22.88
Milk chocolate	1 cup chips	33.6
Milk chocolate coated coffee beans	1 NLEA serving	48
Milk dessert, frozen, fat-free milk, chocolate	1 oz	0.85
Milk shake, thick, chocolate	1 fl. oz	0.568
Pastry, eclair/cream puff, homemade, custard filled w/chocolate	1 oz	0.567
Pie crust, chocolate wafer cookie type, chilled	1 crust, single 9"	11.15
Pie, chocolate mousse, no bake mix	1 oz	0.284
Pudding, chocolate, instant dry mix prep w/reduced fat (2%) milk	1 oz	0.283
Pudding, chocolate, regular dry mix prep w/reduced fat (2%) milk	1 oz	0.567
Pudding, chocolate, ready-to-eat, fat-free	1 oz	0.567
Syrups, chocolate, genuine chocolate flavor, lite, Hershey	2 tbsp	1.05
Topping, chocolate-flavored hazelnut spread	1 oz	1.984
Yogurt, chocolate, nonfat milk	1 oz	0.567
Yogurt, frozen, chocolate, soft serve	0.5 cup (4 fl. oz)	2.16

Source: © 2008 by the American Diabetes Association and the American Dietetic Association. Reproduced with Permission.

Starch List

1 starch choice = 15 g carbohydrate, 0–3 g protein, 0–1 g fat, and 80 cal

Icon Key

☺ = More than 3 g of dietary fiber per serving.

! = Extra fat, or prepared with added fat. (Count as 1 starch + 1 fat.)

🧂 = 480 mg or more of sodium per serving.

Food	Serving Size
Bread	
Bagel, 4 oz	¼ (1 oz)
! Biscuit, 2½" across	1
Bread	
☺ reduced-calorie	2 slices (1½ oz)
white, whole-grain, pumpernickel, rye,	
unfrosted raisin	1 slice (1 oz)
Chapatti, small, 6" across	1
! Cornbread, 1¾" cube	1 (1½ oz)
English muffin	½
Hot dog bun or hamburger bun	½ (1 oz)
Naan, 8" by 2"	¼
Pancake, 4" across, ¼" thick	1
Pita, 6" across	½
Roll, plain small	1 (1 oz)
! Stuffing, bread	⅓ cup
! Taco shell, 5" across	2
Tortilla	
Corn, 6" across	1
Flour, 6" across	1
Flour, 10" across	⅓ tortilla
! Waffle, 4"-square or 4" across	1
Cereals and Grains	
Barley, cooked	⅓ cup
Bran, dry	
☺ oat	¼ c
☺ wheat	½ c
☺ Bulgur (cooked)	½ c
Cereals	½ c
☺ bran	½ c
cooked (oats, oatmeal)	½ c
puffed	1½ c
shredded wheat, plain	½ c
sugar-coated	½ c
unsweetened, ready-to-eat	¾ c
Couscous	⅓ c
Granola	
low-fat	¼ c
! regular	¼ c

Food	Serving Size
Grits, cooked	½ c
Kasha	½ c
Millet, cooked	⅓ c
Muesli	¼ c
Pasta, cooked	⅓ c
Polenta, cooked	⅓ c
Quinoa, cooked	⅓ c
Rice, white or brown, cooked	⅓ c
Tabbouleh (tabouli), prepared	½ c
Wheat germ, dry	3 tbs
Wild rice, cooked	½ c
Starchy Vegetables	
Cassava	⅓ c
Corn	½ c
on cob, large	½ cob (5 oz)
☺ Hominy, canned	¾ c
☺ Mixed vegetables with corn, peas, or pasta	1 c
☺ Parsnips	½ c
☺ Peas, green	½ c
Plantain, ripe	⅓ c
Potato	
baked with skin	¼ large (3 oz)
boiled, all kinds	½ c or ½ medium (3 oz)
! mashed, with milk and fat	½ c
French fried (oven-baked)	1 cup (2 oz)
☺ Pumpkin, canned, no sugar added	1 c
Spaghetti/pasta sauce	½ c
☺ Squash, winter (acorn, butternut)	1 c
☺ Succotash	½ c
Yam, sweet potato, plain	½ c
Crackers and Snacks	
Animal crackers	8
Crackers	
! round-butter type	6
saltine-type	6
! sandwich-style, cheese or peanut butter filling	3
! whole-wheat regular	2–5 (¾ oz)
☺ whole-wheat lower fat or crispbreads	2–5 (¾ oz)
Graham crackers, 2½" square	3

Food	Serving Size	Food	Serving Size
Matzoh	¾ oz	**Beans, Peas, and Lentils**	
Melba toast, about 2" by 4" piece	4 pieces	*(Count as 1 starch + 1 lean meat)*	
Oyster crackers	20	😊 Baked beans	⅓ c
Crackers and Snacks		😊 Beans, cooked (black, garbanzo, kidney, lima, navy, pinto, white)	½ c
Popcorn	3 c	😊 Lentils, cooked (brown, green, yellow)	½ c
❗😊 with butter	3 c	😊 Peas, cooked (black-eyed, split)	½ c
😊 no fat added	3 c	🧂😊 Refried beans, canned	½ c
😊 lower fat	3 c		
Pretzels	¾ oz		
Rice cakes, 4" across	2		
Snack chips			
fat-free or baked (tortilla, potato), baked pita chips	15–20 (¾ oz)		
❗ regular (tortilla, potato)	9–13 (¾ oz)		

Fruit List

1 fruit choice = 15 g carbohydrate, 0 g protein, 0 g fat, and 60 cal
Weight includes skin, core, seeds, and rind.

Icon Key

😊 = More than 3 g of dietary fiber per serving.

❗ = Extra fat, or prepared with added fat.

🧂 = 480 mg or more of sodium per serving.

Food	Serving Size	Food	Serving Size
Apples		Grapes, small	17 (3 oz)
unpeeled, small	1 (4 oz)	Honeydew melon	1 slice or 1 c cubed (10 oz)
dried	4 rings	😊 Kiwi	1 (3½ oz)
Applesauce, unsweetened	½ c	Mandarin oranges, canned	¾ c
Apricots		Mango, small	½ fruit (5½ oz) or ½ c
canned	½ c	Nectarine, small	1 (5 oz)
dried	8 halves	😊 Orange, small	1 (6½ oz)
😊 fresh	4 whole (5½ oz)	Papaya	½ fruit or 1 c cubed (8 oz)
Banana, extra small	1 (4 oz)	Peaches	
😊 Blackberries	¾ c	canned	½ c
Blueberries	¾ c	fresh, medium	1 (6 oz)
Cantaloupe, small	⅓ melon or 1 c cubed (11 oz)	Pears	
Cherries		canned	½ c
sweet, canned	½ c	fresh, large	½ (4 oz)
sweet, fresh	12 (3 oz)	Pineapple	
Dates	3	canned	½ c
Dried fruits (blueberries, cherries, cranberries, mixed fruit, raisins)	2 tbs	fresh	¾ c
Figs		Plums	
dried	1½	canned	½ c
😊 fresh	1½ large or 2 medium (3½ oz)	dried (prunes)	3
Fruit cocktail	½ c	small	2 (5 oz)
Grapefruit		😊 Raspberries	1 c
large	½ (11 oz)	😊 Strawberries	1¼ c whole berries
sections, canned	¾ c		

Food	Serving Size	Food	Serving Size
☺ Tangerines, small ....2 (8 oz)		Grape juice ....⅓ c	
Watermelon ....1 slice or 1¼ c cubes (13½ oz)		Grapefruit juice ....½ c	
		Orange juice ....½ c	
Fruit Juice		Pineapple juice ....½ c	
Apple juice/cider ....½ c		Prune juice ....⅓ c	
Fruit juice blends, 100% juice ....⅓ c			

Milk and Yogurts

1 milk choice = 12 g carbohydrate and 8 g protein

Food	Serving Size	Count as
Fat-free or Low-Fat (1%)		
(0–3 g fat per serving, 100 calories per serving)		
Milk, buttermilk, acidophilus milk, Lactaid	1 c	1 fat-free milk
Evaporated milk	½ c	1 fat-free milk
Yogurt, plain or flavored with an artificial sweetener	⅔ c (6 oz)	1 fat-free milk
Reduced-fat (2%)		
(5 g fat per serving, 120 calories per serving)		
Milk, acidophilus milk, kefir, Lactaid	1 c	1 reduced-fat milk
Yogurt, plain	⅔ c (6 oz)	1 reduced-fat milk
Whole		
(8 g fat per serving, 160 calories per serving)		
Milk, buttermilk, goat's milk	1 c	1 whole milk
Evaporated milk	½ c	1 whole milk
Yogurt, plain	8 oz	1 whole milk
Dairy-Like Foods		
Chocolate milk		
fat-free	1 c	1 fat-free milk + 1 carbohydrate
whole	1 c	1 whole milk + 1 carbohydrate
Eggnog, whole milk	½ c	1 carbohydrate + 2 fats
Rice drink		
flavored, low-fat	1 c	2 carbohydrates
plain, fat-free	1 c	1 carbohydrate
Smoothies, flavored, regular	10 oz	1 fat-free milk + 2½ carbohydrates
Soy milk		
light	1 c	1 carbohydrate + ½ fat
regular, plain	1 c	1 carbohydrate + 1 fat
Yogurt		
and juice blends	1 c	1 fat-free milk + 1 carbohydrate
low carbohydrate (less than 6 g carbohydrate per choice)	⅔ c (6 oz)	½ fat-free milk
with fruit, low-fat	⅔ c (6 oz)	1 fat-free milk + 1 carbohydrate

Sweets, Desserts, and Other Carbohydrates List

1 other carbohydrate choice = 15 g carbohydrate and variable protein, fat, and calories.

Icon Key

🧂 = 480 mg or more of sodium per serving.

Food	Serving Size	Count as
Beverages, Soda, and Energy/Sports Drinks		
Cranberry juice cocktail	½ c	1 carbohydrate
Energy drink	1 can (8.3 oz)	2 carbohydrates
Fruit drink or lemonade	1 c (8 oz)	2 carbohydrates
Hot chocolate		
regular	1 envelope added to 8 oz water	1 carbohydrate + 1 fat
sugar-free or light	1 envelope added to 8 oz water	1 carbohydrate
Soft drink (soda), regular	1 can (12 oz)	2½ carbohydrates
Sports drink	1 cup (8 oz)	1 carbohydrate
Brownies, Cake, Cookies, Gelatin, Pie, and Pudding		
Brownie, small, unfrosted	1¼" square, ⅞" high (about 1 oz)	1 carbohydrate + 1 fat
Cake		
angel food, unfrosted	1⁄12 of cake (about 2 oz)	2 carbohydrates
frosted	2" square (about 2 oz)	2 carbohydrates + 1 fat
unfrosted	2" square (about 2 oz)	1 carbohydrate + 1 fat
Cookies		
chocolate chip	2 cookies (2¼" across)	1 carbohydrate + 2 fats
gingersnap	3 cookies	1 carbohydrate
sandwich, with creme filling	2 small (about ⅔ oz)	1 carbohydrate + 1 fat
sugar-free	3 small or 1 large (¾ oz–1oz)	1 carbohydrate + 1–2 fats
vanilla wafer	5 cookies	1 carbohydrate + 1 fat
Cupcake, frosted	1 small (about 1¾ oz)	2 carbohydrates + 1–1½ fats
Fruit cobbler	½ c (3½ oz)	3 carbohydrates + 1 fat
Gelatin, regular	½ c	1 carbohydrate
Pie		
commercially prepared fruit, 2 crusts	⅙ of 8" pie	3 carbohydrates + 2 fats
pumpkin or custard	⅛ of 8" pie	1½ carbohydrates + 1½ fats
Pudding		
regular (made with reduced-fat milk)	½ c	2 carbohydrates
sugar-free, or sugar-free and fat-free (made with fat-free milk)	½ c	1 carbohydrate
Candy, Spreads, Sweets, Sweeteners, Syrups, and Toppings		
Candy bar, chocolate/peanut	2 "fun size" bars (1 oz)	1½ carbohydrates + 1½ fats
Candy, hard	3 pieces	1 carbohydrate
Chocolate "kisses"	5 pieces	1 carbohydrate + 1 fat
Coffee creamer		
dry, flavored	4 tsp	½ carbohydrate + ½ fat
liquid, flavored	2 tbsp	1 carbohydrate
Fruit snacks, chewy (pureed fruit concentrate)	1 roll (¾ oz)	1 carbohydrate
Fruit spreads, 100% fruit	1½ tbs	1 carbohydrate
Honey	1 tbsp	1 carbohydrate

Food	Serving Size	Count as
Jam or jelly, regular	1 tbs	1 carbohydrate
Sugar	1 tbs	1 carbohydrate
Syrup		
chocolate	2 tbs	2 carbohydrates
light (pancake type)	2 tbs	1 carbohydrate
regular (pancake type)	1 tbs	1 carbohydrate

Condiments and Sauces

Food	Serving Size	Count as
Barbeque sauce	3 tbs	1 carbohydrate
Cranberry sauce, jellied	¼ c	1½ carbohydrates
🧂 Gravy, canned or bottled	½ c	½ carbohydrate + ½ fat
Salad dressing, fat-free, low-fat, cream-based	3 tbs	1 carbohydrate
Sweet and sour sauce	3 tbs	1 carbohydrate

Doughnuts, Muffins, Pastries, and Sweet Breads

Food	Serving Size	Count as
Banana nut bread	1" slice (1 oz)	2 carbohydrates + 1 fat
Doughnut		
cake, plain	1 medium, (1½ oz)	1½ carbohydrates + 2 fats
yeast type, glazed	3¾" across (2 oz)	2 carbohydrates + 2 fats
Muffin (4 oz)	¼ muffin (1 oz)	1 carbohydrate + ½ fat
Sweet roll or Danish	1 (2½ oz)	2½ carbohydrates + 2 fats

Frozen Bars, Frozen Dessert, Frozen Yogurt, and Ice Cream

Food	Serving Size	Count as
Frozen pops	1	½ carbohydrate
Fruit juice bars, frozen, 100% juice	1 bar (3 oz)	1 carbohydrate
Ice cream		
fat free	½ c	1-½ carbohydrates
light	½ c	1 carbohydrate + 1 fat
no sugar added	½ c	1 carbohydrate + 1 fat
regular	½ c	1 carbohydrate + 2 fats
Sherbet, sorbet	½ c	2 carbohydrates
Yogurt, frozen		
fat-free	⅓ c	1 carbohydrate
regular	½ c	1 carbohydrate + 0–1 fat

Granola Bars, Meal Replacement Bars/Shakes, and Trail Mix

Food	Serving Size	Count as
Granola or snack bar, regular or low-fat	1 bar (1 oz)	1½ carbohydrates
Meal replacement bar	1 bar (1⅓ oz)	1½ carbohydrates + 0–1 fat
Meal replacement bar	1 bar (2 oz)	2 carbohydrates + 1 fat
Meal replacement shake, reduced-calorie	1 can (10–11 oz)	1½ carbohydrates + 0–1 fat
Trail mix		
candy/nut-based	1 oz	1 carbohydrates + 2 fats
dried fruit-based	1 oz	1 carbohydrate + 1 fat

Nonstarchy Vegetable List

1 vegetable choice = 5 g carbohydrate, 2 g protein, 0 g fat, 25 cal

Icon Key

☻ = More than 3 g of dietary fiber per serving.

🧂 = 480 mg or more of sodium per serving.

Amaranth or Chinese spinach

Artichoke

Artichoke hearts

Asparagus

Baby corn

Bamboo shoots

Beans (green, wax, Italian)

Bean sprouts

Beets

🧂 Borscht

Broccoli

☻ Brussels sprouts

Cabbage (green, bok choy, Chinese)

☻ Carrots

Cauliflower

Celery

☻ Chayote

Coleslaw, packaged, no dressing

Cucumber

Eggplant

Gourds (bitter, bottle, luffa, bitter melon)

Green onions or scallions

Greens (collard, kale, mustard, turnip)

Hearts of palm

Jicama

Kohlrabi

Leeks

Mixed vegetables (without corn, peas, or pasta)

Mung bean sprouts

Mushrooms, all kinds, fresh

Okra

Onions

Oriental radish or daikon

Pea pods

☻ Peppers (all varieties)

Radishes

Rutabaga

🧂 Sauerkraut

Soybean sprouts

Spinach

Squash (summer, crookneck, zucchini)

Sugar pea snaps

☻ Swiss chard

Tomato

Tomatoes, canned

🧂 Tomato sauce

🧂 Tomato/vegetable juice

Turnips

Water chestnuts

Yard-long beans

Meat and Meat Substitutes List

Icon Key

! = Extra fat, or prepared with added fat. (Add an additional fat choice to this food.)

🧂 = 480 mg or more of sodium per serving (based on the sodium content of a typical 3-oz serving of meat, unless 1 or 2 is the normal serving size).

Food	Amount	Food	Amount
Lean Meats and Meat Substitutes		*Fish, fresh or frozen, plain:* catfish, cod, flounder,	
(1 lean meat choice = 7 g protein, 0–3 g fat,		haddock, halibut, orange roughy, salmon, tilapia,	
100 calories)		trout, tuna . . . . .1 oz	
Beef: Select or Choice grades trimmed of fat:		🧂 *Fish, smoked:* herring or salmon (lox) . . . . .1 oz	
ground round, roast (chuck, rib, rump), round,		*Game:* buffalo, ostrich, rabbit, venison . . . . .1 oz	
sirloin, steak (cubed, flank, porterhouse, T-bone),		🧂 Hot dog with 3 g of fat or less per oz (8 dogs	
tenderloin . . . . .1 oz		per 14 oz package) (*Note: May be high in*	
🧂 Beef jerky . . . . .1 oz		*carbohydrate.*) 1	
Cheeses with 3 g of fat or less per oz . . . . .1 oz		*Lamb:* chop, leg, or roast . . . . .1 oz	
Cottage cheese . . . . .¼ cup		*Organ meats:* heart, kidney, liver (*Note: May be high*	
Egg substitutes, plain . . . . .¼ cup		*in cholesterol*) . . . . .1 oz	
Egg whites 2			

Food	Amount
Oysters, fresh or frozen . . . . .6 medium	
Pork, lean	
🧂 Canadian bacon . . . . .1 oz	
rib or loin chop/roast, ham, tenderloin . . . . . . .1 oz	
Poultry without skin: Cornish hen, chicken,	
domestic duck or goose (well drained of fat),	
turkey . . . . .1 oz	
Processed sandwich meats with 3 g of fat or less	
per oz: chipped beef, deli thin-sliced meats,	
turkey ham, turkey kielbasa, turkey pastrami . . .1 oz	
Salmon, canned . . . . .1 oz	
Sardines, canned . . . . .2 medium	
🧂 Sausage with 3 g or less fat per oz . . . . .1 oz	
Shellfish: clams, crab, imitation shellfish, lobster,	
scallops, shrimp . . . . .1 oz	
Tuna, canned in water or oil, drained . . . . .1 oz	
Veal: Lean chop, roast . . . . .1 oz	

Medium-Fat Meat and Meat Substitutes
(1 medium-fat meat choice = 7 g protein, 4–7 g fat, and 130 calories)

Food	Amount
Beef: corned beef, ground beef, meatloaf,	
Prime grades trimmed of fat (prime rib),	
short ribs, tongue . . . . .1 oz	
Cheeses with 4–7 g of fat per oz: feta, mozzarella,	
pasteurized processed cheese spread,	
reduced-fat cheeses, string . . . . .1 oz	
Egg (*Note: High in cholesterol, limit to 3 per week.*) .1	
Fish, any fried product . . . . .1 oz	
Lamb: ground, rib roast . . . . .1 oz	
Pork: cutlet, shoulder roast . . . . .1 oz	

Food	Amount
Poultry: chicken with skin; dove, pheasant,	
wild duck, or goose; fried chicken;	
ground turkey . . . . .1 oz	
Ricotta cheese . . . . .2 oz or ¼ c	
🧂 Sausage with 4–7 g fat per oz . . . . .1 oz	
Veal: Cutlet (no breading) .1 oz	

High-Fat Meat and Substitutes[a]
(1 high-fat meat choice = 7 g protein, 8+ g fat, 150 calories)

Food	Amount
Bacon	
🧂 pork . . . . .2 slices (16 slices per lb or 1 oz each, before cooking)	
🧂 turkey . . . . .3 slices (½ oz each before cooking)	
Cheese, regular: American, bleu, brie, cheddar,	
hard goat, Monterey Jack, queso, Swiss . . . . . . .1 oz	
🧂 ❗ *Hot dog:* beef, pork, or combination	
(10 per lb-sized package) 1	
🧂 *Hot dog:* turkey or chicken (10 per lb-sized	
package) 1	
Pork: ground, sausage, spareribs . . . . .1 oz	
Processed sandwich meats with 8 g of fat or	
more per oz: bologna, pastrami, hard salami . . . .1 oz	
🧂 *Sausage with 8 g of fat or more per oz:*	
bratwurst, chorizo, Italian, knockwurst,	
Polish, smoked, summer . . . . .1 oz	

[a]These foods are high in saturated fat, cholesterol, and calories and may raise blood cholesterol levels if eaten on a regular basis. Try to eat 3 or fewer servings from this group per week.

Plant-Based Proteins

Because carbohydrate content varies among plant-based proteins, you should read the food label.

Icon Key

😊 = More than 3 g of dietary fiber per serving.

🧂 = 480 mg or more of sodium per serving (based on the sodium content of a typical 3-oz serving of meat, unless 1 or 2 oz is the normal serving size).

Food	Amount	Count as
"Bacon" strips, soy-based	.3 strips	1 medium-fat meat
😊 Baked beans	⅓ c	1 starch + 1 lean meat
😊 *Beans, cooked:* black, garbanzo, kidney, lima, navy, pinto, white	½ c	1 starch + 1 lean meat
😊 "Beef" or "sausage" crumbles, soy-based	.2 oz	½ carbohydrate + 1 lean meat
"Chicken" nuggets, soy-based	.2 nuggets (1½ oz)	½ carbohydrate + 1 medium-fat meat
😊 Edamame	½ c	½ carbohydrate + 1 lean meat
Falafel (spiced chickpea and wheat patties)	3 patties (about 2 inches across)	1 carbohydrate + 1 high-fat meat
Hot dog, soy-based	1 (1½ oz)	½ carbohydrate + 1 lean meat
😊 Hummus	⅓ c	1 carbohydrate + 1 high-fat meat

Food	Amount	Count as
☺ Lentils, brown, green, or yellow	½ c	1 carbohydrate + 1 lean meat
☺ Meatless burger, soy-based	3 oz	½ carbohydrate + 2 lean meats
☺ Meatless burger, vegetable- and starch-based	1 patty (about 2½ oz)	1 carbohydrate + 2 lean meats
Nut spreads: almond butter, cashew butter, peanut butter, soy nut butter	1 tbs	1 high-fat meat
☺ *Peas, cooked:* black-eyed and split peas	½ c	1 starch + 1 lean meat
🧂☺ Refried beans, canned	½ c	1 starch + 1 lean meat
"Sausage" patties, soy-based	1 (1½ oz)	1 medium-fat meat
Soy nuts, unsalted	¾ oz	½ carbohydrate + 1 medium-fat meat
Tempeh	¼ cup	1 medium-fat meat
Tofu	4 oz (½ cup)	1 medium-fat meat
Tofu, light	4 oz (½ cup)	1 lean meat

Fat List

Icon Key

1 fat choice = 5 g fat, 45 cal

🧂 = 480 mg or more of sodium per serving.

Food	Serving Size	Food	Serving Size
Unsaturated Fats— Monounsaturated Fats		Nuts	
Avocado, medium	2 tbs (1 oz)	Pignolia (pine nuts)	1 tbs
Nut butters (trans *fat-free):* almond butter,		walnuts, English	4 halves
cashew butter, peanut butter (smooth or crunchy)	1½ tsp	*Oil:* corn, cottonseed, flaxseed, grape seed,	
Nuts		safflower, soybean, sunflower	1 tsp
almonds	6 nuts	*Oil:* made from soybean and canola oil—Enova	1 tsp
Brazil	2 nuts	Plant stanol esters	
cashews	6 nuts	light	1 tbs
filberts (hazelnuts)	5 nuts	regular	2 tsp
macadamia	3 nuts	Salad dressing	
mixed (50% peanuts)	6 nuts	🧂 reduced-fat (*Note: May be high*	
peanuts	10 nuts	*in carbohydrate.*)	2 tbs
pecans	4 halves	🧂 regular	1 tbs
pistachios	16 nuts	Seeds	1 tbs
Oil: canola, olive, peanut	1 tsp	flaxseed, whole	1 tbs
Olives		pumpkin, sunflower	1 tbs
black (ripe)	8 large	sesame seeds	1 tbs
green, stuffed	10 large	Tahini or sesame paste	2 tsp
Polyunsaturated Fats		**Saturated Fats**	
Margarine: lower-fat spread (30% to 50% vegetable		Bacon, cooked, regular or turkey	1 slice
oil, *trans* fat-free)	1 tbs	Butter	
Margarine: stick, tub (*trans* fat-free), or squeeze		reduced-fat	1 tbs
(*trans* fat-free)	1 tsp	stick	1 tsp
Mayonnaise		whipped	2 tsp
reduced-fat	1 tbs	Butter blends made with oil	
regular	1 tsp	reduced-fat or light	1 tbs
Mayonnaise-style salad dressing		regular	1½ tsp
reduced-fat	1 tbs	Chitterlings, boiled	2 tbs (½ oz)
regular	2 tsp	Coconut, sweetened, shredded	2 tbs

Food	Serving Size	Food	Serving Size
Coconut milk		Lard	.1 tsp
light	⅓ c	*Oil:* coconut, palm, palm kernel	.1 tsp
regular	1½ tbs	Salt pork	¼ oz
Cream		Shortening, solid	.1 tsp
half and half	2 tbs	Sour cream	
heavy	1 tbs	reduced-fat or light	.3 tbs
light	1½ tbs	regular	.2 tbs
whipped	2 tbs		
whipped, pressurized	¼ c		
Cream cheese			
reduced-fat	1½ tbs (¾ oz)		
regular	1 tbs (½ oz)		

Free Foods List

A *free food* is any food or drink that has less than 20 calories and 5 g or less of carbohydrate per serving. Foods with a serving size listed should be limited to three servings per day. Foods listed without a serving size can be eaten as often as you like.

Icon Key

🧂 = 480 mg or more of sodium per serving.

Food	Serving Size	Food	Serving Size
Low Carbohydrate Foods		Salad dressing	
Cabbage, raw	½ c	fat-free or low-fat	.1 tbs
Candy, hard (regular or sugar-free)	.1 piece	fat-free, Italian	.2 tbs
Carrots, cauliflower, or green beans, cooked	¼ c	Sour cream, fat-free, reduced-fat	.1 tbs
Cranberries, sweetened with sugar substitute	½ c	Whipped topping	
Cucumber, sliced	½ c	light or fat-free	.2 tbs
Gelatin		regular	.1 tbs
dessert, sugar-free		**Condiments**	
unflavored		Barbecue sauce	.2 tsp
Gum		Catsup (ketchup)	.1 tbs
Jam or jelly, light or no sugar added	.2 tsp	Honey mustard	.1 tbs
Rhubarb, sweetened with sugar substitute	½ c	Horseradish	
Salad greens		Lemon juice	
Sugar substitutes (artificial sweeteners)		Miso	1½ tsp
Syrup, sugar-free	.2 tbs	Mustard	
Modified Fat Foods with Carbohydrate		Parmesan cheese, freshly grated	.1 tbs
Cream cheese, fat-free	.1 tbs (½ oz)	Pickle relish	.1 tbs
Creamers		Pickles	
nondairy, liquid	.1 tbs	🧂 dill	1½ medium
nondairy, powdered	.2 tsp	sweet, bread and butter	.2 slices
Margarine spread		sweet, gherkin	¾ oz
fat-free	.1 tbs	Salsa	¼ c
reduced-fat	.1 tsp	🧂 Soy sauce, regular or light	.1 tbs
Mayonnaise		Sweet and sour sauce	.2 tsp
fat-free	.1 tbs	Sweet chili sauce	.2 tsp
reduced-fat	.1 tsp	Taco sauce	.1 tbs
Mayonnaise-style salad dressing		Vinegar	
fat-free	.1 tbs	Yogurt, any type	.2 tbs
reduced-fat	.1 tsp		

Drinks/Mixes

Any food on this list—without serving size listed—can be consumed in any moderate amount.

Icon Key

🧂 = 480 mg or more of sodium per serving.

🧂 Bouillon, broth, consommé	Diet soft drinks, sugar-free
Bouillon or broth, low sodium	Drink mixes, sugar-free
Carbonated or mineral water	Tea, unsweetened or with sugar substitute
Club soda	Tonic water, diet
Cocoa powder, unsweetened (1 tbs)	Water
Coffee, unsweetened or with sugar substitute	Water, flavored, carbohydrate free

Seasonings

Any food on this list can be consumed in any moderate amount.

Flavoring extracts (for example, vanilla, almond, peppermint)	Spices
Garlic	Hot pepper sauce
Herbs, fresh or dried	Wine, used in cooking
Nonstick cooking spray	Worcestershire sauce
Pimento	

Combination Foods List

Icon Key

😊 = More than 3 g of dietary fiber per serving.

🧂 = 600 mg or more of sodium per serving (for combination food main dishes/meals).

Food	Serving Size	Count as
Entrées		
🧂 Casserole type (tuna noodle, lasagna, spaghetti with meatballs, chili with beans, macaroni and cheese)	1 c (8 oz)	2 carbohydrates + 2 medium-fat meats
🧂 Stews (beef/other meats and vegetables)	1 c (8 oz)	1 carbohydrate + 1 medium-fat meat + 0–3 fats
Tuna salad or chicken salad	½ c (3½ oz)	½ carbohydrate + 2 lean meats + 1 fat
Frozen Meals/Entrées		
🧂😊 Burrito (beef and bean)	1 (5 oz)	3 carbohydrates + 1 lean meat + 2 fats
🧂 Dinner-type meal	generally 14–17 oz	3 carbohydrates + 3 medium-fat meats + 3 fats
🧂 Entrée or meal with less than 340 calories	about 8–11 oz	2–3 carbohydrates + 1–2 lean meats
Pizza		
🧂 cheese/vegetarian thin crust	¼ of 12" (4½ to 5 oz)	2 carbohydrates + 2 medium-fat meats
🧂 meat topping, thin crust	¼ of 12" (5 oz)	2 carbohydrates + 2 medium-fat meats, + 1½ fats
🧂 Pocket sandwich	1 (4½ oz)	3 carbohydrates + 1 lean meat + 1–2 fats
🧂 Pot pie	1 (7 oz)	2½ carbohydrates + 1 medium-fat meat + 3 fats
Salads (Deli-Style)		
Coleslaw	½ c	1 carbohydrate + 1½ fats
Macaroni/pasta salad	½ c	2 carbohydrates + 3 fats
🧂 Potato salad	½ c	1½ carbohydrates + 1–2 fats
Soups		
🧂 Bean, lentil, or split pea	1 cup	1 carbohydrate + 1 lean meat

Food	Serving Size	Count as
🧂 Chowder (made with milk)	1 c (8 oz)	1 carbohydrate + 1 lean meat + 1½ fats
🧂 Cream (made with water)	1 c (8 oz)	1 carbohydrate + 1 fat
🧂 Instant	6 oz prepared	1 carbohydrate
🧂 with beans or lentils	8 oz prepared	2½ carbohydrates + 1 lean meat
🧂 Miso soup	1 c	½ carbohydrate + 1 fat
🧂 Oriental noodle	1 c	2 carbohydrates + 2 fats
Rice (congee)	1 c	1 carbohydrate
🧂 Tomato (made with water)	1 c (8 oz)	1 carbohydrate
🧂 Vegetable beef, chicken noodle, or other broth-type	1 c (8 oz)	1 carbohydrate

Fast Foods List[a]

Icon Key

😊 = More than 3 g of dietary fiber per serving.

! = Extra fat, or prepared with added fat.

🧂 = 600 mg or more sodium per serving (for fast food main dishes/meals).

Food	Serving Size	Exchanges per Serving
Breakfast Sandwiches		
🧂 Egg, cheese, meat, English muffin	1 sandwich	2 carbohydrates + 2 medium-fat meats
🧂 Sausage biscuit sandwich	1 sandwich	2 carbohydrates + 2 high-fat meats + 3½ fats
Main Dishes/Entrees		
🧂😊 Burrito (beef and beans)	1 (about 8 oz)	3 carbohydrates + 3 medium-fat meats + 3 fats
🧂 Chicken breast, breaded and fried	1 (about 5 oz)	1 carbohydrate + 4 medium-fat meats
Chicken drumstick, breaded and fried	1 (about 2 oz)	2 medium-fat meats
🧂 Chicken nuggets	6 (about 3½ oz)	1 carbohydrate + 2 medium-fat meats + 1 fat
🧂 Chicken thigh, breaded and fried	1 (about 4 oz)	½ carbohydrate + 3 medium-fat meats + 1½ fats
🧂 Chicken wings, hot	6 (5 oz)	5 medium-fat meats + 1½ fats
Oriental		
🧂 Beef/chicken/shrimp with vegetables in sauce	1 c (about 5 oz)	1 carbohydrate + 1 lean meat + 1 fat
🧂 Egg roll, meat	1 (about 3 oz)	1 carbohydrate + 1 lean meat + 1 fat
Fried rice, meatless	½ c	1½ carbohydrates + 1½ fats
🧂 Meat and sweet sauce (orange chicken)	1 c	3 carbohydrates + 3 medium-fat meats + 2 fats
🧂😊 Noodles and vegetables in sauce (chow mein, lo mein)	1 c	2 carbohydrates + 1 fat
Pizza		
🧂 cheese, pepperoni, regular crust	⅛ of 14" (about 4 oz)	2½ carbohydrates + 1 medium-fat meat + 1½ fats
🧂 cheese/vegetarian, thin crust	¼ of 12" (about 6 oz)	2½ carbohydrates + 2 medium-fat meats + 1½ fats
Sandwiches		
🧂 Chicken sandwich, grilled	1	3 carbohydrates + 4 lean meats
🧂 Chicken sandwich, crispy	1	3½ carbohydrates + 3 medium-fat meats + 1 fat
Fish sandwich with tartar sauce	1	2½ carbohydrates + 2 medium-fat meats + 2 fats
Hamburger		
🧂 large with cheese	1	2½ carbohydrates + 4 medium-fat meats + 1 fat
regular	1	2 carbohydrates + 1 medium-fat meat + 1 fat
🧂 Hot dog with bun	1	1 carbohydrate + 1 high-fat meat + 1 fat
Submarine sandwich		
🧂 less than 6 grams fat	6" sub	3 carbohydrates + 2 lean meats
🧂 regular	6" sub	3½ carbohydrates + 2 medium-fat meats + 1 fat

[a]The choices in the Fast Foods list are not specific fast food meals or items, but are estimates based on popular foods. You can get specific nutrition information for almost every fast food or restaurant chain. Ask the restaurant or check its website for nutrition information about your favorite fast foods.

Food	Serving Size	Exchanges per Serving
Taco, hard or soft shell (meat and cheese)	1 small	1 carbohydrate + 1 medium-fat meat + 1½ fats
Salads		
Salad, main dish (grilled chcken type, no dressing or croutons)	salad	1 carbohydrate + 4 lean meats
Salad, side, no dressing or cheese	Small (about 5 oz)	1 vegetable
Sides/Appetizers		
French fries, restaurant style	Small	3 carbohydrates + 3 fats
Medium		4 carbohydrates + 4 fats
Large		5 carbohydrates + 6 fats
Nachos with cheese	Small (about 4½ oz)	2½ carbohydrates + 4 fats
Onion rings	1 serving (about 3 oz)	2½ carbohydrates + 3 fats
Desserts		
Milkshake, any flavor	12 oz	6 carbohydrates + 2 fats
Soft-serve ice cream cone	1 small	2½ carbohydrates + 1 fat

Alcohol List

In general, 1 alcohol choice (½ oz absolute alcohol) has about 100 calories.

Alcoholic Beverage	Serving Size	Count as
Beer		
light (4.2%)	12 fl. oz	1 alcohol equivalent + ½ carbohydrate
regular (4.9%)	12 fl. oz	1 alcohol equivalent + 1 carbohydrate
Distilled spirits: vodka, rum, gin, whiskey, 80 or 86 proof	1½ fl. oz	1 alcohol equivalent
Liqueur, coffee (53 proof)	1 fl. oz	1 alcohol equivalent + 1 carbohydrate
Sake	1 fl. oz	½ alcohol equivalent
Wine		
dessert (sherry)	3½ fl. oz	1 alcohol equivalent + 1 carbohydrate
dry, red or white (10%)	5 fl. oz	1 alcohol equivalent

APPENDIX E   Stature-for-Age Charts

CDC Growth Charts: United States
Stature-for-age percentiles: Boys, 2 to 20 years

Age (years)

in

cm

97th
95th
90th
75th
50th
25th
10th
5th
3rd

Published May 30, 2000.
Source: Developed by the National Center for Health Statistics
in collaboration with the National Center for Chronic
Disease Prevention and Health Promotion (2000).

SAFER · HEALTHIER · PEOPLE™

CDC Growth Charts: United States
Stature-for-age percentiles: Girls, 2 to 20 years

in

78
76
74
72
70
68
66
64
62
60
58
56
54
52
50
48
46
44
42
40
38
36
34
32
30

97th
95th
90th
75th
50th
25th
10th
5th
3rd

200
195
190
185
180
175
170
165
160
155
150
145
140
135
130
125
120
115
110
105
100
95
90
85
80
75

cm

2 3 4 5 6 7 8 9 10 11 12 13 14 15 16 17 18 19 20

Age (years)

Published May 30, 2000.
Source: Developed by the National Center for Health Statistics
in collaboration with the National Center for Chronic
Disease Prevention and Health Promotion (2000).

SAFER · HEALTHIER · PEOPLE™

APPENDIX F Organizations and Resources

Academic Journals

International Journal of Sport Nutrition and Exercise Metabolism
Human Kinetics
P.O. Box 5076
Champaign, IL 61825-5076
(800) 747-4457
www.humankinetics.com/IJSNEM

Journal of Nutrition
A. Catharine Ross, Editor
Department of Nutrition
Pennsylvania State University
126-S Henderson Building
University Park, PA 16802-6504
(814) 865-4721
www.nutrition.org

Nutrition Research
Elsevier: Journals Customer Service
6277 Sea Harbor Drive
Orlando, FL 32887
(877) 839-7126
www.journals.elsevierhealth.com/periodicals/NTR

Nutrition
Elsevier: Journals Customer Service
6277 Sea Harbor Drive
Orlando, FL 32887
(877) 839-7126
www.journals.elsevierhealth.com/periodicals/NUT

Nutrition Reviews
International Life Sciences Institute
Subscription Office
P.O. Box 830430
Birmingham, AL 35283
(800) 633-4931
www.ingentaconnect.com/content/ilsi/nure

Obesity Research
North American Association for the Study of Obesity (NAASO)
8630 Fenton Street, Suite 918
Silver Spring, MD 20910
(301) 563-6526
www.obesityresearch.org

International Journal of Obesity
Journal of the International Association for the Study of Obesity
Nature Publishing Group
The Macmillan Building
4 Crinan Street
London N1 9XW
United Kingdom
www.nature.com/ijo

Journal of the American Medical Association
American Medical Association
P.O. Box 10946
Chicago, IL 60610-0946
(800) 262-2350
http://jama.ama-assn.org

New England Journal of Medicine
10 Shattuck Street
Boston, MA 02115-6094
(617) 734-9800
http://content.nejm.org/

American Journal of Clinical Nutrition
The American Journal of Clinical Nutrition
9650 Rockville Pike
Bethesda, MD 20814-3998
(301) 634-7038
www.ajcn.org

Journal of the American Dietetic Association
Elsevier, Health Sciences Division
Subscription Customer Service
6277 Sea Harbor Drive
Orlando, FL 32887
(800) 654-2452
www.adajournal.org

Aging

Administration on Aging
U.S. Health & Human Services
200 Independence Avenue, SW
Washington, DC 20201
(877) 696-6775
www.aoa.gov

American Association of Retired Persons (AARP)
601 E. Street, NW
Washington, DC 20049
(888) 687-2277
www.aarp.org

Health and Age
Sponsored by the Novartis Foundation for Gerontology &
The Web-Based Health Education Foundation
Robert Griffith, MD
Executive Director
573 Vista de la Ciudad
Santa Fe, NM 87501
www.healthandage.com

National Council on the Aging
300 D Street, SW, Suite 801
Washington, DC 20024
(202) 479-1200
www.ncoa.org

International Osteoporosis Foundation
5 Rue Perdtemps
1260 Nyon
Switzerland
41 22 994 01 00
www.osteofound.org

National Institute on Aging
Building 31, Room 5C27
31 Center Drive, MSC 2292
Bethesda, MD 20892
(301) 496-1752
www.nia.nih.gov

Osteoporosis and Related Bone Diseases National Resource Center
2 AMS Circle
Bethesda, MD 20892-3676
(800) 624-BONE
www.osteo.org

American Geriatrics Society
The Empire State Building
350 Fifth Avenue, Suite 801
New York, NY 10118
(212) 308-1414
www.americangeriatrics.org

National Osteoporosis Foundation
1232 22nd Street, NW
Washington, DC 20037-1292
(202) 223-2226
www.nof.org/

Alcohol and Drug Abuse

National Institute on Drug Abuse
6001 Executive Boulevard, Room 5213
Bethesda, MD 20892-9561
(301) 443-1124
www.nida.nih.gov

National Institute on Alcohol Abuse and Alcoholism
5635 Fishers Lane, MSC 9304
Bethesda, MD 20892-9304
www.niaaa.niri.gov

Alcoholics Anonymous
Grand Central Station
P.O. Box 459
New York, NY 10163
www.alcoholics-anonymous.org

Narcotics Anonymous
P.O. Box 9999
Van Nuys, California 91409
(818) 773-9999
www.na.org

National Council on Alcoholism and Drug Dependence
20 Exchange Place, Suite 2902
New York, NY 10005
(212) 269-7797
www.ncadd.org

National Clearinghouse for Alcohol and Drug Information
11420 Rockville Pike
Rockville, MD 20852
(800) 729-6686
www.health.org

Canadian Government

Health Canada
A.L. 0900C2
Ottawa, ON
K1A 0K9
(613) 957-2991
www.hc-sc.gc.ca/english

National Institute of Nutrition
408 Queen Street, 3rd Floor
Ottawa, ON K1R 5A7
(613) 235-3355
www.nin.ca/public_html/index.html

Agricultural and Agri-Food Canada
Public Information Request Service
Sir John Carling Building
930 Carling Avenue
Ottawa, ON K1A 0C5
(613) 759-1000
www.arg.gc.ca

Bureau of Nutritional Sciences
Sir Frederick G. Banting Research Centre
Tunney's Pasture (2203A)
Ottawa, ON K1A 0L2
(613) 957-0352
www.hc-sc.gc.ca/food-aliment/ns-sc/e_nutrition.html

Canadian Food Inspection Agency
59 Camelot Drive
Ottawa, ON K1A 0Y9
(613) 225-2342
www.inspection.gc.ca/english/toce.shtml

Canadian Institute for Health Information
CIHI Ottawa
377 Dalhousie Street, Suite 200
Ottawa, ON KIN 9N8
(613) 241-7860
www.cihi.ca

Canadian Public Health Association
1565 Carling Avenue, Suite 400
Ottawa, ON K1Z 8R1
(613) 725-3769
www.cpha.ca

Canadian Nutrition and Professional Organizations

Dietitians of Canada
480 University Avenue, Suite 604
Toronto, ON M5G 1V2
(416) 596-0857
www.dietitians.ca

Canadian Diabetes Association
National Life Building
1400-522 University Avenue
Toronto, ON M5G 2R5
(800) 226-8464
www.diabetes.ca

National Eating Disorder Information Centre
CW 1-211, 200 Elizabeth Street
Toronto, ON M5G 2C4
(866) NEDIC-20
www.nedic.ca

Canadian Pediatric Society
100-2204 Walkley Road
Ottawa, ON K1G 4G8
(613) 526-9397
www.cps.ca

Canadian Dietetic Association
480 University Avenue, Suite 604
Toronto, ON M5G 1V2
(416) 596-0857
www.dietitians.ca

Disordered Eating/Eating Disorders

American Psychiatric Association
1000 Wilson Boulevard, Suite 1825
Arlington, VA 22209
(703) 907-7300
www.psych.org

Harvard Eating Disorders Center
WACC 725
15 Parkman Street
Boston, MA 02114
(617) 236-7766
www.hedc.org

National Institute of Mental Health
Office of Communications
6001 Executive Boulevard, Room 8184, MSC 9663
Bethesda, MD 20892
(866) 615-6464
www.nimh.nih.gov

National Association of Anorexia Nervosa and Associated Disorders (ANAD)
Box 7
Highland Park, IL 60035
(847) 831-3438
www.anad.org

National Eating Disorders Association
603 Stewart Street, Suite 803
Seattle, WA 98101
(206) 382-3587
www.nationaleatingdisorders.org

Eating Disorder Referral and Information Center
2923 Sandy Pointe, Suite 6
Del Mar, CA 92014
(858) 792-7463
www.edreferral.com

Anorexia Nervosa and Related Eating Disorders, Inc. (ANRED)
E-mail: jarinor@rio.com
www.anred.com

Overeaters Anonymous
P.O. Box 44020
Rio Rancho, NM 87174
(505) 891-2664
www.oa.org

Exercise, Physical Activity, and Sports

American College of Sports Medicine (ACSM)
P.O. Box 1440
Indianapolis, IN 46206-1440
(317) 637-9200
www.acsm.org

American Physical Therapy Association (ASNA)
1111 North Fairfax Street
Alexandria, VA 22314
(800) 999-APTA
www.apta.org

Gatorade Sports Science Institute (GSSI)
617 West Main Street
Barrington, IL 60010
(800) 616-GSSI
www.gssiweb.com

National Coalition for Promoting Physical Activity (NCPPA)
1010 Massachusetts Avenue, Suite 350
Washington, DC 20001
(202) 454-7518
www.ncppa.org

Sports, Wellness, Eating Disorder and Cardiovascular Nutritionists (SCAN)
P.O. Box 60820
Colorado Springs, CO 80960
(719) 635-6005
www.scandpg.org

President's Council on Physical Fitness and Sports
Department W
200 Independence Avenue, SW
Room 738-H
Washington, DC 20201-0004
(202) 690-9000
www.fitness.gov

American Council on Exercise
4851 Paramount Drive
San Diego, CA 92123
(858) 279-8227
www.acefitness.org

The International Association for Fitness Professionals (IDEA)
10455 Pacific Center Court
San Diego, CA 92121
(800) 999-4332, ext. 7
www.ideafit.com

Food Safety

Food Marketing Institute
655 15th Street, NW
Washington, DC 20005
(202) 452-8444
www.fmi.org

Agency for Toxic Substances and Disease Registry (ATSDR)
ORO Washington Office
Ariel Rios Building
1200 Pennsylvania Avenue, NW
M/C 5204G
Washington, DC 20460
(888) 422-8737
www.atsdr.cdc.gov

Food Allergy and Anaphylaxis Network
11781 Lee Jackson Highway, Suite 160
Fairfax, VA 22033-3309
(800) 929-4040
www.foodallergy.org

Foodsafety.gov
www.foodsafety.gov

The USDA Food Safety and Inspection Service
Food Safety and Inspection Service
United States Department of Agriculture
Washington, DC 20250
www.fsis.usda.gov

Consumer Reports
Web Site Customer Relations Department
101 Truman Avenue
Yonkers, NY 10703
www.consumerreports.org

Center for Science in the Public Interest: Food Safety
1875 Connecticut Avenue, NW
Washington, DC 20009
(202) 332-9110
www.cspinet.org/foodsafety/index.html

Center for Food Safety and Applied Nutrition
5100 Paint Branch Parkway
College Park, MD 20740
(888) SAFEFOOD
www.cfsan.fda.gov

Food Safety Project
Dan Henroid, MS, RD, CFSP
HRIM Extension Specialist and Website Coordinator
Hotel, Restaurant and Institution Management
9e MacKay Hall
Iowa State University
Ames, IA 50011
(515) 294-3527
www.extension.iastate.edu/foodsafety

Organic Consumers Association
6101 Cliff Estate Road
Little Marais, MN 55614
(218) 226-4164
www.organicconsumers.org

Infancy and Childhood

Administration for Children and Families
370 L'Enfant Promenade, SW
Washington, DC 20447
www.acf.dhhs.gov

The American Academy of Pediatrics
141 Northwest Point Boulevard
Elk Grove Village, IL 60007
(847) 434-4000
www.aap.org

Kidnetic.com
E-mail: contactus@kidnetic.com
www.kidnetic.com

Kidshealth: The Nemours Foundation
12735 West Gran Bay Parkway
Jacksonville, FL 32258
(866) 390-3610
www.kidshealth.org

National Center for Education in Maternal and Child Health
Georgetown University
Box 571272
Washington, DC 20057
(202) 784-9770
www.ncemch.org

Birth Defects Research for Children, Inc.
930 Woodcock Road, Suite 225
Orlando, FL 32803
(407) 895-0802
www.birthdefects.org

USDA/ARS Children's Nutrition Research Center at Baylor College of Medicine
1100 Bates Street
Houston, TX 77030
www.kidsnutrition.org

Keep Kids Healthy.com
www.keepkidshealthy.com

International Agencies

UNICEF
3 United Nations Plaza
New York, NY 10017
(212) 326-7000
www.unicef.org

World Health Organization
Avenue Appia 20
1211 Geneva 27
Switzerland
41 22 791 21 11
www.who.int/en

The Stockholm Convention on Persistent Organic Pollutants
11–13 Chemin des Anémones
1219 Châtelaine
Geneva, Switzerland
41 22 917 8191
www.pops.int

Food and Agricultural Organization of the United Nations
Viale delle Terme di Caracalla
00100 Rome, Italy
39 06 57051
www.fao.org

International Food Information Council Foundation
1100 Connecticut Avenue, NW
Suite 430
Washington, DC 20036
(202) 296-6540

Pregnancy and Lactation

San Diego County Breastfeeding Coalition
c/o Children's Hospital and Health Center
3020 Children's Way, MC 5073
San Diego, CA 92123
(800) 371-MILK
www.breastfeeding.org

National Alliance for Breastfeeding Advocacy
Barbara Heiser, Executive Director
9684 Oak Hill Drive
Ellicott City, MD 21042-6321
OR
Marsha Walker, Executive Director
254 Conant Road
Weston, MA 02493-1756
www.naba-breastfeeding.org

American College of Obstetricians and Gynecologists
409 12th Street, SW, P.O. Box 96920
Washington, DC 20090
www.acog.org

La Leche League
1400 N. Meacham Road
Schaumburg, IL 60173
(847) 519-7730
www.lalecheleague.org

National Organization on Fetal Alcohol Syndrome
900 17th Street, NW
Suite 910
Washington, DC 20006
(800) 66 NOFAS
www.nofas.org

March of Dimes Birth Defects Foundation
1275 Mamaroneck Avenue
White Plains, NY 10605
(888) 663-4637
http://modimes.org

Professional Nutrition Organizations

Association of Departments and Programs of Nutrition (ANDP)
Dr. Marilynn Schnepf, ANDP Chair
316 Ruth Leverton Hall
Nutrition and Health Sciences
University of Nebraska-Lincoln
Lincoln, NE 68583-0806
http://andpnet.org

North American Association for the Study of Obesity (NAASO)
8630 Fenton Street, Suite 918
Silver Spring, MD 20910
(301) 563-6526
www.naaso.org

American Dental Association
211 East Chicago Avenue
Chicago, IL 60611-2678
(312) 440-2500
www.ada.org

American Heart Association
National Center
7272 Greenville Avenue
Dallas, TX 75231
(800) 242-8721
www.americanheart.org

American Dietetic Association (ADA)
120 South Riverside Plaza, Suite 2000
Chicago, IL 60606-6995
(800) 877-1600
www.eatright.org

The American Society for Nutrition (ASN)
9650 Rockville Pike, Suite L-4500
Bethesda, MD 20814-3998
(301) 634-7050
www.nutrition.org

The Society for Nutrition Education
7150 Winton Drive, Suite 300
Indianapolis, IN 46268
(800) 235-6690
www.sne.org

American College of Nutrition
300 S. Duncan Avenue, Suite 225
Clearwater, FL 33755
(727) 446-6086
www.amcollnutr.org

American Obesity Association
1250 24th Street, NW, Suite 300
Washington, DC 20037
(800) 98-OBESE

American Council on Health and Science
1995 Broadway
Second Floor
New York, NY 10023
(212) 362-7044
www.acsh.org

American Diabetes Association
ATTN: National Call Center
1701 North Beauregard Street
Alexandria, VA 22311
(800) 342-2383
www.diabetes.org

Institute of Food Technologies
525 W. Van Buren, Suite 1000
Chicago, IL 60607
(312) 782-8424
www.ift.org

ILSI Human Nutrition Institute
One Thomas Circle, Ninth Floor
Washington, DC 20005
(202) 659-0524
http://hni.ilsi.org

Trade Organizations

American Meat Institute
1700 North Moore Street
Suite 1600
Arlington, VA 22209
(703) 841-2400
www.meatami.com

National Dairy Council
10255 W. Higgins Road, Suite 900
Rosemont, IL 60018
(312) 240-2880
www.nationaldairycouncil.org

United Fresh Fruit and Vegetable Association
1901 Pennsylvania Ave. NW, Suite 1100
Washington, DC 20006
(202) 303-3400
www.uffva.org

U.S.A. Rice Federation
Washington, DC
4301 North Fairfax Drive, Suite 425
Arlington, VA 22203
(703) 236-2300
www.usarice.com

U.S. Government

The USDA National Organic Program
Agricultural Marketing Service
USDA-AMS-TMP-NOP
Room 4008-South Building
1400 Independence Avenue, SW
Washington, DC 20250-0020
(202) 720-3252
www.ams.usda.gov

U.S. Department of Health and Human Services
200 Independence Avenue, SW
Washington, DC 20201
(877) 696-6775
www.os.dhhs.gov

Food and Drug Administration (FDA)
5600 Fishers Lane
Rockville, MD 20857
(888) 463-6332
www.fda.gov

Environmental Protection Agency
Ariel Rios Building
1200 Pennsylvania Avenue, NW
Washington, DC 20460
(202) 272-0167
www.epa.gov

Federal Trade Commission
600 Pennsylvania Avenue, NW
Washington, DC 20580
(202) 326-2222
www.ftc.gov

Partnership for Healthy Weight Management
www.consumer.gov/weightloss

Office of Dietary Supplements
National Institutes of Health
6100 Executive Boulevard, Room 3B01, MSC 7517
Bethesda, MD 20892
(301) 435-2920
http://dietary-supplements.info.nih.gov

Nutrient Data Laboratory Homepage
Beltsville Human Nutrition Center
10300 Baltimore Avenue
Building 307-C, Room 117
BARC-East
Beltsville, MD 20705
(301) 504-8157
www.nal.usda.gov/fnic/foodcomp

National Digestive Disease Clearinghouse
2 Information Way
Bethesda, MD 20892-3570
(800) 891-5389
http://digestive.niddk.nih.gov

The National Cancer Institute
NCI Public Inquiries Office
Suite 3036A
6116 Executive Boulevard, MSC 8322
Bethesda, MD 20892-8322
(800) 4-CANCER
www.cancer.gov

The National Eye Institute
31 Center Drive, MSC 2510
Bethesda, MD 20892-2510
(301) 496-5248
www.nei.nih.gov

The National Heart, Lung, and Blood Institute
Building 31, Room 5A52
31 Center Drive, MSC 2486
Bethesda, MD 20892
(301) 592-8573
www.nhlbi.nih.gov/index.htm

Institute of Diabetes and Digestive and Kidney Diseases
Office of Communications and Public Liaison
NIDDK, NIH, Building 31, Room 9A04
Center Drive, MSC 2560
Bethesda, MD 20892
(301) 496-4000
www.niddk.nih.gov

National Center for Complementary and Alternative Medicine
NCCAM Clearinghouse
P.O. Box 7923
Gaithersburg, MD 20898
(888) 644-6226
http://nccam.nih.gov

U.S. Department of Agriculture (USDA)
14th Street, SW
Washington, DC 20250
(202) 720-2791
www.usda.gov

Centers for Disease Control and Prevention (CDC)
1600 Clifton Rd
Atlanta, GA 30333
(404) 639-3311 / Public Inquiries: (800) 311-3435
www.cdc.gov

National Institutes of Health (NIH)
9000 Rockville Pike
Bethesda, MD 20892
(301) 496-4000
www.nih.gov

Food and Nutrition Information Center
Agricultural Research Service, USDA
National Agricultural Library, Room 105
10301 Baltimore Avenue
Beltsville, MD 20705-2351
(301) 504-5719
www.nal.usda.gov/fnic

National Institute of Allergy and Infectious Diseases
NIAID Office of Communications and Public Liaison
6610 Rockledge Drive, MSC 6612
Bethesda, MD 20892
(301) 496-5717
www.niaid.nih.gov

Weight and Health Management

The Vegetarian Resource Group
P.O. Box 1463, Dept. IN
Baltimore, MD 21203
(410) 366-VEGE
www.vrg.org

American Obesity Association
1250 24th Street, NW
Suite 300
Washington, DC 20037
(202) 776-7711
www.obesity.org

Anemia Lifeline
(888) 722-4407
www.anemia.com

The Arc
(301) 565-3842
E-mail: info@thearc.org
www.thearc.org

Bottled Water Web
P.O. Box 5658
Santa Barbara, CA 93150
(805) 879-1564
www.bottledwaterweb.com

The Food and Nutrition Board
Institute of Medicine
500 Fifth Street, NW
Washington, DC 20001
(202) 334-2352
www.iom.edu/board.asp?id-3788

The Calorie Control Council
www.caloriecontrol.org

TOPS (Take Off Pounds Sensibly)
4575 South Fifth Street
P.O. Box 07360
Milwaukee, WI 53207
(800) 932-8677
www.tops.org

Shape Up America!
15009 Native Dancer Road
N. Potomac, MD 20878
(240) 631-6533
www.shapeup.org

World Hunger

Center on Hunger, Poverty, and Nutrition Policy
Tufts University
Medford, MA 02155
(617) 627-3020
www.tufts.edu/nutrition

Freedom from Hunger
1644 DaVinci Court
Davis, CA 95616
(800) 708-2555
www.freefromhunger.org

Oxfam International
1112 16th Street, NW, Suite 600
Washington, DC 20036
(202) 496-1170
www.oxfam.org

WorldWatch Institute
1776 Massachusetts Avenue, NW
Washington, DC 20036
(202) 452-1999
www.worldwatch.org

Food First
398 60th Street
Oakland, CA 94618
(510) 654-4400
www.foodfirst.org

The Hunger Project
15 East 26th Street
New York, NY 10010
(212) 251-9100
www.thp.org

U.S. Agency for International Development
Information Center
Ronald Reagan Building
Washington, DC 20523
(202) 712-0000
www.usaid.gov

ANSWERS TO REVIEW QUESTIONS

Please find answers to Review Questions 11–15 of each chapter on the Companion Website,
www.aw-bc.com/thompson.

CHAPTER 1

1. **d.** micronutrients.
2. **b.** National Institutes of Health.
3. **c.** contain 90 kcal of energy.
4. **d.** "A high-protein diet increases the risk for porous bones" is an example of a hypothesis.
5. **d.** all of the above
6. False. Vitamins do not provide any energy, although many vitamins are critical to the metabolic processes that assist us in generating energy from carbohydrates, fats, and proteins.
7. True.
8. True.
9. True.
10. True.

CHAPTER 2

1. **d.** The % Daily Values of select nutrients in a serving of the packaged food.
2. **b.** provides enough of the energy, nutrients, and fiber to maintain a person's health.
3. **a.** at least half your grains as whole grains each day.
4. **c.** Being physically active each day.
5. **b.** Foods with a lot of nutrients per calorie, such as fish, are more nutritious choices than foods with fewer nutrients per calorie, such as candy.
6. False. There is no standardized definition for a serving size for foods.
7. False. MyPyramid distinguishes low-fat choices and encourages us to consume mostly low-fat foods. It does not emphasize specific low-calorie food choices, but it does emphasize eating low- or non-fat foods to stay within the recommended discretionary calorie level.
8. False. The six exchange lists are starch/bread, meat and meat substitutes, fruits, vegetables, milk, and fats.
9. True. Pasta is listed at the top of the Healthy Eating Pyramid as a food that should be eaten sparingly.
10. False. This program was instituted by the National Institutes of Health.

CHAPTER 3

1. **c.** atoms, molecules, cells, tissues, organs, systems
2. **d.** emulsifies fats.
3. **c.** hypothalamus.
4. **a.** seepage of gastric acid into the esophagus.
5. **c.** small intestine.
6. True.
7. True.
8. False. Vitamins and minerals are not really "digested" the same way that macronutrients are. These compounds do not have to be broken down because they are small enough to be readily absorbed by the small intestine. For example, fat-soluble vitamins, such as vitamins A, D, E, and K, are soluble in lipids and are absorbed into the intestinal cells along with the fats in our foods. Water-soluble vitamins, such as the B vitamins and vitamin C, typically undergo some type of active transport process that helps assure the vitamin is absorbed by the small intestine. Minerals are absorbed all along the small intestine, and in some cases in the large intestine as well, by a wide variety of mechanisms.
9. False. A person with celiac disease cannot tolerate products with gluten, a protein found in wheat, rye, and barley.
10. False. Cells are the smallest units of life. Atoms are the smallest units of matter in nature.

CHAPTER 4

1. **b.** the potential of foods to raise blood glucose and insulin levels.
2. **d.** carbon, hydrogen, and oxygen.
3. **d.** sweetened soft drinks.
4. **a.** monosaccharides.
5. **a.** phenylketonuria.
6. False. Sugar alcohols are considered nutritive sweeteners because they contain 2 to 4 kcal of energy per gram.
7. True.
8. False. A person with lactose intolerance has a difficult time tolerating milk and other dairy products. This person does not have an allergy to milk, as he or she does not exhibit an immune response indicative of an allergy. Instead, this person does not digest lactose completely, which causes intestinal distress and symptoms such as gas, bloating, diarrhea, and nausea.
9. False. Plants store glucose as starch.
10. False. Salivary amylase breaks starches into maltose and shorter polysaccharides.

CHAPTER 5

1. **d.** found in leafy green vegetables, flax seeds, soy milk, and fish.
2. **b.** exercise regularly.
3. **a.** lipoprotein lipase.
4. **d.** high-density lipoproteins.
5. **a.** monounsaturated fats.
6. True.
7. False. Fat is an important source of energy during rest and during exercise, and adipose tissue is our primary storage site for fat. We rely significantly on the fat stored in our adipose tissue to provide energy during rest and exercise.
8. False. A triglyceride is a lipid comprised of a glycerol molecule and three fatty acids. Thus, fatty acids are a component of triglycerides.
9. False. While most *trans* fatty acids result from the hydrogenation of vegetable oils by food manufacturers, a small amount of *trans* fatty acids are found in cow's milk.
10. False. A serving of food labeled *reduced fat* has at least 25% less fat than a standard serving, but may not have fewer calories than a full-fat version of the same food.

CHAPTER 6

1. **d.** mutual supplementation.
2. **a.** Rice, pinto beans, acorn squash, soy butter, and almond milk.
3. **c.** protease.
4. **b.** amine group.
5. **c.** carbon, oxygen, hydrogen, and nitrogen.
6. True.
7. False. Both shape and function are lost when a protein is denatured.
8. False. Some hormones are made from lipids.
9. False. Buffers help the body maintain acid-base balance.
10. False. Depending upon the type of sport, athletes may require the same or up to two times as much protein as nonactive people.

CHAPTER 7

1. **b.** It can be found in fresh fruits and vegetables.
2. **d.** A healthy infant of average weight.
3. **a.** extracellular fluid.
4. **d.** It is freely permeable to water but impermeable to solutes.
5. **b.** Losing weight.

6. False. In addition to water, the body needs electrolytes, such as sodium and potassium, to prevent fluid imbalances during long-distance events such as a marathon. As purified water contains no electrolytes, this would not be the ideal beverage to prevent fluid imbalances during a marathon.
7. False. Our thirst mechanism is triggered by an increase in the concentration of electrolytes in our blood.
8. False. Hypernatremia is commonly caused by a rapid intake of high amounts of sodium.
9. False. Quenching our thirst does not guarantee adequate hydration. Urine that is clear or light yellow in color is one indicator of adequate hydration.
10. False. These conditions are associated with decreased fluid loss or an increase in body fluid. Diarrhea, blood loss, and low humidity are conditions that increase fluid loss.

CHAPTER 8

1. **d.** It is destroyed by exposure to high heat.
2. **b.** an atom loses an electron.
3. **a.** cardiovascular disease.
4. **d.** nitrates.
5. **a.** vitamin A.
6. True.
7. True.
8. False. Vitamin C helps regenerate vitamin E.
9. True.
10. False. Pregnant women should not consume beef liver very often, as it can lead to vitamin A toxicity and potentially serious birth defects.

CHAPTER 9

1. **a.** calcium and phosphorus.
2. **c.** has normal bone density as compared to an average, healthy 30-year-old.
3. **d.** It provides the scaffolding for cortical bone.
4. **c.** a fair-skinned retired teacher living in a nursing home in Ohio
5. **d.** structure of bone, nerve transmission, and muscle contraction.
6. True.
7. True.
8. False. The fractures that result from osteoporosis cause an increased risk of infection and other related illnesses that can lead to premature death.
9. True.
10. False. Our body makes vitamin D by converting a cholesterol compound in our skin to the active form of vitamin D that we need to function. We do not absorb vitamin D from sunlight, but when the ultraviolet rays of the sun hit our skin, they react to eventually form calcitriol, which is considered the primary active form of vitamin D in our bodies.

CHAPTER 10

1. **d.** thiamin, pantothenic acid, and biotin.
2. **b.** vitamin K.
3. **b.** Iron is a component of hemoglobin, myoglobin, and certain enzymes.
4. **c.** an amino acid.
5. **d.** Choline is necessary for the synthesis of phospholipids and other components of cell membranes.
6. True.
7. True.
8. False. Non-heme iron is found in both plant-based and animal-based foods.
9. False. Neural tube defects occur during the first four weeks of pregnancy; this is often before a woman even knows she is pregnant. Thus, the best way for a woman to protect her fetus against neural tube defects is to make sure she is consuming adequate folate before she is pregnant.
10. False. Wilson's disease is a rare disorder that causes copper toxicity.

CHAPTER 11

1. **d.** body mass index.
2. **a.** basal metabolic rate, thermal effect of food, and effect of physical activity.
3. **b.** take in more energy than they expend.
4. **c.** all people have a genetic set-point for their body weight.
5. **a.** hunger.
6. False. It is the apple-shaped fat patterning, or excess fat in the trunk region, that is known to increase a person's risk for many chronic diseases.
7. True.
8. False. Weight-loss medications are typically prescribed for people with a body mass index greater than or equal to 30 kg/m^2, or for people with a body mass index greater than or equal to 27 kg/m^2 who also have other significant health risk factors such as heart disease, high blood pressure, and type 2 diabetes.
9. False. Healthful weight gain includes eating more energy than you expend and also exercising both to maintain aerobic fitness and to build muscle mass.
10. True.

CHAPTER 13

1. **c.** 64 to 90% of your estimated maximal heart rate.
2. **a.** 1 to 3 seconds.
3. **b.** fat
4. **c.** seems to increase strength gained in resistance exercise.
5. **d.** drink a beverage containing carbohydrate and electrolytes both before and during the event in amounts that balance hydration with energy, carbohydrate, and electrolyte needs.
6. True.
7. False. A dietary fat intake of 15 to 25% of total energy intake is generally recommended for athletes.
8. False. Carbohydrate loading involves altering duration and intensity of exercise and intake of carbohydrate such that the storage of carbohydrate is maximized.
9. False. Sports anemia is not true anemia, but a transient decrease in iron stores that occurs at the start of an exercise program. This is a result of an initial increase in plasma volume (or water in our blood) that is not matched by an increase in hemoglobin.
10. True.

CHAPTER 15

1. **b.** bulimia nervosa
2. **a.** increases your risk of developing a psychiatric eating disorder.
3. **d.** disordered eating, menstrual dysfunction, and osteoporosis.
4. **a.** exercise regularly.
5. **b.** I wish I could change the way I look in the mirror.
6. False. People with binge-eating disorder typically do not purge to compensate for the binge; thus, these individuals are usually overweight or obese.
7. False. Although it is suspected that media images of idealized female bodies may contribute to an increase in eating disorders in adolescent girls, there is no scientific evidence to support this suspicion.
8. True.
9. False. People with anorexia typically deny they are hungry and may lie about eating.
10. False. People who suffer from binge-eating disorder may also suffer from chronic overeating behaviors. However, chronic overeating is defined as regularly overeating without losing control, whereas binge-eating involves the loss of control during a binge episode that prevents a person from stopping him- or herself from overeating.

CHAPTER 18

1. **a.** oxygen, heat, and light.
2. **c.** a type of fungus used to ferment foods.
3. **b.** a flavor enhancer used in a variety of foods.
4. **a.** contain only organically produced ingredients, excluding water and salt.

5. **b.** two hours of serving.
6. False. The appropriate temperature for cooking foods varies according to the food.
7. False.
8. True.
9. True.
10. True.

CHAPTER 19

1. **b.** neural tube defects
2. **c.** oxytocin
3. **a.** fiber
4. **b.** women who begin their pregnancy underweight.
5. **d.** iron-fortified rice cereal.
6. False. These issues are most likely to occur in the first trimester of pregnancy.
7. True.
8. True.
9. True.
10. False. If uncontrolled, gestational diabetes can result in a baby that is too large as a result of receiving too much glucose across the placenta during fetal life. It can also result in preeclampsia.

CHAPTER 20

1. **b.** vitamin D
2. **c.** 45 to 65%
3. **d.** allergies
4. **a.** 1/2 cup of iron-fortified cooked oat cereal, two tablespoons of mashed pineapple, and one cup of whole milk
5. **a.** Cigarette smoking can interfere with the metabolism of nutrients.
6. False. Preschool children are able to understand the basic information about which foods are more nutritious and those that should be eaten in moderation. Also, parents are important role models for preschool children.
7. True.
8. False. There are several prescription acne medications that contain vitamin A derivatives, but vitamin A taken in supplement form is not effective in acne treatment and, due to its risk for toxicity, vitamin A should not be used in amounts that exceed 100 percent of the Daily Value.
9. False. In fact, some healthcare providers recommend a limit of one drink per day for older adult males due to the fact that alcohol is metabolized less effectively in older adults.
10. True.

GLOSSARY

24-hour recall A data collection tool that assesses everything a person has consumed over the past 24 hours.

A

absorption The physiologic process by which molecules of food are taken from the gastrointestinal tract into the circulation.

acceptable daily intake (ADI) An estimate made by the Food and Drug Administration of the amount of a non-nutritive sweetener that someone can consume each day over a lifetime without adverse effects.

Acceptable Macronutrient Distribution Range (AMDR) A range of intakes for a particular energy source that is associated with reduced risk of chronic disease while providing adequate intakes of essential nutrients.

acetylcholine A neurotransmitter that is involved in many functions, including muscle movement and memory storage.

acidosis A disorder in which the blood becomes acidic; that is, the level of hydrogen in the blood is excessive. It can be caused by respiratory or metabolic problems.

added sugars Sugars and syrups that are added to food during processing or preparation.

adenosine triphosphate (ATP) The common currency of energy for virtually all cells of the body.

adequate diet A diet that provides enough of the energy, nutrients, and fiber to maintain a person's health.

Adequate Intake (AI) A recommended average daily nutrient intake level based on observed or experimentally determined estimates of nutrient intake by a group of healthy people.

alcohol abuse The act of engaging in inappropriate or dangerous drinking behaviors.

alcohol hangover A consequence of drinking too much alcohol; symptoms include headache, fatigue, dizziness, muscle aches, nausea and vomiting, sensitivity to light and sound, extreme thirst, and mood disturbances.

alcohol poisoning A potentially fatal condition in which an overdose of alcohol results in cardiac and/or respiratory failure.

alcohol Chemically, a compound characterized by the presence of a hydroxyl group; in common usage, a beverage made from fermented fruits, vegetables, or grains and containing ethanol.

alcoholic hepatitis Inflammation of the liver caused by alcohol; other forms of hepatitis can be caused by a virus or toxin.

alcoholism A disease state characterized by chronic dependence on alcohol.

alkalosis A disorder in which the blood becomes basic; that is, the level of hydrogen in the blood is deficient. It can be caused by respiratory or metabolic problems.

alpha-linolenic acid An essential fatty acid found in leafy green vegetables, flaxseed oil, soy oil, fish oil, and fish products; an omega-3 fatty acid.

amenorrhea Lack of menstruation for at least 3 consecutive months in the absence of pregnancy. Primary amenorrhea is the absence of menstruation by the age of 16 years in a girl who has secondary sex characteristics, while secondary amenorrhea is the absence of the menstrual period for 3 or more months after menarche. The presence of amenorrhea is a criterion for the diagnosis of anorexia nervosa.

amino acids Nitrogen-containing molecules that combine to form proteins.

anabolic Refers to a substance that builds muscle and increases strength.

anaerobic Means "without oxygen." Term used to refer to metabolic reactions that occur in the absence of oxygen.

anorexia An absence of the physiologic sensation of hunger; also a serious, potentially life-threatening eating disorder that is characterized by self-starvation, which eventually leads to a deficiency in energy and essential nutrients that are required by the body to function normally. For an individual to be considered to have anorexia nervosa, he or she must be medically diagnosed by a physician and meet specific diagnostic criteria.

antibodies Defensive proteins of the immune system. Their production is prompted by the presence of bacteria, viruses, toxins, allergens, and so on.

antioxidant A compound that has the ability to prevent or repair the damage caused by oxidation.

antiresorptive Characterized by an ability to slow or stop bone resorption without affecting bone formation. Antiresorptive medications are used to reduce the rate of bone loss in people with osteoporosis.

appetite A psychological desire to consume specific foods.

ariboflavinosis A condition caused by riboflavin deficiency.

atom A discrete, irreducible unit of matter. It is the smallest unit of an element and is identical to all other atoms of that element.

atrophic gastritis A condition that results in low stomach acid secretion; is estimated to occur in about 10–30% of adults older than 50.

B

balanced diet A diet that contains the combinations of foods that provide the proper proportions of nutrients.

basal metabolic rate (BMR) The energy the body expends to maintain its fundamental physiologic functions.

Behavioral Risk Factor Surveillance System (BRFSS) The world's largest telephone survey that tracks lifestyle behaviors that increase our risks for chronic diseases.

beriberi A disease caused by thiamin deficiency.

bile Fluid produced by the liver and stored in the gallbladder; it emulsifies fats in the small intestine.

binge drinking The consumption of five or more alcoholic drinks on one occasion.

binge eating Consumption of a large amount of food in a short period of time, usually accompanied by a feeling of loss of self-control.

binge-eating disorder A disorder characterized by binge eating an average of twice a week or more.

bioavailability The degree to which our bodies can absorb and utilize any given nutrient.

blood volume   The amount of fluid in blood.

body composition   The amount of bone, muscle, and fat tissue in the body. Also the ratio of a person's body fat to lean body mass.

body image   A person's perception of his or her body's appearance and functioning.

body mass index (BMI)   A measurement representing the ratio of a person's body weight to his or her height.

bolus   The mass of food that has been chewed and moistened in the mouth.

bone density   The degree of compactness of bone tissue, reflecting the strength of the bones. *Peak bone density* is the point at which a bone is strongest.

brush border   Term that describes the microvilli of the small intestine's lining. These microvilli tremendously increase the small intestine's absorptive capacity.

buffers   Proteins that help maintain proper acid–base balance by attaching to, or releasing, hydrogen ions as conditions change in the body.

bulimia nervosa   A serious eating disorder characterized by recurrent episodes of binge eating and recurrent inappropriate compensatory behaviors (such as self-induced vomiting; misuse of laxatives, diuretics, enemas, or other medications; fasting; or excessive exercise) in order to prevent weight gain.

C

calcitonin   A hormone secreted by the thyroid gland when blood calcium levels are too high. Calcitonin inhibits the actions of vitamin D, preventing reabsorption of calcium in the kidneys, limiting calcium absorption in the intestines, and inhibiting the osteoclasts from breaking down bone.

calcitriol   The primary active form of vitamin D in the body.

cancer   A group of diseases characterized by cells that reproduce spontaneously and independently and may invade other tissues and organs.

carbohydrate   One of the three macronutrients, a compound made up of carbon, hydrogen, and oxygen that is derived from plants and provides energy. Carbohydrates are the primary fuel source for our bodies, particularly for our brain and for physical exercise.

carbohydrate loading   Also known as glycogen loading. A process that involves altering training and carbohydrate intake so that muscle glycogen storage is maximized.

carcinogen   Any substance capable of causing the cellular mutations that lead to cancer, such as certain pesticides, industrial chemicals, and pollutants.

cardiorespiratory fitness   Fitness of the heart and lungs; achieved through regular participation in aerobic-type activities.

cardiovascular disease   A general term that refers to abnormal conditions involving dysfunction of the heart and blood vessels; cardiovascular disease can result in heart attack or stroke.

carotenoids   Fat-soluble plant pigments that the body stores in the liver and adipose tissues. The body is able to convert certain carotenoids to vitamin A.

cash crops   Crops grown to be sold rather than eaten, such as cotton, tobacco, jute, and sugar cane.

cataract   A damaged portion of the eye's lens, which causes cloudiness that impairs vision.

celiac disease   A genetic disorder characterized by an inability to absorb a component of gluten called gliadin. This causes an inflammatory immune response that damages the lining of the small intestine.

cell differentiation   The process by which immature, undifferentiated stem cells develop into highly specialized functional cells of discrete organs and tissues.

cell membrane   The boundary of an animal cell that separates its internal cytoplasm and organelles from the external environment.

cell   The smallest unit of matter that exhibits the properties of living things, such as growth, reproduction, and metabolism.

Centers for Disease Control and Prevention (CDC)   The leading federal agency in the United States that protects the health and safety of people. Its mission is to promote health and quality of life by preventing and controlling disease, injury, and disability.

cephalic phase   Earliest phase of digestion in which the brain thinks about and prepares the digestive organs for the consumption of food.

cholecalciferol   Vitamin D_3, a form of vitamin D found in animal foods and the form we synthesize from the sun.

chronic dieting   Consistently and successfully restricting energy intake to maintain an average or below average body weight.

chylomicron   A lipoprotein produced in the mucosal cell of the intestine; transports dietary fat out of the intestinal tract.

chyme   Semifluid mass consisting of partially digested food, water, and gastric juices.

cirrhosis of the liver   Endstage liver disease characterized by significant abnormalities in liver structure and function; may lead to complete liver failure.

coenzyme   A molecule that combines with an enzyme to activate it and help it do its job. Also the non-protein component of enzymes; many coenzymes are B-vitamins.

cofactor   Any organic or inorganic compound that combines with an enzyme to make that enzyme active.

collagen   A protein that forms strong fibers in bone and connective tissue.

complementary proteins   Two or more foods that together contain all nine essential amino acids necessary for a complete protein. It is not necessary to eat complementary proteins at the same meal.

complete proteins   Foods that contain all nine essential amino acids.

complex carbohydrate   A nutrient compound consisting of long chains of glucose molecules, such as starch, glycogen, and fiber.

constipation   Condition characterized by the absence of bowel movements for a period of time that is significantly longer than normal for the individual. When a bowel movement does occur, stools are usually small, hard, and difficult to pass.

cool-down   Activities done after an exercise session is completed; should be gradual and allow your body to slowly recover from exercise.

cortical bone (compact bone)   A dense bone tissue that makes up the outer surface of all bones as well as the entirety of most small bones of the body.

creatine phosphate (CP)   A high-energy compound that can be broken down for energy and used to regenerate ATP.

cretinism A special form of mental retardation that occurs in infants when the mother experiences iodine deficiency during pregnancy.

cystic fibrosis A genetic disorder that causes an alteration in chloride transport, leading to the production of thick, sticky mucus that causes life-threatening respiratory and digestive problems.

cytoplasm The liquid within an animal cell.

D

DASH diet The diet developed in response to research into hypertension funded by the National Institutes of Health (NIH); stands for "Dietary Approaches to Stop Hypertension."

deamination The process by which an amine group is removed from an amino acid. The nitrogen is then transported to the kidneys for excretion in the urine, while the carbon and other components are metabolized for energy or used to make other compounds.

dehydration Depletion of body fluid that results when fluid excretion exceeds fluid intake.

denature Term used to describe the action of unfolding proteins. Proteins must be denatured before they can be digested.

diabetes A chronic disease in which the body can no longer regulate glucose.

diarrhea Condition characterized by the frequent passage of loose, watery stools.

dietary fiber The nondigestible carbohydrate parts of plants that form the support structures of leaves, stems, and seeds.

Dietary Guidelines for Americans A set of principles developed by the U.S. Department of Agriculture and the U.S. Department of Health and Human Services to assist Americans in designing a healthful diet and lifestyle. These Guidelines are updated every 5 years.

Dietary Reference Intake (DRI) A set of nutritional reference values for the United States and Canada that applies to healthy people.

digestion The process by which foods are broken down into their component molecules, either mechanically or chemically.

disaccharide A carbohydrate compound consisting of two sugar molecules joined together.

discretionary calories A term used in the MyPyramid food guidance system that represents the extra amount of energy you can consume after you have met all of your essential needs by consuming the most nutrient-dense foods that are low-fat or fat-free and that have no added sugars.

diseases of aging Conditions that typically occur later in life as a result of lifelong accumulated risk, such as exposure to high-fat diets, lack of physical activity, and excess sun exposure.

disordered eating General term used to describe a variety of abnormal or atypical eating behaviors that are used to keep or maintain a lower body weight but are not severe enough to make the person seriously ill.

diuretic A substance that increases fluid loss via the urine. Common diuretics include alcohol, some prescription medications, and many over-the-counter weight-loss pills.

docosahexaenoic acid (DHA) A metabolic derivative of alpha-linolenic acid; together with EPA, it appears to reduce our risk of a heart attack.

drink The amount of an alcoholic beverage that provides approximately 0.5 fl. oz of pure ethanol.

dual energy x-ray absorptiometry (DXA or DEXA) Currently the most accurate tool for measuring bone density.

E

eating disorder A psychiatric disorder characterized by severe disturbances in body image and eating behaviors. Anorexia nervosa and bulimia nervosa are two examples of eating disorders for which specific diagnostic criteria must be present for diagnosis.

Eating Disorders Not Otherwise Specified (EDNOS) A group of atypical eating disorders that meet the definition of an eating disorder but not the strict criteria for anorexia nervosa or bulimia nervosa

edema A disorder in which fluids build up in the tissue spaces of the body, causing fluid imbalances and a swollen appearance.

eicosapentaenoic acid (EPA) A metabolic derivative of alpha-linolenic acid.

electrolyte A substance that disassociates in solution into positively and negatively charged ions and is thus capable of carrying an electrical current.

electron A negatively charged particle orbiting the nucleus of an atom.

elimination The process by which the undigested portions of food and waste products are removed from the body.

energy cost of physical activity The energy that is expended on body movement and muscular work above basal levels.

energy expenditure The energy the body expends to maintain its basic functions and to perform all levels of movement and activity.

energy intake The amount of food a person eats; in other words, it is the number of kilocalories consumed.

enteric nervous system The nerves of the GI tract.

enzymes Small chemicals, usually proteins, that act on other chemicals to speed up body processes but are not apparently changed during those processes.

ergocalciferol Vitamin D_2, a form of vitamin D found exclusively in plant foods.

ergogenic aids Substances used to improve exercise and athletic performance.

erythrocytes The red blood cells, which are the cells that transport oxygen in our blood.

esophagus Muscular tube of the GI tract connecting the back of the mouth to the stomach.

essential amino acids Amino acids not produced by the body that must be obtained from food.

essential fatty acids (EFAs) Fatty acids that must be consumed in the diet because they cannot be made by our bodies. The two essential fatty acids are linoleic acid and alpha-linolenic acid.

Estimated Average Requirement (EAR) The average daily nutrient intake level estimated to meet the requirement of half of the healthy individuals in a particular life stage or gender group.

Estimated Energy Requirement (EER) The average dietary energy intake that is predicted to maintain energy balance in a healthy adult.

ethanol A specific alcohol compound (C_2H_5OH) formed from the fermentation of dietary carbohydrates and used in a variety of alcoholic beverages.

evaporative cooling　Another term for sweating, which is the primary way in which we dissipate heat.

Exchange System　Diet planning tool developed by the American Dietetic Association and the American Diabetes Association in which exchanges, or portions, are organized according to the amount of carbohydrate, protein, fat, and calories in each food.

exercise　A subcategory of leisure-time physical activity; any activity that is purposeful, planned, and structured.

extracellular fluid　The fluid outside of the body's cells, either in the body's tissues or as the liquid portion of blood, called *plasma*.

F

famine　A widespread severe food shortage that causes starvation and death in a large portion of a population in a region.

fats　An important energy source for our bodies at rest and during low-intensity exercise.

fat-soluble vitamins　Vitamins that are not soluble in water but are soluble in fat, including vitamins A, D, E, and K.

fatty acids　Long chains of carbon atoms bound to each other as well as to hydrogen atoms.

fatty liver　An early and reversible stage of liver disease often found in people who abuse alcohol and characterized by the abnormal accumulation of fat within liver cells; also called alcoholic steatosis.

female athlete triad　A serious syndrome that consists of three medical disorders frequently seen in female athletes: disordered eating, menstrual dysfunction, especially amenorrhea, and osteoporosis.

ferritin　A storage form of iron in our bodies found primarily in the intestinal mucosa, spleen, bone marrow, and liver.

fetal alcohol effects (FAE)　A set of subtle consequences of maternal intake of alcohol, such as impaired learning and behavioral problems.

fetal alcohol syndrome (FAS)　A set of serious, irreversible alcohol-related birth defects characterized by certain physical and mental abnormalities.

FIT principle　The principle used to achieve an appropriate overload for physical training. Stands for <u>f</u>requency, <u>i</u>ntensity, and <u>t</u>ime of activity.

flexibility　The ability to move a joint through its full range of motion.

fluid　A substance composed of molecules that move past one another freely. Fluids are characterized by their ability to conform to the shape of whatever container holds them.

fluorohydroxyapatite　A mineral compound in human teeth that contains fluoride, calcium, and phosphorus and is more resistant to destruction by acids and bacteria than hydroxyapatite.

fluorosis　A condition marked by staining and pitting of the teeth; caused by an abnormally high intake of fluoride.

food allergy　An inflammatory reaction to food caused by an immune system hypersensitivity.

food insecurity　Situation in which households are uncertain of having, or unable to acquire, enough food to meet the needs of all their members because they have insufficient money or other resources for food.

food intolerance　Gastrointestinal discomfort caused by certain foods that is not a result of an immune system reaction.

free radical　A highly unstable atom with an unpaired electron in its outermost shell.

frequency　Refers to the number of activity sessions per week you perform.

fructose　The sweetest natural sugar; a monosaccharide that occurs in fruits and vegetables. Also called *levulose*, or *fruit sugar*.

functional fiber　The nondigestible forms of carbohydrate that are extracted from plants or manufactured in the laboratory and have known health benefits.

functional food　A food that has been manipulated to provide additional health benefits.

G

galactose　A monosaccharide that joins with glucose to create lactose, one of the three most common disaccharides.

gallbladder　A tissue sac beneath the liver that stores bile and secretes it into the small intestine.

gastric juice　Acidic liquid secreted within the stomach; it contains hydrochloric acid, pepsin, and other compounds.

gastroesophageal reflux disease (GERD)　A painful type of heartburn that occurs more than twice per week.

gastrointestinal (GI) tract　A long, muscular tube consisting of several organs: the mouth, esophagus, stomach, small intestine, and large intestine.

gene expression　The process of using a gene to make a protein.

ghrelin　A protein synthesized in the stomach that acts as a hormone and plays an important role in appetite regulation by stimulating appetite.

glucagon　Hormone secreted by the alpha cells of the pancreas in response to decreased blood levels of glucose. Causes breakdown of liver stores of glycogen into glucose.

gluconeogenesis　The generation of glucose from the breakdown of proteins into amino acids.

glucose　The most abundant sugar molecule, a monosaccharide generally found in combination with other sugars. The preferred source of energy for the brain and an important source of energy for all cells.

glycemic index　Rating of the potential of foods to raise blood glucose and insulin levels.

glycemic load　The amount of carbohydrate in a food multiplied by the glycemic index of the carbohydrate.

glycerol　An alcohol composed of three carbon atoms; it is the backbone of a triglyceride molecule.

glycogen　A polysaccharide stored in animals; the storage form of glucose in animals.

glycolysis　The breakdown of glucose; yields two ATP molecules and two pyruvic acid molecules for each molecule of glucose.

goiter　Enlargement of the thyroid gland; can be caused by either iodine toxicity or deficiency.

grazing　Consistently eating small meals throughout the day; done by many athletes to meet their high energy demands.

H

healthful diet　A diet that provides the proper combination of energy and nutrients and is adequate, moderate, balanced, and varied.

heartburn　The painful sensation that occurs over the sternum when hydrochloric acid backs up into the lower esophagus.

heat cramps Muscle spasms that occur several hours after strenuous exercise; most often occur when sweat losses and fluid intakes are high, urine volume is low, and sodium intake is inadequate.

heat exhaustion A heat illness that is characterized by excessive sweating, weakness, nausea, dizziness, headache, and difficulty concentrating. Unchecked heat exhaustion can lead to heatstroke.

heat stroke A potentially fatal response to high temperature characterized by failure of the body's heat-regulating mechanisms. Symptoms include rapid pulse; reduced sweating; hot, dry skin; high temperature; headache; weakness; and sudden loss of consciousness. Commonly called *sunstroke* or *heatstroke.*

heat syncope Dizziness that occurs when people stand for too long in the heat or when they stop suddenly after a race or stand suddenly from a lying position; results from blood pooling in the lower extremities.

heme The iron-containing molecule found in hemoglobin.

heme iron Iron that is part of the proteins hemoglobin and myoglobin; found only in animal-based foods such as meat, fish, and poultry.

hemoglobin The oxygen-carrying protein found in our red blood cells; almost two-thirds of all of the iron in our bodies is found in hemoglobin.

hemosiderin A storage form of iron in our bodies found primarily in the intestinal mucosa, spleen, bone marrow, and liver.

homocysteine An amino acid that requires adequate levels of folate, vitamin B_6, and vitamin B_{12} for its metabolism. High levels of homocysteine in the blood are associated with an increased risk for vascular diseases such as cardiovascular disease.

hormone Chemical messenger that is secreted into the bloodstream by one of the many glands of the body and acts as a regulator of physiologic processes at a site remote from the gland that secreted it.

hunger A physiologic sensation that prompts us to eat.

hydrogenation The process of adding hydrogen to unsaturated fatty acids, making them more saturated and thereby more solid at room temperature.

hypercalcemia A condition marked by an abnormally high concentration of calcium in the blood.

hyperkalemia A condition in which blood potassium levels are dangerously high.

hypermagnesemia A condition marked by an abnormally high concentration of magnesium in the blood.

hypernatremia A condition in which blood sodium levels are dangerously high.

hypertension A chronic condition characterized by above-average blood pressure readings, specifically, systolic blood pressure over 140 mm Hg or diastolic blood pressure over 90 mm Hg.

hypocalcemia A condition characterized by an abnormally low concentration of calcium in the blood.

hypoglycemia A condition marked by blood glucose levels that are below normal fasting levels.

hypokalemia A condition in which blood potassium levels are dangerously low.

hypomagnesemia A condition characterized by an abnormally low concentration of magnesium in the blood.

hyponatremia A condition in which blood sodium levels are dangerously low.

hypothalamus A region of the forebrain below the thalamus where visceral sensations such as hunger and thirst are regulated.

hypothesis An educated guess as to why a phenomenon occurs

I

impaired fasting glucose Fasting blood glucose levels that are higher than normal but not high enough to lead to a diagnosis of type 2 diabetes.

incomplete proteins Foods that do not contain all of the essential amino acids in sufficient amounts to support growth and health.

inorganic A substance or nutrient that does not contain carbon.

insensible water loss The loss of water not noticeable by a person, such as through evaporation from the skin and exhalation from the lungs during breathing.

insoluble fibers Fibers that do not dissolve in water.

insulin Hormone secreted by the beta cells of the pancreas in response to increased blood levels of glucose. Facilitates uptake of glucose by body cells.

intensity Refers to the amount of effort expended during the activity, or how difficult the activity is to perform.

intracellular fluid The fluid held at any given time within the walls of the body's cells.

intrinsic factor A protein secreted by cells of the stomach that binds to vitamin B_{12} and aids its absorption in the small intestine.

invisible fats Fats that are hidden in foods, such as the fats found in baked goods, regular-fat dairy products, marbling in meat, and fried foods.

ion Any electrically charged particle, either positively or negatively charged.

iron-deficiency anemia A form of anemia that results from severe iron deficiency.

irritable bowel syndrome A bowel disorder that interferes with normal functions of the colon. Symptoms are abdominal cramps, bloating, and constipation or diarrhea.

K

Keshan disease A heart disorder caused by selenium deficiency. It was first identified in children in the Keshan province of China.

ketoacidosis A condition in which excessive ketones are present in the blood, causing the blood to become very acidic, which alters basic body functions and damages tissues. Untreated ketoacidosis can be fatal. This condition is found in individuals with untreated diabetes mellitus.

ketones Substances produced during the breakdown of fat when carbohydrate intake is insufficient to meet energy needs. They provide an alternative energy source for the brain when glucose levels are low.

ketosis The process by which the breakdown of fat during fasting states results in the production of ketones.

kwashiorkor A form of protein-energy malnutrition that is typically seen in developing countries in infants and toddlers who are weaned early because of the birth of a subsequent child. Denied breast milk, they are fed a cereal diet that provides adequate energy but inadequate protein.

L

lactase A digestive enzyme that breaks lactose into glucose and galactose.

lacteal A small lymph vessel located inside of the villi of the small intestine.

lactic acid A compound that results when pyruvic acid is metabolized in the presence of insufficient oxygen.

lactose Also called *milk sugar*, a disaccharide consisting of one glucose molecule and one galactose molecule. Found in milk, including human breast milk.

lactose intolerance A disorder in which the body does not produce sufficient lactase enzyme and therefore cannot digest foods that contain lactose, such as cow's milk.

large intestine Final organ of the GI tract consisting of the cecum, colon, rectum, and anal canal, and in which most water is absorbed and feces are formed.

leisure-time physical activity Any activity not related to a person's occupation; includes competitive sports, recreational activities, and planned exercise training.

leptin A hormone that is produced by body fat that acts to reduce food intake and to decrease body weight and body fat.

leukocytes The white blood cells, which protect us from infection and illness.

limiting amino acid The essential amino acid that is missing or in the smallest supply in the amino acid pool and is thus responsible for slowing or halting protein synthesis.

linoleic acid An essential fatty acid found in vegetable and nut oils; also known as omega-6 fatty acid.

lipids A diverse group of organic substances that are insoluble in water; lipids include triglycerides, phospholipids, and sterols.

lipoprotein A spherical compound in which fat clusters in the center and phospholipids and proteins form the outside of the sphere.

lipoprotein lipase An enzyme that sits on the outside of cells and breaks apart triglycerides so that their fatty acids can be removed and taken up by the cell.

liver The largest auxiliary organ of the GI tract and one of the most important organs of the body. Its functions include production of bile and processing of nutrient-rich blood from the small intestine.

long-chain fatty acids Fatty acids that are fourteen or more carbon atoms in length.

low-intensity activities Activities that cause very mild increases in breathing, sweating, and heart rate.

M

macrocytic anemia A form of anemia manifested as the production of larger than normal red blood cells containing insufficient hemoglobin, which inhibits adequate transport of oxygen; also called megaloblastic anemia. Macrocytic anemia can be caused by a severe folate deficiency.

macronutrients Nutrients that our bodies need in relatively large amounts to support normal function and health. Carbohydrates, fats, and proteins are macronutrients.

macular degeneration A vision disorder caused by deterioration of the central portion of the retina and marked by loss or distortion of the central field of vision.

mad cow disease A fatal brain disorder prompted by consumption of food containing *prions*, which are abnormally folded infectious proteins found in the brains and other organs of infected sheep, cows, and other livestock.

major minerals Minerals that must be consumed in amounts of 100 mg/day or more and that are present in the body at the level of 5 g or more.

malnutrition A state of poor nutritional health that can be improved by adjustments in nutrient intake.

maltase A digestive enzyme that breaks maltose into glucose.

maltose A disaccharide consisting of two molecules of glucose. Does not generally occur independently in foods but results as a by-product of digestion. Also called malt sugar.

marasmus A form of protein-energy malnutrition that results from grossly inadequate intakes of protein, energy, and other nutrients.

maximal heart rate The rate at which your heart beats during maximal-intensity exercise.

meat factor A special factor found in meat, fish, and poultry that enhances the absorption of non-heme iron.

medium-chain fatty acids Fatty acids that are six to twelve carbon atoms in length.

megadose A dose of a nutrient that is ten or more times greater than the recommended amount.

menaquinone The form of vitamin K produced by bacteria in the large intestine.

metabolic water The water formed as a by-product of our body's metabolic reactions.

metabolism The process by which large molecules such as carbohydrates, fats, and proteins are broken down via chemical reactions into smaller molecules that can be used as fuel, stored, or assembled into new compounds the body needs.

metabolites The form that nutrients take when they have been used by our body. For example, lactate is a metabolite of carbohydrate that is produced when we use carbohydrate for energy.

micronutrients Nutrients that are needed in the daily diet in relatively small amounts; vitamins and minerals are micronutrients.

minerals Inorganic substances that are not broken down during digestion and absorption and are not destroyed by heat or light. Minerals assist in the regulation of many body processes and are classified as major minerals or trace minerals.

moderate-intensity activities Activities that cause moderate increases in breathing, sweating, and heart rate.

moderation Eating the right amounts of foods to maintain a healthy weight and to optimize our bodies' metabolic processes.

monosaccharide The simplest of carbohydrates. Consists of one sugar molecule, the most common form of which is glucose.

monounsaturated fatty acids (MUFAs) Fatty acids that have two carbons in the chain bound to each other with one double bond; these types of fatty acids are generally liquid at room temperature.

morbid obesity A condition in which a person's body weight exceeds 100% of normal, putting him or her at very high risk for serious health consequences.

multifactorial disease Any disease that may be attributable to one or more of a variety of causes.

muscle cramps Involuntary, spasmodic, and painful muscle contractions that last for many seconds or even minutes; electrolyte imbalances are often the cause of muscle cramps.

muscular endurance   A subcomponent of musculoskeletal fitness defined as the ability of a muscle to maintain submaximal force levels for extended periods of time.
muscular strength   A subcomponent of musculoskeletal fitness defined as the maximal force or tension level that can be produced by a muscle group.
musculoskeletal fitness   Fitness of the muscles and bones.
mutual supplementation   The process of combining two or more incomplete protein sources to make a complete protein.
myoglobin   An iron-containing protein similar to hemoglobin except that it is found in muscle cells.
MyPyramid   A revised pyramid-based food guidance system developed by the USDA and based on the 2005 Dietary Guidelines for Americans and the Dietary Reference Intakes from the National Academy of Sciences.

N

National Health and Nutrition Examination Survey (NHANES)   A survey conducted by the National Center for Health Statistics and the CDC; this survey tracks the nutrient and food consumption of Americans.
National Institutes of Health (NIH)   The world's leading medical research center and the focal point for medical research in the United States.
neural tube defects   The most common malformations of the central nervous system that occur during fetal development. A folate deficiency can cause neural tube defects.
night blindness   A vitamin A deficiency disorder that results in loss of the ability to see in dim light.
night-eating syndrome   A disorder characterized by intake of the majority of the day's energy between 8:00 PM and 6:00 AM. Individuals with this eating disorder also experience mood and sleep disorders.
nonessential amino acids   Amino acids that can be manufactured by the body in sufficient quantities and therefore do not need to be consumed regularly in our diet.
non-heme iron   The form of iron that is not a part of hemoglobin or myoglobin; found in animal- and plant-based foods.
non-nutritive sweeteners   Also called *alternative sweeteners*, manufactured sweeteners that provide little or no energy.
nucleus   The positively charged, central core of an atom. It is made up of two types of particles—protons and neutrons—bound tightly together. The nucleus of an atom contains essentially all of its atomic mass.
nutrient density   The relative amount of nutrients per amount of energy (or number of calories).
nutrients   Chemicals found in foods that are critical to human growth and function.
nutrition   The science that studies food and how food nourishes our bodies and influences our health.
Nutrition Facts Panel   The label on a food package that contains the nutrition information required by the FDA.
nutrition transition   A shift in dietary pattern toward greater food security, greater variety of foods, and more foods with high energy density; associated with increased incidence of obesity and chronic disease.
nutritive sweeteners   Sweeteners such as sucrose, fructose, honey, and brown sugar that contribute calories (or energy).

O

obesity   Having an excess body fat that adversely affects health, resulting in a person having a weight that is substantially greater than some accepted standard for a given height.
opsin   A protein that combines with retinal in the retina to form rhodopsin.
organ   A body structure composed of two or more tissues and performing a specific function, for example, the esophagus.
organelle   A tiny "organ" within a cell that performs a discrete function necessary to the cell.
organic   A substance or nutrient that contains the element carbon.
osmosis   The movement of water (or any solvent) through a semipermeable membrane from an area where solutes are less concentrated to areas where they are highly concentrated.
osteoblasts   Cells that prompt the formation of new bone matrix by laying down the collagen-containing component of bone that is then mineralized.
osteoclasts   Cells that erode the surface of bones by secreting enzymes and acids that dig grooves into the bone matrix.
osteomalacia   Vitamin D deficiency disease in adults, in which bones become weak and prone to fractures.
osteoporosis   A disease characterized by low bone mass and deterioration of bone tissue, leading to increased bone fragility and fracture risk.
ounce-equivalent   (or oz-equivalent) A term used to define a serving size that is 1 oz, or equivalent to 1 oz, for the grains group and the meats and beans group of MyPyramid.
overhydration   Dilution of body fluid. It results when water intake or retention is excessive.
overload principle   Placing an extra physical demand on your body in order to improve your fitness level.
overnutrition   Malnutrition defined by an absolute excess of calories leading to overweight. Diet may be high quality or poor quality.
overpopulated   Characteristic used to describe a region that has insufficient resources to support the number of people living there.
overweight   Having a moderate amount of excess body fat, resulting in a person having a weight that is greater than some accepted standard for a given height but is not considered obese.
oxidation   A chemical reaction in which molecules of a substance are broken down into their component atoms. During oxidation, the atoms involved lose electrons.

P

pancreas   Gland located behind the stomach; it secretes digestive enzymes.
pancreatic amylase   An enzyme secreted by the pancreas into the small intestine that digests any remaining starch into maltose.
parathyroid hormone (PTH)   A hormone secreted by the parathyroid gland when blood calcium levels fall. It is also known as parathormone, and it increases blood calcium levels by stimulating the activation of vitamin D, increasing reabsorption of calcium from the kidneys, and stimulating osteoclasts to break down bone, which releases more calcium into the bloodstream.

pellagra A disease that results from severe niacin deficiency.

pepsin An enzyme in the stomach that begins the breakdown of proteins into shorter polypeptide chains and single amino acids.

peptic ulcer Area of the GI tract that has been eroded away by the acidic gastric juice of the stomach. The two main causes of peptic ulcers are an *H. pylori* infection or use of nonsteroidal anti-inflammatory drugs.

peptide bonds Unique types of chemical bonds in which the amine group of one amino acid binds to the acid group of another in order to manufacture dipeptides and all larger peptide molecules.

peptide YY (PYY) A protein produced in the gastrointestinal tract that is released after a meal in amounts proportional to the energy content of the meal; it decreases appetite and inhibits food intake.

percent Daily Values (%DV) Information on a Nutrition Facts Panel that identifies how much a serving of food contributes to your overall intake of nutrients listed on the label; based on an energy intake of 2,000 calories per day.

peristalsis Wave of squeezing and pushing contractions that move food in one direction through the length of the GI tract.

pernicious anemia A special form of anemia that is the primary cause of a vitamin B_{12} deficiency; occurs at the end stage of an autoimmune disorder that causes the loss of various cells in the stomach.

pH Stands for percentage of hydrogen. It is a measure of the acidity—or level of hydrogen—of any solution, including human blood.

phospholipids A type of lipid in which a fatty acid is combined with another compound that contains phosphate; unlike other lipids, phospholipids are soluble in water.

photosynthesis Process by which plants use sunlight to fuel a chemical reaction that combines carbon and water into glucose, which is then stored in their cells.

phylloquinone The form of vitamin K found in plants.

physical activity Any movement produced by muscles that increases energy expenditure; includes occupational, household, leisure-time, and transportation activities.

Physical Activity Pyramid A pyramid similar to the previous USDA Food Guide Pyramid that makes recommendations for the type and amount of activity that should be done weekly to increase physical activity levels.

physical fitness The ability to carry out daily tasks with vigor and alertness, without undue fatigue, and with ample energy to enjoy leisure-time pursuits and meet unforeseen emergencies.

phytic acid The form of phosphorus stored in plants.

phytochemicals Compounds found in plants that are believed to have health-promoting effects in humans.

placebo effect An experience of symptom relief, improved athletic performance, or other benefit following administration of a therapy proven to have no scientific value, and thought to be due to a belief that the therapy is effective.

plasma The fluid portion of the blood; is needed to maintain adequate blood volume so that the blood can flow easily throughout our bodies.

platelets Cell fragments that assist in the formation of blood clots and help stop bleeding.

polysaccharide A complex carbohydrate consisting of long chains of glucose.

polyunsaturated fatty acids (PUFAs) Fatty acids that have more than one double bond in the chain, these types of fatty acids are generally liquid at room temperature.

prebiotics Types of fiber that friendly intestinal bacteria thrive on.

probiotics Live beneficial microorganisms in foods that can colonize the intestine and optimize the intestinal bacterial environment. There is promising research suggesting various health benefits from consuming probiotics.

proof A measure of the alcohol content of a liquid; 100 proof liquor is 50% alcohol by volume, 80 proof liquor is 40% alcohol by volume, and so on.

prooxidant A nutrient that promotes oxidation and oxidative cell and tissue damage.

proteases Enzymes that continue the breakdown of polypeptides in the small intestine.

protein digestibility corrected amino acid score (PDCAAS) A measurement of protein quality that considers the balance of amino acids as well as the digestibility of the protein in the food.

protein-energy malnutrition A disorder caused by inadequate consumption of protein. It is characterized by severe wasting.

proteins Large, complex molecules made up of amino acids and found as essential components of all living cells. Also the only macronutrient that contains nitrogen; the basic building blocks of proteins are amino acids.

provitamin An inactive form of a vitamin that the body can convert to an active form. An example is beta-carotene.

purging An attempt to rid the body of unwanted food by vomiting or other compensatory means, such as excessive exercise, fasting, or laxative abuse.

pyruvic acid The primary end product of glycolysis.

R

Recommended Dietary Allowance (RDA) The average daily nutrient intake level that meets the nutrient requirements of 97–98% of healthy individuals in a particular life stage and gender group.

remodeling The two-step process by which bone tissue is recycled; includes the breakdown of existing bone and the formation of new bone.

resistance training Exercises in which our muscles act against resistance.

resorption The process by which the surface of bone is broken down by cells called osteoclasts.

resveratrol A potent phenolic antioxidant found in red wine as well as grapes and nuts.

retina The delicate light-sensitive membrane lining the inner eyeball and connected to the optic nerve. It contains retinal.

retinal An active, aldehyde form of vitamin A that plays an important role in healthy vision and immune function.

retinoic acid An active, acid form of vitamin A that plays an important role in cell growth and immune function.

retinol   An active, alchohol form of vitamin A that plays an important role in healthy vision and immune function.

rhodopsin   A light-sensitive pigment found in the rod cells that is formed by retinal and opsin.

rickets   Vitamin D deficiency disease in children. Symptoms include deformities of the skeleton such as bowed legs and knocked knees.

S

saliva   A mixture of water, mucus, enzymes, and other chemicals that moistens the mouth and food, binds food particles together, and begins the digestion of starch.

salivary amylase   An enzyme in saliva that breaks starch into smaller particles and eventually into the disaccharide maltose.

salivary glands   Group of glands found under and behind the tongue and beneath the jaw that release saliva continually as well as in response to the thought, sight, smell, or presence of food.

saturated fatty acids (SFAs)   Fatty acids that have no carbons joined together with a double bond; these types of fatty acids are generally solid at room temperature.

seizures   Uncontrollable muscle spasms caused by increased nervous system excitability that can result from electrolyte imbalances.

sensible water loss   Water loss that is noticed by a person, such as through urine output and visible sweating.

set-point theory   A theory that suggests that the body raises or lowers energy expenditure in response to increased and decreased food intake and physical activity. This action serves to maintain an individual's body weight within a narrow range.

short-chain fatty acids   Fatty acids fewer than six carbon atoms in length.

sickle cell anemia   A genetic disorder that causes red blood cells to be sickle-, or crescent-, shaped. These cells cannot travel smoothly through blood vessels, rupture easily, and cause inadequate delivery of oxygen to tissues.

simple carbohydrate   Commonly called *sugar*; a monosaccharide or disaccharide such as glucose.

small intestine   The longest portion of the GI tract where most digestion and absorption takes place.

soluble fibers   Fibers that dissolve in water.

solvent   A substance that is capable of mixing with and breaking apart a variety of compounds. Water is an excellent solvent.

sphincter   A tight ring of muscle separating some of the organs of the GI tract and opening in response to nerve signals indicating that food is ready to pass into the next section.

starch   A polysaccharide stored in plants; the storage form of glucose in plants.

sterols   A type of lipid found in foods and the body that has a ring structure; cholesterol is the most common sterol that occurs in our diets.

stomach   A J-shaped organ where food is partially digested, churned, and stored until released into the small intestine.

stunting   Low height for age.

sucrase   A digestive enzyme that breaks sucrose into glucose and fructose.

sucrose   A disaccharide composed of one glucose molecule and one fructose molecule. Sweeter than lactose or maltose.

sustainable agriculture   Techniques of food production that preserve the environment indefinitely.

system   A group of organs that work together to perform a unique function, for example, the gastrointestinal system.

T

teratogen   A compound known to cause fetal harm or danger.

theory   A conclusion drawn from repeated experiments

thermic effect of food (TEF)   The energy expended as a result of processing food consumed.

thirst mechanism   A cluster of nerve cells in the hypothalamus that stimulate our conscious desire to drink fluids in response to an increase in the concentration of salt in our blood or a decrease in blood pressure and blood volume.

thrifty gene theory   A theory that suggests that some people possess a gene (or genes) that causes them to be energetically thrifty, resulting in them expending less energy at rest and during physical activity.

time of activity   How long each exercise session lasts.

tissue   A grouping of like cells that performs a function, for example, muscle tissue.

tocopherol   The active form of vitamin E in our bodies.

tocotrienol   A form of vitamin E that does not play an important biological role in our bodies.

Tolerable Upper Intake Level (UL)   The highest average daily nutrient intake level likely to pose no risk of adverse health effects to almost all individuals in a particular life stage and gender group.

total fiber   The sum of dietary fiber and functional fiber.

trabecular bone (spongy or cancellous bone)   A porous bone tissue that makes up only 20% of our skeleton and is found within the ends of the long bones, inside the spinal vertebrae, inside the flat bones (breastbone, ribs, and most bones of the skull), and inside the bones of the pelvis.

trace minerals   Minerals we need to consume in amounts less than 100 mg per day and of which the total amount in our bodies is less than 5 g.

transamination   The process of transferring the amine group from one amino acid to another in order to manufacture a new amino acid.

transcription   The process through which messenger RNA copies genetic information from DNA in the nucleus.

transferrin   The transport protein for iron.

transgenic crops   Plant varieties that have had one or more genes altered by use of genetic technologies; also called genetically modified organisms, or GMOs.

translation   The process that occurs when the genetic information carried by messenger RNA is translated into a chain of amino acids at the ribosome.

transport proteins   Protein molecules that help to transport substances throughout the body and across cell membranes.

triglyceride   A molecule consisting of three fatty acids attached to a three-carbon glycerol backbone.

T-score   A comparison of an individual's bone density to the average peak bone density of a 30-year-old healthy adult.

tumor Any newly formed mass of undifferentiated cells.

type 1 diabetes Disorder in which the body cannot produce enough insulin.

type 2 diabetes Progressive disorder in which body cells become less responsive to insulin.

U

undernutrition Malnutrition defined by an absolute lack of adequate energy leading to underweight.

underweight Having too little body fat to maintain health, causing a person to have a weight that is below an acceptably defined standard for a given height.

V

variety Eating a lot of different foods each day.

vegetarianism The practice of restricting the diet to food substances of plant origin, including vegetables, fruits, grains, and nuts.

vigorous-intensity activities Activities that produce significant increases in breathing, sweating, and heart rate; talking is difficult when exercising at a vigorous intensity.

viscous Term referring to a gel-like consistency; viscous fibers form a gel when dissolved in water.

visible fats Fat we can see in our foods or see added to foods, such as butter, margarine, cream, shortening, salad dressings, chicken skin, and untrimmed fat on meat.

vitamins Organic compounds that assist us in regulating our bodies' processes.

W

warm-up Also called preliminary exercise; includes activities that prepare you for an exercise bout, including stretching, calisthenics, and movements specific to the exercise bout.

wasting Very low weight for height.

water-soluble vitamins Vitamins that are soluble in water, including vitamin C and the B-complex vitamins.

weight cycling The condition of successfully dieting to lose weight, regaining the weight, and repeating the cycle again.

wellness A multidimensional, lifelong process that includes physical, emotional, and spiritual health.

INDEX

characteristics of, 583
day in the life of a bulimic, 594
family environment and, 585
health risks of, 592–593
peer pressure and, 586–587
prevalence of, 591
symptoms of, 592, *593*
treatment for, *605*, 606–607
warning signs, 592
Bullying Web site, 481
Burger King, 72, *72*
Burger King, nutrient values in food from, A-60 to A-63
Burnout, 573
Butyrate, 121
B vitamins. *See also Names of specific B vitamins*
  alcohol abuse and, 404–405
  for athletes, 545
  as coenzymes, 402–403, *402, 403, 405*
  dental health and, 766
  energy production and, 402–403, *403*
  for older adults, *762*, 766
  for vigorous exercise, *536*

C

1-C metabolism, 411
CACFP (Child and Adult Care Food Program), 769
Caffeic acid, *352*
Caffeine
  bone loss and, 383, 390
  during breastfeeding, 722
  in calorie-burning beverages, 358
  definition of, 652
  effects of, 653
  as ergogenic aid, 551
  foods containing, Appendix C
  ineffective intervention for alcohol, *163*
  irritable bowel syndrome and, 110, *110*
  lethal dose of, 467
  during pregnancy, 715
  weight loss and, 467
Calcidiol, 375, *375. See also* Vitamin D
Calcitonin, 367, *367,* 375, 393
Calcitriol, 375, *375. See also* Vitamin D
Calcium, 366–372
  absorption and transport of, 261, 262, 368–369, 373
  for adolescents, 370, *740,* 755
  blood pressure and, 263
  in bone remodeling, 364, *365*
  during breastfeeding, 719
  for children, 368, *740,* 752
  deficiency of, *258,* 371, *378*
  dental health and, 766
  female athlete triad and, 545–547
  as food additive, 683
  functions of, *258,* 366–368, *367, 378*
  high-protein diets and, 230
  intake quiz, 372, 373
  muscle contraction and, 368, 533
  for older adults, 368, *762,* 763-764
  osteoporosis and, *46*
  during pregnancy, 368, *708,* 709
  recommended intake of, *258,* 368–369, *369, 378, 536,* 709, 741, 755

regulation of blood levels of, 367, *367,* 375
serving sizes of, 370, *370*
sodium and, 390
sources of, *258,* 369–371, *369*
supplements, 374, 764
for toddlers, *740,* 741, 746
toxicity of, *258,* 371, *378*
in vegan diets, 239, *240,* 746
in vigorous exercise, *536*
vitamin D and, 367, *367,* 369, 380
weight loss diets and, 368
Calcium carbonate, 374
Calcium chloride, *682,* 683
Calcium citrate malate, 374
Calcium propionate, 678–679, *682*
Caloric restriction, longevity and, 776–777
Calorie-burning beverages, 357–358
Calories. *See also* Energy
  calculating contribution of macronutrients, 124, 143
  definition of, 9, B-2
  discretionary, 54, *54*
  on food labels, 42, *42, 45*
  in increased serving sizes, 57
  trend in American diets, 188–189, *189*
Campylobacter jejuni, 661, *661, 662*
Canada
  on genetically modified organisms, 697
  nutrition organizations and resources in, F-2
Cancellous (trabecular) bone, 363, *363*
Cancer, 328–334, 797-806
  alcohol intake and, 166, 331
  antioxidants and, 331, 333–334
  basal cell, 332
  beta-carotene supplements and, 320, 333, 353
  bladder, 145
  breast (*See* Breast cancer)
  cervical, 332
  colon (*See* Colon cancer)
  definition of, 328
  development steps in, 328, *329*
  esophagus, 333
  food label claims regarding, *46*
  fruit and vegetable consumption and, 34
  gastric, 333
  high-fat diets and, 203
  high-protein diets and, 250
  infection and, 332
  legumes and, 121
  lung, 320, 328, *329,* 333
  Mediterranean diets and, 62
  mouth, 330, *330*
  obesity and, 331
  omega-3 fatty acids and, 332–333
  physical activity and, 332–333, 487
  phytochemicals and, *352,* 353
  prostate, 133, 203, 333, 353, 688
  risk factors in, 328–333, *330, 332*
  selenium and, 263, 333
  skin, 332, *332*
  squamous cell, 332
  stomach, 332, 333
  tobacco use and, 328–330, *329, 330*
Canning foods, 669, 677-678
Canola oil, 173, 202, 695
Capillaries, 96, *97*
Carageenan, 123, *682*

Caramel, *682,* 683
Carbohydrate Addict's Diet, 462
Carbohydrate-controlled diet, 885–890
Carbohydrate loading, 129–130, 540, *541*
Carbohydrates, 117–152
  for adolescents, *740,* 755
  alternative sweeteners, 143–146, *144, 146,* 331
  in American diets, 134–137, 188, *189*
  for athletes, 129–130, 187, 538–541, *539, 541*
  during breastfeeding, 719
  calculating energy from, 10, 124
  carbohydrate loading, 129–130, 540, *541*
  for children, *740,* 748
  complex (polysaccharides), 120–124, *121, 123,* 126, 137–140, *141*
  definition of, 118
  diabetes and, 127
  digestion of, 91, 95, 128–133, *129, 130, 131*
  energy for daily activity from, 9–11, 124, *531,* 534–535, *534*
  energy for vigorous exercise from, 124–126, *125, 531,* 536
  energy production pathways, 531–533, *532*
  on food labels, *42,* 142, *143*
  gluconeogenesis, 126, 131, *131*
  glycemic index, 132–133, *133,* 540
  hypoglycemia and, 151
  ketoacidosis and, 126, 147, 249
  low-carbohydrate diets, 462, 538–539, *539*
  for older adults, 762
  during pregnancy, 707
  recommended intake of, 50, 134–143, *134*
  simple, 118–120, *120,* 134–137, *141*
  sources of, 11, 140
  timing of intake, 539–540
  for toddlers, *740,* 741
  vitamin B$_6$ and metabolism of, 410
Carbonated water, 278–279
Carcinogens, 239, 328, 333, 797
Cardiopulmonary resuscitation (CPR), 797
Cardiorespiratory fitness, 486–491, 540, *521,* 524–525, *525. See also* Fitness
  aerobics, 489–491
  definition of, 486
  exercise and, 486–488, *486*
  graded exercise test for, 489
  target heart rate zone, 489
Cardiovascular disease (CVD), 334–336, 792–797
  adolescents and, 756
  in anorexia nervosa, 589
  antioxidants and, 335
  chocolate and, 357
  definition of, 193
  dietary fats and, 198–201, *200*
  hormone replacement therapy and, 398–399
  as leading cause of death, 193, *193,* 334
  low-density lipoproteins and, 198, 200, *200*
  omega-3 fatty acids and, 179
  phytochemicals and, *352,* 353
  plaque formation and, 200, *200,* 335
  prevention of, 201–203, *202*

CREDITS

Photo Credits

p. 2-3: Lew Robertson/Jupiter Images; **p. 4:** Lew Robertson/Picture Arts/Corbis; **p. 5:** Lester V. Bergman/Corbis; **p. 9:** Tom Stewart/Corbis; **p. 12:** FoodPix/PictureArts Corporation/Jupiter Images; **p. 13:** Andy Crawford/Dorling Kindersley; **p. 16:** Jon Feingersh/Getty Images; **p. 21:** Stockbyte/Getty Images; **p. 23:** Kristin Piljay; **p. 24:** LA/Tevy Battini/Phototake NYC; **p. 25:** Michael Donne/Photo Researchers; **p. 27 T:** Sean Murphy/Getty Images; **p. 27 M:** Suzy Gorman; **p. 27 B:** Dex Images/Corbis; **p. 28 T:** Kaz Chiba/Getty Images; **p. 28 B:** Ryan McVay/Photodisc/Getty Images; **p 33 L:** Randy Jirtle: **p. 33 R:** Jamey Stillings/Getty Images; **p. 34:** Francesca Yorke/Getty Images; **p. 36-37:** John E. Kelly/Foodpix/Jupiter Images; **p. 37:** Adams Picture Library t/a apl/ Alamy; **p. 39 L:** Duomo/Corbis; **p. 39 R:** Alex Mares-Manton/Asia Images/Getty Images; **p. 41:** Chris Collins/Corbis; **p. 43:** Sky Bonillo/Photo Edit; **p. 44 L:** Dorling Kindersley; **p. 44 R:** KMITU/iStockphoto; **p. 48:** Ryan McVay/Photodisc/Getty Images; **p. 49:** David Sacks/Getty Images; **p. 50 T:** Alexander Walter/Taxi/Getty Images; **p. 50 B:** Andrew Whittuck/Dorling Kindersley; **p. 53:** AGE fotostock; **p. 55:** PLG/Pearson Education/Benjamin Cummings Publishing; **p. 58 TL:** Image Source Pink/Alamy; **p. 58 TR:** Envision/Corbis; **p. 58 BL:** F Schussler/PhotoLink/Getty Images; **p. 58 BR:** Ragnar Schmuck/Getty Images; **p. 59:** Dorling Kindersley; **p. 62:** Andrew Whittuck/Dorling Kindersley; **p. 63 B:** Suzy Gorman; **p. 64:** Creative Digital Visions; **p. 68:** Comstock/Jupiter Images; **p. 71:** Creative Digital Visions; **p. 72:** Joe Raedle/Getty Images; **p. 73 T:** Sigrid Estrada/Getty Images; **p. 73 B:** Koichi Kamoshida/Getty Images; **p. 78:** Pearson Learning Photo Studio; **p. 79 T:** Lars Borges/Getty Images; **p. 79 BL:** Burke/Triolo/Jupiter Images; **p. 79 BR:** Benjamin F. Fink Jr./Jupiter Images; **p. 80-81:** Polka Dot Images/Jupiter Images; **p. 82 T:** Jean Luc Morales/Getty Images; **p. 82 B:** Howard Kingsnorth/Getty Images; **p. 84:** Jon Riley/Getty Images; **p. 85:** Paul Poplis/Foodpix/Jupiter Images; **p. 86:** Ian O'Leary/Dorling Kindersley; p. 87: Suzy Gorman; **p. 91:** Jonelle Weaver/Taxi/Getty Images; **p. 97 L:** Dr. Richard Kessel & Dr. Gene Shih/Visuals Unlimited; **p. 97 R:** Dr. David M. Philips/Visuals Unlimited; **p. 98:** Tim Hawley/Foodpix/Jupiter Images; **p. 100:** SPL/Photo Researchers; **p. 101:** David Sacks/Stone/Getty Images; **p. 102:** Peter Southwick/Stock Boston; **p. 104:** Dr. E. Walker/Science Photo Library/Photo Researchers; **p. 105:** David Murray and Jules Selmes/Dorling Kindersley; **p. 106 T:** Gerald Zanetti /Foodpix/Jupiter Images: **p. 106 B:** Kaz Chiba/Getty Images; **p. 108:** Pramod Mistry/Lonely Planet Images; **p. 110:** Peter Adams/Taxi/Getty Images; **p. 114:** Scott Indermaur/Jupiter Images; **p. 115:** Cordelia Molloy/Photo Researchers; **p. 116-117:** Susan Gottberg/iStockphoto; **p. 118:** Michael Newman / PhotoEdit; **p. 121:** Robert J. Bennett/AGE fotostock; **p. 122 L:** Foodcollection/Getty Images; **p. 122 R:** Envision/Corbis; **p. 123:** Kristin Piljay; **p. 124:** Rob Lewine/Bettmann/Corbis; **p. 125:** Jeff Greenburg/PhotoEdit; **p. 127:** Dorling Kindersley; **p. 132 L:** Steve Shott/Dorling Kindersley; **p. 132 R:** Ryan McVay/Getty Images; **p. 135:** Joe Raedle/Getty Images; **p. 137:** Dorling Kindersley; **p. 139 T to B:** Eduard Andras/iStockphoto; Darja Vorontsova/shutterstock; Jurga Rubinovaite/iStockphoto; Julie Masson Deshaies/iStockphoto; **p. 140:** Sean Murphy/Getty Images; **p. 141:** Creative Digital Visions; **p. 142:** Rebecca Ellis/iStockphoto; **p. 145:** Kristin Piljay; **p. 148:** Roche Diagnostics Corporation; **p. 149:** Scott Camazine / Photo Researchers; **p. 150:** Getty Images; **p. 151:** Suzy Gorman; **p. 152:** Dorling Kindersley; **p. 157:** Brian Buckley/Alamy; **p. 158:** Isifa Image Service s.r.o./Alamy; **p. 159:** Andre Jenny/Alamy; **p. 160:** Supapixx/Alamy; **p. 161:** Kristin Piljay; **p. 162:** Michael Newman/PhotoEdit; **p. 163:** Dex Images/Corbis; **p. 164:** David Young-Wolff/PhotoEdit; **p. 165 L:** CNRI/Science Photo Library; **p. 165 R:** Martin M. Rotker/Photo Researchers; **p. 166:** Paul Conklin/Photo Edit; **p. 167:** George Steinmetz Photography; **p. 170-171:** Goodshoot/Jupiter Images; **p. 171:** AP Wide World Photos; **p. 172:** Dorling Kindersley; **p. 175T:** J.Garcia/Corbis; **p. 175 B:** David Murray/Dorling Kindersley; **p. 177:** AP Wide World Photos; **p. 180:** Maximilian Weinzierl/Alamy; **p. 181:** Andersen Floss/Photodisc/Getty Images; **p. 182:** Doug Pensinger/Getty Images; **p. 183 T:** Odd Anderdsen/Getty Images; **p. 183 B:** Gerald Zanetti/Foodpix/Jupiter Images; **p. 185:** Kip Peticolas/Fundamental Photographs, NYC; **p. 188 T:** Kaz Chiba/Getty Images; **p. 188 B:** Jeff Greenberg/AGE footstock; **p. 189:** Spencer Platt/Getty Images; **p. 192:** James Leynse/Bettmann/Corbis; **p. 195:** Sean Murphy/Getty Images; **p. 197:** Foodfolio/Alamy; **p. 198:** AP Wide World Photos; **p. 200 L:** Ed Reschke/Visuals Unlimited; **p. 200 R:** William Ober/Visuals Unlimited; **p. 203:** Eric Meacher/Dorling Kindersley; **p. 208:** Frances Roberts/Alamy; **p. 209 T:** Dorling Kindersley; **p. 209 B:** Michael Newman/Photo Edit; **p. 210-211:** Ralph Pleasant/Foodpix/Jupiter Images; **p. 212:** Duomo/Corbis; **p. 218 T:** Andrew Syred/Photo Researchers; **p. 218 B:** Foodfolio/Jupiter Images; **p. 219:** Creative Digital Visions; **p. 222 T:** Geri Engberg; **p. 222 B:** Visuals Unlimited; **p. 225:** Ian O'Leary/Dorling Kindersley; **p. 227:** AP Wide World Photos; **p. 231:** Kaz Chiba/Getty Images; **p. 233:** Ranald MacKechnie/Dorling Kindersley; **p. 237:** StockFood/Getty Images; **p. 239:** Jennifer Levy/FoodPix/Jupiter Images; **p. 240:** Dex Images/Corbis; **p. 241:** Dorling Kindersley; **p. 243 L:** Alexandra Avakian/Corbis; **p. 243 R:** AP Wide World Photos; **p. 244:** Oliver Meckes & Nicole Ottawa/Photo Researchers; **p. 249 L:** Lew Robertson/Getty Images; **p. 249 R:** Chris Hondros/Getty Images; **p. 250:** Ryan McVay/Getty Images; **p. 252:** www.blendel1.de/Getty Images; **p. 253 T:** Steve Terrill/Corbis; **p. 253 B:** Dorling Kindersley; **p. 255:** Noe Montes/Foodpix/Jupiter Images; **p. 257 L:** Lisa Hubbard/Botanica/Jupiter Images; **p. 257 R:** Safia Fatimi/Getty Images; **p. 261 T:** James Carrier/Getty Images; **p. 261 B:** Kaz Chiba/Getty Images; **p. 262:** Nancy R. Cohen/Getty Images; **p. 263:** Guy Ryecart and David Jordan/The Ivy Press Limited /Dorling Kindersley; **p. 264-265:** Lily Valde/Pixland/Jupiter Images; **p. 266:** Arthur Tilley/Getty Images; **p. 269:** Theo Allots/Corbis; **p. 274 T:** Randy Sidman-Moore/Masterfile Corporation; **p. 274 B:** Yong Hian Lim/iStockphoto; **p. 275;** Stockbyte/Getty Images; **p. 277:** Corbis; **p. 278:** Kaz Chiba/Getty Images; **p. 280 T:** Network Productions/The Image Works; **p. 280 B:** Masterfile Corporation; **p. 281:** Kristin Piljay, Pearson Benjamin Cummings; **p. 282:** Rachel Weill/Foodpix/Jupiter Images; **p. 284:** Al Bello/Getty Images; **p. 285:** Michael Pohuski/Jupiter Images; **p. 286 T:** Corbis; **p. 286 B:** Spauln/iStockphoto; **p. 287:** Foodcollection/Getty Images; **p. 288:** Shaun Egan/Getty Images; **p. 289 T:** Corbis; **p. 289 M:** istockphoto; **p. 289 B:** Eyewire Collection/Photodisc/Getty Images; **p. 290:** Ryan McVay/Photodisc/Getty Images; **p. 292:** Creatas Images/Jupiter Images; **p. 293:** Stockbyte Platinum/Alamy; **p. 299:** Tobias Titz/Getty Images; **p. 302-303:** Lew Robertson/Getty Images; **p. 303:** Michael Zagaris/Getty Images; **p. 306:** Deborah Davis/Getty Images; **p. 310 T:** Bill Aron/PhotoEdit; **p. 310 B:** Dorling Kindersley; **p. 311 T:** Suzannah Skelton/iStockphoto; **p. 311 B:** Craig Veltri/iStockphoto; **p. 313:** Dorling Kindersley; **p. 314 T:** Steve Gorton/ Dorling Kindersley; **p. 314 B:** Dorling Kindersley; **p. 315 T:** Corbis; **p. 315 B:** Corbis; **p. 316:** Suzy Gorman; **p. 317:** Medical-on-Line/Alamy; **p. 318:** Corbis; **p. 319 T:**

700: David Phillips/The Population Council/Photo Researchers; **p. 704:** Lennart Nilsson/Albert Bonniers Forlag AB; Lennart Nilsson/Albert Bonniers Forlag AB; Neil Bromhall / Photo Researchers; Tom Galliher/Corbis; **p. 705 T:** Ron Sutherland/ Photo Researchers; **p. 705 B:** Ian O'Leary/Getty Images; **p. 708 T:** Biophoto Associates/Science Source/Photo Researchers; **p. 708 B:** Dave King/Dorling Kindersley ; **p. 709:** Carl Tremblay/StockFood Creative/Getty Images; **p. 710:** Allana Wesley White/Corbis; **p. 711:** Brand X Pictures/Photodisc/Getty Images; **p. 713 T:** Dorling Kindersley; **p. 713 B:** Suzy Gorman; **p. 714:** Jim Craigmyle/Corbis; **p. 716:** Phanie/Photo Researchers; **p. 720:** Rick Gomez/AGE fotostock; **p. 723:** Jose Luis Pelaez, Inc./Corbis; **p. 724 T:** Dex Images/Corbis; **p. 724 B:** Mel Yates/Getty Images; **p. 727:** Corbis; **p. 730:** Anne Flinn Powell/Index Stock Imagery; **p. 731:** Dr. Pamela R. Erickson; **p. 736 L:** Philip Gould/Corbis; **p. 736 R:** Darama/Corbis; **p. 737:** Chris Craymer/Getty Images; **p. 738-739:** Ken Fisher/Getty Images; **p. 740:** Michael Newman/PhotoEdit; **p. 743:** Dave King/Dorling Kindersley; **p. 744 T:** Laura Dwight; **p. 744 B:** Roger Phillips/Dorling Kindersley; **p. 746 T:** Travis Amos; **p. 746 B:** Jaume Gual/AGE Fotostock; **p. 748 T:** Laura Murray; **p. 748 B:** Vince Streano/Corbis; **p. 750:** Bob Daemmrich/The Image Works; **p. 751 T:** Gary Buss/Getty Images; **p. 751 B:** Kidnetic.com; **p. 752:** Paul Barton/Corbis; **p. 753:** Sean Murphy/Getty Images; **p. 757:** Tom Stewart/Corbis; **p. 758:** Tome & Dee Ann McCarthy/Corbis; **p. 759:** Richard Koek/Getty Images; **p. 760:** Raymond Gehman/Corbis; **p. 761:** Donna Day/Getty Images; **p. 762:** Don Smetzer/Getty Images; **p. 765 T:** Ryan McVay/Photodisc/Getty Images; **p. 765 B:** Deborah Jaffe/Foodpix/Jupiter Images; **p. 770:** Karen Pruess/The Image Works; **p. 776 L:** Andreas Pollok/Getty Images; **p. 776 R:** Dorling Kindersley; **p. 777 L:** IPS/Jupiter Images; **p. 777 R:** ImageState/Alamy; **p. 778-779:** mediacolor's/Alamy; **p. 779:** Reuters/Corbis; **p. 781:** Geert van Kesteren/Magnum Photos; **p. 783:** Getty Images

Figure and Text Credits

Fig. 1.11 Flow chart based on Bauman, R. *Microbiology*, Figure 1.13 © 2003 Benjamin Cummings. Used by permission of Pearson Education. **Fig. 6.6b** From Germann, W. and Stanfield, C. *Principles of Human Physiology*, Fig. 2.9. Copyright © 2001 Benjamin Cummings. **Fig. 6.6c** From Alberts, Molecular Biology of the Cell, 4/e. Garland Publishers. © 2002 by Bruce Alberts, Alexander Johnson, Julian Lewis, Martin Raff, Keith Roberts, and Peter Walter. **Figure 6.7**

Hemoglobin illustration, Irving Geis. Rights owned by Howard Hughes Medical Institute. Not to be reproduced without permission. **Fig. 8.11** From Marieb, E. *Human Anatomy and Physiology*, 5/e. Fig. 16.7 Copyright © 2003 Benjamin Cummings. Used by permission of Pearson Education, Inc. **Fig. 9.1** From Germann, W. and Stanfield, C. *Principles of Human Physiology*, Fig. 20.14. Copyright © 2001 Benjamin Cummings. **Figure 9.3** Bone illustration, from Germann, W. and Stanfield, C. *Principles of Human Physiology*, Fig. 20.14. Copyright © 2001 Benjamin Cummings. **Figure 10.13** Hemoglobin and myoglobin illustrations, Irving Geis. Rights owned by Howard Hughes Medical Institute. Not to be reproduced without permission. **Fig 13.5** From *Biology: Exploring Life* by Neil Campbell, Brad Williamson, and Robin Heyden. © 2003 by Pearson Education, Inc. Publishing as Prentice Hall. **p. 588** Reprinted with permission from the *Diagnostic and Statistical Manual of Mental Disorders,* Fourth Edition. © 1994 American Psychiatric Association. **p. 592** Reprinted with permission from the *Diagnostic and Statistical Manual of Mental Disorders,* Fourth Edition. © 1994 American Psychiatric Association. **p. 595** Reprinted with permission from the *Diagnostic and Statistical Manual of Mental Disorders,* Fourth Edition. © 1994 American Psychiatric Association. **p. 601** From Otis, et al. 1997. The female athlete triad. *Med Sci Sports.* 29:i-ix. © Lippincott Williams & Wilkins. Used with permission. **p. 607** From *Eating Disorders and Obesity*, 2/e, by N. Piran. Copyright © 2002 Used with permission of The Guilford Press. **Fig. 19.1** Adapted from Germann, W. and Stanfield, C. *Principles of Human Physiology*, 2/e, Fig. 22.20a. Copyright © 2001 Benjamin Cummings. Reprinted by permission of Pearson Education, Inc. **Fig. 19.2** Adapted from Germann, W. and Stanfield, C. *Principles of Human Physiology*, 2/e, Fig. 22.21. Copyright © 2001 Benjamin Cummings. Reprinted by permission of Pearson Education, Inc. **Fig. 19.3** Adapted from Germann, W. and Stanfield, C. *Principles of Human Physiology*, 2/e, Fig. 22.22. Copyright © 2001 Benjamin Cummings. Reprinted by permission of Pearson Education, Inc. **Fig. 19.6** Adapted from Germann, W. and Stanfield, C. *Principles of Human Physiology*, 2/e, Fig. 22.25a. Copyright © 2001 Benjamin Cummings. Reprinted by permission of Pearson Education, Inc. **Fig. 19.9** Adapted from Germann, W. and Stanfield, C. *Principles of Human Physiology*, 2/e, Fig. 22.26a. Copyright © 2001. Reprinted by permission of Pearson Education, Inc. **Fig. 20.6** Adapted from Germann, W. and Stanfield, C. *Principles of Human Physiology*, Figure 20.14. Reprinted by permission of Pearson Education, Inc.

DIETARY REFERENCE INTAKES: RDA, AI*, (AMDR)

	Macronutrients					
Life-Stage Group	Carbohydrate—Total Digestible (g/d)	Total Fiber (g/d)	Total Fat (g/d)	n-6 polyunsaturated fatty acids (linoleic acid) (g/d)	n-3 polyunsaturated fatty acids (α-linolenic acid) (g/d)	Protein and Amino Acids (g/d)[a]
Infants						
0–6 mo	60* (ND[b])[c]	ND	31*	4.4* (ND)	0.5* (ND)	9.1* (ND)
7–12 mo	95* (ND)	ND	30*	4.6* (ND)	0.5* (ND)	13.5 (ND)
Children						
1–3 y	130 (45–65)	19*	(30–40)	7* (5–10)	0.7* (0.6–1.2)	13 (5–20)
4–8 y	130 (45–65)	25*	(25–35)	10* (5–10)	0.9* (0.6–1.2)	19 (10–30)
Males						
9–13 y	130 (45–65)	31*	(25–35)	12* (5–10)	1.2* (0.6–1.2)	34 (10–30)
14–18 y	130 (45–65)	38*	(25–35)	16* (5–10)	1.6* (0.6–1.2)	52 (10–30)
19–30 y	130 (45–65)	38*	(20–35)	17* (5–10)	1.6* (0.6–1.2)	56 (10–35)
31–50 y	130 (45–65)	38*	(20–35)	17* (5–10)	1.6* (0.6–1.2)	56 (10–35)
51–70 y	130 (45–65)	30*	(20–35)	14* (5–10)	1.6* (0.6–1.2)	56 (10–35)
>70 y	130 (45–65)	30*	(20–35)	14* (5–10)	1.6* (0.6–1.2)	56 (10–35)
Females						
9–13 y	130 (45–65)	26*	(25–35)	10* (5–10)	1.0* (0.6–1.2)	34 (10–30)
14–18 y	130 (45–65)	26*	(25–35)	11* (5–10)	1.1* (0.6–1.2)	46 (10–30)
19–30 y	130 (45–65)	25*	(20–35)	12* (5–10)	1.1* (0.6–1.2)	46 (10–35)
31–50 y	130 (45–65)	25*	(20–35)	12* (5–10)	1.1* (0.6–1.2)	46 (10–35)
51–70 y	130 (45–65)	21*	(20–35)	11* (5–10)	1.1* (0.6–1.2)	46 (10–35)
>70 y	130 (45–65)	21*	(20–35)	11* (5–10)	1.1* (0.6–1.2)	46 (10–35)
Pregnancy						
≤18 y	175 (45–65)	28*	(20–35)	13* (5–10)	1.4* (0.6–1.2)	71 (10–35)
19–30 y	175 (45–65)	28*	(20–35)	13* (5–10)	1.4* (0.6–1.2)	71 (10–35)
31–50 y	(45–65)	28*	(20–35)	13* (5–10)	1.4* (0.6–1.2)	71 (10–35)
Lactation						
≤18 y	210 (45–65)	29*	(20–35)	13* (5–10)	1.3* (0.6–1.2)	71 (10–35)
19–30 y	210 (45–65)	29*	(20–35)	13* (5–10)	1.3* (0.6–1.2)	71 (10–35)
31–50 y	210 (45–65)	29*	(20–35)	13* (5–10)	1.3* (0.6–1.2)	71 (10–35)

Source: Reprinted with permission from "Dietary Reference Intakes for Energy, Carbohydrates, Fiber, Fat, Fatty Acids, Cholesterol, Protein, and Amino Acids (Macronutrients)," © 2002 by the National Academy of Sciences, courtesy of the National Academies Press, Washington, DC.

Note: This table is adapted from the DRI reports, see www.nap.edu. It lists Recommended Dietary Allowances (RDAs), with Adequate Intakes (AIs) indicated by an asterisk (*), and Acceptable Macronutrient Distribution Range (AMDR) data provided in parentheses. RDAs and AIs may both be used as goals for individual intake. RDAs are set to meet the needs of almost all (97% to 98%) individuals in a group. For healthy breastfed infants, the AI is the mean intake. The AI for other life stage and gender groups is believed to cover the needs of all individuals in the group, but lack of data prevent being able to specify with confidence the percentage of individuals covered by this intake.

[a] Based on 1.5 g/kg/day for infants, 1.1 g/kg/day for 1–3 y, 0.95 g/kg/day for 4–13 y, 0.85 g/kg/day for 14–18 y, 0.8 g/kg/day for adults, and 1.1 g/kg/day for pregnant (using pre-pregnancy weight) and lactating women.

[b] ND = Not determinable due to lack of data of adverse effects in this age group and concern with regard to lack of ability to handle excess amounts. Source of intake should be from food only to prevent high levels of intake.

[c] Data in parentheses are Acceptable Macronutrient Distribution Range (AMDR). This is the range of intake for a particular energy source that is associated with reduced risk of chronic disease while providing intakes of essential nutrients. If an individual consumes in excess of the AMDR, there is a potential of increasing the risk of chronic diseases and/or insufficient intakes of essential nutrients.

DIETARY REFERENCE INTAKES: RDA, AI*

Life-Stage Group	Vitamins													
	Vitamin A (μg/d)[a]	Vitamin D (μg/d)[b]	Vitamin E (mg/d)[c]	Vitamin K (μg/d)	Thiamin (mg/d)	Riboflavin (mg/d)	Niacin (mg/d)[d]	Pantothenic Acid (mg/d)	Biotin (μg/d)	Vitamin B$_6$ (mg/d)	Folate (μg/d)[e]	Vitamin B$_{12}$ (μg/d)	Vitamin C (mg/d)	Choline (mg/d)
Infants														
0–6 mo	400*	5*	4*	2.0*	0.2*	0.3*	2*	1.7*	5*	0.1*	65*	0.4*	40*	125*
7–12 mo	500*	5*	5*	2.5*	0.3*	0.4*	4*	1.8*	6*	0.3*	80*	0.5*	50*	150*
Children														
1–3 y	300	5*	6	30*	0.5	0.5	6	2*	8*	0.5	150	0.9	15	200*
4–8 y	400	5*	7	55*	0.6	0.6	8	3*	12*	0.6	200	1.2	25	250*
Males														
9–13 y	600	5*	11	60*	0.9	0.9	12	4*	20*	1.0	300	1.8	45	375*
14–18 y	900	5*	15	75*	1.2	1.3	16	5*	25*	1.3	400	2.4	75	550*
19–30 y	900	5*	15	120*	1.2	1.3	16	5*	30*	1.3	400	2.4	90	550*
31–50 y	900	5*	15	120*	1.2	1.3	16	5*	30*	1.3	400	2.4	90	550*
51–70 y	900	10*	15	120*	1.2	1.3	16	5*	30*	1.7	400	2.4	90	550*
>70 y	900	15*	15	120*	1.2	1.3	16	5*	30*	1.7	400	2.4	90	550*
Females														
9–13 y	600	5*	11	60*	0.9	0.9	12	4*	20*	1.0	300	1.8	45	375*
14–18 y	700	5*	15	75*	1.0	1.0	14	5*	25*	1.2	400	2.4	65	400*
19–30 y	700	5*	15	90*	1.1	1.1	14	5*	30*	1.3	400	2.4	75	425*
31–50 y	700	5*	15	90*	1.1	1.1	14	5*	30*	1.3	400	2.4	75	425*
51–70 y	700	10*	15	90*	1.1	1.1	14	5*	30*	1.5	400	2.4	75	425*
>70 y	700	15*	15	90*	1.1	1.1	14	5*	30*	1.5	400	2.4	75	425*
Pregnancy														
≤18 y	750	5*	15	75*	1.4	1.4	18	6*	30*	1.9	600	2.6	80	450*
19–30 y	770	5*	15	90*	1.4	1.4	18	6*	30*	1.9	600	2.6	85	450*
31–50 y	770	5*	15	90*	1.4	1.4	18	6*	30*	1.9	600	2.6	85	450*
Lactation														
≤18 y	1200	5*	19	75*	1.4	1.4	17	7*	35*	2.0	500	2.8	115	550*
19–30 y	1300	5*	19	90*	1.4	1.4	17	7*	35*	2.0	500	2.8	120	550*
31–50 y	1300	5*	19	90*	1.4	1.4	17	7*	35*	2.0	500	2.8	120	550*

Sources: Reprinted with permission from the Dietary Reference Intakes series, National Academies Press. Copyright 1997, 1998, 2000, 2001, by the National Academy of Sciences. These reports may be accessed via www.nap.edu. Courtesy of the National Academies Press, Washington, DC.

Note: This table is adapted from the DRI reports; see www.nap.edu. It lists Recommended Dietary Allowances (RDAs), with Adequate Intakes (AIs) indicated by an asterisk (*). RDAs and AIs may both be used as goals for individual intake. RDAs are set to meet the needs of almost all (97 percent to 98 percent) individuals in a group. For healthy breastfed infants, the AI is the mean intake. The AI for other life stage and gender groups is believed to cover the needs of all individuals in the group, but lack of data prevent being able to specify with confidence the percentage of individuals covered by this intake.

[a] Given as retinal activity equivalents (RAE).
[b] Also known as calciferol. The DRI values are based on the absence of adequate exposure to sunlight.
[c] Also known as α-tocopherol.
[d] Given as niacin equivalents (NE), except for infants 0–6 months, which are expressed as preformed niacin.
[e] Given as dietary folate equivalents (DFE).